Fundamental Skills
and Concepts
in Patient Care

Fundamental Skills and Concepts in Patient Care

Fifth Edition

Barbara Kuhn Timby, R.N.C., B.S.N., M.A.

Nursing Professor
Instructor, Medical-Surgical Nursing
Glen Oaks Community College
Centreville, Michigan

LuVerne Wolff Lewis, M.A., R.N.

Research Associate
Institute of Research and Service in Nursing Education
Teachers College, Columbia University
New York, New York

Formerly Consultant
College of Nursing, Arizona State University
Tempe, Arizona

J. B. Lippincott Company   Philadelphia
New York   London   Hagerstown

Acquisitions Editor: Donna L. Hilton, R.N., B.S.N.
Coordinating Editorial Assistant: Susan Perry
Project Editor: Molly E. Dickmeyer
Indexer: Alexandra Nickerson
Designer: Susan Hermansen
Production Manager: Caren Erlichman
Production Coordinator: William F. Hallman
Compositor: Circle Graphics
Printer/Binder: Courier Westford

5th Edition

Library of Congress Cataloging-in-Publication Data

Timby, Barbara Kuhn.
    Fundamental skills and concepts in patient care / Barbara Kuhn
Timby, LuVerne Wolff Lewis. —5th ed.
        p.   cm.
    Authors' names in reverse order on previous ed.
    Includes bibliographical references and index.
    ISBN 0-397-54848-6
    1. Nursing.   I. Lewis, LuVerne Wolff.   II. Title.
    [DNLM: 1. Nursing Care.   WY 100 T583f]
RT41.L67   1992
610.73—dc20
DNLM/DLC
for Library of Congress   91-14162
                                                                 CIP

Any procedure or practice described in this book should be applied
by the health-care practitioner under appropriate supervision in
accordance with professional standards of care used with regard to
the unique circumstances that apply in each practice situation. Care
has been taken to confirm the accuracy of information presented and
to describe generally accepted practices. However, the authors,
editors, and publisher cannot accept any responsibility for errors or
omissions or for any consequences from application of the
information in this book and make no warranty, express or implied,
with respect to the contents of the book.

Every effort has been made to ensure drug selections and dosages
are in accordance with current recommendations and practice.
Because of ongoing research, changes in government regulations and
the constant flow of information on drug therapy, reactions and
interactions, the reader is cautioned to check the package insert for
each drug for indications, dosages, warnings and precautions,
particularly if the drug is new or infrequently used.

Dedication

To all those who have chosen to light the world by following the example of Florence Nightingale, the lady with the lamp.

Acknowledgments

The authors wish to thank the following people and the agencies for which they work for their help in preparing this text.

- Donna Hilton, Senior Editor, Nursing Division of the J. B. Lippincott Company, Philadelphia, Pennsylvania, for advice, support, and assistance during the development of the revised manuscript.
- Susan Perry, Editorial Assistant, J. B. Lippincott Company, for handling the details of manuscript compilation, tracking permissions, and doing related paperwork.
- Molly Dickmeyer, Project Editor, J. B. Lippincott Company, for editing manuscript and coordinating the related artwork.
- Dr. Philip Ward, President, David Smith, Dean of Instruction, and June DeLong, Director of Nursing, all of Glen Oaks Community College, Centreville, Michigan, for their encouragement to continue this extra-curricular project,
- Marilyn Gosling, Director of the Learning Resource Center of Glen Oaks Community College, and her assistant, Judy Baumeister, for their assistance in locating pertinent reference materials.
- Administrators and personnel from Three Rivers Area Hospital, Three Rivers, Michigan; River Forest Nursing Facility, Three Rivers, Michigan; Fairview Medical Care Facilty, Centreville, Michigan; The Community Health Center, Coldwater, Michigan; and Elkhart General Hospital, Elkhart, Indiana, for extending the use of their facilities when it was requested.
- Ken Timby, whose technical skills in photography helped transform concepts into images.
- Those persons who acted as models and contributed their time and patience while being photographed.
- My children, Jody, Brian, Erin, and Sheila, who had to become more self-reliant and who proved capable of doing so.

Preface

Educators believe that one of the most essential elements for learning involves acquiring a solid foundation of basic information. Once the student has demonstrated an understanding of the fundamentals of a subject, further depth and breadth of knowledge can be introduced.

This principle applies well to nursing education. Regardless of which entry level nursing program the student nurse selects—practical/vocational, associate degree, diploma, or baccalaureate—there is a core of content that is essential for all areas of nursing study. Having mastered these fundamentals, the novice can continue to build on that initial base of knowledge. In addition to serving as an introductory learning tool for beginning nursing students, this textbook has other potential applications. It can be used as a reference for updating the skills of practicing nurses as well as those returning to clinical practice after a period of inactivity.

Before discussing the organization of the fifth edition of Fundamental Skills and Concepts in Patient Care, it is important to identify some of its underlying philosophical concepts.

- The content supports the holistic approach, which is founded on the belief that the human experience is a composite of physiological, emotional, social, and spiritual aspects. Nursing facilitates health and healing in any and all of these component areas.
- The uniqueness of man is emphasized. The best care is individualized to meet each patient's unique needs. Though this text recommends approaches to care, it is up to each nurse to adapt to the circumstances within a specific nurse–patient situation.
- Because patients become temporarily separated from their usual network of support, this text encourages nurses to extend their responsibilities and services to include the patient's family and friends.
- Ethical dilemmas and legal issues continue to increase, and they affect the practice of nursing. Nurses have a duty to practice their profession safely and to protect from harm those committed to their care. Therefore, this text attempts to reinforce the concept that nurses, including student nurses, are accountable for their own clinical decisions and actions.

The information contained in the fifth edition of Fundamental Skills and Concepts in Patient Care could have been arranged in numerous ways. Each arrangement has advantages and disadvantages. The order of presentation is not intended as a rigid course outline; rather, the organization lends itself to easy adaptability within any nursing program.

Several features of this text are designed to help the reader use the fifth edition of Fundamental Skills and Concepts in Patient Care with greater ease.

- To assist in locating information, there is a list of chapters in the contents. A more detailed description is given in the expanded contents. A topical outline of the content is provided on the title page of each chapter.

- Each chapter begins with statements of behavioral objectives. These objectives help alert the student to the expected outcomes, which can be achieved by mastering the content.

- A glossary of terms and definitions is included with each chapter. This helps expand the beginning student's vocabulary and facilitate understanding of the technical language specific to the skills discussed. The glossary terms are re-emphasized with the use of italics when they appear again within the chapter.

- Each chapter includes a bibliography of recent professional literature. Most of the entries refer the reader to periodicals commonly found in most nursing libraries. The bibliographies can be used to help supplement the text's information on a particular topic.

The content revisions and additions in the fifth edition of Fundamental Skills and Concepts in Patient Care were carefully selected to provide the skills and concepts that are most appropriate and practical for beginning nursing students. The information selected for inclusion provides the framework for developing the initial skills required for all subsequent specialty areas of clinical nursing practice. Additionally, this edition incorporates a stronger emphasis on the nursing process, which reflects this important new direction in the National Council Licensure Examination for Practical Nurses.

To remain a reliable resource, changes have been made in virtually every chapter. Once again, the text is organized into five units, each with a specific focus. The first unit introduces the learner to the unique roles and responsibilities of the nurse. Subsequent units present information and nursing skills that apply to individuals with various needs throughout the health continuum—techniques that maintain or improve health, skills that reduce or eliminate health problems, and care for patients who will not recover from an illness. This pattern of organization provides the learner with a logical progression for learning the basic skills associated with patient care.

Each chapter is designed to help the learner grow academically and achieve clinical competence. The content in each chapter reflects the most current concepts and trends in nursing practice. For example, this edition contains the most recent recommendations and guidelines on universal precautions, laser surgery, and autologous blood donations. In one of the new additions, the contributions of representative nursing and non-nursing theorists are discussed in easily understood language. Besides the basic forms of charting, other styles such as focus charting, PIE charting, charting by exception, and computerized charting have been added. New clinical skills and discussions

attempt to reflect the most modern, technical devices being used in patient care, such as the tympanic thermometer, glucometer, patient-controlled analgesia pump, insulin pens, transtracheal oxygen, and a variety of therapeutic beds.

The narrative is generously supplemented with numerous tables and illustrations. Lists of significant facts have been emphasized throughout the text. Specific nursing skills are presented in a step-by-step procedural format emphasizing safety, scientific rationale, and nursing accountability. A list of applicable nursing diagnoses is highlighted in each skill chapter. Sample nursing care plans modeled on the steps in the nursing process have been included to demonstrate the independent autonomy and responsibility of today's practicing nurse. Almost all photographs in the previous edition have been updated. Additional drawings and illustrations have been created as visual aids.

This edition continues to provide special adaptations of basic skills in selected situations. This feature provides the student with suggestions about ways to make individual adjustments when caring for patients in various stages of the life cycle or with special medical problems. This should help students implement new techniques regardless of the characteristics of the patient population within a health care facility.

The patient's length of stay within the health-care agency continues to be brief. This has accentuated the need for nurses to provide health teaching. Therefore, this edition continues to emphasize teaching suggestions in appropriate chapters.

Finally, the pronoun *she* has been avoided in most instances within the text when referring to the nurse. Exceptions occur when the nurse in an illustration is female. We believe that the quality of nursing is enhanced by practitioners of both genders. Therefore, to reflect the increasing numbers of male nurses, an effort has been made to dispel the sexual stereotype that nursing is strictly a career for females. However, we continue to use the pronoun *he* when referring to patients. This reflects traditional English word usage.

The fifth edition of Fundamental Skills and Concepts in Patient Care is accompanied by a complete teaching/learning package. To augment teaching, the Instructor's Manual includes a variety of tools and strategies. The Instructor's Manual is 3-hole punched and the pages are perforated to facilitate the creation of individual lesson plans. To maximize learning, a Study Guide includes chapter summaries, behavioral objectives, a variety of learning excercises with correct answers and rationales, and Performance Checklists. The Performance Checklists follow each step of each nursing skill to provide a complete evaluative tool. These checklists can be used to assist students with examining their technique and to provide a means of self-evaluation or to assist faculty with evaluating student performance. The Study Guide is also 3-hole punched and perforated to facilitate the creation of individual study packets and to allow easy reproduction of the Performance Checklists. Finally, a test bank is available that includes over 850 multiple-choice questions to allow instructors to design their own tests.

It is our sincere hope that this text and its ancillary materials will facilitate learning and, by preparing knowledgeable practitioners, thereby continue to elevate the image of nursing, as well as improve nursing care for the patient.

Contents

Unit I: The Nurse and the Patient

1 Nursing: A Skill-Related Practice 3

2 Patient Services: The Focus of Nursing 15

3 Health: The Goal of Nursing 32

4 The Nursing Process: The Model for Nursing 39

5 Patient Records: Resources for Sharing Information 53

6 Laws and Ethics: The Controls for Nursing 73

Unit II: Nursing Skills for Health Promotion and Maintenance

7 Promoting Personal Hygiene 85

8 Promoting Proper Nutrition 122

9 Promoting Activity and Exercise 158

10 Promoting Comfort, Relaxation, and Sleep 175

Unit III: Nursing Skills Associated With Changing Levels of Wellness

11 Admitting, Transferring, Referring, and Discharging the Patient 201

12 **Promoting Rest and Safety Within the Patient's Environment** 217

13 **Obtaining Vital Signs** 240

14 **Performing Assessment Techniques** 276

15 **Assisting With Examinations and Special Tests** 300

Unit IV: Nursing Skills Related to Health Restoration

16 **Controlling Microorganisms** 327

17 **Preventing the Spread of Communicable Diseases** 353

18 **Caring for the Inactive Patient** 374

19 **Caring for the Patient Undergoing Surgery** 426

20 **Promoting Tissue Healing** 456

21 **Promoting Urine Elimination** 500

22 **Promoting Bowel Elimination** 543

23 **Administering Oral and Topical Medications** 572

24 **Administering Parenteral Medications** 603

25 **Maintaining and Restoring Fluid and Chemical Balance** 639

26 **Caring for the Mechanically Immobilized Patient** 684

27 **Promoting Cardiopulmonary Function** 704

Unit V: Nursing Skills Used During a Dying Experience

28 **Caring for Terminally Ill and Grieving Individuals** 749

Appendix 775

Index 776

Expanded Contents

1 Nursing: A Skill-Related Practice 3

Behavioral Objectives 3
Glossary 3
Introduction 4
Evolution of Nursing Theories 4
Definitions of Nursing 4
Objectives of Nursing Skills 7
Skills Basic to Nursing 8
Basis for Nursing Skills 9
Characteristics of the Practice of Nursing 10
Bibliography 14

2 Patient Services: The Focus of Nursing 15

Behavioral Objectives 15
Glossary 15
Introduction 16
Recipients of Services 16
What Patients Expect as Consumers 16
Components of Patient Services 17
Characteristics of Patient Services 19
The Nurse–Patient Relationship 19
Nursing Skills Related to Patient Services 21
   2-1   Promoting Effective Communication 23
Teaching the Patient 25
   2-2   Providing Emotional Support 26
   2-3   Teaching the Patient 28
Suggested Measures to Provide Patient Services
   in Selected Situations 28
Bibliography 31

3 Health: The Goal of Nursing 32

Behavioral Objectives 32
Glossary 32
Introduction 33
Health 33
Values Associated with Health 34
Trends in Health Promotion 34
Wellness 35
Illness 36
The Health-Care Team 37
Patterns for Administering Patient Care 37
Continuity of Care 38
Bibliography 38

4 The Nursing Process: The Model for Nursing 39

Behavioral Objectives 39
Glossary 39
Introduction 40
The Nursing Process 40

Assessing the Patient's Health Status **41**
Diagnosing the Patient's Health Problems **44**
Planning the Patient's Nursing Care **47**
Implementing the Plan **48**
Evaluating the Results of Nursing Care **49**
4-1 Using the Nursing Process **50**
Bibliography **52**

5 Patient Records: Resources for Sharing Information **53**

Behavioral Objectives **53**
Glossary **53**
Introduction **54**
Uses for Patient Records **54**
Types of Patient Records **55**
Methods of Charting **59**
Allowing Patients Access to Their Records **61**
Protecting Computerized Patient Records **61**
Using Abbreviations **62**
Making Entries on Patient Records **63**
Converting to Military Time **63**
5-1 Making Entries on the Patient's Record **64**
Other Written Forms of Communication **66**
Using Checklists and Flow Sheets **67**
Other Methods for Exchanging Information **68**
Bibliography **71**

6 Laws and Ethics: The Controls for Nursing **73**

Behavioral Objectives **73**
Glossary **73**
Introduction **74**
Laws **74**
Lawsuits **74**
Patients' Rights **75**
Legal Issues **75**
Ethics **78**
Codes of Ethics **78**
Ethical Dilemmas **78**
Ethical Issues **78**
Ethics Committees **79**
Securing Liability Insurance **80**
Preventing Lawsuits **80**
Defense Techniques **80**
Bibliography **82**

7 Promoting Personal Hygiene **85**

Behavioral Objectives **85**
Glossary **85**
Introduction **86**
Structures and Functions of the Skin and Mucous Membranes **86**

Assessment of the Skin and Related Structures **87**
Caring for Healthy Skin **87**
Ordering and Recording Hygienic Care **88**
Providing for a Bath or Shower **88**
7-1 Proving for Tub or Shower Bathing **88**
Tepid Sponging **89**
7-2 Assisting With a Bed Bath **90**
Perineal Care **90**
The Backrub **90**
Shaving **90**
7-3 Giving a Complete Bed Bath **91**
Care of the Teeth and Mouth **94**
7-4 Tepid Sponging **95**
7-5 Administering Perineal Care **97**
7-6 Giving a Backrub **98**
7-7 Shaving a Patient **100**
Care of the Eyes and Visual Aids **100**
7-8 Brushing and Flossing the Teeth **102**
7-9 Performing Oral Hygiene Measures **104**
7-10 Cleansing the Eyes **106**
Care of the Ears and Hearing Aids **107**
7-11 Removing, Cleaning, and Replacing Contact Lenses **109**
Care of the Nose **113**
Care of the Fingernails **113**
Care of the Feet and Toenails **114**
7-12 Inserting a Hearing Aid **114**
Care of the Hair **115**
7-13 Shampooing Hair **116**
Suggested Measures for Hygiene in Selected Situations **117**
Applicable Nursing Diagnoses **117**
Teaching Suggestions for Personal Hygiene **120**
Bibliography **120**

8 Promoting Proper Nutrition **122**

Behavioral Objectives **122**
Glossary **122**
Introduction **123**
Culture and Eating Habits **123**
Human Nutritional Needs **123**
Basic Food Groups **126**
Vegetarianism **126**
Nutritional Assessment **126**
Promoting Weight Gain or Loss **129**
Common Problems That Influence Eating **130**
Measuring and Recording Fluid Intake **132**
Commonly Prescribed Diets **132**
Providing Food for Patients **132**
Alternative Methods of Providing Nourishment **133**

8-1   Serving and Removing Trays   *134*
8-2   Helping the Patient to Eat   *135*
8-3   Inserting, Maintaining, and Removing a Nasogastric Tube   *136*
8-4   Inserting a Small Diameter Feeding Tube   *142*
8-5   Administering a Tube Feeding   *145*
8-6   Irrigating a Nasogastric Tube   *151*
Suggested Measures to Promote Nutrition in Selected Situations   *154*
Applicable Nursing Diagnoses   *154*
Teaching Suggestions to Promote Nutrition   *157*
Bibliography   *157*

9 *Promoting Activity and Exercise*   *158*

Behavioral Objectives   *158*
Glossary   *158*
Introduction   *158*
Maintaining Good Posture   *159*
Principles of Body Mechanics   *160*
Benefits of Activity and Exercise   *162*
9-1   Using Proper Body Mechanics   *163*
Identifying Risk Factors   *166*
Assessing Fitness   *166*
Types of Exercise   *170*
9-2   Planning a Safe Exercise Program   *171*
Suggested Measures to Promote Activity and Exercise in Selected Situations   *172*
Applicable Nursing Diagnoses   *172*
Bibliography   *174*

10 *Promoting Comfort, Relaxation, and Sleep*   *175*

Behavioral Objectives   *175*
Glossary   *175*
Introduction   *176*
The Nature of Pain   *176*
Pain Assessment   *178*
Measures to Relieve Acute Pain   *180*
Measures to Relieve Chronic Pain   *180*
10-1   Relieving Pain   *181*
10-2   Using a Patient-Controlled Analgesia Infuser   *183*
The Nature of Relaxation and Sleep   *186*
10-3   Operating a TENS Unit   *187*
10-4   Facilitating Relaxation   *190*
Assessing Sleep   *193*
Nursing Measures to Promote Sleep   *193*
Common Sleep Disorders   *193*
10-5   Promoting Sleep   *194*
Applicable Nursing Diagnoses   *195*
Suggested Measures Related to Comfort, Relaxation, and Sleep in Selected Situations   *195*

Teaching Suggestions for Comfort, Relaxation, and Sleep   *197*
Bibliography   *197*

11 *Admitting, Transferring, Referring, and Discharging the Patient*   *201*

Behavioral Objectives   *201*
Glossary   *201*
Introduction   *202*
Trends in Health-Care Delivery   *202*
Common Reactions to Hospitalization   *204*
Preparing for Admission   *205*
Admitting the Patient   *206*
Transferring the Patient   *208*
11-1   Admitting the Patient   *209*
Referring the Patient   *209*
Discharging the Patient   *209*
11-2   Transferring the Patient   *211*
Suggested Measures When Admitting and Discharging Patients in Selected Situations   *212*
11-3   Discharging the Patient   *214*
Teaching Suggestions for Admitting and Discharging Patients From a Health-Care Agency   *215*
Applicable Nursing Diagnoses   *216*
Bibliography   *216*

12 *Promoting Rest and Safety Within the Patient's Environment*   *217*

Behavioral Objectives   *217*
Glossary   *217*
Introduction   *218*
The Environment   *218*
The Patient's Room   *218*
Furnishings in the Patient's Room   *219*
12-1   Making an Unoccupied Bed   *220*
12-2   Making an Occupied Bed   *224*
Modifying the Environment   *226*
Sensory Alteration   *227*
Ensuring the Patient's Safety   *227*
12-3   Promoting Sensory Stimulation   *228*
12-4   Applying a Protective Restraint   *231*
When Accidents Occur   *233*
Suggested Measures to Promote a Restful and Safe Environment in Selected Situations   *235*
Applicable Nursing Diagnoses   *237*
Teaching Suggestions to Promote a Restful and Safe Environment   *239*
Bibliography   *239*

13 *Obtaining Vital Signs* 240

Behavioral Objectives *240*
Glossary *240*
Introduction *242*
Body Temperature *242*
    13-1   Cleaning a Glass Thermometer *247*
    13-2   Measuring Body Temperature
            Using a Glass Thermometer *248*
    13-3   Assessing Body Temperature
            Using an Electronic Thermometer *252*
The Pulse *253*
Respirations *257*
    13-4   Assessing the Radial Pulse *257*
Blood Pressure *259*
    13-5   Counting the Respiratory Rate *260*
    13-6   Measuring the Blood Pressure *267*
Frequency of Obtaining Vital Signs *270*
Recording the Vital Signs *270*
Suggested Measures to Obtain Vital Signs
    in Selected Situations *271*
Applicable Nursing Diagnoses *272*
Teaching Suggestions to Obtain Vital Signs *274*
Bibliography *275*

14 *Performing Assessment Techniques* 276

Behavioral Objectives *276*
Glossary *276*
Introduction *277*
Gathering Information About the Patient *277*
Purposes of Physical Assessment *278*
Methods of Physical Assessment *279*
Performing a Physical Assessment *280*
    14-1   Performing a Physical Assessment *283*
    14-2   Assessing Lung Sounds *288*
Applicable Nursing Diagnoses *296*
Suggested Measures to Assess the Patient's
    Health Status in Selected Situations *296*
Teaching Suggestions to Assess the Patient's
    Health Status *298*
Bibliography *298*

15 *Assisting With Examinations and Special Tests* 300

Behavioral Objectives *300*
Glossary *300*
Introduction *302*
Nursing Responsibilities When Special Procedures
    Are Performed *302*
    15-1   Assisting With an Examination *309*
Advancements in Examinations and Tests *310*
Interpreting Terms That Describe Tests *310*
Examinations That Use X-Rays *311*

Examinations of Electrical Impulses *313*
Examinations That Detect Radiation *314*
Examinations That Use Sound Waves *315*
Examinations That Use Endoscopes *315*
Examinations of Body Fluids *316*
Suggested Measures to Assist With Examinations
    in Selected Situations *318*
    15-2   Using a Glucometer *319*
Applicable Nursing Diagnoses *322*
Teaching Suggestions About Tests
    and Examinations *322*
Bibliography *324*

16 *Controlling Microorganisms* 327

Behavioral Objectives *327*
Glossary *327*
Introduction *328*
Characteristics of Microorganisms *328*
Natural Body Defenses *329*
Factors That Weaken Defenses *329*
The Infectious Process Cycle *330*
Description of Asepsis *330*
Common Practices of Medical Asepsis *331*
    16-1   Handwashing *333*
    16-2   Performing a Surgical Scrub *335*
    16-3   Using a Mask *337*
Methods of Disinfection and Sterilization *340*
Principles of Surgical Asepsis *341*
Common Practices Involving Surgical
    Asepsis *342*
    16-4   Donning a Sterile Gown *346*
    16-5   Donning and Removing Sterile
            Gloves *347*
Applicable Nursing Diagnoses *351*
Teaching Suggestions to Practice Medical
    and Surgical Asepsis *351*
Bibliography *351*

17 *Preventing the Spread of Communicable Diseases* 353

Behavioral Objectives *353*
Glossary *353*
Introduction *354*
Progress Toward Infection Control *354*
Limiting the Transmission of Pathogens *355*
Types of Infection Control Practices *355*
Common Transmission Barriers *361*
Confining the Patient and Equipping
    the Room *362*
Wearing Isolation Garments *362*

Disposing of Contaminated Linen, Equipment,
and Supplies *364*
Handling Excretions and Secretions *364*
  17-1   Removing Isolation Garments (Gown,
         Gloves, and Mask) *365*
Additional Infection Control Practices *367*
  17-2   Collecting and Transporting
         a Urine Specimen *368*
Psychological Implications of Communicable
Disease Control *370*
Applicable Nursing Diagnoses *370*
Suggested Measures to Control Communicable
Diseases in Selected Situations *372*
Teaching Suggestions to Control Communicable
Diseases *372*
Bibliography *372*

18 *Caring for the Inactive Patient* 374

Behavioral Objectives *374*
Glossary *374*
Introduction *375*
Dangers of Inactivity *375*
Helping to Prevent Disuse Syndrome *377*
Using Positioning Devices *378*
Using Protective Bed Devices *380*
Using Specialty Beds *382*
Turning and Moving the Patient *384*
Positioning the Patient Confined to Bed *384*
  18-1   Turning the Patient *385*
  18-2   Moving the Patient Up in Bed *392*
Transferring the Patient *395*
  18-3   Positioning the Patient *396*
  18-4   Transferring the Patient To and From
         a Stretcher *400*
Maintaining Joint Mobility *403*
  18-5   Moving the Patient To and From
         a Chair *404*
  18-6   Performing Range-of-Motion
         Exercises *407*
Preparing the Patient for Walking *416*
Suggested Measures to Prevent Inactivity
in Selected Situations *423*
Applicable Nursing Diagnoses *425*
Teaching Suggestions to Prevent Inactivity *425*
Bibliography *425*

19 *Caring for the Patient Undergoing Surgery* 426

Behavioral Objectives *426*
Glossary *426*
Introduction *427*
Types of Surgery *427*
Locations for Surgery *427*
Types of Anesthesia *428*
Identifying Surgical Risk Factors *428*
Informing the Patient *428*
Predonating Blood *429*
Providing Psychological Support *430*
Caring for the Patient Before Surgery *431*
  19-1   Teaching Deep-Breathing
         Exercises *432*
  19-2   Teaching the Patient to Cough *435*
  19-3   Teaching Leg Exercises *436*
  19-4   Using Antiembolism Stockings *438*
Resuming Care After Surgery *441*
  19-5   Preparing the Patient for Surgery *442*
  19-6   Caring for the Postoperative
         Patient *445*
Laser Sugery *446*
Suggested Measures When Giving Preoperative
and Postoperative Care in Selected
Situations *452*
Applicable Nursing Diagnoses *452*
Teaching Suggestions Related to a Surgical
Experience *454*
Bibliography *455*

20 *Promoting Tissue Healing* 456

Behavioral Objectives *456*
Glossary *456*
Introduction *457*
Types of Wounds *457*
The Body's Reaction to Injury *457*
Promoting Skin Integrity *460*
Caring for a Wound *463*
  20-1   Preventing Pressure Sores *465*
  20-2   Changing an Occlusive Dressing *468*
Performing an Irrigation *470*
  20-3   Changing a Gauze Dressing *471*
  20-4   Irrigating a Wound *475*
  20-5   Irrigating an Eye *477*
  20-6   Irrigating an Ear *478*
Caring for a Wound With a Drain *480*
  20-7   Administering a Douche *480*
Packing a Wound *482*
Applying Wet to Dry Dressings *482*
Securing a Dressing *482*
Removing Sutures and Staples *483*
Using Bandages and Binders *484*
  20-8   Applying Bandages and Binders *489*
Understanding the Use of Heat and Cold *490*
  20-9   Applying a Compress *493*
Applicable Nursing Diagnoses *497*
Suggested Measures to Promote Tissue Healing
in Selected Situations *497*

Teaching Suggestions to Promote Tissue
Healing *499*
Bibliography *499*

21 *Promoting Urine Elimination* 500

Behavioral Objectives *500*
Glossary *500*
Introduction *501*
Understanding Urinary Structures
and Function *501*
Factors That Influence Urinary Elimination *502*
Assessing Urinary Function *502*
Toileting the Patient *503*
Managing Incontinence *506*
   21-1   Placing and Removing a Bedpan *507*
Using an External Catheter *511*
   21-2   Managing Incontinence *511*
Using Intermittent Straight Catheterization *512*
   21-3   Applying an External Catheter *512*
Using Urethral Catheterization *514*
   21-4   Inserting an Indwelling Catheter
in the Female Patient *516*
   21-5   Inserting an Indwelling Catheter
in the Male Patient *520*
   21-6   Managing an Indwelling Catheter *525*
   21-7   Irrigating an Indwelling Catheter
Using an Open System *528*
   21-8   Using a Three-Way Catheter
for Irrigation *532*
Eliminating Urine From a Surgical Opening *533*
Obtaining Urine Specimens *535*
   21-9   Collecting a Clean-Catch Midstream
Specimen *536*
Performing Common Urine Tests *537*
Suggested Measures to Promote Urinary
Elimination in Selected Situations *538*
Applicable Nursing Diagnoses *539*
Teaching Suggestions to Promote Urinary
Elimination *541*
Bibliography *541*

22 *Promoting Bowel Elimination* 543

Behavioral Objectives *543*
Glossary *543*
Introduction *544*
Reviewing Bowel Elimination *544*
Understanding Factors Affecting Bowel
Elimination *545*
Assessing Bowel Elimination *545*
Identifying and Relieving Common Alterations
in Bowel Elimination *545*

   22-1   Promoting and Maintaining Bowel
Elimination *548*
   22-2   Inserting a Rectal Tube *551*
Performing Skills That Empty the Bowel *552*
   22-3   Inserting a Rectal Suppository *553*
   22-4   Administering a Cleansing Enema *554*
Eliminating Stool Through a Stoma *558*
   22-5   Changing an Ostomy Appliance *560*
   22-6   Irrigating a Colostomy *561*
Obtaining a Stool Specimen *566*
   22-7   Collecting a Stool Specimen *566*
Suggested Measures to Promote Bowel
Elimination in Selected Situations *567*
Applicable Nursing Diagnoses *568*
Teaching Suggestions to Promote Bowel
Elimination *570*
Bibliography *570*

23 *Administering Oral and Topical Medications* 572

Behavioral Objectives *572*
Glossary *572*
Introduction *573*
Receiving a Medication Order *573*
Implementing the Medication Order *576*
Supplying Medications *577*
Safeguarding Medications *577*
Calculating Dosages *580*
Reviewing the Patient's Health History *581*
Following Basic Guidelines for Administering
Medications *581*
Recording Medication Administration *583*
Reporting Medication Errors *583*
Administering Oral Medications *584*
   23-1   Administering Oral Medications *585*
Administering Oral Medications Through
a Nasogastric Tube *587*
Administering Topical Medications *588*
   23-2   Administering Oral Medications
Through a Nasogastric Tube *589*
   23-3   Applying a Transdermal Patch *590*
   23-4   Instilling Medications Into the Eye
591
   23-5   Instilling Medications Into the Ear *593*
Overcoming Noncompliance *594*
Suggested Measures When Administering
Medications in Selected Situations *594*
   23-6   Administering Nasal Medications *595*
   23-7   Administering Vaginal Medications *596*
Applicable Nursing Diagnoses *597*
Teaching Suggestions for the Administration
of Medications *600*
Bibliography *601*

24 Administering Parenteral Medications 603

Behavioral Objectives **603**
Glossary **603**
Introduction **604**
Selecting Equipment for Parenteral
   Administration **604**
Filling a Syringe with Medication **605**
Reconstituting a Powdered Parenteral
   Medication **608**
Mixing Two Medications in One Syringe **608**
Cleansing the Skin at the Site of Injection **609**
Reducing the Discomfort of an Injection **610**
Disposing of Used Needles and Syringes **610**
Administering an Intramuscular Injection **610**
Administering a Subcutaneous Injection **611**
   24-1   Locating Sites for Intramuscular
            Injections **612**
   24-2   Administering a Subcutaneous
            Injection **617**
   24-3   Using the Z-Track Technique **620**
Administering an Intradermal Injection **623**
Administering Intravenous Medication **623**
   24-4   Administering an Intramuscular
            Injection **624**
   24-5   Administering an Intradermal
            Injection **625**
   24-6   Instilling Intravenous Medication
            Through a Central Venous
            Catheter **630**
Suggested Measures When Administering
   Parenteral Medications in Selected
   Situations **632**
   24-7   Administering Antineoplastic
            Drugs **633**
Teaching Suggestions for the Administration
   of Parenteral Medications **636**
Applicable Nursing Diagnoses **637**
Bibliography **637**

25 Maintaining and Restoring Fluid and Chemical Balance 639

Behavioral Objectives **639**
Glossary **640**
Introduction **641**
Understanding Fluid Balance **641**
Assessing Fluid Balance **643**
Performing Physical Assessments **646**
Common Fluid Imbalances **647**
Correcting Fluid Imbalances **648**
Administering Intravenous Fluids **648**

   25-1   Increasing Oral Fluid Intake **649**
   25-2   Limiting Oral Fluid Intake **650**
   25-3   Starting an Intravenous Infusion **659**
   25-4   Changing Solution Containers **666**
   25-5   Changing Infusion Tubing **668**
   25-6   Adding a Piggyback Solution **669**
Administering a Blood Transfusion **673**
   25-7   Administering a Blood
            Transfusion **674**
Understanding Electrolyte Balance **676**
Understanding Acid–Base Balance **678**
Suggested Measures to Promote Fluid and
   Chemical Balance in Selected Situations **680**
Applicable Nursing Diagnoses **680**
Teaching Suggestions to Promote Fluid and
   Chemical Balance **682**
Bibliography **682**

26 Caring for the Mechanically Immobilized Patient 684

Behavioral Objectives **684**
Glossary **684**
Introduction **685**
General Purposes for Mechanical
   Immobilization **685**
Using Splints **685**
Using Supportive Devices **686**
Caring for the Patient Who Has a Cast **690**
   26-1   Providing Basic Cast Care **691**
   26-2   Petaling a Cast Edge **694**
Caring for the Patient in Traction **695**
   26-3   Caring for the Patient in Traction **697**
Using a Continuous Passive Motion
   Machine **699**
Suggested Measures Related to Mechanical
   Immobilization in Selected Situations **699**
   26-4   Using a Continuous Passive Motion
            (CPM) Machine **700**
Applicable Nursing Diagnoses **701**
Teaching Suggestions Related to Mechanical
   Immobilization **703**
Bibliography **703**

27 Promoting Cardiopulmonary Function 704

Behavioral Objectives **704**
Glossary **704**
Introduction **705**
Clearing the Airway **705**
Suctioning the Airway **706**
   27-1   Promoting Postural Drainage **707**
Relieving Airway Obstruction **709**
   27-2   Suctioning the Upper Airway **710**

Caring for the Patient With an Artificial
Airway   *713*
   27-3   Dislodging an Object From
        the Airway   *713*
   27-4   Suctioning Secretions From a
        Tracheostomy   *718*
Restoring Cardiopulmonary Function   *720*
   27-5   Providing Tracheostomy Care   *720*
   27-6   Administering Oxygen   *728*
   27-7   Maintaining Water-Seal Drainage   *732*
   27-8   Performing Cardiopulmonary
        Resuscitation   *735*
Suggested Measures to Promote Cardiopulmonary
Function in Selected Situations   *740*
Applicable Nursing Diagnoses   *742*
Teaching Suggestions to Promote
Cardiopulmonary Function   *744*
Bibliography   *745*

28 *Caring for Terminally Ill and Grieving Individuals*   *749*

Behavioral Objectives   *749*
Glossary   *749*
Introduction   *750*
Examining Attitudes and Responses
to Dying   *750*

Preparing to Provide Terminal Care   *751*
Informing the Dying Patient   *753*
Identifying Patterns of Emotional Reactions   *755*
Supporting Options for Care   *755*
Responding to Emotional Needs   *758*
Meeting Spiritual Needs   *760*
Attending to Physical Needs   *761*
Recognizing the Signs
of Approaching Death   *763*
Summoning the Family   *764*
Helping Arriving Relatives   *765*
Confirming Death   *765*
Nursing Responsibilities After the
Patient's Death   *765*
Understanding the Grieving Process   *766*
   28-1   Performing Postmortem Care   *767*
   28-2   Facilitating the Process
        of Grieving   *770*
Suggested Measures for Terminally Ill or Grieving
Patients in Selected Situations   *771*
Applicable Nursing Diagnoses   *772*
Teaching Suggestions Involving Terminally Ill
and Grieving Individuals   *772*
Bibliography   *774*

Skill Procedures

2 Patient Services: The Focus of Nursing

2-1   Promoting Effective Communication   **23**
2-2   Providing Emotional Support   **26**
2-3   Teaching the Patient   **28**

4 The Nursing Process: The Model for Nursing

4-1   Using the Nursing Process   **50**

5 Patient Records: Resources for Sharing Information

5-1   Making Entries on the Patient's Record   **64**

7 Promoting Personal Hygiene

7-1   Providing for Tub or Shower Bathing   **88**
7-2   Assisting With a Bed Bath   **90**
7-3   Giving a Complete Bed Bath   **91**
7-4   Tepid Sponging   **95**
7-5   Administering Perineal Care   **97**
7-6   Giving a Backrub   **98**
7-7   Shaving a Patient   **100**
7-8   Brushing and Flossing the Teeth   **102**
7-9   Performing Oral Hygiene Measures   **104**
7-10 Cleansing the Eyes   **106**
7-11 Removing, Cleaning, and Replacing Contact Lenses   **109**
7-12 Inserting a Hearing Aid   **114**
7-13 Shampooing Hair   **116**

8 Promoting Proper Nutrition

8-1   Serving and Removing Trays   **134**
8-2   Helping the Patient to Eat   **135**
8-3   Inserting, Maintaining, and Removing a Nasogastric Tube   **136**
8-4   Inserting a Small Diameter Feeding Tube   **142**
8-5   Administering a Tube Feeding   **145**
8-6   Irrigating a Nasogastric Tube   **151**

9 Promoting Activity and Exercise

9-1   Using Proper Body Mechanics   **163**
9-2   Planning a Safe Exercise Program   **171**

10 Promoting Comfort, Relaxation, and Sleep

10-1   Relieving Pain   **181**
10-2   Using a Patient-Controlled Analgesia Infuser   **183**
10-3   Operating a TENS Unit   **187**
10-4   Facilitating Relaxation   **190**
10-5   Promoting Sleep   **194**

11 Admitting, Transferring, and Discharging the Patient

11-1   Admitting the Patient   **209**
11-2   Transferring the Patient   **211**
11-3   Discharging the Patient   **214**

12 Promoting Rest and Safety Within the Patient's Environment

12-1   Making an Unoccupied Bed   **220**
12-2   Making an Occupied Bed   **224**
12-3   Promoting Sensory Stimulation   **228**
12-4   Applying a Protective Restraint   **231**

13 Obtaining Vital Signs

13-1   Cleaning a Glass Thermometer   **247**
13-2   Measuring Body Temperature Using a Glass Thermometer   **248**
13-3   Assessing Body Temperature Using an Electronic Thermometer   **252**
13-4   Assessing the Radial Pulse   **257**
13-5   Counting the Respiratory Rate   **260**
13-6   Measuring the Blood Pressure   **267**

14 Performing Assessment Techniques

14-1   Performing a Physical Assessment   **283**
14-2   Assessing Lung Sounds   **288**

15 Assisting With Examinations and Special Tests

15-1   Assisting With an Examination   **309**
15-2   Using a Glucometer   **319**

16 Controlling Microorganisms

16-1   Handwashing   **333**
16-2   Performing a Surgical Scrub   **335**
16-3   Using a Mask   **337**
16-4   Donning a Sterile Gown   **346**
16-5   Donning and Removing Sterile Gloves   **347**

17 Preventing the Spread of Communicable Diseases

17-1   Removing Isolation Garments (Gown, Gloves, and Mask)   **365**
17-2   Collecting and Transporting a Urine Specimen   **368**

18 Caring for the Inactive Patient

18-1   Turning the Patient   **385**
18-2   Moving the Patient Up in Bed   **392**
18-3   Positioning the Patient   **396**
18-4   Transferring the Patient To and From a Stretcher   **400**
18-5   Moving the Patient To and From a Chair   **404**
18-6   Performing Range-of-Motion Exercises   **407**

19 Caring for the Patient Undergoing Surgery

19-1   Teaching Deep-Breathing Exercises   **432**
19-2   Teaching the Patient to Cough   **435**
19-3   Teaching Leg and Foot Exercises   **436**
19-4   Using Antiembolism Stockings   **438**
19-5   Preparing the Patient for Surgery   **442**
19-6   Caring for the Postoperative Patient   **445**

20 Promoting Tissue Healing

20-1   Preventing Pressure Sores   **465**
20-2   Changing an Occlusive Dressing   **468**
20-3   Changing a Gauze Dressing   **471**
20-4   Irrigating a Wound   **475**
20-5   Irrigating an Eye   **477**
20-6   Irrigating an Ear   **478**
20-7   Administering a Douche   **480**
20-8   Applying Bandages and Binders   **489**
20-9   Applying a Compress   **493**

21 Promoting Urine Elimination

21-1   Placing and Removing a Bedpan   **507**
21-2   Managing Incontinence   **511**
21-3   Applying an External Catheter   **512**
21-4   Inserting an Indwelling Catheter in the Female Patient   **516**
21-5   Inserting an Indwelling Catheter in the Male Patient   **520**
21-6   Managing an Indwelling Catheter   **525**
21-7   Irrigating an Indwelling Catheter Using an Open System   **528**
21-8   Using a Three-Way Catheter for Irrigation   **532**
21-9   Collecting a Clean-Catch Midstream Specimen   **536**

22 *Promoting Bowel Elimination*

22-1   Promoting and Maintaining Bowel
        Elimination   **548**
22-2   Inserting a Rectal Tube   **551**
22-3   Inserting a Rectal Suppository   **553**
22-4   Administering a Cleansing Enema   **554**
22-5   Changing an Ostomy Appliance   **560**
22-6   Irrigating a Colostomy   **561**
22-7   Collecting a Stool Specimen   **566**

23 *Administering Oral and Topical Medications*

23-1   Administering Oral Medications   **585**
23-2   Administering Medications Through
        a Nasogastric Tube   **589**
23-3   Applying a Transdermal Patch   **590**
23-4   Instilling Medications Into the Eye   **591**
23-5   Instilling Medications Into the Ear   **593**
23-6   Administering Nasal Medications   **595**
23-7   Administering Vaginal Medications   **596**

24 *Administering Parenteral Medications*

24-1   Locating Sites for Intramuscular
        Injections   **612**
24-2   Administering an Intramuscular
        Injection   **617**
24-3   Using the Z-Track Technique   **620**
24-4   Administering a Subcutaneous
        Injection   **624**
24-5   Administering an Intradermal
        Injection   **625**
24-6   Instilling Intravenous Medication Through
        a Central Venous Catheter   **630**
24-7   Administering Antineoplastic Drugs   **633**

25 *Maintaining and Restoring Fluid and Chemical Balance*

25-1   Increasing Oral Fluid Intake   **649**
25-2   Limiting Oral Fluid Intake   **650**
25-3   Starting an Intravenous Infusion   **659**
25-4   Changing Solution Containers   **666**
25-5   Changing Infusion Tubing   **668**
25-6   Adding a Piggyback Solution   **669**
25-7   Administering a Blood Transfusion   **674**

26 *Caring for the Mechanically Immobilized Patient*

26-1   Proving Basic Cast Care   **691**
26-2   Petaling a Cast Edge   **694**
26-3   Caring for the Patient in Traction   **697**
26-4   Using a Continuous Passive Motion
        Machine   **700**

27 *Promoting Cardiopulmonary Function*

27-1   Promoting Postural Drainage   **707**
27-2   Suctioning the Upper Airway   **710**
27-3   Dislodging an Object
        From the Airway   **713**
27-4   Suctioning Secretions
        From a Tracheostomy   **718**
27-5   Providing Tracheostomy Care   **720**
27-6   Administering Oxygen   **728**
27-7   Maintaining Water-Seal Drainage   **732**
27-8   Performing Cardiopulmonary
        Resuscitation   **735**

28 *Caring for Terminally Ill and Grieving Individuals*

28-1   Performing Postmortem Care   **767**
28-2   Facilitating the Process of Grieving   **770**

Unit I

The Nurse and the Patient

1

Nursing: A Skill-Related Practice

Chapter Outline

Behavioral Objectives
Glossary
Introduction
Evolution of Nursing Theories
Definitions of Nursing
Objectives of Nursing Skills
Skills Basic to Nursing
Basis for Nursing Skills
Characteristics of the Practice of Nursing
Bibliography

Behavioral Objectives

When the content of this chapter has been mastered, the learner will be able to:

Define terms appearing in the glossary.

Identify four representative nursing theorists and their theories.

Identify the changes that have occurred in definitions of nursing.

List three objectives of nursing.

Describe four basic skills required of nurses.

List three components that provide a basis for the skills used by nurses.

List 13 characteristics of the practice of nursing.

Glossary

Accountability Responsibility for one's acts.

Active listening Hearing the content of what the patient says as well as the unspoken message.

Activities of daily living Common acts that people carry out each day in the normal course of living.

Art The ability to perform an act skillfully.

Assessment skills Collecting information by interviewing, observing, and examining a patient.

Autonomy The ability to be self-directed.

Caring The concern and attachment that occurs from the close relationship of one human being with another.

Caring skills Those skills that restore or maintain an individual's highest state of functioning.

Comforting skills Those skills that convey to patients that their feelings are understood and accepted.

Continuing education Formal or informal education offered to nurses who have completed a basic educational program.

Counseling skills Skills in communication that involve both talking and listening.

Curative nursing care Care intended primarily to help restore health.

Empathy Detached awareness of what the patient is experiencing.

Health care Services to improve a state of well-being for individuals who are sick or well.

Health practitioner Any individual whose skills improve an individual's state of health.

Health promotion Care intended primarily to help people stay well. Synonym for *preventive nursing care*.

Medical care Care provided or directed by a physician to assist a sick individual in getting well.

Nurse practice acts Laws that regulate the practice of nursing.

Nursing The diagnosis and treatment of human responses to actual or potential health problems.

Nursing process A method of problem solving in which the nurse assesses, diagnoses, plans, implements, and evaluates patient care.

Preventive nursing care Care intended primarily to help people stay well. Synonym for *health promotion*.

Principle An undisputed fact on which certain outcomes can be predicted.

Public health codes Laws that regulate the practice of various health practitioners.

Rehabilitation The art and skill of helping handicapped persons regain function and use remaining abilities in the best way possible.

Rehabilitative nursing care Care intended primarily to prevent further deterioration of or restore physical functions immediately upon a patient's admission.

Science A body of knowledge unique to a particular subject.

Self-image A personal view of oneself.
Supportive nursing care Care intended primarily to offer psychological comfort to the patient.
Sympathy Feeling so similarly to the patient that one's objectivity is lost.
Theory A person's viewpoint.

Introduction

Nurses use specialized skills to care for people who are sick or well. All nurses, regardless of their choice of educational preparation, learn basic skills that are fundamental to the practice of nursing. Nursing practice involves the application of knowledge and the performance of skilled tasks that improve an individual's level of health.

Many individuals, besides nurses, can provide health care. *Health care* consists of services offered to people who are sick or well. Individuals such as nurses, dietitians, respiratory therapists, and physical therapists are called *health practitioners*. Each health practitioner has been educated to provide unique skills that may improve an individual's state of health. Some of those skills may be provided independently of a physician. The regulation of each health practitioner's skills is defined legally by every state.

Health practitioners also work interdependently with the physician and each other as a team. When a doctor requests that a health practitioner carry out a specific task, the term medical care is used. *Medical care* refers to care provided or directed by a physician to assist a sick individual in getting well.

Evolution of Nursing Theories

Since its reformation, nursing has traditionally involved a unique spirit and art. Because Florence Nightingale felt she had a calling to care for the sick, she recruited laywomen and nuns with similar zeal. Nightingale intuitively realized that only individuals who possessed devotion and idealism would accept the discipline and hard work required for caring for the ill, injured, and infirm. Thus, it was and continues to be accepted that a cornerstone of nursing practice is extraordinary dedication and commitment.

An *art* is the ability to perform an act skillfully. The practice of nursing has been considered an art because its skills are acquired under the guidance and direction of other experienced practitioners. The skills are passed on from mentor to student as a result of tradition.

Nursing is now developing into a science. The English word science comes from the Latin word *scio,* which means, "I know." A *science* is a body of knowledge unique to a particular subject. It develops from observing and studying the relation of one phenomenon to another. For instance, one might study the effect of light on the growth

of African violets. The individual who conducts the study identifies a conclusion at the outcome of the study. The conclusion is said to be a theory. Theory comes from a Greek word that means vision. A *theory* is a person's viewpoint or explanation for the outcomes that took place in the study.

Nursing is becoming a science in addition to the spirit and art that have traditionally been hallmarks of its practice. Theories explaining the process called nursing are being identified as a result of the experiences, observations, and studies of pioneer nurses.

Nursing theorists, then and now, examine the interrelationships among man, health, the environment, and nursing. Specific concepts of various nursing theorists are identified in Table 1-1. Nursing theories today are accepted widely by individuals. They are being adopted by entire nursing education programs as a conceptual framework or model for their philosophy, curriculum, and basis for nursing approaches. This is similar to schools of psychology and psychologists who choose Freud's Psychoanalytic Theory or Skinner's Behavioral Theory as a model for their professional practice.

Table 1-2 summarizes some nursing theories and discusses how each theory has been applied to nursing practice. Those selected are only a representative sample of the accumulating theories of nursing. Expanded information on this subject can be researched in more detail in current nursing literature.

Nursing has also adopted and applied theories of nonnurses. Several of these theories and their nursing application are identified in Table 1-3.

Definitions of Nursing

Nursing probably has been practiced since the beginning of human existence. It has changed and will continue to change as theorists refine the science of nursing. It is interesting to note the transitions in definitions of nursing.

Definitions of nursing identify the activities that are unique to nursing. Florence Nightingale, the individual who restored dignity to caring for sick individuals, is also credited with the earliest, modern definition. She proposed that "nursing is putting individuals in the best possible condition for nature to restore and preserve health."

Definitions of nursing have been proposed and revised by others who have come to be recognized as authorities and, therefore, qualified spokespersons on the practice of nursing. One authority is Virginia Henderson. Her definition added a new dimension to previous ones by broadening the description of nursing to include health promotion, not just illness care. She stated in 1966 that

The unique function of the nurse is to assist the individual, sick or well, in the performance of those activities contributing to health or its recovery (or

Table 1-1. Components of Selected Nursing Theories

Theorist	Theory	
Florence Nightingale 1820–1910	**Environmental Theory**	
	Man	Individuals whose natural defenses are influenced by a healthful or unhealthful environment.
	Health	A state in which the environment is optimum for the natural body processes to achieve reparative outcomes.
	Environment	All the external conditions that are capable of preventing, suppressing, or contributing to disease or death.
	Nursing	Putting the patient in the best condition for nature to act.
Virginia Henderson 1897–	**Basic Needs Theory**	
	Man	Individuals with human needs that have meaning and value unique to each person.
	Health	The ability to independently satisfy human needs composed of 14 basic physical, psychological, and social elements.
	Environment	The setting in which an individual learns unique patterns for living.
	Nursing	Temporarily assisting an individual who lacks the necessary strength, will, and knowledge to satisfy one or more of 14 basic needs.
Dorothea Orem 1914–	**Self-Care Theory**	
	Man	An individual who uses self-care to sustain life and health, recover from disease or injury, or cope with its effects.
	Health	The result of practices that individuals have learned to carry out on their own behalf to maintain life and well-being.
	Environment	External elements with which man interacts in his struggle to maintain self-care.
	Nursing	Nursing is a human service that assists individuals to progressively maximize their self-care potential.
Sister Callista Roy 1939–	**Adaptation Theory**	
	Man	A social, mental, spiritual, and physical being who is affected by stimuli in the internal and external environment.
	Health	The ability of an individual to adapt to changes in the environment.
	Environment	Internal and external forces that are in a continuous state of change.
	Nursing	A humanitarian art and expanding science that manipulates and modifies stimuli in order to promote and facilitate man's ability to adapt.

to a peaceful death) that he could perform unaided if he had the necessary strength, will or knowledge. And to do this in such a way as to help him gain independence as rapidly as possible.

In her writing and speaking, Henderson proposed that nursing is more than carrying out medical orders in the care of the sick. It involves a special relationship and service between the nurse and those entrusted for care.

According to Henderson, the nurse acts as a temporary proxy meeting one or more of the basic human needs identified in Display 1-1 for which neither the patient nor his family can provide. All nursing students learn skills that assist patients to meet these needs.

The most recent definition of nursing from the American Nurses Association (ANA; 1980) adds yet another dimension to the practice of nursing. It emphasizes that the nurse has an independent area in which to use nursing

Table 1-2. Nursing Theories and Applications

Theorist	Theory	Summary of Theory	Application to Nursing Practice
Florence Nightingale 1820–1910	Environmental Theory	External conditions such as ventilation, light, odor, and cleanliness are capable of preventing, suppressing, or contributing to disease or death.	Nurses modify unhealthful aspects of the environment to put the patient in the best condition for nature to act.
Virginia Henderson 1897–	Basic Needs Theory	Individuals have 14 basic needs that are components of health. Their significance and value are unique to each individual.	Nurses assist in performing those activities which the patient would if he had the strength, will, and knowledge.
Dorothea Orem 1914–	Self-Care Theory	Individuals learn behaviors that they perform on their own behalf to maintain life, health, and well-being.	Nurses assist patients with self-care to improve or maintain health.
Sister Callista Roy 1939–	Adaptation Theory	Man is a biopsychosocial being. A change in one component results in adaptive changes in the others.	Nurses assess biological, psychological, and social factors interfering with health, alter the stimuli causing maladaptation, and evaluate the effectiveness of the action taken.

Table 1-3. Non-Nursing Theories and Applications

Theorist	Theory	Summary of Theory	Application to Nursing Practice
Abraham Maslow 1908–1970	Human Needs Theory	Human beings have a hierarchial order of needs that, when met, leads to higher levels of wellness.	Nurses use Maslow's hierarchy to set priorities for nursing actions. Problems that have the greatest priority are those that affect first-level needs associated with survival, such as breathing. Once basic needs are met other problems assume greater importance.
Hans Selye 1907–1982	General Adaptation Theory	Biological as well as psychological stressors cause the same physiological changes that lead to disease or death.	Nurses promote health by preventing, modifying, reducing, or removing physical and psychological stressors.
Ludwig von Bertalanffly 1901–1972	General Systems Theory	Systems are composed of individual parts. A system is greater than the sum of its parts. A change in one part of the subsystem affects the whole.	The body is a system of related parts. Illness or injury of one part causes changes to occur in others. A patient is a part of a family and societal group. When illness or injury affects one individual in a group, it also affects others within the group.

Display 1-1. Human Needs

All individuals have basic needs to:
1. Breathe normally.
2. Eat and drink adequately.
3. Eliminate body wastes.
4. Move and maintain desirable postures.
5. Sleep and rest.
6. Select suitable clothing—dress and undress.
7. Maintain body temperature within normal range by adjusting clothing and modifying the environment.
8. Keep the body clean and well groomed and protect the integument.
9. Avoid dangers in the environment and avoid injuring others.
10. Communicate with others in expressing emotions, needs, fears, or opinions.
11. Worship according to one's faith.
12. Work in such a way that there is a sense of accomplishment.
13. Play or participate in various forms of recreation.
14. Learn, discover, or satisfy the curiosity that leads to normal development and health and use of the available health facilities.

Henderson V: The Nature of Nursing. New York, Macmillan, 1966. Copyright © 1966 by Virginia Henderson. Reprinted with permission of the publisher.

---

skills. The position taken by the ANA is that *nursing* is "the diagnosis and treatment of human responses to actual or potential health problems."

These changes in definitions have provided the framework for the addition and elaboration of nursing skills found within the practice of nursing today. As the role of the nurse changes in the future, new definitions of nursing will be developed to describe the functions of the nurse.

Objectives of Nursing Skills

Nursing involves skills that can be beneficial to sick or well individuals. Nurses now provide services in many diverse settings such as schools, industry, hospitals, and home care. The following discussion elaborates and points out the major goals of nursing today.

Nursing Works to Promote Health and Prevent Disease. Nurses today have an increasingly important responsibility to help people stay well. This is often called *preventive nursing care* or *health promotion.*

Promotion of physical health may be seen in the field of nutrition, in which the body's requirements are well known and the results of poor eating have been demonstrated. Nurses have knowledge of normal nutritional needs. Nurses use teaching skills related to nutrition to help people learn how to select, prepare, or modify their diets in order to meet their daily requirements. Eating a variety of foods in the proper amount promotes a healthy state.

Promoting the state of an individual's health will assist in the prevention or reduction in the occurrence of illness. Much work is being done to prevent illnesses that continue to strike humanity. Heart disease and cancer, for example, are being studied in many countries by people of varying professions. Nurses often assist in these studies. The purposes of these programs are to find how these diseases are caused, how they can be treated when present, and how they can be prevented through health promotion measures.

Health practitioners have studied how stress affects health. Based on the findings of researchers, programs that help us deal with stress are making it possible for more people to enjoy better health. Nurses are now assisting those individuals who demonstrate unhealthful physical responses to stress. High blood pressure is a common stress response in the human body. By promoting stress management techniques, nurses can help individuals reduce their blood pressure to safer levels. Maintaining blood pressure at normal levels prevents many potential health problems.

Nursing Is Concerned with Restoring Health. Even with care that promotes health, disease attacks humans. The most basic component of nursing has been the use of skills that help sick people regain health. Nurses take care of the sick by giving aid, comfort, nourishment, protection, and support. This kind of nursing is often called *curative nursing care* and is an important part of nursing practice.

Assisting people to overcome handicaps by helping to return function to a part of the body or by making the best possible use of remaining abilities is often called *rehabilitation.* Until recently, rehabilitation was usually thought of as a specialized field of work done by people who helped severely handicapped patients. Today, nurses plan and use skills that prevent further deterioration of or restore physical functions immediately upon a patient's admission. Some refer to this kind of nursing care as *rehabilitative nursing care.* A nurse gives rehabilitative care when she exercises a partially paralyzed arm to help bring back its normal functioning (Fig. 1-1).

Nursing Is Concerned with Relieving Suffering. Many individuals for whom nurses care may have life-threatening illnesses. Nurses recognize that there is an end to all human life. Health is not a state that can be sustained forever. The nurse continues to provide care for

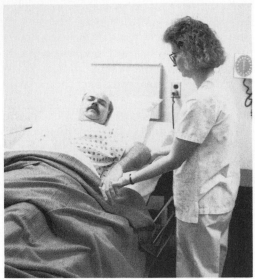

Figure 1-1 The patient is helped to regain full use of his arm as the nurse assists him in moving it through its range of motion.

individuals whose death is a predictable outcome in the near future. The dying patient may present the greatest challenge to the nurse's skills. There is a sensitivity among nurses to the dying person's need for pain relief and physical care, and fear of abandonment. The nurse's presence serves to relieve the burden of lonely suffering (Fig. 1-2).

Skills Basic to Nursing

To provide comprehensive care, the nurse uses skills that are basic to any setting in which nursing is practiced. These skills involve the application of sciences such as anatomy, physiology, sociology, and psychology, which form part of the knowledge base of nursing.

Assessment Skills

Before the nurse can determine what type of care to provide, the needs and problems of the patient must be determined. This requires the use of assessment skills. *Assessment skills* are those acts of interviewing, observation, and examination for the purpose of collecting information. The nurse gathers data from various resources. The patient is the primary source, but the family, the medical record, and verbal information from other health practitioners are also helpful.

The nurse uses verbal skills to interview the patient or family. Certain questions about health and illness can provide facts about the individual's current and past health problems. It is also possible at this time to acquire the patient's view of his health state and expectations for care. Communication with the doctor or others involved with the patient may help the nurse gather information and avoid duplication.

The senses of vision, hearing, touch, and smell can aid in collecting facts about the person's health state through observation. Slurred speech may indicate that the patient has had a stroke; a fruity odor to the breath may indicate a complication of diabetes; bruises may indicate a recent fall; cold skin may mean poor circulation. The nurse uses knowledge of what is normal to analyze that which is abnormal.

Finally, the nurse uses examination skills as part of assessment. Various kinds of equipment such as a thermometer and a stethoscope are used by the nurse to provide information about the patient. The nurse follows a systematic pattern of evaluating the patient from head to toe. Any deviation from normal provides the nurse with

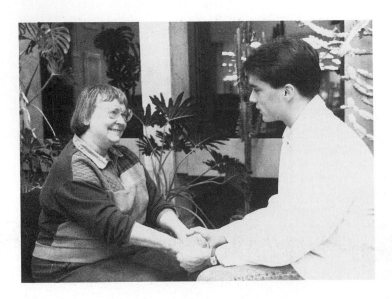

Figure 1-2 Nursing often means being there when the patient needs you. Note that the nurse offers support by touching the patient's hand and by listening to what the patient says.

more clues for identifying the individual's actual or potential health problems. Various nursing skills may be useful in reducing, eliminating, or preventing those identified health problems. Assessment skills are discussed in more detail in Chapters 4 and 14.

Caring Skills

Nurses are and have always been care givers. This has been the most traditional role for nurses. *Caring skills* are those that restore or maintain an individual's highest state of functioning. For some patients this may involve something as minimal as assisting the patient with activities of daily living. *Activities of daily living* is a term used to describe acts that people do in the normal course of living. Such activities include eating, sleeping, elimination, working, moving about, socializing, and so on.

More and more nurses are being required to provide complex care skills such as the monitoring and use of highly technical equipment. This textbook is primarily written about the caring skills that nurses commonly provide in the practice of nursing.

No matter what level of care is provided, the nurse wants the patient eventually to be independent. The nurse who gives too much tender loving care may delay the patient from moving toward wellness and being able to resume normal activities of daily living.

Caring also involves the concern and attachment that occurs from the close relationship of one human being with another. Nurses maintain that their priority is the caring for the patient above all other tasks that may be involved.

Counseling Skills

To promote active participation in decision making, nurses guard against giving advice to patients. Nurses believe that every individual or his family retains the right to make decisions and choices on matters affecting health and illness care. Therefore, nurses use *counseling skills* that involve both talking and active listening.

The nurse provides information to the patient by responding to questions, providing written information, and using charts, models, or diagrams. These activities promote the patient's ability to analyze how his life is affected by his health problem or its treatment. The patient can then choose from several options to decide which is most appropriate for him.

At times counseling involves teaching. While giving care, the nurse finds many opportunities to teach patients how to promote healing processes, stay well, prevent illness, and carry out activities of daily living in the best possible way. People know much more about health and health care today. They expect nurses to share accurate information with them.

Patients do not always ask questions or communicate their concerns. Another counseling skill is the use of empathy. *Empathy* is a detached awareness of what the patient is experiencing. The nurse uses empathy to anticipate the patient's emotional state and his desire or need for information. This skill involves being able to remain impartial in order to evaluate the situation. This quality differs from sympathy. *Sympathy* is feeling so similarly to the patient that the nurse loses objectivity and the ability to help the patient through his problem.

There are times when counseling skills involve active listening. *Active listening* is hearing the content of what the patient says as well as the unspoken message. Patients sometimes appreciate the opportunity to describe their feelings or concerns. This helps the patient organize his thoughts and evaluate the situation more realistically. Often, the only requirements for the nurse are the provision for uninterrupted time with the patient and full attention to what is being said.

Comforting Skills

All individuals possess a personal view of themselves. *Self-image* involves a mental attitude about who and what we are. A state of health is one of the usual characteristics of self-image, since it is the predominant experience for most individuals. When health is threatened, it will usually cause a person to reexamine his self-image. It may cause feelings of insecurity. What the patient assumed about himself, or even took for granted, may no longer be accurate. This change in mental attitude can threaten the foundation on which an individual is able to cope with current and future problems. The patient feels very vulnerable.

It is then that the nurse uses *comforting skills* to convey to the patient that his feelings are understood and accepted. Because the family or other supportive persons may not be continuously available for the patient, the nurse becomes the stabilizing figure during the patient's temporary state of illness. The nurse becomes the guide, companion, and interpreter for the patient during his experiences, thus reassuring him that he is not alone. This type of care, called *supportive nursing care* (Fig. 1-3), produces a trust relationship that reduces the patient's fear and worry.

Basis for Nursing Skills

Nursing began as an extension of nurturing. The early skills were often an accumulation of practices that were handed down from one generation to another. Those who were most successful and willing to assume the functions associated with nursing were entrusted with that responsibility. The present basis for nursing involves more than just apprenticed knowledge.

Scientific Knowledge

The foundation for promoting health is based on information that has been discovered in the sciences. Nursing is said to make use of the applied sciences. Once anatomy and physiology are understood, assessment skills can be applied to identify the characteristics associated with

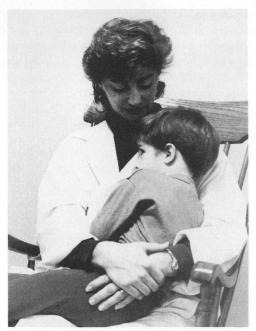

Figure 1-3 This child cried when his parents left for the day. The nurse offers emotional support and demonstrates that she cares by holding the patient securely and by rocking and speaking to him. As a result, having to be hospitalized and away from his family becomes a little easier for the child.

health or disease. Once a knowledge of chemistry and physics is acquired, an understanding of therapeutic treatment such as pharmacology, fluid replacement, and inhalation therapy can be applied. Understanding how organisms grow and multiply through the study of microbiology provides a basis for applying nursing skills that can protect individuals from infection.

Nurses also apply knowledge from the social sciences, such as sociology and psychology. By learning how individuals live and rely on social interaction, nurses can apply skills based on family and group structures. Human behavior has been studied by psychologists. The information from this body of scientists provides information from which the nurse may use skills to help a patient change or modify his behavior.

Research

Nurses have long participated in the research studies of other scientists. Now nurses are designing and conducting their own research. Many inquisitive nurses are not content to implement the skills and practices that have been perpetuated from tradition. Progress in any practice is often the result of challenging long-held beliefs. Many nurses are daring to ask why and why not. This has and will continue to promote the accumulation of scientific knowledge unique to the practice of nursing. It provides a basis for the change or addition of nursing skills that can be used to promote health and to prevent disease.

Nursing journals often publish the written contributions of nurses to promote current skills and knowledge. One

bimonthly periodical, *Nursing Research,* is devoted specifically to nursing research and findings.

Proven Principles

Principles are undisputed facts on which one can predict certain outcomes. Principles usually develop from research. For the findings of research to be considered valid, they must have included a large or long-term test. In addition, the findings must be duplicated by other independent researchers. Once this occurs, the findings are considered proven principles. Nursing skills are based on proven principles. Principles provide nurses with the reasons, or whys, that guide their actions. All skills for patient care reflect a scientific rationale.

Consider the following example. Research has shown that the moist particles, called droplets, expelled during sneezing and coughing can carry live organisms from a person's nose and throat. These droplets are often carried considerable distances, and if someone else inhales them, he may become infected with the microorganisms. However, when the droplets are trapped with a tissue, these microorganisms do not reach others. The suggested nursing action, then, is to teach the patient to cover his nose and mouth when sneezing and coughing. The principle, or reason, for the action is that a tissue forms a physical barrier controlling the transmission of infectious microorganisms.

The nurse selects an appropriate skill based on knowledge of scientific research. The proven principle is the rationale for the nurse's action. Knowing the *why* of one's action and being able to predict its effect is important when implementing nursing skills. Good nursing care requires sound nursing judgment, which becomes possible only when the nurse has knowledge of principles and expected results when performing nursing actions.

Characteristics of the Practice of Nursing

The practice of nursing is unique. The characteristics described in the following discussion are examples of the qualities that distinguish nursing from the work of other health-care practitioners.

Nursing Practice Has a Definable Role. Each state is commissioned within its laws and powers to protect the health and safety of its citizens. State legislatures propose and enact health-related legislation to protect individuals from receiving services from unqualified health practitioners. Legal codes define the skills and limits to which those skills may be used by various health-care workers.

Nursing, which represents the largest group of health-care workers, provides unique skills within the health-care system. Most states regulate nursing through what is referred to as *nurse practice acts* or *public health codes.*

Though the language of each state's nurse practice act is not identical, the intent is similar. The laws describe who may be called a nurse and the boundaries of that practice. The following is an example of the legal language within a nurse practice act that defines practical nursing in the state of Indiana:

"Practical nursing" means the performance of services commonly performed by practical nurses including:

- Contributing to the assessment of the health status of individuals or groups
- Participating in the development and modification of the strategy of care
- Implementing the appropriate aspects of the strategy of care
- Maintaining safe and effective nursing care
- Participating in the evaluation of responses to the strategy of care. (Indiana Public Law #169, passed in 1985).

Indiana's definition of registered nursing is the following:

"Registered nursing" means performance of services which include but are not limited to:

- Assessing health conditions
- Deriving a nursing diagnosis
- Executing a nursing regimen through the selection, performance, and management of nursing actions based on nursing diagnoses
- Advocating the provision of health-care services through collaboration with or referral to other health professionals
- Executing regimens delegated by a physician with an unlimited license to practice medicine, a licensed dentist, a licensed chiropractor, a licensed optometrist, or a licensed podiatrist
- Teaching, administering, supervising, delegating, and evaluating nursing practice
- Delegating tasks that assist in implementing the nursing, medical, or dental regimen
- Performing acts that are approved by the board in collaboration with the medical licensing board of Indiana. (Indiana Public Law #169, passed in 1985).

Nursing Practice Is Valued by Society. Any service that benefits the community at large will be valued. Health is a precious resource of every individual and community. Individuals, such as nurses, who safeguard that resource are appreciated. The worth of that service sustains the practice.

Nursing won its respected position by following the ideals of Florence Nightingale. Before her reforms, those who cared for the sick in England's hospitals were often criminals or paupers. They were ordered by the government to do so in exchange for food and shelter. The quality of care was comparable to the level of the care givers.

As nurses have become formally educated, the hospital has become associated with high-level care. Most people can expect to acquire health rather than die. Today's intensive care is possible through the advanced knowledge and skill of nurses who work all day and night at the patient's bedside.

Nurses are also participating in health education within the community. Illness is less costly to prevent than to treat. Because nursing promotes health, its worth has been valued by the public.

Nursing Practice Involves Unique Competencies. The practice of nursing is based on the nursing process. *Nursing process* is a method of problem solving used by nurses in assessing, diagnosing, planning, implementing, and evaluating patient care. This model provides a foundation for ensuring and improving the quality of individualized care provided for each patient.

The skills implemented by nurses, such as inserting and maintaining a urinary catheter, are not performed by any other health practitioner. Nurses learn principles and practice skills during their educational experience. This book will provide a foundation for those skills that are fundamental for patient care.

Nursing Practice Involves Unselfish Service. The work performed by nurses results in a service to individuals rather than a product. Nursing was once predominantly practiced by men and women in religious orders. Caring for the sick was considered a work of mercy that would be spiritually rewarded.

Nursing is called a helping profession. It continues to involve placing the needs of those committed for care above personal needs. Though the salary compensation for this service is not yet consistent with the responsibilities, nurses gain satisfaction from participating in the healing and health promotion of individuals who need assistance.

Nursing Practice Demonstrates Responsibility and Accountability. Although each state defines the scope of nursing practice, the ANA has identified standards of nursing practice. These identify the direct responsibilities for the services of the nurse to the patient, and they establish the criteria for quality within the practice of nursing. By publishing these standards, the ANA provides its practitioners and the public with a tool for evaluating nursing services. Nurses must show they can be depended on to practice according to these established standards. They also must answer personally for any deviation from those standards.

Nursing Includes Practitioners at Various Educational Levels. Just as individuals experience varying degrees in their health needs, they may require varying levels of assistance, too. The division of labor can be delegated in order to make the best use of each nurse's skills. Table 1-4 identifies the specialized contributions each category of nurse has been educated to provide. Each identified level of practice in the table represents a hierarchy of the other. Each acquires more knowledge, responsibility, and variation in roles as the sequence progresses. For purposes of clarification, a practical nurse is one who has completed a vocational nursing program. A technical nurse is a graduate of an associate degree or hospital diploma program. The professional nurse holds a minimum of a baccalaureate degree in nursing. Many professional nurses go on to acquire graduate nursing degrees.

States currently license both practical or vocational

nurses and registered nurses. Some states may eventually designate another level and title of licensure for graduates from baccalaureate nursing programs. Several types of educational programs prepare nurses for licensure. Most programs that prepare students for practical nursing require a year to 18 months for class work and clinical experience. Individuals who wish to become registered nurses may attend two-year associate degree programs, hospital diploma programs that usually require three years to complete, and four-year baccalaureate programs. Despite variations in length of the last three described programs, all graduates demonstrate high levels of success on licensure examination.

The difference between the various educational programs is the preparation of its graduates for specific entry

Table 1-4. Levels of Responsibilities for the Nursing Process*

	Practical Nurse	Technical Nurse	Professional Nurse
Assessing	Gathers data by interviewing, observing, and performing a basic physical examination of persons with common health problems with predictable outcomes.	Collects data from persons with complex health problems with unpredictable outcomes, their family, medical records, and other health team members.	Identifies the information needed from individuals or groups to provide an appropriate nursing data base.
Diagnosing	Reports problems based on collected abnormal data.	Uses a classification list to write a nursing diagnostic statement including the problem, etiology, signs, and symptoms. Identifies problems that require collaboration with the physician.	Conducts clinical testing of approved nursing diagnoses. Proposes new diagnostic categories for consideration and approval.
Planning	Suggests nursing actions that can prevent, reduce, or eliminate health problems with predictable outcomes. Understands desired outcomes for nursing care.	Sets realistic, measurable goals. Develops a written, individualized plan of care with specific nursing orders that reflects standards for nursing practice.	Develops written standards for nursing practice. Plans care for healthy or sick individuals or groups in structured health-care agencies or the community.
Implementing	Performs basic nursing care under the direction of a technical or professional nurse.	Identifies priorities. Directs others to carry out nursing orders.	Applies nursing theory to the approaches used for resolving actual and potential health problems of individuals or groups of clients.
Evaluating	Shares observations on the progress of the patient in reaching established goals.	Evaluates the outcomes of nursing care on a routine basis. Writes revisions to the plan for care.	Conducts research on nursing activities that may be improved with further study.

*Note that each advanced practitioner can perform the responsibilities of those identified previously. This list is intended to differentiate the additional responsibilities for each level of practice. Responsibilities of practical and technical nurses may overlap depending on the language of each state's nurse practice act.

level positions. The longer the period of time in an educational program, the greater the responsibilities for aspects of the nursing process and staff management. The assignment of patient care is based on the level of the nurse's educational preparation and the acuity of the patient's condition.

Nursing Practice Involves Continuous Learning. *Continuing education* is formal or informal education offered to nurses who have completed a basic educational program in nursing. Nursing responsibilities have increased markedly in the past few decades. This is true for both registered and licensed practical/vocational nurses. In addition, research and science are constantly adding to the body of knowledge concerned with health and illness. The increased use of sophisticated equipment is becoming a routine part of nursing (Fig. 1-4). As these trends continue, nurses find that they must study as they work in order to keep up with changes in their practice. No one educational program is enough to see a nurse through a lifetime of work. Although expertise develops with experience, a need for keeping up with new knowledge and skills continues. Therefore, continuing education has become important, and in many states it is mandated by law.

Nursing Practice Involves Commitment to a Lifetime Career. Nursing traditionally has been associated with females. In years past, women prepared themselves to earn a living, but not with any permanence in mind.

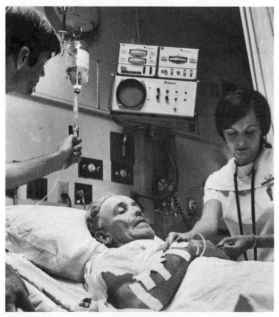

Figure 1-4 Nursing offers many challenges. Practicing nurses are increasingly using continuing education to keep abreast of new equipment and therapy required in the care of their patients. (Rosdahl CB: Textbook of Basic Nursing, 4th ed, p 654. Philadelphia, JB Lippincott, 1985)

Nursing practice was often a temporary pursuit before marriage, after raising children, or in the event of early widowhood.

Nursing is now a lifetime career. More men are choosing to become nurses. These changes in nursing practice have been advantageous for both the nurse and the status of nursing.

Because of the lifetime commitment, nurses are devoting more interest and energy to its advancement. Nurses are becoming social and political activists. The reward has been that nursing is progressing toward higher prestige within the health-care system. As the role and practice of nursing improve, it is attracting more intelligent and assertive male and female practitioners.

Nursing Practice Is Organized to Foster and Ensure the Quality of Its Practice. Any group of individuals that practices common skills must have guidance and direction. Nurses now hold membership in various organizations that are dedicated to improving the quality of the practice of nursing. Two such groups are the ANA and the National League for Nursing. Members of these nursing organizations meet at the district, state, and national levels. The work of both organizations has been referred to in this chapter.

In addition, nurses often join organizations that represent a specialty area of their nursing practice such as the Association of Operating Room Nurses or the American Association of Critical-Care Nurses. Special interests can often be more easily facilitated through group effort.

Nursing Practice Is Guided by Ethical Codes. Living in an orderly society involves respecting various rights and fulfilling obligations. Nurses respect life and direct the performance of skills that protect and preserve life. Nursing requires a high standard of conduct among its practitioners.

Professional organizations such as the ANA and the National Federation of Licensed Practical Nurses have developed written codes of ethics. These codes present certain fundamental guidelines that outline the duties of those who practice nursing. Adhering to these principles helps to ensure a high quality of nursing practice. Examples of ethical codes are presented in Chapter 6.

Nursing Practice Is Self-Regulated. Most states follow similar patterns of appointing nurses to participate on a regulatory board. This group of nurses performs various functions that serve to regulate and ensure the quality of practitioners within that state.

One responsibility of this board involves evaluating nursing educational programs. Curricula and clinical experiences must meet criteria that will promote competency among candidates for licensure examinations.

Each state administers licensing examinations to qualified candidates. If a person licensed by another state petitions to practice, the circumstances and qualifications of the original license must be investigated. If the criteria are met, the nurse may receive a license without reexamination.

The board also investigates allegations of unsatisfactory nursing practice or violation of laws that define nursing practice. The board has the right to suspend, revoke, or reinstate a nurse's license.

Nursing Practice Is Expanding Its Autonomy and Accountability. *Autonomy* refers to the ability to be self-directed. *Accountability* means being responsible for one's actions. Nursing practice has evolved from a historically dependent role to one that has increasing independence.

The well-being of patients depends on collaborative relationships among all members of the health team. Doctors depend on nurses to provide constant care for sick patients. Nurses depend on dietitians to direct the preparation of special diets and pharmacists to supply medications. Yet each contributes a unique function that is not controlled by the other.

Changes in the language of nurse practice acts hold nurses accountable for taking the initiative for more independent responsibilities. The skills of nursing practice are being used to plan and carry out nursing orders. These are compatible with the medical orders but are not entirely dependent on the physician's direction.

Some nurses are finding more autonomy in applying their skills in nonhospital practice. As more people require home care or information on ways to stay well, nurses will find creative outlets for independent application of their unique skills.

Nursing Practice Has Mechanisms for Recognizing and Rewarding the Excellence of Nurses. A special honorary society in nursing, Sigma Theta Tau, has been in existence since 1959. It elects various nurses into its membership, choosing those who have distinguished themselves in nursing and are deserving of national recognition.

Nurses are also recognized for their excellence by being selected for membership as a diplomate in the American College of Nursing Practice. This diplomate status has been developed under the ANA Divisions on Nursing Practice.

Bibliography

Batra C: Nursing theory for undergraduates. Nurs Outlook 35(4):189–192, 1987

Bourgeois PM, Darland NW, Fife BP: Applying a conceptual framework to ADN education. AD Nurse 3(6):25–28, 1988

Carlisle D: A nightingale sings. Nursing Times 85(50):38–39, 1989

Diers D: Learning the art and craft of nursing. Am J Nurs 90(1): 64–66, 1990

Fulton JS: Virginia Henderson: Theorist, prophet, poet. ANS 10(1):1–9, 1987

Gallagher D: A lifetime career. Imprint 35(5):7, 1989

Hanucharunkul S: Comparative analysis of Orem's and King's theories. J Adv Nurs 14(5):365–372, 1989

Herbert M: The value of nursing models. Canadian Nurse 84(11):32–34, 1988

Huch MH: Theory based practice: Structuring nursing care. Nursing Science Quarterly 1(1):6–7, 1988

Jacobson SF: Studying and using conceptual models of nursing. Image: Journal of Nursing Scholarship 19(2):78–82, 1987

Jennings BM: Nursing theory development: Successes and challenges. J Adv Nurs 12(1):63–69, 1987

Kristjanson LJ, Tamblyn R, Kuypers JA: A model to guide development and application of multiple nursing theories. AD Nurs 12(4):523–529, 1987

McWilliams B, Murphy F, Sobiski A: Why self-care theory works for us. Canadian Nurse 84(9):38–40, 1988

Minshull J, Ross K, Turner J: The human needs model of nursing. J Adv Nurs 11(6):643–649, 1986

Powell AH: Good nursing takes more than good intentions. Am J Nurs 89(6):902, 1989

Roy C: An explication of the philosophical assumptions of the Roy adaptation model. Nursing Science Quarterly 1(1):26–34, 1988

Salvage J: Selling ourselves . . . what exactly do nurses do? Nursing Times 85(49):24, 1989

Schlotfeldt RM: Defining nursing: A historic controversy. Nurs Res 36(1):64–67, 1987

Smith CE: Remembering the basics: 14 keys to staff nursing. Nursing 19(11):110, 112, 114, 1989

Wilcoxon CE: A return to the original Nightingale concept. J Nurs Adm 19(3):19, 1989

2

Patient Services: The Focus of Nursing

Chapter Outline

Behavioral Objectives
Glossary
Introduction
Recipients of Services
What Patients Expect as Consumers
Components of Patient Services
Characteristics of Patient Services
The Nurse–Patient Relationship
Nursing Skills Related to Patient Services
Teaching the Patient
Suggested Measures to Provide Patient Services in
    Selected Situations
Bibliography

Skill Procedures

Promoting Effective Communication
Providing Emotional Support
Teaching the Patient

Behavioral Objectives

When the content of this chapter has been mastered, the learner will be able to:

Define terms appearing in the glossary.
Describe the current characteristics of a patient.

List four consumer rights that patients expect in relation to health products and services.
List 10 expectations patients have of nurses.
Identify four types of patient services that are components of holistic nursing.
List five characteristics of patient services.
Discuss three phases of a nurse–patient relationship.
Describe techniques that enhance the nurse–patient relationship.
Differentiate between verbal and nonverbal communications and give examples of each.
Describe and give examples of eight communication techniques.
List six examples of communication barriers.
Describe skills that promote effective communication.
List nine common emotional responses that the nurse may observe in patients.
Describe ways in which the nurse can provide emotional support to the patient.
List and describe six common coping strategies individuals use to relieve stress.
Define five examples of coping mechanisms.
Identify skills that are useful when teaching patients.
List suggested measures for providing patient services in selected situations, as described in this chapter.

Glossary

Advocacy Working indirectly or on behalf of someone.
Client One who actively participates in identifying, planning, and resolving health problems. Synonym for *patient*.
Communication An exchange of information.
Contract An agreement among individuals about the responsibilities each has to the other.
Coping mechanisms Methods that reduce what an individual perceives to threaten his self-concept.
Coping strategies Activities one consciously uses to reduce stress.
Culture Everything a person learns from the groups of people of which he is a part.
Emotion A strong feeling, such as love, hate, or fear.
Emotional services The provision of those nursing skills that encourages the expression of the patient's feelings and an understanding of their significance.
Formal teaching The presentation of preplanned information at a scheduled time.
Holism The concept that all aspects of living—physical, emotional, social, and spiritual—are interrelated and affect the individual as a whole.
Holistic nursing The provision of patient services that integrate the concept that physical functions, emotions, group living, and spirituality all affect health.

Informal teaching The presentation of information given in response to spontaneous questions when they occur.

Nonverbal communication The exchange of information without using words.

Nurse–patient relationship An association between a nurse and a patient in which the desired outcome is health. Synonym for *therapeutic relationship.*

Patient One who actively participates with the nurse in identifying, planning, and resolving health problems. Synonym for *client.*

Patient advocate One who works on behalf of a patient.

Patient services The provision of those physical, emotional, social, and spiritual nursing skills that temporarily assist individuals in resolving health problems that are beyond their capabilities.

Physical services The provision of those nursing skills that assist the body in maintaining or returning to normal functioning.

Product An object that others find useful in their lives.

Psychology A science concerned with the way the mind functions and influences behavior.

Regression Displaying a type of behavior typical of an earlier age.

Relationship An association between people.

Service Skills performed for another.

Social services The provision of those nursing skills that strengthen relationships and mutual support among members of a group.

Sociology A science concerned with relationships among people.

Spiritual services The provision of those nursing skills that promote an understanding and opportunity for the performance of rituals related to a patient's religious belief.

Therapeutic relationship An association between a nurse and a patient in which the desired outcome is health. Synonym for *nurse–patient relationship.*

Verbal communication The exchange of information through the use of words.

Introduction

In a self-sustaining society, there is economic dependence on individuals who can supply needed products and services. A *product* is an object, such as a manufactured farm tool, that others find useful in their lives. *Services* are those skills performed for another. Nurses, teachers, and lawyers are examples of individuals who provide services to the community. The services that are most in demand are those that require special learning or involve a degree of expertise in their performance, which others do not generally have.

All economic endeavors involve a *relationship* between two individuals: those who have a product or a service to provide and those who desire it. The focus of nursing is the provision of *patient services* that temporarily assist individuals in resolving health problems that are beyond their own capabilities. These patient services consist of physical, emotional, social, and spiritual nursing skills.

Recipients of Services

Most nurses refer to the recipients of their services as patients. A patient traditionally has been defined as anyone who is ill and requires care. The term *patient* comes from the word *patience,* which means "to wait." Formerly, a patient tended to accept a passive role and allow others, such as the nurse, to make decisions in his best interest. In the past, nurses spent much time doing things *to* or *for* patients.

Today's relationship between nurse and patient has changed as dramatically as the times have changed. Individuals in present American society are products of the information age spawned first by radio, then television, and now computers. They are more knowledgeable about health and illness than ever before. The level of education among the public has increased. Citizens tend to participate more actively in changing policies that affect them personally.

These circumstances have affected the current interaction between nurses and patients as well. Patients strive to maintain their independence. Patients seek the same rights and responsibilities in relation to their health-care decisions as those they exercise in other decisions affecting their lives.

The trend in nursing is toward encouraging active participation by all persons sick or well. Today, nurses do things *with* the patient. The relationship between the patient and the nurse is characterized as a partnership involved in identifying, planning, and resolving health problems. Each works toward the achievement of the common goal.

Some nurses prefer to use the term *client* when referring to an individual who participates actively in his care. However, *patient,* which is a more common and more familiar term, will be used in this text. The term is not used in its former traditional context, but rather to describe the collaborative nature of the current patient role.

What Patients Expect as Consumers

Health is a valued resource. When threatened by a potential or actual illness, individuals seek health information, products, and services. Patients have come to expect and demand the following consumer rights.

The Right to be Informed. The patient has come to expect that any information about risks and benefits of a product or service be provided.

The Right to Safety. The patient has come to expect that products have been tested and found to be safe before marketing, and that anyone providing a service has met certain minimum qualifications for safe practice.

The Right to Choose. The patient has come to expect that he will be advised of alternatives that may assist him in the accomplishment of a goal.

The Right to be Heard. The patient has come to expect that his evaluation of a product or services will be appreciated and used for the purpose of improvement.

What Patients Expect of Nurses

There have been investigations of what patients expect of nurses. Patients hold nurses responsible for the following:

1. To be current and knowledgeable in the practice of nursing.
2. To be competent in the performance of nursing skills.
3. To be committed to providing patient services.
4. To be available when needed.
5. To ensure privacy.
6. To be courteous and accepting of differences among individuals.
7. To allow participation in decision making.
8. To provide explanations in language that is understandable.
9. To listen to and believe what is said.
10. To teach techniques that will promote improvement of health.

Components of Patient Services

Although the study of man has often described his physical being separately from his emotional, social, and spiritual being, each influences the other simultaneously. The concept that holds that every aspect of man is related one to the others is called *holism.* A diagram depicting holism is illustrated in Figure 2-1. Another way of defining holism is that it is concerned with the relationships between the person's mind and body and between his whole self and his environment.

Nurses recognize that patients have problems—physical, emotional, social, and spiritual—that all have an impact on health. Nurses therefore practice *holistic nursing* by providing services in one or all four of these general areas. As one problem is reduced, it generally has a similar effect on the other aspects of the patient's life.

To understand this concept more fully, consider a factory worker with heart disease who seeks care to overcome his physical disability. Assume that he is the family breadwinner with a wife and five children. He is currently unemployed because of his illness. To provide services that pertain only to his heart problem neglects consideration of the possible emotional, social, and spiritual influ-

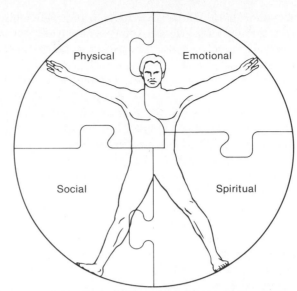

Figure 2-1 This diagram illustrates the integration of the various aspects that affect the total human being. Nurses provide patient services and meet the needs of the whole person.

ences of his illness. How will the family be supported until the patient is employable? Will he need to learn a new type of work when he recovers? How do he and his family feel about his becoming ill? Does the patient feel punished by a higher power? Does the community have services to help the patient? The answers to questions such as these show that physical health and mental health are closely related and that concern with both, as well as with the patient's environment, is important when providing holistic nursing services.

Physical Services

Physical services involve the provision of nursing skills that assist the body in maintaining or returning to normal functioning. Physical services include skills such as providing nourishment and water, maintaining breathing, and promoting urine and bowel elimination.

One of the most basic and most frequently provided services is that related to physical needs. A diagram illustrating a prioritized order of needs for which nurses provide services can be found in Chapter 3 (see Fig. 3-2). Patients primarily associate the nurse with providing physical services. This text emphasizes methods that will prepare nursing students to perform the skills that relate to physical services. This chapter and others, such as Chapter 28, also incorporate skills that make up other holistic aspects of nursing.

Emotional Services

An *emotion* is a strong feeling, such as love, hate, or fear. The nurse often provides services related to the patient's emotional state. In doing so, the nurse applies principles of *psychology,* which is a science that studies the way the mind works and influences behavior. There are common reasons for why people feel, act, and think the way they do.

Terms frequently used to describe *emotional services* include caring, comforting, compassion, and human kindness. These nursing skills encourage the expression of the patient's feelings and an understanding of their significance. Emotional care shows that the nurse has sincere respect, interest, and concern for the patient as a person. Nursing is not really nursing unless it includes these patient services. It includes being there when the patient needs someone. Stated in another way, nursing includes giving a lot of one's heart. There may be times when the nurse does no more than offer the patient comfort with a firm handclasp or a smile. The nurse also shows compassion when allowing a patient the opportunity to express anger or frustration. Taking a few minutes to visit with a lonely patient shows kindness and understanding.

Social Services

Humans live in groups. The most basic unit of society is the family. *Sociology* is a science about relationships among people. Nurses understand that if one member of a group experiences a health-related problem, it will affect all others with whom the patient has a significant relationship. *Social services* involves the provision of nursing skills that strengthen relationships and mutual support among members of a group.

Illness may cause a temporary separation of family members. Providing a cot in a child's room so that parents may stay with a sick child is an example of a patient service that supports social aspects of care.

There may be financial hardships as a result of a health problem. Medical expenses may accumulate, or an individual may experience the loss of a job. The nurse can initiate referrals to various social agencies such as the Department of Vocational Rehabilitation, which may relieve the patient and his family of further worry.

In most instances, services that relate to emotional, social, and spiritual needs are provided after physical needs are met. Although psychosocial needs are described differently, in general they are as follows, in order of priority:

1. Security and survival
2. Affection and a feeling of belonging to a group
3. Recognition and appreciation
4. Self-fulfillment.

Spiritual Services

Religion helps humans understand their relationship with the universe around them. There are countless religious beliefs in the world. In this country, the most commonly practiced religions are Christianity (Protestantism and Roman Catholicism) and Judaism. However, the nurse should expect to care for persons holding other beliefs as well. The nurse can provide *spiritual services* by understanding

and providing opportunities for patients to practice rituals associated with their faith.

Some people do not accept any particular formal religious faith. Yet they may possess a personal belief about their relationship to a spiritual being and a code for moral behavior. They, too, deserve respect for what they choose to believe.

The presence of religious items at the patient's bedside tells the nurse that he is practicing a religious faith. He may wish to spend part of his day in prayer or other religious practices. Because some patients prefer privacy, it is a thoughtful gesture for the nurse to provide this privacy when desired.

Many hospitals have chapels in which patients may worship, such as the one illustrated in Figure 2-2. Patients may be allowed to go to the chapel if their condition permits. Frequently, it is the nurse who can share information with a patient about the availability of a chaplain, a chapel, or scheduled religious services within the hospital. Patients have been known to improve physically and emotionally because of strong faith. Spiritual support is often the key to hope and determination when illness is present.

Although a person's religious faith often appears to help recovery, there are times when beliefs conflict with traditional care. For example, the doctrine of Jehovah's Witnesses does not permit blood transfusions. Certain vegetarians refuse meat, fish, and poultry on religious grounds. If a particular religious practice presents a problem for the patient's care, the nurse may wish to consult with a clergyman, although the patient does have the right to refuse care. A clergyman, however, may very well be the person who can best help the patient accept necessary care. In many hospitals, clergymen of various faiths are available at all times.

The clergyman's visit is usually an important part of the

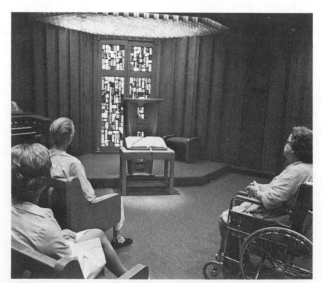

Figure 2-2 The chapel is a place where patients as well as staff may wish to meditate quietly.

patient's day. The thoughtful nurse will help the clergyman locate the patient and see whether he is able to receive the visit. Having the clergyman visit at an unsuitable or inconvenient time is embarrassing to both the patient and the clergyman. The nurse also will provide privacy as desired.

Characteristics of Patient Services

The services that are provided by nurses collectively set an example of the characteristics that make up the nurse–patient relationship.

Patient Services Preserve Human Dignity. Each patient is a human being and thus, in that respect, an equal of the nurse. When providing patient services, the nurse maintains an acceptance that others may be different but that they are no less or more deserving of nursing skills.

Patient Services Uphold the Uniqueness of Each Person. Nurses accept differences in people and, therefore, treat each patient as a unique individual. Although in some ways we are all alike—we need food, water, and oxygen to live, and we need to be able to get rid of wastes from our bodies—each of us is different from every other person. We react differently to events in our lives; we have different levels of intelligence; we play and work in different ways; we believe different things; we have different values; and so on. Understanding people and respecting their beliefs and rights come with experience.

Patient Services are Provided to All Individuals Throughout the Life Cycle. Care is provided regardless of the patient's age, sex, color, creed, or socioeconomic status. It includes the care of the sick and well throughout life. Figure 2-3 illustrates a nurse providing physical services for a healthy newborn infant.

Patient Services Include Advocacy Care. Working indirectly on behalf of someone is called *advocacy,* and the nurse becomes a *patient advocate* when working on behalf of a patient. Nurses usually offer direct services in face-to-face situations. However, there are times when nurses work indirectly on behalf of a patient. For example, a nurse helps a patient receive the services of a social worker when care has become too expensive for the patient and his family. A nurse makes a patient's needs known to the physician or to other health workers. Nurses help promote legislation that benefits health care for patients, usually by working through nursing organizations. These examples illustrate patient advocacy.

Another view of advocacy is that the nurse shares information with the patient so that he can make the best possible decisions for himself. The nurse then supports his decision. This concept of advocacy takes health personnel out of the role as persons "who know best." It recognizes

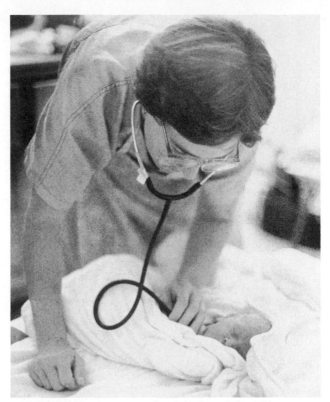

Figure 2-3 This nurse cares for a newborn infant. Nurses care for patients of all ages (Reeder SJ, Martin LL: Maternity Nursing: Family, Newborn, and Women's Health Care, 16th ed, p 548. Philadelphia, JB Lippincott, 1987.)

the right of rational adults to make their own decisions after having appropriate knowledge about courses of action open to them and the consequences of each course of action. However, the advocacy role still recognizes that making a decision for a patient may become necessary in certain emergency situations.

Patient Services Promote Independence. Nurses are teachers. While giving care, the nurse finds many opportunities to teach patients how to promote healing processes, how to stay well, how to prevent illness, and how to carry out activities of daily living in the best possible way. Figure 2-4 shows a nurse teaching a skill that will eventually allow that patient to care for herself at home. Patients expect nurses to share accurate information with them. Nurses teach not only by telling and explaining things to patients, but also by displaying their own behavior. Patients notice what nurses do. Many are heard to say that they do something in a particular manner because they saw a nurse do it that way.

The Nurse–Patient Relationship

The word *relationship* refers to an association between people. To enable the provision of patient services, there must be a relationship between a nurse and a patient. The

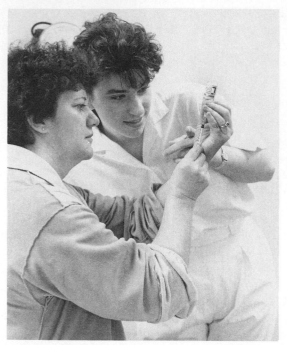

Figure 2-4 Instruction is often necessary for the patient who will be managing at home. This nurse is teaching the patient how to prepare and give herself an injection. Teaching has become especially important because health promotion is now such a key aspect of nursing.

nurse–patient relationship could also be called a *therapeutic relationship,* since the desired outcome of the association is almost always one of moving toward a goal of restored health.

To support the concept that the patient is an active participant in the relationship, some nurses establish a contract with the patient. A *contract* is an agreement among individuals about the responsibilities each has to the other. The contract may be written or verbal. For example, the patient may ask the nurse to help relieve swelling of the feet that appears late in the day. The nurse's responsibilities may include services such as identifying foods that are high in salt that should be restricted, measuring and providing instructions on the use of support stockings, and scheduling a routine for periodic elevation of the legs during the day. In return, the patient would agree to be responsible for following the nurse's instructions so that the goal would be met. Developing a nursing care plan with a patient could also be considered a type of contract. Nursing care plans are discussed in Chapter 4.

Phases of the Nurse–Patient Relationship

Therapeutic relationships ordinarily are not lengthy. They begin with a purpose and end when the goal has been achieved. This type of a relationship is generally described as having three phases: the introductory phase, the working phase, and the terminating phase.

The Introductory Phase. The relationship between a patient and nurse usually begins with a period of getting acquainted. Figure 2-5 shows a nurse using strategies that assist in developing a relationship with a child. Each individual in the relationship usually starts with some preconceived ideas about the other, which eventually will be validated or dismissed. The patient explains the health problems that are interfering with the quality of his life. The nurse uses that information to formulate an understanding of the services the patient desires. During the interaction the patient evaluates whether the nurse can fulfill his expectations. It is important for the nurse to demonstrate behaviors identified earlier—competency, courtesy, active listening, and appropriate communication skills—to ensure that the nurse–patient relationship begins positively.

The Working Phase. When the nurse and patient have reached an agreement on the goals and the steps that can lead to accomplishing those goals, the working phase begins. The working phase sets the plan into action. Both the nurse and the patient participate. Each shares in performing those tasks that will lead to the desired outcome. There may be more than one nurse working within this relationship, which further emphasizes the importance of communication skills.

The Terminating Phase. The nurse and patient should understand that their relationship is a self-limiting one. The ending of a relationship when the problems have been resolved is generally a mutually satisfying experience. However, for some, termination may be difficult.

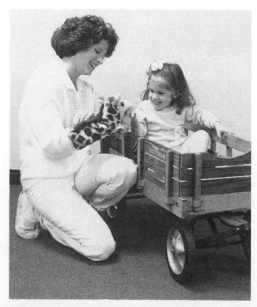

Figure 2-5 Ingenuity and patience are often required to build a good nurse–patient relationship. This nurse found that using a few simple toys and positioning herself near the child helped to put her at ease as she prepared to admit her for hospital care.

Nurses should prepare themselves and patients early for the eventual separation. Some may resist independence, feel rejected, or experience sadness when completion of the work has been accomplished. The nurse must use caring and compassion in facilitating the transition in the relationship.

Nursing Skills Related to Patient Services

There are many intrinsic qualities that the nurse brings to any relationship with a patient. Just as each patient is different, nurses differ, too. Each combination of personalities results in a unique pairing.

It is generally agreed that learning how to get along with others and to respect differences among people begins with knowing oneself. It is a good idea to examine one's attitudes and prejudices. This is not necessarily easy because it means looking closely at shortcomings as well as strengths. As the nurse gains insight, there will also be the acquisition of respect and acceptance of each patient for himself. Some other factors that will be discussed in the remainder of this chapter enhance the nurse–patient relationship and the nurse's ability to provide patient services.

Using Communication Skills

Communication is an exchange of information. Almost everything a person does communicates something. Communication is essential in the development of a nurse–patient relationship because no relationship can exist without it. Communication is a continuous process that occurs with every contact the nurse has with patients.

Verbal Communication. *Verbal communication* is communication that uses words. It includes speaking, reading, and writing. Messages of verbal communication may not be what we think they are. A patient may say that he is not eating because he has no appetite. When the nurse begins to feed him, however, he starts to eat. Does he want the attention of being fed or does he lack the strength to do so?

A word of caution is offered. It would be unwise to assume that everything the patient says must be viewed with suspicion and as a reason for probing and prying to find true meanings. Rather, the nurse will wish to accept what the patient says while being alert to the possibility that the patient may not always be able or willing to say what he really means. Therefore, the nurse will want to observe nonverbal communication carefully while still listening closely to what is said. Some communication techniques the nurse may want to use to achieve a specific purpose are in Table 2-1.

Nonverbal Communication. *Nonverbal communication* is the exchange of information without using words. It is what is *not* said. People communicate nonverbally

Table 2-1. Communication Techniques

Technique	Purpose	Example
Informing	Provides facts.	"Your surgery is scheduled for 9:30 A.M."
Direct questioning	Obtains specific information.	"Are you having any pain?"
Open-ended questioning	Provides a means for the patient to be more descriptive.	"How does your pain feel?"
Reflecting	Provides a means of encouraging the patient to continue and explain more.	PATIENT: "I'm miserable." NURSE: "Miserable?"
Clarifying	Reduces the possibility of misinterpretation.	PATIENT: "Beyond every cloud there's a silver lining." NURSE: "Explain what that means to you."
Confronting	Calls attention to inconsistencies in behavior or verbal statements.	"You say you want to go home but you haven't been doing your exercises."
Silence	Encourages the patient to initiate or continue the conversation.	PATIENT: "It is harder and harder to take care of myself at home." NURSE: (silence) PATIENT: "I get so short of breath climbing stairs."
Summarizing	Restates the areas covered in the conversation in brief form so that progress toward a goal can be identified.	"We've talked about your new diet and the difficulty you have in preparing food. Would you like to think about participating in a community mealsite program?"

through facial expressions, posture, gestures, general physical appearance, mode of dress, grooming, and voice inflections. Crying, laughing, and moaning are also considered nonverbal communication because they do not use a language or words.

A person has less control over nonverbal than verbal communication. Words can be chosen with care, but a facial expression is harder to control. As a result, messages are often communicated more accurately through nonverbal communication. A patient may say he does not feel lonely, but the expression on his face, the way he moves, and the tone of his voice may all show signs of loneliness.

The Role of Touch in Communication. Touching someone carries nonverbal messages. Touch has different meanings to different people and therefore should be used with care. Some people do not like to be touched, and their feelings should be respected. One positive message touch often carries, when used appropriately, is that the person *cares* for the one he touches and is offering him support and comfort.

Touch is common in nursing because of the many times nurses and patients are in close physical contact. The nurse who holds a crying child in her arms gives the child a feeling of security and affection through the sense of touch. Healing has long been associated with hand contact. A patient once said that her nurse gave a backrub that showed "a lot of love." Figure 2-6 illustrates a nurse using touch while speaking with a patient.

The Role of Silence in Communication. Silence is often part of nonverbal communication. Periods of silence may have many different meanings. A patient may use silence as an escape; he may be afraid of an examination and remain silent in order to avoid talking about his fears. A husband and wife may often sit quietly without talking and still be communicating much about their love for one another. A comfortable and happy person may prefer silence to talking as an expression of his contentment. Silence may be used by someone who is exploring his feelings; to interrupt with conversation when someone is deep in thought disturbs his thinking process.

A common obstacle to effective communication is ignoring the importance of silence and talking excessively. Taking the role of silence into account when communicating with patients promotes the development of a nurse–patient relationship.

Communication Barriers to a Therapeutic Relationship. It is important to treat each patient with dignity and respect. There are certain approaches that the nurse should avoid because they belittle the patient. The following approaches will undermine a mutually satisfying relationship:

- Giving orders to the patient
- Threatening the patient
- Shaming or criticizing the patient
- Lecturing the patient
- Giving advice to the patient
- Offering unrealistic reassurance.

The Role of Listening in Communication. Listening involves hearing and interpreting what is heard. A good listener pays close attention to what is said. It is difficult to overstress the importance of listening to patients when communicating with them. During the course of a busy day, it is easy to think about what must be done and to forget to listen to the patient. Many important signs of the patient's condition and how he feels are missed because a nurse fails to listen when a patient speaks.

Most people quickly learn when someone is pretending to listen. They usually can tell also when the listener is

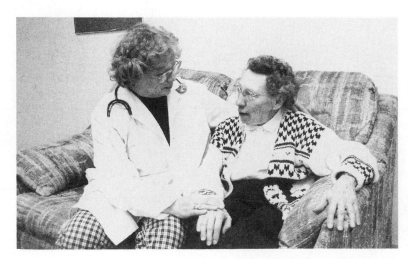

Figure 2-6 This nurse uses touch as she talks with her patient. The nonverbal communication conveys mutual feelings of trust and understanding.

bored or impatient to get on with something else. For example, a nurse may look out a window, interrupt a patient, or have a faraway look while a patient speaks. It is easy to see that if the nurse becomes careless and does not listen, a productive nurse–patient relationship cannot be expected to develop.

A learned person once said that all wise men share one trait—the ability to listen. It is a comment worth every nurse's consideration.

Techniques to Help Promote Communication. Various techniques may be used to promote effective communication between nurse and patients. They are described in Skill Procedure 2-1.

Understanding the Patient's Responses to Illness

All individuals are unique. Each patient brings to the relationship a different set of experiences and values that affect the significance he attaches to a certain situation. The more accurately the nurse interprets the patient's responses to his illness, the more appropriately the patient services can be adapted for the individual.

Culture and Illness. Cultural factors often influence an experience with illness. *Culture* is everything that an individual learns from the groups of people of which he is a part. In the United States, health, in general, is highly valued and illness is considered unpleasant and undesir-

Skill Procedure 2-1. Promoting Effective Communication

Suggested Action	Reason for Action
Have a purpose for a conversation with the patient.	So-called idle talk may serve as an opener in a conversation, but having a purpose in mind for a conversation helps prevent drifting from important subjects into irrelevant chatter.
Identify the amount of time you can spend.	The patient will not misinterpret the reason for leaving.
Be knowledgeable about the subject being discussed with the patient.	The patient is very likely to realize when you are unfamiliar with the topic of conversation and to lose confidence in his care-giver.
Admit not knowing about something and offer to obtain the information for the patient.	It is impossible to know everything. Trust and confidence can be maintained by making an effort to seek unknown facts.
Focus a conversastion on the patient and his needs and problems.	Communication has little value in terms of giving the patient needed care when attention is focused on you or on an activity you are performing for the patient.
Show interest in what the patient is saying.	Showing interest can be demonstrated by techniques such as using eye-to-eye contact (without staring) with the patient, thinking before talking, sitting down when convenient while conversing with the patient, relaxing while conversing, and listening to the patient. Most patients soon recognize when you pretend to be listening, and they then lose confidence in you.
Provide privacy while communicating with a patient.	Communication will usually be blocked if the patient thinks what he is saying will be overheard by others.
Assure the patient that a conversation with you will be held in confidence.	Although it is important to assure confidentiality, it is equally important to explain that you will have to share information with other health personnel if, in your judgment, what he tells you can influence his medical or nursing care. Serious problems may arise if you promise the patient you will tell no one about what he says. When the information is important for other health personnel to know, you will lose the patient's trust and confidence if you break your promise not to tell.

(continued)

Skill Procedure 2-1. Continued

Suggested Action	Reason for Action
Keep your mind open and do not prejudge the patient.	Failing to keep your mind open obstructs communication because you may fail to receive correct messages.
Be as clear and concise as possible and use language the patient understands.	Most patients are unfamiliar with nursing and hospital jargon and there will be no communication if you describe things in a way that the patient does not understand.
Avoid giving the patient false reassurance.	Statements such as "Everything will be all right," must be avoided. No one can predict or guarantee outcomes. False reassurance can result in mistrust and loss of confidence.
Do not probe for information.	Probing for information puts the patient on the defensive and he is likely to stop a conversation with you.
Do not give advice.	The patient has a right to information so that he can make up his own mind.
Observe while you converse with a patient and use silence and touch appropriately.	The appropriate use of observation, silence, and touch are discussed in the text.

able. In some cultures, illness is regarded with much less concern, almost as an acceptable way of life.

Trying to understand a patient's cultural background helps the nurse understand that individual's behavior. The nurse who feels a certain cultural background to be the best is biased and will tend to judge others with a certain amount of prejudice. Efforts to develop a helping nurse–patient relationship in such instances are almost certain to fail.

Common Emotional Responses. An actual or potential illness is a form of stress that presents a threat to an individual's survival. Because the mind and body are interrelated, the nurse can expect changes in the patient's usual emotional state. The nurse can anticipate certain common emotional reactions in those for whom services are provided. Some common responses are identified in Table 2-2. The nurse in Figure 2-7 uses a technique that helps a child overcome the fear of unfamiliar equipment.

Not all patients experience these emotions to the same degree. The extent to which some patients become distressed depends on the unique personality of the patient, past experiences related to illness, the severity of the health problem, and whether the patient is simultaneously

Table 2-2. Common Emotional Responses to Illness

Emotional Response	Definition
Anxiety	An emotional state characterized by feelings of uneasiness about the unknown.
Worry	A mild form of anxiety characterized by preoccupation with a problem.
Fear	An emotional state characterized by expected harm or unpleasantness.
Depression	An emotional state characterized by unhappiness.
Anger	An emotional state characterized by feelings of resentment due to a real or supposed injury to oneself or others.
Overdependence	An emotional state characterized by feelings of helplessness beyond what is considered normal.
Self-pity	Feeling sorry for oneself.
Regression	Displaying a type of behavior typical of an earlier age.
Apathy	An emotional state characterized by indifference to what is happening.

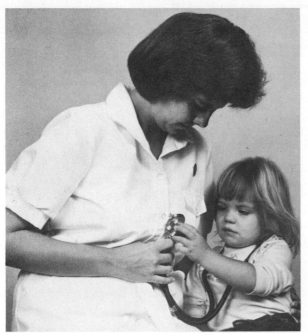

Figure 2-7 After this child was given time to use a stethoscope, she gladly cooperated in removing her clothing so that the nurse could examine her.

experiencing other problems. Nurses may relieve some of the emotional discomfort of patients by following the suggested actions in Skill Procedure 2-2.

Most individuals use methods to relieve their discomfort. The methods used are those that have been previously successful in relieving stress during an individual's life. These techniques are called coping strategies and coping mechanisms. *Coping strategies* are activities one consciously uses to reduce stress. Some commonly used strategies include the following:

1. Turning to a supportive person for reassurance
2. Talking about problems with others
3. Working at a physical activity such as racquetball
4. Eating to restore a feeling of contentment associated with a full stomach
5. Sleeping to avoid dealing with a problem
6. Using a symbolic object such as rabbit's foot or religious medal.

Coping mechanisms are methods, usually outside one's conscious awareness, that reduce what an individual perceives to threaten his self-concept. Some common coping mechanisms, their definitions, and examples can be found in Table 2-3.

Teaching the Patient

One of the most important nursing skills is the promotion of the patient's independent ability to meet his own health needs. One way this can be achieved is through health teaching. An old proverb that reinforces how education promotes self-sufficiency says, "Give a man a fish and he will eat for a day; teach a man to fish and he will eat for a lifetime."

High-quality nursing includes providing the patient with information or skills that will allow him to remain healthy, regain his health, or cope with his illness or injury. Teaching is no longer an optional patient service. Many state nurse practice acts legally require it. Nurses have been sued when discharged patients are readmitted or harmed because they were uninformed. Medical records must document the teaching that was done and the evidence that learning took place. Limited hospitalization

Table 2-3. Common Coping Mechanisms

Coping Mechanism	Definition	Example
Repression	Forgetting about situations that produced stress.	Being unable to remember the circumstances of a tragic traffic accident.
Denial	Refusing to believe information.	Not accepting a diagnosis despite medical evidence.
Rationalization	Minimizing a disappointment by finding something positive in the outcome.	Believing that it was better to have been passed over for a job promotion because the raise would have placed one in a higher tax bracket.
Compensation	Redirecting a desire for something unobtainable into efforts toward achieving or acquiring something similar.	Being unsuited to be a great athlete, and becoming a sports journalist instead.
Displacement	Redirecting anger toward one person onto an object or different person.	Kicking a wastebasket after being criticized by a supervisor at work.

Skill Procedure 2-2. Providing Emotional Support

Suggested Action	Reason for Action
Watch for signs of stress such as rapid heart rate, crying, excessive cigarette smoking, excessive sleep or insomnia, loss of appetite, or excessive eating.	Responses to stress are manifested through the sympathetic and parasympathetic nervous systems, which cause a speeding up or slowing down of body functions.
Sit in a relaxed position at eye level with the patient.	Power, authority, and control can be communicated in physical height and distance from the patient. The nurse can convey a nonjudgmental attitude by assuming a position similar to that of the patient.
Allow the patient to bring his emotions to the surface.	Identifying one's feelings and emotions is the first step in dealing with them. If the nurse chooses to ignore this aspect of care, holistic services are not provided.
Protect the patient from being overheard.	Most adults feel that admitting to feeling scared is a sign of weakness. Protecting the patient's public image reinforces a therapeutic relationship.
Share information with the patient.	The unknown can be fantasized beyond proportion and can escalate fear.
Indicate attention by gestures such as nodding the head at appropriate times.	Active listening involves concentration and participation in what is being said.
Don't dismiss or make light of what the patient is experiencing with statements like "Don't worry, everything will be all right."	Each person attaches significance to a situation from his own experience. Being told by another that this is unnecessary overlooks that each patient is unique.
Allow time for discussing feelings.	Feelings are usually expressed with more difficulty than facts. Feeling pressed for time or being rushed may be interpreted as disinterest.
Allow the patient to express emotions such as anger and hostility without retaliation.	Patients usually do not mean to direct their feelings at the nurse personally. All behavior has meaning, and the nurse may uncover it after the anger has been expressed.
Tolerate crying and protect the patient from being observed.	Crying is a result of feeling hurt and helpless. It is also associated with feeling out of control. The nurse who allows this reaction shows acceptance and a desire to stay and help the patient gain control.
Spend time with the patient at times other than when providing physical services.	Some patients may feel that the only reason a nurse spends time with them is because it is part of a job. Being with a patient at other times reinforces that he is important as an individual.

time has demanded that nurses begin teaching as soon as possible after admission rather than waiting until discharge.

Assessing Learning Needs

The best teaching and learning takes place when it is individualized. To be most efficient and personalized, the nurse needs to gather pertinent information from the patient. Second guessing what the patient wants and needs to know often leads to a futile expenditure of time and effort.

The following are techniques the nurse can use to assess the patient's learning needs from his own perspective.

What does being healthy mean to you?
What things in your life interfere with being healthy?
What don't you understand as fully as you would like to?
What activities do you need help with?
What do you hope to accomplish before being discharged?
How can we help you at this time?

Assessing the Learner

For teaching to be effective the nurse must consider many variables that affect each individual, such as the capacity to learn, motivation for learning, and readiness to learn.

Assessing the Capacity to Learn. In order for the mind to receive, remember, analyze, and apply new information, a certain amount of intellectual ability must exist. Because concepts are interpreted through language, the nurse should determine the patient's cultural background and ability to understand and speak English as a primary or second language. Another friend, family member, or nursing team member may be needed as an interpreter if language presents a barrier to learning.

Besides a common language, the nurse should consider the patient's ability to see, hear, and read. The latter may be the most difficult to assess because many illiterate or functionally illiterate people are not apt to volunteer this information. However, the patient has an opportunity to protect his self-esteem by indicating a method other than reading if the nurse asks, "How do you learn best?" If the patient needs to learn a motor skill, the nurse should appraise the patient's strength, stamina, and coordination.

The patient's attention and concentration should be evaluated. The individual's ability to remain attentive and focused on the subject content will affect the numbers and length of teaching sessions.

Assessing Motivation. Optimum learning takes place when an individual has a purpose for acquiring new information. The relevance for learning is also an individual variable. The desire for new learning may be to satisfy intellectual curiosity, restore independence, prevent complications, or facilitate discharge and return to the comfort of home. Other, less desirable reasons for learning are to please others and to avoid criticism.

Assessing Readiness. When the capacity and motivation for learning exist, the final component of learning readiness must be determined. Readiness refers to the patient's physical and psychological well-being. A person who is in pain, uncomfortably warm or cold, having difficulty breathing, feeling depressed, or fearful, for example, is not in the best condition for learning to take place.

Types of Learning

There are generally three domains of learning. Learning facts is referred to as the cognitive domain. Learning a neuromuscular skill is in the psychomotor domain. Ac-

quiring or changing an attitude or value is in the affective domain. Table 2-4 identifies behaviors that result from learning in the various domains.

Principles of Learning

Once the nurse identifies the content, domain, and learning style of the patient, it is important to use principles that enhance learning. Many of these are incorporated within Skill Procedure 2-3. For the sake of completeness, they are identified in more detail in Display 2-1.

Formal and Informal Teaching

Teaching may be *formal* in that preplanned information is presented at a scheduled time. For example, couples often attend prenatal classes with planned weekly lessons when they are expecting a baby. But teaching can also be *informal,* occurring spontaneously at the patient's bedside.

Formal teaching requires a plan. Without a plan, teaching becomes haphazard. The potential for reaching goals, providing adequate information, and ensuring the patient's comprehension are jeopardized unless there is some organization of time and content.

The student nurse may work with a staff nurse or instructor in developing a teaching plan. Usually one or more nurses carry out certain specific parts of a teaching plan. This is the most desirable approach so that a patient is not overwhelmed with processing volumes of new information or learning skills that are difficult for a novice to perform. Skill Procedure 2-3 can be used as a model when the nurse identifies that a patient needs teaching.

Methods for Teaching

Some patients learn better by reading, listening, watching, or doing. Various teaching methods accommodate the instructional presentation with the patient's learning style. The following is a list of techniques to consider when planning to teach a patient: lecture, panel presentation, group discussion, demonstration, games and simulations, pamphlets and other printed materials, audiovisual formats, role playing and role modeling. Eventually many people will have access to computers and will be able to use software programs and interactive videos for learning. These are currently being implemented on a small scale at community health fairs or classes.

Table 2-4. Behaviors Associated With Various Learning Domains

Cognitive Domain		Psychomotor Domain		Affective Domain	
List	Label	Remove	Fill	Advocate	Promote
Identify	Summarize	Change	Assemble	Support	Refuse
Locate	Select	Empty	Add	Accept	Defend

Skill Procedure 2-3. Teaching the Patient

Suggested Action	Reason for Action
Find out what the patient wants to know.	Learning is facilitated when there is some personal interest.
Determine what the patient should know if he is to remain healthy.	Patients are not always aware that there is information that is vital to continued health and safety.
Teach when the patient appears ready and interested in learning.	Patients who are very ill or who are visiting with friends or relatives need to have teaching postponed.
Provide an environment that promotes learning.	Learning takes place best in a room that is well ventilated, well lighted, and of a comfortable temperature. Distractions and interruptions interfere with concentration.
Adjust teaching to a level the patient understands.	It is of little value to use terms that are not familiar to the patient, or to teach in such depth that he becomes confused.
Divide information into manageable amounts.	The patient may be overwhelmed by the amount of information and will not retain it.
Use different teaching aids, such as pamphlets, diagrams, models, and demonstrations.	People learn in a variety of ways. The more senses that can be stimulated, the more probable that the information will be learned.
Review previous information briefly.	Repetition increases retention of information.
Evaluate the patient's learning by asking the patient to make a list, draw a picture, or demonstrate a skill.	It is best to devise some method for assessing the patient's comprehension. The ability to recall with accuracy is proof that learning took place.
Document on the patient's record the information that has been taught and the patient's level of comprehension.	Following a teaching plan and reinforcing weak areas reduces duplication of efforts and facilitates goal achievement.

Suggested Measures to Provide Patient Services in Selected Situations

When the Patient Is an Infant or Child

Expect an infant to demonstrate emotional responses when his needs are not met with crying, kicking, thrashing about, and irritability. An infant responds emotionally to cuddling, rocking, touching, and soothing sounds, including the sound of your voice.

Remember that youngsters need emotional support and display many of the same emotional responses to illness as do adults: fear, anger, worry, and so on. The nurse is a parent substitute during hospitalization of youngsters and must gain a child's confidence and trust.

Expect that many children regress when ill. *Regression* means that a person displays a type of behavior typical of an earlier age. For example, a child that has been toilet trained regresses and soils himself or a child able to drink from a cup demands a bottle. Show respect for the child's need for extra dependence during illness and hospitalization, and help parents understand this temporary change in the child's behavior.

Just as with adults, learn to accept a child's emotional outbursts, even when they are directed against you. Recognize that there is a cause for his behavior. Patience and understanding help you to find reasons for behavior; problems can then be better handled in a constructive manner.

Do not attack the behavior, but attack its cause when behavior becomes destructive.

Offer explanations of what you are going to do in ways a child can understand. Using dolls or puppets can be effective when explaining and gaining cooperation.

Keep in mind that from birth to maturity, a person is developing his own unique behavior. He has feelings and is learning to cope with problems through methods that will eventually prepare him for adulthood.

Take into account that among the strongest influences in the life of an adolescent is that of his peers. While he strives for individuality, he also

---

Display 2-1.
Techniques for Effective Teaching

Collaborate with the client on content, goals, and a realistic time for accomplishing the task.

Develop a written plan that builds from
• familiar to unfamiliar
• simple to complex
• normal to abnormal.

Select teaching methods and resources that are compatible with the patient's preferred style for learning.

Arrange an appropriate location for the learning to take place that will be comfortable and free from distractions.

Make sure the patient is wearing sensory aids, such as a hearing aid, glasses, or contact lenses, if he has need of them.

Review any information covered during earlier teaching sessions.

Assess the patient's interest and level of comfort at periodic intervals during the teaching session.

Postpone or discontinue a teaching session if the patient is not physically or emotionally ready.

Inform the patient as to when and how his learning will be evaluated.

Use vocabulary that is within the patient's level of understanding, neither beneath nor above it.

Build on the patient's prior knowledge and experiences.

Involve the patient actively through sharing ideas and handling equipment.

Stimulate a variety and as many of the senses as possible.

Use sophisticated language or vocabulary unless it leads to misunderstanding and a potential for harm.

Allow time for questions and answers.

Use equipment similar to equipment the patient will need to use.

Arrange an opportunity for the patient to use or apply the new information as soon as possible after it was taught.

Provide written information or sample equipment that the patient can use for practice or review.

Summarize the key points that were covered during the current period of teaching.

Review the progress toward reaching goals.

Evaluate the need for further teaching.

Establish the time, place, and content for the next teaching session.

---

wants to be like his peers. Failing to respect an adolescent's feelings in this regard does little to promote a therapeutic relationship.

Protect the parent–child relationship. Understand that parents are also under tension and often suffer feelings of guilt when a child is ill. Include the family in the child's care, to the greatest extent possible, and include family members in your teaching also.

When the Patient Is Elderly

Take into account that a person's sensory system tends to fail with advanced age. Modified techniques that will subsequently be described may need to be adapted when providing patient services.

Use touch but use it appropriately. Touch has been found to help make up effectively for other sensory losses in the elderly.

Show genuine respect and warmth with the elderly patient. Avoid using titles such as "granny," "gramps," "auntie," and the like, unless the patient wishes you to use them. You also show respect by talking to and treating the elderly as adults, not as children.

Give the patient opportunities to control whatever aspects of his life he can, such as the planning of his care and self-care. Dependence is often difficult for elderly patients to accept. Being allowed to maintain independence to the greatest extent possible is gratifying for them and promotes a helping relationship.

Allow the patient to self-pace his care when possible. This technique requires more time, but rushing the elderly often results in frustration, anger, and resentment.

Listen to the patient and allow him to reminisce. A conversation can be related to the present by gradually drawing attention to today's events.

Use family members as indicated for teaching purposes, for helping to strengthen family relationships, and for promoting a nursing relationship with people who are important to the patient.

When the Patient Is Blind or Has Impaired Vision

Identify yourself as you approach a blind patient and tell him when you are leaving. Explain to him what you are going to do while with him.

Explain your reason for touching a patient when you do. Avoid touching a blind patient suddenly because it is likely to frighten him.

Speak in a normal tone of voice. A blind person is not necessarily hard of hearing.

Be sure that the patient has his call signal handy and that he knows exactly where it is and how to use it.

Explain typical noises the patient can expect to hear that will be strange to him. Also familiarize the patient with the room's arrangement and furnishings.

Use the following techniques when the patient is not blind but has some impaired vision: have adequate light available; remove obstacles over which he could fall; and, when possible, provide him with a magnifying glass for reading.

Obtain reading material that uses oversized print; avoid glossy paper; select black print on white paper in order to obtain maximum contrast.

When the Patient Is Deaf or Hard of Hearing

Use such devices as a magic slate, chalk board, flash cards, and writing pads to communicate.

Be thoughtful by keeping reading material handy for the patient.

Walk toward the patient slowly and allow him to see you as you approach. The patient will be frightened easily if someone suddenly appears in his line of vision.

Determine if the patient prefers a night light in order to enhance his sensory perception.

If the patient reads lips, talk slowly, use simple language, and speak in a quiet, natural tone of voice.

Make sure that a person who lip reads and requires glasses is wearing them.

Avoid standing in front of a bright light or window. A lip reader will avoid the glare and not be able to watch the speaker's mouth.

Use gestures as much as possible.

When the patient is hard of hearing, the following techniques are recommended:

Encourage the patient to wear his hearing aid if he has one.

Reduce background noises, such as a television.

Avoid communications involving a group of people. A hearing-impaired person may be able to focus on one voice but may not readily adapt to rapid changes in other voices.

Establish eye contact.

Enunciate clearly, but do not exaggerate lip movements when pronouncing words because this may confuse someone who reads lips.

Lower the pitch of the voice. A lower pitch improves hearing and may explain why some hard-of-hearing persons understand whispers and male voices better than female.

Rephrase rather than repeat when the patient does not understand. Words with "f," "s," "k," and "sh" are high-pitched sounds. They are difficult for the hearing-impaired person to discriminate.

Try to use a stethoscope when the patient is hard of hearing; the patient wears the earpieces while you speak clearly with a low voice into the bell.

Identify that the patient is hearing impaired by using a sticker or notation on the nursing Kardex.

Respond to the hard-of-hearing person's call light in person rather than use an intercom.

When the Patient Cannot Read

Patients who cannot read may be visually impaired or have a learning disability. Individuals with low literacy levels are not necessarily intellectually below average. They may speak and understand effectively. Use the following guidelines for teaching these individuals:

Use a verbal and visual mode when providing information.

Be brief and as simple as possible.

Give directions in the same sequence that the patient will need to follow when repeating.

Request that the patient repeat the information at frequent intervals to assess comprehension and retention.

Be consistent. Always use the same word for a particular object or concept, such as "shot," rather than using the words "injection" and "hypo."

Promote self-worth through positive reinforcement and constructive feedback, because nonreaders often have low self-esteem.

Provide diagrams or an audiotape for future review.

When the Patient Has a Short Attention Span

Attempt to discover the cause for being inattentive. Distractability can be due to simple things like stress, fatigue, boredom, or even a need to urinate.

Determine if the patient has any visual or hearing deficits that interfere with his ability to follow instructions or communicate.

Discuss how long the teaching session will last. For instance, say, "Let's spend ten minutes practicing how to fill a syringe," to indicate that the task is limited. Knowing that the activity will not last indefinitely may help. If a timeframe is established, the nurse must conform to it.

Write directions or information down for the patient. This will assist in future review and recall.

When the Patient Cannot Speak

Use special devices to communicate.

1. A magnetic "talk board" contains common phrases that the patient can select to communicate something. Phrases such as "I am thirsty" and "I have pain" are common.

2. A "magic slate" is a device on which one can write a message with a stylus. The message is removed by lifting specially treated paper, and the slate can then be used again.

3. Flash cards are cards of about 3 by 5 inches on which common phrases are written or symbols are drawn. The patient selects the appropriate phrase or symbol to convey a message. Extra cards or a writing pad on which the patient writes additional messages may also be used.

Use nonverbal communication to the greatest extent possible. For example, gestures and facial expressions carry a variety of messages. If the patient cannot move, use prearranged signals such as finger movements or eye blinking to convey a message.

Talk to a patient even though he cannot answer, and explain what you are going to do. It is a thoughtful gesture and also conveys caring and interest in the patient. Speak slowly, keep to one subject, use simple language, keep eye contact with the patient, use gestures, use consistent wording, and give the patient plenty of time to receive your message.

Be sure to keep a call signal handy for a patient who cannot talk and cannot call out for help.

Praise patients who are relearning how to talk as they make progress. Help the patient to relax and to speak slowly during reeducation.

When the Patient Is Unconscious

Be careful about what is said in the presence of an unconscious patient. Hearing is believed to be the last sense lost; therefore, the patient may hear what is being said even though he cannot respond.

Assume that the patient can hear, and continue to talk with him as you normally would when giving care.

Speak to the patient before touching him; keep in mind that touch is an effective means of communication, although the patient cannot respond.

Keep noises in the room at a low level so that the patient can focus on conversation if it seems that he is receiving messages.

When the Patient Is From a Different Culture

Make a concerted effort to learn as much as possible about the belief systems of the patient.

Make it as easy as possible for a hospitalized patient to carry out his cultural practices as long as they do not disturb others.

Modify care so that the patient's cultural practices and beliefs are not violated. To ignore them may result in his refusing care.

Use an interpreter when possible. Often a member of the patient's family can help. Also, a dictionary that translates one language into another is helpful.

Use gestures or pictures to demonstrate messages.

Be alert to nonverbal communication. Most nonverbal communication is universal and understood by everyone.

Prepare cards with a word in English on one side and its equivalent in the language the patient speaks on the other. The nurse and the patient can then select a particular card to convey a message to one another.

Bibliography

Armstrong ML: Orchestrating the process of patient education: Methods and approaches. Nurs Clin North Am 24(3):597–604, 1989

Brown S: How to create patient education tools. RN Magazine 52(2):77–78, 1989

Burard P: Meaningful dialogue. Nursing Times 83(20):43–45, 1987

Casserly DM, Strock E: Educating the older patient. Caring 7(11):60–64, 66–67, 1988

Chovaz D: Nursing the hearing impaired patient. Canadian Nurse 85(3):34–36, 1989

Doak C, Doak L, Root J: Teaching Patients with Low Literacy Skills. Philadelphia, JB Lippincott, 1985

Drayton–Hargrive S, Mandzak–McCarron K: Respiratory rehabilitation for the tracheotomized patient. Rehabilitation Nursing 12(4):193–195, 1987

Foster SD: The role of education in discharge planning. American Journal of Maternal Child Nursing 13(6):403, 1988

Gessner BA: Adult education: The cornerstone of patient teaching. Nurs Clin North Am 24(3):589–595, 1989

Harding M: I can't hear you: Caring for deaf patients. Registered Nurses' Association of British Columbia News 18(6):9–12, 1986

Harrison LL: Interacting with videodisc technology. American Journal of Maternal Child Nursing 14(3):173, 1989

Harrison LL: The patient education bridge. American Journal of Maternal Child Nursing 14(1):51, 1989

Honsinger MJ, Yorkston KM, Dowden PA: Communication options for intubated patients. Respiratory Management 17(3):45–46, 48–49, 51–52, 1987

Lange JW: Developing printed materials for patient education. Dimensions in Critical Care Nursing 8(4):250–258, 1989

Luker K, Caress AL: Rethinking patient education. J Adv Nurs 14(9):711–718, 1989

Merritt SL: Patient self-sufficiency: A framework for designing patient education. Focus on Critical Care 16(1):68–73, 1989

Montgomcry C: How to say "I care" when you have no time to talk. RN Magazine 50(5):21, 1987

Rankin SH, Stallings KD: Patient Education, 2nd ed. Philadelphia, JB Lippincott, 1990

Ruzicki DA: Realistically meeting the educational needs of hospitalized acute and short stay patients. Nurs Clin North Am 24(3):629–637, 1989

Smith CE: Patient teaching: It's the law. Nursing 17(7):67, 1987

Spink LM: Six steps to patient rapport. AD Nurse 2(2):21–23, 1987

Tanner G: A need to know. Nursing Times 85(31):54–56, 1989

Trapp–Reimer T, Afifi LA: Cross cultural perspectives on patient teaching. Nurs Clin North Am 24(3):613–619, 1989

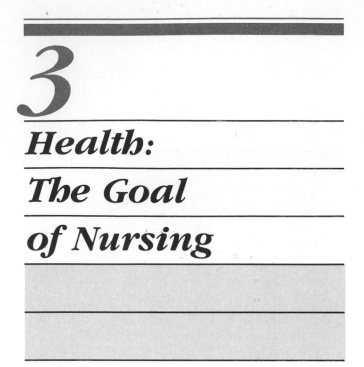

3

Health:
The Goal
of Nursing

Chapter Outline

Behavioral Objectives
Glossary
Introduction
Health
Values Associated With Health
Trends in Health Promotion
Wellness
Illness
The Health-Care Team
Patterns for Administering Patient Care
Continuity of Care
Bibliography

Behavioral Objectives

When the content of this chapter has been mastered, the learner will be able to:

Define terms appearing in the glossary.

Discuss the aspects of well-being that characterize health.

Describe various ways that well-being is interpreted.

Identify ways that nurses work toward the well-being of patients.

List and discuss three beliefs that Americans have about health.

Identify four trends that have influenced attitudes for health promotion.

Differentiate the terms health, wellness, and illness.

Explain the concept of a health–illness continuum.

Discuss how individuals with varying levels of health may each experience high-level wellness.

Describe the usefulness of a hierarchy of human needs to nurses.

Describe where and how nurses function within the health-care system.

Describe how nursing care is administered when the following methods are used: functional nursing, case method, team nursing, primary nursing, nurse-managed care.

Discuss the importance of continuity of care when providing patient services.

Glossary

Acute illness An illness that comes on quickly and lasts a relatively short time.

Case method A pattern for administering patient care in which one nurse is responsible for all the care for each assigned patient.

Chronic illness An illness that comes on slowly and lasts a relatively long time.

Continuity of care A continuum of health care.

Continuum A continuous whole.

Emotional well-being A state in which one feels good about life.

Exacerbation A period during an illness when the symptoms become worse.

Functional nursing A method of administering care in which each person performs specific tasks.

Germ theory The proposition that organisms too small for human vision could cause diseases among people.

Health A state of physical, emotional, social, and spiritual well-being.

Health-care system The network of institutions and agencies that provide assistance to individuals with varying levels of wellness.

Health–illness continuum States of health and illness that fluctuate within a whole.

Health team People who help patients overcome illnesses and stay well.

Hierarchy A series arranged so as to rank from a lower to a higher order.

High-level wellness A state of health in which the body is functioning at its best level in relation to the person's abilities.

Ill Having a disease. Synonym for *sick*.

Need A component of living that is necessary for life.

Nurse-managed care The nursing care planned by a nurse manager for a group of patients based upon their medical diagnosis.

Nursing team A group of nursing personnel who have the responsibility of providing patient services.

Physical well-being A state in which the body organs are functioning normally.

Primary nursing A method for administering nursing care in which a patient's total 24-hour needs are the responsibility of one nurse.

Remission An interval during an illness when the disease seems to have disappeared.

Resource A possession that is valuable because its supply is limited and it has no substitute.

Right A privilege that one can expect others to provide.

Sick Having a disease. Synonym for *ill*.

Social stigma A mark of disapproval against an individual due to the violation of a group's value system.

Social well-being A state in which one feels safe, well liked, and productive.

Spiritual well-being A state in which an individual experiences an inner peacefulness in relation to himself and the meaning of life.

Team nursing A method of administering care in which all nursing personnel divide the work and complete it together.

Value A treasured, personal belief.

Value system A group of beliefs that form the framework for one's attitudes and behavior.

Well-being A state in which one is experiencing an acceptable quality of life.

Introduction

A predictable characteristic of being human is that there will be changes in health. It is impossible to be well and stay well, or get well and remain well forever. Health is a goal to which nursing is committed. All the patient services that nurses provide through the skills they perform are directed toward assisting individuals to improve their health.

How each person defines health is varied and personal. In the preamble of its constitution, the World Health Organization defined *health* as "a state of complete physical, mental, and social [most nurses would also add the word spiritual] well-being and not merely the absence of disease or infirmity." The term *well-being* means that a person is experiencing an acceptable quality of life as he defines it. It is important to discover what each individual identifies as a healthy state and not impose the nurse's standards on the patient.

Today, well-being is generally accepted as the right of everyone. A *right* is a privilege that one can expect others to provide. Maintaining or acquiring health cannot always be done alone. Nurses pledge themselves to assist individuals who require help from time to time in reaching their highest potential for health.

Health

The fact that humans have physical, emotional, social, and spiritual needs was discussed in Chapter 2. Nurses provide patient services to meet the individual's needs in each of those four components. Health, the goal of nursing, could be measured by the patient's physical, emotional, social, and spiritual well-being.

Physical Well-Being

Perhaps the most expected assistance from health personnel is an improvement in physical well-being. For most, *physical well-being* is a state in which the body organs are functioning normally. Remember that definitions of health are different among different people. For some, an ability to function without experiencing symptoms may fit the definition for physical well-being. For example, a diabetic whose disease is controlled with proper diet, exercise, or medication may also consider himself physically well. For others, physical well-being may mean possessing the highest resistance against disease, which is perhaps the most desirable definition of all. It may include living a life-style that reduces a potential for illness. An individual with this concept of physical well-being may seek assistance from the nurse to stop smoking, maintain a desirable weight for his height, and develop a schedule of regular, appropriate exercise.

Emotional Well-Being

How one feels emotionally is also a part of health. Most would agree that a desirable life would include more than just normal physical functioning. A vegetative state is not usually associated with quality of life. Feelings add another dimension to life and are what distinguish being human.

There are common feelings that could be characterized as positive or desirable, such as happiness, contentment, joy, and humor. Negative or undesirable feelings would include anger, sadness, fear, and loneliness. Life involves feeling both negative and positive kinds of emotions. One would not know the value of happiness without having experienced sadness. An emotionally healthy individual is often able to find some bittersweet lesson in even the worst feelings. An example of this is the old saying, "Better to have loved and lost than never to have loved at all."

Emotional well-being is a state in which one feels good about life. Again, keep in mind that there are variations in the interpretation of this definition. Some may view emotional well-being as simply an attitude that life involves a mixture of feelings while others may seek opportunities for experiencing them. The nurse may support or provide coping strategies and mechanisms, discussed in Chapter 2, that help to restore balance to the patient's emotional state.

Social Well-Being

Social well-being is a state in which one feels safe, well liked, and productive. Entire communities were once made up of lifelong friends and relatives. Generally the entire group experienced supportive interrelationships. As individuals have become increasingly mobile, their feelings of belonging to a group and receiving group support have been affected. More people see their social role as protecting their own personal territory rather than working toward the good of the group. In this age of nuclear accidents and terrorism, it should be easy to see that we are all world citizens rather than citizens of a geographical area.

Nurses treat each patient as someone of personal worth. There are some diseases that carry a *social stigma;* that is, there is some shame attached to an individual with a physical condition because it somehow violates a group's value system. A *value system* is a group of beliefs that form the framework for one's attitudes and behavior. Examples of these conditions may include alcoholism, venereal disease, or obesity. The nurse promotes social well-being by conveying to the patient and coworkers that the patient deserves the same efforts and care for these diseases as for other illnesses.

Spiritual Well-Being

Spiritual well-being is a state in which an individual experiences an inner peacefulness in relation to himself and the meaning of life. This aspect of man's health provides a feeling that despite hardships there is a purpose for one's existence. Nurses promote health when they accept the patient's spiritual attitudes and beliefs. The definition of spiritual well-being is perhaps the most personal of all.

Values Associated With Health

Values are treasured, personal beliefs. They are likely to be shared by others within a group. Nurses value health and life, a value similarly held by many Americans. Beliefs associated with health among Americans include that health is a resource, a right, and a personal responsibility.

Health Is a Resource

Health is a valued resource. A *resource* is a possession that is valuable because its supply is limited and it has no substitute. Although health is an intangible substance, it is nonetheless considered precious. People often say, "as long as you have your health, you have everything," and "health is wealth." Nurses are committed to protecting, preserving, and replenishing this personal resource by providing services aimed at health promotion—keeping healthy people well.

Health Is a Right

This country was established on the foundation that all men are equal and entitled to life, liberty, and the pursuit of happiness. If this premise is accepted, then it follows that each individual, regardless of age, social position, or

wealth, is entitled to health. Rights are also discussed in Chapters 2 and 6.

Rights are always counterbalanced with obligations to others. If all are deserving of health, it follows that individuals are required to behave in such a way as to safeguard one another's health. This responsibility could be taken further to include a duty to protect and preserve the health of those who may be unable to assert this right for themselves. Nurses must always be prepared to act as advocates for the health of others.

Health Is a Personal Responsibility

Health requires continuous personal effort in order to be maintained. There is always as much potential for illness as there is for health. Everyone has the capacity to be instrumental in the outcome. The choice rests within each individual.

Once the choice has been made in the direction of health, others such as nurses stand ready to provide assistance. Pilch (1981) said, "No one can do wellness to or for another; you alone do it, but you don't do it alone." For too long patients expected their health to be restored or improved through the efforts of doctors, nurses, drugs, and machines. The personal power within the human spirit to change the body's function is currently being researched, promoted, and tested in areas such as biofeedback, meditation, and guided imagery.

Trends in Health Promotion

Given the choice, no matter what the period of history, all individuals would agree that they desired health. Life was short more often than not regardless of any hope otherwise. There was a feeling that little if anything could be done to alter the course of events. Now circumstances have changed. There are several reasons for the growing movement to promote health.

Extended Life Expectancy

One of the most common causes of early death in the past was contagious disease. Diseases currently associated with aging were uncommon because individuals died before their organs began to dysfunction. With medical and scientific advances, life expectancy has increased. Infants born today can expect to live on an average into their late seventies. The focus now is toward promoting health so that there is a quality to life that matches the extended quantity.

The Relationship of Lifestyle to Illness

Early in this century the *germ theory* was advanced. This theory proposed that organisms too small for human vision could cause diseases. People felt themselves to be helpless victims. Scientists tried to apply the germ theory to many diseases whose causes could not be explained. It was easy but not always accurate to blame illness on something microscopic.

With the discovery of antibiotics and vaccines, health could be dramatically restored or maintained. There was a common assumption that these powerful drugs and those who were knowledgeable in their use could cure any illness. Individuals did not feel a need for personal health promotion because the diseases they most feared were treated successfully.

Today there is increasing evidence that many disabling and fatal diseases are caused by people, not microscopic germs. Their prevention involves changing unhealthful behaviors, thus doing so is within each individual's control. Many people are seeking assistance to alter their lifestyles to promote a lifetime of health. Steps that can be adopted to promote health include the following:

- Eat fewer calories, especially foods high in fat or refined sugars.
- Eliminate the use of tobacco.
- Exercise regularly.
- Schedule physical and dental examinations on a regular basis.
- Perform self-breast or self-testicular examinations monthly.
- Wear seat belts.
- Cultivate friendships among individuals who are supportive.
- Participate in an activity that provides a sense of creativity and self-fulfillment.
- Explore concepts that provide explanations for the meaning of life.

Increased Knowledge, Technology, and Services

More scientific data are available now than ever before. Computers possess vast memory storage. They have the ability to process information and calculate mathematically in microseconds. This facilitates the transfer of information about health and disease prevention among scientists and eventually to the public.

Technology has made possible the application of machines with early diagnostic capabilities and efficient treatment of diseases that would have meant certain death in other eras. People are needed to operate this high technology. Various ways are being tried to bring health services to everyone—those living in the city, in the suburbs, on farms, and in rundown neighborhoods. Nurses and others are branching out into extensions of their careers, such as with emergency helicopter flight services, to provide an access for health.

Escalating Costs

As the sophistication of medical care increases, costs related to the treatment of illness have skyrocketed. Few can afford direct payment for medical care. Health promotion is far less expensive in the long run than the treatment of disease. Given this rationale, many individuals are seeking methods to protect and maintain their health.

Wellness

Wellness is more than just the absence of physical symptoms. It is a full and satisfying integration of all the aspects of well-being already discussed in this chapter. There can be variations in wellness; all of us experience changes from time to time. The goal is always the highest level of wellness that can be achieved. Guidelines for the components of wellness, known as human needs, direct us to areas that lead to higher and higher states of health.

The Health–Illness Continuum

Although most people think of themselves as being well when they are not sick, health and illness usually fluctuate within a wide range. In other words, well-being may not necessarily be constant in nature. At times people who are considered healthy may not feel as well as they do at other times. For example, you may have a headache and not do as well as usual in school. Although you may not feel "tops," you probably do not think of yourself as being sick unless your headache continues or returns frequently. Likewise, people who are sick may find that they feel better at times and can do more for themselves than they can at other times. However, they still may be considered sick and unable to go to work or school.

A *continuum* is a continuous whole. Changes in health and illness can be described on a *health–illness continuum,* as illustrated in Figure 3-1. As can be seen, there is no exact point at which health ends and illness begins. Health and illness are different for each person, and there

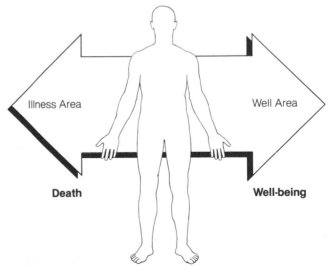

Figure 3-1 The health–illness continuum shows that there is no one point at which illness or wellness begins or ends.

may be a considerable range within which any one person may be considered ill or well.

High-Level Wellness

High-level wellness means that a person is functioning at his best level in relation to his abilities. Helping patients reach and stay at high-level wellness is the goal of every health practitioner.

Two situations may clarify this. During a patient's yearly checkup she tells the nurse that she is not sleeping well at home. She works as a waitress and consumes coffee throughout the day while waiting on customers. The loss of sleep is causing her to feel tired during the day. In another situation, a patient cannot move about because his left side has been weakened by a stroke. Both have experienced a change in a previous state of wellness, and neither is functioning at his or her highest level.

Suggesting to the waitress that she eliminate her intake of coffee or switch to a decaffeinated type may restore her ability to sleep. Working with the stroke patient to strengthen muscles and eventually use a cane may restore his ability to be mobile again. Both may achieve high-level wellness though one's level of functioning is higher than the other's.

Hierarchy of Needs

Human beings have needs that must be met. A *need* is a component of living that is necessary for life. Maslow (1970) identified and organized human needs in order of importance. Kalish (1973) expanded on the components within Maslow's original list. This series is referred to as a *hierarchy* because it is arranged from a lower to a higher rank. This tiered arrangement is illustrated in Figure 3-2.

Nurses sometimes use this sequence of needs as a guide for identifying the priority area in which patients require nursing assistance. The components on the lowest level

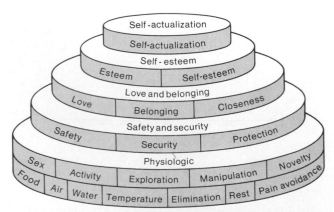

Figure 3-2 Maslow's hierarchy of needs and Maslow's needs as adapted by Kalish. (From Kalish RA: The Psychology of Human Behavior, 5th ed. Copyright © 1966, 1970, 1973, 1977, 1983 by Wadsworth, Inc. Reprinted by permission of Brooks/Cole Publishing Company, Monterey, CA.)

require attention before others. For example, the need for air is more important to life than shelter. Once the needs at one level are satisfied, the focus can be directed at the next higher level. Usually, once the lower or basic level of needs is met the patient can become more independent of the nurse's services.

Illness

Being *sick* or *ill* means that the person has some disease. A sickness or illness may be physical, affecting primarily a physical process; or it may be due to an accident or injury. It may be a mental disease, affecting primarily a mental process. Although a person may be considered either mentally or physically ill, his body still functions holistically. Hence, a person with a mental illness often has physical problems, and a physical illness influences most patients emotionally in some way.

Acute Illness

An *acute illness* is one that comes on quickly and lasts a relatively short time. Since the discovery of antibiotic drugs, many acute illnesses, such as streptococcal sore throats (strep throats), are treated with relative ease. Nevertheless, many acute illnesses, such as infectious hepatitis, an acute illness that affects the liver, and the common cold still remain difficult to treat, and science continues to look for their cure.

Chronic Illness

A *chronic illness* is one that comes on slowly and lasts a relatively long time. Arthritis, a joint disease, is an example. The number of elderly people in our population is increasing, and these people especially tend to suffer with chronic diseases. The more we learn about chronic illnesses, the more we can do to prevent them. When they do appear, every effort is being made to start early treatment so that their effects on the body can be decreased.

Remission. Some patients with chronic diseases experience periods of remission. A *remission* is an interval during which the disease seems to have disappeared. This does not mean the disease has been cured. The disease is likely to be remanifested; when it may reappear is unpredictable. Multiple sclerosis, a chronic disease of the nervous system, is an example of a condition in which periods of remission may occur.

Exacerbation. Patients with chronic diseases may also undergo exacerbation of their disease. An *exacerbation* is a period during which the symptoms of a disease become worse. A patient with emphysema, a chronic lung disease, may find his symptoms become worse when he catches a cold.

The Health-Care Team

The nurse may find various opportunities for employment within the health-care system. The *health-care system* is the network of institutions and agencies available to provide assistance to individuals with varying levels of wellness.

Most nurses work in hospitals. Wherever they provide patient services they are considered members of the health team. The *health team* consists of people who help patients overcome illnesses and stay well. These team members include physicians, dietitians, pharmacists, social workers, occupational therapists, physical therapists, clinical psychologists, and students in these various fields. If each group worked independently, there would be utter chaos in giving services, and the patient would probably rarely have complete and total care.

There are also groups of nursing personnel who work together to provide direct patient care. This group is called the *nursing team*. Figure 3-3 illustrates a nursing team, of which the center of attention is the patient and his family.

Hospitals are not the only places within the health care system where nurses work. Because nurses possess skills that assist the healthy or dying and all those at stages in between, there are many opportunities for providing the skills and services that patients need. Nurses work in health maintenance organizations, physical fitness centers, diet clinics, public health departments, home health agencies, and hospices to name a few.

Patterns for Administering Patient Care

When nursing personnel work together, one of several methods may be used to promote efficiency in providing patient care. Each method—functional nursing, case method, team nursing, primary nursing, and nurse managed care—has advantages and disadvantages. Students may encounter one or all of these methods while acquiring clinical experience.

Functional Nursing

One method for administering nursing care is the *functional method*. When this pattern is used, each nurse on a patient unit is assigned specific tasks. For example, one is assigned to give all the medications to the patients and another is assigned to do the treatments. This pattern is becoming the least used since its focus tends to be more on completing the task rather than treating the patient.

Case Method

Providing nursing care by the *case method* involves assigning one nurse to administer all the care a patient needs for a shift or some other designated period of time. This pattern of providing patient care is used in home health nursing, critical care, and in clinical assignments for nursing students.

Team Nursing

In *team nursing* many nursing personnel divide the patient care and all work until it is completed. The nursing team is headed by a nurse called the team leader. The team leader has assistants, such as other registered nurses, licensed practical/vocational nurses, students from various nursing programs, nursing assistants, nursing aides, clerical assistants, volunteers, and possibly others.

The leader, with the assistance of other members of the team, identifies the type of care each patient requires. The team, under the leader's direction, plans the kinds of skills that will be needed to solve the patient's health problems. The nurse who is the leader may assist with, but usually supervises, the care that other team members provide. It is the responsibility of the team leader to evaluate whether the goals of patient care are being met.

Conferences are an important part of team nursing. Conferences may cover a variety of subjects, but they are planned with certain goals in mind. Examples of goals include determining the best approaches to each patient's health problems, increasing the team members' knowledge, and promoting a cooperative spirit among nursing personnel.

Primary Nursing

Primary nursing is described as a method for administering nursing care whereby a patient's total 24-hour care is the responsibility of one nurse. The patient's total care is planned in writing. The primary nurse is responsible for making certain that the plan of care is followed around the clock. When the primary nurse is off duty, other nurses are designated to implement the patient's plan of care. How-

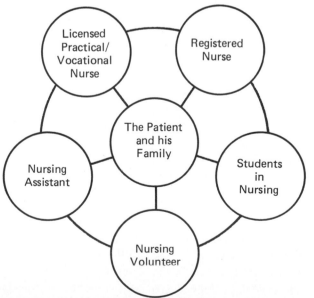

Figure 3-3 This figure illustrates the nursing team, whose members work cooperatively to help meet the patient's needs.

ever, the primary nurse continues to remain responsible and accountable.

If others, in the absence of the primary nurse, identify new patient problems or determine that the plan for patient care requires modification, the primary nurse is consulted. The duties of the primary nurse include seeing how the patient responds to the nursing care he receives and making adjustments as needed.

Nurse-Managed Care

A new type of nursing-care delivery system is being implemented in pilot studies in several areas of the United States. It is called nurse-managed care by some and case management by others.

This innovative system was developed in response to several current crises affecting the delivery of health care today, such as the nursing shortage and the need to balance the costs of medical care within limited reimbursement systems. Nurse-managed care is similar to the principles practiced by successful businesses. In the business world, corporations pay executives to forecast trends and facilitate the best strategies for making profits. In *nurse-managed care,* a professional nurse is a case manager. The nurse manager plans the nursing care of a group of patients based upon their type of case, or medical diagnosis. Predictable outcomes are forecast and evaluated on a daily basis. By meeting the outcomes or revising the care in a timely manner, the patient is ready for discharge before or by the time designated by prospective payment systems.

In some cases, nurse managers are salaried rather than paid according to clock hours. The number of hours that are worked depends on the changing needs of a nurse's cases. The nurse is allowed creativity and flexibility in arranging a work schedule. The design of this model relieves the nurse from performing non-nursing tasks. It also provides more autonomy in clinical practice, a characteristic of professionalism. Using nurses more efficiently and preventing burnout increases retention.

Pilot studies found that overtime costs were reduced. Practitioners felt an increase in job satisfaction. Standards of care continued to be met. Hospitals were able to decrease their losses and operate within their budgets. Most importantly, patients felt they received more personalized attention by having their care planned by one nurse.

Continuity of Care

Continuity of care is a continuum of health care. It is important that the services provided to patients not be fragmented. It is also equally important that an individual, whether healthy or ill, not feel isolated or abandoned when in need of health-care services.

Continuity of care requires the smooth transfer and periodic follow-up of patients among health practitioners and health agencies. It means that all levels of care pro-

viders work together, making their services available to everyone as needed.

Chapters 5 and 11 explain how nurses communicate among themselves so that the patient's nursing care is both continuous and complete. There is also discussion of how nurses assist in referring patients from one health agency to another, or from one unit in an agency to another, so that continuity of care is possible.

Bibliography

Anderson D: Opportunity knocks at last . . . the time is ripe for the nursing profession to assert its value. RN Magazine 52(10):52–56, 59–60, 63, 1989

Blixen CE: Aging and mental health care. Journal of Gerontological Nursing 14(11):11–15, 1988

Castledine G: A question of health. Geriatric Nursing & Home Care 8(2):8, 1988

Clark M: Patient/client advocates. J Adv Nurs 14(7):513–514, 1989

Colantonio A: Lay concepts of health. Health Values 12(5):3–7, 1988

Collins HL: How well do nurses nurture themselves? RN Magazine 52(5):39–41, 1989

Davis GC: Nursing values and health care policy. Nurs Outlook 36(6):289–292, 1988

del Bueno DJ, Leblanc D: Nurse managed care: One approach. J Nurs Adm 19(11):24–25, 1989

Dellasega C: Health in the sandwich generation. Geriatr Nurs 10(5):242–243, 1989

Dimond M: Health care and the aging population. Nurs Outlook 37(2):76–77, 1989

Duffy ME: Determinants of health promotion in midlife women. Nurs Res 37(6):358–362, 1988

Field PA: Brenda, Beth and Susan . . . three approaches to health promotion. Canadian Nurse 85(5):20–24, 1989

Kelly LS: Wild cards in a new health care game. Nurs Outlook 37(2):71, 1989

Mitchell GJ: Man–living–health: The theory in practice. Nursing Science Quarterly 1(3):120–127, 1988

Mitchell L: Whose health for all? Nursing Times 85(34):48–50, 1989

Moch SD: Health within illness: Conceptual evolution and practice. ANS 11(4):23–31, 1989

Moran MJ: Access to care for the elderly. Nursing/Connections 2(3):3–5, 1989

Nyamathi A: Comprehensive health seeking and coping paradigm. J Adv Nurs 14(4):281–290, 1989

Olivas GS, Del Togno–Armanasco V, Erikson JR, Harter S: Case management: A bottom line care delivery model. Part 1: The concept. J Nurs Adm 19(11):16–20, 1989

Pilch JJ: Your Invitation to Full Life. Minneapolis, Winston Press, 1981

Pollock SE: The hardiness characteristic: A motivating factor in adaptation. ANS 11(2):53–62, 1989

Smith DL: Health promotion for older adults. Health Values 12(5):46–51, 1988

Solovy A: Health care in the 1990s: Forecasts by top analysts. Hospitals 63(14):34–36, 38–40, 42, 1989

Stillwaggon CA: The impact of nurse managed care on the cost of nurse practice and nurse satisfaction. J Nurs Adm 19(11):21–27, 1989

Ulin PR: Global collaboration in primary health care. Nurs Outlook 37(3):134–137, 1989

4

The Nursing Process: The Model For Nursing

Chapter Outline

Behavioral Objectives
Glossary
Introduction
The Nursing Process
Assessing the Patient's Health Status
Diagnosing the Patient's Health Problems
Planning the Patient's Nursing Care
Implementing the Plan
Evaluating the Results of Nursing Care
Bibliography

Skill Procedures

Using the Nursing Process

Behavioral Objectives

When the content of this chapter has been mastered, the learner will be able to:

Define the terms appearing in the glossary.
List the five parts of the nursing process in the order in which they are performed.
List seven characteristics of the nursing process.
Describe each of the steps in the five parts of the nursing process and give an example that illustrates each step.

Glossary

Actual health problem A health problem that currently exists.

Analysis A process in which information is examined in order to identify patterns.

Assessment An action that involves collecting information.

Collaborative problem A potential health problem that would require the cooperative treatment efforts of the nurse and the physician if it occurred.

Data Information from which conclusions can be drawn.

Database assessment The collection of facts that cover aspects of the patient's physical, emotional, social, and spiritual health.

Etiology The cause or basis of a problem.

Evaluation The process of measuring how well a goal or objective is reached.

Focus assessment A limited collection of a few specific, related facts.

Goal An expected or desired outcome; the desired end result for which one works. Synonym for *objective*.

High risk for problem A health problem that is likely to occur in the future. Synonym for *potential problem*.

Long-term goal A desired outcome that may take a few weeks or months to accomplish.

Need A necessity or a requirement.

Nursing diagnosis A statement describing a health problem that has the possibility of being resolved totally through nursing measures.

Nursing orders Specific, detailed directions for accomplishing goals.

Nursing process An organized sequence of steps that nurses use to solve the health problems of patients.

Objective An expected or desired outcome; the desired end result for which one works. Synonym for *goal*.

Objective data Information that can be measured.

Organization A process of grouping related information.

Pathophysiology The science that deals with the physical changes that occur when there is an altered state of health.

Possible problem A situation in which some but not enough data have been collected to confirm the presence of a health problem.

Potential problem A health problem that is likely to occur in the future. Synonym for *high risk for problem*.

Problem Something that stands in the way of meeting a need; an unmet need.

Process A set of actions leading to a particular goal.

Short-term goal A desired outcome that may be accomplished within a few days or a week.

Subjective data Information that only the patient can experience and describe.

Validation A process of making sure information is factual.

Introduction

In the past, nursing practice involved actions that were based mostly on common sense and the examples set by older, experienced nurses. The actual care of patients tended to be limited according to the medical orders given by a physician. Nurses today continue to work interdependently with other health practitioners. However, now nurses are directing patient care more independently. In even stronger terms, nurses are being held responsible and accountable for providing appropriate patient care that reflects current accepted standards for nursing practice.

This change in attitude and practice occurred through the development of the nursing process. The nursing process is a problem-solving method. When nursing practice is based on the components of this method, the patient receives quality care within a minimum of time and at a maximum of efficiency.

The nursing process is widely used in all areas of clinical nursing practice. The head nurse, a team leader, or a primary nurse is usually responsible for seeing to it that the nursing process is fully carried out. However, it is necessary for all the members of the nursing team to understand and contribute to the activities associated with the nursing process.

The Nursing Process

A *process* is a set of actions leading to a particular goal. The *nursing process* is an organized sequence of steps that nurses use to solve the health problems of patients. The goal of the nursing process is to provide care that will help a patient reach and maintain high-level wellness.

The nursing process, at one time, was described as consisting of a sequence of four steps:

1. Assessing the patient's health
2. Planning the patient's nursing care
3. Giving the patient care
4. Evaluating the results of nursing care.

One of the most recent definitions of nursing, given in Chapter 1 as "the diagnosis and treatment of human responses to actual or potential health problems," has led to the addition of a fifth step to the nursing process. This new step, which comes after assessing the patient's health status, is diagnosing health problems. The parts of the nursing process are illustrated in Figure 4-1.

Characteristics of the Nursing Process

The nursing process is an effective method of problem solving. The actions necessary for solving problems are somewhat universal. A baker may seek to determine why a batch of bread does not rise; a scientist may seek a cure for AIDS. Nurses help to solve health problems. They deal with people, not objects or diseases. The nursing process,

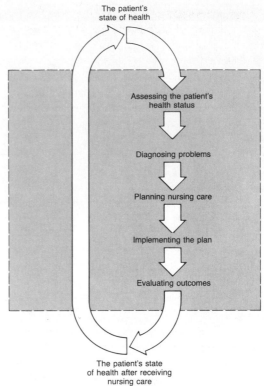

Figure 4-1 This diagram illustrates the five steps of the nursing process. The broken lines indicate that information can enter the process at any time and influence the decisions about nursing care.

as a problem-solving method, contains some distinct characteristics. The nursing process is:

Within the legal scope of nursing. The definitions of nursing in nurse practice acts are expanding to describe nursing in terms of a more independent problem-solving role.

Based on knowledge. Nurses are increasing the depth and breadth of their knowledge. The ability to solve problems using the nursing process involves the application of the laws of science to patient care. Nurses now use their increased knowledge base to correlate a patient's health problem with the use of certain nursing skills to achieve a fairly predictable effect.

Planned. The steps of the nursing process are organized and systematic. One step leads to the next in an orderly fashion.

Patient centered. Each patient is the unique product of physical, emotional, social, and spiritual components. The nursing process involves a comprehensive appraisal of each patient. Nurses encourage patients to become involved as active participants in various problem-solving steps.

Goal directed. It is important that the patient and the nurse understand the final expected outcome. The nursing process involves the cooperative efforts of the patient and nurse toward a target.

Prioritized. A hierarchy of needs was discussed in Chapter 3. When the nursing process is used, some problems need to be solved before others. Those that are life threatening require immediate attention. First solving the problems that present the greatest potential for harm provides a strategy leading to improved health.

Dynamic. The health status of any patient is constantly changing. One problem is often related to another; as one problem changes, so may the other. The nursing process is like a continuous loop; when the last step has been completed, there is a need to begin all over again.

Assessing the Patient's Health Status

The nurse begins the nursing process by performing an assessment. *Assessment* is an action that involves collecting and organizing information, or *data*. The purpose of assessment is to identify past, current, and possible future health problems. Assessment is ongoing, and by comparing changes in information, the nurse may evaluate whether there is progress toward a goal.

Collecting Data. The information may be gathered in different ways, such as by asking the patient or family questions, making observations while examining the patient, reading the patient's record, and asking other health workers about their observations of the patient. Information that is measurable, such as the patient's blood pressure, is called *objective data*. Information that only the patient can experience and describe, such as pain, is called *subjective data*. The opinions of others may also be called subjective because they are based on personal assumptions from within their own experience.

Gathering a Database. For the nursing process to be useful, the assessment must be thorough and accurate. It is important that data cover a wide variety of information about the patient's physical, emotional, social, and spiritual health. This comprehensive collection of facts is often referred to as a *database assessment*. It is often obtained during the first meeting with the patient. Many hospitals have a printed form that prevents the nurse from accidentally omitting anything. A database assessment generally includes questions about the patient's life, a health history, and review or examination of each system of the body.

It is important that this base of information reflect the individuality of the patient. The nursing process loses its value if it is not patient centered. Nurses may prefer to use some tool as a guide for asking questions during the database assessment. Many nurses use a framework, such as one reflecting functional health patterns, to help maintain the personal focus on the patient. This type of comprehensive list of categories helps the nurse gather information about the physical, emotional, social, and spiritual views, habits, and routines that are part of the patient's lifestyle. A list of health patterns can be found in Table 4-1 along with the types of information each category includes. This helps the nurse to assess health from the patient's perspective. Figure 4-2 shows an example of how these functional health patterns have been adapted within a hospital admission form.

Adding to the Database. The process of assessment is continuous. Nurses gather information frequently throughout the nurse–patient relationship. The database assessment is broad and time consuming. The initial information may be superficial. The nurse may need to explore some aspects of the data base in more depth at a later time. This is called a *focus assessment*. It involves gathering a limited amount of specific information. This information expands the original database. A focus assessment may also be performed when specific information must be obtained frequently at short intervals of time. For example, after a patient returns from surgery a type of focus assessment generally includes gathering information about the patient's ability to breathe, blood pressure and pulse, skin color, condition of the incision or dressing covering it, volume, rate, and type of intravenous fluids, level of consciousness, and amount of pain. The nurse uses the trend of information to determine if problems are developing that may require use of further nursing skills.

Ensuring Accuracy. The nurse should have a good picture of the patient and his present state of health if data have been gathered appropriately and accurately. To reduce the chance of interpreting the data incorrectly, the nurse should make sure the information is factual. This is often called *validation*. In other words, the nurse should make sure that questionable information was not misinterpreted or collected with faulty equipment. The nurse may need to continue double-checking information in a variety of ways, making sure it is correct.

Organizing Data. Interpretation of data is easier if the information is organized. *Organization* involves placing groups of related information into certain categories in much the same way that a cook files recipes. Some nurses use Maslow's or Kalish's hierarchy, identified in Chapter 3, to organize related information.

Recognizing Needs or Problems. While organizing data, the nurse may be thinking in terms of whether a need or problem exists. This requires the knowledge to recognize what is normal from abnormal. A *need* is a necessity

(*Text continues on page 44*)

Table 4-1. Functional Health Patterns

Health Pattern	Type of Information
Health-perception/health-management pattern	Includes information about the patient's view of his health, the actions the patient has used in the past while healthy or ill, and his feelings about how his health care should be managed.
Nutritional–metabolic pattern	Includes information about the patient's habits of eating and drinking: amounts, types, times, use of supplements, and physical characteristics that relate to the quantity and quality of food consumption.
Elimination pattern	Includes information about the patient's elimination of stool and urine; some data would include the frequency, amounts, appearance, changes, and any use of medications or equipment that has been required.
Activity–Exercise pattern	Includes information about the patient's daily routine, both work and recreation; facts relating to what he is able to do, would like to do, and reasons for any differences between the two.
Cognitive–perceptual pattern	Includes information about the patient's use of language and his mental status; it also includes the patient's sensory abilities and the use of any artificial aids such as a hearing aid or glasses.
Sleep–rest pattern	Includes information about the patient's routine of sleep and inactivity; it would involve data related to the usual time for retiring and rising, and any customs or rituals the patient follows when preparing for sleep.
Self-perception/self-concept pattern	Includes information on the patient's attitudes about his personal strengths and weaknesses; any behavior that correlates with this, such as speaking with confidence, would also be included.
Role–relationship pattern	Includes information on how the patient interprets his functions and responsibilities within the group of people who are significant to him; this may include relatives, friends, and coworkers.
Sexuality–reproductive pattern	Involves information about the patient's analysis of the adequacy or inadequacy of his sexual behavior; also common reproductive information such as number of pregnancies or status of menstruation would be included.
Coping–stress–tolerance pattern	Involves information about the methods the patient uses when faced with problems and whether they assist him to a satisfactory outcome.
Value–belief pattern	Includes information about the patient's beliefs about the meaning and purpose of life; any applications to these beliefs related to health and illness would be especially appropriate.

Adapted from Gordon M: Manual of Nursing Diagnosis 1988–1989. St. Louis, CV Mosby, 1989. Reprinted with permission of the publisher.

**Community Health Center
of Branch County**

ADMISSION ASSESSMENT RECORD

RESPIRATION

[ ] PROBLEM	HISTORY OF	[ ] CHEST PAIN [ ] PNEUMONIA [ ] BRONCHITIS [ ] ASTHMA [ ] EMPHYSEMA

SHORTNESS OF BREATH
[ ] YES   [ ] WITH EXERCISE   [ ] WITHOUT EXERCISE
[ ] NO

COUGH
[ ] YES   [ ] PRODUCTIVE   [ ] NON-PRODUCTIVE   [ ] SPUTUM COLOR
[ ] NO

BREATH SOUNDS (DESCRIBE)

RATE	RHYTHM	QUALITY	SKIN COLOR
		[ ] LABORED [ ] SHALLOW	[ ] PINK [ ] PALE [ ] CYANOTIC

ACCESSORY MUSCLES

COMMENTS

[ ] PROBLEM
[ ] POTENTIAL FOR REFERRAL

CIRCULATION

[ ] PROBLEM	HISTORY OF	[ ] BLOOD CLOTS [ ] EDEMA [ ] ABNORMAL EKG [ ] NUMBNESS [ ] TINGLING [ ] POOR CIRCULATION [ ] FATIGUE [ ] HYPERTENSION

APICAL RATE	APICAL RATE [ ] REGULAR [ ] IRREGULAR	RHYTHM

NECK VEIN DISTENSION [ ] PRESENT [ ] ABSENT	NAIL BEDS [ ] PINK [ ] PALE [ ] CYANOTIC

PEDAL EDEMA	[ ] PRESENT [ ] ABSENT

PEDAL PULSES	LEFT [ ] PRESENT [ ] WEAK [ ] ABSENT RIGHT [ ] PRESENT [ ] WEAK [ ] ABSENT

COMMENTS

[ ] POTENTIAL FOR REFERRAL

NUTRITIONAL/METABOLIC

[ ] PROBLEM	HISTORY OF	[ ] DIABETES [ ] HYPOGLYCEMIA [ ] THYROID PROBLEMS	NUTRITIONAL STATUS [ ] WELL NOURISHED [ ] EMACIATED [ ] OBESE

MEALS PER DAY	DIET AT HOME	DIET PREFERENCE	LAST MEAL [ ] A.M. [ ] P.M.	RECENT WEIGHT CHANGES

NUTRITIONAL DISTURBANCES
[ ] VOMITING   [ ] NAUSEA   [ ] ANOREXIA   [ ] CHEWING PROBLEMS   [ ] OTHER (DESCRIBE)

JAUNDICE PRESENT [ ] YES [ ] NO	DENTAL HYGIENE (DESCRIBE)	TEETH [ ] OWN [ ] DENTURES	TONGUE CONDITION [ ] DRY [ ] COATED [ ] MOIST [ ] SWOLLEN	ORAL MUCOSA [ ] DRY [ ] MOIST	COLOR

COMMENTS

[ ] POTENTIAL FOR REFERRAL

ELIMINATION

[ ] PROBLEM	BOWEL HABITS COLOR [ ] SOFT FORMED [ ] CONSTIPATED LAST BOWEL MOVEMENT STOOLS PER DAY _____ [ ] DIARRHEA [ ] USE LAXATIVE

BLADDER [ ] URGENCY [ ] CALCULI [ ] HEMATURIA [ ] DYSURIA [ ] NOCTURIA [ ] FREQUENCY [ ] PROSTATE PROBLEM	BOWEL SOUNDS [ ] PRESENT [ ] ABSENT OSTOMIES OR TUBES (DESCRIBE)

ABDOMEN [ ] TENDER [ ] SOFT [ ] FIRM [ ] DISTENDED [ ] NOT DISTENDED	URINARY DEVICES (DESCRIBE)

COMMENTS

[ ] POTENTIAL FOR REFERRAL

COGNITIVE/PERCEPTUAL

[ ] PROBLEM	HISTORY OF	[ ] SEIZURES [ ] FREQUENT [ ] INFREQUENT [ ] HEADACHES [ ] FREQUENT [ ] INFREQUENT	LIMITATION OR RESTRICTION RELATED TO [ ] HEARING - IMPAIRED [ ] YES [ ] NO [ ] VISION - IMPAIRED [ ] YES [ ] NO

LEVEL OF CONSCIOUSNESS
[ ] ALERT   [ ] LETHARGIC   [ ] CONFUSED   [ ] LISTLESS   [ ] RESPONDS TO PAIN   [ ] UNRESPONSIVE

ORIENTED TO [ ] TIME [ ] PLACE [ ] PERSON	AFFECT [ ] CALM [ ] WITHDRAWN [ ] APPREHENSIVE	[ ] OTHER (DESCRIBE)

BEHAVIOR [ ] COOPERATIVE [ ] UNCOOPERATIVE	PUPILS [ ] EQUAL [ ] REACTIVE	[ ] OTHER (DESCRIBE)

COMMUNICATION
[ ] SPEAKS ENGLISH   [ ] ABLE TO READ   [ ] ABLE TO WRITE   [ ] COMMUNICATES ADEQUATELY

AWARENESS
[ ] NO PROBLEM WITH MEMORY   [ ] PROBLEM WITH MEMORY

DISCOMFORT/PAIN [ ] YES [ ] NO	WHERE	TYPE	PAIN MANAGEMENT	POTENTIAL RISK OF FALLS [ ] YES [ ] NO

COMMENTS

[ ] POTENTIAL FOR REFERRAL

Figure 4-2 This hospital admission assessment form is organized according to functional health patterns. Only one page is shown here. Using this form as a data-gathering tool helps the nurse to collect comprehensive information. (Courtesy of the Community Health Center of Branch County, Coldwater, MI.)

or a requirement. Man has certain basic physical needs. For example, the needs for oxygen, food, water, and elimination are basic to life. Well-being requires that a person also meet his needs for security, love, self-esteem, and self-actualization.

A *problem* is something that stands in the way of meeting a need. It is an unmet need. For example, to survive, a person must have oxygen. A person who is choking on food has a problem because his need for oxygen cannot be met. People have a need for self-respect. A problem arises when a person dislikes himself. A problem in which a health need is not being satisfied ordinarily brings a person to seek help from health workers.

Learning to use the words *need* and *problem* correctly helps a nurse understand areas in which the patient has a strength, or a need that is being met. It also helps to identify a problem, or deficit, indicating that a need is not being met.

The assessment of a patient's health status may be summarized as having the following four steps:

1. Collect information about a patient.
2. Check all data for accuracy.
3. Organize information under a list of categories.
4. Analyze the needs or problems of the patient by comparing the information about the patient with what is considered to be normal.

Diagnosing the Patient's Health Problems

As discussed in Chapter 1, the ANA's definition of nursing is "the diagnosis and treatment of human responses. . . ." Human responses fall into one of nine patterns, described in Table 4-2. They are integrated into chart form in Figure 4-3.

Analyzing Data

Analysis is a process in which information is examined in order to identify patterns. Nurses analyze the responses of the patient looking for relations between the data. The abnormal findings are sorted into groups. Using knowledge and experience, the nurse then interprets their meaning.

Determining Patient Problems

Nurses do not make medical diagnoses of diseases. Nurses identify alterations that occur within normal patterns of human responses. These alterations or the patient's problems may currently exist or occur in the future as a consequence of the trend in current findings. For example, while assessing an adult patient, the nurse determines that the patient is unable to walk. The ability to move is an alteration in a normal, essential, human activity. At the moment this patient has a mobility problem. If the patient remains inactive, the nurse understands that the patient

Table 4-2. Human Response Patterns

Pattern	Description
Exchanging	Mutually giving and receiving
Communicating	Sending messages
Relating	Establishing bonds
Valuing	Assigning relative worth
Choosing	Selecting from alternatives
Moving	Involving activity
Perceiving	Receiving information
Knowing	Acquiring meaning with information
Feeling	Involving subjective awareness of information

Conceptual base for identifying and classifying nursing diagnoses. Approved by NANDA General Assembly, 1986.

has the potential for future problems, such as losing the ability to maintain his independence.

Making a Nursing Diagnosis

Doctors use standardized terms to identify the titles of diseases that represent a group of symptoms. There is consensus on the names given to diseases that consist of a group of related symptoms. For instance, if a physician says the patient has diabetes, other medical doctors understand the definition of this term, its cause, and some of the symptoms the patient is likely to have.

Nurses, like physicians, have also developed a definition of a nursing diagnosis and a list of nursing diagnoses to facilitate a uniform, standardized language for the types of patient problems nurses identify. The North American Nursing Diagnosis Association (NANDA) is the group that defines these problems and compiles the list of altered, impaired, deficient, and ineffective human responses. Display 4-1 gives the definitions of actual, high-risk, and of wellness diagnoses. The current list of accepted nursing diagnoses is located in Appendix A. Each skill chapter includes a list of NANDA-approved nursing diagnoses that may be applicable to patients requiring the procedures discussed in these chapters. Diagnoses previously labeled "Potential for" are labeled "High Risk for" throughout this book.

Writing a Diagnostic Statement

A nursing diagnosis generally is a three-part statement. It contains the diagnostic category or problem, the cause of the problem or *etiology,* and the signs and symptoms that the patient with a particular diagnosis is experiencing. This is often referred to as the PES: problem + etiology + signs and symptoms. The third part of the statement may be documented elsewhere in some clinical agencies. It

CC
CC **Community Health Center**
of Branch County

274 East Chicago Street
Coldwater, MI 49036-2088
(517) 278-7361

DISCHARGE ASSESSMENT - MATERNAL / INFANT   **PART II**

MOTHER			INFANT		
EXCHANGING	YES	NO	**EXCHANGING**	YES	NO
VITAL SIGNS: TEMP. <99°F. (0), BP>90/60 <140/90, PULSE <100, RESP. >12			FONTANELS — SOFT, FLAT (ANTERIOR AND POSTERIOR)		
			HEAD: ABSENCE OF ABRASIONS, BRUISING, CEPHALOHEMATOMA		
LABS: HGB. >10, gm/dl HCT. >30%			EYES, EARS, NOSE, THROAT: ABSENCE OF ABNORMAL		
ADEQUATE FOOD AND FLUID INTAKE			DRAINAGE, SECRETIONS OR		
ELIMINATION: BOWEL-ABSENCE OF CONSTIPATION, DIARRHEA, INCONTINENCE. BLADDER-ABSENCE OF BURNING, FREQUENCY, INCONTINENCE.			STRUCTURAL ABNORMALITIES		
			ABDOMEN: SOFT, ROUND, ACTIVE BOWEL SOUNDS		
LOCHIA: MINIMAL TO MODERATE			NEUROLOGIC: ABSENCE OF SEIZURES, TREMORS, ERRATIC MOVEMENTS		
CARDIO/RESP: ABSENCE OF CARDIAC OR RESPIRATORY COMPROMISE			SKIN/TISSUE: PINK, WARM, DRY, ABSENCE OF LESIONS, PUSTULES, BLEEDING, CORD DRY AND FREE OF SIGNS OF INFECTION, CIRCUMCISION CLEAN AND DRY		
SKIN: ABSENCE OF SKIN OR TISSUE IMPAIRMENT					
COMMUNICATING / CHOOSING / VALUING	YES	NO			
ABSENCE OF NEED FOR ADDITIONAL SPIRITUAL SUPPORT			WEIGHT: LOSS WITHIN 10% OF BIRTH		
EFFECTIVE/UNCOMPROMISED INDIVIDUAL OR FAMILY COPING			FEEDING: ABSENCE OF FEEDING PROBLEMS, VOMITING, REGURGITATION, EXCESSIVE MUCUS		
APPROPRIATE VERBAL/NON-VERBAL COMMUNICATION					
RELATING / PERCEIVING	YES	NO	OXYGENATION: SYMMETRICAL CHEST; ABSENCE OF STERNAL RETRACTIONS; NASAL FLARING; GRUNTING; APNEA		
ADEQUATE FAMILY SUPPORT SYSTEM					
APPROPRIATE INTERACTION BETWEEN MOTHER, FATHER, INFANT			CIRCULATION: ABSENCE OF CYANOSIS; EXTREMITIES AND TRUNK COLOR - PINK; NORMAL HEART SOUNDS		
VERBALIZES POSITIVE FEELINGS TOWARD SELF AND INFANT					
REFERS TO INFANT BY NAME			VITAL SIGNS: TEMP >97<99 F. (AX), RESP. >30<60 MIN., APICAL > 110 <160		
MAKES EYE CONTACT, HOLDS AND TOUCHES INFANT					
VERBALIZES SATISFACTION WITH INFANT			ELIMINATION: NORMAL STOOL AND VOIDING PATTERN ESTABLISHED		
MOVING	YES	NO	LABS: PHYSICIAN NOTIFIED OF BILIRUBIN > 5 AT 24 HOURS OR > 10 AT 48 HOURS; PHYSICIAN NOTIFIED OF OTHER OUTSTANDING OR ABNORMAL RESULTS		
NO ACTIVITY/EXERCISE RESTRICTIONS					
FEELS RESTED			**RELATING/PERCEIVING**	YES	NO
ABLE TO CARRY OUT ACTIVITIES OF DAILY LIVING			APPROPRIATE AUDIO/VISUAL RESPONSES TO LIGHT, SOUND OR OTHER STIMULI		
FEELING	YES	NO			
INCISION: HEALING, ABSENCE OF REDNESS, SWELLING, HEMATOMA, DISCOLORATION			**MOVING**	YES	NO
			SMOOTH, EXTREMITY MOVEMENTS x 4, POSITIVE BABINSKI, MORO, ROOTING, SUCKING, GRASPING AND STEPPING REFLEXES		
COMFORT: MINIMAL PAIN THAT IS RELIEVED WITH TYLENOL OR EQUIVALENT MILD ANALGESIA AND/OR SITZ BATH AND/OR ICE PACK			GOOD MUSCLE TONE AND STRENGTH		
ABSENCE OF BREAST ENGORGEMENT, NIPPLE SORENESS, REDNESS			ABNORMALITIES: ABSENCE OF ABNORMALITIES OF HANDS, FEET, HIPS, SPINE		
ABSENCE OF SIGNS OF DEPRESSION-WITHDRAWAL/ CONFUSION/GRIEVING			AWAKE/SLEEP: NORMAL SLEEP/WAKE PERIODS		
IF ADDITIONAL COMMENTS ARE NECESSARY ON ANY OF THE FIELDS COVERED HEREIN, PLEASE DO SO BELOW. ▼ ▼			**FEELING**	YES	NO
			COMFORT: ABSENCE OF PAIN, NORMAL CRYING ACTIVITY (VIGOROUS, RHYTHMATIC)		

NURSE'S SIGNATURE	DATE
COMMENTS	
SIGNATURE	DATE

FORM U-385 (6/89)   **DISCHARGE ASSESSMENT-MATERNAL/INFANT**

CHART

Figure 4-3 The darker headings on this form are labeled according to human response categories. (Courtesy of the Community Health Center of Branch County, Coldwater, MI.)

Display 4-1. NANDA Definitions of Nursing Diagnoses

Nursing Diagnosis

A nursing diagnosis is a clinical judgment about individual, family, or community responses to actual or potential health problems and life processes. Nursing diagnoses provide the basis for selection of nursing interventions to achieve outcomes for which the nurse is accountable.

Wellness Nursing Diagnosis

A wellness nursing diagnosis is a clinical judgment about an individual, family, or community in transition from a specific level of wellness to a higher level of wellness. The term "Potential for Enhanced" will be the designated qualifier. Enhanced is defined as made greater, increased in quality, or more desired.

High-Risk Nursing Diagnosis (NANDA-approved diagnoses previously designated as "Potential" will now be labeled "High Risk for")

A high-risk nursing diagnosis is a clinical judgment that an individual, family, or community is more vulnerable to develop the problem than others in the same or similar situation. High-risk nursing diagnoses are supported by risk factors that guide nursing interventions to reduce or prevent the occurrence of the problem.

North American Nursing Diagnosis Association. Classification of Nursing Diagnoses: Proceedings of the Ninth Conference, March 1990.

1. Sleep pattern disturbance = problem
2. Related to excessive intake of coffee = etiology
3. As manifested by difficulty in falling asleep, feeling tired during the day, and irritability with others = signs and symptoms

Figure 4-4 This shows the three parts of a nursing diagnosis statement. It is also an example of an actual problem because it is one that currently exists.

Some human responses to illness or injury may not yet exist, but are likely to occur unless preventive nursing measures are taken. In this case the nurse would begin the diagnostic statement with the words "*High Risk for;*" for example, "High Risk for Impaired Skin Integrity related to immobility." This would mean that the skin may break down and develop sores because the patient is not moving around enough to relieve the pressure from his body weight; the skin, however, is currently intact. NANDA's decision to replace the words "Potential for" with "High Risk for" in all its approved diagnoses was made in order to reinforce the fact that the diagnosis should only be used for patients who are especially vulnerable to developing the problem because of their unique health status.

At times the nurse may suspect that a problem exists but may not have gathered enough data to be sure. In this case the nurse would use the term *possible* before the diagnostic statement; for example, possible social isolation related to facial burn scars. In other words, the nurse thinks that perhaps the patient is avoiding going anywhere or being with anyone because he is self-conscious about his disfigurement. This may take more careful assessment; with more data the nurse may discover that this patient has felt satisfied with only a few close friends and has never cared to go to public places. The suspected diagnosis would thus not be appropriate in this case.

Note that any diagnostic statement that indicates a potential or possible health problem only contains two parts: the problem and the cause. This is because the patient has not demonstrated any or enough signs that relate to it.

Identifying a Collaborative Problem. A *collaborative problem* is a potential complication that would require the cooperative efforts of the nurse and the physician if it occurred. Figure 4-5 shows this interdependent relation. The definitive treatment of a collaborative problem is outside the legal scope of nursing. The nurse must be aware that certain patients are prone to developing disease or treatment complications. This requires the knowledge of pathophysiology. *Pathophysiology* is the science that deals with the physical changes that occur when there is an altered state of health.

may be a hospital's policy to include the assessed signs and symptoms on a focus assessment sheet or in the nurse's charting.

The PES parts of a diagnostic statement are illustrated in Figure 4-4. Using this example you should be able to understand that the second step of the nursing process, diagnosis, has followed from the first step of assessment. The nurse collected information that was valid. It was categorized under a basic physiologic need. The nurse used knowledge about the quality and quantity of this patient's sleep compared with that of an average adult and the relation to chemicals in coffee. The nurse was then able to determine that the need for sleep was being unmet. Sleeplessness is a human response, not a disease. It can be reduced or eliminated through certain nursing actions. It therefore fits the definition of a nursing diagnosis.

Differentiating Actual, Potential, and Possible Health Problems. An *actual health problem* is one that currently exists. An example of this is the statement in Figure 4-4.

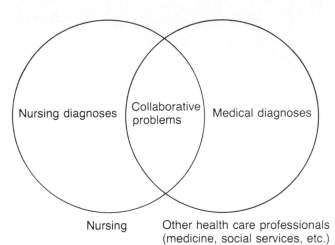

Nursing   Other health care professionals
(medicine, social services, etc.)

Figure 4-5 These two overlapping circles illustrate that the nurse independently treats nursing diagnoses. Doctors, other health professionals, and nurses work together on collaborative problems. (Carpenito LJ: Nursing Diagnosis, Application to Clinical Practice, 3rd ed, p 28. Philadelphia, JB Lippincott, 1989)

The nurse must monitor the patient to detect these complications and notify the physician if they occur. For all nursing personnel to be aware of the need to assess certain data, the nurse will write a statement that identifies the collaborative problem. Carpenito (1989) recommends labeling a collaborative problem by writing "Potential Complication:" followed by the specified problem. For example, "Potential Complication: Hemorrhage." The nurse and other members of the nursing team would be aware and informed that this complication is possible. They would make certain observations, looking for signs of blood loss, and they would take precautions against any potential injury that would lead to bleeding. If signs of blood loss occurred, nurses would be expected to use certain first-aid techniques to control bleeding. The physician would need to be consulted about administering drugs or replacing any blood that may have been excessively lost. Nurses may not legally prescribe medications, alter a dosage, or administer fluids such as blood without a written medical order.

The actions associated with the diagnostic aspect of the nursing process may be summarized as follows:

1. Analyze which problems can be solved by the nurse and which problems need cooperation with the physician.
2. Write statements that clearly identify the problem, its cause, and, when applicable, the manifestations found in the patient.

Planning the Patient's Nursing Care

The nurse develops a plan for care. The care plan can be handwritten, standardized, or computer generated. The nurse can make additions or deletions to printed care plans to individualize the care of a specific patient.

The patient should agree that the problems identified by the nurse do indeed exist. He may even have suggestions about how some problems may be solved. At the very least, he should be informed as to what the nurse will be trying to accomplish during his hospitalization. In some clinical agencies, nurses share the completed plan with the patient. The patient signs the care plan to indicate that he has been informed.

Setting Priorities. Not all of the patient's problems may be resolved during the short time in the institution. Therefore, it is important to determine which ones require the most attention.

There are several ways to determine priorities. The first is to think in terms of the hierarchy of needs. Those problems that are interfering with the lower-level needs must be considered significant. The ranking of needs can be reviewed in Chapter 3. Another way to set priorities is to evaluate which problems can be solved or reduced in a short time. For an alternate strategy, the nurse could analyze which problems, if changed, would result in a change in others. These criteria are used in the prioritized list of problems found in Table 4-3. Ultimately, the most effective method for determining priorities is to consult with the patient.

Establishing Goals. A *goal* or *objective* is an expected or desired outcome, or the desired end result for which one works. The nurse may begin planning nursing care by stating one overall goal. However, there should be an additional goal for each problem identified. The goals may be short term, perhaps accomplished in a few days or certainly before the patient will be discharged from the hospital. Or the goal may be long term, taking weeks or months to complete. The written goals should indicate some specific, measurable fact showing that the patient's problem has been or is becoming resolved. It should also indicate an estimated target date for completion. The following are two examples of goal statements that show how a patient's improvement will be measured:

1. The patient will be able to walk ten steps without assistance by July 30.
2. The patient will be able to comb her own hair by August 3.

Having no goal for nursing care can be compared with buying an airline ticket without having a destination. Stating goals is an essential part of the process of planning nursing care with each patient.

Writing Nursing Orders. After the goals are clearly stated, the nurse selects measures that are most likely to help the patient reach those goals. The plan is based on the knowledge that certain actions will produce a desired

Table 4-3. Prioritized Listing of Problems

Nursing Diagnosis	Reason for Priority
Altered Nutrition: less than body requirements related to fatigue associated with physical activity as manifested by eating only a few bites per meal, a weight loss of 5 pounds in three days, and a below-normal hemoglobin level.	Eating is a basic human need. Without adequate nutrition, cells die and death may occur. Until the nutrition is improved, the patient will not have the energy to move about.
Self-Care Deficit related to muscle weakness and fatigue as manifested by an inability to bathe, comb hair, or walk to the toilet without assistance.	The inability to carry out these activities while in the hospital will not be a threat to survival. It may interfere with what the patient feels is the quality of life. It may affect his self-esteem, a higher level need. Improving nutrition may result in the patient's ability to care for himself.
High Risk for Impaired Skin Integrity related to inactivity.	This problem has not yet occurred. It may be prevented with certain nursing measures. Certainly if the previous two problems are changed, they will also affect this problem.

effect, which in turn will lead to accomplishing the goal. Any nurse who develops or contributes to the plan demonstrates accountability by signing each entry.

The activities that are planned are written on the patient's plan of care. They are called *nursing orders,* which are directions for the care that is to be carried out with the patient. Nursing orders are specific, detailed statements that direct who, what, when, where, and how much of an action should be done. They may also incorporate the activities that the doctor has indicated the nurse should perform. They must not be general or vague statements. The following is an example of a specific nursing order: "Position from side to side every two hours on the even hours. Place pillows between legs and upper arm for support. Place a small bath blanket under lower leg to keep the ankle from rubbing on the sheet." A vague statement would be one that states: "Turn frequently." This could be interpreted differently and carried out inconsistently.

Communicating the Plan. Goal achievement depends on consistency and continuity of care. The nurse must share the plan with the patient, his family, and other members of the nursing team. The written plan becomes a permanent part of the record. The record and its contents may be reviewed by hospital accrediting representatives or committees within the hospital to evaluate the quality of care that patients receive.

Planning nursing care for a patient may be summarized in the following five steps:

1. Write the goals or objectives of nursing care.
2. Rank the problems in order of their priority.
3. Select actions that are most likely to help the patient reach goals of care.
4. Enter nursing orders on the care plan.

5. Discuss the plan with the patient and share it with other members of the nursing team.

Implementing the Plan

During the next part of the nursing process, the nursing care plan is put into effect by carrying out the nursing orders. Some nurses refer to this as nursing intervention or implementation. Skills that the nurse uses during the implementation of the nursing orders are the subject of this book. These technical skills must be combined with the caring, comforting, and counseling skills described in Chapter 1 so that the patient is treated holistically.

The term *nursing implementation* may be somewhat of a misnomer. Sometimes the nurse may carry out the activities alone, especially when a patient is very ill. However, the nurse encourages patients to participate to whatever extent possible. Thus, some activities may be carried out by the patient independently; others may require that the nurse and the patient work cooperatively. For instance, the nurse may teach the patient how to do certain leg exercises; the patient would then do the exercises ten times every hour while awake. This is an example of the partnership that has been discussed between the nurse and patient.

Making Pertinent Observations. When giving nursing care, a nurse observes the patient to see how well or poorly he is responding to his care. There may be new information about the patient that has not been identified before. Assessment is a continuous process.

Charting the Care. Charting is called documentation by some. The techniques of charting are discussed in more detail in Chapter 5. The chart is a legal record of observations and activities related to the care of each patient. Everything written in the chart must be legible and accurate. If something is not recorded, it is assumed that it did not occur. To prove that the planned care was subsequently implemented, the nurse's charting of what took place should correlate with the plan. If there is a discrepancy between the plan and what is charted, the nurse is responsible for determining its cause. This is another example of how nursing assumes accountability for patient services. This principle of accountability for carrying out nursing orders should not be any less than the accountability nurses demonstrate when carrying out the doctor's orders.

The charting should also indicate the patient's level of participation. It should note any progress or regression that may have occurred as the plan was carried out. Quoting what the patient says at times during an interaction helps identify what is occurring from the patient's point of view. It safeguards individuals from making incorrect assumptions.

Carrying out the plan may be summarized as having the following three steps:

1. Put the plan into action.
2. Observe the patient's responses to nursing care.
3. Record the care provided and the patient's responses on the patient's chart.

Evaluating the Results of Nursing Care

Evaluation is the process of measuring how well a goal or objective is reached. In terms of the nursing process, evaluation provides information on the degree to which a goal is being met through the use of specific nursing measures. Like assessment, it is an ongoing part of the nursing process.

Evaluation is more or less a scheduled event. Recall that the goal associated with each problem has an expected date for completion. As that date arrives, the nurse compares the patient's level of achievement with the measurable goal. Or, the nurses on a particular unit may establish a policy that all care plans will be reviewed on a certain routine. In other words, perhaps the care plans on all patients may be reviewed on Mondays and Fridays. Each nurse would write on the care plan that it had been reviewed for its current appropriateness.

There are three possible results of evaluation:

1. A goal of nursing care has been met; therefore, nursing orders to accomplish that goal are discontinued. *Example:* It is observed that a patient is using his crutches well and correctly; nursing orders about teaching and assisting him with crutch walking are discontinued.

2. A goal of nursing care has been unmet, but progress toward it has occurred; therefore, the nursing orders described in the plan should continue. *Example:* It is observed that a patient remains inactive but is free of bedsores; nursing orders to turn him and massage his back and bony prominences at regular times are continued.

3. A goal for nursing care is not being met; therefore, modifications and revisions in nursing care are necessary. *Example:* After a week of teaching a diabetic patient with reading and illustrated materials, it is observed that he is unable to select proper foods for his prescribed diet while using the exchange system. A modification in the nursing orders must be made.

Consulting With the Patient and Team Members

It is important to discuss the progress toward goal achievement with the patient. In this way both the nurse and the patient can speculate on what activities need to be discontinued, added, or changed. Other health team members who are familiar with a particular patient or problems similar to those of the patient may offer their expertise on those actions that have been previously successful for others. The evaluation of a patient's progress may be the subject of a nursing team conference. Some progressive units even invite the patient and his family to attend and participate.

Revising the Plan

Unfortunately, not all patient problems are solved with the nursing care that was originally planned. It is important to identify the factors that are interfering with goal achievement. Some patients may have developed new problems. It may take some longer than expected. Some goals may be unrealistic. Some nursing orders may not be as effective as first hoped. Changing the goal, extending the date of expected accomplishment, or revising the nursing orders may result in improving the progress toward an improved state of health.

Evaluation can be summarized as having the following three steps:

1. Determine if goals have been met, partially met, or remain unmet.
2. Consult with the patient and other health team members about measures to accomplish partially met and unmet goals.
3. Revise the written plan for care.

The nursing process is generally accepted as an important method for planning and giving appropriate and competent nursing care. More detailed discussions of the nursing process can be found in specialty texts and in some of the bibliographic entries at the end of this chapter. Skill Procedure 4-1 describes the steps for using the nursing process.

Skill Procedure 4-1. Using the Nursing Process

Suggested Action	Reason for Action
Collect information about the patient.	The nurse must determine what past, current, and potential health problems exist.
Validate all information.	Incorrect data may result in errors in the identification of problems.
Group information into categories.	Organizing related data simplifies the process of analysis.
Compare information about the patient to norms.	Using standards for comparison helps identify any deviations that represent the patient's needs or problems.
State the nursing diagnoses and collaborative problems.	Clear identification of health problems directs the nurse to select skills that will improve the patient's health.
Determine how a successful outcome will be measured.	Meeting certain criteria will determine when nursing actions no longer need to be continued.
Rank problems in the order of their importance.	Working and solving some problems are more important than others for the patient's overall health to improve.
Select nursing measures that are most likely to meet the goals of nursing care.	Scientific knowledge about the purpose of certain actions makes it possible for nurses to predict an expected effect.
Write directions for the care of the patient.	Written information can provide consistency and continuity of care throughout each 24-hour period.
Discuss the plan with the patient, his family, and other nursing team members.	Communicating with everyone involved promotes cooperative efforts leading to success.
Put the plan into action.	Work produces results.
Observe the patient for his responses to the activities.	Any changes in the patient will affect each step of the nursing process.
Write down the activities that were carried out and the patient's responses.	Recording correlates the plan with the actions and verifies that it is being carried out.
Compare the patient's level of accomplishment with the identified criteria for a successful outcome.	There should be progress toward the goal if all the planning and care have been appropriate.
Discuss the progress or lack of it with the patient, his family, and health-team members.	Pooling resources often results in better ideas for future plans.
Change the plan in areas that are no longer appropriate.	Alternative methods may be more successful in solving a problem.
Continue to gather information.	The nursing process is a continuous sequence of actions that is repeated until the patient and nurse are satisfied that the goals have been met.

Nursing Care Plan 4-1 and other care plan examples within this book use a nursing process approach. This format was selected in order to reinforce the essential steps in every nurse–patient interaction. The value of the nursing process, and the true measure of learning, is its application rather than memorization. Repetition provides a mechanism for imprinting the pattern for its use.

Each sample care plan presents a realistic patient scenario beginning with subjective and objective assessments to coincide with the first step in the nursing process. The assessments that are described reflect the supporting data for the diagnosis that is made. The second step, diagnosis, is represented by identifying the problem using the current approved terms in the NANDA taxonomy. The problem is coupled with the addition of its etiology. The planning step is demonstrated through the principles of a good goal statement—one that is patient centered, realistic, measurable, and time oriented. The plan for care is written

NURSING CARE PLAN

4-1. Altered Oral Mucous Membrane

Assessment	**Subjective Data** States, "My dentures slip when I chew and it's beginning to hurt."
	Objective Data 78-year-old woman transferred from the hospital for extended, skilled nursing care following surgery to relieve a bowel obstruction. Patient has lost 20 lbs. since surgery. There is a 1/2-in, round, red lesion on the right, upper, posterior gum. Bleeding from same lesion when wiped with a cotton tipped applicator.
Diagnosis	Altered Oral Mucous Membrane related to mechanical trauma from dentures.
Plan	**Goal** The oral mucosa will be pink, moist, intact, and free of discomfort by 9/13.

Orders: 9/9

1. Assess gums every morning and evening.
2. Provide a mechanically soft diet; omit citrus and spicy foods.
3. Remove dentures after meals and at bedtime for the following mouthcare:
   - Clean dentures after eating with toothbrush and toothpaste.
   - Swish mouth with 1:4 dilution of hydrogen peroxide and water.
   - Follow with a normal saline rinse.
   - Replace dentures during awake hours as desired._____ J. HALL, RN

Implementation (Documentation)

9/10

0715	Oral mucosa pink, moist, intact except for 1/2-in, round, reddened lesion on R upper, posterior gum._____ D. BORDON, SN
0730	Dentures inserted for breakfast._____ D. BORDON, SN
0745	Ate cream of wheat, apple juice, sliced pears, and muffin with whole milk._____ D. BORDON, SN
0815	Dentures removed and cleansed. 1:4 hydrogen peroxide solution used as mouthwash followed by saline rinse._____ D. BORDON, SN

Evaluation (Documentation)

0815	Sm. amt. of blood noted in expectorated rinse. States "I can't say that my mouth feels any better yet."_____ D. BORDON, SN

in the form of nursing orders. Most care planning books provide numerous general suggestions for care. Students often imitate these examples failing to write specific directions. Or, they include measures that will not help prevent, reduce, or eliminate the etiology of the problem. The student is helped to experience the fourth step of implementation by reading narrative charting. This method was used to exemplify how the nurse is accountable for carrying out the written nursing orders. Using sample charting also benefits the student by providing phrasing and terminology techniques for recording pertinent information. The last step, evaluation, is based upon the responses of the patient to the interventions. Quality assurance and agency accreditation require that this information appear in the patient's record. Therefore, the results of the implemented care are shown as part of the documentation. The ultimate decision to continue, revise, or discontinue the orders is determined by comparing the patient outcome with the criteria established in the goal statement.

The nursing diagnosis used in the first sample care plan is Altered Oral Mucous Membrane. This diagnosis is defined in the NANDA Taxonomy (1989) as, "The state in which an individual experiences disruptions in the tissue layers of the oral cavity."

Bibliography

Alfaro R: Application of Nursing Process: A Step by Step Guide. Philadelphia, JB Lippincott, 1986

Andersen JE, Briggs LL: Nursing diagnosis: A study of quality and supportive evidence. Image: The Journal of Nursing Scholarship 20(3):141–144, 1988

Anthony ML, Williams A, Hoagland B: Nursing interventions: Independent or not? Nursing Management 19(12):14–15, 1988

Brooking JI: A scale to measure use of the nursing process. Nursing Times 85(15):44, 46, 48–49, 1989

Bulechek GM, McCloskey JC: Nursing interventions: What they are and how to choose them. Holistic Nursing Practice 1(3):36–44, 1987

Carlson C, Davis K, Marks S: Nursing process how-to's. AD Nurse 2(1):24–27, 1987

Carpenito LJ: Nursing Diagnosis: Application to Clinical Practice, 3rd ed. Philadelphia, JB Lippincott, 1989

Castledine G: The nursing process evaluated. Geriatric Nursing & Home Care 7(1):8, 1987

Donnelly GF: The promise of nursing process: An evaluation. Holistic Nursing Practice 1(3):1–6, 1987

Goodall C: How should we teach the nursing process? Nursing Times 84(48):47–49, 1988

Henderson V: Nursing process—A critique. Holistic Nursing Practice 1(3):7–18, 1987

Johnson CF, Hales LW: Nursing diagnosis anyone? Do staff nurses use nursing diagnosis effectively? Journal of Continuing Education in Nursing 20(1):30–35, 1989

McHugh MK: Has nursing outgrown the nursing process? Nursing 17(8):50–51, 1987

Moss AR: Determinants of patient care: Nursing process or nursing attitudes. J Adv Nurs 13(5):615–620, 1988

Peterson M: Time and nursing process. Holistic Nursing Practice 1(3):72–80, 1987

Polaski AL, Vitron SK, Carrier BJ: A multidimensional teaching–learning strategy for the nursing process. Nursing Education 13(4):19–23, 1988

Richards DA, Lambert P: The nurse process: The effect on patients' satisfaction with nursing care. J Adv Nurs 12(5):559–562, 1987

Rew L, Barrow EM: Nurses' intuition: Can it coexist with the nursing process? AORN J 50(2):353–354, 356, 358, 1989

Sawton V: Carry-out care plans. Nursing Times 84(13):66, 68, 1988

5

Patient Records: Resources for Sharing Information

Chapter Outline

Behavioral Objectives
Glossary
Introduction
Uses for Patient Records
Types of Patient Records
Methods of Charting
Allowing Patients Access to Their Records
Protecting Computerized Patient Records
Using Abbreviations
Making Entries on Patient Records
Converting to Military Time
Other Written Forms of Communication
Using Checklists and Flow Sheets
Other Methods for Exchanging Information
Bibliography

Skill Procedure

Making Entries on the Patient's Record

Behavioral Objectives

When the content of this chapter has been mastered, the learner will be able to:

Define terms appearing in the glossary.
Discuss seven uses for patient records.

Summarize the differences between traditional records and problem-oriented records.
List and describe five methods of charting.
Explain the reasons for using approved abbreviations.
Describe recommended practices for making entries on patient records and the reason for each practice.
Convert common expressions of time to military time; give two advantages for using military time.
Discuss how computers are being used in relation to patient care.
Describe the differences between a nursing care plan and a nursing Kardex.
List ways in which health practitioners exchange information.

Glossary

Auditors Inspectors who examine patient records.
Bias The interpretation of an observation that is affected by an individual's personal beliefs.
Chart The sum total of forms related to one patient's care. Synonym for *health-care record*.
Charting The act of making entries on the patient's chart. Synonym for *documenting* or *recording*.
Charting by exception A method of charting that documents care but only requires that the nurse describe information that deviates from established standards.
Checklist A form for documenting routine care.
Database The part of a problem-oriented record on which all the health information about the patient is recorded.
Documenting The act of making entries on the patient's chart. Synonym for *charting* or *recording*.
Flow sheet A form for recording frequently repeated assessments.
Focus charting A modification in the SOAP method of charting that describes data, actions, and responses of the patient.
Health-care record The sum total of forms related to one patient's care. Synonym for *chart*.
Initial plan The part of a problem-oriented record used to record the overall care that health practitioners will use to help the patient overcome his health problems.
Mainframe computer A large computer that can process, store, and retrieve more information than any other type of computer.
Military time A method for expressing time that uses a different four-digit number for each hour and minute of the 24-hour day.
Narrative charting A method of charting about the patient using a chronological order.
Nurses' notes A form within a traditional record used by nurses to describe observations about the patient, the

nursing care, and events that took place during the patient's care.

Nursing care plan A plan written by a nurse describing the actions that should be performed when providing care to a patient.

Nursing Kardex A short, summarized version of the current basic care for a patient listed on a form the size of a large index card.

Physician's orders A form used in a traditional record on which the doctor writes the kinds of medical interventions that apply to a patient's care.

Physician's progress notes A form used in a traditional record by a doctor to describe the patient's response to the medical treatment.

PIE charting A method of charting similar to SOAP charting that addresses the patient's problems, interventions, and evaluation.

Problem list Numbered statements within a problem-oriented record describing those aspects that interfere with the patient's well-being.

Progress notes and follow-up The part of a problem-oriented record that describes the patient's response to the measures that were carried out and identifies what remains to be done.

Recording The act of making entries on the patient's chart. Synonym for *charting* or *documenting*.

SOAP charting A method of charting subjective and objective data, an assessment of the problem, and the plan for care on the progress notes of a problem-oriented record.

Terminal Computer equipment used only for entering and retrieving information from a computer that is located in another area.

Introduction

When the patient requires care from health practitioners, records will be kept. These records contain many different printed forms on which information about a patient and his care is written. The collection of forms is usually placed in a binder or folder. Some agencies use the word *chart* or *health-care record* to describe the sum total of forms related to one patient's care. The process of making entries on those forms is called *recording, charting,* or *documenting*.

Specific requirements on the frequency for charting vary from agency to agency and within different clinical areas of practice. For instance, in an intensive care unit (ICU) charting is almost continuous, but in a nursing home it may be done only once a week. Despite the differences in the frequency of charting, each nurse is, nevertheless, required to record information about a patient and his care.

The nurse must be able to communicate health-care information clearly, concisely, and accurately. This chapter will describe various written and spoken forms of health communication. A general overview of the skills related to nursing responsibilities for record keeping and reporting will be discussed.

Uses for Patient Records

A patient's record serves a variety of purposes.

Providing a Permanent Account of a Patient's Health Care

A patient's chart provides a record of information describing the patient's health and the care that was given. Entries on a patient's record are dated and written in the sequence of time in which observations or actions occurred. This practice helps personnel to understand the patient's health status, the type of care or treatment that was administered, and the patient's responses. The patient's health-care record is filed and kept for future reference.

Keeping Health Personnel Informed

Entries on the patient's record are made by all health practitioners according to their area of expertise. For example, nurses, physicians, physical therapists, respiratory therapists, dietitians, social workers, and discharge coordinators may make entries on forms within the chart. All are interested in the contributions of others concerning the patient's care and condition. Thus, a patient's written record helps to share information among personnel such as the doctor and nurse in Figure 5-1 who are involved in a patient's care.

Ensuring Safety and Continuity in the Patient's Care

Sharing of information prevents duplication and helps reduce the chance of error or omission. For example, if a

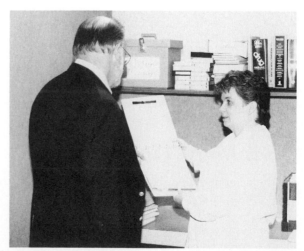

Figure 5-1 The nurse and doctor discuss information recorded on the patient's record.

patient requests medication for pain, the nurse will check the patient's chart to determine when he last received a pain-relieving drug. If another nurse gave this type of drug earlier, the time of its administration would be noted. Having this information available helps in making decisions that affect the patient's care. It prevents the chance that the medication will be administered too frequently or unnecessarily withheld. Keeping records on immunizations given to an infant in a pediatric clinic or office ensures that they will be administered according to an appropriate schedule from one appointment to the next. This is another example of how maintaining patient records promotes continuity.

Serving as Legal Documents

Patient's records are admissible as evidence in courts of law in this country. They are a basis for proving or disproving allegations concerning a patient's care. Therefore, it is essential that entries on the records be *objectively written, accurate, complete,* and *legible.* Descriptions and notations should not include personal conclusions. A written statement, such as "Asking for pain medication more frequently than needed," shows bias. *Bias* means that an interpretation of an observation was affected by an individual's personal belief.

Each person who makes an entry is responsible for the information that is recorded. The person who signs a recorded entry may be called upon as a witness to testify concerning what has been written. Any writing that cannot be clearly read, or is vague, scribbled through, whited out, written over, or erased can be misinterpreted or leave room for doubts, making for a poor legal defense.

A consent form, one of the parts of a patient's record, has important legal implications as discussed in Chapter 6. A consent form that is kept with the other records relating to a patient's care is legal proof of the patient's permission to carry out certain procedures. Other forms such as those indicating a release from responsibility, when a patient leaves against medical advice or refuses siderails, may help to prove a health practitioner's guilt or innocence if lawsuits occur.

Collecting Data for Research

Some types of clinical research are difficult to conduct. There may not be enough people available to participate or test facilities may be limited. Patient records contain an abundance of information. When these data are collected, it may contribute to the statistics of research projects.

Only authorized persons should have access to patient records. Formal permission must be obtained from the health agency's administrator or other authority whenever a patient's record will be used for a purpose other than record keeping, such as research.

If health workers use patient records for a class assignment, conference, or a written clinical report, the identity of the patient must be concealed. When this practice is not observed, health workers run the risk of legal problems concerning the patient's right to privacy.

Determining Reimbursement

The costs of most patients' hospital and home care are billed to third-party payers such as Medicare and private insurance companies. Charts and bills are surveyed by auditors. *Auditors* are inspectors who examine patient records. They determine if the care that was provided meets established criteria for reimbursement. Undocumented, incomplete, or inconsistent documentation of care may result in a denial for reimbursement.

Obtaining Agency Accreditation

Health-care institutions seek and maintain licensure or certification from various organizations. One accrediting organization is the Joint Commission on Accreditation of Healthcare Organizations. Accreditation indicates to the public that an institution has met specific regulations concerning acceptable standards of care. Institutions may also need to meet other requirements to qualify for Medicare and Medicaid funds.

Besides meeting minimum standards in the building's structure and staffing, approval by various organizations is based on evaluation of the quality of the care that is provided. To evaluate the quality of care delivered in a hospital, patient records are reviewed to compare how frequently the written standards for care are actually reflected in the charting. A high rate of similarity between the two provides supporting evidence that patients are receiving high-quality care.

Types of Patient Records

The patient's health-care record is maintained in a manner in which information can be identified for quick and easy access. Chart forms may be color coded and labeled according to their use. There are two common methods for organizing the patient's health records. Each health agency will use one of the methods.

The Traditional Record

A traditional record is organized according to the source of information. It contains multiple forms; examples include separate forms for the patient's health history as obtained by the physician, a health history and physical assessment obtained by the nurse on admission, findings of the physician during a physical examination, the physician's orders, the physician's progress notes, graphic sheets for vital signs, nursing notes, and laboratory and x-ray test results. Further explanations of some of these forms follow.

Physician's Orders. This form within a traditional record is used by a doctor to request diagnostic tests, prescribe medications and their administration, and advise nurses of special care that the physician feels should be carried out. An example of a form showing physician's orders is illustrated in Figure 5-2.

Physician's Progress Notes. This part of the traditional record, shown in Figure 5-3, is used by the physician to describe the findings of that day's physical examination and to evaluate the patient's response to medical treatment. It may indicate ideas about the future possibilities for medical care.

Nursing Notes. This is an area in the patient's chart where the nurse records assessments of the patient's condition and the events that occurred as part of a patient's care. Figure 5-4 shows a sample form used by nurses for documenting information in a traditional record.

Because some of these forms are used by only one type of health practitioner and similar information may be found in various places within a traditional record, a criti-

cism has been that the care seems to be fragmented. That is, common goals and plans for the patient's care are not cooperatively set.

The Problem-Oriented Record

A record that is organized according to a patient's specific health problems is being used in some health agencies. It is called a problem-oriented record (POR). The POR is a method in which all the pertinent information about a patient's problems is organized and recorded in one place. All health-care personnel record on the same forms rather than on separate forms.

There are four major parts to a POR as compared with the many included in a traditional record. They are as follows:

Database. The database consists of the overall health information about the patient, including his present state

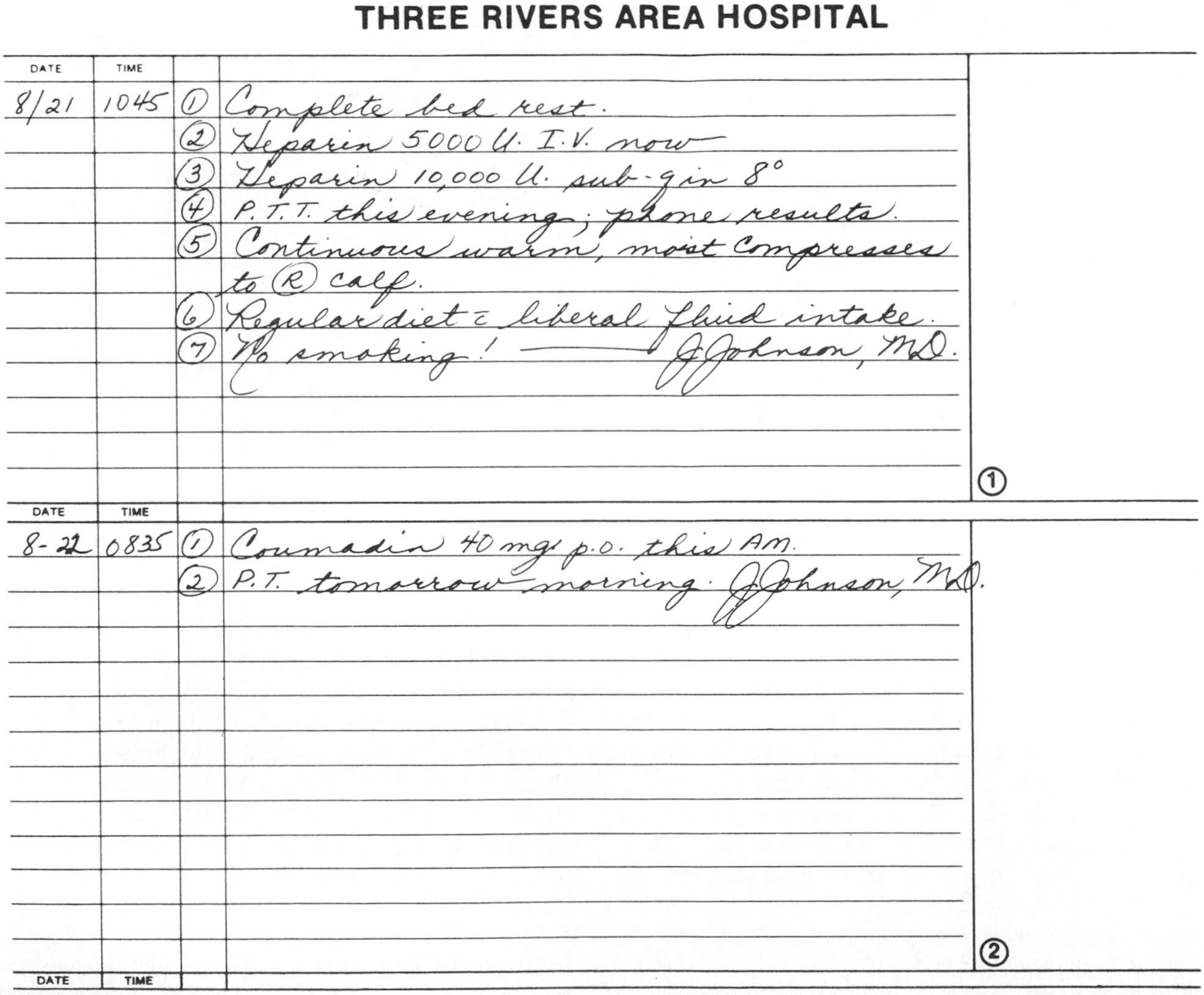

THREE RIVERS AREA HOSPITAL

DATE	TIME		
8/21	1045	①	Complete bed rest.
		②	Heparin 5000 U. I.V. now
		③	Heparin 10,000 U. sub-q in 8°
		④	P.T.T. this evening; phone results.
		⑤	Continuous warm, moist compresses to ⓡ calf.
		⑥	Regular diet c̄ liberal fluid intake.
		⑦	No smoking! — J. Johnson, MD.

DATE	TIME		
8-22	0835	①	Coumadin 40 mg. p.o. this AM.
		②	P.T. tomorrow morning. J. Johnson, MD.

Figure 5-2 The physician uses this form in a traditional record for writing medical orders. (Courtesy of Three Rivers Area Hospital, Three Rivers, MI.)

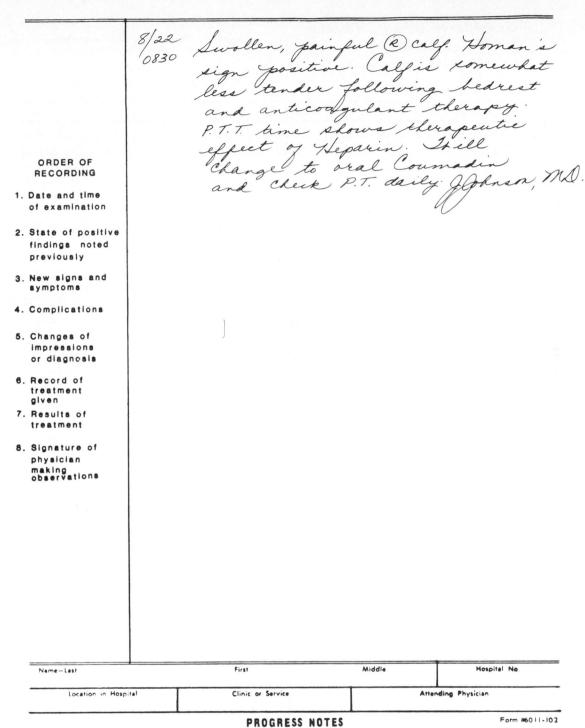

8/22
0830

Swollen, painful ® calf. Homan's sign positive. Calf is somewhat less tender following bedrest and anticoagulant therapy. P.T.T. time shows therapeutic effect of Heparin. Will change to oral Coumadin and check P.T. daily. J.Johnson, M.D.

ORDER OF RECORDING

1. Date and time of examination

2. State of positive findings noted previously

3. New signs and symptoms

4. Complications

5. Changes of impressions or diagnosis

6. Record of treatment given

7. Results of treatment

8. Signature of physician making observations

Name—Last	First	Middle	Hospital No.
Location in Hospital	Clinic or Service	Attending Physician	

PROGRESS NOTES   Form #6011-102

Figure 5-3 The physician is the only person who uses this type of form in a traditional record. It is used to note the progress of the patient to the medical treatment. (Courtesy of Three Rivers Area Hospital, Three Rivers, MI.)

of health, the physical examination findings, the health history, and so on.

Problem List. The problem list contains numbered statements describing those aspects that interfere with the patient's well-being. All health practitioners contribute to the list.

Initial Plan. The initial plan describes the overall care that will be used to help the patient overcome his health problems. The plan reflects a multi-professional approach; each health practitioner suggests problem-solving methods within his or her area of expertise. Planning, regardless of the way it is recorded, should always be done with the patient.

Three Rivers Area Hospital

214 SPRING STREET
THREE RIVERS, MICHIGAN 49093

ROOM NO._____

NAME_____

NURSING NOTES

DOCTOR_____

Date Time	NURSES REMARKS Signature	Date Time	NURSES REMARKS Signature
1330	states "I'm having chest pain. It's like an elephant is sitting on me."——B. Zook, RN		transfer.——B. Zook, RN
		1440	Family notified of transfer.——B. Zook, RN
1340	BP 150/90, P-122 and irregular. Skin is pale and moist. O₂ started at 5L/min. Nitroglycerin I tab. administered sublingually.——B. Zook, RN.		
1350	Dr. Johnson notified of the change in condition. EKG ordered. 1000 cc. 5% D/W started IV c̄ #20 gauge angiocath in (L) arm. IV running at 20 gtts/minute.——B. Zook, RN.		
1410	EKG obtained. BP 142/88 P-110 and still irregular, skin pink but moist. No relief from Nitroglycerin. States "It's still pretty bad." B. Zook, RN.		
1420	Morphine 10 mg. administered sub-q for chest pain and anxiety.——B. Zook, RN		
1430	Transferred to CCU per bed. Clothing, dentures, and eye-glasses accompanied		

Figure 5-4 Narrative charting involves writing information in the order in which it occurred. (Courtesy of Three Rivers Area Hospital, Three Rivers, MI.)

Progress Notes and Follow-Up. This part of a problem-oriented record describes the patient's responses to what has been done. It identifies what still remains to be done. The format for completing a progress note on a POR contains several parts. These parts were once defined as subjective information, objective information, assessment, and plan for care (SOAP). It has since been expanded to include intervention and evaluation (SOAPIE), and even more recently revision was added (SOAPIER). The SOAP-IER format is described in Table 5-1.

Persons using a POR find it to be logical and flexible. Many believe it facilitates continuity of patient care and provides better communication and cooperation among health workers. It also tends to result in the recording of

Table 5-1. Using the Acronym **SOAPIER** *in a Problem-Oriented Record*

Letter	Explanation	Example of Recording
S = Subjective information	Information reported by the patient.	S— "I'm cold."
O = Objective information	Observations made by health personnel.	O— Temperature 102.4°F, pulse 96, respirations 24. Skin is pale. Blanket pulled up to chin.
A = Assessment	Analysis of the problem.	A— Abnormally elevated temperature.
P = Plan for care	Measures that will be used to restore health.	P— Give 50 mL of liquids every 2 hours. Provide additional warmth until chilling stops.
I = Intervention	Specific activity that was carried out.	I— 75 mL of ginger ale taken. Two blankets applied.
E = Evaluation	Effectiveness of the intervention.	E— States, "I feel warmer now." Temperature 101°F, pulse 90, respirations 20. Skin is warm and flushed.
R = Revision	Changes that will be made in the original plan.	R— Increase minimum fluid intake to 100 mL every 2 hours. Remove blankets unless chilling recurs.

more pertinent information from which the quality of care can be compared with certain standards.

Methods of Charting

There are a variety of styles used to record information on the patient's record. Examples of charting methods include narrative notes, SOAP charting, focus charting, PIE charting, and charting by exception.

Narrative Charting

Narrative charting involves writing information about the patient and his care in chronological order. It is used primarily in traditional records. Each person involved in a patient's care, such as the doctor, nurse, or physical therapist writes information on separate forms in the patient's chart. This adds bulk to the medical record and tends to fragment the information. Figure 5-4 is an example of narrative charting.

One criticism of narrative charting is that nurses need to make frequent entries, which is time consuming. Without frequent entries, others may not have access to the most current information about the patient. The nursing shortage has resulted in increased numbers of very sick patients being assigned to fewer nurses. Charting sometimes becomes less of a priority. Nurses tend to jot down information on scrap paper to help jog their memory for narrative charting at a later time. Transcribing notes a second time continues to deprive the nurse of time to provide patient care.

Narrative charting has other disadvantages. It is often difficult to read through what is written to find specific information. It also has been noted that insignificant information is recorded.

SOAP Charting

The corresponding terms for the letters in SOAP, SOAPE, SOAPIE, and SOAPIER stand for subjective, objective, assessment, plan, implementation, evaluation, and revision. Health-care agencies may elect to use any one of these variations. *SOAP charting* is one method for charting on the progress notes of a problem-oriented record. An example can be found in Table 5-1.

When a SOAP format is used, every member of the health team writes entries on the same form. This reduces the amount of paper in a chart. It promotes interdisciplinary cooperation. The content of information tends to center on the patient's significant problems and progress.

Focus Charting

Focus charting is a modified form of SOAP charting. It substitutes "focus" rather than "problem," which carries negative connotations. A focus can refer to a patient's current or changed behavior, significant events in the patient's care, or even a NANDA nursing diagnosis category. Instead of making entries using the SOAP format, a data, action, and response (DAR) framework is used. When notations refer to each of these three aspects, the documentation reflects the nursing process.

PIE Charting

PIE charting is very similar to a SOAPIE format of charting. PIE is the acronym for problem, intervention, and evaluation. However, when using the PIE method for charting, assessments are documented on a separate form. The patient's problems may be entered once on the nursing care plan and given a corresponding number. The number is subsequently used in daily charting when referring to the interventions and responses associated with each problem. Figure 5-5 shows an example of PIE charting.

Charting by Exception

Nurses have always tried to be comprehensive and complete in charting. It is often said that "if it isn't charted, it hasn't been done." Now some health-care agencies are adopting a new method of charting. It is called *charting by exception*. It is a method of documenting the care, but limits the amount of writing to information that is abnormal or deviates from written standards. This does require that the institution develop comprehensive documents describing norms and standards before using charting by exception. However, once that task is done, the nurse primarily uses check lists. Narrative charting is used only to describe how the patient and his care have differed.

Most chart forms are kept at the bedside allowing for timely entry of information. Making entries in the patient's room rather than at a nursing station keeps the nurse in close contact with patients. Nurses have long complained that doing paperwork and non-nursing tasks have distanced them from caring for patients.

Besides being time-efficient, those who chart by exception say this method provides quick access to abnormal findings because normal and routine information need not be described. Charting is, therefore, brief. Lengthy duplication is avoided when assessments or care are performed repeatedly without any changes.

Computerized Charting

Computers are gradually finding their way onto hospital units and the patient's bedside. Nursing units are being equipped with terminals that link patient-care areas to other areas in the agency. A *terminal,* shown in Figure 5-6, is a device that looks like a personal computer. A terminal includes a monitor, which looks like a television, and a keyboard that resembles a typewriter. The terminal is connected electronically to a large *mainframe computer* located in another area that processes, stores, and retrieves information. The terminal allows information to be exchanged more swiftly and accurately than any other method of communication.

Computer applications are beginning to help nurses with nursing. Systems are available for patient monitoring, as shown in Figure 5-7. They help to analyze numeric data. Staffing patterns can be developed based upon the numbers of patients on a unit and their acuity levels. Generic nursing care plans can be stored and printed when needed.

Most nurses like using computers that help with charting. Nurses make entries frequently on patient records. Nurses' documentation is the most frequently used data in the chart. Having a computer do that task quickly and accurately is a welcomed form of assistance. Though each system varies, charting is done by selecting statements from a list of choices. The nurse reads the information on the monitor screen. When satisfied, the entry is printed and added to the chart. Figure 5-8 shows an example of computerized charting.

Computerized charting has many advantages. It is always legible. The abbreviations and terms are consistent

NURSING NOTES   DOCTOR _____

Date Time	NURSES REMARKS Signature	Date Time	NURSES REMARKS Signature
6/19 0750	P#1 Crackles heard on inspiration in the bases of R and L lungs. ———		
	I#1 Incision splinted with pillow. Instructed to breathe deeply, open mouth, and cough at the end of expiration ———		
	E#1 Lungs clear with coughing. ——————— *a. Walker, LPN*		

Figure 5-5 In PIE charting all entries concerning interventions or evaluation are paired with a numbered problem. Assessments and problems are documented on separate forms. (Courtesy of Three Rivers Area Hospital, Three Rivers, MI.)

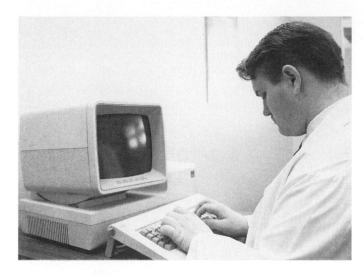

Figure 5-6 This nurse uses a computer terminal. Information is entered and retrieved very rapidly.

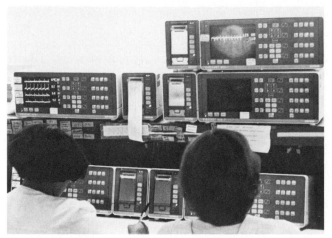

Figure 5-7 These nurses monitor cardiac data on several patients within a coronary care unit. Computer microchips are programmed to detect abnormal changes and instantly sound alarms.

with agency-approved lists. Trivia is eliminated. Nurses are likely to continue adding and expanding the use of computers in patient care.

Allowing Patients Access to Their Records

Historically, patients were not allowed to see their health-care record. Certain federal laws have now changed that practice. These laws have been passed as a result of the movement to restore and protect human rights, which include freedom of information.

Health agencies have developed written policies that describe the guidelines by which patients may read their record. Policies range from complete, unrestricted access upon the patient's written request to requiring written permission from the patient's physician or the hospital

administrator. The nurse must follow whatever policies have been established.

The Patient's Bill of Rights, described in Chapter 6, does not state that a patient has the right to read his record. However, it clearly indicates that he is entitled to be told about the information contained in that record. Now, more than ever before, the patient is being informed about his state of health and methods of care.

Protecting Computerized Patient Records

Patient information must be kept confidential. This is a little more difficult to do when the data are stored within a computer's memory. The nurse cannot monitor the access to computerized patient records as effectively as written records.

Health agencies are adopting methods to ensure protection of computerized patient records. Some techniques include:

- Assigning an access password to authorized personnel. This password must be kept secret and must be changed frequently.
- Issuing a plastic card or key that must be used by authorized personnel to retrieve information.
- Using a fingerprint or voice-activation device for gaining access to patient information. This eliminates the possibility of anyone but the authorized person using the access method.
- Locking some information from various departments and their personnel. In other words, the laboratory may be able to retrieve information for the medical orders but will be locked from accessing the information on the patient's personal history.
- Automatically identifying the time and location of a terminal from which information from the patient's record was accessed.

Washington Hospital Center

Requested by   Page — 1

RoutneNurseCare

DATE (1990)	6/18	6/19		6/20	6/21		
TIME	2200	0400	1300	2200	0200	2000	2310
Bath Care	Complt	None	Partl	Complt	Partl	Complt	None
Oral Care	q4h	q8h	q4h	q2h	q4h	q4h	q4h
Skin Care	Yes	Yes	Yes	Yes	Yes	Yes	Yes
Freq. Turned	q2h	q2h	q2h	q2h	q2h	q2h	q2h
ROMq4	Ys-Act	No	Ys-Act	Ys-Pas	Ys-Pas	Ys-Pas	
Decubitus care	None	None	None			None	None
Foly/Texs Care	Yes	Yes	Yes	Yes	Yes	Yes	Yes
Line Dressing	Ok	Ok	Ok	None	None	Ok	Ok
IV tubing	Ok	Ok	Chnged	Ok	Chnged	Chnged	Chnged
HeprinLk Flush	None	None		Yes	None		None
OOB	Assist	Bedrst	Assist			Assist	Bedrst
OOB-hrs	>1hr		>2hr			>1hr	
Slept-hrs	1–4hr	>4hr	1–4hr			<1hr	>4hr
Nares Care	q8h	q8h		q8h	q8h	q8h	q8h
ET/Trach Care	q8h	q8h	q8h	q8h	q8h	q4h	q8h
Chest PT	q6h	q6h		q6h	q6h	q6h	q6h
Restr.check q2		Yes	None				
Pulse check q8	Palp	Palp	Palp	Palp	Palp	Palp	Palp
NG/Dobpatentq4	Yes	Yes	Yes	Yes	Yes	Yes	Yes
BowelSounds q8	Normal	Normal	Normal	Normal	Normal	Normal	Normal
Wound Dressing						Ok	
Daily Wght (kg)			66.1	65.5			
Alrmlmitchk q4	Yes	Yes	Yes	Yes	Yes	Yes	Yes
Stop cock chk					No	Yes	
CXR done			No	No	No		Yes
12 Lead EKG			No	No	No		
Pt.Clasificati	B	B	B	B	B	B	B

Critical Care Data	Date: 6/22/90	Patient :
RoutneNurseCare		Hosp. No.:
		Location : 4G08

Figure 5-8 This page from a patient's chart is an example of charting that the nurse has done with a computer.

Using Abbreviations

Regardless of the type of record that a health agency uses, the nurse must be brief when writing entries on a patient's chart. This prevents the accumulation of excessive volumes of paper that must be eventually filed and stored. Brevity, however, should not take priority over complete and accu-rate documentation. It is better to write at length than to omit information or make entries that are vague.

Abbreviations are a method of shortening what is writ-ten. Shortening the task of writing can also reduce the time the nurse is away from the actual bedside of the patient. Many abbreviations have common meanings that are inter-preted the same in all regions of the United States. Examples of these are provided occasionally in the definitions of glossary terms and discussions within this text.

However, the nurse cannot assume that *all* abbreviations will be interpreted the same universally. Some may have one meaning in one locale or agency and may mean something different or be unfamiliar in another. To avoid confusion, each health agency provides its employees with a written list of acceptable abbreviations and their meanings. The nurse may only use those abbreviations found on the approved list when recording on the patient's chart. Abbreviations that are commonly used are listed in Table 5-2.

Making Entries on Patient Records

Each health agency sets certain policies about making entries on a patient's health record. Examples include policies about the personnel who are responsible for writing on each form, the frequency for recording information, and whether routine nursing care, such as giving a bath, is recorded. It is important that the nurse follow the policies of each particular health agency. The policies are often based on principles for ensuring the protection of the agency and its personnel from legal liabilities. Because entries are made by numerous people, there must be uniform compliance to the standards for record keeping. Deviation from an agency's charting policies reduces an individual's protection if the record is legally questioned. Common practices for making entries that are recommended by most agencies are described in Skill Procedure 5-1.

Converting to Military Time

Some hospitals use military time on health-care records. *Military time* is a method of expressing time, using a different four-digit number for each hour and minute of the 24-hour day. The first two of the four digits indicate the hour; the last two digits indicate the minute(s). This avoids confusion, since no number is ever duplicated. It also (*Text continues on page 66*)

Table 5-2. Commonly Used Abbreviations

Abbreviation	Meaning	Abbreviation	Meaning
Abd.	Abdomen	OD	Right eye
AM	Before noon	OOB	Out of bed
AMA	Against medical advice	OR	Operating room
Amt.	Amount	OS	Left eye
Approx.	Approximately	OU	Both eyes
BM	Bowel movement	Per	By or through
BRP	Bathroom privileges	PO	By mouth
$\bar{c}$	with	Postop.	Postoperative, meaning after surgery
CCU	Cardiac care unit		
DC	Discontinue	Preop.	Preoperative, meaning before surgery
ER	Emergency room		
Exam.	Examination	pt.	Patient
H_2O	Water	PT	Physical therapy
I & O	Intake and output	R, Rt., or Ⓡ	Right
L, Lt., or Ⓛ	Left	$\bar{s}$	Without
NKA	No known allergies	SS	Soap suds
NPO	Nothing by mouth	Via	By way of
NSS	Normal saline solution	WC	Wheelchair
O_2	Oxygen	WNL	Within normal limits
OB	Obstetrics	Wt.	Weight

Skill Procedure 5-1. Making Entries on the Patient's Record

Suggested Action	Reason for Action
Use a pen to make entries; use the color of ink determined by agency policy.	Entries made in pencil can be erased; ink is permanent. If parts of a chart need to be duplicated, blue ink does not photocopy well.
Never record information for someone else.	Each person is accountable for the information that is written. Recording for another places an individual in a position of being held responsible for care and observations that were not personally carried out.
Write or print information so it can be read with ease.	Illegible entries become questionable information in a court of law. The entry loses its value for exchanging information if it is unreadable.
Enter the month, day, and year at midnight. Indicate the hour and minute of each entry. Some agencies use military time.	Legal implications may depend on the accurate date and time of entries.
Record the information in the sequence in which it occurred.	The recorded information should show the actual assessments and care as they took place.
Do not rely on memory. Record as promptly as possible or make notes for later use.	Errors and omissions are likely when information is gathered on many individuals.
Chart frequently. Follow the agency's policies for the minimum interval between entries.	Many agencies require that entries be made at least every two hours. This helps to prove that the patient was not unattended or unobserved for long periods of time.
If information is accidently omitted, make the entry as soon as possible. Record the current time of the entry, but identify the actual time the action or observation took place within the notation.	Every effort should be made to avoid omissions. When it does occur, being sure to identify the time when something happened helps to provide order and logic in understanding what took place.
Fill all the space on each line of the form. Draw a line through all the blank space that remains in a line that is not used (as shown in Figure 5-4).	Leaving empty space or lines could result in someone else adding words, thus making them appear as part of the original entry.
Follow agency policy concerning whether routine hygienic care, such as giving a bath, is recorded.	When providing hygienic care is a policy of the agency, unless there is something unusual about the care, it is generally assumed that it was carried out.
Record the actions that correspond to carrying out the physician's orders and the nursing orders.	The charting verifies that the medical plan and the nursing plan were carried out. If these actions are not recorded, it is assumed that they are omitted.
Document when a patient is transferred, discharged, or leaves and returns to the unit from another department.	Nurses are responsible for knowing the whereabouts of patients. The charting indicates the time and order of events taking place during the day.
Record information that is significant to the patient's condition and state of health.	The nurse's charting should reflect competent, knowledgeable care. Entries such as "no complaints" are meaningless.
Omit words such as a, an, or the.	Extra words add length to the entry.
Omit stating the patient's name or using pt. as an abbreviation.	Each page of a chart form is labeled with the patient's name and identifiable information. It is understood that all the entries on that page refer to that particular patient.
Use abbreviations, but only those approved for use by the agency.	Not all abbreviations have the same meaning. Using acceptable abbreviations prevents confusion and misinterpretation.

(continued)

Skill Procedure 5-1. Continued

Suggested Action	**Reason for Action**
Do not use ditto marks.	The danger of ditto marks is that someone may write over them or they may represent information in an inaccurate way.

Do not erase or scribble through words. Rather, draw a single line through the mistake; put the word *error* above it, and continue the recording with the correct information, as in the following:
 	
                  error
1:30 P.M. Wheezes heard in ~~lt. base of lung.~~
                                     R. Smith, R.N.
1:30 P.M. Wheezes heard in the base of Rt. lung.
                                     R. Smith, R.N.
	Correcting an error must be done in such a way that the words first recorded can be clearly read. This is especially important when a record is being used as legal evidence. Erasures or obliterated words can cause others to suspect that an effort was made to conceal or change an entry to alter evidence associating the writer with negligence or malpractice.

Avoid writing personal opinions about a patient's behavior. Quote the patient whenever possible, especially when it relates to his mental status and emotional feelings.	Facts should be recorded. The nurse's interpretation may be incorrect. Uncomplimentary or false written statements about a patient may be grounds for libel.
Avoid phrases such as "appears to be" or "seems to be."	Phrases implying uncertainty about what was observed suggest that the nurse lacks reasonable knowledge.
Avoid labeling. For example, the word *depressed* may suggest various types of behavior to different people. Describe how a patient acts.	Terms may not mean the same to all people. Reporting the characteristics of behavior is a much more accurate and objective method than using a general label.
Describe only care that has been given; do not record care that is yet to take place.	Making early entries can cause legal problems, especially if the patient's condition suddenly changes. It would be difficult to explain why the nurse would chart "2:00 A.M. Taking sips of water," and then explain why the same patient had been pronounced dead at 12:45 A.M.
Record the safety measures that were associated with a patient's care.	A patient may claim he was injured. The court may use the nurse's notes to determine if reasonable precautions were taken to avoid harm.
Record any adverse reactions; include what measures were taken to manage them.	If adverse reactions are described but the actions taken are not included, the patient could claim that his safety was jeopardized by substandard care.
Record when a physician or supervising nurse is called about a patient's condition. Include the reason for the notification and the result of the exchange of information.	The nurse ultimately is held responsible for the patient's care. Recording this information indicates that the nurse acted wisely and reasonably to ensure a patient's safety. This may reduce or eliminate the nurse's personal liability if harm should come to a patient. The nurse should never hesitate to call other individuals of authority if there is a lack of response to a plea of help.
Describe teaching. State what was taught, when, and how. Describe the patient's reaction. Include an evaluation of the patient's progress at learning.	When a chart is audited, the nursing care may be viewed as substandard if teaching is not recorded. Documenting teaching helps others with the continuity of care. Entries on the record indicate what still needs to be done.
Sign each entry according to agency policy. Most require that the first initial, the last name, and the abbreviation for one's title be used. A student nurse would use the initials S.N.	Identification of the person making the entry is important so that there is no question about who gave care or made an assessment. If the record is used for legal purposes, an unsigned entry is considered questionable evidence.

eliminates the need to always add the labels A.M., P.M., midnight, and noon.

When military time is used, one must think in terms of a 24-hour clock. A zero is placed before each number when indicating the hours from one until ten. After noon, twelve is added to each hour. For example, the first hour, or one o'clock in the morning, is 0100 hours; 10 A.M. is 1000; and midnight is 2400 hours. These numbers would be stated "O-one hundred hours," "ten hundred hours," and "twenty-four hundred hours," respectively. All the hours in between are numbered according to their sequence from 0100. Figure 5-9 is a drawing that identifies military time on the face of a clock.

The minutes in military time are identified in numbers from 1 to 59, each representing a separate, sequential number. Table 5-3 illustrates examples converted to military time.

Other Written Forms of Communication

In addition to the patient's record, there are several other commonly used written forms that are prepared and maintained by nurses. These include the nursing care plan and the nursing Kardex.

The Nursing Care Plan

A *nursing care plan* is a plan written by a nurse, describing the actions that should be performed when providing care for a patient. A nursing care plan is written on a standard form developed for use within the health agency. It is a nursing responsibility to complete a nursing care plan for each patient who is admitted. It is revised frequently as the patient's condition changes. Entries on the patient's chart should correlate with both the medical and the nursing orders. This correlation may be evaluated during an audit of patient records.

A nursing care plan usually has columns for writing the nursing diagnosis, goal statements, and nursing orders. Nursing orders are sometimes called measures or approaches. Some health-care agencies use a multidisciplin-

Table 5-3. Examples of Military Time Conversions

Time	Equivalent in Military Time
1:00 A.M.	0100
2:00 A.M.	0200
9:00 A.M.	0900
12:00 noon	1200
1:00 P.M.	1300 (12 + 1)
2:00 P.M.	1400 (12 + 2)
9:00 P.M.	2100 (12 + 9)
12:00 midnight	2400 (12 + 12)
12:01 A.M.	0001
3:15 A.M.	0315
7:59 P.M.	1959

ary team approach to planning patient care. A form that illustrates this concept is shown in Figure 5-10.

It is important that the orders be specific in order to guide others to carry out the plan. Display 5-1 gives a list of verbs that are useful for writing directions in nursing orders. The principles and style for writing the nursing diagnosis, goal statements, and nursing orders have been described in Chapter 4.

The nursing care plan may be kept separate from the chart during the time that an individual is a patient. This is so the nurse can refer to it quickly and easily. However, when the patient is discharged, all current and revised nursing care plans are added to the other forms in the chart. The nursing care plan is considered part of the chart, and thus a legal document.

The same kinds of principles for charting also apply to writing a nursing care plan. Entries should be clear, concise, and legible. All orders and revisions should be dated. Only approved abbreviations should be used. The nurse who writes the orders should sign them.

The Nursing Kardex

The *nursing Kardex,* sometimes just called Kardex, is a short, summarized version of the current basic care for a patient. The form is frequently the size of a large index card. The Kardex form is often something as simple as an itemized list of multiple choices within broad categories of routine care. The nurse may make checks by items that apply to the patient or may write single words that are easily interpreted. An example of a nursing Kardex form is illustrated in Figure 5-11.

A Kardex form is prepared for each patient at the time of admission. The forms on all patients are kept collectively in a holder that allows flipping from one to another. They are

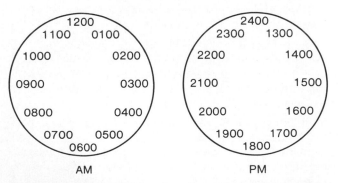

Figure 5-9 These clock faces represent the numbering of the hours within a day when using military time.

PATIENT CARE PLAN

NAME _____ DIAGNOSIS _____ ROOM _____

DISCHARGE PLAN

Date

_____ 1. _____

_____ 2. _____

_____ 3. _____

_____ 4. _____

Date	Problem Number	Problem/Need	Goal	Target Date	Approach	Responsible Discipline	Patient Outcome

ROOM	NAME	AGE	ADM. DATE	DIAGNOSIS: ALLERGIES:

Figure 5-10 This form facilitates a team approach in planning patient care. (Courtesy of Fairview Medical Care Facility, Centreville, MI.)

usually filed in the sequence of the room numbers on a nursing unit.

The entries on a Kardex may be changed frequently, sometimes daily or even several times in one day. Information on the form is written in pencil so that it can be erased. *This is the only form on which this may be done.*

A Kardex may be used to:

- Identify the patient by name and room number
- Identify the patient's doctor and medical diagnosis
- Provide a quick check for current medical orders
- Serve as a reference for a change-of-shift report
- Serve as a guide when making nursing assignments
- Check quickly on a patient's type of diet
- Alert nursing personnel to scheduled tests or test preparations

---

Display 5-1. Examples of Verbs that Direct Actions

Ambulate	Instill
Apply	Irrigate
Cleanse	Measure
Empty	Position
Feed	Turn
Give	Wrap

- List activities that a patient should perform and those that are restricted
- Identify comfort or assistive measures the patient may require
- Provide a tool for estimating the personnel-to-patient ratio of staff that should be assigned to a nursing unit.

Using Checklists and Flow Sheets

It is rather obvious that information in a patient's record is sometimes difficult to locate. It may involve a great deal of reading time in various places within the record before obtaining particular data. Therefore, many hospitals are developing checklists and flow sheets.

A *checklist* is a form that can be used to document routine types of care, such as bathing and mouth care. The checklist is a part of the permanent record. It saves writing time because all that is required is a check showing that a routine of patient care was performed. This charting technique is especially helpful in long-term care facilities where the care is similar each day and the patient's condition may not differ much for extended periods of time.

A *flow sheet* is a chart form that was recommended for use by the Joint Commission on Accreditation of Healthcare Organizations. It contains sections for recording frequently repeated assessments. There is often room for recording numbers or brief descriptions. A flow sheet

BATH:	DIET:	BOWEL/BLADDER:	PHYSICAL TRAITS:
_____ Complete	_____ NPO	_____ Catheter	_____ Left handed
_____ Partial	_____ Hold Brkfst	_____ Commode	_____ Right handed
_____ Self	_____ Feed	_____ Incontinent	_____ Paraplegic
_____ Tub	_____ Liquid	_____ Ostomy	_____ Hemiplegic
_____ Shower	_____ Soft	Type: _____	L ___ R ___
	_____ General		_____ Blind
ACTIVITY:	_____ Special	SAFETY MEASURES:	L ___ R ___
_____ Bed Rest		_____ Siderails	_____ Deaf
_____ BRP only	FLUIDS:	_____ Restraints	L ___ R ___
_____ Dangle	_____ I & O	Jacket: _____	_____ Speech Imp.
_____ Ambulate	_____ Restrict to:	Wrist: _____	_____ Other (list)
_____ Change pos.	_____	Ankles: _____	
_____ Up as tol.	_____ Increase to:	Constant: _____	
	_____	When OOB: _____	ALLERGIES (in red) If
HYGIENE:	_____ IV	Night only _____	none, so state:
_____ Dentures		_____ Supervise	
_____ Oral Care	VITAL SIGNS:	Smoking	_____
_____ Special	_____ TPR	_____ Other (list)	_____
_____	_____ BP	_____	_____

DIAGNOSIS: OPERATION: DATE: RELIGION:

ROOM: NAME: AGE: DOCTOR:

Figure 5-11 A Kardex form provides a quick summary of current information about the care of a patient. (Courtesy of Fairview Medical Care Facility, Centreville, MI.)

helps members of the health team find certain data all on one form. With the collective information in one location, trends can be interpreted at a glance.

Other Methods for Exchanging Information

The patient's record, nursing care plan, and the Kardex are not the only means for communicating health information. Other commonly used methods are change-of-shift reporting, filling out assignment sheets, participating in conferences, making rounds, and using the telephone and computer. The nurse may be involved in exchanging information through all or several of these methods.

Change of Shift Reports

When a new nursing team arrives to assume the care of patients on a nursing unit, a reporting session takes place. A report includes a summary of the admissions, transfers, discharges, and deaths. It is followed by a discussion of each patient's condition and the significant events that took place since that team last cared for them. This overview of current information is necessary for providing continuity of patient care. In most agencies the report takes place in a meeting as shown in Figure 5-12.

In some agencies the report is tape recorded, as shown in Figure 5-13. A taped report saves time because there are no interruptions or digressions during the report. The

tape can be replayed if there is a need to have information repeated. The greatest disadvantage is that it does not facilitate immediate questions and answers on information contained or omitted on the taped recording.

The following are suggested practices when a report is given.

1. Be prompt so that a report can start and end on time.
2. Do not socialize during reporting sessions.
3. Be prepared to take notes on the information that is reported. The nurse who provides the report should also have notes or use a Kardex as a guide.
4. Listen to information regarding the response of the patient to his care, any remaining problems, and plans for resolving them. This is reported as each patient is identified.

Assignment Sheets

During or following a change-of-shift report, assignment sheets are given to nursing personnel. A nurse makes out an assignment sheet for each member of the team. The assignment sheet identifies the patients that each person will care for and includes a description of the work they are to do. The time that each person is scheduled for a meal and break may be indicated on the assignment sheet. This planning is important so that not all personnel are gone from a unit at the same time. Times for breaks are somewhat flexible, since unforeseen circumstances do occur. A nursing team member has a responsibility for the care and

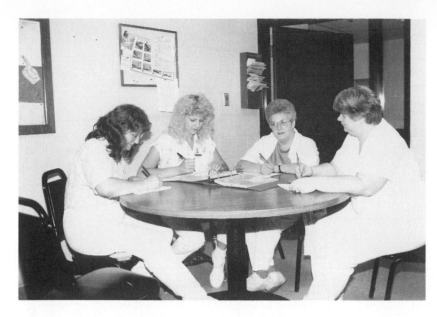

Figure 5-12 A group of nurses begin their shift by receiving a report on their patients.

safety of patients, which is more important than leaving for a scheduled break. Special duties that are necessary to keep the nursing unit efficient may also be assigned occasionally. Equipment may need to be checked and restocked, or the supply of emergency drugs may need to be inventoried. An example of a nursing assignment sheet is illustrated in Figure 5-14.

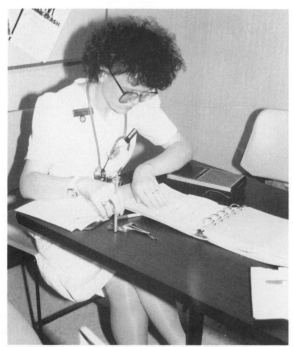

Figure 5-13 A nurse reads information on a patient's chart before using the tape recorder for report.

Conferences

Conferences are commonly used for exchanging information. Informal conferences occur when other health practitioners, such as the doctor, dietitian, and physical therapist, meet with nursing team members.

Nursing conferences are held frequently. During these conferences information about patient care problems may be exchanged, problem-solving approaches may be discussed, new equipment or treatment methods may be explained, or changes in policies, procedures, or routines may be introduced.

Team conferences may include many more individuals than just the nursing team. These are usually scheduled for exchanging information about one particular patient. All those who are involved with the patient, and even the patient himself, may be invited to attend. Individuals who attend a team conference may be doctors, nurses, clergy, social workers, personnel from community agencies, the patient, and relatives or friends of the patient. Usually one person organizes and directs the conference. Responsibilities for certain outcomes that result from the team conference may be delegated to various members who attend the meeting.

Rounds

Nursing and health teams sometimes use rounds to exchange information. Team members visit patients' bedsides in a group, and the patient may be asked to participate in the discussion of his care.

Some nurses use walking rounds for a change-of-shift report. The nurse who is leaving gives a summary report to the nurse who is arriving. The report includes identifying the care that has been given, trends in assessment data,

NURSING ASSIGNMENT SHEET

TEAM MEMBER Jane Doe L.P.N.	BREAK 9:15 AM. CONFERENCE 10:30 AM. LUNCH 12:00 N. DATE:
TEAM LEADER Mary Black RN	ASSIGNMENT Filling and distributing water carafes on the Northwing

ROOM	PATIENT	BATH	ACTIVITY	DIET	FLUIDS	TO BE CHECKED	TREATMENTS	SPECIMEN	COMMENTS
296¹	Flora Brown Duodenal Ulcer	BED SELF * SHOWER TUB SITZ	BED DANGLE B R P B R P · HELP AMB AMB · HELP WALKER CRUTCHES W C	REGULAR SOFT SURG LIQ FULL LIQ SPECIAL Bland III FASTING TUBE FEEDING	FORCE N P O LIMIT SIPS WATER ICE CHIPS I V DIST WATER	BLOOD PRESSURE 8A T P R 8A TEST URINE A C & HS SLIDING SCALE I & O LEVIN TUBE CHEST TUBE FOLEY OXYGEN	ENEMA DOUCHE PERI CARE · LIGHT WEIGH ORAL HYGIENE SPECIAL BACK CARE PREPARE FOR SURG PREPARE FOR X-RAY O T · P T · E C T	STOOL OB URINE SPUTUM BLOOD CULTURE TISSUE	
296²	Mary Green Coronary	BED SELF * SHOWER TUB SITZ	BED DANGLE B R P B R P · HELP AMB AMB · HELP WALKER CRUTCHES W C	REGULAR SOFT SURG LIQ FULL LIQ SPECIAL 2Gm Na FASTING TUBE FEEDING	FORCE N P O LIMIT SIPS WATER ICE CHIPS I V DIST WATER	BLOOD PRESSURE 8-12 T P R 8-12 TEST URINE A C & HS SLIDING SCALE I & O LEVIN TUBE CHEST TUBE FOLEY OXYGEN 4L/M -1hr pc + HS	ENEMA DOUCHE PERI CARE · LIGHT WEIGH 8A ORAL HYGIENE SPECIAL BACK CARE PREPARE FOR SURG PREPARE FOR X-RAY O T · P T · E C T	STOOL URINE SPUTUM BLOOD CULTURE TISSUE	
298¹	John Snapp C.O.P.D.	BED SELF * SHOWER TUB SITZ	BED DANGLE B R P B R P · HELP AMB c̄ O2 AMB · HELP WALKER CRUTCHES W C	REGULAR SOFT SURG LIQ FULL LIQ SPECIAL FASTING TUBE FEEDING	FORCE N P O LIMIT SIPS WATER ICE CHIPS I V DIST WATER	BLOOD PRESSURE T P R TEST URINE A C & HS SLIDING SCALE I & O LEVIN TUBE CHEST TUBE FOLEY OXYGEN 1L/M CONT.	ENEMA FLEETS DOUCHE PERI CARE · LIGHT WEIGH ORAL HYGIENE SPECIAL BACK CARE PREPARE FOR SURG PREPARE FOR X-RAY O T · P T · E C T	STOOL URINE SPUTUM BLOOD CULTURE TISSUE	1000cc 5% D/W c̄ 500mg Aminophyllin @ 100cc/hr CONT.
298²	Tom Henry C.H.F.	BED SELF * SHOWER TUB SITZ	BED DANGLE B R P B R P · HELP AMB AMB · HELP WALKER CRUTCHES W C	REGULAR SOFT SURG LIQ FULL LIQ SPECIAL ½Gm Na FASTING TUBE FEEDING	FORCE N P O LIMIT 300/8h SIPS WATER ICE CHIPS I V DIST WATER	BLOOD PRESSURE q2h T P R q2h TEST URINE A C & HS SLIDING SCALE I & O LEVIN TUBE CHEST TUBE FOLEY OXYGEN 4L/M CONT.	ENEMA DOUCHE PERI CARE · LIGHT WEIGH 8 ORAL HYGIENE 8-12 SPECIAL BACK CARE PREPARE FOR SURG PREPARE FOR X-RAY O T · P T · E C T	STOOL URINE SPUTUM BLOOD CULTURE TISSUE	Change Position q 2hr.
299	Jim Smith Diabetes Mellitus	BED SELF * SHOWER TUB SITZ	BED DANGLE B R P B R P · HELP AMB AMB · HELP WALKER CRUTCHES W C	REGULAR SOFT SURG LIQ FULL LIQ SPECIAL 1800 Cal Diabetic FASTING TUBE FEEDING	FORCE N P O LIMIT SIPS WATER ICE CHIPS I V DIST WATER	BLOOD PRESSURE T P R 8 TEST URINE A C & HS SLIDING SCALE I & O LEVIN TUBE CHEST TUBE FOLEY OXYGEN	ENEMA DOUCHE PERI CARE · LIGHT WEIGH ORAL HYGIENE SPECIAL BACK CARE PREPARE FOR SURG PREPARE FOR X-RAY O T · P T · E C T	STOOL URINE SPUTUM BLOOD CULTURE TISSUE	
		BED SELF * SHOWER TUB SITZ	BED DANGLE B R P B R P · HELP AMB AMB · HELP WALKER CRUTCHES W C	REGULAR SOFT SURG LIQ FULL LIQ SPECIAL FASTING TUBE FEEDING	FORCE N P O LIMIT SIPS WATER ICE CHIPS I V DIST WATER	BLOOD PRESSURE T P R TEST URINE A C & HS SLIDING SCALE I & O LEVIN TUBE CHEST TUBE FOLEY OXYGEN	ENEMA DOUCHE PERI CARE · LIGHT WEIGH ORAL HYGIENE SPECIAL BACK CARE PREPARE FOR SURG PREPARE FOR X-RAY O T · P T · E C T	STOOL URINE SPUTUM BLOOD CULTURE TISSUE	
		BED SELF * SHOWER TUB SITZ	BED DANGLE B R P B R P · HELP AMB AMB · HELP WALKER CRUTCHES W C	REGULAR SOFT SURG LIQ FULL LIQ SPECIAL FASTING TUBE FEEDING	FORCE N P O LIMIT SIPS WATER ICE CHIPS I V DIST WATER	BLOOD PRESSURE T P R TEST URINE A C & HS SLIDING SCALE I & O LEVIN TUBE CHEST TUBE FOLEY OXYGEN	ENEMA DOUCHE PERI CARE · LIGHT WEIGH ORAL HYGIENE SPECIAL BACK CARE PREPARE FOR SURG PREPARE FOR X-RAY O T · P T · E C T	STOOL URINE SPUTUM BLOOD CULTURE TISSUE	
		BED SELF * SHOWER TUB SITZ	BED DANGLE B R P B R P · HELP AMB AMB · HELP WALKER CRUTCHES W C	REGULAR SOFT SURG LIQ FULL LIQ SPECIAL FASTING TUBE FEEDING	FORCE N P O LIMIT SIPS WATER ICE CHIPS I V DIST WATER	BLOOD PRESSURE T P R TEST URINE A C & HS SLIDING SCALE I & O LEVIN TUBE CHEST TUBE FOLEY OXYGEN	ENEMA DOUCHE PERI CARE · LIGHT WEIGH ORAL HYGIENE SPECIAL BACK CARE PREPARE FOR SURG PREPARE FOR X-RAY O T · P T · E C T	STOOL URINE SPUTUM BLOOD CULTURE TISSUE	

CODE

*	You wash back and legs	W C	Wheelchair	E C T	· Electrical Convulsive Therapy
B R P	Bathroom privileges	B P	Blood pressure	O T	· Occupational Therapy
AMB	Ambulatory	N P O	Nothing by mouth	P T	· Physical Therapy
I & O	Intake and output	DIST	Distilled water		

Figure 5-14 This is a nursing assignment sheet describing the team member's responsibility for the day. Note the definitions of abbreviations at the bottom of the form, which eliminates the danger of misunderstandings.

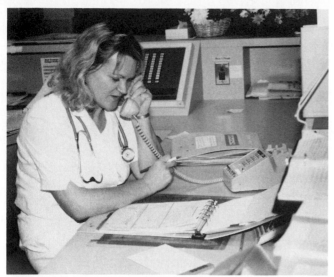

Figure 5-15 The nurse uses the phone to consult with another health practitioner about a patient's care.

and a check of the equipment being used. This provides for on-the-spot clarification through direct communication. The patient is a witness to and participant in the interaction. This type of reporting boosts the patient's level of confidence in the transition of care.

Telephone

Using the telephone as shown in Figure 5-15 is a convenient way to exchange information when it is difficult for people to get together. For example, the nurse may call various departments in a health agency, such as the laboratory, x-ray department, and the operating room. Using the telephone saves time in many instances. Common courtesies when using a telephone are as follows:

- If an incoming call occurs, answer the telephone as promptly as possible and speak in a normal tone of voice.
- Identify yourself by name and title and indicate the department or unit on which you are located when making or receiving a telephone call.
- Obtain or state the reason for the call.
- Carefully identify the patient about whom information is required. Spell the patient's name if there is any chance of confusion.
- Keep calls as short as possible to avoid tying up the telephone and wasting people's time.
- Converse in a courteous and businesslike manner.
- Do not use the business phone in a health agency for personal matters.

The telephone may be used to notify a physician about a change in a patient's condition. Always write the informa-

tion that was given and the instructions that were received in the patient's record. The reporting nurse may ask a second nurse to listen on another line so that instructions are not misinterpreted. The nurse should contact the nursing supervisor or head of the medical department if unable to reach the patient's physician in an emergency. These same people should also be informed if the nurse feels that the physician has not responded in a safe manner to the information that was given.

Bibliography

Burke LJ, Murphy J: Charting by Exception: A Cost-Effective, Quality Approach. New York, Wiley & Sons, 1988

Cline A: Streamlined documentation through exceptional charting. Nursing Management 20(2):62–64, 1989

Coles MC, Fullenwider SD: Documentation: Managing the dilemma. Nursing Management 19(12):65–66, 70, 72, 1988

Courtright G: Unofficial charting: Make it work for you. Nursing Management 19(1):62, 1988

Creighton H: Legal significance of charting. Part 1. Nursing Management 18(9):17, 20, 22, 1987

Creighton H: Legal significance of charting. Part 2. Nursing Management 18(10):14–15, 1987

Eggland ET: Charting: How and why to document your care daily—and fully. Nursing 18(11):76–79, 81–84, 1988

Fracassi J: ICU flowsheets: Are they cost effective? Nursing Management 18(12):66–67, 1987

Gropper EI: Does your charting reflect your worth? Geriatr Nurs 9(2):99–101, 1988

Hanna DV, Wyman NB: Assessment + diagnosis = care planning: A tool for coordination. Nursing Management 18(11):106–109, 1987

Kerr AH: How the write stuff can go wrong. Nursing 17(1):48–50, 1987

Lampe SS: Focus charting: Streamlining documentation. Nursing Management 16(7):43–46, 1985

Montemuro M: CORE documentation: A complete system for charting nursing care. Nursing Management 19(8):28–32, 1988

Morrissey–Ross M: Documentation: If you haven't written it, you haven't done it. Nurs Clin North Am 23(2):363–371, 1988

Murphy J, Bellinger JE, Johnson B: Charting by exception: Meeting the challenge of cost containment. Nursing Management 19(2):56–58, 62, 64, 1988

Murphy J, Burke LJ: Charting by exception: A more efficient way to document. Nursing 20(5):65, 68–69, 1990

Newton GA: A better way to chart IV therapy. RN Magazine 51(7):26–28, 1988

Northrop CE: Filling in charting gaps . . . in court. Nursing 17(9):43, 1987

Omhahl D: Home care charting do's and don'ts. Am J Nurs 88(2):203–204, 1988

Petrucci KE, McCormick KA, Scheve AAS: Documenting patient care needs: Do nurses do it? Journal of Gerontological Nursing 13(11):34–38, 46–48, 1987

Philpott M: 20 rules for good charting. Nursing 16(8):63, 1986

Richard JA: Walking rounds: A step in the right direction. Nursing 18(6):63–64, 1989

Rich PL: Make the most of your charting time. Nursing 17(5):68–73, 1987

Rich PL: With this flow sheet, less is more. Nursing 15(7):25–29, 1985

Rutkowski B: How DRGs are changing your charting. Nursing 15(10):49–51, 1985

Scher BB: Are checklists replacing good care? Nursing 19(1):47, 1988

Sterns L: Nursing diagnosis: An assessment form. Nursing Management 19(4):101–102, 1988

Tamelleo AD: Who can change a nurse's notes? RN Magazine 51(5):75–76, 1988

Vandenbosch TM: How to use a pain flow sheet effectively. Nursing 19(8):50–51, 1988

6

Laws and Ethics: The Controls for Nursing

Chapter Outline

Behavioral Objectives
Glossary
Introduction
Laws
Lawsuits
Patients' Rights
Legal Issues
Ethics
Codes of Ethics
Ethical Dilemmas
Ethical Issues
Ethics Committees
Securing Liability Insurance
Preventing Lawsuits
Defense Techniques
Bibliography

Behavioral Objectives

When the content of this chapter has been mastered, the learner will be able to:

Define the terms appearing in the glossary.
Discuss laws that control and protect nurses.
Discuss the legal position of student and licensed nurses in relation to the care of patients.
List the elements that must be proven in a negligence or malpractice lawsuit.
Identify a reference that describes the rights of patients.
Identify five legal issues that affect patient care.
Describe the purpose of a code of ethics.
List ways that nurses may be guided in making ethical decisions.
Identify five ethical issues that affect patient care.
List criteria that should be investigated when selecting a professional liability insurance policy.
Describe methods for preventing lawsuits.
List three written records that can be used in court during a negligence or malpractice suit.
Discuss actions that may be helpful if a nurse is summoned to testify in court.

Glossary

Allocation of scarce resources An ethical issue involving decisions as to who will receive certain health-care measures and who will be denied.

Anecdotal note A written report that records the facts about a particular event.

Assault A threat to harm another person.

Battery Making bodily contact without the person's consent.

Code of ethics A list of written statements describing ideal behavior for members of a particular group.

Competency A legal term for the ability to understand information and the consequences of a decision.

Confidentiality An ethical issue that refers to the right of an individual to have personal information protected from public knowledge.

Defendant The accused person in a trial.

Ethics A system of moral or philosophical principles that directs actions as being either right or wrong.

False imprisonment Unjustifiable restraint or prevention of movement of a person without proper consent.

Good Samaritan law A law that gives persons legal protection when they give aid to someone in an emergency.

Incident sheet A written report of an event that caused harm or could eventually cause harm.

Informed consent Permission given by one person to another based upon acquired information or knowledge.

Invasion of privacy An illegal act that violates the right of a person to avoid public attention.

Law A rule of conduct established and enforced by the government of a society.

Lawsuit A legal action in a court.

Liable Accountable, responsible, or answerable for an act.

Libel An untruthful written statement about a person that subjects him to ridicule or contempt.

Living will A statement of a person's wishes about how he wants to or wants not to be treated medically if no longer able to speak for himself.

Malpractice Harm caused by a professional when his action, or lack of action, differs from that of other professionals.

Mandatory nurse practice act A law requiring a nurse to be licensed in order to practice nursing.

Negligence Harm caused to someone because an action that was taken, or not taken, differs from that of other reasonable persons.

Nurse practice acts Laws passed by each state that protect the public from persons considered unfit to practice nursing.

Permissive nurse practice act A law that allows an individual to be called a licensed practical nurse or a registered nurse if the state's requirements for licensure have been met.

Plaintiff The person who brings charges in a trial.

Right to die An ethical issue involving witholding or withdrawing consent for treatment.

Slander An untruthful oral statement about a person that subjects him to ridicule or contempt.

Tort A legal action involving any act or its omission that harms somebody.

Truth-telling An ethical issue that refers to the duty of physicians and nurses to tell a patient the truth about matters concerning his health.

Whistle-blowing An ethical issue that refers to publicly reporting incompetent or unethical practices.

Will A statement of a person's wishes about what shall be done with his property after his death.

Introduction

A full discussion of legal and ethical aspects of nursing is usually undertaken near graduation. Laws, rights, and duties, however, affect nursing students from the time they begin their clinical experience. This chapter gives a brief overview of some major legal and ethical issues as they apply to nursing.

Laws

A *law* is a rule of conduct established and enforced by the government of a society. Laws are intended primarily to protect the rights of people

Laws Controlling Nursing Practice

Laws that affect nursing have been enacted. *Nurse practice acts,* for example, are laws passed by each state that protect the public from persons considered unfit to practice nursing. They control the requirements for nursing and the acts nurses may perform.

The first law dealing with the practice of nursing in this country was enacted in North Carolina in 1903. At present, there are nurse practice acts in all 50 states, the District of Columbia, Guam, Samoa, Puerto Rico, and the Virgin Islands.

The laws vary considerably from state to state. In some states, the law requires that nurses be licensed to practice. Such a law is called a *mandatory nurse practice act.* In other states, the law allows an individual to be called a licensed practical nurse (licensed vocational nurse) or registered nurse if the state's requirements for licensure have been met. This law is called a *permissive nurse practice act.*

Laws Protecting Nurses

Laws have been enacted to protect nurses when they administer care. Laws also have been passed to extend to nurses the same benefits as those of other laborers.

Good Samaritan Laws. *Good Samaritan laws* protect nurses when they administer emergency care as a citizen outside their place of employment. They are named after a traveler, described in the Bible as the good Samaritan, who helped a stranger who had been beaten and robbed. These laws vary from state to state. Nurses are not covered by this legislation in all states.

Because good Samaritan laws offer protection, they tend to encourage persons to give assistance at the scene of an emergency. However, they do not make it legally necessary to do so. Vermont's law is the only exception to this. When health practitioners do assist, they are expected to administer safe care based upon what others would do in similar circumstances. If the emergency care can be shown to be unsafe, a good Samaritan law will not necessarily provide protection from a lawsuit.

Laws Affecting Employment. Nurse Practice Acts and good Samaritan laws are passed by state legislatures. Many additional federal laws affect nurses specifically or indirectly. The list in Table 6-1 is not complete. These laws were enacted to afford laborers, including nurses, protection of their rights. Some of these rights include:

- The right to a just wage
- The right to participate in decisions that affect working conditions
- The right to work in a safe and healthful environment
- The right to opportunities for career and educational mobility
- The right to political activity
- The right to organize professionally.

Lawsuits

Accountability is defined in Chapter 1. The word *liable* means accountable, responsible, or answerable for an act. A *lawsuit* is a legal action in a court of law. An accused person is called the *defendant.* The person bringing the

Table 6-1. Laws That Affect Nursing Employment

Federal Law	Application to Nursing
Workmen's Compensation Act	Requires employers to subscribe to insurance that would cover the cost of illness or injury, such as a fall or needle puncture acquired while at work.
Occupational Safety and Health Act	Protects nurses as well as other workers from working conditions that endanger health or safety.
Comprehensive Drug Abuse Prevention and Control Act (The Controlled Substances Act)	Regulates the control of abused drugs and protects the nurse from being charged with a crime while administering prescribed narcotics.
The Civil Rights Act; Title VII: The Equal Employment Opportunity Law	Forbids discrimination in hiring or promotion on the basis of sex, age, race, or religion.
Nonprofit Health Care Amendment to the Taft-Hartley Act	Prohibits an employer from taking action against nurses who unionize.
Hazard Communication Standard (Right-to-Know Legislation)	Provides that an employee be informed about any potentially hazardous chemicals in the workplace and instructions on how to avoid or treat exposure to them.

suit against a defendant is called the *plaintiff.* A defendant has a basic right to defend himself in court and is presumed innocent until proven guilty.

Nurses are liable for their acts when they give patients nursing care. Students are not relieved of personal liability if they cause injury to patients. Courts have held students accountable to the same standards as a licensed nurse. It may seem severe to hold a student responsible; the patient, however, should be able to expect safe care no matter who provides it. If a student feels that an assignment is beyond his ability, the supervising nurse should be consulted before attempting to carry it out.

Most of the legal actions involving nurses are torts. A *tort* is any action or its omission that harms somebody. Negligence and malpractice suits are torts. *Negligence* involves harm to a patient because an action that was taken, or not taken, differs from what other reasonable persons would do in the same circumstance. Members of a jury use their own judgment for determining what a reasonable person would do. Malpractice involves being held accountable to a higher standard of care. *Malpractice* involves harm caused by a professional because the action, or lack of action, differs from that of other professionals. To inform the court of the accepted standard, jurors listen to the testimony of expert witnesses.

In a nursing negligence or malpractice case the following must be proven:

- A standard of care existed
- The standard was not met
- Harm occurred
- The harm resulted directly from not meeting the standard.

Display 6-1 provides common causes of nursing lawsuits.

Display 6-1. Common Causes of Nursing Lawsuits

- Medication errors
- Falls
- Inadequate patient assessment
- Unperformed care
- Errors in transfers
- Failure to communicate with other nurses or physicians.

Patients' Rights

In order to avoid lawsuits nurses should be familiar with the patient's rights. Patients' rights have legal and, in some instances, ethical implications. Many statements of patient rights have been published. One, which follows in Display 6-2, has been prepared by the American Hospital Association. It is widely distributed to patients. It may even be posted in public areas of health-care agencies.

Legal Issues

Some situations, unless clearly understood, may place the nurse in legal jeopardy.

Assault and Battery. *Assault* is a threat to harm another person. *Battery* occurs when bodily contact is made without the person's consent. Every person is protected by law from bodily contact with another. This is the basis for obtaining the patient's signature on a consent form before performing certain medical procedures, such as surgery

---

Display 6-2. A Patient's Bill of Rights

1. The patient has the right to considerate and respectful care.
2. The patient has the right to obtain from his physician complete current information concerning his diagnosis, treatment, and prognosis in terms the patient can be reasonably expected to understand. When it is not medically advisable to give such information to the patient, the information should be made available to an appropriate person in his behalf. He has the right to know, by name, the physician responsible for coordinating his care.
3. The patient has the right to receive from his physician information necessary to give informed consent prior to the start of any procedure and/or treatment. Except in emergencies, such information for informed consent should include but not necessarily be limited to the specific procedure and/or treatment, the medically significant risks involved, and the probable duration of incapacitation. Where medically significant alternatives for care or treatment exist, or when the patient requests information concerning medical alternatives, the patient has the right to such information. The patient also has the right to know the name of the person responsible for the procedures and/or treatment.
4. The patient has the right to refuse treatment to the extent permitted by law and to be informed of the medical consequences of his action.
5. The patient has the right to every consideration of his privacy concerning his own medical care program. Case discussion, consultation, examination, and treatment are confidential and should be conducted discreetly. Those not directly involved in his care must have the permission of the patient to be present.
6. The patient has the right to expect that all communications and records pertaining to his care should be treated as confidential.
7. The patient has the right to expect that within its capacity a hospital must make reasonable response to the request of a patient for services. The hospital must provide evaluation, service, and/or referral as indicated by the urgency of the case. When medically permissible, a patient may be transferred to another facility only after he has received complete information and explanation concerning the needs for and alternatives to such a transfer. The institution to which the patient is to be transferred must first have accepted the patient for transfer.
8. The patient has the right to obtain information as to any relationship of his hospital to other health care and educational institutions insofar as his care is concerned. The patient has the right to obtain information as to the existence of any professional relationships among individuals, by name, who are treating him.
9. The patient has the right to be advised if the hospital proposes to engage in or perform human experimentation affecting his care or treatment. The patient has the right to refuse to participate in such research projects.
10. The patient has the right to expect reasonable continuity of care. He has the right to know in advance what appointment times and physicians are available and where. The patient has the right to expect that the hospital will provide a mechanism whereby he is informed by his physician or a delegate of the physician of the patient's continuing health care requirements following discharge.
11. The patient has the right to examine and receive an explanaton of his bill regardless of source of payment.
12. The patient has the right to know what hospital rules and regulations apply to his conduct as a patient.

---

or diagnostic tests. Written consent is legal protection from a lawsuit involving battery, provided it meets all the criteria for informed consent.

Informed Consent. *Informed consent* means that a person has received adequate information for making a decision. Informed consent has both ethical and legal implications for the patient and health practitioners. The patient is legally protected from procedures that he does not agree to or does not understand. Having the patient's consent legally protects the hospital and its employees from claims that the patient did not give his permission. Consent forms are discussed further in Chapter 19.

Those who may give consent include the following:

1. Any competent adult.

2. Any parent or legal guardian of a minor. In a few instances, persons are referred to as emancipated minors and their signatures are accepted on a consent form. These are individuals who live separately from and independently of their parents or legal guardian.
3. Any legal guardian of an incompetent adult.

Competency is a legal term. It refers to the ability of an individual to understand information and the consequences of his decision. Use of alcohol and drugs, severe pain, and overwhelming grief or fear may affect an individual's competence temporarily.

Information must be provided to the patient in terms he can understand. The content should include the following:

1. The risks and benefits of a procedure
2. Any alternatives for treatment
3. The consequences of the procedure or its alternatives.

If a nurse believes the patient does not understand or has misunderstood information, it should be reported to the physician or supervising nurse promptly.

Slander and Libel. *Slander* is an untruthful oral statement about a person that subjects him to ridicule or contempt. *Libel* is the same, except that the statement is in writing, signs, pictures, or similar visuals. Untrue statements that indicate someone is not fit to practice his profession may be held as slander or libel. Nurses who gossip or make false statements about their patients or coworkers in public run the risk of being sued for slander or libel.

False Imprisonment. Preventing the movement of a person without proper consent can constitute *false imprisonment*. Such a wrong would be committed if any person were forcibly held in a health agency. If an adult patient is competent, he may leave a health agency even if health practitioners believe he should remain for additional care. In these instances, health agencies provide a form for the patient to sign. The signature of the patient indicates that he is leaving of his own will and against medical advice. This form is discussed in Chapter 11. Some mentally ill patients and patients with certain communicable diseases may legally be kept in a health agency against their will if it can be shown that they present a danger to society.

Protective restraints are discussed in Chapter 12. Using them unnecessarily may constitute battery or false imprisonment.

Invasion of Privacy. Everyone has the right to withold himself from public exposure. If a person is exposed to the public either personally or through pictures without his consent, the person responsible for such exposure could be sued for *invasion of privacy*.

Exposure that is necessary while caring for a patient does not constitute an invasion of privacy. However, nurses should recognize that a failure to cover patients, pull privacy curtains, or close doors to rooms may violate privacy laws.

Health practitioners who discuss information about patients with anyone who is not involved in the patient's care may be charged with invasion of privacy even if the information is true. Information on patients' records is considered confidential and should not be divulged to any unauthorized person. Students who prepare class assignments (oral or written) are advised not to reveal the identity of patients, which could be considered invasion of privacy. Talking about patients with classmates, coworkers, and others is an unwise, illegal, and unethical practice.

Wills. A *will* is a statement of a person's wishes about what should be done with his property after his death. There are occasions when a patient may wish to initiate or revise a will. It is best to notify the nursing supervisor or agency administrator who will help facilitate the legal aspects of this act. Individuals employed by the agency, such as the business office or public relations department, may be designated to act as a witness during the signing of the document.

At times, the nurse may be required to participate as a witness. There are certain guidelines concerning a will and the witnessing of its signing with which nurses should be familiar:

- The witness should feel sure that the person signing the will is of sound mind (that is, that he knows what he is doing and is free of the influence of medications that could likely change his thinking processes).
- The witness should feel sure that the person signing the will is acting voluntarily and is not being pressured in any way concerning the terms of his will.
- Witnesses should see the person signing his will and they should sign in the presence of one another. State law indicates how many witnesses must acknowledge the signature on a will. Two or three witnesses are most commonly required.
- Witnesses to the signing of a will need not read it, but they should be sure that the document being signed is a will and not some other type of document.
- In most states, a person who receives money or property from a will is not eligible to act as a witness to the signing of the will.

A *living will* is another type of will. It is a description of how one wishes to be treated or not treated medically when he is no longer competent to speak for himself. This advanced directive helps the family and doctor make ethical decisions for the patient. Living wills are not legal in all states. They are discussed again in Chapter 28.

Ethics

The word *ethics* comes from the Greek word *ethos,* meaning customs or modes of conduct. Ethics may be described as a system of moral or philosophical principles that directs actions as being either right or wrong.

Ethics involves identifying the rights of individuals, respecting those rights, and performing certain obligations, called duties, which protect rights. Ethics often arise from social customs and religious traditions. Ethics may describe ideal standards that may present conflicts in certain situations. Some ethical standards have been models for legal applications, which are discussed later in this chapter.

There was a time when making decisions about health-care issues was quite simple. Today, certain issues present health practitioners with difficult ethical decisions, primarily because of the increased use of sophisticated equipment, new techniques in health care, and a change in national values toward health care. Nurses may find themselves facing dilemmas when personal codes of conscience conflict with those being used as a standard. Examples of situations in which an ethical dilemma may arise include abortion on demand, test-tube fertilization, and the prolongation of life with various types of equipment.

Codes of Ethics

Various organizations representing nurses have developed ethical codes. A *code of ethics* is a list of written statements describing ideal behavior for members of a particular group. A code of ethics is used as a model for professional practice.

The National Association for Practical Nurse Education and Services (NAPNES), and the National Federation for Licensed Practical Nurses (NFLPN), and the International Council of Nurses (ICN) are examples of organizations that have composed codes of ethics. Display 6-3 is a current code of ethics that was revised in 1985 by the ANA. The written codes of the other nursing organizations are similar. They can be obtained by writing to the respective organizations.

Ethical Dilemmas

Decisions affecting health care are often guided by ethical or legal standards. However, there are situations in which an action considered legal may be ethical or unethical and an action considered ethical may be legal or illegal.

There is often no one easy answer to every situation. Some guidelines may be helpful in making ethical decisions including the following:

- Make sure that whatever is done is in the patient's best interest.
- Preserve and support the Patient's Bill of Rights.

Display 6-3. Code for Nurses

1. The nurse provides services with respect for human dignity and the uniqueness of the client, unrestricted by considerations of social or economic status, personal attributes, or the nature of health problems.
2. The nurse safeguards the client's right to privacy by judiciously protecting information of a confidential nature.
3. The nurse acts to safeguard the client and the public when health care and safety are affected by incompetent, unethical, or illegal practice by any person.
4. The nurse assumes responsibility and accountability for individual nursing judgments and actions.
5. The nurse maintains competence in nursing.
6. The nurse exercises informed judgment and uses individual competency and qualifications as criteria in seeking consultation, accepting responsibilities, and delegating nursing activities.
7. The nurse participates in activities that contribute to the ongoing development of the profession's body of knowledge.
8. The nurse participates in the profession's efforts to implement and improve standards of nursing.
9. The nurse participates in the profession's efforts to establish and maintain conditions of employment conducive to high-quality nursing care.
10. The nurse participates in the profession's effort to protect the public from misinformation and misrepresentation and to maintain the integrity of nursing.
11. The nurse collaborates with members of the health professions and other citizens in promoting community and national efforts to meet the health needs of the public.

Reprinted with permission from Code for Nurses With Interpretive Statements, Kansas City, American Nurses Association, 1985.

- Work cooperatively with the patient and other health practitioners.
- Follow written policies, codes of ethics, and laws.
- Follow your conscience.

Ethical Issues

Conflicts that develop from ethical dilemmas are not always easily solved. How can nurses best deal with these situations? Certainly, the first obligation for a nurse is to be well informed about the issues that may arise and present personal controversy. Better understanding comes through study and discussion of ethics in a classroom. It also develops through understanding one's own values. In addition, nurses benefit when ethical issues are openly discussed and when specialists in ethical and legal aspects of nursing are used as consultants. The only certainty about issues that are not clearly legal or ethical is that the nurse will be held accountable for whatever personal action is taken.

Telling the Truth. The issue of honesty is somewhat related to informed consent. *Truth-telling* refers to the duty of physicians and nurses to tell a patient the truth about matters concerning his health. The usual circumstance that challenges this ethical issue involves situations in which a patient is terminally ill and does not yet know it. The conflict centers on (1) whether the patient should be told and (2) who should tell the patient.

Many health practitioners agree that the majority of individuals who ask and are told about their impending death seem to adjust. However, patients do not always ask direct questions about their condition. Working closely with the patient allows nurses to analyze the patient's statements to determine their desire to know information.

It is the physician's responsibility to inform the patient. The nurse should try not to divulge this information prematurely. It may undermine the united and supportive relationship that the patient will need to adjust to his situation. In some cases a physician may be reluctant or may refuse to talk honestly with the patient. The nurse may feel more allegiance to the nurse–patient relationship than to the physician–nurse relationship. Following one's conscience may result in frustrating consequences.

Confidentiality. The foundation of any relationship is trust. *Confidentiality* is a principle that directs nurses and other health practitioners to prevent private information about a patient from becoming public. Any health information that the patient confides should not be divulged without his written permission.

The expanding health-care delivery system and increased population have required that much information about patients now be stored and retrieved with computers. With the increase in the numbers of people accessing personal files, there is another aspect to this moral obligation. It requires that the nurse protect the patient's health history from others not only through overheard spoken communication but also through written or electronic data.

Whistle-Blowing. *Whistle-blowing* refers to publicly reporting incompetent or unethical practices. As the name implies, someone calls attention to an unsafe or potentially harmful situation. For instance, a nurse may report another nurse or doctor who cares for patients while under the influence of controlled substances such as alcohol or cocaine. The decision to "blow the whistle" usually presents a grave dilemma. Health-care workers depend on one another for support and respect. Breaking silence can result in the loss of friendship and even employment. However, the nurse's first allegiance is to the patient.

The Right to Die. The *right to die* is an ethical issue involving witholding or withdrawing consent for treatment. Any competent adult has the right to refuse treatment even if it will eventually result in his death. Conflict arises when a patient is no longer competent or able to make decisions for himself. Then others, such as the next of kin or a physician, may institute treatment because its omission violates his or her own value system. Many patients discuss their philosophy of death and dying with their physician. Some hospitals routinely ask patients about their desire for resuscitative measures even during routine admissions. Still others draw up living wills.

A spokesperson may be selected by a patient. This person then acts on the patient's behalf. The spokesperson makes sure that the patient's wishes are carried out should he become unconscious or unable to express himself. Ethical problems concerning the right to die can develop. This is especially the case when a patient becomes incompetent and has never expressed his wishes regarding prolonging life.

Allocation of Scarce Resources. Though many believe that health care is a right, there may be times when the demand exceeds the supply. *Allocation of scarce resources* means that a decision has to be made to distribute the available equipment or procedures to only one or a few of several who could benefit from it. Some will receive the health-care services and others will be denied. Benefitting one results in harm to the others. This is a classic example of an ethical dilemma. It is a win/lose situation. Ethicists use various strategies to make this type of hard decision. They may elect a "first come/first serve" approach. Or the choice may be made by trying to project which recipient would result in the most good for the most number of people. However, forecasting the future is humanly impossible.

Ethics Committees

Ethical decisions are complex. It is especially difficult to apply justice when facing all the different personalities and variables of each situation. Making a substitute judgment for another is a weighty responsibility. Sometimes many heads are better than one. For this reason ethics committees have been formed. They are composed of groups of people with various backgrounds. Ethics committees are best used in a policy-making capacity before any specific dilemma occurs. These committees also may be called on to offer advice to protect a patient's best interests and to avoid legal battles.

Securing Liability Insurance

Health agencies carry liability insurance to protect themselves and their employees in case of a lawsuit. It is recommended that nurses carry additional malpractice insurance separate from that of an employer. This is especially important if the nurse practices in high-risk areas, such as obstetrics, the emergency department, surgery, or postanesthesia reacting areas. Liability or malpractice insurance is available through the NFLPN, the National Student Nurses' Association, the ANA, and other private insurance companies.

Before purchasing insurance, the nurse should compare policies. The cost of the policy should not be a priority in choosing insurance. Look for a high monetary coverage per professional claim. A professional claim is one that occurs in the performance of nursing acts occurring on or off the job. Check to see if there is also personal liability protection to cover lawsuits involving a non-nursing situation, for instance, if someone slipped on an icy home sidewalk. Read or ask if the insurance covers lawsuits filed in the future although the insurance may not be current at the time the lawsuit is filed. The best policies provide future protection for claims that occurred while the policy was in effect. Statutes of limitations make it possible for lawsuits to be filed long after they actually occurred. Finally, the best types of insurance policies cover defense costs and provide partial reimbursement for lost wages while the lawsuit is in process.

Preventing Lawsuits

The best protection from lawsuits is competent nursing. Competency can be demonstrated by participating in continuing education programs, taking nursing courses at a college or university, and becoming certified. These approaches help the nurse deliver patient care that is safe, adequate, and appropriate. Defensive nursing practice also involves thorough and objective documentation.

Probably the best defense against a lawsuit is to administer care compassionately. The "golden rule" of doing unto others as you would have them do unto you is a good principle to follow. Patients who perceive the nurse as caring and concerned tend to be satisfied with their care. These techniques will communicate a caring attitude:

- Smile.
- Introduce yourself by name.
- Call the patient by the name he prefers.
- Touch the patient appropriately to demonstrate concern.

- Respond quickly to the call-light.
- Communicate the time you will be leaving the unit, how long you will be detained, and inform the patient of your return.
- Provide the name of the person to whom you have delegated his care.
- Spend time with the patient other than performing required care.
- Be a good listener.
- Explain everything so a patient can understand it.
- Be a good host or hostess; offer visitors extra chairs, snacks and beverages, directions for the restrooms and parking areas.
- Accept justifiable criticism without becoming defensive.
- Say "I'm sorry."

The patient can sense when the nurse really wants to do a good job rather than just do a job. The relationship that develops is apt to reduce the potential for a lawsuit, even if harm occurs.

Defense Techniques

Not every lawsuit can be avoided. Physicians are sued 500 times as often as nurses. However, each year nurses continue to be sued with more and more frequency.

The best legal defense is well-written documentation. This applies both to the patient's health record and a factually written incident sheet. An *incident sheet,* shown in Figure 6-1, is a written report of an event that caused harm or could eventually cause harm. It is not a part of the patient's health record. That does not mean, however, that it cannot be used in court by the prosecuting or defense attorneys.

Incident sheets are reviewed by a risk management committee. The main purpose for incident sheets is to determine how similar situations can be prevented. Secondarily, they are used as a reference for any future litigation. The incident sheet should document the who, what, when, where, and how of an event. It should identify all witnesses involved by name. Any pertinent statements made by the injured party before or after the incident should be quoted.

The nurse may choose one other approach. An anecdotal note may be written. An *anecdotal note* is a written report that records the facts about a particular event. This may be compared with making an entry in a personal journal or diary. The anecdotal note should be kept and safeguarded for future retrieval. It can be helpful later for refreshing one's memory. It can also be used as an item of court evidence on advice of one's attorney.

The legal advice in Display 6-4 may be useful if and when a nurse becomes involved in a lawsuit.

INCIDENT REPORT

PERSON INVOLVED:
(Last Name)   (First Name)   (M. I.)

DATE of incident: TIME of incident: SEX: BIRTHDATE:

	Pt. Condition Before Incident:				Room Number
PATIENT	Normal Senile Disoriented Sedated Other				
	Bed Rails:	Height of Bed Adjustable:			Release/Order:
	Up Down	Yes No Up Down			Yes No
	Restraints:				
	Not ordered Ordered Restrained Unrestrained Restraint Removed				

EMPLOYEE   Department   Job Title   Physician Services Offered:
                                                                                                    Accepted   Declined

VISITORS   Home Address   Occupation   Home Phone
                                                                                                 (   )

Witnessed: Yes   No   By Whom: Reason for Presence at This Facility:
  * Describe on back of report

Property Involved: Equipment Involved: Person Authorized to be in Location:
  Describe: Yes   No

Describe incident including injuries in detail. Exactly how person was found.

_____

_____

_____

VITAL SIGNS: B/P   Temp.   Pulse   Resp.   Type of footwear:

Person Seen By a Physician?   WHEN: WHERE: PHYSICIAN'S NAME:
  Yes   No

First Aid Administered?   WHEN: WHERE: BY WHOM:
  Yes   No

Person Taken to a Hospital?   WHEN: WHERE: BY WHOM:
  Yes   No

Date of Report   Title & Signature of Person Preparing Report   Nurse's Signature

Indicate on Diagram Location of Injury

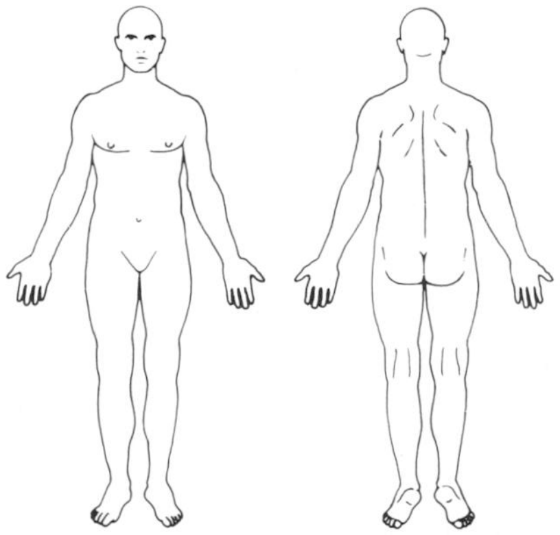

FOR ADMINISTRATIVE USE ONLY
Follow-up:
_____

TYPE OF INJURY

1. Laceration   _____
2. Hematoma   _____
3. Abrasion   _____
4. Burn   _____
5. None Apparent   _____
6. Other: Specify

_____
_____
_____
_____
_____
_____

_____
Reviewed by Director of Nursing   Date

_____
Reviewed by Administrator   Date

Family Notified?   DATE: TIME: WHO: BY WHOM:
  Yes   No
   If No, give reason

Physician's Comment/Signature

Remedial Action Taken:

Figure 6-1 An incident sheet is completed whenever a patient, employee, or visitor is injured. (Courtesy of River Forest Nursing Care Center, Three Rivers, MI.)

Display 6-4. Legal Advice

1. Notify the claims agent of your professional liability insurance company.
2. Contact the National Nurses Claims Data Base through the American Nurses' Association in Kansas City, Missouri. This confidential service provides information that supports nurses involved in litigation.
3. Discuss the particulars of the case only with your attorney.
4. Tell your attorney everything.
5. Avoid giving public statements.
6. Reread the patient's record, incident sheet, and your anecdotal note before testifying.
7. Ask to reread information again in court if it will help to refresh your memory.
8. Dress conservatively in a businesslike manner. Avoid excesses in makeup, hairstyle, or jewelry.
9. Look directly at whomever asks a question.
10. Speak in a modulated but audible voice that can be heard easily by the jury and others in the court.
11. Tell the truth.
12. Use language you are comfortable with. Do not try to impress the court with legal terms.
13. Say as little as possible in court under cross-examination.
14. Answer the prosecuting lawyer's questions with "Yes" or "No"; limit answers to only the questions that are asked.
15. If you do not know or can not remember information, say so.
16. Wait to expand on information if asked by your defense attorney.
17. Remain calm, objective, and cooperative.

Bibliography

Arbeiter J: A buyer's guide to malpractice insurance. RN Magazine 49(5):22–26, 1986

Brown CE: The law and your profession. Journal of Practical Nursing 39(3):14–15, 1989

Code for Nurses with Interpretive Statements. Kansas City, American Nurses' Association, 1985

Cournoyer CP: Protecting yourself legally after a patient's injured. NursingLife 5(2):18–22, 1985

Cushing M: Incident reports: For your eyes only? Am J Nurs 85(8):873–874, 1985

Cushing M: Malpractice: Are you covered? Am J Nurs 84(8):985–986, 1984

Cushing M: When the courts define nursing: What it is, what it does. Am J Nurs 87(6):773–774, 1987

Flight MR: Law, Liability, and Ethics. Albany, Delmar, 1988

Forkner DJ: Expert advice on becoming an expert witness. Nursing 17(6):69–71, 1987

Hardy GR: Ensuring clinical competence. Nursing Management 19(12):46–47, 1988

Hollowell EE, Eldridge JE: The nurse's role in informed consent. Journal of Practical Nursing 39(3):28–31, 1989

Hollowell EE, Eldridge JE: The nursing shortage: The increased risk of legal liability and how to avoid it. Journal of Practical Nursing 39(2):28–31, 1989

Klein CA: Preventing malpractice suits. Nursing Practice 11(3):78, 80, 82, 1986

Kremerer AA: Nurse Practice Acts. AD Nurse 4(2):29–33, 1989

Mancini M: Charting: Keeping it professional so your care can't be faulted. NursingLife 4(5):50–51, 1984

Mandell M: How to defend yourself against lawyer's attacks. NursingLife 7(3):25–29, 1987

Mandell M: Preventing injury. What you don't do can land you in court. NursingLife 7(1):26–28, 1987

Mandell M: Ten legal commandments for nurses who get sued. NursingLife 6(3):18–21, 1986

Murphy EK: Legal aspects of whistle-blowing. AORN J 49(2):480, 482, 484, 1989

Murphy JF, Connel CC: Violations of the state's nurse practice act: How big is the problem? Nursing Management 18(9):44–46, 48, 1987

Northrup CE: Filling in charting gaps . . . in court. Nursing 17(9):43, 1987

Northrup CE: Student nurses and legal accountabilities. Imprint 32(4):16, 18–20, 1985

Pohlman KJ: Privacy, confidentiality, and privilege. Focus on Critical Care 15(6):60–61, 1988

Rabinaw J: Where you stand in the eyes of the law. Nursing 19(2):34–42, 1989

Rhodes AM: Contents of nurses' detailed notes. Maternal and Child Nursing 12(1):61, 1987

Scrivenger M: Nursing ethics and the law. Nursing Times 83(42):28–29, 1987

Stabler–Haas S: A strategy for avoiding a lawsuit. Critical Care Nurse 9(2):12–13, 1989

Weeks LC, Gleason VR, Reiser S: How can a hospital ethics committee help? Am J Nurs 89(5):651–652, 1989

Wright RA: Human Values in Health Care. New York, McGraw–Hill, 1987

Unit II

Nursing Skills for Health Promotion and Maintenance

7

Promoting Personal Hygiene

Chapter Outline

Behavioral Objectives
Glossary
Introduction
Structures and Functions of the Skin and Mucous
    Membranes
Assessment of the Skin and Related Structures
Caring for Healthy Skin
Ordering and Recording Hygienic Care
Providing for a Bath or Shower
Tepid Sponging
Perineal Care
The Backrub
Shaving
Care of the Teeth and Mouth
Care of the Eyes and Visual Aids
Care of the Ears and Hearing Aids
Care of the Nose
Care of the Fingernails
Care of the Feet and Toenails
Care of the Hair
Suggested Measures for Hygiene in Selected Situations
Applicable Nursing Diagnoses
Teaching Suggestions for Personal Hygiene
Bibliography

Skill Procedures

Providing for Tub or Shower Bathing
Assisting With a Bed Bath
Giving a Complete Bed Bath
Tepid Sponging
Administering Perineal Care
Giving a Backrub
Shaving a Patient
Brushing and Flossing the Teeth
Performing Oral Hygiene Measures
Cleansing the Eyes
Removing, Cleaning, and Replacing Contact Lenses
Inserting a Hearing Aid
Shampooing Hair

Behavioral Objectives

When the content of this chapter has been mastered, the learner will be able to:

Define the terms appearing in the glossary.

Discuss briefly the variations in the location of nursing orders and the recording of hygienic care.

List at least four reasons for bathing.

Identify four methods of bathing a patient.

List three modifications of bathing that occur in various health agencies.

Discuss the components of healthy skin, mucous membranes, nails, hair, vision, and hearing.

Describe how to care for the patient's perineal area, teeth and mouth, including dentures and bridges, and for the eyes, ears, nose, fingernails, feet, toenails, and hair.

Discuss the care of eyeglasses, contact lenses, artificial eyes, and hearing aids.

List suggested measures for promoting personal hygiene in selected situations, as described in this chapter.

Summarize suggestions for patient teaching offered in this chapter.

Glossary

Acne A skin eruption due to inflammation and infection of oil glands in the skin.

Antiperspirant A preparation for reducing the amount of perspiration on the skin.

Bridge A dental appliance that replaces one or several teeth.

Callus A thickening of the outer layer of the skin.

Caries The decay of teeth with the formation of cavities.

Cerumen The waxlike substance found in the external canal of the ear.

Ceruminous glands Glands in the skin that secrete cerumen.

Decibel A measurement of sound.

Denture A dental appliance of artificial teeth that replaces the person's own upper, lower, or all teeth.

Deodorant A preparation to mask or diminish body odors.

Emollient An agent to soften, smooth, and protect the skin.

Eye fatigue The discomfort experienced from poor lighting or prolonged focusing on an object.

Feedback The loud, shrill noise from a hearing aid that is not fitted snugly into the ear canal.

Field of vision The ability to see images in all directions.

Generalist A nurse who carries out the nursing process with a broad cross-section of patients.

Gingivitis Inflammation of the gums.

Hygiene The establishment and preservation of well-being through personal care.

Integument A covering; refers to the skin.

Integumentary system The skin and its parts including mucous membranes, hair, and nails.

Mucus The slimy substance secreted by glands in the mucous membranes.

Perineal care Cleansing the genital and anal areas.

Periodontitis Severe inflammation of the gums and bone tissue around the teeth. Synonym for *pyorrhea*.

Plaque A mass of bacteria covering teeth, causing cavities and gum disease.

Podiatrist A specialist on care of the feet.

Prosthesis A manmade object that replaces a natural body part.

Pyorrhea Severe inflammation of the gums and bone tissue around teeth. Synonym for *periodontitis*.

Sebaceous glands Glands in the skin that secrete sebum.

Sebum A thick, fatty substance secreted by the sebaceous glands.

Specialist A nurse who has obtained advanced education and usually cares for a specific category of patients.

Visual acuity The ability to see words or objects that are near or far both clearly and comfortably.

Introduction

Hygiene deals with the establishment and preservation of well-being through personal care. This chapter discusses common practices that contribute to well-being through cleanliness, grooming, and care of vision and hearing.

A person's health values and health perception can be associated with his degree of self-care including personal hygiene, dental care, and care of vision and hearing. People differ in their practices of personal health management. For example, some people prefer bathing to showering; some brush their teeth after every meal and others just in the morning and evening; some keep regular appointments when their vision or hearing becomes impaired, while others live with their losses.

A primary concern for nurses is that personal care be carried out in a manner that promotes health. Personal care does not have to be carried out in an identical fashion among all people. In fact, to do so would ignore the individuality among people in relation to their age, inherited characteristics, and cultural background. The exact way it is done is less important than the fact that it meets the health needs of the individual. The nurse must become tolerant of personal preferences and adapt to the differences among people.

The nurse should reinforce and encourage appropriate hygiene practices among healthy individuals. There may be opportunities to teach patients and their families new or modified practices that may improve established hygiene patterns. For those who are ill, the nurse may substitute the care that a patient is unable to perform. The nurse may be one of the first to detect deficits in hearing and vision. Referrals may be made to other health practitioners who can help improve an individual's overall health and quality of life.

Structures and Functions of the Skin and Mucous Membranes

The word *integument* means a covering. The largest organ that covers the body is the skin. The main components of the *integumentary system* include the skin, its various parts such as hair and nails, and mucous membranes.

Within the skin there are specialized glands and cells that support the healthy functions of this system. *Sebaceous glands* secrete *sebum,* a thick, fatty substance that oils the skin and keeps it supple. Sebum also lubricates the hair. Sweat glands secrete perspiration. *Ceruminous glands* secrete *cerumen,* a waxlike substance found in the external canal of the ear.

The mucous membranes are continuous with the skin. They line body passages that open to the outside of the body. These passages include the digestive, respiratory, urinary, and reproductive systems. The conjunctiva of the eye is also lined with mucous membrane. Goblet cells in the mucous membranes secrete *mucus,* which is the slimy substance that keeps the membranes soft and moist.

The skin has a variety of functions, including the following:

- It protects the body.
- It helps regulate body temperature.
- It assists with the body's fluid and chemical balance.
- It has nerve endings that are sensitive to pain, temperature, touch, and pressure.
- It produces vitamin D with the help of sunlight, and the vitamin D is then absorbed from the skin into the body.
- It provides a basis for personal identification.

Assessment of the Skin and Related Structures

Most beginning nurses are generalists. *Generalists* are nurses who are expected to carry out the nursing process with a broad cross-section of patients. They gather data to maintain and improve a healthy state as well as to identify alterations associated with common diseases. The assessment skills that are discussed in this book are those geared for a generalist. A *specialist* is a nurse who has obtained additional education that includes the performance of advanced assessment techniques. A specialist nurse usually limits clinical practice to the care of a specific category of patients, such as coronary care, care of emergency and trauma patients, or care of high-risk infants.

Assessment techniques as performed by a nurse generalist are discussed in more depth in Chapter 14. The following will help lay the foundation for the hygiene skills that are the subject of this chapter.

Characteristics of Healthy Skin and Mucous Membranes. There are general features of the skin that are important to evaluate. One of the first concerns should be whether the skin is intact. Its very protective nature depends on this quality. The color of the skin should be uniform and reflect the ethnic origin of the patient. The texture, or feel, to the skin should be warm, soft, smooth, and easily moved. Mucous membranes should be pink, moist, and smooth.

Characteristics of Healthy Hair. Hair generally covers similar parts of each adult male or female. There are hereditary factors that may affect its distribution, color, and texture. Some individuals may alter these characteristics cosmetically. The nurse should evaluate the cleanliness and luster of hair when assessing the individual's personal hygiene.

Characteristics of Healthy Nails. Fingernails and toenails are hardened extensions of the skin. They should be thin, pink, and smooth. A free margin should extend from the end of each nail. The skin around the nail should be intact.

Characteristics of Healthy Teeth. Adults normally have 32 permanent teeth. The color of teeth generally is a result of inheritance. Some drugs, food and beverages, and tobacco may discolor teeth. Teeth should be firm in the gums without open spaces. Any malposition, missing teeth, or offensive breath odor may reflect information about the oral hygiene of the patient.

Characteristics of Normal Vision. Vision depends on normally functioning structures of the eyes. Each eye should be assessed separately. Normal vision includes the ability to identify words or objects without straining. Vision should be comfortable both at a maximum distance of 20 feet and as close as one would hold a book for reading. This is called *visual acuity.* The ability to see without effort, especially for close or fine work, becomes increasingly difficult as individuals age. Glasses may be worn by persons over 40 to restore adequate vision.

Another normal characteristic of vision is the ability to identify colors correctly. Most individuals can inform the nurse about any problems they may have in color perception. It is also normal for individuals to see images in all directions within a full circle. This is called the *field of vision.*

Characteristics of Normal Hearing. Just as vision changes with age, so does hearing. Hearing should be adequate to understand words spoken with a normal voice at a conversational distance. Most can also distinguish a whisper at two feet in a quiet room. Each ear should be assessed separately. Any hearing, visual, or dental aids that replace and restore normal functioning should be noted on a patient's record.

Caring for Healthy Skin

One of the primary practices associated with personal hygiene is regular bathing. Cleansing the skin helps remove bacteria, oils, and dirt. These substances are responsible for body odor and the potential for infection. *Deodorants* mask or diminish body odor; *antiperspirants* contain a chemical to close or clog pores, thus reducing perspiration on the skin. Bathing should always precede the use of any cosmetic product.

The following are examples of practices that protect unbroken and healthy skin. There may be times when the nurse will need to perform skills that meet the hygiene needs of a patient when the individual cannot do so independently.

Bathing is an important part of hygiene whether accomplished in a tub or shower. It serves various purposes:

- The bath cleans the skin and gives a feeling of refreshment.
- The warmth of bath water and the massage associated with washing and drying the skin aid relaxation.
- Circulation of blood is stimulated as a result of the friction created by washing and drying the skin.
- The activity involved when giving a bath acts as a muscle toner and body conditioner. Sometimes, it may even help stimulate the appetite.
- The bath often helps improve self-image and morale.
- Discomfort is often relieved by bathing. Moist heat is soothing to sore muscles. Some medications can be added to bath water to treat skin conditions, skin dryness, or itching.

Ordering and Recording Hygienic Care

Health agency policies differ concerning hygienic care. Most often, a nursing team leader or primary nurse takes the responsibility for writing nursing orders for hygienic care. These usually appear on the nursing care plan. Some hygienic care may require a physician's order. An example is cutting the toenails. It is important that the nurse follow orders on the nursing care plan or consult the supervising nurse if there are doubts about what may or may not be done.

Agency policies also differ about what hygienic care is recorded and where. Many agencies no longer require recording routine hygienic care, such as bathing a patient. Others may require that certain hygienic care, such as giving a shampoo, be recorded. Still others may record all hygienic care. The nurse should observe policies about writing orders and recording in the agency where the care is given.

Providing for a Bath or Shower

Skilled nursing procedures are described throughout this chapter and text. All procedures should be explained by the nurse to the patient. The nurse should always begin and end each procedure with hand-washing. The equipment should be put away and the patient returned to a comfortable position. These steps will not necessarily be repeated in each skill that is discussed, but they always represent necessary components whenever a skill is performed.

Skill Procedure 7-1 describes a suggested method for the nurse to follow when the patient is well enough to perform his own tub bath or shower. The nurse should encourage as much independence and participation from the patient as possible not only in relation to hygiene but also with any care that is planned.

Sometimes the patient cannot go to a bathroom, but can bathe most of his body at the bedside with a minimum of assistance. The description for a bed bath taken by a patient can be found in Skill Procedure 7-2.

Skill Procedure 7-1. Providing for Tub or Shower Bathing

Suggested Action	Reason for Action
Clean the tub or shower.	Use of a common tub or shower is a way that bacteria can be transferred among patients.
Assemble supplies and clean garments near the shower or tub.	Organizing equipment prevents the patient from becoming tired or chilled once the bath has begun.
Use a nonskid bathmat or strips in tubs or showers. A bath towel may be used as a substitute if a mat is not available.	The floors of tubs and showers are slippery. Modifying the surface may prevent falls.
Regulate the temperature of the water to between 40° C to 43° C (105° F to 110° F) or adjust water in the shower to the appropriate temperature. To prevent burning, do not turn on hot water while the patient is in the tub except with extreme caution.	The temperature of the water should be warm but not hot enough to burn the skin. Agitate the water well to equalize the water temperature.
Fill the tub approximately half full.	Water is displaced when the patient sits in a tub. Filling a tub half full prevents spilling, which could be a safety hazard.
Escort the patient to the shower or tub.	If the patient becomes weak, the nurse will be there for assistance.
Place a DO NOT DISTURB sign on the door.	The nurse is responsible for protecting the patient from invasion of privacy.
If necessary, help the patient into the tub or shower; place your hands in his armpits or place a chair next to the tub.	Supporting the weight of the patient helps provide stability for maintaining balance.
Have the patient ease himself from the chair to the edge of the tub, pivot, place his feet in the tub, and then lower his body.	Using slow, simple instructions will promote safety through the coordinated efforts of the patient and the nurse. More falls take place in the bathroom than any other location.

(continued)

Skill Procedure 7-1. *Continued*

Suggested Action	Reason for Action
Encourage the patient to use handrails while in the shower.	Installed rails provide a permanent safety device that prevents falls.
A stool may be placed in the shower.	If the patient becomes tired or weak, the stool may be used for both comfort and support.
Remain with the patient if he appears weak, faint, or fearful.	The nurse may be held liable for any injury that may occur because of poor judgment or negligence.
Provide the patient with a means to summon the nurse.	The patient may appear capable of bathing without assistance but may develop problems later.
Adult patients may be left alone, but stay close at hand and check the patient frequently.	The nearer the nurse, the quicker assistance may be provided. Children should never be left alone in a tub or shower.
The nurse may make the bed while the patient is in the tub or shower if the patient can be left alone.	The patient may wish to go directly to bed following bathing. A bed with clean linen extends the feeling of refreshment from the bath.
Offer to assist the patient with bathing.	There may be some parts of his body, such as his back, that he cannot reach but would appreciate to have washed.
Assist the patient out of the tub or shower onto a dry bath mat.	Wet, slippery floors can lead to falls.
Help the patient, as necessary, with drying and putting on a gown or pajamas.	Some patients may have used considerable energy in bathing and appreciate assistance with getting dressed.
Help the patient back to a clean bed and give the patient a backrub following the suggestions in Skill Procedure 7-6.	A backrub can further contribute to a feeling of relaxation while at the same time it stimulates the circulation to the skin.
When the patient is comfortable, return to the bathroom, remove all soiled and wet linen, and restore the room for the next patient's use.	Leaving the bathroom in the same way it was found is one way that nurses work as a conscientious team.

There may be times when the patient is too ill or weak to bathe by himself. The nurse may need to bathe the patient. Skill Procedure 7-3 describes and illustrates a suggested way to give a bed bath. However, agency procedures do vary. Variations in the bathing procedure are usually of little significance. The important thing is to accomplish the purposes for which the bath is given.

Some agencies schedule routines during which baths are given during morning hours; others may schedule bathing at other times of the day. Some agencies offer complete baths every day; others schedule them two or three times weekly. Table 7-1 describes other common bathing modifications that may be practiced in various health agencies.

Giving a bed bath offers the nurse an excellent time to become better acquainted with a patient and to work on developing a helping relationship with him. Other nursing contacts with the patient tend to be more brief than the time involved in giving a bath. Good opportunities for assessment and health teaching usually arise while bathing

a patient. Giving a patient a bath demonstrates caring, an important aspect of the nurse–patient relationship.

Tepid Sponging

The skin has many protective and regulatory functions. Bathing is a hygienic measure for removing dirt, bacteria, and oily secretions. Intact, clean skin prevents infection.

The skin also helps to regulate body temperature. Shivering increases heat production. Perspiration promotes heat loss through evaporation. It is a more effective mechanism in adults than in children. Children perspire much less in comparison.

Bathing has another therapeutic use. Tepid sponging is a therapeutic bath for reducing a dangerously high fever in infants, and children. Children have a large proportion of body surface area. They have less body fat. This means that their blood vessels lie very near the skin. By substituting bathing for perspiration, it is possible to reduce a fever. Fevers that exceed 104°F (40°C) increase the risk for sei-

Skill Procedure 7-2. Assisting With a Bed Bath

Suggested Action	Reason for Action
Roll the head of the bed to a sitting position or help the patient sit on the edge of the bed.	The patient will use less energy in reaching the equipment and parts of his body in this position.
Pull the curtains around the patient's bed.	This protects the patient's privacy and prevents chilling from drafts.
Assemble the following equipment: basin with warm water between 40° C to 43° C (105° F to 110° F), towels, bath blanket, soap, shaving equipment, mirror, oral hygiene supplies, cosmetics, and clean bed clothes.	Organizing equipment prevents fatigue, delay, and chilling during a bath.
Remove the top linens and replace them with a bath blanket.	A bath blanket absorbs water and is likely to provide more warmth than sheets.
Allow the patient to bathe himself; assist him as necessary.	Most patients prefer to be alone while bathing. There may be some areas of the body with which the patient may appreciate assistance, such as the back, buttocks, lower legs, and feet.
Change the water frequently.	The water may become cool and soapy.
Remove the bath water and make the patient's bed. A method for bedmaking can be found in Skill Procedure 12-1.	Removing the water prevents any spilling on the floor. The patient will feel more refreshed with a clean change of linen.
Give the patient a backrub. Suggestions for giving a backrub can be found in Skill Procedure 7-6.	Following the activities of bathing and bedmaking with a backrub will restore a feeling of relaxation and rest.
Clean and put away all the patient's personal hygiene items to their proper place.	A sense of orderliness will contribute to relaxation, and the patient will know where to look for his bathing supplies when needed again.

zures. Methods for assessing body temperature are described in Chapter 13. Skill Procedure 7-4 explains the steps in performing tepid sponging for an infant or child. Alcohol and cool water baths for adults with more serious heat-regulating conditions are discussed in Chapter 20.

Perineal Care

There are times when the patient cannot wash his own genital and anal areas at the time of a bath, or this type of hygiene may require more skill than the patient can provide. The special care of this area is called *perineal care.* The nurse should not ignore or omit cleansing this area because many bacteria and secretions located there could lead to unpleasant odors or infection. The method for administering perineal care is described in Skill Procedure 7-5.

The Backrub

A backrub is ordinarily given after a patient is bathed. It acts as a general body conditioner and promotes relaxation and comfort. If given briskly, it can also act as a stimulant. A good backrub should take a minimum of 4 to 6 minutes to complete. It is the rare patient who does not enjoy, appreciate, and remember a good backrub.

The nurse should know the patient's diagnosis before giving a backrub. It is usually contraindicated, for example, for patients who have fractured ribs, have had back surgery, or have had a heart attack. Skill Procedure 7-6 describes how to give a backrub.

Shaving

In the United States, a common hygiene routine for men is to remove, clean, or groom facial hair. Most men prefer to be clean shaven. American women shave the hair from their legs and underarms. Many prefer to shave at the time of bathing. The patient should be consulted about his preferences for this personal practice.

On the basis of the nurse's knowledge some modifications for shaving may need to be made. For instance, patients who have blood disorders or take medications that increase the tendency to bleed should use electric razors. Also, use of a razor with a blade by a confused or depressed person should be forbidden to prevent accidental or self-inflicted injury. Those receiving oxygen may use safety or battery-operated razors to reduce electrical hazards and the possibility of combustion.

(Text continues on page 94)

Skill Procedure 7-3. Giving a Complete Bed Bath

Suggested Action	Reason for Action
Preparing for the Bath	

Suggested Action	Reason for Action
Bring articles needed for hygiene and bedmaking to the bedside and arrange them in order of their use on the bedside table, overbed table, or a chair. The bathwater should be comfortably warm, about 40° C to 43° C (105° F to 110° F). Include equipment for shaving and oral hygiene. If the patient uses a safety razor, he will need a basin of hot water, a mirror, and a good light.	Bringing everything to the bedside conserves time and energy. Arranging items conveniently and in order of their use saves time and helps prevent stretching and twisting of the nurse's muscles. Warm water is comfortable and relaxing for the patient.
Pull curtains or shut the door.	The patient's privacy and warmth are maintained from unnecessary exposure.
Place an adjustable bed in the high position and lower the siderails.	Having the bed in a high position and removing the bed siderails prevent strain on the nurse's back.
Loosen top linen where it is tucked under the mattress. Fold the spread and blankets individually from top to bottom and in half again (in fourths). Drape them over the back of a chair if they are to be reused. If not, fold them again one or two times and place them in a laundry hamper. Keep linens away from the uniform while handling them.	Folding linen in place and as it is removed avoids stretching of the arms and saves time and energy when putting it back on the bed later. Keeping linens away from the uniform help prevent the spread of organisms.
Place a fanfolded bath blanket over the patient's chest and have the patient hold the top edge of the bath blanket. Grasp the bottom of the bath blanket and the top edge of the sheet; pull the sheet and bath blanket together to the foot of the bed. Remove the sheet and place it in a hamper.	The patient is not exposed unnecessarily as the top sheet is removed, thus avoiding drafts.
Assist the patient to the side of the bed where you will work. Have him lie on his back.	Having the patient positioned near the nurse helps prevent unnecessary stretching and twisting of muscles.
Assist the patient with oral hygiene, as necessary, and as described in the text.	Oral hygiene is an important part of helping to keep the mouth and teeth clean, healthy, and refreshed.
Remove the patient's gown by slipping it off under the bath blanket. Remove all but one pillow and place the bed in a flat position.	Keeping the bath blanket in place avoids exposure and chilling. Having the patient flat in bed with one pillow is comfortable for most patients and convenient for the nurse.

| General Techniques to Observe During the Bathing Procedure | |

Suggested Action	Reason for Action
Protect the bed linens with a towel while bathing each part of the body.	Keeping the linens protected with a towel prevents the patient from feeling uncomfortable in a damp or wet bed.
Expose, wash, rinse, and dry one part of the body at a time.	Exposing, washing, rinsing, and drying one part of the body at a time avoids unnecessary exposure and chilling.
Fold the washcloth like a mitt on the hand so that there are no loose ends.	Having loose ends of cloth drag across the patient's skin is uncomfortable for the patient. Loose ends cool quickly and will feel cold to the patient.
Keep the washcloth wet enough to wash, lather, and rinse well but not so wet that it drips.	Dripping water from the washcloth is uncomfortable for the patient and will dampen the bed. Too little moisture on the cloth makes thorough washing and rinsing difficult.

(continued)

Skill Procedure 7-3. Continued

Suggested Action	Reason for Action

General Techniques to Observe During the Bathing Procedure

Wash, rinse, and dry the skin well. Change the water as necessary if it becomes dirty or too soapy for thorough washing and rinsing.	Thorough cleaning removes dirt, oil, and many organisms. Soap or moisture left on the skin is uncomfortable and may irritate the skin.
Do not leave the soap in the bathwater.	The soap will become soft and water becomes too soapy for good rinsing.
Use firm but gentle strokes while washing and drying the patient. Use strokes as long as the body part allows.	Friction helps remove dirt, oil, and organisms and helps dry the skin. Friction stimulates circulation and muscles. Too much friction may injure tender skin. Long, firm strokes are relaxing and more comfortable than are short, uneven strokes.
Pay particular attention to these areas: under the breasts; axillae; between fingers and toes; in any folds of the skin, such as in the groin or on the abdomen of a patient who is obese; behind the ears; and the umbilicus.	Organisms and dirt are lodged in areas where skin touches skin; if these areas are not washed, rinsed, and dried well, they will become irritated, and injury to the skin will eventually occur.

Bathing the Patient

With no soap on the washcloth, wipe one eye from the inner part of the eye near the nose to the outer part near the forehead, as illustrated in Figure 7-1. Rinse or turn the cloth before washing the other eye. Bathe the patient's face, neck, and ears, avoiding soap on the face if the patient prefers.	Bathing one eye and then the other prevents spreading organisms from one to the other. Soap is irritating to the eyes. Moving from the inner to the outer aspect of the eye prevents carrying debris toward the lacrimal duct, from which it may enter the nose.

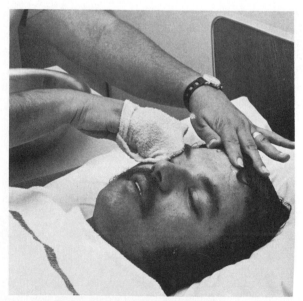

Figure 7-1 The patient lies near the side of the bed where the nurse works. The nurse washes the patient's eye by moving from the inner aspect of the eye outward to the area near the temple.

(continued)

Skill Procedure 7-3. *Continued*

Suggested Action	**Reason for Action**

Bathing the Patient

Bathe the patient's arms, the one farther from the nurse and then the other, as illustrated in Figure 7-2 . The axillae may be bathed with the arms or with the chest, which is bathed after the arms and hands are finished.

If the nearer arm is washed first, the water may accidentally drip on the clean arm as the nurse reaches to do the other.

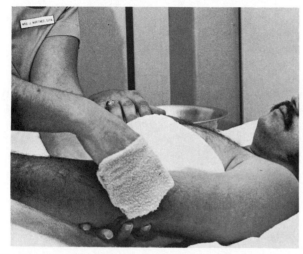

Figure 7-2 The arm farther from the nurse is washed before the one that is closer. A towel protects the bed.

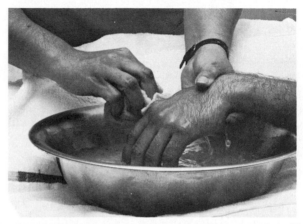

Figure 7-3 The patient's hand is washed by being placed in a basin of water.

Place the hands in the wash basin for bathing, as illustrated in Figure 7-3.

Placing the hands in the basin of water to bathe them is comfortable and relaxing for the patient and allows for a thorough washing of the hands and the areas between the fingers.

Bathe the leg, thigh, and groin area farther from the nurse first, as illustrated in Figure 7-4. The front of the thighs and the groin may be washed with the abdomen, and the back of the thighs with the back if desired.

If the nearer leg is washed first, water may accidentally drip on the clean leg as the nurse reaches across to do the other.

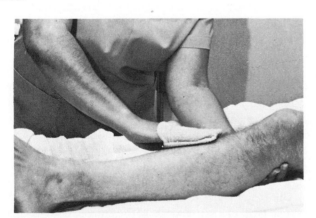

Figure 7-4 The leg farther from the nurse is washed before the leg that is nearer. A towel protects the bed.

(*continued*)

Skill Procedure 7-3. Continued

Suggested Action	**Reason for Action**

Bathing the Patient

Place the feet in the wash basin while supporting the ankle and heel in your hand and the leg on your arm. Bathe the feet. Groom the toenails after bathing and drying the feet. Change the water or wash the feet after the genital area is washed in the manner described below.	Supporting the foot and leg helps reduce strain and discomfort for the patient. Placing the feet in a basin of water to bathe them is comfortable and relaxing for the patient and allows for a thorough cleaning of the feet and the areas between the toes.
Leave the patient at this time, if safe, after placing the wash basin, washcloth, and towel within easy reach so that he can wash the genital and anal areas. If the patient requires assistance, use Skill Procedure 7-5 as a guide.	
Discard the used washcloth, towel, and water. Obtain fresh water. Have the patient lie on his abdomen or on his side, facing away from the nurse. Tuck the clean towel under the length of the back. Wash the back of the neck, shoulders, back, and buttocks. Expose and wash the upper back only, and then the lower back, if the patient is likely to become chilled.	The washcloth, towel, and water are considered highly contaminated after washing the genital and anal areas. Changing to clean supplies decreases the spread of organisms.
The genital and anal areas may be washed after the back, thus eliminating the need to change the washcloth, towel, and water. Follow agency procedure.	

The nurse may need to shave patients from time to time. Some patients may be unable to shave because they are too ill or because an arm is immobilized in a cast or traction. Skill Procedure 7-7 describes suggestions for shaving that the nurse may find helpful.

Care of the Teeth and Mouth

General good health is important for keeping the mouth and teeth healthy. Unfortunately, dental diseases are common primarily because of poor oral hygiene, lack of dental care, and general poor eating habits. Another point of concern to nurses is that many persons who observe good practices of oral hygiene when well often become careless and unmotivated in carrying out oral hygiene when ill.

Benefits of Good Oral Hygiene. The following are some benefits of good oral hygiene:

- Most persons report that they enjoy the aesthetic effects of having the mouth and teeth well cared for and clean.
- Proper oral hygiene and the prevention of mouth diseases help improve a person's self-image.
- Because the process of digestion starts in the mouth, sound practices of oral care promote digestion.

- The pleasure of eating and the taste of food is improved when practices of oral hygiene are observed.
- Proper mouth and tooth care decrease various infections and the decay of teeth.

The decay of teeth with the formation of cavities is called *caries.* One of the leading contributors to dental caries is accumulated plaque. *Plaque* is a mass of bacteria that covers teeth, and it can extend to the roots of teeth, thus causing cavities and gum disease. Plaque can be removed with daily dental care. Figure 7-10 illustrates the chain of events that leads to dental caries. Breaking the chain with oral hygiene techniques can reduce their formation.

There are several commonly recommended ways to help prevent caries: cutting down on sweets, such as soft drinks, candy, gum, and pastries; brushing the teeth often and as soon after eating and snacking as possible; if brushing is not convenient, rinsing the mouth well with water after eating; using a toothpaste, powder, or rinse containing fluoride; and visiting the dentist regularly, at least once or twice a year.

The major cause of tooth loss in adults is gum disease. *Gingivitis* is an inflammation of the gums; a common cause is trench mouth, properly called Vincent's disease. Severe inflammation of the gums, including the bone tissue around the teeth, is called *periodontitis,* or *pyorrhea.* Regu-

Table 7-1. Modifications of the Bath Procedure

Modification	Description
Partial bath	Follow Skill Procedure 7-3, but omit bathing the chest, abdomen, legs, thighs, and feet. Give the patient a backrub. Tighten the bottom linens securely before replacing top linens.
Early A.M. care, given before daytime activities begin or breakfast is served	Offer the bedpan or urinal.
	Supply water, soap, washcloth, and a towel for the patient to wash his hands and face. Assist the patient as necessary.
	Give the patient equipment and supplies to care for his teeth, mouth, and hair. Assist the patient as necessary.
	Straighten bed linens and assist the patient to a position in bed so that he is ready for breakfast.
P.M. or H.S. (Hour of Sleep) care, carried out in preparation for sleep	Assist the patient as necessary with the care of the teeth, mouth, and hair. Offer the patient a bedpan or urinal.
	Wash the patient's face and hands. Wash the patient's back and give him a backrub. Fanfold top linens to the foot of the bed if a bath blanket is used. Straighten and tighten the bed linens.
	Prepare the patient for sleep: arrange his pillows comfortably; offer an extra blanket; lower an adjustable bed; put up the bed siderails; adjust the temperature and ventilation as necessary; and darken the room.

Skill Procedure 7-4. Tepid Sponging

Suggested Action	Reason for Action
Assess the child's temperature as described in Chapter 13.	Sponging is not appropriate unless the body temperature is 102° F (38.8° C) or higher.
Notify the doctor if the temperature is above 102° F (38.8° C).	The doctor may advise additional measures for reducing the fever such as administering medications.
Close the privacy curtains and the door in the room used for bathing.	Drafts may cause shivering, which counteracts the purpose of tepid sponging.
Fill a tub or basin with water. Water may need to be warmer than tepid, over 93° F (33.9° C) initially. A beginning temperature of 98.6° F (37° C) may be more tolerated until the child adjusts to lower temperatures as the water cools.	The water must be warm enough to prevent chilling but cooler than the child's body temperature to promote heat loss.
Omit the addition of alcohol to the water.	Alcohol speeds evaporation, but in a small child gradual heat loss is safer than producing a rapid change in body temperature.
Get a supply of face cloths and towels. Protect the bed with waterproof material and an absorbent bath towel or bath blanket if a basin rather than tub will be used.	A child should not be left alone once sponging begins. Having all the supplies together saves time.
Remove the child's clothing.	Clothing acts as insulation. Exposing body surface promotes heat loss.
Place the child in the tub of water or lay the child on the bed.	Sponging can take ½ hour or longer. The choice of using a tub or basin depends upon the availability of each, the size of the child, and what is convenient for the nurse.

(continued)

Skill Procedure 7-4. *Continued*

Suggested Action	Reason for Action
Observe the child's reaction to the temperature of the water. Remove the child and add warm water if shivering occurs.	Water that is too cool will have the opposite effect. Shivering produces heat and is an undesirable response while administering a tepid sponge bath.
Use a sponge or saturated wash cloth and squeeze the water over exposed skin in the tub.	The immersed body will cool from contact with the tepid water. Skin that is not immersed will cool as the water evaporates from its surface.
In bed, apply moist face cloths or hand towels bilaterally to the axilla and groin.	Large arteries are located superficially in these areas. Cooling the skin will cool the blood and reduce the internal temperature of the child.
Reapply the cloths as they become warm.	Warmed cloths need to be replaced to continue promoting heat loss.
Wipe, but do not rub, the surface of each extremity, the back, and buttocks with damp cloths.	Rubbing causes friction and produces heat.
Concentrate on each area for approximately 3–5 minutes.	Chilling may occur with heat loss from multiple or large areas of the body surface.
Cover half of the body with a light towel or bath blanket.	Partial covering can prevent or relieve chilling.
Reassess body temperature in 15 minutes to ½ hour. Record each assessment.	A trend toward a gradual decrease in body temperature is an indication that tepid sponging is therapeutically effective.
Continue bathing until the temperature is below 102° F (38.8° C) and appears to be stabilized.	A stabilized temperature indicates there is less likelihood that it will drift to dangerously higher levels. Sponging is no longer neessary once a fever remains below 102° F (38.8° C).
Pat the skin dry. Dress in light, loose-fitting clothing or just a diaper or underwear.	Air currents passing over the body continue to promote heat loss.
Protect the child's safety in a crib or playpen while disposing of the wet linen and other equipment.	A child with a fever is often irritable and drowsy. Safety needs must be considered.
Replace oral liquids that may have been lost due to fever and increased metabolism.	Maintaining adequate fluid intake prevents dehydration.
Continue to monitor the temperature frequently and renotify the doctor if the high fever returns.	Additional fever-reducing measures may be necessary. Brain damage or death can occur when body temperature remains dangerously high.

lar dental care and good oral hygiene are the best ways to prevent periodontitis.

Brushing the Teeth. A toothbrush should be small enough to reach all teeth. The bristles should be firm enough to clean well, but not so firm that they are likely to injure tissues. Many dentists recommend a soft-textured, multitufted toothbrush with a flat brushing surface. Others recommend brushes with widely spaced tufts. When tufts are widely spaced, the brush is easier to keep clean and dry. Electric or battery-operated toothbrushes have been found to be as good as hand brushes.

Opinion differs on the best way to brush the teeth. Some dentists recommend that the brush be placed at a 45° angle at the area where the teeth and gums meet, with the tufts facing in the direction of the gums. Other dentists recommend that the brush be placed at the same angle but with the tufts facing away from the gum line. When assisting and teaching patients, the nurse will wish to follow the preference of the patient's dentist.

Flossing the Teeth. Many bacteria in the mouth become lodged between the teeth. The toothbrush cannot reach these areas well. Therefore, flossing several times a day is recommended. The practice not only removes what the brush cannot, but also helps to break up groups of bacteria between teeth. There are no significant differences between the ability of waxed and unwaxed dental floss to remove plaque. Waxed floss is thicker than unwaxed, making it slightly harder to insert into narrow

Skill Procedure 7-5. Administering Perineal Care

Suggested Action	Reason for Action
For Female Patient	
Bring equipment and supplies to the bedside, including soap or solution for cleaning, clean washcloths or cotton balls, and plain water for rinsing. The solution should be about 40° C (105° F).	Bringing everything to the bedside saves time and energy. A warm solution will be comfortable for the patient.
Place the patient on her back and cover with a bath blanket. Fanfold the top linens to the foot of the bed.	Proper draping prevents unnecessary exposure and chilling of the patient.
Place a towel beneath the buttocks or place the patient on a bedpan.	These measures provide for the collection or absorption of water.
Bend the patient's knees and spread her legs.	This exposes the area that will be washed.
Wear gloves if an infection or blood may be present.	Gloves act as a transmission barrier between microbes and the nurse.
Separate the folds of the labia and wash from the pubic area toward the anal area. Use a clean area of the washcloth or a separate cotton ball for each stroke.	Care is taken to avoid introducing secretions and bacteria into the opening through which urine is released. This could cause a urinary tract infection.
Rinse the area, following the same steps described above, with a clean washcloth, cotton balls, and water, or water may be poured from a height of 15 cm (6 in) over the area.	Rinsing removes loosened dirt, organisms, and soap.
Dry the area well.	Drying prevents skin irritation and injury.
Turn the patient to the side. Wash away from the genital area. Rinse and dry well.	Cleaning an area where there are fewer organisms before an area with many helps prevent spreading them to cleaner parts of the body.
For Male Patient	
Follow the same general instructions described previously with the following modifications.	The differences in male and female genital anatomy call for some modifications.
Place a towel under the penis in addition to the one under the buttocks.	Male patients are generally not placed on a bedpan, and the extra towel will absorb any excess.
Grasp the shaft of the penis; if the patient is not circumcised, carefully pull back the foreskin.	Secretions collect within the loose folds of the skin that covers the tip of an uncircumcised penis.
Clean the end of the penis toward the pubic area with circular motions made with cotton balls or the washcloth. Never go back over an area once it has been cleaned.	Washing toward the pubis prevents dirt and secretions from being introduced into the opening from which urine is released.
Rinse and dry the penis. Replace the foreskin to its original position covering the penis.	Replacing the foreskin prevents injury to the penis.
Spread the patient's legs and wash, rinse, and dry the scrotum and skin folds of the crotch area.	Thorough washing and rinsing remove dirt and organisms that cause skin irritation and unpleasant odors.
Proceed with washing the anal area as described for a female.	

Skill Procedure 7-6. Giving a Backrub

Suggested Action	**Reason for Action**
Raise the bed to the level of the nurse's waist.	Raising the bed, rather than leaning over a patient, maintains good posture, which will decrease muscle strain.
Use the preparation of the agency's choice for the backrub. Alcohol followed by powder may be used when the skin is oily. Lotions and creams are better when the skin is dry. Warm the solution in the hands before applying it to the back, or allow it to warm by placing the bottle in the bathwater while washing the back.	Alcohol feels refreshing and tends to toughen skin. Alcohol has a drying effect on the skin, and lotions and creams help prevent drying. A warm solution feels comfortable and relaxing for the patient.
With the patient on his side or abdomen, move the hands, placed on either side of the lower spine, up the length of the back, across the shoulder blades, and along the patient's sides. Use the entire surface of your hands, as illustrated in Figure 7-5. Move with long, circular strokes followed by long, vertical strokes. Use firm strokes but end the rub with lighter strokes. Maintain touch on the skin at all times.	A backrub stimulates circulation, tones muscles, and helps the patient relax and feel comfortable when firm, smooth, even strokes are used. Short, uneven strokes are uncomfortable. Strokes that are directed in general toward the heart assist the circulation to carry blood toward the heart and away from the extremities.
	Ending with lighter strokes gives the patient a relaxing sensation. Removing the hands and then reapplying them during the rub is not as comfortable and relaxing as when touch is maintained.

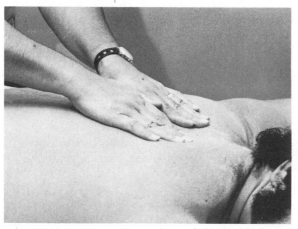

Figure 7-5 Using the entire surface of the hand, the nurse strokes the length of the patient's back. This technique is sometimes referred to as *effleurage.*

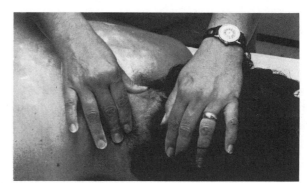

Figure 7-6 The nurse massages the cervical spine.

Rub the neck to the hairline. Place the fingers on one side of the spine in the neck and the thumb on the other side, as illustrated in Figure 7-6. Use a circular motion and move the fingers and thumb toward the hairline.	
Use stimulating strokes if the patient desires and if they are appropriate in view of the patient's condition:	For patients who enjoy the extra stimulation, the strokes described here are effective and especially useful as a muscle toner and as a stimulant to blood circulation.
Move the hands in a circular motion; move rapidly and firmly over the buttocks, over the length of the back, and across the shoulders.	
Strike the back, but not the spinal cord, with the sides of the hands, as illustrated in Figure 7-7, being careful not to strike with enough force to cause discomfort.	

(continued)

Skill Procedure 7-6. *Continued*

Suggested Action	Reason for Action

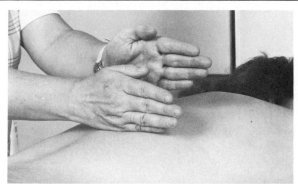

Figure 7-7 The nurse alternately strikes the back with the sides of her hands. This technique is referred to as *tapotement.*

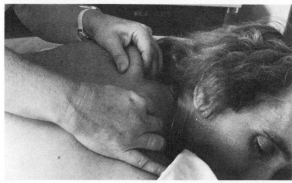

Figure 7-8 The nurse grasps skin on the patient's back. The sequence of movements is from up the back to either side of the spine, then along the shoulders. This technique is referred to as *petrissage.*

Pick up areas of skin between the fingers, as illustrated in Figure 7-8, while moving up either side of the spinal cord and along the shoulders.

Rub the buttocks, using the palm of the hand and a circular motion. Use the heel of the hand to massage the area at the base of the spine.

End the backrub by using long strokes up the length of the back while gradually lightening the pressure as you move your hands. However, use sufficient pressure to prevent a tickling sensation.

Long, soothing strokes with increasingly less pressure promote relaxation and a sense of comfort.

Wipe off any excess lotion with a fresh towel.

Excess lotion that remains on the skin is sticky and uncomfortable. It may also create moist bed linen.

---

spaces. Unwaxed floss frays somewhat more quickly. The choice of dental floss is a personal preference. Skill Procedure 7-8 describes a recommended way to brush and floss teeth.

Oral Irrigating Appliances. Appliances that generate pulsating jet streams of water under pressure are available to assist with oral hygiene. They are particularly helpful for flushing debris that accumulates around stationary bridges and braces attached to the teeth. However, if too much pressure is used, damage to gum tissues may occur. Also, debris may be forced into tissue pockets, where a local infection can then develop. Because of these disadvantages, a dentist should be consulted before their use is recommended.

Giving Oral Hygiene. Measures for oral hygiene may need to be modified for certain patients. If the patient is able to assist with his mouth care, he should be offered the necessary materials on awakening in the morning, before

bedtime, after each meal, and between meals, as indicated. If he is helpless, the nurse should give oral hygiene as often as necessary to keep the mouth and teeth clean and moist. Skill Procedure 7-9 describes how to give oral hygiene to a patient.

The Care of Dentures and Bridges. Mouth care is equally important for a person with false teeth. The word *denture* refers to a dental appliance of artificial teeth that replaces the person's upper, lower, or entire set of teeth. A *bridge* is a dental appliance that replaces one or several teeth. A bridge may be fixed to other teeth so that it cannot be removed, or it may be removable and fasten to adjoining teeth with a clasp. Dentures and removable bridges should be taken from the mouth and cleaned with a brush as shown in Figure 7-22. There are commercial solutions available in which to soak dentures and bridges, if the patient prefers.

Many dentists recommend that dentures and bridges remain in place except while they are being cleaned.

Skill Procedure 7-7. Shaving a Patient

Suggested Action	Reason for Action
Determine the patient's usual shaving routine.	The nurse should attempt to follow the patient's grooming patterns as closely as possible.
Gather the equipment the patient prefers to use; modify any equipment for potential safety hazards.	The nurse may need to substitute safety, battery, or electric razors in certain situations.
If possible, place the patient in a sitting position.	Being upright is a similar position to one a patient would assume himself. It also promotes eye contact and communication between the patient and nurse.
Wash the patient's face with warm, soapy water.	Removing oil helps to raise the hair shaft, promoting its removal. Soap removes bacteria that can enter tiny cuts from the razor.
Inspect the face for elevated moles, birthmarks, or lesions.	Scraping or cutting can cause bleeding, irritation, or infection.
Lather the face with shaving cream or soap.	Lathering softens the beard and helps the razor slide over the skin without nicking or cutting.
Using short strokes with the razor, shave in the direction of the hair growth as illustrated in Figure 7-9. Start from the upper face and lip and extend to the neck. The patient may tilt his head to help shave in hollow or curved areas.	Shaving in the direction of the hair shaft will produce a closer shave without irritating the underlying skin.

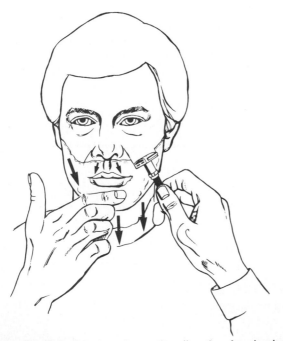

Figure 7-9 This drawing shows the direction for shaving a patient's face.

Use the hand without the razor to pull the skin below the area being shaved.	Pulling flattens and firms the skin surface, promoting uniform shaving.
Rinse the razor after each stroke.	Rinsing removes hair from between the blade and blade guard so the cutting edge remains clean.
Rinse and dry the face when completely finished.	Final rinsing removes remnants of lather and shaved hair.

(continued)

Skill Procedure 7-7. Continued

Suggested Action	Reason for Action
Apply the patient's choice of lotion or cologne.	Most after-shave preparations contain scented alcohol. The alcohol acts as an antiseptic in any microabrasions. As the alcohol evaporates, it causes a cooling sensation that feels refreshing.
Return all shaving equipment to its proper location. Discard any dulled disposable razors or razor blades in a special safety container.	The nurse must take care that others will not be accidentally injured by sharp objects.

Keeping dentures and bridges out for long periods of time permits the gum lines to change, affecting the fit.

If the patient has been instructed to remove dentures or bridges while sleeping, a disposable, covered cup is convenient and easy to use. For aesthetic reasons, it is better not to use cups, drinking glasses, or other dishes used for eating. Plain water is most often used to store dentures and bridges. Some persons add mouthwash to the water; this practice results in a pleasant taste when dentures and bridges are returned to the mouth.

Care should be taken when cleaning dentures and bridges. They are expensive, and damage or loss can create problems. They should be cleaned over a basin of water or a soft towel so that they will not drop onto a hard surface, should they accidentally slip from the nurse's hands. Warm water is used because hot water may warp the plastic material from which many dentures and bridges are made.

Care of the Eyes and Visual Aids

It is not true that using one's eyes will lead to a decrease in the ability to see. As much as anyone may protest, it is impossible to ruin the eyes from reading. It is true that certain factors can cause eye fatigue. *Eye fatigue* is the discomfort experienced from poor lighting or prolonged focusing on an object. To reduce eye fatigue, observe the following directives.

- Use adequate light such as daylight or a minimum of 75-watt light bulbs when reading.

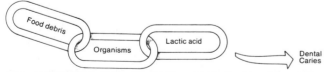

Figure 7-10 This chain illustrates events that lead to caries. Debris remaining in the mouth after eating (especially sfter eating concentrated carbohydrates, such as sweets) accumulates on and between the teeth. This debris is attacked by organisms in the mouth, which feed on it and produce lactic acid. Lactic acid destroys tooth enamel causing cavities. Proper oral hygiene breaks the chain by removing debris and by breaking up colonies of organisms.

- Adjust the light source so it comes from above rather than from the side of printed material.
- Lamps should be on while one watches television. There is too much contrast in a completely dark room.
- Glance about the room at frequent periods while reading or doing fine work. Muscles that must remain contracted to hold an image in focus become strained.

Ordinarily the eyes are so well protected naturally with eyelashes, tearing, and a split-second blink reflex that they do not require special care. In spite of this, eyes occasionally become irritated. They may require special lenses to help focus images sharply, or they may become diseased or injured, thus requiring removal. The nurse may then need to provide special eye-care skills. If a patient does not shut his eyes or blink, which is the case of some unconscious patients, the eyes need to be medicated, closed, and patched. They should be inspected and cleansed several times a day to make sure there are no signs of infection.

Cleansing the Eyes. The eyes can become irritated from wind, smoke, dust, bacteria, or exposure to a source of allergy. In response to these irritants, the eyes increase mucus production and other secretions that trap and remove the irritating substances. This can lead to an accumulation of dried or liquid material. Discharges from the eyes should be removed carefully and as frequently as necessary to keep eyes clean. Skill Procedure 7-10 provides suggestions for cleansing eyes.

Care of Eyeglasses. Many patients wear eyeglasses, which represent a considerable financial investment. They are not quickly or easily replaced. The nurse should use every effort to prevent glasses from being broken, scratched, or lost. Eyeglasses should be cleaned as follows:

- Work over a basin of water or a towel so that if the glasses accidentally slip from your hands they will not fall on a hard surface and break.
- Allow warm water to flow over the lenses and frames. Hot water may damage plastic lenses and frames. Use a little soap or detergent with the water if there is

(Text continues on page 106)

Skill Procedure 7-8. Brushing and Flossing the Teeth

Suggested Action	**Reason for Action**

Position the brush with the bristles at the junction of the teeth and gums as in Figure 7-11.

This position helps clean debris away from the margin of the gums.

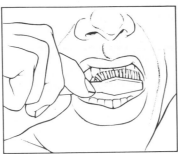

Figure 7-11 A soft-bristled toothbrush allows the flexibility to reach every tooth. (Adapted from How to Brush and Floss. Chicago, The American Academy of Periodontology, 1989)

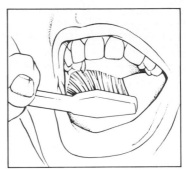

Figure 7-12 Change the position of the brush to reach and clean all tooth surfaces. (Adapted from How to Brush and Floss. Chicago, American Academy of Periodontology, 1989)

Move the brush back and forth gently several times using small circular strokes.

Clean the inside of the back teeth, shown in Figure 7-12, using the same method.

Hold the brush vertically, shown in Figure 7-13, and brush back and forth over each tooth.

Light pressure helps clean between teeth; excess pressure can cause discomfort and gum injury.

All surfaces of all teeth need brushing.

Holding the brush vertically cleans the inside surfaces of the upper and lower teeth.

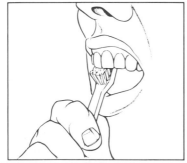

Figure 7-13 Make back-and-forth strokes over each tooth and its surrounding gum tissue. (Adapted from How to Brush and Floss. Chicago, American Academy of Periodontology, 1989)

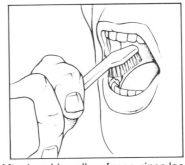

Figure 7-14 After brushing all surfaces, rinse loosened debris from the mouth. (Adapted from How to Brush and Floss. Chicago, American Academy of Periodontology, 1989)

Position the toothbrush parallel to the back teeth, as in Figure 7-14, and brush with circular strokes.

Wrap floss around the middle fingers of each hand as shown in Figure 7-15.

Insert the floss between two teeth guiding it toward the gumline as shown in Figure 7-16.

Move the floss up and down on the side of each tooth, with the middle fingers approximately 1/2″ apart.

This technique cleans the biting and chewing surfaces of the teeth.

Threading the floss helps to insert, move, and wind the used portion after each use.

Forcing the floss can cause discomfort.

The floss removes particles of food and plaque that cannot be removed with a toothbrush.

(continued)

Skill Procedure 7-8. Continued

Suggested Action	Reason for Action

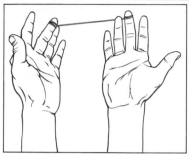

Figure 7-15 Wrap approximately 18 inches of dental floss between the two middle fingers. (Adapted from How to Brush and Floss. Chicago, American Academy of Periodontology, 1989)

Turn the floss from one middle finger to the other as it becomes frayed or soiled.

Repeat the technique on all the upper and lower back teeth, shown in Figures 7-17 and 7-18.

Finish flossing with the back side of the last tooth, shown in Figure 7-19.

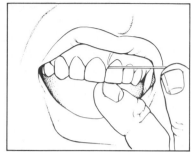

Figure 7-16 Curve the floss into a C shape against one tooth. Slide it into the space between the gum and the tooth until meeting resistance. (Adapted from How to Brush and Floss. Chicago, American Academy of Periodontology, 1989)

Using a clean, intact section of floss ensures maximum cleansing.

Thorough flossing helps to prevent periodontal disease.

Flossing is complete when the outside margin of the last tooth is finished.

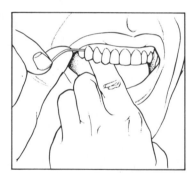

Figure 7-17 The fingers controlling the floss should be no more than ½ inch apart. (Adapted from How to Brush and Floss. Chicago, American Academy of Periodontology, 1989)

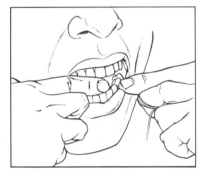

Figure 7-18 Guide the floss using the forefingers of both hands. (Adapted from How to Brush and Floss. Chicago, American Academy of Periodontology, 1989)

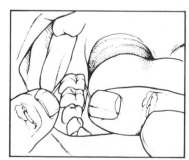

Figure 7-19 Dental care costs can be kept to a minimum with regular and thorough brushing and flossing. (Adapted from How to Brush and Floss. Chicago, American Academy of Periodontology, 1989)

Adapted from Effective Oral Hygiene. Chicago, American Academy of Periodontology.

Skill Procedure 7-9. Performing Oral Hygiene Measures

Suggested Action	Reason for Action
For cleansing use toothpaste or, if the patient prefers, a mouthwash solution. Plain water may also be used, although it does not have the cleansing ability that many other agents do. Additional cleansing agents are described below.	The choice of cleansing agents is largely personal, but the agent should be one that does not injure or irritate oral tissues.
Use a solution of half water and half hydrogen peroxide, especially if sordes are present. Sordes are the dry, crustlike particles of mucus and secretions that collect and stick on the teeth and around the lips.	Hydrogen peroxide releases oxygen and causes a froth that helps to break up dried and sticky particles.
Avoid the prolonged use of hydrogen peroxide.	Hydrogen peroxide may damage tooth enamel if used over a long period of time.
Consider using milk of magnesia to clean the mouth and teeth.	Milk of magnesia reduces oral acidity, dissolves film on the teeth, tends to increase the flow of saliva, and soothes oral lesions.
Consider using normal saline or a solution of soda bicarbonate if hydrogen peroxide and milk of magnesia are unsatisfactory.	Normal saline and a solution of soda bicarbonate are effective cleansing agents if other agents cause nausea or if the taste of other agents is unappealing to the patient.
Consider using half hydrogen peroxide and half ginger ale as still another cleansing agent. Be sure to rinse the mouth well after using a ginger ale solution.	A solution of hydrogen peroxide and ginger ale has been reported to be an effective cleansing agent, especially if there is blood in the mouth. The sugar in ginger ale tends to promote dental caries.
Use a toothbrush for cleansing the mouth and teeth as shown in Figure 7-20. Run hot water over the tufts of the brush if they are stiff.	A toothbrush is an effective device for cleansing the mouth and teeth. Hot water helps soften stiff tufts on a toothbrush, thereby decreasing the danger of injuring oral tissues.

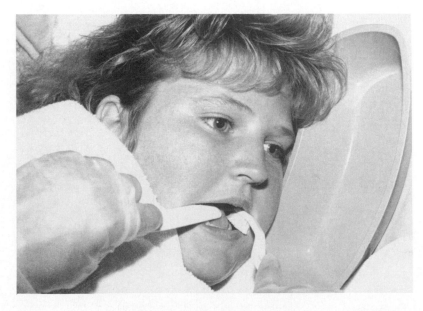

Figure 7-20 The mouth is held open with a padded tongue blade.

If a toothbrush cannot be used, try cleaning with a tongue blade wrapped with gauze or commercially prepared mouth swabs. Large cotton applicators may be used. Be sure the cotton or gauze is secured *well* so that it does not come off in the patient's mouth.	Gauze and cotton are less irritating than a toothbrush. However, if gauze or cotton becomes dislodged in the mouth, the patient may choke on it. Commercial mouth swabs are safer and more convenient, but they are more expensive than the other supplies.

(continued)

Skill Procedure 7-9. Continued

Suggested Action	Reason for Action
Use a padded tongue blade to open the patient's mouth if he is unconscious or too ill to open his mouth. Do not try to open the mouth with your fingers.	A human bite can be a dangerous wound because of the many organisms normally found in the mouth.
Place the unconscious or very ill patient on either side with his head resting over the edge of a pillow while giving him oral hygiene. If gauze or applicators are used, be sure they are not dripping wet. Use suction equipment to remove rinsing solution and oral secretions as in Figure 7-21. Allow the suction tip to remain in the mouth while giving oral hygiene if there is any danger of the patient's choking.	The positioning described allows for drainage from the mouth. Continuous suctioning helps prevent choking. Even small amounts of liquid can cause choking in an unconscious or very ill patient.

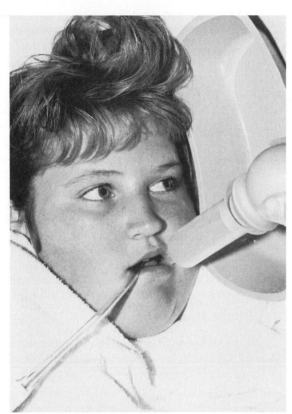

Figure 7-21 The mouth is rinsed and simultaneously suctioned.

Moisten the mouth and lips after cleaning all areas. Swabs moistened with glycerin and lemon juice are often used. Do not use them over a prolonged period of time. Petrolatum jelly or a cream can also be used to protect the lips. Oral tissues may be moistened with water or by having the patient suck ice chips, if this is permitted.	The skin on the lips is very thin and evaporation of moisture from them occurs rapidly unless they are covered with a protective coating. Glycerine absorbs water and causes the oral tissues to become dry if used over a period of time (*i.e.,* more than several days).
Remember that caring for the mouth and teeth is important for a patient's well-being and should be carried out as often as necessary to keep them clean and moistened.	Studies have shown that the procedure for cleansing the mouth and teeth appears more important than the agent used. The nurse is responsible for seeing to it that the patient receives proper oral hygiene.

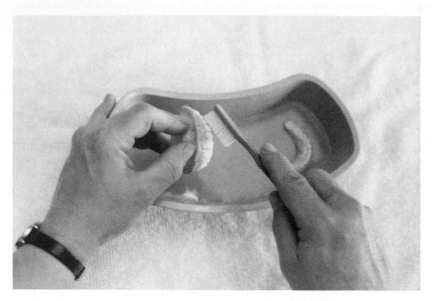

Figure 7-22 All the surfaces of dentures are brushed for the patient who is unable to care for himself.

dried material on the glasses. Commercial glass cleaners may be used also.
- Rinse the glasses well. Soap or detergent is likely to streak the glasses if not rinsed off well.
- Dry glasses with a soft, clean cloth, such as a cotton handkerchief. Tissues are not recommended. They

are made of wood pulp and have been found to scratch lenses, especially when the lenses are made of plastic material.
- Do not clean eyeglasses without washing them first. The dirt and dust on the lenses are likely to scratch when a cloth is wiped across dirty glasses.

Skill Procedure 7-10. Cleansing the Eyes

Suggested Action	Reason for Action
Tap water or normal saline should be warmed to near body temperature. For eyes that are extremely irritated or infected, the solution and its container may need to be sterile.	Warm water is soothing to the eye and promotes the patient's comfort. Sterile solutions prevent adding bacteria to the eye.
Wash·hands well. If an infection or blood is present, the nurse may need to wear sterile gloves for self-protection.	The hands contain many bacteria that could cause an infection in the eye. If an infection is already present, gloves act as a barrier for their transfer to the nurse.
Place a towel or a basin to the side of the patient's face.	The towel and basin will collect any solution that may drain downward and prevent having to change bed linen.
Position the patient on the side with the eye that will be cleansed, or the patient may sit and tilt his head to the side.	Water will flow downward due to gravity. Turning toward the side will prevent solution that may also contain some of the discharge material from flowing into the opposite eye or down the face.
Moisten cotton balls in the solution. Wipe once with each cotton ball from the corner of the eye near the nose toward the other side near the temple.	The movement of the cotton ball toward the temple prevents solution from entering the nose through the lacrimal duct.
Use each cotton ball only once while cleansing the eye and then discard it.	This practice helps prevent carrying debris back over the eye.
Clean the other eye in a similar manner if necessary. If each eye is infected with different bacteria, all equipment, solutions, and gloves will need to be changed.	Care must be taken to avoid transferring any organisms from one eye to the other.

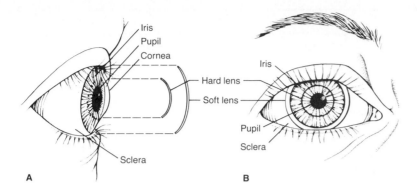

Figure 7-23 (*A*). This side view of the eye shows various eye structures. The cornea is clear. It is located in front of the iris and pupil. Contact lenses cover the cornea. Soft lenses are slightly larger than hard lenses. (*B*). A frontal view shows how soft contact lenses extend beyond the cornea.

Plastic lenses have become popular because they are considerably lighter in weight than are glass lenses. Plastic lenses have one disadvantage, however: they are very easily scratched. All glasses that are not being worn should be stored in a case or resting on the frame.

Caring for Contact Lenses. Contact lenses are small plastic disks worn directly on the cornea. The cornea is the clear layer of tissue that lies over the iris, the colored part of the eye. A diagram identifying these structures is shown in Figure 7-23. Contact lenses are used in place of eyeglasses to improve vision. They are usually worn in each eye. Some patients who have had cataract surgery in one eye may wear a single contact lens. Eyeglasses may also be worn in addition to a single contact lens. For this reason the nurse should not assume that a patient who wears eyeglasses does not use a contact lens.

There are several types of contact lenses available. Contact lenses may be hard, soft, or gas permeable. The type of lenses is prescribed by the ophthalmologist or optometrist after considering many individual factors about each patient. Ordinarily, the type of contact selected depends on which one will provide the most improvement of the patient's vision with the least risk for complications. All contact lenses, except the new disposable type, require removal for cleaning and eye rest, periodic disinfection, and proper storage. Patients who are not dedicated to following a routine for the care of their contact lenses risk infection, abrasion, and eye damage. Table 7-2 lists some advantages and disadvantages among the various types of contact lenses.

The patient or someone in his family usually cares for contact lenses. However, a patient's condition may require the nurse's assistance. If the patient indicates that he wears contact lenses but one or both cannot be found with simple inspection, the eyelids may need to be everted. Eversion facilitates inspection in the folds under the lids.

It is best that a nurse who wears contact lenses demonstrate to other staff how to remove, clean, store, and replace contact lenses. Several techniques and products may be used depending on the type that are worn. Skill Procedure 7-11 can be used for general guidelines.

Care of an Artificial Eye. Any man-made object that replaces a natural body part is called a *prosthesis*. An artificial eye, leg, and arm are examples of prosthetic devices. Artificial eyes are primarily plastic; rarely, the nurse may encounter an older prosthetic eye made of glass. Artificial eyes are custom made to match the patient's remaining eye.

Most people think that an artificial eye is round like a marble. Actually it is shaped like a shell, as illustrated in Figure 7-30. An object called an implant is permanently inserted within the bony orbit at the time of the eye's removal. It is impossible to remove an implant.

An artificial eye is used strictly for cosmetic reasons; there is no way of restoring vision once the eye is removed. The artificial eye may need to be removed and cleaned from time to time. The patient wearing an artificial eye will generally wish to care for it himself. If the patient is unable to remove the eye, the nurse will need to do so using the following techniques:

- Have the patient lie down so that the artificial eye will not fall to the floor accidentally while it is being removed.
- Depress the patient's lower lid until the lower edge of the artificial eye slides out and into your hand.
- Clean the artificial eye well with soap and water by washing it with your fingers. Chemicals and alcohol are not used on an artificial eye because they are likely to damage its surface.
- Rinse the prosthetic eye before replacing it so that any remaining soap does not irritate the tissue on which it rests.
- The cavity of the eye may be irrigated before reinsertion of the artificial eye, following the suggested actions in Chapter 20.

Care of the Ears and Hearing Aids

The outer ears are the collectors of sounds. The ability to hear sounds is important to survival and the appreciation of life. Too much sound or unpleasant sound has been referred to by some as "noise pollution."

Table 7-2. Types of Contact Lenses

Type	Description	Advantages	Disadvantages
Hard	Discs made from rigid plastic	Durable Provides clear, sharp vision Care is simpler and cheaper	Interferes with oxygen supply to the cornea Must be removed overnight and after 12–14 hours of wear Causes discomfort while the patient adjusts to wearing them
Soft	Flexible discs made from water-absorbing plastic	Larger and more comfortable Quick adjustment to wearing	Cleaning is more complicated and expensive Easily torn with replacement needed on the average of every 9–12 months
Daily Wear Soft	Removed each evening	Permits oxygen to reach the cornea	Increased incidence of eye infection and irritation
Extended Wear Soft	Can be worn overnight; longer than one week is not recommended	Quickly replaced without delay in refitting	Does not produce the quality of vision compared with hard or gas permeable lenses
Disposable Soft	Worn continuously for one week, then replaced with new lenses	No cleaning or disinfection required Safer than other lenses because they are not reused	In an attempt to economize, wearers may reuse rather than discard disposable lenses Reuse increases risk of infection and eye injury
Gas Permeable	Semi-rigid discs made of air-breathing fluoropolymers	Some brands designed for daily wear or one week extended wear Better vision than with soft lenses More oxygen reaches the eye than with some soft lenses	Tend to develop surface deposits from natural eye secretions that reduce comfort and clarity

The ability to hear decreases with age. The process can be speeded by exposure to loud sounds. Noise levels are measured in *decibels* (dB). According to the Environmental Protection Agency permanent damage to hearing begins to occur at 90 decibels. Table 7-3 shows the decibel levels of various common sounds.

Healthy ears only need to be washed, rinsed, and dried when a patient is given a bath. No object should be placed into the ear canal because of the danger of injuring the eardrum. If the ear becomes plugged with cerumen, or wax, it may be necessary for a physician to remove it by using a looped instrument. Nurses may irrigate the ear, using the procedure in Chapter 20. Some nurses have found that using a pulsating stream of water produced by an oral irrigating appliance is useful to help remove wax

and debris from the ear canal. When using this type of appliance; it is very important to be sure that the tympanic membrane is intact and that the stream of water is set at its *lowest* setting.

Some people require the use of a hearing aid, which increases the ability to hear sounds. These devices do not replace the complete quality of hearing but can be an adequate substitute for some people. They can be worn on the body, but more often they are fitted into eyeglasses, worn behind the ear, or placed completely within the ear. The individual in Figure 7-31 is wearing a hearing aid that fits behind the ear. The nurse should know about hearing aids when caring for a patient who uses one. Note the following important information:

(Text continues on page 113)

Skill Procedure 7-11. Removing, Cleaning, and Replacing Contact Lenses

Suggested Action	**Reason for Action**
Prepare a separate container for each lens that can be covered and sealed like the one in Figure 7-24.	Contact lenses are small and may become lost or broken.

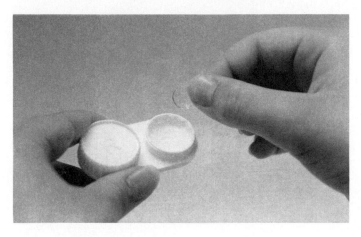

Figure 7-24 Contact lenses are stored in a labeled container when not being worn.

Label one container "right" and one "left."	The lens prescription may differ in each eye. Labeling prevents misidentification.
Have the patient sit up or lie down.	Either position provides access to the lens. The nurse may find that one, more than the other, works better.
Place a soft towel or cloth beneath the patient's face.	If the lens is dropped, the cloth may protect it from damage and aid in finding it.
Wash hands.	Handwashing deters the spread of microorganisms.
Fingernails should be smooth and trimmed short.	Long fingernails could injure the eye or damage a soft lens during removal or reinsertion.

Removing a Contact Lens

Removing a Soft Lens

Slide the soft lens onto the sclera, the white area of the eye shown in Figure 7-25.	Moving the lens facilitates grasping the lens without injuring the sensitive cornea.
Compress the lid margins toward the edges of the contact lens.	Soft lenses will bend when compressed. Bending lets air enter beneath the lens and releases it from the surface of the eye.
Gently pick up the loosened lens between the thumb and forefinger.	Pinching the lens between the thumb and forefinger is safe provided the fingernails do not contact the lens or eye.
Clean and store the soft lens in a soaking solution. Repeat for the other lens.	Soft lenses dry and crystallize if exposed to air. Rehydrating a lens may not be possible.

Removing a Hard Lens Using the Blink Method

With the patient sitting up, place a towel beneath the patient's face.	The towel helps to catch and protect a free lens.
Place a thumb or finger on the center of the upper and lower lids.	The opposing thumbs or fingers help to break the seal that holds the lens in place.
Gently press inward while instructing the patient to blink.	Air enters beneath the lens when the patient blinks and separates it from the cornea.

(continued)

Skill Procedure 7-11. *Continued*

Suggested Action	Reason for Action

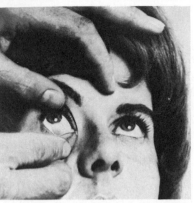

Figure 7-25 A soft lens can be moved off the cornea onto the sclera for removal. (Contact Lens Emergency Care Information & Instruction Packet. St. Louis, American Optometric Association Committee on Contact Lenses)

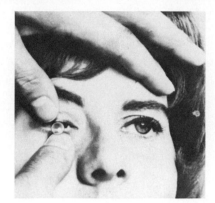

Figure 7-26 A hard lens can be compressed between the thumbs if the patient cannot remove it. (Contact Lens Emergency Care Information & Instruction Packet. St. Louis, American Optometric Association Committee on Contact Lenses)

Remove the loosened lens as shown in Figure 7-26.	Handling one lens at a time prevents misidentification later.
If unsuccessful, a suction cup, shown in Figure 7-27, may be used to remove a hard lens.	A suction cup is a tool that may assist with the safe removal or insertion of a contact lens when a patient is unconscious or cannot assist.

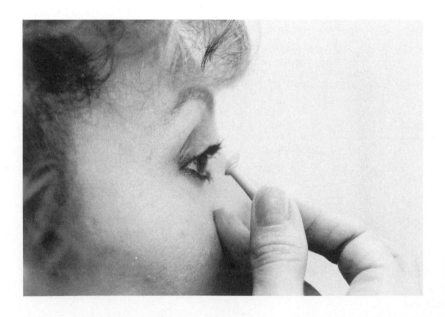

Figure 7-27 One end of this tool is used for removal of a hard lens. The other is used for insertion. It is only used with hard lenses.

Moisten the suction cup.	Moisture provides slight surface tension when it is touched to the contact lens.
Position the suction cup in front and parallel to the lens.	In this position, the suction cup is more apt to make contact with the lens than the eye.
Touch the cup to the lens and apply gentle pressure.	Pressure causes the lens to adhere to the cup.
Lift the cup and attached lens from the eye.	As long as the suction is applied, the lens will remain attached.

(continued)

Skill Procedure 7-11. Continued

Suggested Action	Reason for Action
Slide the lens sideways from the suction cup.	Sliding the lens breaks the vacuum and separates its attachment.
Clean and soak each lens in its respective container.	Cleaning and soaking reduces the risk of infection. When hard lenses are removed, oxygen can be resupplied to the cornea.

Cleaning Contact Lenses

Wash hands with an oil-free soap such as Ivory, and rinse well.	Handwashing deters the spread of microorganisms. Emollients leave a residue that may not be completely removed with rinsing.
Dry hands with a clean, lint-free towel.	Cloth fibers could damage the eye if they adhere to the lens.
Protect the work surface with a clean, soft cloth.	A soft cloth prevents damage or loss of dropped contact lenses.
Place the lens in the palm of the hand with the cup side of the lens up, shown in Figure 7-28.	The cup of the lens and the palm act as a container for the cleaning solution.

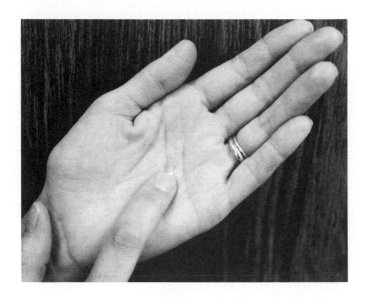

Figure 7-28 The palm of the hand is a convenient area for cleansing contact lenses. The finger is used to make circular strokes.

Pour a small amount of cleaning solution into the cup of the lens and palm of the hand.	Excessive amounts of solution are unnecessary and may lead to loss of the lens if solution runs from the hand.
Rub the cleaning solution over the inner and outer surfaces of the contact lens for 30 seconds on each side.	Friction and the cleaning solution remove organisms and eye secretions from the surface of the lens, reducing the potential for infection and irritation.
Rinse and store the lens in a soaking solution.	Lenses may become warped, dehydrated, or support the growth of microbes if not kept in solution. Soaking solutions contain chemicals that interfere with the growth of microorganisms.
Clean soft lenses with an enzyme product weekly and rinse before reinsertion.	Enzyme solutions remove protein deposits that are not removed with daily cleansing. Rinsing removes chemical enzymes that can irritate the eye.

(continued)

Skill Procedure 7-11. Continued

Suggested Action	**Reason for Action**

Replacing Contact Lenses

Replacing Soft Lenses

Wash hands thoroughly.

Washing the hands continues to reduce the transfer of organisms onto the surface of the contact lens.

Rinse the soft lens with normal saline solution.

Soft lenses absorb liquids. Normal saline is compatible with the tissues of the eye and will not cause irritation.

Verify that the lens is not turned inside out as shown in Figure 7-29.

Vision and comfort will be affected if the lenses have been accidently inverted.

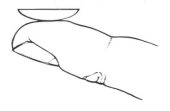 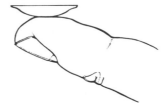

Figure 7-29 (*A*). This lens is bowl shaped and is in the correct position for reinsertion. (*B*). The edges of this lens point outward, which indicates it is inside out.

Position the lens cup side up on the tip of the index or middle finger.

It is easier to insert the lens by just touching it to the surface of the eye.

Separate the patient's lids and have him look up or to the side.

Not looking directly at the approaching lens prevents the patient from blinking while it is being applied.

Place the lens on the eye, release the lids, and instruct the patient to blink.

This combination of actions tends to center the lens automatically.

If the lens is not centered, have the patient close his eyelids. Use a finger over the closed lid to move the lens about the eye until it is in place.

A soft lens is flexible and can glide easily into place.

Replacing Hard Lenses

Perform thorough handwashing.

Washing the hands continues to reduce the transfer of organisms onto the surface of the contact lens.

Rinse the contact lens in tap water.

Hard lenses do not absorb liquids so saline is not needed.

Position the lens cup side up on the tip of the index or middle finger.

It is easier to insert the lens by just touching it to the surface of the eye.

Drop wetting solution into the cup of the lens.

A wetting solution helps provide a film of fluid that will help hold the lens to the cornea.

Separate the patient's lids and have him look up or to the side.

Not looking directly at the approaching lens prevents the patient from blinking while it is being applied.

Touch the lens to the cornea.

Contact with the cornea transfers the lens from the fingertip.

Ask the patient to close his eyelids without squeezing or blinking.

This adjusts the position of the contact lens. Squeezing or blinking may move or release the contact lens.

The opposite end of a suction cup can be used as an alternative for inserting a moistened hard lens.

The tool acts as a substitute for the finger when inserting a contact lens.

Inspect the eye to verify that the contact lens is in place over the cornea. Assess vision and eye comfort.

Vision and comfort will be affected when a contact lens is placed incorrectly.

(continued)

Skill Procedure 7-11. Continued

Suggested Action	Reason for Action
Remove and attempt to reapply if the lens is uncomfortable or the vision is distorted.	Eye damage can occur if a hard lens is applied incorrectly.
Wash containers used for soaking lenses daily with hot water.	Containers can be a source of microbial growth if they are not emptied and cleaned.
Dry upside down on a clean cloth or paper towel.	Removing moisture interferes with the growth of microbes.
Boil the case once a week for 20 minutes and let air dry or soak the case in a 1:10 bleach and water solution for 10 minutes. Rinse thoroughly with hot water.	Heat or chemical sterilization kill microorganisms.

- Avoid exposing the hearing aid to extreme heat, water, cleaning chemicals, or hair spray.
- The outside of a hearing aid should be cleaned with just a dry, soft cloth or tissue. Some hearing aids that are molded to fit within the ear come with a special tool for removing any wax that may accumulate around the hearing aid.
- Turn the hearing aid off when not being worn to prolong the life of the battery.
- Store the hearing aid, when not in use, where it will not fall. A cracked case can cause variations in the sound level.
- Lack of sound or poor sound may indicate a need for a new battery. Use fresh batteries that are specific for each type of hearing aid. Old batteries can be recycled.

Most patients or their families are instructed on the care and use of hearing aids. They may continue to care for their hearing aid while being hospitalized for other reasons. If the nurse does need to help the patient insert a hearing aid, suggestions in Skill Procedure 7-12 may be helpful.

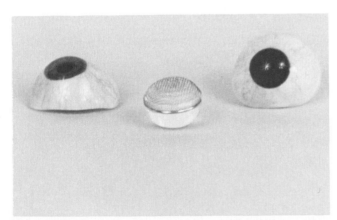

Figure 7-30 Front and side views of the shell-shaped artificial eye are shown. The round device is the implant that is inserted permanently within the eye at the time of surgery.

Care of the Nose

The best way to clean the patient's nose is to have him blow it *gently* while allowing both nostrils to be open. Blowing while closing one nostril carries the danger of forcing debris into the eustachian tube. Occasionally, secretions may dry around the outside of the nose, especially when the patient is receiving oxygen or has a tube inserted through the nose. Washing with soap and water may be sufficient to remove these secretions. Cream, lotions, or ointments may be applied to the area to keep the skin moist.

Care of the Fingernails

The nails are a structure of the skin. They are composed of flat, hard, keratin cells. Keratin is an insoluble protein material. The root of the nail lies in a groove where the nail grows and is nourished by the bloodstream. Nursing measures to care for fingernails include the following:

- Care for the nails at the time of the bath; this is usually convenient for the patient and the nurse. Soaking the nails before grooming will soften them and prevent injury.

Table 7-3. Common Sound Levels

Common Sounds	Decibel Level
Air raid siren	140
Discotheque	130
Stereo	up to 120
Chain saw	100
Riding mower	90–95
City traffic	90
Noisy restaurant	70
Living room	40
Library	30

Courtesy of the Environmental Protection Agency.

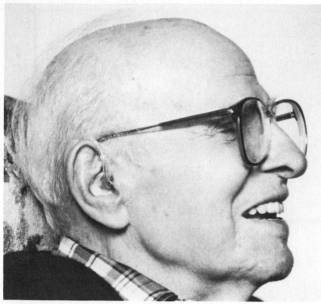

Figure 7-31 This man is wearing a hearing aid that fits behind the ear. It is the most common type used. The part that fits within the ear is custom fitted from a mold of the ear canal.

- Groom the nails by filing or cutting. The nails should not be trimmed too far down on the side because of the danger of injury to the cuticle and the skin around the nail. Nail scissors should be used with great care to avoid injuring the skin.
- After washing the hands, push the cuticle back gently to prevent hangnails, which are dried and broken pieces of cuticle. Once present, they may be removed with cutting. This should be done with great care to prevent injury to the cuticle.
- Clean under the nails with a blunt instrument, such as an orange stick or the large end of a flat toothpick. The

nurse will wish to be careful to avoid injuring the area under the nail where it is attached to the skin.
- Finish care by lubricating the hands with a cream or lotion to prevent drying and chapping of the skin. Massage the hands from the fingertips toward the wrists to help prevent congestion of blood in the hands.

Care of the Feet and Toenails

Patients who have diabetes or vascular diseases should have orders from a physician for cutting toenails. Many people, especially the elderly who may have diminished vision, strength, or coordination may utilize the services of a podiatrist. A *podiatrist* is an individual with special training in caring for feet. The services of a podiatrist are covered by Medicare funds.

The following measures are important for proper foot care:

- Start foot care by cleaning the feet well. An important part of the bed bath is to soak the feet, rinse off the soap well, and dry the feet thoroughly.
- Use frequent bathing and foot powder when the feet tend to perspire freely. Odors can usually be controlled by these measures. Changing stockings regularly also helps keep the feet clean and dry. Shoes may be rotated on a daily basis to allow for moisture to evaporate.
- Trim straight across the toenails with nailclippers (Figure 7-32) or scissors. Be sure to check agency policy before doing so, because a physician's order is sometimes required to trim toenails. Cutting or digging deeply at the sides of the nails predisposes the patient to ingrown nails and injury. Patients with in-

---

Skill Procedure 7-12. Inserting a Hearing Aid

Suggested Action	Reason for Action
Inspect the external ear and clean it if cerumen has accumulated.	Accumulation of cerumen can interfere with sound conduction.
Test the ability of the hearing aid to function by turning it on.	A functioning hearing aid produces a continuous whistle when not being worn.
Make sure the hearing aid is off and the volume is turned down before insertion.	A sudden loud level of sound can be annoying and uncomfortable for a patient who uses one.
Insert the hearing aid in the external ear. The earlobe should be pulled downward while pressing the hearing aid inward.	The hearing aid is custom molded to fit snugly so that sound does not escape. *Feedback,* a loud, shrill noise, occurs when a hearing aid is not positioned correctly.
Turn the hearing aid on and gradually increase the volume.	The patient can best judge the volume that is most comfortable.
Turn the hearing aid off when it is removed from the ear.	The life of the hearing aid battery can be prolonged by turning the device off during periods of nonuse.

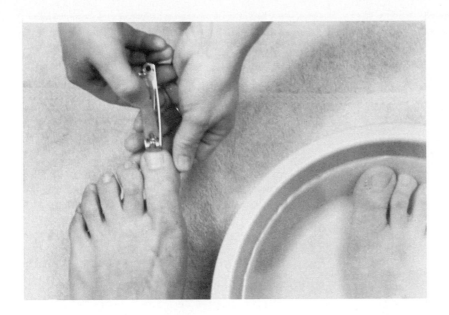

Figure 7-32 Soaking the feet softens the nails. They are trimmed straight across.

grown toenails may need medical attention. The area under the toenails is cleaned in the same manner as that under the fingernails.

- Soak the feet of the patient before trimming brittle, thick toenails. If a basin of water is not convenient for soaking, the feet may be wrapped in damp cloths and each foot placed in a plastic bag for a period of time.
- Massage the feet with cream or lotion after trimming the nails. Begin with the toes and move toward the ankles to prevent congestion of blood in the feet. If the skin is not dry or if the feet are perspiring, use plain powder.
- Do not try to cut off a *callus,* which is a thickening of the outer layer of the skin due to pressure and friction. A pumice stone is frequently recommended to remove a callus if it becomes troublesome.
- Be aware of foot problems the patient may have, such as infections, inflammations, ingrown nails, breaks in the skin, corns, warts, and bunions. Such conditions require a physician's attention.

Care of the Hair

Hair grows on most parts of the body. Each hair has a shaft with its root in a hair follicle. There are small muscles attached to hair follicles that contract, causing the hair to stand on end (gooseflesh) when a person is shivering or very frightened.

Good general health is important for attractive hair. Cleanliness helps keep hair attractive. Poor nutrition and illness affect hair. Patients with elevated temperatures may need frequent care of the hair. Perspiration and sebum may mat the hair as the body attempts to regulate heat loss. Some drugs used for cancer treatment cause temporary loss of hair. The cancer patient may appreciate a nurse's

creative efforts to design turbans or provide hats to compensate for the change in body image.

Grooming the Hair. The following are recommended measures for grooming the hair:

- Try to use the hairstyle of the patient's preference. The patient feels more comfortable about his appearance when this is done.
- Brush the hair slowly and carefully to avoid damaging the hair follicles. Brushing keeps hair clean and distributes oil along the shafts. A comb cannot do this. Brushing also stimulates scalp circulation, which helps bring nourishment to the hair follicles.
- If the hair is tangled, use a wide-toothed comb and pull, starting at the ends of the hair rather than from the crown downward. Forcing and pulling on a tangled mass may break large numbers of hairs. Sometimes alcohol will loosen a tangle.
- Use a comb for arranging the hair after it has been brushed. Sharp and irregular teeth may scratch and injure the scalp and should be avoided. A large-toothed comb is recommended for very thick, curly hair.
- Wash the comb and brush periodically.
- Use oil on the hair if it is dry. There are many preparations on the market, but pure castor oil, olive oil, and mineral oil are satisfactory. Coarse, curly hair tends to be dry, and, therefore, oil is usually necessary. If the hair is oily, more frequent shampooing is necessary.
- Do not neglect the hair of ill persons who may beg to have their hair left undisturbed. This can become a problem, especially if the hair is long. If the patient's hair is not combed even for one day, hours of careful combing of small sections of hair will become necessary.

Skill Procedure 7-13. Shampooing Hair

Suggested Action	Reason for Action
Assemble the shampoo and towels near a source of running water if possible.	Being close to water will help to keep the water at a regulated, comfortable temperature of 40° C (105° F).
Move the patient to a stretcher if permitted.	The bed is protected from becoming wet if the patient can be transferred to a stretcher.
Protect the bottom sheets of the stretcher or bed with moisture-proof pads or several thicknesses of towels.	The patient may become chilled and uncomfortable as water drips toward the back.
Use a plastic tray with a water trough such as the one illustrated in Figure 7-33 if available. Consider using a fracture bedpan if a commercial tray is not available. Pad the lip of the pan before placing it under the nape of the patient's neck.	The water drains from the tray down the trough and into a receptacle on the floor. The bedpan can collect a small volume of water before emptying is necessary.

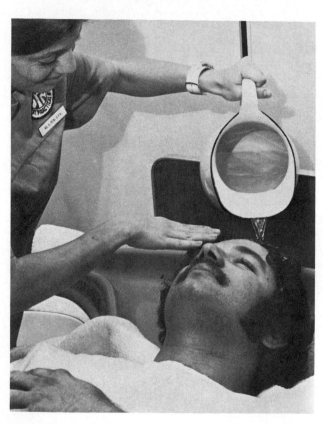

Figure 7-33 The nurse is using a plastic tray with a trough that carries water to a receptacle on the floor. Note how the patient's neck is supported with a towel on the edge of the tray.

Suggested Action	Reason for Action
Place a towel over the patient's chest and shoulders.	A towel can be used to wipe away any water that splashes the patient's face or ears.
Wet the hair thoroughly and apply shampoo.	The wet hair dilutes the shampoo, forming suds.
Work the shampoo into a lather.	The shampoo must be distributed throughout the hair to get it uniformly clean.
Rinse the hair with clean, running water.	Shampoo that remains on the hair and scalp may cause irritation.
Wrap the head with dry towels.	Towels absorb water, beginning the process of drying while allowing the patient to assume a more comfortable position.
Fluff the hair with towels, and comb out the hair.	Loosening and combing the hair prepares it for styling.
Braid, blow dry, or set the hair.	Most prefer to work with the hair following a shampoo in order to make it more attractive.

- If the patient does not object, braid the hair in two braids on either side of the head to prevent tangling or matting. The patient then does not have to lie on one heavy braid. Bobby pins or hair clips should be avoided because they may injure the scalp.
- Be sure to obtain the patient's or family's permission if the hair is hopelessly tangled and cutting it seems advisable.

Shampooing the Hair. Hair is exposed to the same dirt and oil as the skin. It should be washed as often as necessary to keep it clean. A weekly shampoo is sufficient for most persons but more or less shampooing may be indicated for others.

Shampooing the hair may be done in the shower when the patient bathes or in a basin in the bathroom if he is allowed out of bed. Some health agencies employ or arrange with a beautician or barber to provide patients with their hair-care needs. However, there may be circumstances in which the nurse will need to shampoo the patient's hair. The nurse may be responsible for shampooing the hair, especially when the patient cannot get out of bed. Skill Procedure 7-13 provides suggestions for shampooing the hair of a patient who is confined to bed.

Suggested Measures for Hygiene in Selected Situations

When the Patient Is an Infant or Child

Remember that the skin and mucous membranes of an infant or child are easily injured. Therefore, offer personal hygiene while handling infants and children gently and with care.

Newborns have difficulty regulating their temperature. The temperature of the room should be increased and there should be adequate protection from drafts during bathing.

Until the umbilical cord of a newborn comes off, bathing should be restricted to sponge bathing. Use warm water, no hotter than 40° C (105° F). Soaps should be used sparingly and rinsed off well before an infant is dried because of the irritating effects of soap remnants.

Use appropriately sized tubs for bathing a newborn after the cord comes off, and for bathing an infant. Be sure to hold the infant firmly across the back of the shoulders with one arm and hand so that the infant's head is well out of water.

Pat newborns and infants dry to prevent injury to the skin.

Check the temperature of water for an infant's or child's bath with a bath thermometer. They may not be able to indicate to the nurse when water is too hot or too cold. Children under 5 years of age are at the greatest risk.

Discourage the use of bubble baths for female children. The chemicals have been known to irritate the mucous membranes of the urinary system and cause burning when the child urinates.

Remember that children also need eye examinations and parents should be taught their importance. Many times, early detection of vision problems can prevent the occurrence of later problems that are more difficult to handle.

Infants should not be given bottles of milk or juice at night once the teeth have erupted. The sugar from the milk or juice remains in the mouth and can cause cavities. Water may be given or the mouth rinsed after a bottle of milk or juice.

Assist children under 3 years of age with oral hygiene. After about age 3, the youngster should be helped to learn how to perform his own oral hygiene.

Be sure to keep mouthwashes out of the reach of toddlers and young children. The color and taste are appealing but some mouthwashes contain substances that, if swallowed in large amounts, could threaten a youngster's life.

Teach parents how to help prevent dental caries in children. A fluoride solution is used by many dentists who also recommend using a toothpaste containing fluoride. Some dentists recommend a fluoride supplement for all children up to about 14 years of age. Sealants may be applied by some dentists to cover uneven surfaces of teeth in order to prevent their decay.

Applicable Nursing Diagnoses

Patients who require assistance with personal hygiene may have nursing diagnoses such as
- Bathing/Hygiene Self-Care Deficit
- Dressing/Grooming Self-Care Deficit
- Activity Intolerance
- High Risk for Impaired Skin Integrity
- Unilateral Neglect
- Impaired Home Maintenance Management

Nursing Care Plan 7-1 is an example for a patient with a nursing diagnosis of Bathing/Hygiene Self-Care Deficit. This category is defined in the NANDA Taxonomy (1989) as, "A state in which the individual experiences an impaired ability to perform or complete bathing/hygiene activities for oneself."

NURSING CARE PLAN

7-1. Bathing/Hygiene Self-Care Deficit

Assessment	**Subjective Data** States "I can't bathe myself and I need help brushing my teeth." **Objective Data** 52-year-old woman admitted for the repair of fractures sustained as a result of falling down the basement stairs of home. Arm cast on right. Right hand is dominant. Uses exposed right thumb and fingers for grasping objects like toothpaste. Right elbow not enclosed within cast and has full range of motion. Left arm in traction and suspension.
Diagnosis	Bathing/Hygiene Self-Care Deficit related to musculoskeletal impairment as manifested by the inability to use hands effectively for performing hygiene independently.

Plan	**Goal**
	The patient will report feeling clean and refreshed following assistance with daily bathing and mouth care.
	
	Orders: 6/2
	1. Bathe in bed after breakfast and before 1000.
	2. Use patient's own castile soap.
	3. Place small towel in rt. hand for assisting with drying face and chest.
	4. Provide a gown with sleeves that fasten with snaps.
	5. Apply deodorant and powder to underarms daily.
	6. Turn toward the arm in traction for washing back and buttocks.
	7. Provide mouth care after each meal as follows:
	   • Wrap and tape washcloth around handle of toothbrush so patient can grasp it with fingers and thumb of right hand.
	   • Apply toothpaste to toothbrush.
	   • Set emesis basin and glass of water with straw on overbed table. ___ V. MILLER, RN

Implementation (Documentation) 6/3	0845 Brushed own teeth after breakfast. _____ L. COOK, LPN 0900 Complete bed bath administered using castile soap. Able to assist with drying upper body. Hair under arms shaved. Deodorant and powder applied in axillae. Skin is pink, warm, and intact. No redness around edges of cast. Able to turn without difficulty to left side for back care. _____ L. COOK, LPN
Evaluation (Documentation)	0930 States, "I feel so much better about seeing my doctor and visitors after I've gotten cleaned up in the morning." _____ L. COOK, LPN

When the Patient Is an Adolescent

Help the adolescent who has *acne,* which is a skin eruption caused by inflammation and infection of oil glands in the skin. At present, acne cannot be cured or prevented, but teaching the adolescent the following hygienic skin care may help control it:

1. Wash the area where acne is present, usually the face, upper back, and chest, two to four times daily with soap and hot water to keep the skin clean and free of oils.
2. Shampoo the hair frequently to control oiliness.
3. Avoid using oily cosmetics.
4. Do not eat foods that make the condition worse. Other than avoidance of foods that aggravate the condition, dietary restrictions have not been found helpful in the control of acne.
5. Use preparations available on the market for con-

trolling acne according to directions, but do not use them if they irritate the skin.

6. Do not pick and squeeze pimples. These practices cause scarring and spread of infection, making matters worse.

7. Teach that exposure to the sun tends to help control acne, but stress the importance of avoiding overexposure that may cause burning and predispose the patient to precancerous lesions.

8. Seek medical attention if these conservative measures are unsuccessful.

When the Patient Has Diabetes Mellitus

Teach diabetic persons the importance of observing good practices of hygiene, since they may encounter serious problems with healing when the skin and mucous membranes are irritated or injured.

Stress the importance of proper foot care. Because diabetics tend to have circulatory and nerve deficits, especially in the legs and feet, they should learn to take special precautions to help prevent injury and irritation.

1. Inspect the feet daily. Use a mirror to look at the bottom of the feet if unable to lift and rotate them for inspection. Be sure to check between the toes for injury and infection.

2. See a physician or a podiatrist to remove corns and calluses. Do not try to remove them, and explain to the patient that he should not use commercial preparations or sharp instruments to remove them.

3. Refer the patient to a physician when there is infection or inflammation on the skin of the feet.

4. Avoid cutting toenails with a scissors. Nails should be trimmed only with a file and with great care to prevent injuring the skin around the nails.

5. Teach the diabetic person to avoid placing heating pads or hot-water bottles at the feet. The patient often is unaware of burning until damage to the skin has occurred. Serious problems may arise when the feet have been burned.

6. Teach the patient to avoid stockings with elastic tops or round garters. Garters and elastic tend to decrease normal circulation in the legs and feet, which is often already impaired in persons with diabetes.

7. Recommend that the patient prop up his feet several times a day to encourage good blood return to the heart.

8. Recommend that a diabetic person not cross his legs at the knees when he is sitting down. This practice tends to decrease circulation to the lower legs and feet.

9. Teach the diabetic person that he should avoid going barefoot to prevent injury to the feet.

10. Instruct the patient to keep his feet dry and warm and to wear stockings and shoes that are clean and fit well. The diabetic person should be taught to break in new shoes gradually to avoid blisters and skin injury.

When the Patient Is Elderly

Remember that the elderly person's skin is thin, has little elasticity, is wrinkled because of little subcutaneous fat, and is dry because of a decrease in the secretions of sebum. These characteristics make the skin easily susceptible to injury, and, therefore, all hygienic measures should be carried out with gentleness.

Take into account that the elderly have a decreased sense of temperature. Therefore, bathwater should be checked with a bath thermometer so that the skin is not burned. This is especially important for the patient who is mentally or physically handicapped.

Be sure to thoroughly rinse soap or detergent from the skin, especially between fingers and toes. Remnants of soap or detergent irritate the skin.

Assist the elderly who take showers or tub baths. Be sure the water is of a proper temperature, obstacles over which they may fall are removed, and the light is of good intensity to help prevent accidents. Do not use bath oils in the water because they make the surfaces of tubs and showers very slippery.

Use an *emollient,* which is an agent to soften, smooth, and protect dry skin. Cocoa butter, petrolatum jelly, and lanolin are often present in skin creams and lotions that serve as good emollients. Encourage the patient's fluid intake to help prevent dry skin.

Give careful foot care to the elderly person. In addition to measures described earlier in this chapter in relation to foot care, these measures should also be observed and taught:

1. Soak the feet for as long as 10 minutes and encourage the patient to wiggle and stretch his toes. Pat the feet dry, being careful to dry between the toes, and use an emollient when the skin is dry.

2. Refer the patient to a physician or podiatrist if the nails are deformed or corns or calluses are present.

3. Clean under the nails with great care to avoid injury. Bits of cotton may be placed under nails that tend to grow down and over the ends of the toes.

Be sure oral hygiene is used for the elderly who have dentures. Check the mouth for lesions and evidence of ill-fitting dentures and report abnormal findings.

Use a soft toothbrush to prevent injury to oral tissues when mouth care is given.

Use shampoos infrequently when the hair is dry. Brushing the hair regularly is recommended. Clean sections of hair by stroking them with cotton balls moistened in a mouthwash solution. This measure cleans the hair when a shampoo cannot be given and leaves the hair with a pleasant, clean odor.

Teach the dangers of overexposure to the sun, which may cause burning. The elderly are especially sensitive to overexposure to the sun. Some medications used for daytime sedation also increase sensitivity to sunlight.

High environmental temperatures and the diminished ability of the elderly to perspire predispose to heat stroke.

Encourage as much hygienic self-care as possible. This practice helps promote independence and improves morale.

Teaching Suggestions for Personal Hygiene

Suggestions for teaching when carrying out measures of personal hygiene have been described in this chapter. They are summarized below:

Recommended measures that promote personal hygiene should be included in patient-teaching plans when the nurse notes that a patient is careless about hygiene, uses poor or incorrect techniques, or misuses products intended for personal hygiene.

The sketch in Figure 7-10 illustrates the chain of events that leads to the development of dental caries. It can be used to explain to patients and family members how the chain can be broken and cavity formation prevented through proper brushing and flossing of the teeth.

Teaching about oral care should include recommendations for regular dental care and emphasis on the importance of preventive dental care for persons of all ages. Patients with dentures and bridges need the continued services of a dentist.

The person with diabetes mellitus who is well educated about proper self-care is less likely to develop complications. Proper foot care is especially important for every diabetic, a point that should be stressed in a diabetic's teaching plan.

Families of patients being cared for at home should be taught how to carry out hygienic measures that the patient cannot manage on his own.

It has been rather clearly demonstrated that overexposure to the sun can lead to serious skin problems, such as skin cancer. If people wish to be or must be in the sun for long periods, they should use a good sunscreen on the skin to help prevent damage.

Bibliography

Alberti PW, Ginsberg IA, Goode RL: Managing adult hearing loss. Patient Care 22(3):54–58, 63, 67, 1988

Arentsen JJ: A review of complications associated with soft contact lenses. Journal of Ophthalmic Nursing and Technology 6(6):230–233, 1987

Auld EM: Oral health. Geriatr Nurs 9(6):340–341, 1988

Badger F: What gets a bath? . . . Who should carry out this very necessary service. Community Outlook 15–17, March 1989

Bucholz K: When dental care is up to you. RN Magazine 51(2):42–44, 1988

Carbary LJ: What did you say? Caring for the patient who has a hearing impairment. Journal of Practical Nursing 38(3):36–39, 1988

Care of the perianal area. Patient Care 20(5):178, 1986

Chovaz C: Nursing the hearing impaired patient. Canadian Nurse 85(3):34–36, 1989

Contact lenses: What to consider. Consumer Reports 54(6):411–415, 1989

Cotgraeve JT, Patch TM, Perten CE: Part of your daily routine: Teaching good contact lens care. Professional Nurse 4(9):446–449, 1989

Danielson KH: Oral care & older adults. Journal of Gerontological Nursing 14(11):6–10, 1988

Daschner FD: Useful and useless hygienic techniques in intensive care units. Intensive Care Med 11(6):280–283, 1985

Donahue AM: Tepid sponging. Journal of Emergency Nursing 9(2):78–82, 1983

French S. Understanding partial sight. Nursing Times 84(3):32–33, 1988

Gleason C, Hops S, Macmillan K: Dental care for disabled adults. Canadian Nurse 84(3):21–23, 1988

Hearing loss: Basic anatomy of the ear. Hospital Medicine 22(7):160, 162–165, 1986

How to remove contact lenses. NursingLife 6(4):14–15, 1986

Joyner M: Hair care in the black patient. Journal of Pediatric Health Care 2(6):281–287, 1988

Kovach T: Controlling infection as part of the bathing care process. Provider 14(12):43–44, 1988

Lindell ME, Olsson HM: Lack of care givers' knowledge causes unnecessary suffering in elderly patients. J Adv Nurs 14(11):976–979, 1989

Meckstroth RL: Improving quality and efficiency in oral hygiene. Journal of Gerontological Nursing 15(6):38–44, 1989

Mulhall A, Chapman R, Crow R: Meatal cleansing. Nursing Times 84(4):66, 69, 1988

Page JC: Selecting a hearing protective device. AORN J 36(1):40–41, 1988

Parrott TE: Care of long hair. AD Nurse 2(5):8–10, 1987

Pesci BR: When the patient's problem is really poor vision. RN Magazine 49(10):22–25, 1986

Petrowski DD: Care of an artificial eye after enucleation. Journal of Ophthalmic Nursing and Technology 5(4):135–138, 1986

Rakow PL: Disposable lenses: A Pandora's box. Journal of Ophthalmic Nursing and Technology 7(2):72, 74, 1988

Rakow PL: RGP (Rigid gas permeable) lenses: Proceed with caution. Journal of Ophthalmic Nursing and Technology 7(3):108–110, 1988

Rakow PL: Soft lens cleaning and disinfection. Journal of Ophthalmic Nursing and Technology 4(5):36, 38, 1985

Renn N: Oral health and hygiene for the elderly. Home Healthcare Nurse 7(3):37–39, 1989

Verma S: Caring for nursing home residents means caring for their vision. Nursing Homes 34(6):39–40, 1985

Wagnild G: Convey respect during bathing procedures. Journal of Gerontological Nursing 11(12):6–10, 1985

Walsh C: Common sense nursing care for the patient with poor vision. RN Magazine 49(10):24–25, 1986

Wright L: Bathing by towel. Nursing Times 86(4):36–37, 39, 1990

8

Promoting Proper Nutrition

Chapter Outline

Behavioral Objectives
Glossary
Introduction
Culture and Eating Habits
Human Nutritional Needs
Basic Food Groups
Vegetarianism
Nutritional Assessment
Promoting Weight Gain or Loss
Common Problems That Influence Eating
Measuring and Recording Fluid Intake
Commonly Prescribed Diets
Providing Food for Patients
Alternative Methods of Providing Nourishment
Suggested Measures to Promote Nutrition in Selected
　Situations
Applicable Nursing Diagnoses
Teaching Suggestions to Promote Nutrition
Bibliography

Skill Procedures

Serving and Removing Trays
Helping the Patient to Eat
Inserting, Maintaining, and Removing a Nasogastric
　Tube
Inserting a Small Diameter Feeding Tube
Administering a Tube Feeding
Irrigating a Nasogastric Tube

Behavioral Objectives

When the content of this chapter has been mastered, the learner will be able to:

Define the terms appearing in the glossary.

List examples of food and eating habits influenced by culture.

Describe the basic nutritional needs of man.

Identify two guides that may be used to plan well-balanced diets. Discuss ways in which vegetarians remain healthy with the use of little or no animal protein.

List information that is useful for a nutritional assessment.

List suggestions for gaining or losing weight.

Discuss measures that may reduce or relieve anorexia, nausea, vomiting, and stomach gas.

Describe actions the nurse could take when feeding patients, or when providing alternative nourishment through a nasogastric tube, nasointestinal tube, gastrostomy tube, jejunostomy tube, or by hyperalimentation.

Discuss methods for inserting, maintaining, irrigating, and removing a nasogastric tube.

Describe techniques for inserting a small-diameter feeding tube.

List suggested measures for promoting nutrition in selected situations, as described in this chapter.

Summarize suggestions for patient teaching offered in this chapter.

Glossary

Anorexia Loss of appetite or lack of desire for food.

Aspiration The entry of fluid into the air passages and lungs.

Belching The discharge of gas from the stomach through the mouth. Synonym for *eructation*.

Bolus feeding The instillation of a large volume of liquid nourishment at one time.

Cachexia A condition in which there is general wasting away of body tissue.

Calorie The amount of heat necessary to raise the temperature of 1 g of water 1°C.

Continuous feeding The instillation of a small volume of liquid nourishment without any interruption.

Emesis Vomited contents from the stomach. Synonym for *vomitus*.

Eructation The discharge of gas from the stomach through the mouth. Synonym for *belching*.

Flatus Intestinal gas released from the rectum.

Gastric gavage Introduction of nourishment into the stomach with a tube inserted through the nose and esophagus.

Gastric residual The volume remaining in the stomach.

Gastrostomy A surgical opening into the stomach through the abdominal wall.

Gavage Introducing nourishment through a nasogastric or nasointestinal tube.

Intermittent feeding The instillation of liquid nourishment over a period of 30 to 60 minutes.

Jejunostomy tube A method for instilling liquid nourishment into the midportion of the small intestine.

Junk food Food that adds large amounts of calories without contributing much to nutrition.

Malnutrition A condition resulting from a lack of proper nutrients in the diet.

Megadose An amount of a substance that exceeds that which is recommended to sustain health.

Metabolic rate The rate at which the body burns calories.

Nausea The feeling of sickness with a desire to vomit.

Nutrition The process whereby the body uses foods and fluids to reach and maintain health.

Obesity A condition in which there is an excess amount of body fat.

Parenteral hyperalimentation A method to supply all the necessary nutrients the body needs when other methods are no longer adequate. Synonym for *total parenteral nutrition.*

Patent A state in which a tube remains unobstructed.

Projectile vomiting Vomiting with great force.

Protein complementation The act of combining two or more plant proteins at the same meal in order to supply the same amino acids present in animal protein.

Recommended dietary allowance The average daily amount of a nutrient that is felt to be adequate to meet health needs.

Regurgitation The act of bringing the stomach contents to the throat and mouth without vomiting effort.

Retching The act of vomiting without producing vomitus.

Total parenteral nutrition A method to supply all the necessary nutrients the body needs when other methods are no longer adequate. Abbreviated TPN. Synonym for *parenteral hyperalimentation.*

Vegetarian An individual who avoids eating meat and animal products.

Vomiting The act of forcing the contents of the stomach out through the mouth.

Vomitus Vomited contents from the stomach. Synonym for *emesis.*

Introduction

More and more data support the fact that food intake, or the lack of it, influences health and well-being. Modifying and regulating food has been a standard technique used in the treatment of diseases. Now, there is an emphasis on improving nutrition in order to prevent diseases and im-

prove a state of wellness. Healthy people in general are becoming selective about the quantity and quality of their daily food consumption. Nurses must be able to advise people about what to eat in order to meet normal needs, discourage food fads and unsafe dieting, and perform skills that affect the patient's nutrition and digestive processes.

Most nursing students study nutrition in a separate course. Therefore, only a brief review of some of the basic knowledge from the field of nutrition is presented. This chapter primarily deals with nursing care that will help people maintain normal nutrition. It also provides suggestions for skills that may be necessary when normal nutrition or digestion is affected.

Culture and Eating Habits

Eating is one of man's basic needs. If an individual is deprived of food for a length of time, health will be affected or life may be endangered. Most eating habits are learned early in life and vary from culture to culture.

Religious practices often influence eating habits. For instance, many Jews and Moslems avoid pork, and fasting is practiced in certain religions. Some persons, because of religious or personal reasons, are vegetarians and eat no meat.

Specific kinds of food are associated with certain nationalities. Hamburgers and hot dogs are associated with Americans; pasta, such as spaghetti, has been popularized by Italians; and baklava, a dessert, is a favorite among Greeks.

Some people prefer the largest meal of the day at noon. Others prefer this meal in the evening.

Family get-togethers are often centered around a holiday meal, such as Thanksgiving and Christmas dinners.

Certain beverages and foods are associated with festive occasions. Champagne is the traditional wedding beverage, turkey is served for Thanksgiving, and candy is a popular St. Valentine's Day gift.

Eating utensils differ. Americans use knives, forks, and spoons; Far Easterners eat with chopsticks; and Arabs use bread to dip foods from serving containers.

Despite variations in preferred foods and eating customs, all humans have the same basic nutritional needs for health. The nurse should respect cultural differences while helping individuals meet nutritional requirements.

Human Nutritional Needs

Nutrition is defined as the process in which the body uses food and fluids to reach and maintain health. The science of nutrition has identified the body's needs for calories, water, proteins, carbohydrates, fats, vitamins, and minerals.

Calories

Man has discovered that various substances can be converted into energy. Coal, oil, wood, steam, and alcohol are energy sources for machines. Food is the source of energy for humans. It provides the means by which the body carries out its functions.

Energy sources can be measured; in this way their effectiveness as a fuel can be determined. This is done by comparing a certain volume or weight of the energy source with its ability to produce heat.

The energy equivalent of foods is measured in calories. A *calorie* is the amount of heat necessary to raise the temperature of 1 gram of water 1° C. Protein, fats, and carbohydrates have caloric value; they furnish energy to the body. Foods are usually combinations of proteins, fats, and carbohydrates. Water, vitamins, and minerals do not contain calories, although they are essential for health.

Needs for calories vary and depend on factors such as age, activity, body temperature, and gender. Most average adults need between 2000 and 3000 calories per day according to the National Research Council of the National Academy of Science.

Water

Approximately 45% to 75% of our body weight is water. The normal amount depends mostly on age. Infants have the largest amount and the elderly have the least in relation to body weight. Individuals can live longer without food than water. Water must be maintained at a fairly constant level to maintain health. Therefore, sufficient water intake is an essential part of wellness. Nursing skills for maintaining fluid balance will be discussed further in Chapter 25.

Proteins

The body uses proteins to build, maintain, and repair body tissue. Protein can be used for energy. It provides 4 calories per gram. The body spares protein for energy use as long as calories are available from carbohydrates and fats.

Protein is constantly being formed or broken down in order to maintain a healthy state. The body cannot supply its own raw source of protein. Food sources of protein supply amino acids, the ingredients that the body refashions into types of proteins it requires. As long as the dietary intake of protein is adequate, the body can function at a fairly optimum level.

Proteins come from animal and plant sources of food. Animal sources of protein contain all the essential amino acids, or building blocks, the body needs for growth and repair. However, if certain plant sources are eaten together, each contributes some of these amino acids. *Protein complementation,* the act of combining two or more plant sources at the same meal, may supply the same total amino acids found in a single animal source. This will be discussed further in relation to vegetarian diets later in the chapter.

People who are poorly nourished almost always consume foods that are poor in protein content. The other extreme may also be unwise; diets that are exclusively protein are also dangerous. Protein food, especially from animal sources, is likely to be the most expensive nutrient in the diet. Individuals on low incomes who do not understand the principle of combining cheaper plant sources of protein are likely to be malnourished. *Malnutrition* is a condition resulting from a lack of proper nutrients in the diet. This is a common problem among people in poorer, developing countries. In the United States, however, certain groups of people tend to be under nourished, such as the socially isolated elderly living on fixed incomes, children of economically deprived parents, and people with alcoholism. Even those who eat mostly convenience and fast foods may be marginally nourished.

The following are examples of protein foods: milk, meat, fish, poultry, eggs, legumes (peas, beans, peanuts), nuts, and components of grains.

Carbohydrates

Carbohydrates are the chief component of most people's diets. Plants are the main source of carbohydrates; they are often referred to as sugars and starches. Carbohydrates supply 4 calories of energy per gram. Carbohydrates are used primarily as a quick energy source. They make the diet more tasty and attractive.

Carbohydrates, however, are important for more than just their calories. For example, the undigestible fiber found in the stems, skins, and leaves of many fruits and vegetables gives the diet bulk that helps elimination. Some claim that various diseases can be prevented by increasing dietary fiber. People in the United States tend to eat precooked or excessively cooked and refined carbohydrates. As a health measure, many are increasing their consumption of fresh fruits, vegetables, and whole grains.

The following are examples of good sources of carbohydrates: cereals and grains, such as rice, wheat and wheat germ, oats, barley, corn and corn meal; fruits and vegetables; molasses, maple and corn syrups, honey, and common table sugar.

Fats

Dietary fats come from both animal and plant sources. Fats have a higher energy value than other nutrients; they yield 9 calories per gram. This is 2½ times the amount of either proteins or carbohydrates. For this reason alone, their consumption should be limited especially by those who have a tendency to be overweight. Alcoholic beverages, though they are not fats, are also high in calories. Alcohol provides 7 calories per gram; these calories and the chemical, alcohol, are unnecessary and even damaging to the health of some people.

Though fats are high in calories, they should not be totally eliminated. Fats provide energy and are necessary for many chemical reactions in the body. Some vitamins are absorbed with dietary fats. They add to the flavor of food and, because they leave the stomach slowly, they promote a feeling of having satisfied appetite and hunger.

In general, Americans eat more fats than do people in most other countries. The influence of fat consumption in relation to diseases is being studied. There seems to be a direct link between the intake of certain types of fat and heart disease. Being over-weight, usually from excess calorie consumption, is being investigated as having a relationship with some types of cancer. Results that link cancer with fat are not yet conclusive. In 1982, in an effort to improve the health of the nation, the Committee on Diet, Nutrition, and Cancer of the National Academy of Science's Research Council recommended that Americans should reduce their present fat intake from 40% of the day's calories to 30%.

The following foods are rich in fat: red meat, such as beef and pork; butter, margarine, and vegetable oils; egg yolk; whole milk and cheese; peanut butter; salad dressings; avocados; chocolate; and nuts.

Minerals

There are substances in food, other than the calories in nutrients, that are necessary for health. These substances are minerals and vitamins. Minerals are chemical substances, such as calcium, sodium, potassium, chloride, and so on. When these substances are dissolved in the body, they are called electrolytes. These chemicals do not supply the body with energy, but they are necessary ingredients of cells, body tissue, and body fluids. They play a role in the regulation of many of the body's chemical processes, such as blood clotting and the conduction of nerve impulses. Table 8-1 lists some of the major and trace minerals of the body, their chief functions, and common dietary sources.

Table 8-1. **Common Minerals Needed by the Body, Their Chief Functions, and Dietary Sources**

Mineral	Chief Functions	Common Dietary Sources
Sodium	Maintenance of water and electrolyte balance	Table salt
		Processed meat
Potassium	Maintenance of electrolyte balance	Bananas
	Neuromuscular activity	Oranges
	Enzyme reactions	Potatoes
Chloride	Maintenance of fluid and electrolyte balance	Table salt
		Processed meat
Calcium	Formation of teeth and bones	Milk
	Neuromuscular activity	Milk products
	Blood coagulation	
	Cell-wall permeability	
Phosphorus	Buffering action	Eggs
	Formation of bones and teeth	Meat
		Milk
Iodine	Regulation of body metabolism	Seafoods
	Promotion of normal growth	Iodized salt
Iron	Component of hemoglobin	Liver
	Assistance in cellular oxidation	Egg yolk
		Meat
Magnesium	Neuromuscular activity	Whole grains
	Activation of enzymes	Milk
	Formation of teeth and bones	Meat
Zinc	Constituent of enzymes and insulin	Seafoods
		Liver

Vitamins

Vitamins are unique chemical substances. They are not components of cells or tissue, but they are necessary in minute amounts for normal growth, maintenance of health, and functioning of the body. Many deficiency diseases have been associated with diets in which specific foods, rich in a source of a vitamin, have been lacking. For example, scurvy, a disease associated with vitamin C (ascorbic acid) deficiency, frequently occurred among British sailors who did not eat fresh fruits and vegetables. When limes were eaten while at sea, this disease did not occur. Hence, to this day British sailors are referred to as "limeys."

Vitamins were first named according to the sequence of letters in the alphabet. Numbers were subsequently added to some letters as more were identified. Chemical names are now replacing the letter-number system of identification.

Vitamins are dissolved in the water and fat of the body. The former require daily replacement because they are lost along with the water, which is eliminated from the body. The other fat-soluble vitamins are stored as a reserve for future needs. With the exception of vitamin K (menadione) and biotin, vitamins cannot be manufactured by the body. They are usually consumed within the food that is eaten. Cooking, processing, and lack of refrigeration can deplete the content of some vitamins in food.

Some prefer to take vitamin and mineral supplements, but they are not necessary for most people as long as they eat a well-balanced diet consisting of a variety of foods. Some foods have been enriched with vitamins and minerals to ensure that most individuals consume adequate daily amounts. Table 8-2 lists vitamins required by the body, their chief functions, and common dietary sources.

Consuming *megadoses* of vitamins, amounts exceeding those considered adequate for health, can be dangerous. Some people with terminal diseases follow unconventional diets and take large doses of vitamins in a desperate attempt to restore their health. There is no conclusive evidence that this approach cures their condition.

Basic Food Groups

Much research has been done on how much of each nutrient an individual should consume to stay healthy. The Food and Nutrition Board of the National Academy of Science publishes advice about food and nutrition. Some of its recommendations are referred to in this chapter.

One of the first standards for good nutrition was a list of *Recommended Dietary Allowances* (RDAs). These are average daily amounts of nutrients felt to be adequate to meet the health needs for practically all people. Because individuals are unique, these amounts are useful only as a guide.

The RDA amounts are difficult for average individuals to interpret and use. Therefore, a simpler system was developed to help individuals consume a variety of foods in appropriate amounts to prevent deficiency diseases. It originally was called the Basic Seven, which was simplified to what is now referred to as the *Basic Four.* This serves as a guide for planning a well-balanced, daily diet for the average adult. These food groups and recommended daily servings are described in Figure 8-1. Snack foods, such as soft drinks and potato chips, are often called *junk food* because they add so many calories without contributing much to nutrition.

Modifications in the recommended amounts still need to be made for individual differences. Children, adolescents, pregnant women, and breast-feeding mothers require more servings per day of certain groups, particularly the milk group. Some adult women and children need to eat more to consume adequate amounts of iron.

Vegetarianism

Individuals who for religious or personal reasons do not eat animal sources of food are called *vegetarians*. A strict vegetarian is one who not only does not consume animal food, like meat, but also avoids eating any products from animals, such as milk or eggs. There are variations among the practices of vegetarians. Lacto-ovovegetarians eat milk and eggs; lactovegetarians drink milk and eat milk products but avoid eggs and meat. Because meat, eggs, and milk products are recommended sources of daily nutrients, deficiency diseases may be a potential nutritional problem. A strict vegetarian is wise to take vitamin B_{12} (Cyanocobalamin) supplements because the main sources of this vitamin are found in animal substances.

Those who omit eating meat as part of an organized religion or ethnic tradition, such as the Seventh Day Adventists and Moslems, usually have developed dietary substitutions for meat that are essentially healthful. There may be difficulty in obtaining appropriate foods or a variety of them while these individuals are patients. Nurses should make the effort to accommodate dietary choices rather than permit a patient to refuse eating. Family members are often willing to provide special food.

Those who arbitrarily choose to become vegetarians may need to learn how to combine plant sources to ensure that they are consuming adequate amounts of all the essential amino acids. Table 8-3 shows the types of incomplete proteins appropriate for protein complementation. All plant sources, if eaten daily with small amounts of dairy products or eggs, should be adequate for health.

Nutritional Assessment

Because eating is a basic need, it is important for the nurse to identify any current or potential problems from inadequate nutrition. One place to begin is to obtain a diet

Table 8-2. Common Vitamins Needed by the Body, Their Chief Functions,
and Common Dietary Sources

Vitamin	Chief Functions	Common Dietary Sources
A (Retinol) Not destroyed by ordinary cooking temperatures	Growth of body cells Promotion of vision, healthy hair and skin, and integrity of epithelial membranes Prevention of xerophthalmia, a condition characterized by chronic conjunctivitis	Animal fats: butter, cheese, cream, egg yolk, whole milk Fish liver oil and liver Green leafy and yellow fruits and vegetables
B$_1$ (Thiamine) Not readily destroyed by ordinary cooking temperatures	Carbohydrate metabolism Functioning of nervous system Normal digestion Prevention of beriberi, a condition characterized by neuritis	Fish Lean meat and poultry Glandular organs Milk Whole grain cereals Peas, beans, and peanuts
B$_2$ (Riboflavin) Not destroyed by heat except in presence of alkali	Formation of certain enzymes Normal growth Light adaptation in the eyes	Eggs Green leafy vegetables Lean meat Milk Whole grains Dried yeast
B$_3$ (Niacin)	Carbohydrate, fat, and protein metabolism Enzyme component Prevention of appetite loss Prevention of pellagra, a condition characterized by cutaneous, gastrointestinal, neurologic, and mental symptoms	Lean meat and liver Fish Peas, beans Whole grain cereals Peanuts Yeast Eggs Liver
B$_6$ (Pyridoxine) Destroyed by heat, sunlight, and air	Healthy gums and teeth Red blood cell formation Carbohydrate, fat, and protein metabolism	Whole grain cereals and wheat germ Vegetables Yeast Meat Bananas Black strap molasses
B$_9$ (Folic acid)	Protein metabolism Red blood cell formation Normal intestinal-tract functioning	Green leafy vegetables Glandular organs Yeast
B$_{12}$ (Cyanocobalamin)	Protein metabolism Red blood cell formation Healthy nervous system tissues Prevention of pernicious anemia, a condition characterized by decreased red blood cells	Liver and kidney Dairy products Lean meat Milk Saltwater fish and oysters

(continued)

Table 8-2. Continued

Vitamin	Chief Functions	Common Dietary Sources
C (Ascorbic acid) Readily destroyed by cooking temperatures	Healthy bones, teeth, and gums Formation of blood vessels and capillary walls Proper tissue and bone healing Facilitation of iron and folic acid absorption Prevention of scurvy, a condition characterized by hemorrhagic condition and abnormal bone and teeth formation	Citrus fruits and juices Tomato Berries Cabbage Green vegetables Potatoes
D (Calciferol) Relatively stable with refrigeration	Absorption of calcium and phosphorus Prevention of rickets, a condition characterized by weak bones	Fish liver oils, salmon, tuna Milk Egg yolk Butter Liver Oysters Formed in the skin by exposure to sunlight
E (Alpha-tocopherol) Heat stable in absence of oxygen	Red blood cell formation Protection of essential fatty acids Important for normal reproduction in experimental animals (*i.e.,* rats)	Green leafy vegetables Wheat germ oil Margarine Brown rice
Pantothenic acid	Metabolism	Liver Egg yolk Milk
H (Biotin) Heat sensitive	Enzyme activity Metabolism of carbohydrates, fats, and proteins	Egg yolk Green vegetables Milk Liver and kidney Yeast
K (Menadione)	Production of prothrombin	Liver Eggs Green leafy vegetables Synthesized in the gastrointestinal tract by bacteria

history. The nurse should ask questions about the following:

- The amounts of specific foods eaten on an average day. The foods within the basic four groups may be used as a guide. It may be helpful for the patient to use household measurements, such as a cup, glass, or bowl, when describing the amounts.

- The amounts of non-nutritional foods eaten on an average day, including sweets, soft drinks, snack foods, coffee, and alcohol.
- Food likes, dislikes, and beliefs.
- Vitamin or mineral supplements that are taken routinely and why.
- Food supplements or restrictions and the reason for them.

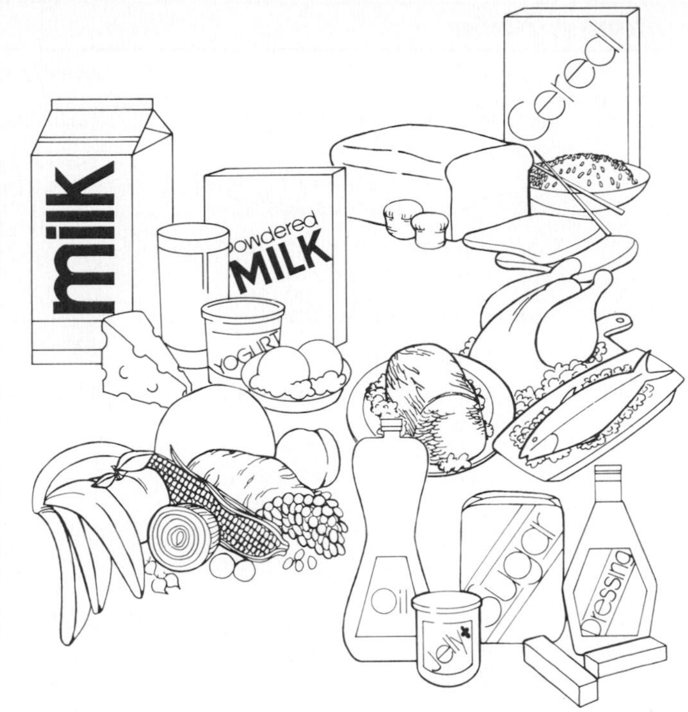

Milk Group
Some milk for everyone
Children under 9 . . . 2 to 3 cups
Children 9 to 12 . . . 3 or more cups
Teenagers . . . 4 or more cups
Adults . . . 2 or more cups

Vegetable Fruit Group
4 or more servings
Include—
A citrus fruit or other fruit or
vegetable important for vitamin C
A dark-green or deep-yellow
vegetable for vitamin A—at
least every other day
Other vegetables and fruits,
including potatoes

Bread Cereal Group
4 or more servings
Whole grain, enriched, or
restored

Meat Group
2 or more servings
Beef, veal, pork, lamb, poultry,
fish, eggs
As alternatives—dry beans, dry
peas, nuts

Other Foods
To round out meals and meet
energy needs, most everyone
will use some foods not
specified in the Four Food
Groups. Such foods include
breads, cereals, flours, sugars,
butter, margarine, other fats.
These often are ingredients in a
recipe or added to other foods
during preparation or at table.
Try to include some vegetable
oils among the fats used.

Figure 8-1 Food for Fitness: A Daily Food Guide. (Adapted from Leaflet 424, US Department of Agriculture, Institute of Home Economics.)

- Current or previous special diets that have been medically or self-prescribed.
- Any problems with eating, digestion, or elimination.

One of the easiest, though not always the most accurate, assessments related to an individual's nutritional state is body weight. Various growth charts and height-age-sex graphs may be used. A quick determination of the ideal weight of an adult with an average frame can be made if the following formula is used.

For women: 100 pounds for the first 5 feet + 5 pounds for each additional inch.
For men: 106 pounds for the first 5 feet and 6 pounds for each additional inch.*

An average frame exists if the index finger and thumb meet when they encircle the wrist.

A more significant factor is the ratio of lean body mass to fat. Many an athlete weighs more than charts indicate is healthy, yet the body is composed primarily of lean, muscular tissue.

Cachexia is a condition in which there is general wasting away of body tissue. Most people in America do not manifest this except when extremely ill. More often the nurse is

likely to find that individuals are obese. *Obesity* is a condition in which there is an excessive amount of body fat, usually over 20% of the ideal weight. Being able to "pinch an inch," as a famous cereal advertisement describes, is probably a good indication of excess weight. Measuring skin-fold thickness with a special instrument called calipers is a more objective measurement. This would also be a better method for comparing any future changes in the amount of body fat.

Other assessments also include the characteristics of healthy skin, mucous membranes, and hair and nails, as discussed in the previous chapter. Laboratory tests such as hemoglobin and blood fat levels also contribute information to the database about nutrition.

Promoting Weight Gain or Loss

It is important that individuals who are dissatisfied with their appearance actually have a need to lose or gain weight. A desire to change one's weight may be based on wanting to resemble an unrealistic cultural ideal. Individuals who are extremely underweight or overweight should be referred to a physician to determine if any physical or emotional problems are contributing to the person's weight.

Measures to Promote Weight Gain. The nurse may find some of the following suggestions useful for a patient who is only slightly underweight.

*Hamwi GJ: Therapy: Changing dietary concepts. In Danowski TS, Hamwi GJ (eds): Diabetes Mellitus: Diagnosis and Treatment, pp 73–78. New York, American Diabetes Association, 1964. Reproduced with permission from the American Diabetes Association, Inc.

Table 8-3. Protein Complementation

Plant Combinations	Types	Serving Suggestions
Legumes + cereal grains	Legumes: peas (chickpeas, split peas, green garden peas), beans (soy, kidney, black, pinto, navy; not green beans) peanuts, lentils	Bean soup with corn bread
		Peanut butter sandwich on whole wheat bread
	Cereal grains: rice, wheat, barley, oats, corn, millet, etc.	Nonmeat chilli served over rice or macaroni
Legumes + seeds or nuts	Seeds: sunflower, sesame	Tofu and sunflower seeds in a tossed green salad
	Nuts: cashews, walnuts, pecans	
Grains + nuts + nonmeat animal protein	Nonmeat animal protein: milk, cheese, yogurt, eggs	Granola with milk

Lappe FM: Diet for a Small Planet, 10th anniversary ed. Ballantine, New York, 1985. Reprinted by permission of Frances Moore Lappe and her agents, Raines & Raines. Copyright © 1971, 1975, 1982, 1985 by Frances Moore Lappe.

- From each of the basic four food groups, select foods that are higher in calories than those usually eaten.
- Eat slightly larger servings than previously eaten, especially if the daily schedule includes a lot of hard work or recreational exercise.
- Eat with others. Sometimes people don't bother to eat, or they eat very little, if they are the only ones eating.
- Snack on high-calorie but nutritious foods such as hard cheese, milk shakes, and nuts.

Measures to Promote Weight Loss. More often than not, the nurse will be asked for suggestions on ways to lose weight. The nurse should emphasize that a gradual loss of about 1 to 2 pounds a week will probably result in longer maintenance of weight loss. The nurse must advise individuals against the hazards of unsupervised weight loss techniques like fasting, fad diets, or diet drugs. To lose weight safely, use the following guidelines.

- From each of the basic four food groups, select foods that are lower in calories than those usually eaten.
- Omit junk food.
- Eat several small meals. Any nutrients not used from large meals are stored as fat.
- Sit at the table to eat, and do not do other things, such as reading, while you eat. Distraction often fools the brain's awareness that eating has taken place.
- Increase fiber in the diet from fresh fruits, vegetables, and whole grains. Fiber is not digested and may provide a full feeling without large numbers of calories.
- Participate in some regular, active form of exercise. Exercise raises the *metabolic rate,* the rate at which calories are used, while actually suppressing the appetite. Information on activity and exercise can be found in Chapter 9.

Common Problems That Influence Eating

Anorexia is a loss of appetite or a lack of desire for food. There are many factors that may produce anorexia. Some are illness, general lack of interest in food, and feeling tense and worried. If the symptom continues and the patient is eating poorly, the physician may need to prescribe measures that will help the patient receive adequate nourishment. An example is to provide the patient with nourishment intravenously (*i.e.,* to instill solutions directly into his veins). Nursing skills for administering intravenous solutions are discussed further in Chapter 25.

Nausea is a feeling of sickness with a desire to vomit. It may be associated with feeling faint or weak. Often, dizziness, perspiration, skin pallor, a rapid pulse rate, and a headache are present. *Retching,* which is the act of vomiting without producing vomitus, may also be present.

Vomiting results when the contents of the stomach are forced out through the mouth. The vomited content is called *emesis* or *vomitus.* Nausea is usually present before vomiting occurs.

Projectile vomiting is vomiting with great force. Nausea may be present but often is not. Projectile vomiting is often noted in certain disease conditions, such as increased pressure on brain tissues or when gastrointestinal bleeding is present.

Bringing stomach contents to the throat and mouth without the effort of vomiting is called *regurgitation.* It occurs quite commonly among infants after eating.

Eructation or *belching* is a discharge of gas from the stomach through the mouth. It often occurs when the patient swallows air while eating. Some foods such as beans, onions, cucumbers, and vegetables in the cabbage family may increase a tendency to cause gas. *Flatus* is gas that is formed in the intestine and released from the rectum. Methods to relieve the distension from intestinal gas are discussed in Chapter 22.

Overcoming Anorexia and Nausea. The following guidelines are often helpful when anorexia and nausea are present.

- Check to see if something as simple as an annoying odor or sight has produced anorexia, nausea, and even vomiting.
- Have the individual take several deep breaths to help overcome feelings of nausea.
- Avoid abrupt movements and limit activities. Moving about increases feelings of nausea.
- Limit the intake of food and fluid temporarily until signs of nausea subside. Then offer fluids in small sips.
- Avoid making negative comments about food. Such comments tend to increase anorexia and nausea.
- Offer a light but nutritious breakfast. Often, the condition worsens during the course of the day but the appetite may be good for the first meal of the day.
- Offer bland foods when a person is nauseated. Spicy foods and greasy foods tend to increase nausea. Carbonated beverages, especially colas, often help to relieve nausea. Sucking on ice chips also helps to relieve nausea.
- Consult the physician when anorexia and nausea continue. Certain medications may help relieve these conditions.

Controlling Vomiting. The following nursing measures are recommended when a person vomits.

- Temporarily limit the intake of food. Adding contents to an already upset stomach may prolong episodes of vomiting.
- Use measures to prevent choking or having vomitus enter the lungs (*aspiration*) when a person is vomiting. Lean the head forward over a container or the toilet.
- If vomiting is frequent, a person is usually more comfortable lying down, rather than remaining in a sitting position.
- Adjust the light, sound, ventilation, and temperature to a comfortable level. Reducing stimulation may reduce the urge to vomit.
- Provide a cool washcloth to the forehead or back of the neck. Vomiting may be accompanied by an increase in perspiration and a clammy feeling to the skin.
- Rinse the mouth, offer mouthwash, or provide mouthcare as soon as possible after vomiting. Gastric acid is harmful to the enamel of teeth. Emesis usually produces an unpleasant aftertaste in the mouth.

Individuals who are patients in a health agency present other challenges to the nurse because they are often weak and helpless. They may have other conditions that vomiting can complicate. Further suggestions in these situations include the following.

- Turn an unconscious or weak patient onto his abdomen or side. This helps emesis drain from the mouth rather than the throat, where it may be aspirated into the lungs.
- Use a suction machine to clear vomitus from the mouth and throat of a weak or unconscious patient to prevent choking and aspiration.
- Provide firm support with the hands or a pillow to abdominal incisions. Strong muscle contractions may pull on stitches and increase pain and discomfort. An abdominal binder may also offer support.
- Help reduce tension as much as possible. The patient may appreciate a face cloth or a backrub.
- Remove the container of emesis from the patient's bedside as soon as possible. The appearance and odor may stimulate more vomiting. Provide ventilation to remove any lingering odors.
- Observe the characteristics of the emesis. Note the amount, color, and any unusual odor, such as the odor of fecal material or alcohol. Send a specimen to the laboratory if ordered. Save a specimen or delay flushing if the characteristics are unusual. Have another nurse check the vomitus if there are any questions.
- Measure the amount of emesis if the patient's fluid intake and output are being totaled.
- Consult with the physician when vomiting continues. It may be necessary to use prescribed medications to relieve it.

Relieving Stomach Gas. Gas normally forms during digestion. It only becomes a problem when it forms excessively and accumulates. The following suggestions may be used when the patient experiences discomfort from an accumulation of gas in the stomach.

- Suggest that the patient chew food with his mouth closed. Laughing and talking while eating contributes to the amount of air that is swallowed with food.
- Avoid using a straw. Each swallow of liquid also contains the air present in the straw.
- Avoid eating foods that are gas formers.
- When under tension avoid eating. Emotions delay the stomach's emptying. Any gas that is present will be prevented from being distributed to the intestine.
- Walking about may help the gas rise to its highest point in the stomach, making it easier to be belched through the mouth.
- Some may prefer to use medications that absorb gas from the stomach. Care should be taken that all package directions are followed.
- Patients who are unable to release gastric gas or vomit continuously may need to have a tube passed into the stomach to remove the gas and fluid with suction.

Measuring and Recording Fluid Intake

An important means of identifying a potential fluid problem is to measure and record the amounts of all liquids consumed or instilled into the body. This includes those foods that are liquid at room temperature, such as ice cream, Jello, and sherbet. It also includes thin, cooked cereals. If fluid balance exists, the total intake should approximate the total output. In health agencies, intake and output are often abbreviated as I and O. More information on assessing and maintaining fluid balance is discussed in Chapter 25.

Health agencies generally have lists readily available to tell the nurse the amount of fluid contained in common serving dishes, glasses, cups, and water containers. The unit of measure is a milliliter, abbreviated mL.

Agency policies are followed concerning the measurement and recording of I and O. Each institution usually supplies a special form that contains spaces where entries can be made throughout the day. The patient should be helped to understand why his intake and output are to be measured and recorded and why it is important to do so accurately. The amounts are usually totaled at 8- and 24-hour periods by the nurse or some other person assigned to this task. The nurse is responsible for evaluating the amounts. When communicating with others who will be responsible for the patient's care on other shifts, fluid intake and output are part of the information that is reported. Figure 8-2 is an example of a form used to record the patient's intake.

Measuring and recording I and O are often done carelessly, yet they are very important nursing duties. Much of the patient's care may be affected by these figures. If the patient appears not to be taking enough fluids, for example, the physician may order a solution to be given intravenously. Inattention to this important nursing responsibility represents poor quality care.

For home care, the nurse may need to teach an individual or a family member how to measure and record fluid intake. While using a common household measuring cup, the fluid content of that person's cup, glass, soup dish, or other container used at home can be determined. Then it becomes an easy matter to measure and record the intake. Home measurement is usually stated in ounces.

INTAKE CHART

7:00 A.M. ______ TO 7:00 A.M. ______

		INTAKE				
	ORAL	I.V.		BLOOD	OTHER	COMMENTS
7-8	370ml					
8-9						
9-10						
10-11	100 ml					
11-12						
12-1	350ml					
1-2	75ml					
2-3	200ml					
8 HR. TOT.	1095ml					
3-4						
4-5	50ml					
5-6						
6-7	400ml					
7-8	200ml					
8-9	125ml					
9-10	100ml					
10-11						
8 HR. TOT.	875ml					
11-12						
12-1						
1-2	50 ml					
2-3						
3-4						
4-5						
5-6	75ml					
6-7	125ml					
8 HR. TOT.	250ml					
24 HR. TOT.	2220ml					

TOTAL INTAKE

923-12-76-I

Figure 8-2 This is an example of a form used to record oral intake. Note that there are three 8-hour totals as well as the 24-hour total.

Commonly Prescribed Diets

Most patients eat a well-balanced diet planned by a dietitian while they are in a health agency. Many are permitted to select from various choices on a prepared daily menu.

Some commonly ordered diets for patients are given in Table 8-4. Each is used to meet the specific needs of particular patients. The nurse should know the prescribed diet for each patient and why the diet was ordered. The patient needs to understand why he is receiving the diet. Care should be taken that the patient does not accidentally receive foods that are to be excluded.

Some individuals may need to continue a special diet or generally eat well-balanced meals when they leave the health agency. Local organizations in some areas provide food services both by home delivery and at community meal sites. Also, some commercial vendors, even hospital food services, serve special meals for minimal fees to discharged individuals at home. In places where such services are not available, the nurse may be of help in teaching ways to meet nutritional needs at home.

Providing Food for Patients

Patients are usually served food at their bedside. Some hospitals have cafeterias for patients who are up and about. Nursing homes often have a large dining room where patients eat together in small groups.

Table 8-4. Common Types and Characteristics of Prescribed Diets

Type of Diet	Characteristics
Regular or general	This diet is usually a selective diet and is allowed for persons who do not require a therapeutic diet. The basic diet provides about 1400 calories and foods usually selected by the patient are added as necessary to meet total caloric needs.
Light or convalescent	This diet differs from a regular diet primarily in the method of preparing foods. The foods are simply cooked. Fried foods, rich pastries, fat-rich foods, gas-forming foods, and raw foods are typically omitted. The diet may include all types of food served in soft and liquid diets.
Soft	This diet contains foods that are soft in texture and liquids and semi-liquids. The diet is low in residue, is readily digested, contains few or no spices or condiments, and has fewer fruits, vegetables, and meats than a light diet.
Mechanical soft	This diet resembles a light diet but is used for persons with poor or no teeth or with dentures that they will not or cannot wear. Vegetables and fruits are cooked and whole meats are avoided.
Full liquid	Fruit, vegetable juices, and soups are strained or blended. Milk, ices, ice cream, gelatin, junket, custards, and usual beverages are included in this diet.
Clear liquid	This diet consists of water, clear broth, clear fruit juices, plain gelatin, tea, and coffee. Carbonated beverages may or may not be permitted.
Special therapeutic	There is a wide variety of therapeutic diets that are prepared to meet special needs. These are a few examples of therapeutic diets: high-caloric, low-caloric, diabetic, restricted-sodium, low-fat, low-protein, high-protein, and low-roughage diets.

Nursing responsibilities for food service vary among health agencies. Most hospitals have a dietitian and centralized food service. However, nurses are still generally responsible for ordering and canceling diets for patients, for assisting with serving of meals, for helping patients to eat, and for recording information about how well the patient is eating.

Serving and Removing Trays. Nurses and dietary personnel must work cooperatively in delivering food to the patient. The food should have been prepared in a clean, sanitary environment. It should be transported during delivery to the patient unit in such a way as to retain its appropriate serving temperature. Skill Procedure 8-1 provides suggested actions for the nursing responsibilities associated with serving and removing trays.

Helping the Patient to Eat. Some patients will need the nurse's help with eating. The suggestions offered in Skill Procedure 8-1 on serving food still apply. The recommendations in Skill Procedure 8-2 are also suggested.

Alternative Methods of Providing Nourishment

Patients are not always able to take fluid or food by eating normally. Other methods are used to maintain nutrition. Giving solutions intravenously has already been mentioned. Another method is feeding the patient liquid nutrients through a tube leading from the nose to the stomach or intestine. Other than being inserted into the nose, a tube for feeding can be inserted through the skin and tissue of the abdomen and secured within gastrointestinal structures. This method is used when an alternative to eating will be needed for an extended period of time. Finally, special nutrient solutions can be instilled through a polyethylene catheter that is threaded through a vein into the heart or one of its major blood vessels.

Types of Nasal Feeding Tubes

Nasal feeding tubes differ in their diameter, length, and composition material. The outside diameter of tubes and catheters is measured using the French scale. This is indicated by a number followed by the letter "F." Each number on the French scale is the approximate equivalent of 0.33 millimeters (mm). Feeding tubes used for adults range from 16 F to 8 F. The larger the number, the larger the diameter. Gastric tubes, such as the Levin tube, are shorter because they terminate in the stomach. Levin tubes are made of rubber or polyvinyl chloride. Smaller diameter feeding tubes are made of polyurethane or silicone. They can remain in the same nostril for up to four weeks. Some are long enough to reach the small intestine.

Large-sized tubes are less likely to become plugged. They are more difficult for patients to swallow. Most pa-

Skill Procedure 8-1. Serving and Removing Trays

Suggested Action	Reason for Action
Be available when trays arrive from the dietary department.	Delay in serving food alters the serving temperature of food.
Clear the area where the patient will eat.	Clutter is likely to cause the tray or the patient's belongings to fall or become misplaced.
Check the general appearance of the tray for spilled liquids, missing items, or ordered food that is missing.	The tray should be complete, orderly, and tidy so that eating can be enjoyed.
Compare the name on the tray with the name on the patient's identification bracelet.	A tray served to the wrong patient can be a serious error.
Make sure that patients who are undergoing special tests have food withheld or provided according to the test directions.	Some tests require that patients fast or eat specific types of foods, such as a fat-free meal.
Check to see that the patient is not being served foods to which he is allergic or cannot tolerate.	A patient's condition may be made worse by eating foods that his system cannot tolerate.
Place the tray so that it faces the patient, and remove the food covers.	Positioning the tray and removing covers allow easy access for the patient.
Open milk cartons and cereal boxes, butter toast, cut up meat, and otherwise assist as necessary.	It may be difficult for the patient to do these simple tasks even if he is not disabled.
Serve trays that have been kept warm to those patients who need help with eating last.	It is unappetizing and often annoying for the patient to have cold food waiting at his bedside.
Note the kinds and amounts of food the patient is not eating.	Substitutes for uneaten food may be ordered, or the nurse may need to solve other problems, such as loose dentures, which are interfering with eating.
Observe whether the patient feels satisfied with the amounts of food he is served.	Servings need to match appetites. Serving large portions to an individual with a minimal appetite may reduce food consumption.
Follow agency policies about serving food brought from home. Be sure the food is covered, labeled, and refrigerated or stored properly.	As long as the food is appropriate for the patient's diet, there usually is no problem. Spoiled or misplaced food offends those who made special efforts to prepare it.
Be considerate and visit with the patient on a special diet who may be denied food he likes because of a health problem.	The patient needs the nurse's help, support, and understanding with unwanted changes in lifestyle.
Encourage individuals to eat, but do not scold those who feel they cannot.	Insisting that the patient eat or implying that he is uncooperative is not a good nursing approach.
Remove trays as soon as possible, and restore the cleanliness of the eating area.	It is pleasant for the patient to be left clean and comfortable after eating.
Assist or offer the patient an opportunity to brush and floss his teeth.	Oral hygiene after eating helps prevent caries.
Record how the patient ate and enter the amounts of fluids consumed if appropriate.	Nurses need to evaluate if the nutritional and fluid needs of the patient are being met.

tients experience nose and throat discomfort with larger tubes. Prolonged pressure can lead to skin breakdown. Large tubes can dilate the esophageal sphincter, a circular muscle between the esophagus and the stomach. A partial opening of this ring can allow a reflux of gastric secretions and feeding formula. The reverse movement of liquid could enter the airway and lungs and interfere with respiratory function.

Smaller tubes are not free of disadvantages. They tend to curl during insertion because they are so flexible. Checking the placement of the distal end is more difficult. A tube with a smaller diameter becomes obstructed more easily. Despite the problems associated with maintenance, however, small-diameter are preferred for their comfort. They are ideal for providing a continuous infusion of nourishment into the small intestine.

Skill Procedure 8-2. Helping the Patient to Eat

Suggested Action	Reason for Action
Complete or delay care that will interfere with eating.	Food should be eaten at its appropriate serving temperature.
Provide a period of rest or quiet before meals.	A tired or excited patient is usually in no mood to eat.
Offer the patient a bedpan or urinal before mealtime.	It is uncomfortable for the patient to eat when he needs to go to the bathroom.
Provide the patient an opportunity for handwashing and offer mouth care before eating.	Soiled hands can carry bacteria to the mouth. A fresh mouth improves the appetite.
Remove any soiled articles or clutter from the room.	An unattractive enviornment tends to decrease the desire to eat.
Make the patient comfortable for eating; use pain relief techniques if needed.	Food can be enjoyed more if the patient is comfortable.
Raise the head of the bed to a sitting position if possible.	The sitting or semi-sitting position usually makes swallowing easier and choking less likely than does the lying position.
Cover the patient's upper chest with a napkin or towel.	Use of an absorbent substance protects the bedclothes and linen from becoming soiled.
Sit beside the patient. Avoid appearing rushed or hurried.	Tension interferes with chewing and digestion. The time spent should be relaxing and should provide an opportunity to gather more data or do informal teaching.
Encourage the patient to take part in his eating as much as possible and to the extent his condition permits.	Developing independence is a goal of nursing. Most adults feel childlike when they are fed by someone else.
Provide a flexible straw for patients unable to use a cup or glass.	A straw helps a patient direct liquids into his mouth at a pace and amount that match his ability to swallow.
Serve manageable amounts of food with each bite.	Even patients sitting up may choke when the amounts of food are too large.
For a stroke patient, direct the food toward the side of the mouth that is not paralyzed.	The stroke patient is better able to chew and swallow food placed where he has feeling and muscle control.
Serve the food in the order of the patient's preference.	Feeding should stimulate the manner in which a patient would eat by himself.
Give the patient time to chew thoroughly and swallow his food.	Chewing aids the first step of digestion by breaking up food and mixing it with saliva and enzymes in the mouth.
Modify utensils and the texture of food if the patient must remain flat while eating. Use a baby's training cup or a large syringe with a flexible rubber tube. Puree or grind foods if necessary.	A flat position decreases the ability to control food in the mouth and increases the risk of choking.
If you have begun to feed a patient, do not leave until he has finished eating.	A meal should be uninterrupted. Food and beverages change temperatures with delays, thus making them unappealing.
Talk with the patient about pleasant subjects.	Eating is a social situation. Focusing on problems may interfere with the patient's appetite.
Use the suggested actions that refer to removing a tray in Skill Procedure 8-1.	

Using Gavage

Gastric gavage means introducing nourishment through a nasogastric or nasointestinal tube. It is used when the patient has no alterations in stomach or intestinal function. An example is the patient who has had extensive mouth surgery. A patient who has difficulty swallowing because of a stroke may also receive nourishment through a tube. An unconscious patient or patients who are too weak to eat or drink can be kept nourished by administering gavage feedings.

In some agencies, a registered nurse may be responsible for inserting feeding tubes. Skill Procedure 8-3 describes how to insert, maintain, and remove a nasogastric (Text continues on page 141)

Skill Procedure 8-3. Inserting, Maintaining, and Removing a Nasogastric Tube

Suggested Action	Reason for Action
Inserting the Tube	
Assemble the following equipment: tube, glass of water and straw, towel, lubricant, tissues, tape, emesis basin, flashlight, and stethoscope.	Organization contributes to efficient time management.
Explain the procedure to the patient.	Informing the patient reduces fear and aids in obtaining his cooperation.
Wash hands.	Handwashing reduces the spread of microorganisms.
Place the nasogastric tube on ice chips if it is very flexible. Place it in warm water if it is very inflexible.	The tube must be directed down and around curved structures, as shown in Figure 8-3. Changing its resiliency ensures better control.

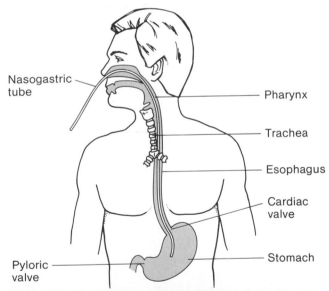

Figure 8-3 A nasogastric tube is inserted through curved passages of the nose and throat, or pharynx.

Suggested Action	Reason for Action
Assist the patient to a sitting position and protect the patient's chest, bedclothing, and linen. Have the patient remove dentures.	The patient may retch or vomit during the procedure. The sitting position facilitates the tube's passage. The patient may choke on dentures if they become dislodged.
Place the tip of the tube at the end of the nose; the earlobe; and finally to the xiphoid process of the sternum, as shown in Figure 8-4.	This is referred to as the NEX (nose–earlobe–xiphoid) measurement. It approximates the length of tubing required to reach the stomach.

(continued)

Skill Procedure 8-3. Continued

Suggested Action	Reason for Action

Inserting the Tube

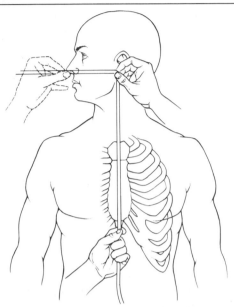

Figure 8-4 The distance from the nose (N) to the earlobe (E) to the xiphoid (X) is called the NEX measurement. It is used to determine the approximate distance to the stomach. An alternative, and in some cases more accurate, formula is:

$$\frac{NEX - 50 \text{ cm (20 in)}}{2} + 50 \text{ cm} = \text{length for gastric insertion.}$$

Mark the tube using the permanent felt-tip pen at the distance from the nose to ear and add a second mark at the xiphoid measurement, as shown in Figure 8-5.

These marks will be used as landmarks when inserting the tube. Tubes that are premarked may not correlate exactly with each patient's measurements.

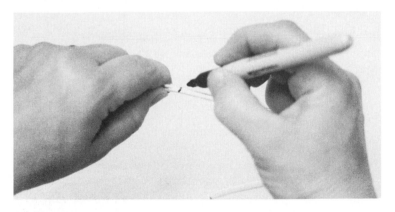

Figure 8-5 If the NEX measurement does not correspond with a premarked tube, the nurse identifies the length for insertion with a marking pen.

Lubricate the tube with a water-soluble jelly for 15 to 20 cm (6–8 inches).

Lubrication reduces friction and reduces the chance of injury during insertion.

(continued)

Skill Procedure 8-3. *Continued*

Suggested Action	Reason for Action

Inserting the Tube

Use Xylocaine® ointment for lubrication if policy permits and the patient is not allergic to it.

Xylocaine® ointment is a water-soluble, topical anesthetic. It can reduce sensation and discomfort in the nose and pharynx.

Evaluate the size and shape of the passageway of each nostril. Have the patient exhale while one nostril is closed.

Using the nostril that is larger and allows freer movement of air will make passage of the tube easier.

After asking the patient to lift his head, as illustrated in Figure 8-6, insert the tube into the nostril while directing the tube backward and downward until the first measurement mark is at the tip of the nose.

Following the normal contour of the nasal passage while inserting the tube reduces irritation and possible injury.

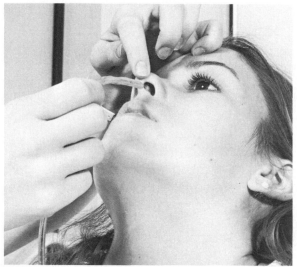

Figure 8-6 The end of the tube has been lubricated. The nurse inserts the tube into the patient's nostril.

Using a small light, look for the tip of the tube at the top and back of the throat.

Advancing the tube only this short distance gives the patient a chance to prepare for the remaining insertion. The tube should be located high enough that it should not cause gagging.

Have the patient lower his chin to his chest and instruct him to swallow sips of water as the tube is advanced to the second measurement mark.

Bringing the head forward helps close the trachea and open the esophagus. Swallowing helps advance the tube and causes the epiglottis to cover the opening of the trachea.

Do not force the tube. Rotate if there is some resistance.

Forcing the tube may injure mucous membrane, coil the tube, or cause gagging.

Discontinue the procedure and remove the tube if there are signs of distress, such as gasping, coughing, a bluish skin color, or the inability to speak or hum.

These signs usually mean that the tube is not in the esophagus or stomach and is probably in the airway or lungs.

Once the tube is passed without problems to the second mark on the tube, determine that the tube is in the patient's stomach:

Validating placement ensures the safety of the patient.

(continued)

Skill Procedure 8-3. Continued

Suggested Action	**Reason for Action**

Inserting the Tube

1. Aspirate fluid with a syringe. Compare its characteristics with those of stomach secretions.

   No other anatomic structures in this area should contain secretions that are clear brownish-yellow or green and test between a pH of 1 to 3.

2. Listen over the stomach with a stethoscope while 10 mL of air are instilled into the tube through a syringe, as shown in Figure 8-7.

   The whooshing sound of air can be heard when the air enters the stomach through the tube.

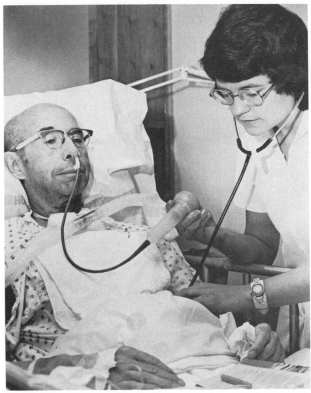

Figure 8-7 The nurse checks to be sure that the gavage tube is in the patient's stomach before instilling nourishment.

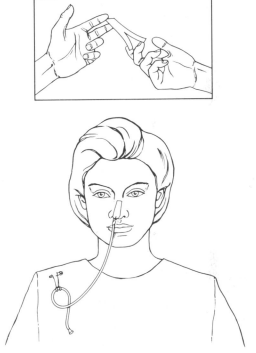

Figure 8-8 The nasogastric tube is taped to the nose so there is no pulling on the sides of the nostrils causing sores to form. Providing a loop of tubing between the nose and where it is pinned to the gown gives some freedom for head movement.

3. Place the end of the tube into a glass of water.*

   The tube is in the respiratory passages if bubbles appear at regular intervals as the patient exhales. False results are possible with this technique.

Secure the tube with tape to the patient's nose as illustrated in Figure 8-8. Use a clamp or pin to fasten the tube to the patient's gown or bed linen.

This allows the patient to move without danger of the tube being pulled out of place.

If the tube will not be used for immediate feeding, clamp the tube.

Clamping prevents the tube from possibly becoming a siphon through which stomach contents could drain.

Connect a tube that will be used to remove stomach fluid to a suction machine on low, intermittent settings, unless ordered otherwise.

A low setting prevents excessive negative pressure from pulling on the lining of the stomach. Intermittent suction prevents excess depletion of stomach acid and other chemicals.

(continued)

Skill Procedure 8-3. *Continued*

Suggested Action	Reason for Action

Maintaining the Tube

If the tube is used to remove stomach contents, ensure that the patient does not receive anything by mouth other than sips of water or crushed ice if ordered.	Fluids and nutritional balance must be maintained by alternate means, such as intravenous therapy. Water and ice must be measured and recorded as fluid intake.
Give special care to the mouth, lips, and nose.	Mouth care prevents drying of the mucous membranes and relieves thirst. Preventing and removing the accumulation of secretions promotes comfort.
Offer the patient analgesic throat lozenges. Lidocaine (Xylocaine) viscous solution may be gargled or applied to the back of the throat with a doctor's order.	In cases in which ice does not relieve the irritation of the throat, prescribed medications may be necessary.
Note and record the fluid intake and output every 8 hours and the total amount every 24 hours.	The nurse must evaluate the fluid balance of the patient.
Change the tube and the drainage receptacle according to agency policy.	A tube that remains for a prolonged period of time may cause sores to form. Equipment should be cleaned and changed periodically for sanitary reasons.

Removing the Tube

Remove the tape from the patient's skin.	The tube will need to move freely.
Don clean gloves or protect hands with a towel.	The tube will be coated with mucus and stomach secretions.
Clamp or pinch the tube.	Clamping prevents secretions from leaking as the tube is withdrawn.
Coil the tube around the gloved hand as it is steadily removed, as shown in Figure 8-9.	Coiling aids in controlling the tube and concealing its appearance from the patient.

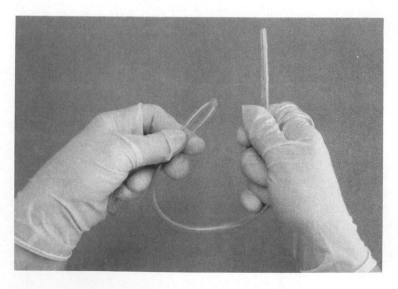

Figure 8-9 Coiling the tube around the gloved hand helps to control the slack as it is withdrawn from the stomach.

Cover the tube with the towel or pull the glove over the tube, as shown in Figure 8-10.	The appearance of the coated tube may make some patients feel ill.

(continued)

Skill Procedure 8-3. *Continued*

Suggested Action	Reason for Action

Removing the Tube

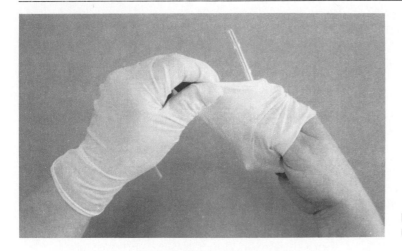

Figure 8-10 The nurse encloses the tube while removing a glove.

Offer oral hygiene after the tube is removed.	Mouth care will help to remove any disagreeable tastes from the patient's mouth.
Remove the equipment from the patient's room. Care for the soiled equipment according to the agency's policies.	Nurses are often responsible for the initial cleaning of soiled equipment before returning it for more thorough cleansing and storage.

*This is the least accurate testing method since the tube could be coiled or kinked or stomach gas could exit from the tube.

tube. The technique for inserting a small-diameter feeding tube differs somewhat from a large-sized nasogastric tube. Skill Procedure 8-4 explains those differences.

Bolus Tube Feedings. A *bolus feeding* is the instillation of a large volume of liquid nourishment into the stomach at one time using a syringe. Approximately 250 to 400 mL of formula are given within a few minutes. The bolus feeding is repeated four to six times a day. This mimics, to some extent, the natural filling and emptying of the stomach. Bolus feeding permits an ambulatory patient to clamp the tube and move about freely doing other activities. Some patients experience discomfort from the rapid delivery of this quantity of fluid. Patients who are unconscious or who have delayed gastric emptying are at greater risk for vomiting and aspiration using this method of administration.

Intermittent Tube Feedings. An *intermittent feeding* is the instillation of liquid nourishment into the stomach in the time most people would spend eating a meal. Usually the volume is 250 to 400 mL. It is given by gravity drip from a suspended container over a period of 30 to 60 minutes. Feedings are scheduled four to six times a day. Gradual filling of the stomach at a slower rate reduces the bloated feeling experienced with bolus feedings.

Continuous Tube Feedings. A *continuous feeding* is the instillation of a small volume of liquid nourishment without any interruption. Approximately 1.5 mL/minute are administered. An electric feeding pump is used to regulate the infusion. The small amount does not need to be held in the reservoir of the stomach. It can be delivered directly into the small intestine. Instilling small amounts of fluid beyond the valves in the stomach and esophagus reduces the danger for vomiting and aspiration. Continuous feeding does, however, create some inconvenience. The pump goes wherever the patient goes. Skill Procedure 8-5 gives suggestions for administering tube feedings.

Common Problems With Gastric Feedings. There are several common problems associated with providing nourishment through a nasogastric tube. When they occur, they should be reported promptly. These problems and common ways to prevent and handle them are described in Table 8-5.

(Text continues on page 144)

Skill Procedure 8-4. Inserting a Small Diameter Feeding Tube

Suggested Action	Reason for Action
Assemble the following equipment: tube, glass of water and straw, 50-mL syringe, flashlight, marking pen, towel, emesis basin, tissues, tape, and stethoscope.	Organization contibutes to efficient time management.
Explain the procedure to the patient.	Informing the patient reduces fear and aids in obtaining his cooperation.
Wash hands.	Handwashing reduces the spread of microorganisms.
Spread the towel over the patient's chest.	The towel protects the patient from moisture and soiling.
Inspect the nose to determine which nostril will be used.	A nostril that has structural alterations such as a deviated septum or polyps should be avoided if possible.
Obtain the NEX measurement and add 9 inches (23 cm) for intestinal placement. Mark each measurement on the tube with a permanent marker.	Nine inches in addition to the NEX provides extra length to pass from the stomach through the pyloric valve and into the small intestine.
Follow the manufacturer's suggestions for activating the tube's bonded lubricant.	Small-diameter feeding tubes are coated either internally or externally with bonded lubricant. Dipping the tip in water or instilling water through the tube transforms the dry bond to a gelatinous consistency.
Secure the stylet within the feeding tube.	A stylet, optional with some tubes, is a wire guide within the tube that provides more rigidity during its passage.
Have the patient hyperextend his neck. Insert the tube through the selected nostril to the point of the first mark.	Hyperextension helps the nurse to guide and direct the tube.
Look for the tip of the tube at the back of the throat using a flashlight.	Visualization indicates that the tip has advanced through the curve of the nasopharynx. Some tubes have a weighted tip that helps them travel through gastrointestinal structures.
Have the patient bring his head forward until his chin rests on his chest.	Flexing the neck closes the trachea and opens the esophagus.
Instruct the patient to swallow water and advance the tube to the next marking.	Swallowing helps advance the tube into the stomach rather than the respiratory tract.
Verify the location of the tube as described for a nasogastric tube when it is advanced to the second mark. Use a 50-mL syringe for aspiration as shown in Figure 8-11.	Using a large-volume syringe helps reduce the negative pressure during aspiration. Lower pressure lessens the tendency for the sides of the narrow tubing to collapse.
Use caution if aspiration and auscultation do not yield definite results.	Even with the best technique, it is difficult to assess location by these methods when the tube is a small diameter.
Confirmation by x-ray may be required and is recommended for patients who are unconscious or lack a gag reflex.	X-ray is the most accurate method for verifying the location of a small-diameter feeding tube.
Tape a 9-inch loop of tubing loosely to the cheek if intestinal placement is desired. Position the patient on his right side.	Advancement into the small intestine may take several hours. A loop provides slack while it progresses the remaining distance. Lying on the right side facilitates the forward movement of the tube.
Observe the mark on the tube at intervals. Secure the tube to the patient's nose with tape when the third mark reaches the tip of the nose.	Taping the tube securely prevents advancement of the tube further within the intestinal tract.

(continued)

Skill Procedure 8-4. *Continued*

Suggested Action	Reason for Action

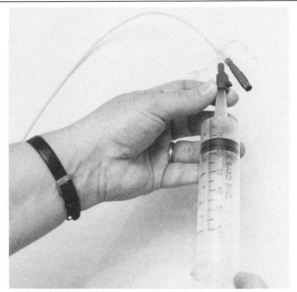

Figure 8-11 A syringe is inserted into a special port when checking placement. The port is capped at other times.

Use gentle traction, as shown in Figure 8-12, or follow the manufacturer's suggestions to remove the stylet once the tube is in its proper location.	Various techniques help to remove the stylet without displacing the tube to a higher level.

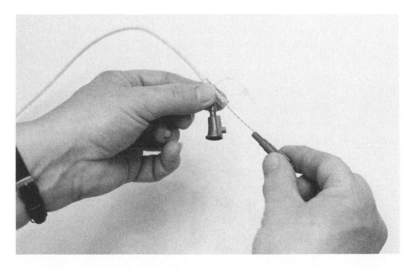

Figure 8-12 The thin wire stylet is removed from the feeding tube.

Store the stylet within the tube wrapper at the patient's bedside.	Saving the stylet prevents the expense of using a new tube if the current tube is pulled out and needs reinsertion.
Never reinsert the stylet while the tube is in the patient.	The stylet can puncture the flexible tube and injure the body structures where it protrudes.
Flush small-diameter feeding tubes with a 50-mL syringe every 4 hours even when a patient is receiving continuous feedings.	Small-diameter feeding tubes are prone to obstruction. Using a syringe smaller than 50 mL may create enough pressure during flushing to burst the walls of the tube.

(continued)

Skill Procedure 8-4. Continued

Suggested Action	Reason for Action
Flush feeding tubes with tap water before and after each administration of medication, and each time a feeding pump is stopped.	Frequent flushing maintains patency.
Remove the tape securing the tube to the nose daily or more often if it becomes loose or soiled. Retape the tube after assessment and cleansing.	Assessment of the skin and hygiene are part of daily care.
Note that the mark is visible at the junction of the tube and the tip of the nose.	A change in the location of the measuring mark would indicate that the tube has slipped up or down from its original position.
Replace a small-diameter feeding tube at least every 4 weeks. Use the alternate nostril if possible.	Periodic replacement maintains a tube in functional condition.
Give mouth and nose care at least twice a day.	Patients with nasal tubes tend to be mouthbreathers. Their oral mucous membranes become dry and irritated. The nasal passages tend to fill with additional dried mucus in response to the presence of the tube.

Keeping a Nasogastric Tube Patent. Nasogastric tubes and other kinds of tubes can get plugged. The nurse must assess whether the tube is remaining *patent,* or unobstructed. If a tube becomes plugged, it cannot serve its function for either instilling or draining fluids. Filling the nasogastric tube with water and clamping it after each tube feeding is a method to ensure its continued patency.

Nasogastric tubes used as drains have a tendency to become obstructed. Thick mucous secretions can collect within the tube. Giving a patient ice chips or small sips of water, which shortly become suctioned out the tube, helps to dilute the secretions. Thinning secretions usually keeps the tube draining freely.

Occasionally, the nurse may need to instill solution through the tube to maintain its function. A doctor's order is always required. Some patients who have had recent stomach surgery should not have a tube irrigated. Skill Procedure 8-6 describes a suggested method for irrigating a nasogastric tube.

Administering Nourishment Through a Gastrostomy

A *gastrostomy* is an opening into the stomach through the abdominal wall. Some gastrostomies are created surgically. A new technique, percutaneous endoscopic gastrostomy (PEG), makes it possible to insert a gastrostomy tube with local anesthesia. In this procedure, the gastrostomy tube is inserted using an endoscope. An endoscope is a flexible tubular instrument that allows internal visualization of body structures. The endoscope is inserted through the patient's mouth and into the stomach. The gastrostomy tube is attached to the endoscope. It is pulled into the stomach and out a cannula that pierces the abdominal wall.

Gastrostomy tubes are generally used when a patient requires an alternative to oral feeding for longer than a month. Bolus or intermittent feedings are usually administered through a gastrostomy tube. The tube is clamped between feedings. The tube can be covered with a gauze dressing and clothing when not in use. Concealment allows the patient to socialize in public without being concerned about personal appearance.

Gastric secretions sometimes leak from the stomach through the channel with the tube. The acid and enzymes in stomach secretions can break down the skin. The nurse needs to inspect and cleanse this area with warm soapy water. After the skin is dry, a skin barrier product, such as zinc oxide or Stomahesive, can be placed around the tube where it exits from the skin. The site and tube are covered with a small gauze dressing.

To administer a bolus or an intermittent feeding:

- Attach a syringe to the gastrostomy tube.
- Release the clamp.
- Aspirate the gastric residual.
- Hold the syringe perpendicular to the abdomen and 3 to 6 inches above it.
- Refeed the residual by gravity.
- Flush the tube with 1 to 2 ounces of water.
- Instill the formula by gravity, shown in Figure 8-22.
- Rinse the tubing with water following the feeding.
- Clamp the tubing.
- Cover with a dry dressing.
- Keep the patient in an upright position.

Some gastrostomy feedings are performed by inserting a tube through a healed opening or plug. When the nurse

(Text continues on page 152)

Skill Procedure 8-5. Administering a Tube Feeding

Suggested Action	Reason for Action
Bolus Feeding	
Listen to the abdomen with a stethoscope.	Gurgling and growling sounds indicate a functioning bowel. Introducing a feeding when the bowel is not active can lead to abdominal distention.
Notify the doctor if no sounds are heard after listening for 1 minute.	Bowel sounds are only considered absent if they cannot be heard anywhere on the abdomen during 1 minute.
Check that the tube is located in the patient's stomach by following the methods described in Skill Procedure 8-3.	The far end of the tube could become displaced into the air passages. Verifying that it is still in the stomach prevents fluid from being placed into the lungs.
Warm refrigerated nourishment to room temperature in a basin of warm water before instilling it through the tube.	The patient may become chilled with cold solutions. Cold nourishment may also cause abdominal cramping and diarrhea.
Place the patient in a sitting position between a 30° and 90° angle.	A sitting position helps prevent regurgitation of the nourishment.
Empty the stomach of its contents, called the gastric residual, with a syringe. Measure the amount.	*Gastric residual* is the volume of liquid remaining in the stomach. It should be less than half of the previous hour's gastric tube feeding infusion. Overfilling the stomach can cause vomiting and aspiration.
Refeed the removed formula by pouring it back into the syringe, as shown in Figure 8-13.	The contents from the stomach contain partially digested formula and important chemicals that should not be thrown away.

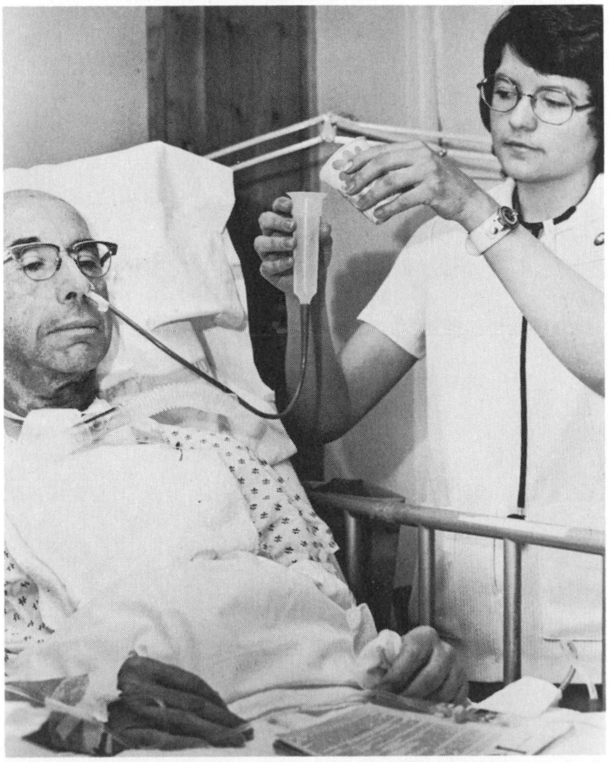

Figure 8-13 The nurse returns the aspirated volume. Bolus formula is administered in the same way. The height of the syringe affects the rate of instillation.

(*continued*)

Skill Procedure 8-5. Continued

Suggested Action	Reason for Action

Bolus Feeding

Suggested Action	Reason for Action
Do not administer any fresh formula if 100 to 150 mL remain from a previous feeding.	Consult with the doctor or follow the agency's policies to avoid overfeeding the patient.
Wait 1 hour and recheck the gastric residual. If it still measures 100 mL or more, notify the physician.	The residual generally lessens with time. Additional measures may be necessary if the volume remains high.
Begin tube feedings with a small volume of formula, approximately 100 mL, or follow written policy.	Diarrhea can occur when a large volume of full-strength liquid formula is instilled for the first time.
Allow the nourishment to flow into the stomach steadily by gravity.	Pushing formula in may cause cramping and distension from rapid filling.
Regulate the rate of flow by raising or lowering the syringe.	Raising will speed the flow; lowering will slow the flow.
Do not let the syringe completely empty when adding more nourishment.	Air should not be allowed to enter the stomach. It can cause distension and discomfort.
Follow policy for diluting the first feedings. Some recommend a 1:1 ratio of formula to water.	Diluting highly concentrated formula can prevent the onset of diarrhea during early tube feedings.
Gradually increase the volume and strength of the formula according to policy and the patient's tolerance.	The patient will be more likely to adapt to gradual changes in the liquid diet.
When the formula is instilled, add 1 or 2 ounces of tap water.	Water washes the remaining nourishment in the tube into the stomach, prevents obstruction with coagulated formula, and adds to a patient's daily intake of water.
Plug or clamp the tube between feedings.	Occluding the tube prevents air from entering the tube with each feeding.
Keep the head of the bed elevated for at least 30 minutes after feeding.	Gravity helps keep the formula within the stomach.
Wash and dry the feeding equipment. Return them to the bedside.	Clean equipment can be reused.
Provide oral hygiene at least twice daily.	The mouth requires extra care to prevent drying and irritation.
Record the total amount of fresh formula and water that was instilled.	Recording I and O aids in determining if the patient's fluid requirements are being met. Caloric intake can be calculated based on the daily volume of instilled formula.
Monitor capillary or urine glucose. Record and report abnormally high or low levels to the physician.	High caloric formulas may affect blood sugar levels and require temporary treatment with insulin.

Intermittent Feeding

Suggested Action	Reason for Action
Follow the previous instructions for assessing, positioning, and checking gastric residual.	Safety principles remain the same.
Replace formula containers and administration tubing every 24 hours.	Daily replacement reduces the potential for bacterial growth in the tubing and container. Contaminated equipment can cause diarrhea.
Fill the feeding container with room temperature formula.	Cold formula causes gastric discomfort.
Cover, label with the date and time, then refrigerate any unused formula.	Opened formula that is properly labeled and refrigerated can be used up to 24 hours.

(continued)

Skill Procedure 8-5. Continued

Suggested Action	**Reason for Action**

Intermittent Feeding

Purge the air from the tubing by gradually opening the clamp on the tubing.

Filling the tubing with formula prevents distending the stomach with air.

Connect the tubing to the nasogastric tube as shown in Figure 8-14. Adjust the flow to 10 mL/minute as shown in Figure 8-15, or follow written policy.

An intermittent feeding is given at a slow, steady rate over approximately 30 to 60 minutes.

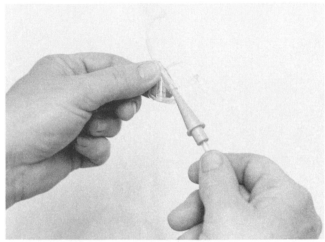

Figure 8-14 A cone-shaped tip from the administration tube is inserted into the proximal end of the feeding tube.

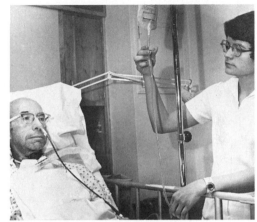

Figure 8-15 The rate of flow is regulated with a clamp on the administration tubing.

Check the infusion frequently.

Checking ensures that the feeding is infusing at the prescribed rate.

Flush the tubing with 1 to 2 ounces of tap water when the formula is completely instilled.

Water washes the remaining formula into the stomach, prevents obstruction, and adds to a patient's daily intake of water.

Wash, dry, and store cleaned equipment for up to 24 hours of reuse.

Washing and drying reduces growth of microorganisms. Continued reuse increases the potential for contamination.

Provide oral hygiene at least twice daily.

The mouth requires extra care to prevent drying and irritation.

Record the total amount of fresh formula and water that was instilled.

Recording I and O aids in determining if the patient's fluid requirements are being met. Caloric intake can be calculated based on the daily volume of instilled formula.

Monitor capillary or urine glucose. Record and report abnormally high or low levels to the physician.

High caloric formulas may affect blood sugar levels and require temporary treatment with insulin.

Continuous Feeding

Follow the previous instructions for assessing the patient and tube placement.

Safety principles remain the same.

Check gastric residual every 4 hours if the tube is in the stomach following the suggestions identified in the bolus feeding discussion.

Because the feeding infuses continuously, a routine must be scheduled for checking gastric residual.

(continued)

Skill Procedure 8-5. Continued

Suggested Action	Reason for Action

Continuous Feeding

Suggested Action	Reason for Action
Observe patients with small-diameter feeding tubes for nausea, abdominal distention, or cramps.	Small-diameter tubes may collapse with aspiration. Assessing for delayed emptying requires more indirect methods.
Attach a time tape to a formula container as shown in Figure 8-16.	A time tape facilitates quick assessment during the hours that formula is infusing.

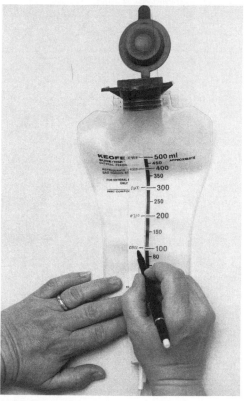

Figure 8-16 The nurse marks the time corresponding to the desired hourly volume on a strip of tape.

Figure 8-17 The machine electronically monitors the continuous infusion of formula as it passes through the drip chamber.

Suggested Action	Reason for Action
Flush a new container and tubing with water.	Coating the inner surface with water promotes the passage of large protein molecules through the equipment.
Fill the feeding container with no more than 8 hours' worth of formula. Do not prewarm refrigerated formula.	Limiting the time that formula hangs reduces the growth of microorganisms. The formula will warm itself as a result of the slow rate of infusion.
Purge the tubing of air.	Air contributes to distention of the stomach.
Thread the tubing within the feeding pump according to the manufacturer's directions. An example is shown in Figure 8-17.	A feeding pump mechanically compresses the tubing at programmed intervals in order to regulate the continuous instillation of formula.
Connect the tubing to the patient. Set the prescribed rate as shown in Figure 8-18. Continuous feedings infuse on the average of 100 mL/hr once the patient adjusts to progressively increased concentrations and volumes.	Formulas are rapidly absorbed from the intestine. High volumes are not as easily tolerated when tube feedings are first begun.

(continued)

Skill Procedure 8-5. Continued

Suggested Action	Reason for Action

Continuous Feeding

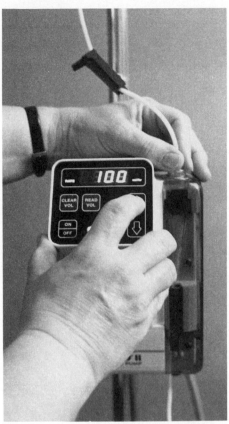

Figure 8-18 The nurse sets the rate in milliliters per hour by pressing touch-sensitive controls.

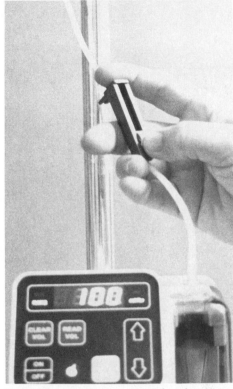

Figure 8-19 When the feeding pump has been programmed, the clamp is released so the formula can be instilled.

Open the clamp, shown in Figure 8-19, and start the pump.	The fluid will not infuse until the machine is activated.
Flush the tubing with 1 to 2 ounces of water every 4 hours after checking residuals, before and after medications and before adding new formula.	Small-diameter feeding tubes are especially susceptible to becoming obstructed.
Do not add new formula to formula that has been hanging.	The longer formula remains outside the body, the greater the potential for contamination.
Provide oral hygiene at least twice daily.	The mouth requires extra care to prevent drying and irritation.
Record the total amount of fresh formula and water that was instilled.	Recording I and O aids in determining if the patient's fluid requirements are being met. Caloric intake can be calculated based on the daily volume of instilled formula.
Monitor capillary or urine glucose. Record and report abnormal levels to the physician.	High caloric formulas may affect blood sugar levels. The caloric content may need to be adjusted. Some patients are treated temporarily with insulin.

Table 8-5. Common Problems Associated With Tube Feedings

Problem	Common Cause	Usual Care
Diarrhea	Highly concentrated formula	Dilute to between ¼ to ½ initial strength.
	Rapid administration	Start continuous drip feedings at 25 mL/hr and increase by 25 mL every 12 hours.
	Bacterial contamination	Wash hands.
		Do not hang more than 4 to 8 hours' worth of formula.
		Refrigerate unused formula.
		Change feeding bag and tubing every 24 hours.
	Inadequate protein content of formula	Raise serum albumin levels with TPN solutions containing supplemental protein or administer albumin intravenously.
	Food allergy or lactose intolerance	Switch to a lactose-free formula or a milk-free product.
Nausea and vomiting	Rapid feeding	Instill bolus and intermittent feedings by gravity.
	Overfeeding	Delay feeding until gastric residual is less than 100 mL.
		Maintain sitting position for at least 30 minutes following the feeding.
		Administer continuous feedings into the small intestine with a small-diameter feeding tube.
	Air in stomach	Keep tubing filled with formula or water.
Aspiration	Incorrect tube placement	Check placement before instilling formula or water.
	Vomiting	Utilize measures to prevent vomiting listed previously.
Constipation	Lack of fiber	Change formula; use measures to assist with bowel elimination.
	Dehydration	Increase supplemental volume of water.
Elevated blood sugar	Undiluted or rapidly infused feeding	Slowly instill diluted formula; gradually increase concentration, then volume.
Weight loss	Inadequate calories	Increase caloric content.
		Increase rate or frequency of feeding.
		Supplement with TPN.
Elevated electrolytes	Dehydration	Increase volume of water when flushing tube.
Dry oral and nasal mucous membranes	Mouthbreathing	Frequent mouth and nose care.
	Dried nasal mucus	
Acute middle ear inflammation	Obstruction of eustachian tube from feeding tube	Turn from side to side every 2 hours.
		Use a small-diameter feeding tube.
Sore throat	Pressure and irritation from tube	Use a small-diameter feeding tube.
		Gargle with dilute salt water.
		Suck on medicated lozenges.

(*continued*)

Table 8-5. Continued

Problem	Common Cause	Usual Care
Plugged feeding tube	Administering medication through the feeding tube	Use liquid medications.
		Crush tablets and dilute with warm water.
		Flush the tubing after each administration of medication.
	Large molecules in formula	Dilute formula.
		Flush tubing frequently with water.
		Use a large-diameter feeding tube.

Skill Procedure 8-6. Irrigating a Nasogastric Tube

Suggested Action	Reason for Action
Place a towel under the tube and over the sheets where the tube will be separated.	Sometimes solution or stomach contents may drip and soil the linen.
Disconnect the nasogastric tube from the suction machine. Take care that the end of the tubing from the machine does not fall to the floor.	Although the stomach is not a sterile area, the cleanliness of the equipment should be maintained.
Check the location of the far end of the nasogastric tube, using the methods described in Skill Procedure 8-3.	Irrigating solution could be instilled into the lungs if the tube is not in the stomach.
Fill an Asepto syringe or an irrigating syringe, such as the one the nurse is using in Figure 8-20, with 30 to 60 mL of a normal saline solution.	Normal saline contains sodium and chloride, which help to maintain the body's electrolyte balance.

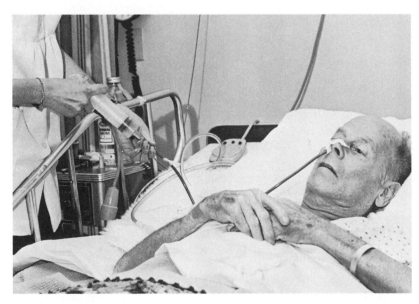

Figure 8-20 The nurse irrigates a gastric tube. The amount instilled is recorded as intake.

Allow the solution to flow in by gravity, or gently apply pressure.	Never use force.
If the solution fails to enter the tube, change the patient's position.	The tip of the tube may be against the wall of the stomach. Moving the patient may cause the tip of the tube to move.

(continued)

Skill Procedure 8-6. *Continued*

Suggested Action	Reason for Action
If there still is resistance, unfasten the tape from the nose and move the tube up or down a few inches. Recheck and verify that it continues to be located in the stomach.	Valves are located at the top and bottom of the stomach. The tip of the tube may have become located just above or within these valves.
Reattach the tube to the nose, and proceed with instilling the irrigating solution.	Taping helps to ensure that the tube remains in the stomach.
Following the instillation, withdraw and measure an amount approximately equal to the amount instilled. Report any signs of bleeding.	Withdrawing fluid will reveal whether secretions can move freely through the tube.
Reconnect the nasogastric tube to the suction machine.	The suction machine will continue to remove stomach gas and contents on an automatic cycle.
Record the amount of fluid instilled and withdrawn on the I and O sheet.	Measurements provide the nurse with data for evaluating the patient's total fluid balance.
Check the drainage regularly to note its characteristics and amount as the nurse is doing in Figure 8-21.	Drainage that continues to increase in appropriate amounts is an indication that the tube is remaining open.

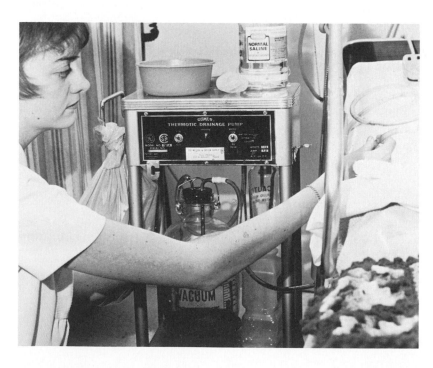

Figure 8-21 After irrigating, the nurse checks the flow of drainage through the tube.

Follow the agency policies about recording the procedure and its outcome.	The nurse should describe the action and the patient's response on the agency's forms.

inserts the tube, it is generously lubricated and inserted 4 to 6 inches.

Administering Nourishment Through a Jejunostomy

Feeding directly into the jejunum, the midportion of the small intestine, can be done through the use of a *jejunostomy tube.* Figure 8-23 shows how this tube is inserted

through a gastrostomy device. This route provides the least risk for aspiration.

Continuous feedings of predigested formula are administered through a jejunostomy tube using a pump. The small intestine tends to be intolerant of the high caloric content of concentrated formulas. It is best to administer dilute solutions initially and increase their strength if diarrhea does not occur. If loose stools occur, consult with the

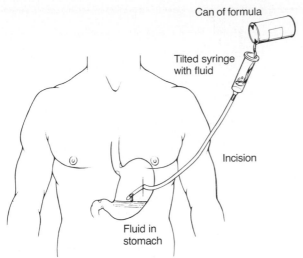

Figure 8-22 Tilting the barrel of the feeding syringe permits air displaced by formula to escape. This helps to reduce gastric distention.

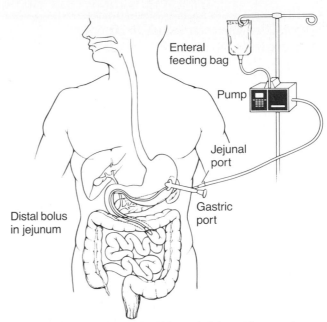

Figure 8-23 A feeding tube is inserted through a mushroom-shaped gastrostomy tube. The formula is deposited within the jejunum by a continuous drip infusion. (Courtesy of IVAC Corporation, San Diego, CA, 1990).

doctor. An antidiarrheal medication may be needed. The best dietary approach is to return to the dilution strength administered before the diarrhea. Continue with the pre-diarrhea concentration for several days until normal bowel function is restored. The strength of the formula can then be increased gradually until it meets the nutritional needs of the patient without causing cramping and frequent stools.

Nourishing the Patient by Parenteral Hyperalimentation

Still another way to provide a patient with nutrients is to use *parenteral hyperalimentation,* which provides total nutrition directly into the bloodstream. The term *total parenteral nutrition* (TPN) is a synonym. This method is used when the patient is not able to eat, digest, or absorb nutrients adequately through the gastrointestinal tract.

Simple intravenous therapy supplies neither sufficient calories nor enough protein when alternative nutrition is needed quickly or for long periods. TPN supplies a concentrated solution of carbohydrate in the form of glucose, along with protein, vitamins, and minerals. Some solutions contain fats.

The pharmacy usually prepares nutritional solutions for parenteral hyperalimentation if commercial preparations are not used. The tubing, called a central venous catheter, is used to infuse the solution. It is guided through a needle into a vein where blood flow is high. This helps to dilute the solution quickly in the blood. The preferred vein is the subclavian vein, which leads to the superior vena cava. Inserting the catheter is the responsibility of a physician. Nurses may assist during the procedure and are responsible for maintaining its patency and care of the site. The guidelines for these actions are provided in Chapter 25. Figure 8-24 illustrates the location of the catheter.

The nursing care plan or written standards for the care of a patient receiving total parenteral nutrition usually includes the following:

- Assessment of the insertion site
- Volume, solution, and rate of infusion
- Frequency and directions for changing the dressing and equipment
- Measures for keeping the catheter patent
- Specific patient assessments to evaluate the response of the patient, such as weight, I and O, and blood or urine glucose levels.

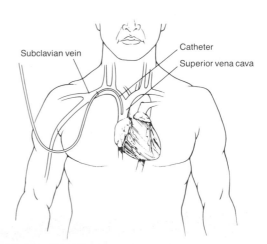

Figure 8-24 A nutrient solution is instilled into a large vein near the heart. This alternative is used when the gastrointestinal tract is not an adequate route for nutrition.

Suggested Measures to Promote Nutrition in Selected Situations

When the Patient Is an Infant or Child

Observe the same procedure for inserting a gavage tube in an infant as described earlier in this chapter, with these exceptions: Use a small tube, a size 8 being common.

Place an infant's head over a rolled-up towel or diaper placed under the head. This positioning helps in the insertion of the tube by straightening the esophagus.

Plan that it may be necessary to start the flow of nourishment by using a very gentle push on the syringe barrel or plunger. Use gravity to continue the flow.

Bubble the infant after giving nourishment to help remove air from the stomach, and position him in a crib on his right side.

Offer an infant being gavaged a pacifier at regular intervals to satisfy his sucking reflex.

Infants born prematurely are often fed by gavage to conserve their strength until they have matured sufficiently to suck well.

Observe the following techniques when an infant has a cleft palate:

Follow agency policy concerning the type of equipment to use for feeding. A medicine dropper, a small spoon, or a syringe may be used, or a nipple can be slit and then placed in the mouth with the slit running vertically. It is helpful when the nipple can be placed between the tongue and the existing palate to promote successful sucking.

Hold the infant in a sitting position while feeding him to help avoid choking and aspiration.

Feed the infant very slowly to avoid choking and aspiration.

Bubble the infant several times during and after feedings. A child with a cleft palate tends to swallow large quantities of air.

Be sure to check the temperature of formula before offering it to an infant. The formula should feel comfortably warm, but not hot, when a few drops are allowed to fall on the inner aspect of the nurse's wrist.

Alternate the sides on which the infant is held for bottle feedings, as with a nursed baby, to promote bilateral stimulation and coordination.

Hold an infant when he is nursing from a bottle. Do not prop a bottle. The infant needs the touch and cuddling offered while holding him, and he may choke on a bottle propped in place.

Applicable Nursing Diagnoses

Several nursing diagnoses may be made when a patient has nutritional problems. Some of these include

- Health-Seeking Behavior: Improve Nutrition
- Altered Nutrition: Less than Body Requirements
- Altered Nutrition: More than Body Requirements
- Knowledge Deficit: Proper Nutrition
- Feeding Self-Care Deficit
- Altered Health Maintenance
- Impaired Swallowing
- High Risk for Aspiration
- Altered Oral (and Nasal) Mucous Membranes
- Fluid Volume Deficit
- Diarrhea
- Constipation
- Colonic Constipation

Nursing Care Plan 8-1 is an example of how a patient with Impaired Swallowing may be helped by the nurse. This diagnostic category is defined in the NANDA Taxonomy (1989) as, "The state in which an individual has decreased ability to voluntarily pass fluids and/or solids from the mouth to the stomach."

Offer finger foods to mature infants and toddlers up to about age 3. Then cut up food finely for them. Young children enjoy helping themselves to food but cannot manage utensils with ease. Unbreakable spoons are best when a child shows readiness to handle them.

Use small plastic cups partially filled with beverage for children learning to use a cup to help prevent spilling. Training cups are available and will also help prevent spilling when children are learning to use a cup.

Plan that, in terms of body weight, the infant or preschooler requires more calories than does the school-age child, whose body is growing at a slower rate. During adolescence, total caloric requirements increase because of a growth spurt.

Enlist the help of parents, when possible, for helping with feeding their children and also when children are on increased or restricted fluid intake. This helps parents feel that they can do something to help care for their child. They can also help make selections from a menu because they know what foods their child enjoys.

Offer the following items, which children generally enjoy, when fluids are to be encouraged:

Popsicles of various flavors

Ice cream

NURSING CARE PLAN

8-1. *Impaired Swallowing*

Assessment	**Subjective Data**
	States "I'm losing weight. I've almost given up trying to eat. I get more on me than in me since my stroke."

Objective Data

67-year-old woman recovering from a cerebral vascular accident (CVA). Gag reflex is present upon stimulating the throat with a cotton-tipped swab. Produces an audible cough on request. Food lodges in pockets of left cheek. Drools from left side of mouth when attempting to swallow.

Diagnosis

Impaired Swallowing related to neuromuscular impairment.

Plan

Goal

The patient will demonstrate swallowing techniques that result in an empty mouth and maintenance of present weight of 110 lb. by 2/5.

Orders: 2/1

1. Weigh every day on standing scale at 0730 wearing slippers, patient gown, and cotton robe.
2. Maintain suction machine, suction catheter, and oxygen per mask at the bedside in case of choking.
3. Seat in a high-backed chair for meals.
4. Cover chest with towel.
5. Assist to open sealed dietary containers.
6. Sit with patient and remain throughout meals.
7. Remind to place food on the unaffected (right) side of the mouth and chew well.
8. Repeat the following instructions for swallowing:
   - Work the food to the back of mouth
   - Lift tongue up to the roof of mouth
   - Close lips tightly
   - Lower chin toward chest
   - Swallow once and repeat
9. Give patient a hand mirror for inspecting the mouth.
10. Have patient use a finger to clear food from the cheek and repeat instructions for swallowing. ———————————————————————— T. BERENSON, RN

Implementation (Documentation)

2/2   0745   Weighed 109 lbs. using standing scale. Up in chair for breakfast. Places food on R. side of mouth with spoon. Given instructions for swallowing as identified in care plan. ———————————————————————— V. HILL, RN

Evaluation (Documentation)

0830   Mouth suctioned twice. Food still under tongue after several swallowing attempts. States, "I can't feel were the food's at." Used a mirror to visualize retained food. Able to swallow food after finger sweep. Ate half of breakfast. States, "I'm so discouraged. I don't think I'll ever be able to eat in public again." ———————————————————————— V. HILL, RN

Gelatin—often especially attractive to children when molded in various shapes and sizes

Soda pop and various fruit drinks

Place a stethoscope on a child and allow him to listen to the gurgling sound of liquids in his stomach. This technique often helps encourage drinking when children are to have a generous fluid intake.

Use game techniques to encourage fluid intake. For example, taping a picture on the bottom of a glass often interests a child in drinking so that he can see the picture. Also, stars may be placed on the side of a glass or cup as a reward for reaching certain goals.

Offer a child on restricted fluid intake an occasional popsicle or a little gelatin. These items help relieve thirst while still helping to keep the fluid intake low.

Use highchairs and small tables and chairs for children able to be out of bed. Children also like to eat in groups.

Use straws for children old enough to use them. If there is a problem with spilling, liquids can be placed in a bottle that is capped with a nipple; cut slits in the nipple in the form of an X, and place the straw through the slit.

When the Patient Is Pregnant or Lactating

Note in a nursing history whether a pregnant or lactating woman is receiving sufficient calcium and iron in her diet. These two minerals are likely to be deficient when the mother's diet is inadequate.

For most pregnant women, expect that the total number of calories necessary to support the developing fetus must be increased by approximately 300 daily.

For most lactating mothers, plan that several hundred additional calories per day are necessary to supply adequate nutrition for the infant. The lactating mother's diet should be rich in milk, in foods high in proteins, and in minerals and vitamins. The lactating mother should have a generous daily fluid intake.

When the Patient Is Blind or Has His Eyes Patched

The suggestions given earlier in this chapter to help a patient eat should be observed when feeding a patient who is blind or whose eyes are patched. These additional techniques are recommended:

Tell the patient what you are offering him with each mouthful.

Use a system, such as a hand touch, to indicate when the patient is ready for more food or beverage or when there is another bite ready for him.

If the patient can help, consider using dishes with rims if spilling is a problem. Place the food in

identical positions for each meal. The place of food on his tray can be described by using a clock. For example, a beverage is placed in the position of 1 o'clock, a vegetable is placed at 3 o'clock, etc.

When the Patient Is Elderly

Remember that the elderly lose their sensitivity to taste and smell. Herbs and spices often help perk up a poor appetite. Foods and beverages with an aroma and flavors that are relatively intense often appeal more than bland foods. There appears to be a decrease in sensitivity to salty and bitter tastes but not to sweet and sour.

Remember also that the sense of temperature decreases with age. Therefore, be especially careful to avoid serving very hot foods with which the elderly could be burned without their realizing it.

Consult the elderly patient about supplemental vitamins if his eating habits are poor. The need for vitamins does not change with age, but vitamin intake is often reduced. The vitamins most often lacking in the diet of the elderly include thiamine and vitamins A and C. Foods high in vitamin B, such as grain cereals, meat, poultry, and fish, should be encouraged because vitamin B helps stimulate the appetite.

Take into consideration that the need for calories decreases with age, as people become more sedentary. As a general rule, the elderly person needs about one-third fewer calories than do young and middle-aged adults.

Take into account that the person with dentures or without teeth cannot chew well. Foods should be finely chopped or ground, as indicated.

If the patient has difficulty swallowing, position his head slightly forward when offering foods and fluids. This technique helps prevent choking and aspiration.

Consider using double-strength milk if the patient is undernourished. The protein and vitamin content of milk can be increased without increasing the fat content by reconstituting dry skimmed milk with whole milk.

Be sure that the elderly patient receives good oral hygiene. A clean, moist mouth, free of debris and irritation, helps improve the appetite and the desire to eat.

Be prepared to teach the elderly about common food fads. Many fad diets tend to make the elderly patient believe falsely that they will regain youth by using them.

Allow the elderly to dine in groups when possible. They ordinarily enjoy the social interaction and company of others when eating.

Teaching Suggestions to Promote Nutrition

The nurse should use opportunities to teach patients, their families, and the parents of children about the importance of proper nutrition. The team leader usually collects information about the patient's eating habits when obtaining the nursing history. From this history, the nurse can identify areas where teaching is indicated. Including families in health teaching is especially important when the patient is a child or when he is elderly or too incapacitated to understand.

Patients requiring special diets need the nurse's help in learning how to select appropriate foods and understanding why the special diet is important for health. A diet low in sodium content (low salt or salt free) is commonly prescribed. If the patient uses a salt substitute, the patient's potassium level should be monitored because many salt substitutes contain potassium. A high blood level of potassium can endanger health.

Advertising has been relatively effective in leading people to use fad diets and foods. The nurse can play an important part in helping patients understand the nutritional dangers of these products through proper teaching.

There are various services available in most communities for serving meals to shut-ins. Some of these services bring meals to the home; others have programs where people gather for meals served to them. The nurse should be familiar with these services and inform those who could benefit from them.

A variety of suggestions has been offered in this chapter to help patients meet nutritional needs, including suggestions in selected situations. These suggestions should be shared with patients and families as situations indicate.

Bibliography

Birdsall C: Clinical savvy, when is TPN safe? Am J Nurs 85(1):73, 1985

Castiglia PT: Obesity in adolescence. Journal of Pediatric Health Care 3(4):221–223, 1989

Cerrato PL: Fast action for a tube-fed patient's diarrhea. RN Magazine 51(3):89–90, 1989

Cerrato PL: Spotting the patient who looks healthy but isn't. RN Magazine 52(3):81–82, 1989

Conant MJ, Fiesleler ME: Healthy eating for the 1980s and 1990s. Holistic Nursing Practice 3(1):75–85, 1988

Curtas S, Chapman G, Meguid MM: Evaluation of nutritional status. Nurs Clin North Am 24(2):301–313, 1989

D'Agostino NS: Managing nutrition problems in advanced cancer. Am J Nurs 89(1):50–56, 1989

Dietz WH, Mirkin GB, Schmitt BD: Feeding strategies for children. Patient Care 23(5):131–135, 1989

Donahue PA: When it's hard to swallow: Feeding techniques for dysphagia management. Journal of Gerontological Nursing 16(4):6–9, 1990

Farley JM: Current trends in enteral feeding. Critical Care Nurse 8(4):23–27, 1988

Finn SC: Alzheimer's disease and nutrition. Caring 8(8):32–25, 1989

Groth K: Age-related changes in the gastrointestinal tract. Geriatr Nurs 9(5):278–280, 1988

Hennessy K: Nutritional support and gastrointestinal disease. Nurs Clin North Am 24(2):373–382, 1989

Johndrow PD: Making your patient and his family feel at home with T.P.N. Nursing 18(10):65–69, 1988

Konstantinides N, Shronts E: Tube feedings: Managing the basics. Am J Nurs 83(9):1312–1320, 1983

Metheny N, Eisenberg P, McSweeney M: Effect of feeding tube properties and three irrigants on clogging rates. Nurs Res 37(3): 165–169, 1988

Orr ME: Nutritional support in home care. Nurs Clin North Am 24(2):437–445, 1989

Pritchard V: Tube feeding-related pneumonias. Journal of Gerontological Nursing 14(7):32–36, 1988

Spence RL: Nutrition in hospice care. Caring 7(8):50–51, 1988

Starkey JF, Jefferson PA, Kirby DF: Taking care of a percutaneous endoscopic gastrostomy. Am J Nurs 88(1):42–45, 1988

Steinborn PA: Home enteral nutrition. Caring 7(9):20–23, 1988

Vickery CE, McAneny B, Daicar E: Nutrition assessment in the adult day care center. Geriatr Nurs 9(5):292–295, 1988

Williams PJ: How do you keep medicines from clogging feeding tubes? Am J Nurs 89(2):181–182, 1989

9

Promoting Activity and Exercise

Chapter Outline

Behavioral Objectives
Glossary
Introduction
Maintaining Good Posture
Principles of Body Mechanics
Benefits of Activity and Exercise
Identifying Risk Factors
Assessing Fitness
Types of Exercise
Suggested Measures to Promote Activity and Exercise in
    Selected Situations
Applicable Nursing Diagnoses
Bibliography

Skill Procedures

Using Proper Body Mechanics
Planning a Safe Exercise Program

Behavioral Objectives

When the content of this chapter has been mastered, the learner will be able to:

Define the terms appearing in the glossary.
Identify characteristics of good posture in a standing, sitting, or lying position.
Identify principles of body mechanics that should be maintained using various activities as examples, such as ironing, gardening, carrying groceries, and so on.
List seven benefits of exercise.
Discuss factors that indicate risks to certain individuals who impulsively begin an exercise program.
Describe three types of data that are useful when assessing an individual's fitness.
Compare isotonic exercise with isometric exercise.
Describe ways that exercise may be performed safely.
List examples of exercises that are considered leisure-time activities.
List suggested measures to promote activity and exercise in selected situations, as described in this chapter.

Glossary

Active exercise A form of exercise performed by a person without the assistance of another.
Activity Movement.
Aerobic exercise A form of active exercise that challenges the heart and lungs.
Body composition The ratio of lean mass to fat mass.
Body mechanics The efficient use of the body as a machine.
Exercise Movement intended to increase strength, stamina, and overall body tone.
Fitness An increased capacity to perform work with greater ease.
Flexibility The ability to move joints through their normal range of motion.
Isometric exercise A form of active exercise that alternates contraction and relaxation of skeletal muscles with little or no movement.
Isotonic exercise A form of active exercise that involves movement and work.
Musculoskeletal system The structures of the body used for support and movement.
Osteoporosis A condition in which the bones lose calcium and become less dense.
Passive exercise An exercise in which one person moves the body parts of another.
Posture The position of the body or the way in which it is held.
Range of motion The amount of movement that is possible in the joints of the body.
Stamina The ability to sustain effort.
Strength The potential for power.
Stress electrocardiogram A test that records the activity of the heart during exercise.
Tone The potential to respond when stimulated to work.

Introduction

Movement of the body is necessary for work and play. The need to move about is directly related to the quality of life.

Yet, science and technology continue to develop devices that decrease physical activity. What was once a long day's work at hard, manual labor has subsequently been lightened and reduced by time and labor-saving machines.

People in the United States, as a whole, have become physically unfit. The President's Council on Physical Fitness and Sports estimates that only slightly half of all adults exercise, and of those who do, most do not exercise enough to improve their health. Though not everyone is destined to become an athlete, even maintaining good posture and using proper body mechanics for normal musculoskeletal function will help individuals look and feel better.

There is currently a renewed interest and awareness of the importance for exercise. This has led many Americans to participate in some increased physical activity. The nurse can do much to identify the multiple physical and emotional benefits associated with a more active lifestyle. In addition, the nurse may be called upon to teach methods for avoiding exercise-related complications. This chapter may help the nurse assess the fitness of individuals and promote safe aspects of movement and exercise so that more people may find enjoyment and improved health through independent, group, or team activities.

Activity is movement. For most people, each day is filled with reaching, lifting, stooping, pulling, pushing, sitting, standing, and so on. *Exercise* is movement intended to increase strength, stamina, and overall body tone. *Fitness* is the result of exercise; it is an increased capacity to perform work with greater ease.

The *musculoskeletal system* of the body consists of structures that the body uses for support and movement. The manner in which these structures are used affects the efficiency with which the tasks are accomplished. A preliminary step to fitness is preventing strain and injury through the development of good posture and body mechanics.

Maintaining Good Posture

Posture refers to the position of the body or the way in which it is held. Posture requires energy to overcome gravity. Without this energy, the body would become entirely limp and fall to the floor.

Having good posture means positioning the body so that there is good body alignment and good balance. In this position, the musculoskeletal system can be used in the best way possible. Good posture makes it possible for other systems of the body to work more efficiently. For example, slouching when standing or sitting makes breathing difficult. There is also a quality of attractiveness about a person when the body is positioned appropriately.

Standing

The following is a description of good posture in the standing position:

- Keep the feet parallel, at right angles to the lower legs, and about 10 cm to 20 cm (4 to 8 in) apart. Distribute weight equally on both feet. This position of the feet gives the body a good base of support.
- Bend the knees slightly. This position of the knees avoids the strain of "locked knees" and acts as a shock absorber for the entire body.
- Pull in the buttocks and hold the abdomen up and in. This position is often referred to as "putting on an internal girdle." It will help to keep the back straight by preventing swayback; this, in turn, keeps the spine properly aligned. This position supports the abdominal organs and reduces strain on both back and abdominal muscles.
- Hold the chest up and slightly forward and extend or stretch the waist. This position is often described as "putting on a long midriff." It gives internal organs, such as the lungs, the greatest amount of space possible for effective work. It also helps maintain good alignment of the spine by preventing a humped back. The shoulders may be relaxed but held back slightly.
- Hold the head erect with the face forward and with the chin in slightly. In a sense, the head is balancing at the top of the spine in this position. The position also helps keep the spine in good alignment by preventing a curve in the neck area. Correct and incorrect standing positions are illustrated in Figure 9-1.

Sitting

A good sitting position is like that just described for standing, except the buttocks and upper thighs become the base of support on the chair and the knees are bent. The legs should not be crossed at the knees when sitting because that position interferes with proper circulation of blood. The area under the knees, the popliteal area, should be free from the edge of the chair. Pressure in the popliteal area interferes with circulation in the legs and may cause damage to nerves in the area. Figure 9-2 shows poor and proper posture when sitting.

Lying Down

It is also important to have good posture when lying down. The muscles are in a state of relaxation when resting or sleeping. Unless the parts of the body are properly supported, the body will respond to gravity and fall out of good alignment. Poor alignment makes it difficult for the body to function effectively. Descriptions of ways to support the body of a patient in proper alignment when lying down are given in Chapter 18. Correct and incorrect positions when lying down are illustrated in Figure 9-3.

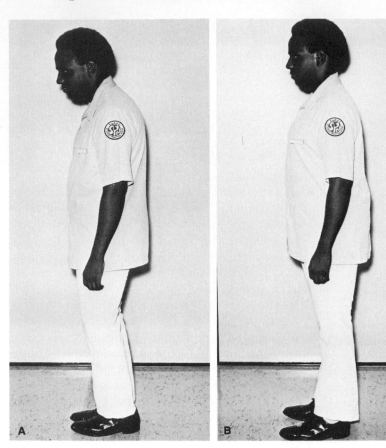

Figure 9-1 (*A*). Slouching is a result of relaxed abdominal muscles. It places the body in poor alignment. (*B*). This nurse is in a good standing position.

Principles of Body Mechanics

Body mechanics is defined as the efficient use of the body as a machine. Using good body mechanics is as important to the nurse as it is for others. Basic principles of body mechanics are illustrated in this chapter, which uses the nurse as an example. However, the principles can be applied regardless of the worker or the task. Common terms used when speaking of body mechanics are defined in Table 9-1. Figure 9-4 illustrates some of the terms.

General principles for good use of the musculoskeletal system are described as follows:

- *Use the longest and strongest muscles to provide the energy needed for the task.* It is best to use the long and strong muscles in the arms, legs, and hips whenever possible. Smaller, weaker muscles will strain and injure quickly if forced to work beyond their capacity. One of the most common injuries affects the muscles in the lower part of the back. It is a painful injury and usually slow to heal, but it is preventable when proper body mechanics are used.

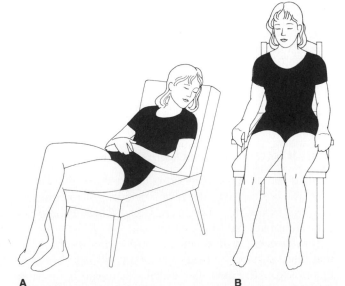

Figure 9-2 (*A*). Muscles are quickly strained when the weight is not distributed over the center of gravity. (*B*). Sitting with uncrossed legs helps blood to flow. (Courtesy of Lowren West, New York, NY.)

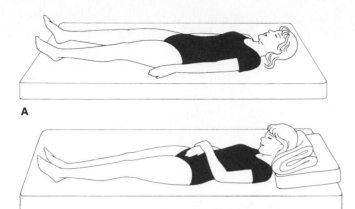

A

B

Figure 9-3 (*A*). The line of gravity passes through the body as though the person were standing. (*B*). Flexion of the neck and arms interferes with breathing and proper alignment. (Courtesy of Lowren West, New York, NY.)

- *Use the internal girdle and make a long midriff to protect the muscles of the abdomen and pelvis.* This technique overcomes slouching and uses muscles properly to prevent strain and injury to the abdominal wall.
- *Push, pull, or roll objects whenever possible, rather than lift them.* It takes more effort to lift something against the force of gravity. Use body weight as a lever

to assist with pushing or pulling an object. This reduces the strain placed on a group of muscles.
- *Keep feet apart for a broad base of support.* If the feet are close together, weight is distributed over a small area. Balance can be upset in this position when there is even a slight tilt of the body.
- *Bend the knees and keep the back straight when lifting an object, rather than bending over from the waist with straight knees.* This position makes best use of the longest and the strongest muscles in the body. It also improves balance by keeping the weight of the object being lifted close to the center of gravity.
- *Avoid twisting and stretching muscles during work.* These movements strain muscles and usually occur when there has been failure to bring the work as close to the body and its center of gravity as possible. The result is that the line of gravity falls outside the body's base of support.
- *Rest between periods of exertion.* Muscles that are overused or misused build up chemicals that accentuate fatigue. Muscles work more effectively by resting them occasionally after working or exercising strenuously.

These principles are emphasized in the actions and illustrations in Skill Procedure 9-1. If the principles of good posture and body mechanics are practiced, the result will be good balance, increased muscle effectiveness, less

Table 9-1. Basic Terminology of Body Mechanics

Term	Definition	Example
Gravity	A force that pulls objects toward the center of the earth.	The pull of gravity causes objects, such as an item dropped from the hand, to fall to the ground. It causes water to drain to its lowest level.
Energy	The capacity to do work.	Energy is used to move the body from place to place. Energy is required to overcome the force of gravity.
Balance	Having a steady position with weight distributed equally on the base of support.	A person falls when he is off balance as gravity pulls him out of position and to the ground.
Center of gravity	The point at which the mass of an object is centered.	The center of gravity for a standing person is the center of the pelvis and about halfway between the umbilicus and the pubic bone.
Line of gravity	An imaginary, vertical line that passes through the center of gravity.	The line of gravity in a standing person is a straight line from the head to the feet that passes through the center of gravity of the body.
Base of support	The area on which an object rests.	The feet are the base of support when a person is in a standing position.
Alignment	Having parts of an object in proper relationship to one another.	The body is in good alignment in a position of good posture.

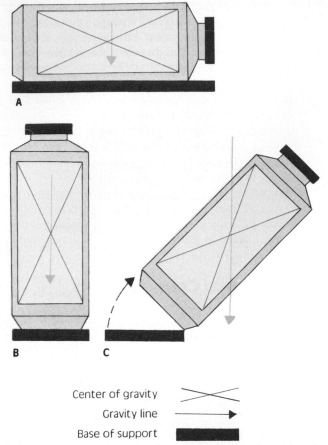

Center of gravity
Gravity line
Base of support

Figure 9-4 Body mechanics are affected by gravity and one's base of support. (*A*). The line of gravity passes through the wide base of support. The wider the base, the greater is the stability. Spreading one's feet apart is a way of widening the base. (*B*). This base is narrower, but gravity is still centered. There is a potential for instability. (*C*). The line of gravity is not centered over the base of support. A body in this position is extremely unstable. The ability to work without injury is reduced. (Taylor C, Lillis C, LeMone P: Fundamentals of Nursing, The Art and Science of Nursing Care, p 623. Philadelphia, JB Lippincott, 1989)

fatigue or injury to the musculoskeletal system, and an attractive appearance.

Benefits of Activity and Exercise

Besides feeling and looking better, increasing exercise can lead to many positive effects. Exercise has a holistic effect; both physical and emotional well-being are improved.

Improved Cardiopulmonary Function. The heart and the lungs work together to provide cells with oxygen and to remove wastes. The heart is a muscle. Any muscle that is exercised increases its tone. *Tone* is a term referring to the ability to respond when stimulated to work. Eventually the exercised muscle of the heart will be able to pump more blood with less effort. Athletes generally have low pulse rates, but their cells are adequately oxygenated. Similarly, the lungs take in more oxygen with each breath.

The circulation of blood is also improved with exercise. Blood in the veins of the legs, arms, and lower body must travel back to the heart against gravity. Muscle movement helps to move blood out of these areas. People who sit or stand for long periods may experience swollen feet and ankles.

Improved Muscle Strength and Stamina. The muscles of the body become strengthened with use. *Strength* is the potential for power. *Stamina* is the ability to sustain effort. Most people who exercise develop increased endurance. The *body composition,* the ratio of lean mass to fat mass, also changes. Physically fit individuals appear sleek and coordinated.

Maintenance of Joint Mobility. Joints move in various directions. The amount of movement that is possible is called *range of motion.* The range that is available in each joint is referred to as *flexibility.* When joints are not moved, the normal range is reduced. Activity and exercise help promote the flexibility of joints. Table 9-2 describes and illustrates some of the common terms used to describe body positions when joints are flexible.

Increased Bone Density. One of the chief minerals that allows bones to be strong and compact is calcium. Activity and exercise promote the deposit and retention of calcium. A common problem for bedridden individuals and inactive elderly people is a softening of the bones called *osteoporosis.* Women are at higher risk for this when they age, since a decrease in estrogen, a female hormone, is thought to be a contributing factor. Figure 9-11 shows the difference in height due to a loss of bone density. The effects of this condition can be reduced by increasing the intake of dairy products or using calcium supplements, and by exercise.

Promotion of Bowel Elimination. Stool forms throughout the intestine as nutrients and water are absorbed. Gravity and muscle movement help move stool toward the rectum, from which it is eventually passed. Activity and exercise promote this process.

Aid to Sleep. Fatigue is the body's signal for rest. Sleep restores the sense of well-being. It is enhanced by the stimulation from physical and mental activity. More on promoting rest and sleep can be found in Chapter 10.

Reduction of Tension. Separating oneself from the usual daily stressors has been a technique frequently used
(Text continues on page 166)

Skill Procedure 9-1. Using Proper Body Mechanics

Suggested Action	Reason for Action
Maintain good posture.	Good posture reduces strain and helps prevents injury to the musculoskeletal system. It helps maintain balance and keeps the body in good alignment.
When stooping, place one foot in front of the other; lower the body while bending the knees. Keep the body weight on the front foot and the ball of the back foot (Fig. 9-5). Keep the back as straight as possible. Return to the standing position by lifting the body with the muscles in the thighs and hips while using an internal girdle and a long midriff.	These movements make use of the longest and strongest muscles of the body and reduce strain on the back. They provide for a good base of support, proper back alignment, and balance.

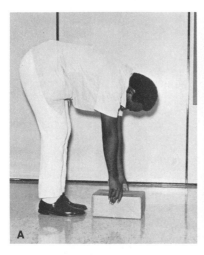 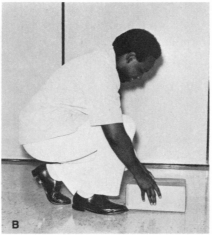

Figure 9-5 (*A*). The nurse reaches down to pick up the package. This results in poor body alignment and strain on back muscles. (*B*). The nurse stoops down to pick up the package, using long, strong muscles to lift the package and to raise himself into the standing position.

Keep the work area as close to the body as possible (Fig. 9-6).	Stretching and twisting fatigue muscles quickly. When stretching or twisting, balance will be poor as the line of gravity falls outside the body's base of support.

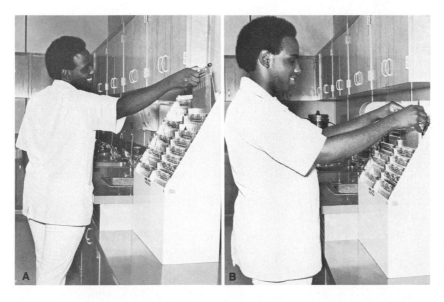

Figure 9-6 (*A*). Stretching and twisting place the nurse's body in poor alignment and strain muscles. (*B*). Keeping the work area close to the body minimizes stretching and twisting.

(continued)

Skill Procedure 9-1. Continued

Suggested Action	**Reason for Action**
Face the work area.	A position that requires twisting strains and tires muscles.
Pivot to turn the body. When pivoting, keep the feet apart and the body weight on the ball of each foot (heels slightly raised), turn in the desired direction. Keep the body straight (Fig. 9-7).	Twisting the body causes strain on the muscles. Turning is easier when the weight is off the heels and helps prevent twisting the knees.

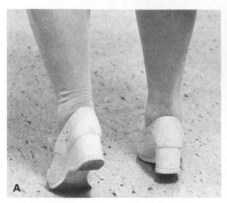 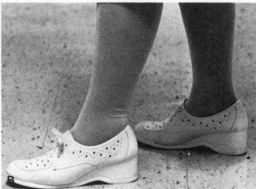

Figure 9-7 (*A*). Before pivoting, the nurse places weight on the ball of each foot by raising the heels slightly. (*B*). This is the position of the feet after the pivot.

Carry objects close to the body but without touching the uniform. Put on an internal girdle and a long midriff (Fig. 9-8).	Carrying objects close to the body helps place the line of gravity within the body's base of support. Stretching the arms outward while carrying an object strains arm muscles. Putting on an internal girdle and a long midriff helps protect abdominal organs and reduces strain.

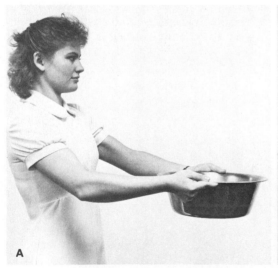 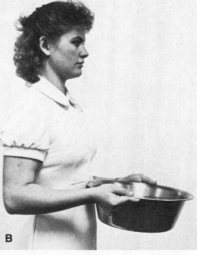

Figure 9-8 (*A*). The nurse strains the arms carrying the wash basin in this manner. The line of gravity is not within the base of support, which results in poor balance. (*B*). By bringing the line of gravity closer to the base of support, the nurse improves balance and reduces the strain on arm muscles.

Keep the work area at a comfortable height, as illustrated in Figure 9-9.	Body alignment and balance are easier to maintain when the work is at a comfortable height. When a work area is too high, arm muscles are strained by stretching. When the work area is too low, back muscles are strained by bending over the work.

(*continued*)

Skill Procedure 9-1. Continued

Suggested Action	**Reason for Action**

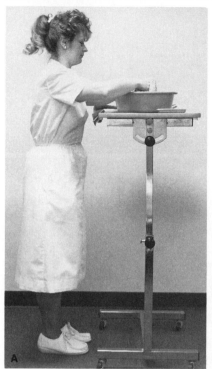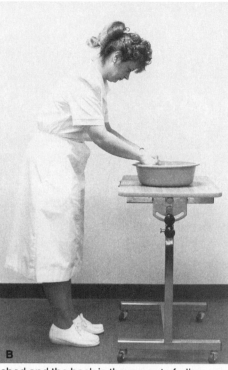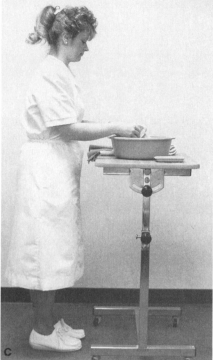

Figure 9-9 (*A*). The nurse's arms are stretched and the back is thrown out of alignment when using a high work area. (*B*). Bending over the work area strains back muscles. (*C*). Having the work area at a comfortable height prevents the strain of bending and stretching.

Lean toward objects being pushed and away from objects being pulled. Use the muscles of the legs as much as possible, and use the internal girdle and a long midriff (Fig. 9-10).

Body weight adds force to muscle action when pushing or pulling. Using the long and strong muscles of the legs relieves strain on the arms and back. Using the internal girdle and a long midriff protects abdominal organs and reduces strain.

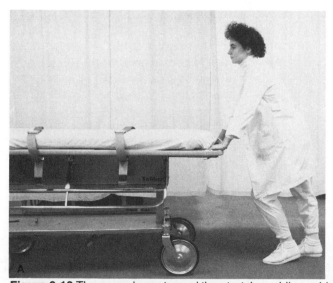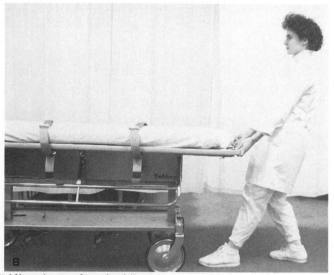

Figure 9-10 The nurse leans toward the stretcher while pushing it (*A*) and away from it while pulling (*B*). The body weight assists muscles in moving the stretcher.

(*continued*)

Skill Procedure 9-1. *Continued*

Suggested Action	Reason for Action
Roll an object rather than lift it whenever possible.	Rolling an object requires less muscle work than does lifting an object.
Use the longest and strongest muscles of the body when possible.	These muscles are less likely to become strained and injured than smaller muscles.
Use a sturdy stepstool when obtaining articles out of easy reach.	Stretching causes strain on muscles. As the center of gravity is raised while in the stretching position, the body is placed in poor balance.
Move muscles smoothly and evenly while working.	Jerky movements produce more strain on muscles and are uncomfortable for the nurse and the patient.

to reduce tension. Some do this by meditating; some participate in leisure-time activities; some exercise. Research suggests that during activity the body releases chemicals that elevate one's mood and promote a feeling of well-being.

Identifying Risk Factors

Even though most people are reasonably active, not all should make rash decisions to suddenly change their lifestyle by exercising. Caution should be used. Even some experienced athletes have died suddenly and unexpectedly during exercise. Factors that make some more prone than others to complications include:

- *Inactivity.* Those whose jobs require that they are stationary and those individuals whose leisure time is filled with sedentary activities such as playing card games or watching television may not be able to adapt to the increased physical demands associated with exercise.
- *Obesity.* Those who are over 20% of their ideal weight are generally obese. Food that is not used for energy is converted to fat. A logical analysis is that fat people are inactive people.
- *Aging.* As age increases so do changes in the functioning of vital organs such as the heart, lungs, and blood vessels. These organs may function adequately during rest and inactivity, but may not be able to meet the changes required during exercise.
- *Smoking.* The use of tobacco affects the heart and lungs, making an individual even more susceptible to exercise-related complications. Nicotine causes the heart rate to increase. The walls of blood vessels become smaller, thus elevating the blood pressure. This interferes with the circulation of oxygen-rich blood to cells. Mucus increases in lungs and makes it more difficult for gases to be exchanged. Long-term smoking causes even more serious, irreversible changes in lung tissue. One of the most healthful

changes, even more healthful than exercise, is to stop smoking.
- *High blood pressure.* Elevated blood pressure usually means that the heart must work especially hard to pump blood through narrowed blood vessels. During exercise, cells need even more oxygen than at rest. When a vital organ, such as the heart, cannot receive the oxygen it needs, life-threatening complications can occur.
- *Heredity.* Otherwise healthy individuals who have a family history of deaths or diseases associated with the heart should be careful. Some of these diseases may be so subtle that they do not cause obvious signs or symptoms until dangerously advanced. Exercise may trigger the first experience with symptoms, which may be so severe that they cause death.

Assessing Fitness

There are ways that an individual's readiness for or response to exercise may be evaluated. It is best to use the results of several methods to be sure of the findings.

Measuring Body Composition. The inaccuracies of height and weight charts were discussed in Chapter 8. One of the better assessments is body composition. Body composition can be determined by measuring skinfold thicknesses. Skinfold thickness is a measurement of the amount of fat in areas of the body. The fleshy part of the upper arm, below the shoulder blade, the lower abdomen, and the upper thigh are measured with calipers. Excess amounts are usually an indication of overeating or lack of exercise, or both. The individual in Figure 9-12 is measuring skinfold thickness.

Recording Vital Signs. Temperature, pulse, respirations, and blood pressure are referred to as vital signs. They have acquired this name because they provide so much information about life. *Vita* is the Latin word for life.

Table 9-2. Terms Commonly Used to Describe Body Positions and Movements

Term	Description/Example	Term	Description/Example
Abduction (verb: abduct)	The act of moving a body part away from the center of the body.	Flexion (verb: flex)	The act of moving so that the angle between adjoining parts is reduced; bending.

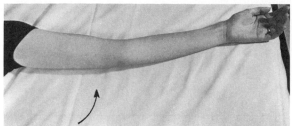

Abduction of arm

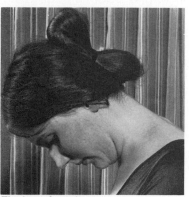

Flexion of neck

Term	Description/Example	Term	Description/Example
Adduction (verb: adduct)	The act of moving a body part toward the center of the body.	Hyperextension (verb: hyperextend)	The act of moving so that the angle between adjoining parts is made larger than its normal or average range, or more than 180 degrees.

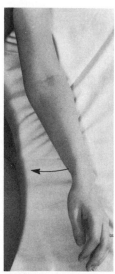

Adduction of arm

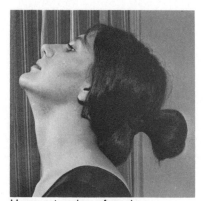

Hyperextension of neck

Term	Description/Example	Term	Description/Example
Extension (verb: extend)	The act of straightening or increasing an angle that brings parts into or toward a straight line.	Rotation (verb: rotate)	The act of turning: the head is rotated when it is turned from side to side.
		External rotation	The act of turning outward: the leg is rotated outward when the toes point outward.
		Internal rotation	The act of turning inward: the leg is rotated inward when the toes point inward.

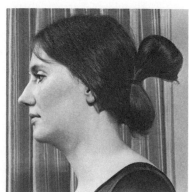

Extension of neck

(continued)

Table 9-2. Continued

Term	Description/Example	Term	Description/Example
Pronation (verb: pronate)	The act of positioning the forearm so that the palm of the hand faces downward; also, the act of positioning the body so that the person lies on his abdomen, as shown below.		

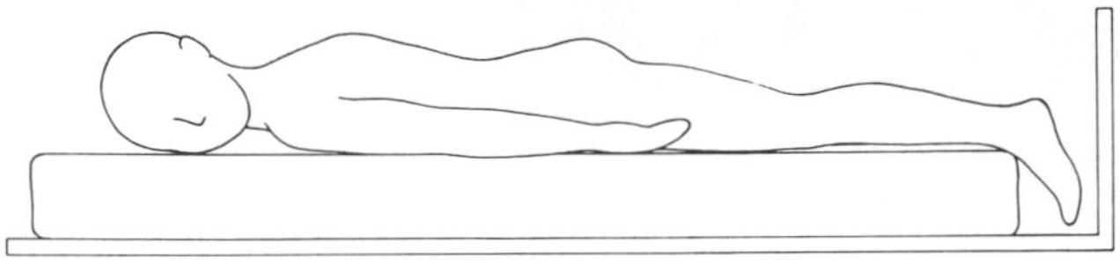

Prone position

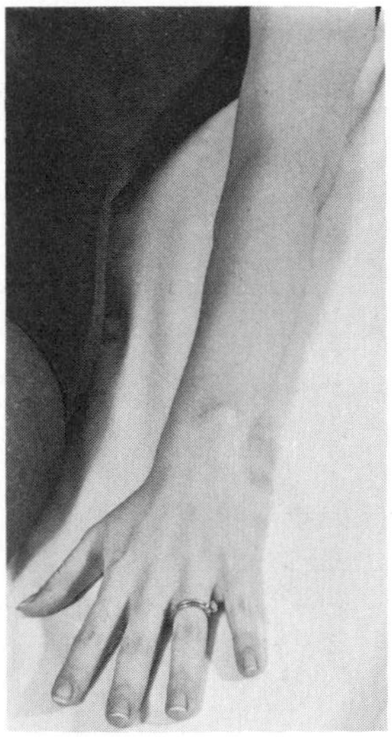

Supination

Pronation

Term	Description/Example	Term	Description/Example
Supination (verb: supinate)	The act of positioning the forearm so that the palm of the hand faces upward; also, the act of positioning the body so that the person lies on his back, as shown below.	Distal	Farthest from the center of the body: the foot is distal to the knee, the hand is distal to the elbow.
		Proximal	Nearest the center of the body: the knee is proximal to the foot, the elbow is proximal to the hand.
		Active exercise	An exercise performed by a person without assistance: a person rotates his head without assistance, a person flexes and extends his elbows and knees without assistance.
		Passive exercise	An exercise in which one person moves the body parts of another: a person rotates another person's head, a person flexes and extends another person's elbows and knees.

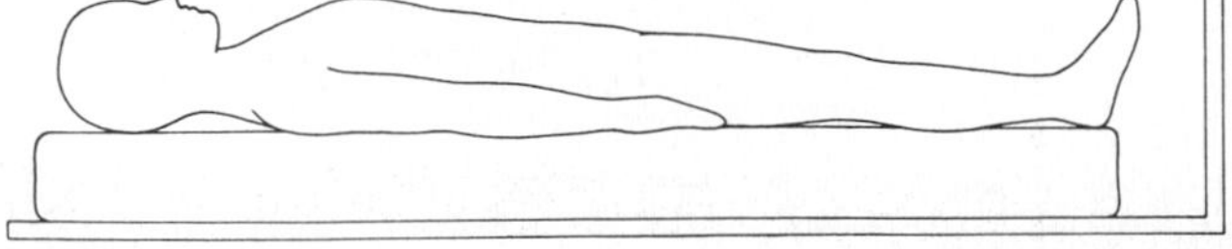

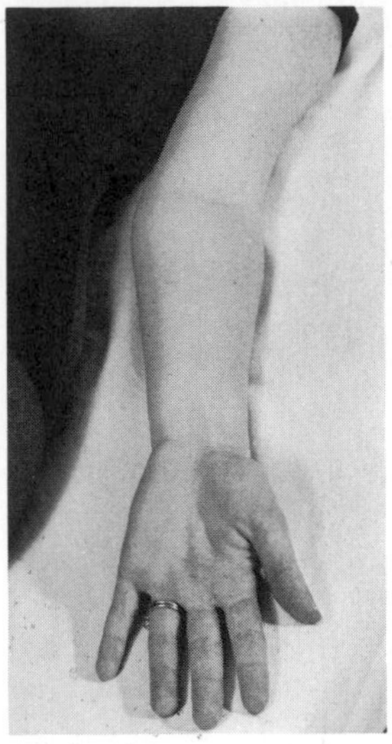

Supine position

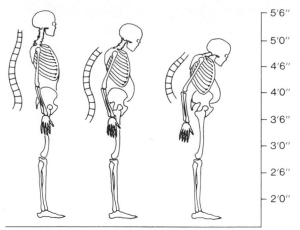

Figure 9-11 These figures show the potential change in height from young adulthood through middle age to old age as a result of the loss in bone density. (Statistics on Height Due to Bone Loss. Tallahassee, Nutrition Company, 1983)

When vital signs fluctuate above or below normal, it is often an ominous sign that a person's life is in danger. More information can be found on vital signs in Chapter 13. If vital signs are above normal at rest, the individual may be unfit to exercise vigorously. Exercise usually will increase these measurements even more. Further testing and evaluation should be performed by a physician. After a period of regular but modified exercise, a person may condition himself so that these measurements will become lowered.

Fitness Tests. Some tests are useful in evaluating an individual's current ability to exercise. These are impor-

tant for determining the potential for life-threatening complications associated with exercise after a period of inactivity.

A *stress electrocardiogram* is often recommended for middle-aged and older individuals. It is a test that records the activity of the heart during the time that an individual exercises. Figure 9-13 shows an individual undergoing a stress electrocardiogram. The heart rate, respirations, blood pressure, and any symptoms such as chest pain are also recorded. Any irregularities or abnormal values may be reason to stop the test. Individuals can still exercise, but the level and length of time may require careful planning.

A test that requires less sophisticated equipment is the Three-Minute Step Test. Despite its simplicity, during the test life-threatening risks are still possible. The test should be used with caution and where medical assistance is available when an individual is middle aged or older, has been inactive, or is overweight. If the person develops any discomfort or fatigue, the test should be stopped, and he should be checked by a doctor.

When conducting the step test, the individual alternates going up and down two steps. The rate per minute should average approximately 26 to 27 steps. The pulse is counted at one-minute intervals after the exercise for three successive times. The rates for all three recordings are added. Values that reflect a state of fitness are listed in Table 9-3.

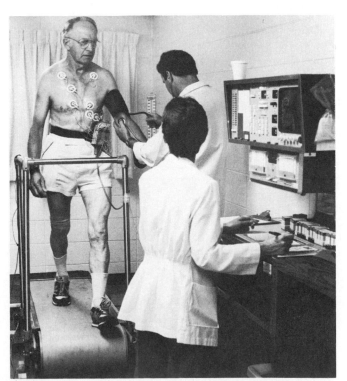

Figure 9-13 Walking a treadmill, which moves at a progressively faster pace while the heart's activity is recorded, is a way of determining the heart's ability to adapt to increased work during exercise. (Courtesy of Borgess Medical Center, Kalamazoo, MI.)

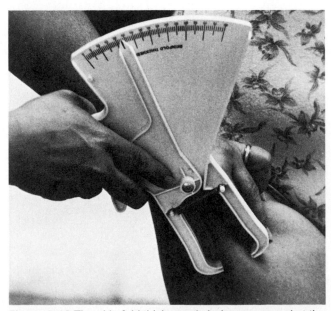

Figure 9-12 The skin fold thickness is being measured at the thigh. Various other areas of the body should also be measured.

Table 9-3. The Three-Minute Step Test Recovery Index

	Cumulative Pulse Rate	
	Men	Women
Excellent	132 or less	135 or less
Good	150–133	155–136
Average	165–149	170–154
Fair	180–164	190–171
Poor	Above 180	Above 190

From Getchell B: Physical Fitness: A Way of Life, 3rd ed. New York, Macmillan, 1983. Reprinted with permission of Macmillan Publishing Company.

Types of Exercise

The preferred type of exercise is *active exercise.* This is a form of exercise performed by a person without assistance. People who are ill may need the assistance of another to move. This would be considered *passive exercise.* Passive exercise and other forms of exercise that are considered therapy for patients are described in Chapter 18. Healthy people may choose to perform several types of active exercise.

Isotonic Exercise. These exercises involve movement and work. One of the best examples is *aerobic exercise,* a type of active exercise that challenges the heart and lungs. Eventually these organs may perform at peak levels. To evaluate that the exercise is sufficient to accomplish this, certain guidelines must be met. An individual should exercise every other day for 20 minutes while sustaining a target heart rate. The target heart rate may be computed using the following formula:

$$220 - age \times 70\% = target\ heart\ rate$$

At this rate an individual should still be able to talk comfortably with another person. Exercise that is more frequent, less intensive, and of longer duration may also be beneficial.

Isometric Exercise. These exercises involve contracting and relaxing muscle groups with little, if any, movement. An example of this type of active exercise is that used for weight training and body sculpting. These exercises increase the mass and definition of skeletal muscles, but they do not increase the capacity of the heart and lungs to perform.

Exercising Regularly. Health risks can be reduced through regular exercise. Display 9-1 shows the national objectives for fitness and exercise for citizens of the United States. Many individuals, such as those in Figure 9-14, are finding ways to add or increase regular exercise into their weekly routine.

When it has been determined that an individual can exercise safely, the nurse can offer health teaching tips. The object of exercise should be to promote health while avoiding injury or complications from overexertion. Skill Procedure 9-2 describes suggestions that may be beneficial.

Leisure-Time Activities. Few people care to do one thing all day long; most enjoy some variety. Recreation and leisure-time activities can be more than just having fun. They can contribute to both physical and mental well-being.

Some spend a portion of their leisure time in exercise or sports activities. For various reasons many prefer group activities to solitary exercise. Fitness centers are now located in almost every city. The competition among them is resulting in attractive, affordable memberships. Even some health maintenance organizations provide frequent, daily physical exercise programs to fit various work schedules. Businesses are offering supervised exercise periods for those workers who perform relatively inactive jobs. Corporate fitness programs keep employees healthy and productive.

Sports provide an opportunity for exercise. Not all schools require physical education, but many do. Children seem to be as unfit as adults. Community recreation programs extend sports from the school-aged to larger numbers of people of all ages. Many businesses sponsor employee teams that compete with one another. Some annual races or walks are open to amateurs who solicit money for charitable causes.

There are many opportunities to add exercise to one's life.

Display 9-1. National Objectives for Physical Fitness and Exercise in the 1990s

Over 90% of children and adolescents ages 10 to 17 will participate in regular physical activity.

Over 60% of children and adolescents will participate in daily school physical education programs.

Over 60% of adults age 18 to 65 will participate in vigorous physical exercise.

One-half of all adults 65 or over will be engaging in appropriate physical activity.

Adapted from MMWR Progress toward achieving the 1990 national objectives for physical fitness and exercise. 38(26): 449–453, 1989

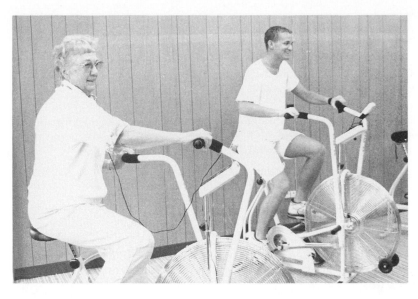

Figure 9-14 Americans of all ages are exercising regularly.

Skill Procedure 9-2. Planning a Safe Exercise Program

Suggested Action	Reason for Action
Assess the level of fitness.	Serious complications can occur in individuals who are not able to adapt to the increased demands associated with exercise.
Find a partner who also exercises.	Exercising with someone can provide motivation and support when the best-intentioned person loses interest or becomes discouraged.
Set a time during each day for exercise.	An activity that is scheduled is more often given priority.
Dress for the climate; wear layers of clothing. Clothing should be wind resistant and absorbent.	The body heats during exercise. Perspiration is a method for cooling. Being able to take clothing off or on may prevent overheating or cooling.
If exercising in areas of traffic, wear reflective clothing. Walk or run against the traffic; cycle in the same direction as traffic.	Reflective clothing is more readily seen by drivers. Following these directions reduces the potential for being injured.
Eat complex carbohydrates rather than high sugar food before exercising.	Foods such as oatmeal, granola, or pasta take longer to digest and will sustain energy needs longer.
Drink or have access to a source of water or other liquids, such as orange juice or Gatorade.	The body loses water and electrolytes in perspiration. On days of high humidity there may be a problem in maintaining fluid balance.
Avoid drinking alcohol.	Alcohol dilates blood vessels. This contributes to the loss of body heat. It may also interfere with the good sense to rest or discontinue the activity.
Caution should be used when wearing radio headphones.	Music acts as a distraction from the effort of exercise, but it also reduces a person's awareness of the sounds that warn of hazards.
Begin performing some mild form of exercise daily, such as walking.	The heart and other structures of the body need a period of conditioning to avoid injury.
Determine the target heart rate.	Exercising at less than maximum intensity still promotes cardiopulmonary performance while preventing overexertion.

(continued)

Skill Procedure 9-2. Continued

Suggested Action	Reason for Action
Warm up for at least 5 minutes before attempting to reach the target rate. Stretch the muscles or walk at a progressively faster pace.	Gradually increasing the need for the body organs to perform avoids injury.
Use as many muscle groups as possible while exercising. Aerobic dancing, cross-country skiing, swimming, and brisk walking are several examples.	Using a variety of muscles promotes overall distribution of work. It also develops and strengthens the body more uniformly.
Sustain the target rate for 20 minutes three times a week or every other day.	This level and frequency of exercise promotes many benefits for cardiopulmonary fitness.
Be attentive to body responses such as pain, difficult breathing, abdominal cramps or nausea, and feeling faint.	Exceeding one's tolerance or not compensating for weather conditions can lead to serious complications.
Cool down for approximately the same amount of time and in the reverse order of the warm-up routine. Fainting commonly occurs as the brain suddenly has a decrease in its blood supply.	The aim of the cool-down is to help the body adjust gradually to the changing levels of activity.

Finding a leisure-time activity may open the door to developing a lifelong habit that is pleasurable and healthful.

Suggested Measures to Promote Activity and Exercise in Selected Situations

When the Individual Is an Infant or Child

Use toys and play activity to promote exercise and activity.

Select toys that are appropriate for the age of the child and choose them carefully with safety in mind. Toys with small, removable parts should be avoided because of the danger of their being swallowed. Also, toys with sharp edges or points should be avoided. Interesting and inexpensive toys can be made from common objects found in the home.

Select play activity with safety in mind. Play activity should be supervised at all times.

Select play activities that are appropriate for the age of the child. For example, young children may play next to each other but rarely play with each other. Activities involving groups of children become more appropriate among school-age children.

Use television with discrimination for leisure-time activity. Watching television promotes minimal activity and does little to stimulate a child's imagination and ingenuity.

Plan activities with the knowledge that children have a short interest span and become bored easily when there is little variety.

When the Individual Is Pregnant

Consult an obstetrician early in pregnancy in order that a realistic assessment of health and fitness may be obtained.

There is no common agreement on the effects of exercise during pregnancy, since research studies have not provided sufficient data.

Applicable Nursing Diagnoses

Patients who are inactive or unable to move about while performing desired activities may have one or more of the following nursing diagnoses:

- Decreased Cardiac Output
- Ineffective Airway Clearance
- Ineffective Breathing Pattern
- High Risk for Disuse Syndrome
- High Risk for Impaired Skin Integrity
- Social Isolation
- Impaired Physical Mobility
- Fatigue
- Impaired Home Maintenance Management
- Bathing/Hygiene Self-Care Deficit

Nursing Care Plan 9-1 provides an example of actions that help a patient with Activity Intolerance. Activity Intolerance is defined in the NANDA Taxonomy (1989) as, "A state in which an individual has insufficient physiological or psychological energy to endure or complete required or desired daily activities."

NURSING CARE PLAN

9-1. Activity Intolerance

Assessment	**Subjective Data**
	States, "I feel weak as a cat. I want to take care of myself, but I no more start and I'm exhausted."
	Objective Data
	35-year-old man admitted with a history of a chronic bleeding ulcer. Reports vomiting blood recently as well as passing black tarry stools. Hemoglobin 9.2 g%. Heart rate 120 beats/minute during ambulation. Respirations become rapid (32/minute) when getting out of bed.
Diagnosis	Activity Intolerance related to imbalance between oxygen supply and demand.
Plan	**Goal**
	The patient's heart rate will remain ≤100 and respiratory rate ≤24/minute when performing activity by 3/10.

Orders: 3/6
1. Monitor apical heart rate following 15 minutes of rest q shift and while performing activities of daily living.
2. Administer oxygen at 36% by nasal cannula 15 minutes prior to and during bathing, and any other activity during which the heart rate exceeds 110 or the respiratory rate exceeds 28.
3. Stop activity when heart rate >110 bpm.
4. Discontinue oxygen when pulse rate is <100 bpm.
5. Space activities between at least 30 minutes of rest. _____ G. SLENTZ, RN

Implementation (Documentation)

3/7

0730 Resting apical heart rate 96 bpm. O_2 @ 4 L (36%) by nasal cannula prior to hygiene. _____ P. VALE, LPN

0745 Able to complete oral hygiene and wash face while maintaining heart rate <100. Heart rate accelerates to 122 when washing arms. _____ P. VALE, LPN

Evaluation (Documentation)

0815 Heart rate of 100 following 5 minutes of rest. Bath completed with assistance. _____ P. VALE, LPN

0900 Rested 15 minutes. Heart rate 94 bpm. Oxygen discontinued. _____ P. VALE, LPN

Strenuous exercise is as unwise for the unfit pregnant woman as it is for any unfit woman.

A previous complication of pregnancy should be considered a risk factor for any extreme in behavior, including exercise.

The American College of Obstetricians and Gynecologists (ACOG) has identified its position and recommendations on exercise during pregnancy. A pregnant woman could ask her obstetrician for these guidelines or write the organization directly.

The ACOG has produced videocassette and audiocassette exercise programs, "Pregnancy Exercise Program" and "Postnatal Exercise Program," which are available at costs comparable to other commercial cassettes. Information on these can be obtained by calling (800) 762-2264 or by writing to ACOG Exercise Programs, 3575 Cahuenga Boulevard West, Suite 440, Los Angeles, CA, 90068.

When the Individual Is Elderly

Many elderly people have little opportunity to participate in exercise programs. The nurse has an important opportunity and responsibility to initiate or encourage exercise.

Some elderly persons are reluctant to participate in exercise and activity programs. Gaining their cooperation often requires ingenuity, but concerted efforts are well worthwhile to prevent the serious complications of inactivity.

Take every precaution to prevent falls when promoting exercise and activity. Complications of falls are leading causes of death in the elderly. Safe walking shoes with nonskid soles, stable furniture, low beds, and an environment kept free of clutter are especially important.

Use rocking chairs as one means of promoting activity. Rocking a chair requires an activity most elderly persons can carry out with ease. Also, most enjoy using a rocking chair.

Work with the knowledge that elderly persons tend to have decreasing sensory perceptions. These factors make it especially important to plan exercises and activities that are appropriate and safe.

Bibliography

Aldana SG, Silvester LJ: The relationships of physical activity and perceived stress. Health Values 13(5):34–37, 1989

Bockmon DF: Facilitating health pattern change in exercise. Journal of Holistic Nursing 6(1):21–24, 1988

Brannon M: A hands-on rehab technique that really works. RN Magazine 52(11):65–66, 68, 1989

Carlisle D: Moving with the times. Nursing Times 85(45):46–47, 1989

DeMarco T, Sidney K: Enhancing children's participation in physical activity. J Sch Health 59(8):337–340, 1989

Fitzmaurice JB: Nurses' use of cues in the clinical judgment of activity intolerance. Classification of nursing diagnoses, pp 315–323. Proceedings of the Seventh Conference of the NANDA, 1987

Heeschen SJ: Getting a handle on patient mobility. Geriatr Nurs 10(3):146–147, 1989

James B, Parker AW: Active and passive mobility of lower limb joints in elderly men and women. Am J Phys Med Rehabil 68(4):162–167, 1989

Laurent C: Fit for nursing: Let's get physical. Nursing Times 85(27):64–65, 1989

Leerhsen C, DeLaPena N: To live longer, take a walk: A new study shows a little exercise goes a long way. Newsweek 114(20):77, 1989

Lemonick MD, Purvis A: Take a walk—and live: A new study says even mild exercise can postpone death. Time 134(20):90, 1989

Moore SR: Walking for health: A nurse-managed activity. Journal of Gerontological Nursing 15(7):26–28, 35–36, 1989

Papazoglou N, Kolokouri–Dervou E, Fanourakis I: Jogging in place: Evaluation of a simplified exercise test. Chest: The Cardiopulmonary Journal 96(4):840–842, 1989

Paul GH, Fafoglia BA: Exercise, sports and asthma. School Nurse 5(3):39–40, 42, 1989

Petosa R: Adolescent wellness: Implications for effective health education programs. Health Values 13(5):14–20, 1989

Progress toward achieving the 1990 national objectives for physical fitness and exercise. MMWR 38(26):449–453, 1989

Rickert L: Benefits of exercise. Journal of Urological Nursing 8(4):758–759, 1989

Seligmann J, Robins K, Barish EB: Fitness boom vs. baby boom: Pregnancy with sweat. Newsweek 114(24):79, 1989

Sinaki M, Wahner HW, Offord KP: Relationship between grip strength and related regional bone mineral content. Arch Phys Med Rehabil 70(12):823–826, 1989

Swaffield L: Fit for nursing: Entering the gym jungle. Nursing Times 85(29):45–47, 1989

Tanji JL: The exercise prescription: Promote fitness and prevent injury. Consultant 28(6):57–60, 63, 1988

Thompson TC: Rehabilitation: Option or requirement? Rehabilitation Nursing 14(6):344, 1989

Trevelyan J, Cullen D: Fit for nursing: How healthy are you? Nursing Times 85(32):25–30, 1989

Walsh R: Human kinetics: Good movement habits. Nursing Times 84(37):59–61, 1988

Wilson RW, Patterson MA, Alford DM: Services for maintaining independence. Journal of Gerontological Nursing 15(6):31–37, 43–44, 1989

10

Promoting Comfort, Relaxation, and Sleep

Chapter Outline

Behavioral Objectives
Glossary
Introduction
The Nature of Pain
Pain Assessment
Measures to Relieve Acute Pain
Measures to Relieve Chronic Pain
The Nature of Relaxation and Sleep
Assessing Sleep
Nursing Measures to Promote Sleep
Common Sleep Disorders
Applicable Nursing Diagnoses
Suggested Measures Related to Comfort, Relaxation, and
    Sleep in Selected Situations
Teaching Suggestions for Comfort, Relaxation, and
    Sleep
Bibliography

Skill Procedures

Relieving Pain
Using a Patient-Controlled Analgesia Infuser
Operating a TENS Unit
Facilitating Relaxation
Promoting Sleep

Behavioral Objectives

When the content of this chapter has been mastered, the learner will be able to:

Define terms appearing in the glossary.
Describe at least 10 characteristics of pain.
Explain why identifying and relieving pain is a difficult task.
Discuss the differences among types of pain.
List the information that should be obtained when assessing an individual's pain.
Describe methods for relieving pain.
Guide another person through a relaxation session.
List some examples of situations that can interfere with a person's biorhythms.
Discuss facts that are associated with the characteristics of sleep.
Outline the stages of sleep.
Discuss at least five factors that influence sleep.
Describe the effects of sleep loss.
Discuss the information that is essential for assessing an individual's sleep.
Describe nursing measures that may be useful for promoting sleep.
List and describe five common sleep disorders.
List suggested measures for promoting comfort, relaxation, and sleep in selected situations as discussed in this chapter.
Summarize suggestions for instructing the patient.

Glossary

Acupressure A technique in which simple pressure on various body parts is used to reduce pain.

Acupuncture A technique that uses long, thin needles inserted into the body parts to produce insensitivity to pain.

Acute pain Discomfort of short duration, up to 6 months, that is expected to end.

Biofeedback A method for controlling and altering various undesirable symptoms, such as pain.

Biorhythms Body functions that occur in cycles.

Chronic pain Discomfort lasting 6 months or longer.

Circadian rhythm Events that are repeated every 24 hours.

Endorphins Natural chemicals in the body with properties similar to morphine.

Enuresis A type of sleep disorder in which there is nightly bedwetting.

Gate-control theory A theory that a gating mechanism in the spinal canal can be closed, thus preventing pain stimuli from reaching the brain.

Hypnosis A technique to produce a subconscious state through suggestion by a hypnotist.

Infradian rhythm Events that repeat monthly.

Insomnia A sleep disorder characterized by difficulty in falling or remaining asleep.

Intermittent pain Discomfort that comes and goes.

Intractable pain Discomfort that is constant.

Mantra A Hindu word for a sound that is repeated during prayer and meditation.

Meditation A relaxation technique in which a person excludes disturbing thoughts for those that have a calming effect.

Narcolepsy A condition characterized by an uncontrollable onset of sleep.

Night terrors A childhood sleep disorder in which the child seems to be awake and in a state of panic, yet has no memory of the experience.

Nonrapid eye movement A broad category referring to four distinct stages of sleep in which little movement, including eye movement, can be observed. Abbreviated NREM.

Pain A sensation of physical and/or mental suffering.

Pain threshold The point at which the sensation of pain becomes noticeable.

Pain tolerance The ability of an individual to endure pain.

Phantom limb pain Pain that is felt in a missing arm or leg.

Placebo An inactive substance given as a substitute for drug therapy.

Placebo effect A positive response to a pain-relieving technique that is enhanced through the power of suggestion.

Psychogenic pain Discomfort that is mental or emotional in origin rather than due to a physical cause.

Rapid eye movement The dream stage of sleep that is associated with characteristic darting of the eyes beneath the eyelids. Abbreviated REM.

Referred pain Discomfort in a location distant from the part of the body that is diseased or injured.

Relaxation A state in which the body is less rigid and tense.

Sleep A state of relative unconsciousness.

Sleep apnea Periods that occur during sleep when a person does not breathe.

Somnambulism A sleep disorder characterized by sleep-walking.

Transcutaneous electrical nerve stimulation The administration of electrical stimuli to the skin for the relief of pain. Abbreviated TENS.

Ultradian rhythm Events that repeat several times within a 24-hour period.

Yoga A special type of relaxation exercise involving bending and stretching of the body.

Introduction

Chapter 9 discussed activity and exercise. The logical counterpoint to this is rest and sleep. Ensuring that individuals receive adequate rest and sleep is an important component of health and well-being. Pain interferes with relaxation. Relieving a person's pain may be the first step in promoting his ability to rest and sleep. This chapter discusses techniques for pain relief and measures that promote relaxation, rest, and sleep.

The Nature of Pain

A state of comfort is highly personal, as are methods that promote it. Pain is an example of discomfort. The nurse may interact with people who have varying degrees of pain. *Pain* has been defined in many ways. This text defines pain as a sensation of physical and/or mental suffering and hurting that causes misery or agony. Encouraging individuals to describe their state of discomfort and exploring methods that may relieve it are important nursing skills.

Characteristics of Pain

Pain is currently a subject of much research because its qualities are so puzzling and complex. Studies of pain have revealed that wide variations in the characteristics of pain can occur. Treating individuals in pain is a challenge to health practitioners because of the following diverse characteristics.

Pain is subjective in nature. It can be described only by the person who feels it and knows how much it hurts.

All pain is real to the patient, regardless of its cause and even when the cause is unknown.

Responses to pain vary widely. The *pain threshold,* the point at which the sensation of pain becomes noticeable, appears to be about the same among healthy persons. But for whatever reasons, people accept and bear the sensation of pain differently. The ability of an individual to endure the discomfort from pain is called his *pain tolerance.* Those who endure more pain than others without efforts to relieve it are said to have a high pain tolerance; those who endure less have a low pain tolerance.

Pain may or may not be associated with damage to body tissues. The pain of grief when a loved one dies causes mental suffering that does not involve tissue damage. Although there may be neither tissue damage nor nerves to conduct pain impulses, a patient with an amputation may experience discomfort, called *phantom limb pain,* in the missing limb.

The amount of pain is not necessarily in proportion to the amount of damage occurring in the body. For example, a patient may not complain of pain until a malignant growth is beyond hope of cure. A person with a migraine headache may be in severe pain with no damage to brain tissue.

Some degree of consciousness and attention are necessary to experience pain. With loss of consciousness, as in the case of a deeply comatose patient, there may be no response to something that should produce pain, such as pinching the skin. Nor may there be any memory of it. On the other hand, an athlete hurt while playing football may not be aware of pain until after the game, when attention is directed toward the injury.

Pain has cultural implications. In some cultures, people learn to bear pain bravely and behave as though it is hardly present, even when it is severe. In other cultures, people learn to express emotions and to show great concern and anxiety about pain. There are also differences in responses to pain between the sexes in the same culture. Although cultural implications should be taken into account, one should never prematurely expect persons from a particular culture to express responses to pain in the same way. Even within the same culture, individuals respond differently to discomfort.

Pain is a demanding sensation. Dealing with it requires physical and emotional energy. This may drain the individual of the necessary resources to carry out his usual activities of daily living.

Anxiety and fear are common emotions accompanying pain. They usually intensify the discomfort. Anticipating the pain associated with activities, such as going to the dentist, may lead some to postpone necessary medical or dental care. As illogical as it may seem, some may experience satisfaction or enjoyment from pain—the person, for example, who uses pain to seek attention or to avoid an unpleasant task.

Responses to pain may be physical and emotional. Both verbal and nonverbal means are used to express pain. Figure 10-1 illustrates what the nurse may observe. These data may indirectly indicate that an individual is experiencing pain.

The body does not adapt to pain, as it does, for example, to heat, cold, noise, and odors.

Types of Pain

Pain can be described in many ways. One of the more common methods is to categorize pain as either acute or chronic. *Acute pain* is physical discomfort of short duration. Short duration is defined as existing less than six months; for most, it is much shorter than this. It is usually severe, and associated with some current injury or disease. Generally it can be reduced by treating its cause and by using medications. *Chronic pain* is physical discomfort

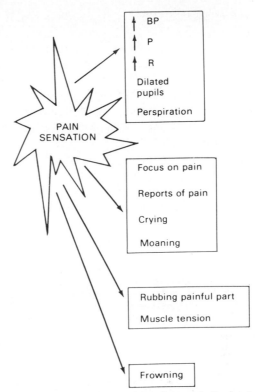

Figure 10-1 Several observable signs of discomfort exist. Symptoms of pain are those reported by the patient. (Adapted from Brunner LS, Suddarth DS: Textbook of Medical–Surgical Nursing, 6th ed, p 291. Philadelphia, JB Lippincott, 1988)

that usually has lasted longer than six months. It persists out of proportion to its initial cause. It does not respond in the same way to the techniques and medications used to relieve acute pain. *Intermittent pain* may be acute or chronic pain that comes and goes. *Referred pain* is pain in another location some distance from the part of the body that is diseased or injured. Though heart pain is classically felt in the chest, it may be referred to the arms, the neck, and even the jaw.

Two other types of pain that present a challenge to health practitioners are intractable pain and psychogenic pain. *Intractable pain* is a type of pain that is constant. It is usually associated with conditions that are not likely to be cured. Surgical procedures may be performed in an effort to relieve extreme cases. *Psychogenic pain* is pain that is from some mental or emotional origin. The pain, nevertheless, is real and experienced in the same manner as that from a physical disease or injury.

Most nurses deal with people who have acute pain. Special physical, emotional, and social skills are necessary to understand and care for people who live with constant, long-term pain. The nursing skills described in this text are those that deal primarily with people in acute pain.

Pain Assessment

Health practitioners have no instruments that can measure the presence or the amount of pain directly. Nurses tend to evaluate pain on the basis of the way individuals describe or react with it. Margo McCaffrey, a renowned nursing authority on pain and its management, described pain as "whatever the person says it is and exists whenever the person says it does" (1979).

As a result of the inadequacy with which one person tries to interpret the experience of another, the nurse must rely on identifying certain characteristics of pain. Assessment involves gathering data about the quality, intensity, location, and duration of the patient's pain. Table 10-1 describes these components in more detail. When assess-

ing pain, the nurse should also ask the person what symptoms accompany the pain, such as nausea or shortness of breath, and what helps to relieve the pain.

Some special treatment units or centers that specialize in the treatment of pain ask their clients to complete a self-questionnaire. An example of one such questionnaire is shown in Figure 10-2. The person scores his own present pain intensity (PPI) by selecting a word with an associated numerical value. The pain rating index (PRI) is determined by the words selected from various groups. The words in groups 1 to 10 describe sensory (S) components of pain; groups 11 to 15 describe affective (A), or emotional components of pain; evaluative (E) terms are in group 16; and groups 17 to 20 are miscellaneous terms. Combinations of words can be identified, M(S) and M(AE), and the entire

---

Table 10-1. Components of Pain Assessment

Feature of Pain	Description
Quality	There are no specific terms to describe the quality of pain. Adjectives, such as stabbing, throbbing, and others that appear in Figure 10-2 within the McGill–Melzack Pain Questionnaire are often used.
Intensity	The following words are commonly used to describe the intensity of pain.
	Slight or mild—The discomfort is noticeable but interferes little with activities of daily living.
	Moderate—The discomfort is definitely noticeable and interferes with activities of daily living.
	Severe or excruciating—The discomfort makes persistent demands for attention and makes it impossible to carry out most activities of daily living.
Location	The location of pain is described according to where in the body the person has discomfort, such as in the stomach, in the knee, and so on.
	Diffuse—Discomfort that covers a large area of the body, such as the entire abdomen or back.
	Shifting—Discomfort that moves from one area of the body to another, such as from the lower abdomen to the chest.
	Referred—Discomfort distant from the diseased or injured area, such as when a person with gallbladder disease feels pain in the upper back or shoulder area
Duration	The length of time that discomfort lasts is described by the person in pain in terms of a clock or calendar, such as in seconds, minutes, hours, days, weeks, or months. Health personnel also often use the following terms when describing the duration of pain:
	Acute—Discomfort of short duration from which relief is expected; up to 6 months in duration.
	Chronic—Discomfort lasting 6 months or longer.
	Intermittent—Discomfort that comes and goes.

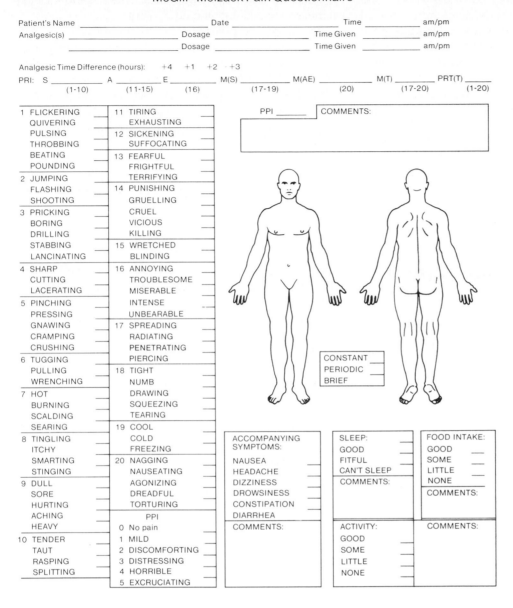

McGill - Melzack Pain Questionnaire

Patient's Name _____ Date _____ Time _____ am/pm
Analgesic(s) _____ Dosage _____ Time Given _____ am/pm
_____ Dosage _____ Time Given _____ am/pm

Analgesic Time Difference (hours):   +4   +1   +2   +3
PRI: S _____ A _____ E _____ M(S) _____ M(AE) _____ M(T) _____ PRT(T) _____
         (1-10)   (11-15)   (16)   (17-19)   (20)   (17-20)   (1-20)

PPI _____   COMMENTS:

1 FLICKERING	11 TIRING
QUIVERING	EXHAUSTING
PULSING	12 SICKENING
THROBBING	SUFFOCATING
BEATING	13 FEARFUL
POUNDING	FRIGHTFUL
2 JUMPING	TERRIFYING
FLASHING	14 PUNISHING
SHOOTING	GRUELLING
3 PRICKING	CRUEL
BORING	VICIOUS
DRILLING	KILLING
STABBING	15 WRETCHED
LANCINATING	BLINDING
4 SHARP	16 ANNOYING
CUTTING	TROUBLESOME
LACERATING	MISERABLE
5 PINCHING	INTENSE
PRESSING	UNBEARABLE
GNAWING	17 SPREADING
CRAMPING	RADIATING
CRUSHING	PENETRATING
6 TUGGING	PIERCING
PULLING	18 TIGHT
WRENCHING	NUMB
7 HOT	DRAWING
BURNING	SQUEEZING
SCALDING	TEARING
SEARING	19 COOL
8 TINGLING	COLD
ITCHY	FREEZING
SMARTING	20 NAGGING
STINGING	NAUSEATING
9 DULL	AGONIZING
SORE	DREADFUL
HURTING	TORTURING
ACHING	PPI
HEAVY	0 No pain
10 TENDER	1 MILD
TAUT	2 DISCOMFORTING
RASPING	3 DISTRESSING
SPLITTING	4 HORRIBLE
	5 EXCRUCIATING

CONSTANT
PERIODIC
BRIEF

ACCOMPANYING SYMPTOMS:	SLEEP:	FOOD INTAKE:
	GOOD	GOOD
NAUSEA	FITFUL	SOME
HEADACHE	CAN'T SLEEP	LITTLE
DIZZINESS	COMMENTS:	NONE
DROWSINESS		COMMENTS:
CONSTIPATION		
DIARRHEA		
COMMENTS:	ACTIVITY:	COMMENTS:
	GOOD	
	SOME	
	LITTLE	
	NONE	

Figure 10-2 To help in pain assessment, a patient checks the words that best describe what he is feeling. The words have a numerical value. The score quantifies the severity of the patient's pain. (Courtesy of the Pain Research Foundation of the International Association for the Study of Pain, Seattle, WA.)

number can be totaled, PRI(T). By comparing changes in the selections on subsequent questionnaires, an individual's improvement, or the reverse, can be determined.

Guidelines for Relieving Pain

There are some basic guidelines the nurse should use when caring for someone in pain:

- Building a helping relationship is essential. In Chapter 2, skills in effective communication and providing emotional support were discussed. Many people have said that having a caring person at hand who will just listen and show interest in their plight helps to relieve discomfort. Experience has shown that most individuals who have confidence in their health practitioners need less treatment for the relief of pain than do those who have little confidence in those caring for them.

- It is recommended that the nurse involve the person in pain as much as possible. Nurses have found that discussing pain with the individual and having him help select methods to relieve it produce better results. This approach reinforces the person's sense of control over his pain rather than the reverse. It also supports the person's ability to cope.

- People should be taught about their pain. For example, explain why the person has pain; help him understand that pain is a common experience. Assure him that it is normal and acceptable to show he has pain.

• It is important to accept the individual as he is and with a nonjudgmental attitude. Remember that all people bring a lifetime of living to a painful experience. Each responds in his own way with behavior that is consciously or unconsciously meaningful to him.

Measures to Relieve Acute Pain

The nurse is frequently called upon to use skills for relieving pain such as those discussed in Skill Procedure 10-1. Medications are also commonly used to relieve pain. Analgesic drugs must be ordered by a physician. Chapters 23 and 24 discuss nursing responsibilities for administering medications. When nursing measures are used with pain medication, they may increase the effect of drugs. That is, a person may experience more relief than he would with only medication.

Patient-Controlled Analgesia (PCA)

A new approach in controlling pain is to use a machine, called a patient-controlled analgesia (PCA) infuser. It allows the patient to self-administer his own pain medication intravenously. Using a PCA infuser, the patient can give himself a very low dose of a narcotic at frequent intervals when he feels uncomfortable. Use of the PCA infuser has several advantages to both the patient and the nurse.

Pain relief is rapidly experienced because the drug is delivered directly into the bloodstream.

Pain is controlled within a constant tolerable level, as illustrated in Figure 10-3.

Less total narcotic is actually used because the discomfort rarely falls below a tolerable range.

The patient avoids the additional discomfort of multiple injections into muscle or subcutaneous tissue.

Anxiety is reduced because the patient's pain does not intensify while waiting for the nurse to administer medication.

Extremes in drug side effects, such as sedation and respiratory depression, are avoided with lower dosages.

Complications associated with immobility, such as blood clots and pneumonia, are reduced because the patient ambulates or moves about more.

The patient takes an active role in his own treatment.

The patient's sense of control and independence are preserved.

Use of a PCA infuser frees the nurse to provide other adjunctive pain-relieving measures.

PCA infusers are used in hospitals primarily to relieve acute pain following surgery. They are being manufactured, however, in small sizes for use in home-health settings by patients who have cancer and require pain control. Compact mini-infusers allow individuals to be ambulatory and carry out their activities without being tethered to cumbersome equipment.

The nurse is responsible for preparing the machine with the medication, instructing the patient, and monitoring his use. Several companies market PCA infusers. Skill Procedure 10-2 explains how one machine is prepared and used. The principles for using other infusers are similar.

Measures to Relieve Chronic Pain

Various other measures used to control pain appear to be gaining popularity in selected situations. These methods are usually used in cases of chronic pain or when acute pain is not relieved with ordinary measures.

Acupuncture and Acupressure. *Acupuncture* is a technique that has been practiced for some time in China. Long, thin needles are inserted into various parts of the body to produce insensitivity to pain. *Acupressure* is a technique in which simple pressure on various body parts is used to reduce pain. The exact nature in which acupuncture and acupressure work has not been definitely determined. The gate-control theory, discussed in Skill Procedure 10-1, is used by some to explain their effectiveness. Others believe that acupuncture and acupressure may stimulate the body's production of *endorphins,* chemicals produced by the body, that have pain-relieving qualities.

Biofeedback. *Biofeedback* consists of a training program that helps a person become aware of certain body changes. The individual then learns to alter these physical responses. This promotes active participation of the individual in overcoming a particular health-related problem. Among other things, biofeedback has been particularly helpful for many persons in controlling the pain of migraine headaches by redirecting blood flow from the head to the hands. Biofeedback also may be used to distract attention from pain and help the person to relax.

Hypnosis. *Hypnosis,* which produces a subconscious state made possible by suggestions from a hypnotist, has also been used to control pain. Hypnosis and biofeedback serve as examples of a mind-body connection that can produce effective results. Hypnosis is generally used along with other pain-relief techniques. Those who practice hypnosis have received special training and generally are certified members of hypnosis societies.

Placebos. A *placebo* is an inactive substance given as a substitute for drug therapy. Studies have shown that placebos can be effective pain relievers when not used on a continuous basis and when the patient has confidence in his health-care providers. It is a fallacy to assume that a patient relieved of pain with placebos is a malingerer or is

Skill Procedure 10-1. Relieving Pain

Suggested Action	Reason for Action
Assess the nature of the individual's pain.	Measures for pain relief may be incorrect or inadequate unless the nurse determines the type of pain and its characteristics.
Use words other than "pain," such as "discomfort," during assessment.	Certain words are accompanied by mental meanings. Their very use may intensify the experience for some individuals.
Decrease or remove any factors that may contribute to discomfort. Some of the following are examples: Loosen a tight binder if this is not contraindicated; relieve a full urinary bladder; change an uncomfortable position.	Minor discomforts potentiate the experience of pain. In some cases, altering these discomforts may reduce pain to a tolerable level.
Assist an individual to rest. Speak with family and friends whose constant presence could be tiring. Visits may be scheduled for fewer people and for shorter periods of time.	Energy is required to endure pain. Fatigue depletes the individual's resources for coping with pain.
Provide food or water when the individual feels the need for them.	Hunger and thirst contribute to discomfort. Basic needs for food and water continue to require priority attention.
Regulate the temperature and ventilation of the room.	A room that is too hot, cold, stuffy, or breezy stimulates the individual's awareness of his discomfort.
Use techniques discussed later in this chapter to promote relaxation and sleep.	Anxiety that accompanies pain stimulates the mind and body. It tends to cause an exaggerated state of muscle contraction and interferes with sleep.
Use distraction to take attention away from pain. Some examples include: • Reading • Listening to the radio • Watching television • Discussing enjoyable memories • Breathing rhythmically • Visualizing pleasant experiences	The brain must be aware of pain in order for it to be experienced. Diverting the brain's attention from the pain to something else tends to reduce the individual's awareness.
Use measures that prevent pain impulses from reaching the brain, such as: • Providing a backrub • Applying cold or warm substances to body parts • Massaging the body part opposite to the painful one	The *gate-control theory* suggests that pain and other sensations of the skin and muscles travel the same pathways through large nerves in the spinal canal. If other cutaneous stimuli are being transmitted, the "gate" through which the pain impulse must travel is temporarily blocked. The brain cannot perceive the pain while it is kept busy with interpreting the other stimuli.
Use humor, within reason, to promote laughter. Some have watched videocassettes of favorite comedians in order to stimulate laughter.	Laughing is thought to release normal substances in the body called *endorphins,* which act similar to morphine.
Use techniques that reduce depression such as tender touching. Implement pet therapy if possible.	Enduring pain can wear down an individual's spirit. Touching conveys a message of caring. It communicates understanding and a willingness to share the burden. Pets respond affectionately to attention. The companionship and bonding that occur may improve the morale of someone in pain.

(continued)

Skill Procedure 10-1. *Continued*

Suggested Action	Reason for Action
Give prescribed medications for pain when other nursing measures are not enough. Use judgment about this. Do not wait to give something until the person is miserable.	Using drugs as a substitute for good nursing care or withholding needed medication is not considered high-quality practice.
Project a positive and hopeful attitude about the outcome for a pain-relief technique.	The power of suggestion may facilitate or potentiate a positive response to a pain-relieving technique. This is called the *placebo effect.*
Stay with the person in pain or make frequent checks. Encourage selected family or friends to stay quietly at the bedside.	Closeness of another person relieves the fear of desertion and isolation.
Make regular observations of the person in pain.	Evaluation is an essential part of the nursing process.
Record the measures and the response of the individual to the care that has been given.	Written information can serve as a communication tool to others who may be assisting with pain-relieving techniques.
Evaluate the care in terms of its success or failure to relieve pain.	Alternative courses of action may need to be planned and carried out when a nursing measure fails to help.
Consult with other health personnel for help when the skills being used are not producing adequate results.	There are more sophisticated and complex methods that may be necessary to relieve the pain experienced by some individuals.

imagining his pain. A theory now being studied is that a placebo possibly helps release endorphins that, among other things, can alter a person's perception of pain.

Placebos must be prescribed. They are ordinarily used when other measures have been ineffective or when addiction to drugs is a problem. Members of the health team are consulted before a coordinated effort of use is implemented.

Transcutaneous Electrical Nerve Stimulation.
Transcutaneous electrical nerve stimulation, abbreviated *TENS,* consists of administering electrical stimulation to the skin for the relief of pain. External electrodes are taped to the skin. A battery-powered stimulator produces the electrical stimuli, which are perceived by the person as a pleasant tapping, tingling, or massaging sensation. TENS

(Text continues on page 186)

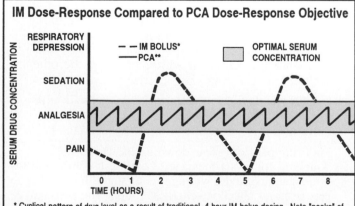

IM Dose-Response Compared to PCA Dose-Response Objective

* Cyclical pattern of drug level as a result of traditional 4-hour IM bolus dosing. Note "peaks" of analgesia/sedation preceded and followed by "valleys" of inadequate analgesia levels.
** Individual patient/PCA-maintained drug levels tend to define the range of optimal analgesic dosing and avoid blood level concentrations that are subtherapeutic or sedative. Superior individualization of anagesic regimen is thus achieved.

Figure 10-3 The large wavy line represents the peaks and valleys in pain control when the patient receives injections from the nurse at four-hour intervals. The jagged line within the wide band shows the uniform level of controlled pain without sedation when the patient self-administers his own medication with a PCA infuser. (Adapted from White PF. Use of a patient controlled analgesia infuser for the management of postoperative pain. In: Hormer M, Rosen M, Vickers MD, eds. Patient-controlled analgesia. St. Louis: CV Mosby (Blackwell Scientific), 1985)

Skill Procedure 10-2. Using a Patient-Controlled Analgesia Infuser

Suggested Action	Reason for Action
Obtain the following equipment: infuser, PCA tubing with Y-connector, prefilled medication container, IV solution and tubing, IV pole, and equipment for starting an IV.	Gathering all supplies in advance promotes efficient time management.
Check the wristband of the patient.	Accurate identification of the patient helps to prevent medication errors.
Check that the IV solution is compatible with the prescribed drug.	Incompatible solutions can cause precipitates to form and travel into the bloodstream.
Attach the infuser to the IV pole.	The infuser may be separate. It can be attached manually but requires a key for removal.
Plug the power cord into the wall outlet.	Using a power source preserves the battery for portable use.
Wash hands before preparing the equipment.	Handwashing deters the spread of microorganisms.
Attach the PCA tubing to the assembled syringe as in Figure 10-4.	The medication in the vial is released into the PCA tubing.

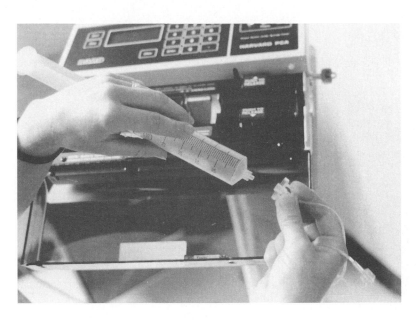

Figure 10-4 The syringe and administration tubing are connected without touching the uncapped openings.

Suggested Action	Reason for Action
Fill the tubing with medication up to the Y-connection. Clamp that section of tubing.	Solution must fill the tubing to avoid injecting air into the bloodstream.
Open the cover or the door of the infuser. Load the medication into its cradle shown in Figure 10-5, making sure that the tubing is not kinked.	The cradle holds and stabilizes the syringe within a pumping mechanism. Kinked tubing would obstruct the flow of medication.
Attach the IV solution with its tubing connecting it to the PCA tubing at the Y-connection.	The patient's vein is kept open between administrations of medication by the slow infusion of IV solution.
Flush the air from the empty tubing as the nurse is doing in Figure 10-6.	Filling the tubing with solution prevents instilling the air into the bloodstream.
Clamp the tubing and perform a venipuncture described in Chapter 25, if one does not presently exist.	The solution and medication flows through a needle or flexible catheter inserted into a vein.

(continued)

Skill Procedure 10-2. *Continued*

Suggested Action	Reason for Action

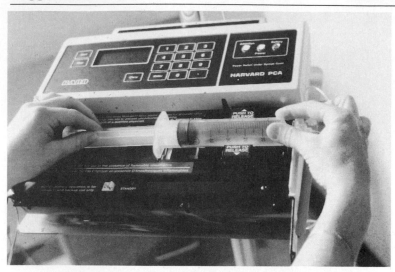

Figure 10-5 The syringe is inserted into the machine.

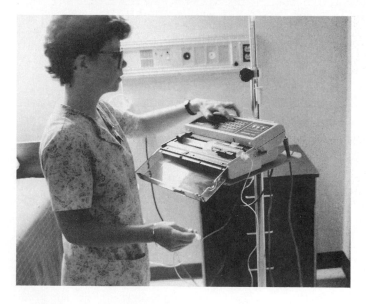

Figure 10-6 The nurse purges air from the tubing by filling it with medication from the syringe.

Connect the PCA tubing to the venipuncture device and begin infusing the IV solution.	The movement of solution prevents blood from clotting and obstructing the passageway for the medication.
Open the slide clamp on the PCA tubing.	Medication cannot be released while the tube remains clamped.
Assess the characteristics of the patient's pain.	A baseline of information will assist in evaluating the effectiveness of intermittent medication administration.
Set the volume for the prescribed loading or bolus dose and administer it to the patient.	A slightly higher than usual dose is administered initially to establish an acceptable serum level of the drug and provide pain reduction.
Program the infuser with a 1- or 4-hour limit, the dose volume, and lockout interval for patient administration.	These amounts are ordered by the physician. Setting limits prevents overdosing. The capacity of these limits varies with manufacturers.

(continued)

Skill Procedure 10-2. Continued

Suggested Action	Reason for Action
Close the security cover and lock it with a key, as the nurse in Figure 10-7 is doing.	Locking the machine and control keys safeguards the medication from theft and keeps the settings tamperproof.

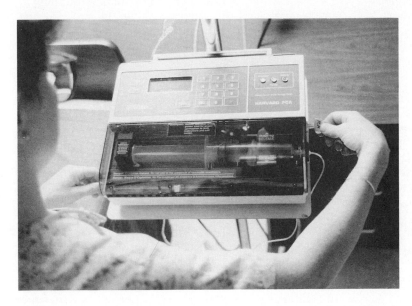

Figure 10-7 To prevent unauthorized access to the medication syringe, it is locked within the machine. Alarms sound when the cover is open.

Hand the control device, shown in Figure 10-8, to the patient. Instruct the patient to press and then release the button when he desires pain medication.	Medication is administered only when the button is pressed and released as long as the patient has not exceeded the frequency for its administration.

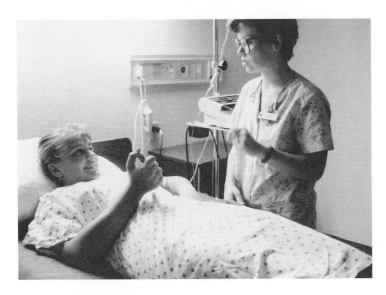

Figure 10-8 The nurse explains how the patient can administer her own pain medication.

Explain that an audible sound will occur when the infuser is used.	Hearing a bell indicates that medication has been released. The patient receives sensory reinforcement that the machine is functioning.

(continued)

Skill Procedure 10-2. Continued

Suggested Action	Reason for Action
Assess the change in pain characteristics at periodic intervals.	The medication should reduce the intensity of pain. If not, the doctor needs to be informed to increase the dose volume or administer an additional bolus dose.
Check the total volume and number of doses administered at the end of the shift. Then clear the amount.	Each nurse should document and communicate how much medication the patient is using.
Replace the vial of medication when an attention alarm sounds.	An alarm, different from that heard with drug administration, sounds when there is a low reserve of medication left in the machine.
Change the IV solution every 24 hours.	Fluid that is open and does not completely infuse within 24 hours has the potential to grow microorganisms.

may be used intermittently as the patient feels a need for it, or on a continuous basis. A qualified nurse or technician ordinarily teaches how to use it.

TENS has been used for patients with chronic pain for some time. More recently, surgical patients are using it. Reports of its results range from useless to fantastic. No one is sure how TENS works. Some think the gate-control theory explains its effectiveness. Supposedly the transmission of electrical stimuli takes precedence over the pain stimuli. In this way, TENS decreases or eliminates the perception of pain in the brain. Others think TENS stimulates the body to increase endorphins. Others feel that a placebo effect is partially responsible for the results.

TENS has several advantages. It is a nonnarcotic, noninvasive agent without toxic effects. It is contraindicated for pregnant individuals because its effect on the unborn has not been determined. Individuals using cardiac pacemakers, especially the demand type of pacemaker, patients prone to irregular heartbeats, and those having had previous heart attacks are not candidates for the use of TENS. Skill Procedure 10-3 describes the use of a TENS unit.

The Nature of Relaxation and Sleep

Relaxation is a state in which the body becomes less rigid and tense. The entire body, including the muscles, respond to stress. Life is full of stressors. As a result, many people experience stress-related health problems. These include migraine headaches, high blood pressure, ulcers, anxiety, and depression. The effects of stress are compounded for patients. They must deal with illness and its consequences. Display 10-1 identifies and ranks stress-producing events associated with a hospital visit. Some of these stressful events, such as not having questions answered by staff, can be eliminated with good nursing care.

Relaxation precedes sleep. *Sleep* is a state in which a person is seemingly unconscious, yet can be aroused easily. During sleep, a person's perception and activity are reduced. Adequate, high-quality sleep is essential for health.

Promoting Relaxation

Relaxation is necessary in order to feel rested. It facilitates sleep. If relaxation is achieved for even brief periods during the day, it may be sufficient to restore an individual's mental and physical resources. A person may be better able to deal with the responsibilities of life and the physical work associated with it. Skill Procedure 10-4 describes some techniques that may be useful in achieving a relaxed state. *Yoga,* which is a special type of relaxation exercise, involves bending and stretching of the body. It is often combined with *meditation,* in which a person excludes disturbing thoughts for those that have a calming effect.

Biologic Cycles

The patterns for sleep and some other physical functions seem to recur in rather predictable cycles. The physical cycles often correlate with cycles in nature. They are collectively referred to as *biorhythms.* Phenomena that recur every 24 hours are said to be cycling in a *circadian rhythm.* The sleep-awake pattern is an example that corresponds to the cycling of night followed by day. Events that repeat monthly, such as menstruation, are on an *infradian rhythm,* similar to the monthly cycling of the moon. *Ultradian rhythm* is the term given to those physical occurrences that take place frequently in a repeated sequence during a 24-hour period. For instance, scientists now know that there are sleep cycles that recur in repeated patterns during sleep. The stages during sleep will be described later in this chapter.

When biorhythms become disturbed, people often feel poorly. Situations that can disturb these cycles include working the night shift and rapidly changing from one time zone to another, which produces "jet lag." Patients in intensive care units who are exposed to constant artificial

Skill Procedure 10-3. Operating a TENS Unit

Suggested Action	Reason for Action
Obtain the following equipment: TENS control unit, electrodes, conductive jelly, and tape if the electrodes are not precoated and self-adhesive.	Gathering all supplies in advance promotes efficient time management.
Read the patient's history to determine if there is any cardiac disease or if pregnancy is possible.	TENS is contraindicated for patients with pacemakers, abnormal heart rhythms, and pregnancy.
Explain the meaning of TENS and the theories associated with the principles of pain relief.	An explanation promotes understanding and cooperation. A positive belief system facilitates pain relief.
Consult the physician or physical therapist on the location for electrode placement. Variations include: • On or near the painful site • Over superficial peripheral nerves • On either side of an incision • Over nerve roots along the spine • Over a joint • Along acupuncture meridians • Over muscle-trigger points that correlate similarly to acupuncture points	Electrode placement varies with each patient's anatomy and the location of pain. Adjustments may be made if the initial placement proves ineffective.
Spread conductive jelly on electrodes that are not self-adhesive.	The jelly provides a medium for delivering electrical current through the skin to the neuromuscular system.
Position each electrode flat against the skin, shown in Figure 10-9.	Contact with the skin is necessary for maximum effectiveness.

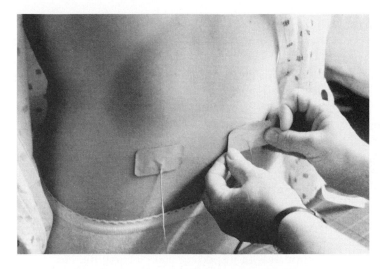

Figure 10-9 Self-adhesive electrodes are applied to the back of this patient.

Suggested Action	Reason for Action
Space the electrodes the width of one from the other.	The skin may be burned if the electrodes are too close to each other.
Use strips of tape to hold the electrodes in place, if they do not have an adhesive property.	Tape secures the electrodes once they are in the desired position.
Make sure all the settings on the unit are off while the machine is turned on.	An initial unpleasant sensation may discourage the patient from continuing its use.
Assess the patient's comfort as settings are made. Expect the patient to describe feeling a tingling, buzzing, or vibrating sensation.	The calibration of the unit is unique for each patient.

(continued)

Skill Procedure 10-3. Continued

Suggested Action	Reason for Action
Gradually increase the amplitude (intensity) of the stimulation to the point at which the patient experiences a mild or moderately pleasant sensation, as the nurse in Figure 10-10 is doing.	A high intensity may not necessarily provide the most pain relief; in fact, it can produce increased discomfort, muscle contractions, or itching.

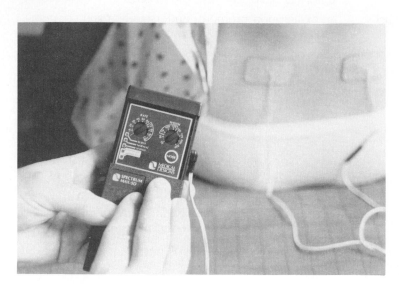

Figure 10-10 The nurse adjusts the intensity, rate, and pulse width of electrical stimulation.

Suggested Action	Reason for Action
Set the rate (pulses per second) at a low range and increase it gradually as the patient becomes adjusted to the sensations.	A high rate may be more effective, but the patient may protest the initial unpleasantness associated with rapid pulsations.
Set the pulse-width dial (if one is available) at a low number of microseconds.	The pulse-width dial regulates the duration of each impulse. Small muscle areas respond better to lower pulse widths, at least initially.
Lock or tape over the settings on the TENS unit when the final settings are made.	The settings should be left unchanged until a sufficient trial evaluation is made.
Adjust the electrode placements and settings according to the response of the patient.	Changes may be made in order to produce maximum comfort. It may take from a few days to a week to determine what works best for the patient.
Document the combinations of settings and the amount of time and response of the patient to the adjustments.	A written record avoids repeating previous unsatisfactory settings.
Turn off the unit before removing the electrodes for bathing and as ordered by the physician.	Hazards exist when electricity and water are combined. Removal aids in inspecting and cleaning the electrode sites. TENS units are not generally used during the night.
Slightly change the position of the electrodes, use hypoallergenic tape, or substitute medicated cream for the conduction jelly if skin irritation is apparent.	With continuous or long-term electrode application, the skin may become irritated and require alternative skin care measures.
Replace or recharge the batteries as needed.	Batteries wear down with continued use.

Display 10-1. Stress-Producing Events in the Hospital

Rank	Event	Rank	Event
1	Thinking you might lose your sight	27	Being cared for by an unfamiliar doctor
2	Thinking you might have cancer	28	Not being able to call family or friends on the phone
3	Thinking you might lose a kidney or some other organ	29	Having to eat cold or tasteless food
4	Knowing you have a serious illness	30	Worrying about your spouse being away from you
5	Thinking you might lose your hearing	31	Thinking you might have pain because of surgery or test procedures
6	Not being told what your diagnosis is		
7	Not knowing for sure what illness you have	32	Being in the hospital during holidays or special family occasions
8	Not getting pain medication when you need it	33	Thinking your appearance might be changed after your hospitalization
9	Not knowing the results or reasons for your treatment	34	Being in a room that is too cold or too hot
10	Not getting relief from pain medications	35	Not having friends visit you
11	Being fed through tubes	36	Having a roommate who is unfriendly
12	Missing your spouse	37	Having to be assisted with a bedpan
13	Not having your questions answered by the staff	38	Having a roommate who is seriously ill or cannot talk with you
14	Not having enough insurance to pay for your hospitalization	39	Being aware of unusual smells around you
15	Not having your call light answered	40	Having to stay in bed or the same room all day
16	Having a sudden hospitalization you were not planning	41	Having a roommate who has too many visitors
17	Being hospitalized far away from home	42	Not being able to get newspapers, radio, or TV when you want them
18	Knowing you have to have an operation		
19	Not having family visit you	43	Having to be assisted with bathing
20	Feeling you are getting dependent on medications	44	Being awakened in the night by the nurse
21	Having nurses or doctors talk too fast or use words you cannot understand	45	Having strange machines around
		46	Having to wear a hospital gown
22	Having medication cause you discomfort	47	Having to sleep in a strange bed
23	Thinking about losing income because of your illness	48	Having to eat at different times than you usually do
24	Having the staff be in too much of a hurry		
25	Not knowing when to expect things that will be done to you	49	Having strangers sleep in the same room with you
26	Being put in the hospital because of an accident		

Adapted from Volcier BJ, Bohamon MW: A hospital stress rating-scale. Nurs Res 24(5):352–359, 1975.

---

light and monotonous noise may experience disturbed sleep patterns. Some develop emotional problems. These disappear when the natural pattern of sleep is restored.

Biologic cycles can work to an individual's advantage. Some people can predict the time of day, or month, during which they are at the peak of productivity. Research is being carried out on plotting biorhythms to promote health.

Characteristics of Normal Sleep

The need for sleep varies throughout life at various ages. Table 10-2 shows the various amounts of sleep required during different stages within the life cycle. Other facts about sleep follow:

- The exact purpose and mechanism of sleep are not clearly understood. However, the importance of rest and sleep for well-being is clearly established.
- Rest and sleep generally occur best when a person is relaxed and relieved of tension and worry. One can relax without sleeping. However, sleep rarely occurs until one relaxes.
- The depth of unconsciousness during sleep varies. During certain periods of sleep, the person can be awakened easily. During others, it is difficult to do so. The depth of unconsciousness affects sensory perception. For example, the sense of smell is the least perceived of the sensory experiences during sleep. This may explain why home fires gain headway because

Skill Procedure 10-4. Facilitating Relaxation

Suggested Action	Reason for Action
Find a room that is not associated with work or tension and that will be free from momentary distractions.	Relaxation involves altering one's state of consciousness. Decreasing stimuli helps in the transition from heightened awareness to one that is described as peaceful.
Assume a relaxed position. The correct postures for sitting or lying down that were illustrated in Chapter 9 may be useful.	Allowing an object, such as a chair or the floor, to support the body frees a person from the muscle activity needed to overcome gravity.
If a quiet room is unavailable, close the eyes and consciously focus within oneself or think about a relaxing location.	Blocking visual stimuli and using the imagination may compensate for the inability to change one's location.
Listen to soothing music or the sounds of nature that produce a personal calming effect. Some hum a repetitive sound called a *mantra*.	The functions of the body tend to become synchronized with the slow, repetitive sounds.
Breathe slowly and deeply through the nose; concentrate on the rising and falling of the abdomen.	Tension restricts breathing. As the breathing becomes slower with concentration, the heart and other muscles will tend to follow the pattern.
Let the muscles of the body loosen as though becoming weightless. Focus on relaxing each limb and body part from the toes to the head.	Any effort to hold the muscles in a state of contraction inhibits total body relaxation.
Enjoy the feeling that relaxation produced.	Training oneself to recognize how a relaxed state feels may help to promote the same effect again with less effort.
At the end of the period of relaxation, gradually increase movement and awareness.	The calming effect should produce an increase in the ability to cope mentally and perform physically.

sleeping occupants do not smell the smoke. Pain and sounds seem to be perceived easily. This explains why ill persons experience sleeplessness when pain is present. Strange noises may disturb the sleep of hospitalized persons. Parents tend to wake easily to the cries of their children. Alarm clocks use sound to wake most individuals from sleep.

- Eight hours of sleep daily is generally recommended for adults, yet some people need more to feel refreshed and some require less. Factors such as metabolic rate, age, physical condition, type of work, and amount and kind of exercise influence the amount of sleep people need. Despite these differences, healthy adults average seven to nine hours of sleep daily.

Table 10-2. Age Variations in Total Sleep Needs

Age	Total Sleep Needs
Neonate (Up to 1 month)	16–20 hours
Infant (Up to 1 year)	10–12 hours plus 2–3 naps
Toddler (1–3 years)	10–12 hours plus 1–2 naps
Preschooler (3–5 years)	9–11 hours plus 1 nap or rest period
School-age child (6–12 years)	9–11 hours
Adolescent (13–18 years)	9–11 hours
Adult (over 18 years)	7–8 hours

Bellack J, Bamford P: Nursing Assessment, p. 457. Wadsworth Health Sciences, 1987. Reprinted with permission of Jones and Bartlett Publishers, Inc.

• Refreshing sleep can occur during any period of the day or night. Most people work during the day and sleep during the night. However, many nighttime workers learn to sleep well during the day. Some people tend to work best during early morning hours; others prefer working later. There is no indication that any one of these patterns is better than another.

Stages of Sleep

The total number of hours are spent cycling through various stages. Sleep is broadly separated into two major stages described as *nonrapid eye movement,* abbreviated NREM, and *rapid eye movement,* abbreviated REM.

There are four stages within NREM sleep. The first two stages consist of light sleep. During the third and fourth stages, the person sleeps deeply, hardly moving. Ordinarily, more sleep occurs in the fourth stage of NREM sleep in the first half of the night, especially if the person is tired.

During REM sleep, dreams take place. The eyes appear to dart about beneath closed lids. The person appears close to being awake because there is a great deal of body movement. However, it is more difficult to awaken a person during REM sleep than during NREM sleep. The cycling patterns of the stages of sleep are illustrated in Figure 10-11. Additional characteristics of NREM and REM sleep are summarized in Table 10-3.

Factors That Influence Sleep

The amount and quality of sleep can be affected by various factors.

Age. The amount of sleep required for well-being varies with age. The younger the person, the more sleep is required, until adulthood, when the amount of sleep necessary for well-being remains quite constant for the rest of life.

Activity. Activity, especially exercise, increases fatigue and the need for sleep to restore well-being. It appears that activity increases both REM and NREM sleep, but especially the deep sleep of the fourth stage of NREM.

Environment. Most people sleep best in their usual home environment. Certain habits that develop and conditions associated with bedtime seem to contribute to sleep. Preferences for sleepwear, the type of pillow, the numbers of blankets, room temperature and ventilation, and even lighting are factors that promote sleep. Individuals even tend to adapt to the unique sounds of their residence, such as traffic, trains, and the hum of appliance motors or furnaces. When these conditions change, as they may if a person goes on vacation or is hospitalized, the ability to fall asleep and feel rested may be affected.

Motivation. When there is no particular reason to stay awake, sleep generally occurs easily. But if the desire to remain awake is strong, such as when a person wishes to participate in something interesting or important to him, sleep can be delayed.

Emotions. The level of awareness and the ability to sleep are influenced by many naturally occurring chemicals released as a result of emotional stimulation. Those

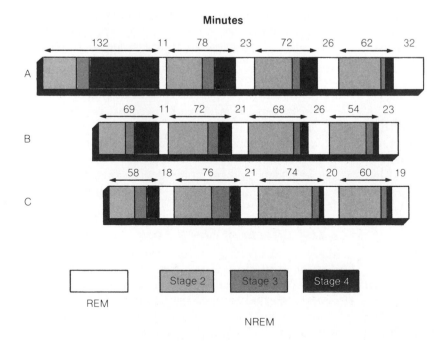

Figure 10-11 These graphs show sleep patterns during four cycles among sleep research participants. Variations occurred among (*A*) children, (*B*) young adults, and (*C*) normal elderly persons. Note that dreaming, which occurs during REM sleep, lasts longer as sleep cycles progress. (Wolff L, Weitzel MH, Zornow RA, Zsohar H: Fundamentals of Nursing, 7th ed, p 482. Philadelphia, JB Lippincott, 1983)

Table 10-3. Stages of Sleep*

Stage	Characteristics
Sub-Stage I	This stage is a transition stage between wakefulness and sleep.
	Great relaxation is present.
	Muscle jerking may occur and awaken the person.
	The stage lasts only a few minutes.
	Arousal is easy.
Sub-Stage II	A state of sleep exists.
	Arousal is relatively easy.
Sub-Stage III	The depth of sleep increases.
	Arousal becomes increasingly difficult.
Sub-Stage IV	This stage is one of deep (delta) sleep.
	Arousal is difficult.
	Brain waves are slow, pulse and respiratory rates are decreased, blood pressure decreases, metabolism slows, and body temperature is low.
REM Stage	Dreams occur during this stage.
	Respirations are irregular; apnea may sometimes occur.
	The pulse rate is rapid and occasionally irregular.
	The blood pressure increases or fluctuates.
	Gastric secretions, metabolism, and body temperature increase.
	Arousal is difficult.

* Normally, persons are observed to go through four or five sleep cycles each night, and each cycle lasts approximately 90 minutes to 100 minutes.

that interfere with sleep are generally produced by worry or anxiety. However, even anticipating a pleasant future event, such as a vacation, may stimulate production of these chemicals, which will cause sleeplessness.

Food and Fluids. A constituent in protein (L-tryptophan), found especially in milk and other dairy products, is believed to promote sleep. A diet lacking in sufficient protein may interfere with normal sleep. Alcoholic beverages, in moderation, appear to promote sleep in some people. Excessive amounts reduce normal REM and deep sleep. Beverages containing caffeine, which is a central nervous system stimulant, tend to cause wakefulness. Caffeine is present in coffee, tea, chocolate, and most cola drinks.

Illness and Drugs. The stress and anxiety commonly associated with illness disturb sleep, as does the pain that accompanies many illnesses. In the hospital many conditions interfere with the sleep of patients. These include the noise from equipment, which tends to be constant and monotonous; being interrupted with nursing and medical measures; unfamiliar sounds associated with hospital activity, such as elevators, dietary carts, and housekeeping equipment. Interrupting the rest and sleep of a hospitalized person may seem unimportant when the patient appears to have little to do except rest and sleep; however, it represents poor-quality care because it interferes with well-being.

Sleep is influenced by certain drugs other than just caffeine and alcohol. Most drugs used to promote sleep, relieve anxiety, and overcome depression interfere with REM sleep. The individual may sleep but not feel rested.

The Effects of Sleep Loss

Most individuals can lose sleep on occasion without experiencing ill effects. However, if sleep loss occurs regularly, or when an individual is totally deprived of sleep over an extended period of time, serious physical and emotional changes occur. Some of the facts that have been identified with sleep loss include the following:

- The feelings of pleasantness, reassurance, and buoyancy that occur with adequate sleep are replaced by diminished energy and enthusiasm. Judgment becomes dull and normal performance of activities of daily living fades. There are lapses in attention, memory, and the ability to concentrate.
- Unpleasant sensations, such as blurring of vision, itching of the eyes, nausea, and headache are common signs of tiredness.
- There may be an attitude of not caring what happens and of feeling irritable and depressed with fatigue.
- Inability to recognize reality, even experiencing hallucinations, is likely when sleep loss is prolonged. There is research being done to determine if the chemicals that become imbalanced during sleep loss are the same ones that may contribute to certain mental illnesses such as schizophrenia. The symptoms are remarkably similar.
- A person normally attempts to "catch up" on the sleep that has been lost. The fourth stage of NREM sleep generally tends to be extended when sleep occurs following sleep loss.
- When REM sleep is reduced, as occurs with the use of some drugs, the dream stage is shortened. These individuals tend to have an increased sensitivity to pain, poor judgment, and increased irritability. Normal relationships with others suffer, and depression becomes common. When REM sleep finally recurs, the body appears to try to make up for its loses with excessive dreaming. Nightmares are also reported among those who dream after REM sleep deprivation.

Assessing Sleep

The need for sleep can vary from person to person. Before planning and providing measures to promote sleep, it is important to obtain information that is particular to the individual person. The following are types of information the nurse should gather and analyze:

- Learn the person's usual sleep pattern. Ask about his usual times for retiring and arising. Inquire about napping and the type of environment the patient prefers for sleep.
- Determine the individual's bedtime habits. For example, some like a snack before bedtime; others may prefer a beverage. Reading, listening to a radio, or watching television can be a relaxing activity. For many, preparations for sleep include brushing the teeth, washing the hands and face, and going to the bathroom. A bath or shower may be preferred by some at night rather than in the morning.
- Ask about relaxation techniques the individual has found to promote sleep. Inquire about what activities of daily living, such as dietary habits and daily exercise, influence his sleep.

- Determine whether the person is experiencing any sleep disorders. Various disorders are described later in this chapter.
- Learn if and how often the person uses drugs, including alcohol, to promote sleep. Determine the name of the products used.
- Observe the person's energy level. There may be other information than this required to validate that a person is experiencing insufficient sleep. However, this plus other signs associated with fatigue, such as short concentration, yawning, and "nodding off" to sleep may be characteristics associated with sleep loss.
- If the individual is hospitalized, the nurse can determine how the patient's sleep may be influenced by his illness, medications, and therapy.

Nursing Measures to Promote Sleep

As the nurse begins to know and appreciate the importance of sleep and the problems that can result with sleep loss, there should be a great deal of effort to help promote rest and sleep. Skill Procedure 10-5 provides suggested actions that may relieve restlessness and sleeplessness.

Common Sleep Disorders

Many unusual patterns of sleep can be observed. Some are not necessarily dangerous to the person. Others are quite serious sleep disorders and require for affected individuals special treatment. Those sleep disorders that occur with some frequency in the general population are discussed here in more depth.

Insomnia. Difficulty in falling asleep, waking during sleeping hours, and early awakening from sleep describe *insomnia.* The condition may lead to such distress that further wakefulness occurs. There are some physical conditions that cause wakefulness, but insomnia is usually noted to occur during a period of personal stress and when the person is a worrier.

Having a patient keep a sleep log is helpful to assess insomnia. Studies have shown that insomniacs tend to underestimate the time they sleep and overestimate the time it takes them to fall asleep. However, these findings do not relieve the distress that most insomniacs suffer. When a person says he has insomnia, steps to promote rest and sleep should be taken.

In addition to the suggestions in Skill Procedure 10-5, the following are recommended for helping overcome insomnia:

- Advise the person to lie down for sleep only when he feels sleepy, not when he feels wakeful.

Skill Procedure 10-5. Promoting Sleep

Suggested Action	Reason for Action
Assess the individual's sleep pattern.	Sleep is a basic need. An individual's customary sleep routine, if adequate, should be maintained in order to promote well-being.
Simulate as much as possible the person's usual sleep environment and rituals.	Human beings are creatures of habit. Slight deviations from personal routines may result in a disturbed sleep pattern.
Respect the person's usual time for retiring regardless of how it differs from one's own.	The time for retiring is not as critical as the total amount of sleep. Interfering with a personal biorhythm may cause sleeplessness.
Provide the person with a glass of milk or other dairy product.	Milk is a source for L-tryptophan, a component of a chemical within the body that promotes sleep.
Avoid any excess intake of foods or beverages that contain caffeine. Diet medications should also be taken with caution.	Drugs such as caffeine and those found in appetite control medications are stimulants. They may interfere with the ability to sleep.
Help the person assume a comfortable position in bed.	Good posture in a lying position and support for the musculoskeletal system facilitate comfort.
Use techniques that promote relaxation discussed earlier in Skill Procedure 10-4.	Relaxation is a preliminary step to sleep.
Use measures described earlier in this chapter to relieve pain, if that is a problem for the individual.	Pain causes anxiety. An aroused state is associated with worry, tension, and fear.
Give prescribed medications for sleep when other measures have failed.	Medications should be used with good judgment and not as a substitute for good nursing care.
Advise those individuals such as hospitalized patients who have sleep medications ordered that the medication is available if needed.	Knowing that a medication is available may provide enough reassurance that relaxation and sleep occur naturally.
Be conscientious about controlling loud or unfamiliar noises.	Sleep may be interrupted most easily through the sense of hearing.
Use every effort not to awaken or disturb an individual who is sleeping.	It is important that the stages of sleep cycle in an uninterrupted fashion.
Evaluate the quality of the person's sleep by asking questions that reflect the night that just passed.	Nurses must be careful not to assume that a person is asleep just because his eyes are closed.
Discuss alternative courses of action that may promote sleep if other measures have failed.	Involving a person contributes to an individual's sense of personal control.
If the nurse is caring for a hospitalized patient, write any helpful directions that promote sleep on the nursing orders.	Specific communication promotes continuity of care. Other nurses and the patient benefit from successful prior experiences.
Consult other health personnel for help when it seems that current efforts are insufficient to promote rest and sleep.	Some people suffer from sleep disorders that may require elaborate testing and complex treatment in order to restore natural sleep.

- If sleep does not occur within 20 minutes of retiring, suggest that the individual get up and do something to keep himself busy and occupied until he feels sleepy.
- Instruct the person to try to wake up and get out of bed at the same time every morning and to take no naps during the day.
- Avoid using the bed for other activities, such as reading or sewing. The bed should be used only for sleeping.
- Recommend daily exercises, but not before bedtime.

Many insomniacs tend to self-medicate themselves with drugs that do not require prescriptions. Temporary relief may be obtained, but prolonged use of these drugs may not prove beneficial. Some may go from doctor to doctor accumulating prescription drugs that they take in amounts other than directed. Caution must be advised about the dangers of substance abuse and misuse with this class of drugs.

Somnambulism. *Somnambulism* is sleepwalking. It is seen more commonly in children than in adults. The danger of this disorder is that the person may suffer injury. Measures to provide safety include having secure locks on doors. If a sleepwalker is admitted to the hospital, a record should be made of this and proper precautions taken to prevent injury. The cause of sleepwalking is unknown but it has been found that certain medications taken at bedtime, such as those to control depression, most tranquilizers, and some antihistamines may lead to sleepwalking.

Snoring and Sleep Apnea. A person who snores is a noisy nuisance to anyone sharing the same room. Snoring occurs most commonly when the person lies on his back with his head tipped forward. This position causes a narrowing of the air passageways, which, when added to complete relaxation of the soft palate and uvula, results in the snoring sound. A collar worn at the neck, similar to that used by persons with injuries in the cervical area of the spine, is often helpful in preventing snoring.

Snoring itself is not a disorder, but sleep apnea, which often accompanies it, is a disorder. *Sleep apnea* refers to periods during sleep when a person does not breathe. It is most common among overweight, middle-aged men. During long periods of apnea, the patient's body suffers from lack of sufficient oxygen and an accumulation of carbon dioxide. Then, starved for air, the patient usually resumes breathing with snoring. Sleep apnea may be repeated hundreds of times a night in some people. For some, it can become life threatening and fatal if the apnea is not interrupted. Awakening the person will restore breathing.

Sleep Talking. From observations, it appears that almost everyone talks in his sleep at some time. It rarely presents a problem unless the talking disturbs persons sharing the same room.

Narcolepsy. *Narcolepsy* is a neurologic disorder. Its primary symptom is an uncontrollable onset of sleep. The danger is that the person with the condition may fall asleep while carrying out potentially dangerous activities, such as driving a car or swimming. Persons with narcolepsy need to be watched closely so that they do not suffer injury. Fortunately, drugs that cause wakefulness have been used effectively for controlling the condition. However, the drugs must be taken faithfully throughout an affected person's lifetime to avoid a return of symptoms.

Suggested Measures Related to Comfort, Relaxation, and Sleep in Selected Situations

When the Individual Is an Infant or Child

Use distraction when caring for an infant or child in pain. Using mobiles over a crib and encouraging play with favorite toys often distract attention from pain. Singing, tapping a homemade instrument, or clapping with a song may also be tried.

As soon as a child is old enough to understand, explain when something will hurt. Saying that a procedure will not cause pain when it will is deceptive. A child will quickly lose confidence in his caretakers.

Tell a child that it is all right to cry if he hurts. This technique often relieves tension and makes the child feel that he is being accepted even though he cries.

Expect that newborns and young infants sleep most of the time. It is best to rotate their sleeping position from side to side. It is difficult for regurgitated and vomited material to leave the mouth when the infant is in the back-lying position. It is generally recommended that an infant not be placed on his abdomen for sleep unless he is old enough to raise his head. This prevents danger of suffocation. Pillows are not recommended for infants because of the danger of suffocation.

Applicable Nursing Diagnoses

Patients who have problems with comfort, relaxation, or sleep may have nursing diagnoses such as:

- Fatigue
- Sleep Pattern Disturbance
- Pain
- Chronic Pain
- Anxiety
- Fear
- Ineffective Individual Coping
- Knowledge Deficit: Pain-Relieving Techniques
- Health-Seeking Behaviors: Stress Management

Nursing Care Plan 10-1 may be used as an example of the care planned for a patient with a nursing diagnosis of Pain. Pain is defined in the NANDA Taxonomy (1989) as, "A state in which an individual experiences and reports the presence of severe discomfort or an uncomfortable sensation."

NURSING CARE PLAN

10-1. Pain

Assessment	**Subjective Data**
	States, "It feels like a semi-truck is parked on my chest. I know I must be having a heart attack." Indicates that pain measures 10 on a scale of 1 to 10.
	Objective Data
	55-year-old man brought to Emergency Department from work. Holds hands over L. precordial area. Rubs L. arm. Perspires profusely. Startles with loud noise of staff entering room. Pulse is 108 beats/min and irregular. Blood pressure is 148/92. Respirations are 30/min. Elevated ST segment on cardiac rhythm strip.
Diagnosis	Pain related to reduction in oxygen to myocardium.
Plan	**Goal**
	The patient will report that his pain is reduced to ≤7 using a 1–10 scale by 9/20.
	Orders: 9/19
	1. Maintain bedrest.
	2. Administer 50% oxygen continuously by mask.
	3. Explain all procedures and routines before being performed.
	4. Allow wife to remain at bedside as desired.
	5. Administer prescribed analgesic as needed. ———————————— R. VERCLER, RN

Implementation (Documentation)

9/19

1400	Face mask applied and oxygen administered at 6 liters per minute. Respirations 28 and labored. Placed in high Fowler's position. ——————— N. DUNN, RN	
1415	States, "I feel tightness and aching from my chest into my neck and L. arm. It's still a 10; please do something." ——————— N. DUNN, RN	
1420	Nitroglycerin tab given sublingually. Instructed to let tablet remain under tongue for absorption. Explained there may be tingling in the area of the tablet, a headache, and a warm, flushed feeling associated with absorption, but the medication will help more blood get to the heart muscle. Advised to remain in bed for the time being. Wife at bedside holding hands. ————— N. DUNN, RN	
1435	1000 mL D5W started IV in L. hand with a #18 angiocath. Running at a keep open rate. No pain relief from nitroglycerin. ——————— N. DUNN, RN	
1445	Morphine sulfate 4 mg given IV push for chest pain. ————— N. DUNN, RN	

Evaluation (Documentation)

1500	States, "My pain is starting to ease up. It's about an 8½ right now." ——————————————————— N. DUNN, RN

Expect that the amount of sleep children require decreases with age. Children ordinarily take naps until about school age.

Newborns and infants may manifest sleep apnea, which some believe is a factor in infant crib deaths. Sleep monitors are available for children who have sleep apnea. These monitors sound alarms if the child stops breathing.

Cuddle and rock infants and toddlers to promote relaxation and sleep.

Some children experience nightmares and night terrors. Parents may find that avoiding stories or television programs that are apt to suggest fears to the child are helpful in preventing nightmares. *Night terrors* are a type of childhood sleep disorder in which the child seems to be awake and in a state of panic. The child does not seem to respond to questions by concerned family members trying to soothe the child. The child generally has no memory of the episode. It is more frightening to the family than to the child.

Enuresis is involuntary urination and is often called bed-wetting. Because enuresis occurs at night, it is commonly considered a disorder of sleep. Children who experience frequent bed-wetting should always be examined by a physician to make sure that no urinary problems are the cause. The greatest problem with bed-wetting is the damage that can occur to a child's self-esteem. Enuresis is an uncommon disorder among healthy adults.

When the Individual Is Elderly

Carefully observe the elderly person whose sense organs may have diminished with age. This person may have tissue damage without the usual sensation of pain.

Be aware that the sleep patterns of the elderly vary widely but that they tend to sleep less at night and do more napping than younger adults. Some persons state that elderly persons require less sleep than younger persons because of less activity and exercise.

Take into account that elderly people typically require more time to fall asleep, find it more difficult to change sleep patterns, are awake more often during sleeping hours, retire and awaken earlier, and show more concern about sleep than do younger adults.

Assess an elderly person's diet in relation to protein when sleep is poor. A combination of a low-protein intake and poor absorption of nutrients in the elderly may account for unsatisfactory sleep.

In planning, remember that the elderly prefer a warmer room in which to sleep than do younger adults. Use extra covers as necessary for their comfort.

Teaching Suggestions for Comfort, Relaxation, and Sleep

Suggestions for teaching when carrying out measures to promote comfort, relaxation, and sleep have been described in this chapter. They are summarized as follows:

Very few people understand pain. Therefore, an important responsibility for nurses is to explain its cause and the reasons behind measures used to relieve it. From an understanding of pain, people are in a better position to help cooperate in its control.

Many remedies are available to help control pain. Unfortunately, most people turn to the use of medications immediately. Nurses have an important role in helping people explore other measures to relieve pain.

Sleep also is poorly understood by most people. As with pain, teaching about sleep helps individuals cooperate more fully when using measures to promote rest and sleep. This type of teaching will also facilitate an understanding of normal changes in sleep patterns so that people do not become unduly concerned when there are sleep changes during the life cycle.

There are many measures to help promote relaxation and sleep, as this chapter demonstrates. Individuals should be taught about alternative ways to overcome sleeplessness so that they are less likely to use medications unnecessarily.

It is a fallacy that everyone needs 8 hours of sleep every night. The fact is that sleep is a highly individual matter. It has been demonstrated that for some, more or less than 8 hours of sleep promotes well-being.

A great variety of medications for relieving pain and sleeplessness is available. Sleeping medications have been observed to lose their effectiveness after a week or two of use. Using medications that do not require a prescription may delay a person from seeking medical attention.

Drug abuse is a serious problem in this country. It is not limited to illegal drugs. High-quality nursing includes teaching about the danger of the careless use of all drugs, including those for relieving pain and sleeplessness.

Bibliography

Beebe A, McBride RE, Gol P: Pain: Its assessment and treatment. Journal of Practical Nursing 39(2):17–27, 1989

Beyerman K: Etiologies of sleep pattern disturbance in hospitalized patients. Classification of nursing diagnoses, pp. 193–198. Proceedings of the Seventh Conference of the NANDA, 1987

Dalton JA: Nurses' perceptions of their pain assessment skills, pain management practices, and attitudes toward pain. Oncology Nursing Forum 16(2):225–231, 1989

Fitzgerald JJ: Let your patient control his analgesia. Nursing 17(7):48–51, 1987

Gast PL, Baker CF: The CCU patient: Anxiety and annoyance to noise. Critical Care Nursing Quarterly 12(3):39–54, 1989

Gaysek J: IV team management of patient controlled analgesia. Journal of the National Intravenous Therapy Association 10:142, 1978

Guzzetta CE: Effects of relaxation and music therapy on patients in a coronary care unit with presumptive acute myocardial infarction. Heart and Lung: Journal of Critical Care 18(6):609–616, 1989

Hobbie C: Relaxation techniques for children and young people. Journal of Pediatric Health Care 3(2):83–87, 1989

Insomnia in the elderly. Nursing Times 85(47):32–22, 1989

Jones L, Neiswender JA, Perkins M: PCA: Patient satisfaction, nursing satisfaction, and cost-effectiveness. Nursing Management 20(1):16–17, 1989

Klein LS, Bruce NP: Night shift work in nursing and biorhythms. Imprint 36(4):112, 115, 1989

Kucharski KC, Zuckerman IH: Pain management and symptom control. Caring 7(8):45–47, 1988

Lange MP, Dahn MS, Jacobs LA: Patient-controlled analgesia versus intermittent analgesia dosing. Heart and Lung: Journal of Critical Care 17(5):495–498, 1988

McCaffery M: Nursing Management of the Patient with Pain, 2nd ed. Philadelphia, JB Lippincott, 1979

Pigeon HM, McGrath PJ, Lawrence J: How neonatal nurses report infants' pain. Am J Nurs 89(11):1529–1530, 1989

Procedures for your practice: Patient-controlled analgesia. Patient Care 23(20):145–146, 1989

Rauen KK, Ho M: Children's use of patient controlled analgesia after spine surgery. Pediatric Nursing 15(6):589–593, 1989

Reimer M: Sleep pattern disturbance: Nursing interventions perceived by patients and their nurses as facilitating nocturnal sleep in hospital. Classification of nursing diagnoses, pp 372–376. Proceedings of the Seventh Conference of the NANDA, 1987

Riordan MP: Validation of the defining characteristics of the nursing diagnosis, alteration in comfort: Pain. Classification of nursing diagnoses, pp 221–228. Proceedings of the Seventh Conference of the NANDA, 1987

Shaver JLF, Giblin EC: Sleep. Annu Rev Nurs Res 7:91–93, 1989

Smith J, Bulich RG, New PB: High-tech advances in the treatment of chronic cancer pain. Caring 8(10):8–10, 12, 1989

Trevelyan J: Now I lay me down to sleep . . . mysteries surrounding sleep. Nursing Times 85(47):34–35, 1989

Trevelyan J: Prevailing over pain . . . psychological management of pain. Nursing Times 84(33):45–47, 1988

Turton P: Touch me, feel me, heal me . . . therapeutic effects of massage and the laying on of hands. Nursing Times 85(19):42–44, 1989

Walsh M, Brescia FJ: Pain and symptom consult: Comfort for patients with advanced cancer. Am J Nurs 90(1):112, 1990

Walsh M, Ford P: Rituals in nursing: "It can't hurt that much!" . . . nurses' reactions to patients' pain, part 2. Nursing Times 85(42):35–38, 1989

Willis J: A good night's sleep. Nursing Times 85(47):28–29, 31, 1989

Unit III

Nursing Skills Associated With Changing Levels of Wellness

11

Admitting, Transferring, Referring, and Discharging a Patient

Chapter Outline

Behavioral Objectives
Glossary
Introduction
Trends in Health-Care Delivery
Common Reactions to Hospitalization
Preparing for Admission
Admitting the Patient
Transferring the Patient
Referring the Patient
Discharging the Patient
Suggested Measures When Admitting and Discharging
  Patients in Selected Situations
Teaching Suggestions for Admitting and Discharging
  Patients from a Health Care Agency
Applicable Nursing Diagnoses
Bibliography

Skill Procedures

Admitting the Patient
Transferring the Patient
Discharging the Patient

Behavioral Objectives

When the content of this chapter has been mastered, the learner will be able to:

Define terms appearing in the glossary.

List at least three health-care delivery methods that are being used to prevent or decrease the time spent as a patient within a hospital.

Describe at least four common emotional reactions that occur during a hospitalization or admission to a nursing home.

Discuss ways that a nurse can reduce or eliminate the emotional effects associated with admission to a health agency.

Identify the nurse's responsibilities during admission to a health agency.

Discuss the nursing actions that are important during the transfer of a patient within a health agency or to another health agency.

Discuss the purpose of a referral and typical information included in a referral.

Describe how a nurse should prepare a patient for discharge, and the actions associated with discharging a patient.

Indicate the usual procedure the nurse should follow when a patient chooses to leave a hospital against advice.

List suggested measures for admitting and discharging patients in selected situations, as described in this chapter.

Summarize suggestions for instructing the patient.

Glossary

Admission The process of entering a health agency for care and treatment.

Continuity of care Providing uninterrupted care among various health practitioners and agencies without disrupting a patient's progress.

Discharge A process that occurs when a patient leaves a health agency.

Extended-care facility A nursing home or medical-care agency that cares for individuals with long-term or rehabilitation problems.

Family birthing units Short-stay maternity services provided by hospitals in a homelike setting.

Gatching Positioning the bed so as to bend the knees.

Home health care Nursing care provided within a person's home.

Immediate care center A health-care facility, open 24 hours, which treats people with minor illnesses without any prior appointments.

Orientation The act of providing a person with new information.

Outpatient A sick or injured person who travels back and forth to a health agency for testing or treatment.

Personal space The invisible area around one's body in which an individual feels safe.

Referral The process of sending or guiding someone to another place for assistance.

Rooming in A service allowing a parent to share a room with his or her child.

Separation anxiety The uncomfortable feeling associated with leaving familiar people and surroundings.

Step-down unit A special area in the hospital for patients who are recovering from serious conditions, but who no longer require intensive nursing observation and care.

Transfer The process of discharging a patient from one unit or health agency and admitting him to another.

Introduction

Unfortunately, everyone experiences changes in health. Some become ill suddenly; some sustain an injury; others may have felt poorly for some time. All may need some form of care and treatment for their needs. This care may require entry into a health agency such as a hospital or a nursing home.

Most nurses are employed by health agencies that care for sick people. Illnesses or injuries that require admission to a health agency are likely to cause a person to feel overwhelmed. The nurse faces the challenge of carrying out agency policies for admission, transfer, referral, or discharge while helping an individual maintain his dignity and sense of control.

The information in this chapter is intended to help the nurse understand and respond to typical reactions that occur when a person is admitted to a hospital or nursing home. The skill procedures describe general routines when an individual enters or leaves a health agency.

Trends in Health-Care Delivery

People being admitted to health agencies require skilled treatment now more than ever before. There are various options available to reduce the amount of time an individual must be away from home while receiving health care. Creative alternatives for the services commonly associated with hospital care are being established. The trend is to provide care in the most economical way possible. Even when hospitalization is necessary, the amount of time spent there is brief. The cost-effectiveness of many of these new programs is due to the manner in which nurses are applying their knowledge and skills.

Immediate Care Centers

Immediate care centers are small, health-care facilities created to care for individuals with minor illnesses without any prior appointment. These centers, staffed by doctors and nurses, are open 24 hours. They limit the use of a hospital's emergency room as a substitute for a doctor's office. Costs to the individual, or his insurance company, are less than the same service provided by a hospital. Early treatment, before a condition worsens, also usually means less cost in the long run. Many people appreciate this type of access to health care because they do not have to miss work or school.

Outpatient Services

An *outpatient* is a sick or injured person who continues to live at home but travels back and forth to a health agency for testing or treatment. Outpatient services have been available for laboratory testing, physical therapy, and respiratory therapy for some time. Many types of surgery are now being performed on this model. Nurses play a major role in teaching and preparing a person for the procedure. They monitor the immediate postsurgical period for several hours until the person can safely go home. Finally, nurses phone or reexamine the person the next day to ensure that all is progressing well.

Family Birthing Units

Family birthing units are special maternity facilities within hospitals with a homelike atmosphere. Couples not faced with a high-risk pregnancy may seek this alternative to the traditional obstetrical experience. The mother may be joined during labor or delivery by those she feels are meaningful for the birth. Children are allowed to be present. Many mothers stay only 24 hours, and return later with the infant for additional teaching and examinations. Nurses remain in close contact by phone or personal visits to ensure the health and safety of the mother and the newborn.

Home Health Care

Home health care is the care provided by nurses within a person's home. Some individuals may only need temporary or brief assistance with technical procedures. Providing nursing services within the home may prevent admission to a hospital or nursing home, or it may shorten the time spent recovering in the hospital. This extension of the nurse's knowledge and skills maintains a person's independence and helps control health-care costs. Table 11-1 lists common community services that assist persons with declining health or physical disabilities.

Extended-Care Facilities

As the population ages, more people are having difficulty remaining independent. The need for geriatric nurse practitioners and specialized agencies for the care of the elderly is increasing. The majority of those hospitalized are people over the age of 65. The reimbursement for hospital care is time limited. Therefore, many community agencies are being burdened with an increasing need for extended service.

Table 11-1. Common Community Services

Organization	Service
Commission on Aging	Assists elderly with transportation to medical appointments, outpatient therapy, and community meal sites
Hospice	Supports the family and terminally ill individuals who choose to stay at home
Visiting Nurses' Association	Offers intermittent nursing care to homebound persons
Meals on Wheels	Provides one or two hot meals per day, delivered either at home or a community meal site
Homemaker Services	Sends adults to the home to assist in shopping, meal preparation, and light housekeeping
Home-Health Aid	Assists with bathing, hygiene, and medication supervision
Adult Protective Services	Makes social, legal, and accounting services available to incompetent adults who may be victimized by others
Respite Care	Provides short-term, temporary relief to fulltime caregivers of homebound persons
Older Americans' Ombudsman	Investigates and resolves complaints made by, or on behalf of, nursing home residents; at least one fulltime ombudsman is mandated for each state

An *extended-care facility* may also be called a nursing home. It is an agency that cares for persons with chronic or rehabilitative health needs. Some people require extended care before hospitalization. Others are transferred after acute care for temporary or long-term nursing care.

Nursing homes are licensed in the type of care they are authorized to provide. They may deliver either skilled, intermediate, or residential care, or all three.

Skilled nursing care involves 24-hour nursing services. A person who needs skilled care requires the continuous skills, judgment, and knowledge of a licensed nurse. Examples of skilled care include caring for wounds, suctioning, tube feeding, and continuous oxygen therapy.

Intermediate care, sometimes called basic, helps individuals with activities of daily living. A licensed nurse performs a periodic assessment, plans care to meet identified needs, and evaluates the outcomes. The actual care may be provided by a nursing assistant under the supervision of a nurse. Basic care can include positioning, preventive skin care, help with toileting, and assistance with ambulation.

Residential care usually implies that a person's room and board are provided. There is access to daily supervision. Social and recreational activities are made available in residential care. Nursing services and medical care are not provided. Transfer to a basic or skilled-care facility is available if a person's health needs change. Display 11-1 lists information that one should obtain when selecting an extended-care facility for a family member.

Medicare, a federal health insurance program, only pays for up to 100 days of skilled care. Medicaid, a federal public assistance program, pays for both basic and skilled care. Recipients of Medicaid funds, however, must meet financial need eligibility requirements. Medicaid is only granted to people with low incomes who have completely exhausted their own resources. Unfortunately, this often includes depleting a spouse's income and assets as well. Reform of this aspect is being addressed.

Extended-care facilities try to duplicate a homelike environment for residents who may be there for months or years. Meals are served to groups. Lounge areas for socializing and recreation are available. Contracts are made with beauticians and barbers for hair care at the agency. Social activities, such as the one in Figure 11-1, and religious services are scheduled on a routine basis. As many people as possible are encouraged to participate.

Display 11-1. Guidelines for Selecting an Extended-Care Facility

- Find out if the agency provides the type of care (skilled, intermediate, or residential) needed.
- Ask if the facility is Medicare and Medicaid approved.
- Review inspection reports on specific homes. This information is available on a charge per page basis from the state's Department of Public Health.
- Ask others in the community for recommendations.
- Visit nursing homes with, and again without, a prior appointment. Go at least once during a mealtime.
- Look for or ask about the institution's current license.
- Request brochures that identify medical care, nursing services, rehabilitation therapy, social services, activities programs, religious observances, rights, and privileges.
- Clarify charges and billing procedures.
- Analyze if your overall impression of the agency is positive.

Common Reactions to Hospitalization

Despite methods to prevent or reduce the time spent away from home when a person is ill, admission to a health agency may be inevitable. The need to leave home for care compounds the stress of physical illness. The exact effects are unique to each individual, but some common reactions can be anticipated.

Separation Anxiety

Separation anxiety is the uncomfortable feeling associated with leaving familiar people and surroundings. The need for love and belonging are higher level needs described by Maslow and Kalish. Children and parents are mutually sensitive to being separated. The child in Figure 11-2 would be much more frightened if his father were not with him. Elderly people may become depressed, confused, and disoriented when they must leave home. The nurse must be aware of the effects on all of the people who are involved—not just the patient.

Loneliness

Loneliness occurs when an individual misses the company of others. Individuals can feel lonely even if they are surrounded by other people. The nurse can never take the place of those who are significant to a patient. However, the nurse can spend time with lonely patients. Many hospitals and nursing homes have liberal visiting hours to counteract loneliness. Age restrictions are also being lifted in order to allow children to visit sick relatives. Parents are now permitted and encouraged to stay with their sick children.

Insecurity

The hospital environment and routine are generally unfamiliar to most people. Fear of the unknown creates insecurity and anxiety. The nurse may relieve some of the patient's anxiety by orienting the patient to the nursing unit and his room. A simple explanation of the time for meals, visiting hours, and equipment within the room is important when a person is first admitted for care.

Decreased Privacy

Humans establish real and imaginary boundaries for themselves and their possessions, creating an area that identifies ownership and provides a feeling of safety. There is a tendency to protect and defend this territory when it becomes threatened. When a person is admitted to a hospital or nursing home, a new territory must be established. Closed doors or pulled curtains indicate that a person wishes to be alone; the nurse should always knock or ask permission to enter.

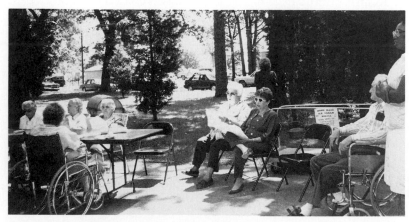

Figure 11-1 The staff and residents of an extended-care facility enjoy a songfest before their picnic in the park.

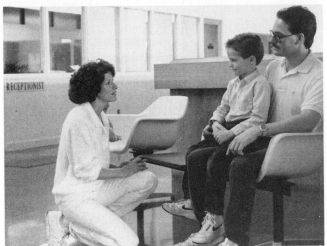

Figure 11-2 A child needs the support of a parent when entering an unfamiliar setting such as the hospital.

There is even an invisible body area that an individual considers private. For most, it is just beyond an arm's length. Entry into this area, called one's *personal space*, may cause an individual to feel threatened. This space often becomes invaded in the course of health care and treatment. Nurses should respect the individual's personal space by explaining what will be done during a procedure, especially when it involves close contact with the person's body. The patient should also be protected from the view of others when care is given.

Loss of Identity

All people have a need for esteem and recognition. It is enhanced by objects, such as clothing, and personal effects. When a person is admitted to a health agency, the symbols of his identity may be left behind. Providing patients with institutional gowns increases an impersonal attitude toward the person. It may even be some time before all the staff are familiar with a new patient's name. The nurse should always learn and call the patient by name. First names should only be used if the patient asks that this be done. Efforts should be made to display the patient's family pictures or other personal objects that reinforce the unique aspects of each individual's life.

Preparing for Admission

Admission is a process that takes place when a person enters a health-care agency for care and treatment. Each health agency has a procedure for admitting, transferring, referring, and discharging patients. Most admissions are for physical illnesses. That is the focus of the discussion in this chapter. Special types of admissions exist, however for patients with mental illness. They are identified in Table 11-2.

Special procedures were developed for the mentally ill to protect the public and the disturbed individual from harm. The rights of the person with emotional problems are also protected within mental health admission legisla-

Table 11-2. Types of Psychiatric Admissions

Type	Description	Length
Voluntary	A person petitions a psychiatrist for admission. If admitted, the patient retains his right to sign himself out of the institution.	Varies with response to treatment
Involuntary	A person legally petitions that another person be admitted for psychiatric assessment. The patient always retains the right to have his case reviewed.	Determined by individual state law
Emergency Admission	The petitioner alleges that the patient is dangerous to himself or others.	Generally automatically expires after 48 to 72 hours
Temporary Admission	During a court hearing, the psychiatrist discusses the reasons for needing continued hospitalization. The patient is represented by legal counsel and can testify in his own behalf.	Ranges on average of up to 60 days
Extended Admission	Court reconvenes and hears testimony from the psychiatrist and patient about the need for longer treatment. The law demands that a patient be confined in the least restrictive environment for treatment.	Range varies from 60 to 180 days

tion. Past history shows that some people were institutionalized for long periods of time in psychiatric facilities. Some were not mentally ill, but were held against their will as a result of unsubstantiated accusations.

The Admitting Department

Most hospitals have an admitting department where clerical personnel begin to gather information. The patient's record is started in the admitting department. Forms are prepared with the patient's address, place of employment, insurance company and policy numbers, and other data. This information is used primarily by the hospital's business office for record keeping and future billing.

A plastic card similar to a credit card may be prepared. This card is attached to forms that are delivered to the nursing unit. The card is used to identify all the pages within the chart during the patient's hospitalization.

Preparing an identification bracelet for the patient is one of the first components of the admission routine. Someone in the admitting department types identifying information on the bracelet, such as the patient's name, the patient's identification number, the name of the physician caring for the patient, and the patient's room number. The bracelet is usually applied by someone in the admitting department. An identification bracelet is illustrated in Figure 11-3. It is important for the patient's safety that the bracelet remain on throughout his time in the hospital. The patient is then escorted to the unit and room where he will be cared for.

Preparing the Patient's Room

When the nurse learns that a patient will be arriving, the room should be prepared. The patient should feel that everyone on the nursing unit is prepared and ready for his admission. If the patient feels that he is unexpected or is an inconvenience to the personnel, it is likely to make a rude first impression.

Before the patient is escorted to the unit, the nurse should check the room and replace any missing items from the bedside stand. If the patient is known to need special equipment, such as oxygen, it should be at his bedside upon his arrival.

The bed should be in a low position if the patient can walk. If the patient is arriving by stretcher, the bed is placed in a high position to facilitate moving the patient onto the bed. Moving helpless patients is described in Chapter 18. Some wait to unfold the top sheets and spread until after the patient is inside the room. This shows that the room is neat, clean, and orderly. The patient will need a hospital gown or, if the agency policy permits, he may use his own bed-clothes.

Admitting the Patient

Nursing responsibilities that are common with these routines will be discussed, but it is recommended that the policies and procedures of each health agency be followed. One of the most important steps in the admission procedure is to make the patient feel welcome. The nurse in Figure 11-4 is greeting a patient who has just arrived on the unit. Being treated as an expected guest helps put the patient at ease.

Orienting the Patient

Orientation is the act of providing a person with new information. To help the patient feel more secure, several explanations should be made. The nurse should point out the following locations: the nurse's work area in relation to the patient's room; the toilet; the shower or bathing area if

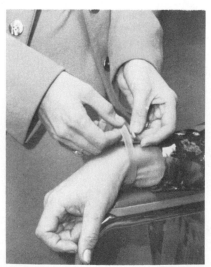

Figure 11-3 A clerk in the admitting department applies an identification bracelet to a patient's wrist.

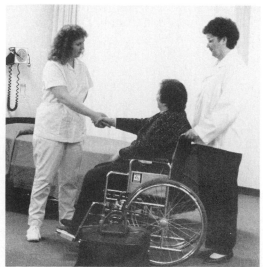

Figure 11-4 Admitting a patient sincerely and with courtesy helps her feel welcome and at ease.

not located with the toilet; and any lounge area that may be used by the patient and his family.

In the room, the nurse who is admitting the patient should explain:

- How to contact a nurse. This may be done, with a signal light. If an intercommunication system is available between the nurse and the patient, this should also be explained and demonstrated.
- Directions for changing the position of the bed. Any position that is restricted, such as not gatching the knees, should be explained. *Gatching* is a term that describes bending the bed at the knees. This may be contraindicated for a patient who has had abdominal surgery. Any patient prone to blood clots should not have the knees gatched.
- How phone calls may be made or received. Some hospitals divert calls during the night through the switchboard to the nursing unit. This policy avoids disturbing the rest and sleep of patients.
- The use of remote controls for operating a television.

The daily routine and activities that will affect the patient should also be explained. The nurse should identify the times for meals, when the doctor may be expected, when surgery is scheduled, and when laboratory tests or x-rays may be performed. Some hospitals provide booklets with general information for newly admitted patients. Many patients are anxious when they are admitted. Anxiety interferes with the ability to remember. A booklet acts as a reminder for what was explained. Booklets should never take the place of the nurse's explanations.

Handling the Patient's Valuables and Clothing

It is preferable for admitting personnel to give the patient's valuables, such as jewelry and money, to family members to take home. If this is not possible, admitting personnel may temporarily place the patient's valuables in a safe. There should be a note made on the patient's record about how valuables were handled.

When the nurse is responsible for handling the patient's valuables and clothing, *the agency's policies must be carefully observed.* Losing personal items belonging to a patient can have serious legal implications for both the nurse and the health agency. The patient may sue, claiming his belongings were lost or stolen because they were handled carelessly. It is best to have a second nurse or a representative from the hospital's administrative staff present when a nurse receives valuables for safekeeping. An inventory is made. The nurse and the patient may cosign the inventory. One copy is given to the patient, while another is attached to the chart. Problems occur when in the course of hospitalization other valuable items are brought in without subsequent documentation. Figure 11-5 illustrates one type of clothing and valuables checklist used by a nursing home.

Agencies have facilities in the patient's room for the proper storage of street clothing. The nurse should also note any supplies or equipment the patient brings with him, such as glasses, crutches, a wheel-chair, or other items. Items that are similar to those owned by the hospital should be labeled with the patient's name. This identification will help if the items become mixed with hospital equipment.

Helping the Patient Undress

There will be times when a patient is unable to undress without the nurse's help. Methods for helping the patient are as follows:

- Provide privacy.
- Have the patient sit on the edge of the bed, which has already been lowered.
- Remove the patient's shoes.
- Assist the patient to turn on the bed and help him into the lying position if he is weak and tired.
- Slip off the patient's clothing in a manner least disturbing to him after fasteners, such as zippers and buttons, are opened. For example, fold or gather a garment in your hands as you work it up the body. Have the patient lift his hips, if he can, to slide clothes up or down.
- Lift the patient's head so garments can be guided over the head.
- Roll the patient from side to side to remove clothes that fasten up the front or back, after removing arms from sleeves.
- Cover the patient with a bath blanket after removing the outer clothing.
- Gather a stocking, sliding it down the leg and over the foot.
- Put on the patient's gown after he is undressed.

Gathering Information

At the time of admission, the nurse begins assessment and collecting information for the database. Assessment skills are discussed in more depth in Chapters 13 and 14. The nurse ordinarily obtains the patient's temperature, pulse and respiratory rates, and blood pressure. The patient is weighed on the hospital's scales. A specimen of urine may be obtained. Observations of the patient's general condition are made. All known allergies are noted. Collecting specimens and obtaining vital signs are discussed in subsequent chapters.

The physician is ordinarily notified when a patient for whom he is caring has been admitted. The physician may have sent forms with the patient. In some cases, physicians' orders and a copy of a medical history and physical examination are brought with the patient's forms from the

CLOTHING LIST:

(Please check articles of clothing with patient and describe.)

Dress *1 - BLUE & WHITE*   Pants_____

Slip *1 - WHITE (½ SLIP)*   Shirt_____

Bra *1 - WHITE*   Undershirt_____

Panties *1 - WHITE*   Undershorts_____

Hose_____   Socks_____

Girdle_____   Tie_____

Slippers *1 - PINK*   Shoes *1 - WHITE*

Nightgown *1 - BLUE, 1 - PINK*   Pajamas_____

Suit_____   Robe_____

Sweater_____   Coat_____

Slacks_____   Truss_____

Blouse_____   Backsupport_____

Shorts_____   Belt_____

Skirt_____   Hat_____

Other items not listed:

_____

_____

Check valuables below and describe if necessary:

Watch_____   Earrings_____

Medals_____   Rings - Type & Number *1 - YELLOW METAL, PLAIN BAND*

Other Jewelry_____

Dentures - Yes ✔ No_____   Prosthesis - Yes_____ No ✔

Contact Lenses - Yes_____ No ✔   Glasses - Yes ✔ No_____

Removed - Yes_____ No_____   Hearing Aid - Yes_____ No ✔

Wallet ✔ Color *RED* With Pt. ✔ In Safe_____ To Family or Friend_____

Purse ✔ Color *WHITE* With Pt. ✔ In Safe_____ To Family or Friend_____

Cash *$25.00* With Pt._____ In Safe ✔ To Family or Friend_____

Checks/Check Book_____ With Pt._____ In Safe_____ To Family or Friend_____

The above list is correct:

Patient's signature *Helen Jones*   Witness *Nancy Smith, L.P.N.*

Clothing taken home by_____

Relationship_____

Witness_____

Received by on Nursing Unit_____

Figure 11-5 This form is commonly used in health agencies for listing the patient's clothing and valuables. It is completed at the time the patient is admitted to the health agency.

admitting department. The nurse should check to determine whether there are orders that are to be carried out at the time of admission.

Skill Procedure 11-1 describes a summary of the steps in admitting a patient to a health agency's unit. More specific details depend largely on the patient's condition and agency policies. A description of the admission and initial database assessment information must be entered on the patient's record within the first 24 hours.

Transferring the Patient

A *transfer* involves discharging a patient from one unit or agency and admitting him to another. A transfer takes place when a patient's condition changes for better or worse. Not all facilities are equipped to handle the conditions of patients brought to emergency rooms. Transferring critically ill patients as rapidly as possible, as in Figure 11-6, affects the outcome. Transferring a recovering patient elsewhere frees space for the services another may require.

The move usually provides some advantage to the patient. It may reduce health-care costs, such as going from a hospital to a nursing home. It may locate the patient on a unit where nurses and staff have special experience and skills in caring for particular types of patients. Examples include the intensive care unit, cardiac care unit, surgical unit, even a step-down unit. A *step-down unit* is a term given to an area that cares for patients recovering from serious conditions, who no longer need intensive nursing observation or care.

Skill Procedure 11-1. Admitting the Patient

Suggested Action	Reason for Action
Greet the patient and relatives. Introduce yourself to the patient and the patient to his roommate(s).	Calling the patient by name, extending common courtesies, and welcoming the patient and relatives often help them feel at ease and less frightened.
Check the patient's identification bracelet to be sure it contains complete and accurate information.	The safety of the patient often depends on being accurately identified before tests are performed or medications are given.
Explain use of the bathroom and of agency equipment, such as the call system, adjustable bed, television, telephone, and so on. Explain agency routines, such as mealtimes and visiting hours.	Explaining agency routines and how to use equipment helps put the patient at ease. Knowing how to use equipment helps prevent anger, frustration, and accidents.
Make provisions for privacy. Ask the patient if he wishes relatives to remain or leave while the rest of the admission procedure is carried out.	Providing privacy shows respect and interest in the patient as a person. The patient often wants his family present as a source of security and emotional support.
Help the patient to undress and to get into a comfortable position.	Helping the patient to undress conserves his strength, can prevent accidents such as falling, and prepares the patient for receiving care. It also gives the nurse an opportunity to assess his skin and ability to move.
Take care of the patient's clothing and valuables. Follow agency procedure.	Losing items is upsetting to the patient and can result in serious legal problems.
Place the signal device and other equipment so that it will be convenient for the patient to use.	Being unable to call for help is unsafe, and can result in accidents. When equipment is handy for patients, accidents are less likely to occur.
Obtain the patient's temperature, pulse, respiratory rate, and blood pressure. If indicated, obtain a urine specimen at a time that is convenient during the admission procedure.	Collecting this information is an important part of the patient's beginning database.
If the patient's relatives left the room earlier, indicate that they may return to the patient's bedside.	Relatives have worries and fears, too. They usually feel better when they know the patient is admitted, settled, and comfortable.
Do necessary recording on the patient's record, following agency policy.	The information is an important part of the permanent record. It is the description of the beginning of the patient's care.

A transfer is similar to an admission and discharge. A patient is received on the new unit in a manner much the same as that used for his admission. Skill Procedure 11-2 describes general suggestions for transferring a patient. When the patient is moving within the same agency, financial arrangements do not have to be transacted. Also, the patient does not dress in street clothes.

Referring the Patient

A *referral* is the process of sending or guiding someone to another place for assistance. A patient may be referred by a nurse in a hospital to a community service agency that provides home health care. A school nurse may refer a student who does not see well to an eye-care specialist. An example of a referral form used when a patient was moved from a hospital to a nursing home appears in Figure 11-7.

Thinking about a referral is often a part of good dis-

charge planning. The nurse should begin to anticipate what kind of care the patient may require before it is time for him to leave. Planning, coordination, and communication take time in order to ensure that patients receive *continuity of care.* This term means that a patient's care is uninterrupted among various health practitioners and agencies. This avoids disrupting any progress that has been made.

Discharging the Patient

A *discharge* is a process that occurs when a patient leaves a health agency. Preparing a patient for discharge actually should begin when he is admitted. The purpose of his stay is to help him reach an improved state of wellness, and this begins at the time of admission.

Planning for a patient's discharge requires that the specific needs of a patient be identified. One group of nurses

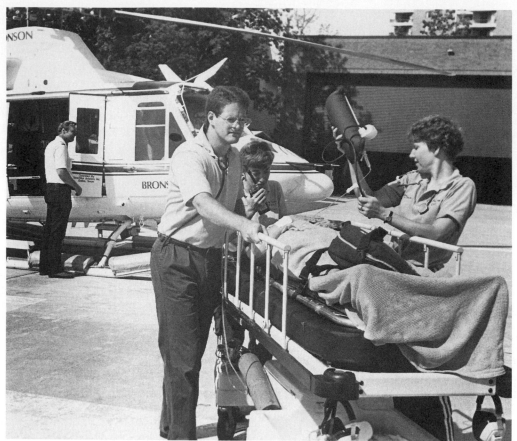

Figure 11-6 Transferring a patient as rapidly as possible often makes the difference between life and death. (Courtesy of Bronson Methodist Hospital, Kalamazoo, MI.)

prepared an assessment guide (Fig. 11-8) to identify the discharge needs of a patient. The guide can be adapted to identify patients with treatments or conditions that are commonly seen in a particular hospital unit.

Another group of nurses, who emphasized a need for a good teaching plan to prepare patients for discharge, used the acronym METHOD as a guide.

M——Medications. The patient should have thorough knowledge of the medications he should continue taking after discharge.

E——Environment. The environment to which the patient will be going after discharge from a hospital should be safe. The patient should also have whatever services are necessary for continuing care in that environment.

T——Treatments. The nurse should be sure that treatments to be continued after discharge can be carried out by the patient or a member of his family. If this is not possible, arrangements should be made so that someone can come into the home to give skilled care.

H——Health teaching. The patient being prepared for discharge should be taught how to maintain well-

being. This includes which signs and symptoms indicate that additional health care is required.

O——Outpatient referral. The patient should be familiar with services from the hospital or other community agencies that will promote his continued care and progress.

D——Diet. The patient should be taught about any restrictions in his diet. He should be able to select an appropriate diet for himself.

As is true when a patient is admitted, certain policies are carefully observed when he is discharged. Skill Procedure 11-3 describes discharging a patient from a health agency.

Leaving Against Medical Advice

There are times when a patient leaves a health agency against medical advice (sometimes abbreviated AMA). In such instances, he is asked to sign a special form, which states that he is leaving without being discharged by his doctor. It indicates that the individual will not hold the doctor, the hospital, or hospital personnel responsible for

Skill Procedure 11-2. Transferring the Patient

Suggested Action	Reason for Action
Be sure the patient and his family receive information about the transfer.	Communication promotes cooperation when dealing with the changes in a patient's condition.
Be sure that the patient has all his personal belongings.	Carelessness can lead to loss of the patient's clothing or valuables.
Notify receiving-unit personnel that arrangements are being made for a patient transfer.	Other personnel should be allowed time to plan and adjust their schedules so the transferred patient will feel welcomed and unhurried.
In a brief summary to new personnel, list significant information, such as medical diagnosis, treatment, nursing diagnoses, care, tests, and medications.	New personnel may not have time to read the chart thoroughly before assuming responsibility for the patient's care.
Review the current written nursing and medical orders with the nurse taking over the patient's care.	Reviewing the patient's current records together avoids overlooking aspects of the patient's care. Serious errors have occurred when there was insufficient communication between nurses during a patient's transfer.
Explain procedures, policies, and equipment that will be new to the patient.	Surroundings that are new to the patient may continue to cause fear and worry.
Introduce the patient to those who will be caring for him, as well as to his new roommate(s) if he shares a room.	Learning the names of other patients and personnel conveys a feeling of belonging.
Take the patient, if his condition permits, on a tour of the new unit.	Not all hospital units are exactly similar.
Record the circumstances and condition of the patient when transferred. The nurse who assumes care for the patient should also record a brief summary of assessments about the condition of the patient upon his arrival.	The chart is a record of all the care and responses of the patient throughout hospitalization.
Notify other departments within the hospital of the patient's change in location.	Services such as mail and phone calls will need to be redirected. Other personnel will experience less delay in their schedules when they must locate the patient.
Visit the transferred patient from time to time.	It is a courteous and thoughtful gesture to remain in contact with a patient. This promotes a feeling of self-esteem and recognition of their personal worth.

anything that may happen to him as a result of his leaving. If the patient refuses to sign the form, he may not be detained from leaving. The refusal should be noted within the patient's hospital record.

The nurse responsible for the patient's care should be sure the physician is notified and aware of the patient's wishes to leave. Unsuccessful attempts to locate the doctor should be noted on the patient's record. The hospital's nursing supervisor may also be notified. Health practitioners should share information with the patient about the risks his decision involves, but the patient cannot be forcefully detained when he is a rational adult. The only exception to this is the case of a patient admission that has been ordered by a judge. This usually only occurs when a patient has a mental illness. It may also occur if the patient

has a contagious disease and has refused measures that would prevent its spread among other susceptible people. In all other cases, detaining a patient against his wishes invites serious legal problems. A health practitioner and the hospital could be sued for false imprisonment.

Cleaning the Room and Equipment

Cleaning a patient's room and equipment after discharge is ordinarily a housekeeping responsibility. However, in some instances, a nurse may be required to do this job. The nurse is referred to Chapter 16, in which recommended techniques for cleaning, disinfection, and sterilization techniques are discussed.

PATIENT TRANSFER FORM
(INTER-AGENCY REFERRAL)

1. PATIENT'S LAST NAME	FIRST NAME	MIDDLE	2. SEX	3. HEALTH INSURANCE CLAIM NUMBER
Carver	Anna	B	☐ M ☒ F	66585-83-2G

4. PATIENT'S ADDRESS (Street number, City, State, Zip Code)	5. DATE OF BIRTH	RELIGION
358 W. York Three Rivers MI 49093	9/03/17	Protestant

7. DATE OF THIS TRANSFER	8. FACILITY NAME AND ADDRESS TRANSFERRING TO
12/5/87	Twin Oaks Nursing Home, 215 Riverside, Sturgis, MI

11. Dates of qualifying stay	12-A. FACILITY NAME AND ADDRESS TRANSFERRING FROM
FROM 12 5 87	Three Rivers Area Hospital 1111 Broadway, Three Rivers, MI
THRU 1 5 88	12-B. QUALIFYING AND OTHER PRIOR STAY INFORMATION (Including Medical Record Numbers)

EMPLOYMENT RELATED	MEDICAID ELIGIBLE
☐ YES ☒ NO	☐ YES ☒ NO

13. INSURING ORGANIZATION OR STATE AGENCY NAME AND ADDRESS	14. POLICY OR MEDICAL ASSISTANCE NO.
Medicare (Blue Cross of Michigan)	311425609

CLINIC APPOINTMENT DATE	TIME	ATTACH CLINIC APPOINTMENT CARD	DATE OF LAST PHYSICAL EXAMINATION	WEIGHT
1/10/88	10 AM		12/3/87	167

ATTENDING PHYSICIAN INFORMATION

1. NAME AND ADDRESS OF PHYSICIAN AT NEW FACILITY

Chester Sweder MD (Sturgis)

2. FINAL DIAGNOSIS(ES), OR PROTOCOPY ATTACHED ☐

PRIMARY:

Fractured Ⓡ hip

ALL OTHER CONDITIONS:

CHF

3. SURGICAL PROCEDURE(S) AND DATE(S) OR, CHECK NONE ☐

Open reduction c̄ Ⓡ hip pin 11/15/87

4. PHYSICIAN ORDERS ON TRANSFER:

Low Na (0.5Gm) Soft diet
Lanoxin 0.25mg daily
Diupres 250 mg B.I.D.

5. ESTIMATED MEDICALLY NECESSARY STAY:
30 DAYS ____ WEEKS OR ____ MONTHS

6. DRUG SENSITIVITIES OR, CHECK NONE ☐

Allergic to Penicillin

7. DIETARY REGIMEN:

see above #4

8. PHYSICIAN'S SIGNATURE   Chester Sweder MD   DATE 12/3/87

NURSING EVALUATION

	NORMAL	Impaired			
9. SPEECH	NORMAL ☒	Impaired ☐		Unable To Speak ☐
10. HEARING	NORMAL ☒	Impaired ☐		Deaf ☐
11. SIGHT	NORMAL ☐	Impaired ☒		Blind ☐
12. MENTAL STATUS	ALWAYS ALERT ☒	Occasionally Confused ☐		Always Confused ☐
13. FEEDING	INDEPENDENT ☒	Help With Feeding ☐		Cannot Feed Self ☐
14. DRESSING	INDEPENDENT ☐	Help With Dressing ☒		Cannot Dress Self ☐
15. ELIMINATION	INDEPENDENT ☐	Help To Bathroom ☐	Bedpan or Urinal Required ☒	Incontinent ☐
16. BATHING	INDEPENDENT ☐	Bathing With Help ☒	Bed Bath With Help ☒	Bed Bath ☐
17. AMBULATORY STATUS	INDEPENDENT ☐	Walks With Assistance ☒	Help From Bed To Chair ☒	Bed Bound ☐

18. DRESSINGS AND BANDAGES: OR, CHECK NONE ☒

19. APPLIANCES OR SUPPORTS: OR, CHECK NONE ☐

Uses walker; only partial weight bearing on Ⓡ leg

20. NURSING ASSESSMENT AND RECOMMENDATIONS:

Incision healed
Wears glasses and dentures
Help with shoes
Likes to take pills with apple juice rather than water
Needs reassurance and encouragement with ambulation

SUMMARY ATTACHED ☐ Yes ☒ No

21. SIGNATURE	TITLE	DATE
Laurie Highfield LPN		12/3/87

SOCIAL EVALUATION

22. NAME AND ADDRESS OF PERSON TO CONTACT:

Thomas Carver, 110 Armitage, Three Rivers, MI

RELATIONSHIP TO PATIENT: Son
TELEPHONE NUMBER: 279-6013

23. PATIENT LIVES:
ALONE ☒   WITH FAMILY ☐   WITH SPOUSE ☐   OTHER ☐   EXPLAIN:

24. PATIENT ATTITUDE:

Motivated and Cooperative

25. SUMMARY ATTACHED SOCIAL/EMOTIONAL FACTORS ☐ YES ☒ NO

26. POST STAY PLANS:

Family + neighbors will check daily

27. SIGNATURE	DATE	TITLE
Susan Adams	12/3/87	Discharge Planner / Coordinator

0880-5 FEB. 75

TRANSFERRING HOSPITAL

Figure 11-7 This form is used when patients are referred from one health agency to another. It illustrates the type of information the receiving agency needs to make continuity of care possible.

Suggested Measures When Admitting and Discharging Patients in Selected Situations

When the Patient Is an Infant or Child

Remember that a hospital admission is a difficult experience for most children and their parents. No admission to a hospital is routine for them. Therefore, every effort should be taken to offer explanations, give emotional support, and orient both the child and his parents to the hospital environment.
Parents of very young, hospitalized infants often require more nursing support than the patient. Their protective and nurturing role is threatened, and they feel helpless.
Permit a parent to help undress a child and help with other admission and hospital procedures as much as possible. This practice helps to reduce a child's fears and anxieties.

Discharge Planning Assessment Guide

Patient's Name _____ Date _____
Directions: Check all items that apply

CONSIDER NEED FOR CONTINUING CARE when patient is:
__ Elderly (living alone or spouse ill)
__ Admitted from nursing home
__ Served by home health-care agency
__ Known to social service community agencies
__ Indigent
__ Emotionally/psychologically unstable
__ Alcohol dependent
__ Drug dependent
__ Victim of child abuse
__ Victim of violent crime
__ Functionally handicapped
__ Single parent with newborn child
__ Terminally ill
__ Premature infant

ANTICIPATE POTENTIAL DISCHARGE PROBLEMS when patient has:
__ Multiple diagnoses
__ Complicated treatment/medication regimens
__ Dietary restrictions
__ Wound infection
__ Contagious disease
__ Recurrent hospital admissions
__ Major surgery
__ Alteration of body function/image (e.g., ostomy, amputation, mastectomy)
__ Chronic/debilitating/immobilizing disease process

INITIATE DISCHARGE PLANNING when patient is admitted with:
__ Myocardial infarction
__ Diabetes (uncontrolled, newly diagnosed, new prescription)
__ Arthritis (exacerbation, joint replacement)
__ Chronic pulmonary disease
__ Chronic heart disease
__ Cerebrovascular accident
__ Congestive heart failure
__ Hypertension
__ Cancer
__ Tuberculosis
__ Burns
__ Kidney failure
__ Fractures

Figure 11-8 This form provides a checklist to help the nurse assess a patient's specific needs so that discharge planning is facilitated. (Reprinted with permission from the July issue of Nursing 81. Copyright © 1981, Springhouse Corporation, 1111 Bethlehem Pike, Springhouse, PA 19477. All rights reserved.)

Parents should be told if a hospital permits *rooming in,* a service that allows a parent to share a room with their child. It has been found that hospitalization and separation from parents are extremely difficult for young children, especially if the child is under 4 or 5 years of age. When rooming in is permitted, children can be saved from much emotional trauma.

When a child is very young, obtain information about a child and his illness from a parent. The nurse should also ask a parent to describe how the child may feel about his illness. It is best to interview parents out of the child's hearing. This protects the child from hearing something he cannot understand, which may be extremely frightening to him.

If the child is old enough, ask the child to explain how he feels and how his illness is affecting him. Ignoring that a child can participate in the conversation conveys a message to the child that his contributions are not important.

Preschool children can often cope with the experiences of hospitalization by using dolls. The dolls may represent models of themselves and other hospital personnel. Playing provides an opportunity for acting out conflicts and a means to their resolution.

Encouraging the early school-age child to draw a picture about the hospital and discuss it may help the nurse assess the significance of hospitalization to a child.

Be sure that the parents are aware when a child is

Skill Procedure 11-3. Discharging the Patient

Suggested Action	Reason for Action
Check to see that the patient has a discharge order.	It is the physician's responsibility to discharge the patient.
If the patient is leaving without a physician's consent, request that the patient sign a certain agency form.	The patient cannot legally be held in an agency against his wishes except in certain circumstances. Having the patient's signature on a form identifies that the patient assumes responsibility for the consequences of leaving the health agency.
Notify the family or responsible person who will provide transportation from the health agency.	A discharged patient should not sit in the lobby or wait for a long period of time for someone who will drive him home.
Check to see that the patient or a relative has had discharge instructions, such as instructions about diet or medications.	The patient or a relative will be able to continue with necessary care safely after discharge when properly instructed.
Check to see that all necessary equipment and supplies, such as prescriptions and dressings, are ready for the patient to take with him. Locate missing items.	Having equipment and supplies ready saves the time and annoyance of having to wait for them when the patient is ready to leave.
Write down the date, time, and location of the next appointment with the physician.	Some patients may be unfamiliar with the office locations of doctors who have provided care. Writing down appointment information will help the patient maintain continued follow-up.
Refer family members or the patient to the business office.	Seeing that proper financial arrangements have been made helps maintain accurate records for billing.
Check the patient's belongings with the clothing and valuables list. Some agencies require that the patient sign the form if he agrees that he can account for all the items that were listed.	Following the agency's policy may help to avoid legal problems in the future.
Help the patient to dress and to pack his belongings. Some disposable hospital equipment, such as the soap dish and water pitcher, may be taken home by the patient.	Assisting the patient conserves his strength. Such assistance is courteous and helps the patient feel that personnel are interested in his welfare.
Transport the patient and his belongings to a car and help him into the car if necessary.	Hospital personnel are responsible for the patient's safety until he has left the hospital grounds. The hospital is liable for any personal injury that occurs on its property.
Record essential information on the patient's chart.	Information concerning discharge is important because it indicates the patient's condition at the time of his release on the permanent record.

to be discharged and that they have been properly instructed about continuing care after discharge.

When the Patient Is Elderly

Do not misjudge an elderly patient as being senile when he is admitted to a hospital until you have sufficient evidence. Very often, the elderly person is so concerned about a physical problem with which he is trying to cope that he becomes confused and sometimes disoriented, especially when admitted to the strange environment of a hospital.

Be prepared to expect that an elderly patient may be fearful of discharge from a hospital and may wish to stay. Many are very concerned about their care after discharge, especially if they live alone or with a spouse who has limited ability to give necessary care. The nurse should work toward helping the elderly patient become as self-sufficient as possible during hospitalization so that he can better cope with his care at home.

Allow a patient to decorate or display personal items within the room. This promotes a feeling of security and familiarity within a strange environment.

NURSING CARE PLAN

11-1. Anxiety

Assessment	**Subjective Data** States, "Ever since my doctor told me I had to come to the hospital for this test, I've felt like a rubberband that's stretched to the limit." **Objective Data** 35-year-old woman admitted for heart catheterization. Heart rate 105, flushed, pacing about room. Twists hair with fingers. Asks that admission questions be repeated. Stares out window. Crying off and on during interview.
Diagnosis	Anxiety related to charge in health status.
Plan	**Goal** The patient will demonstrate reduced anxiety as evidenced by identifying one resolution of a problem caused by hospitalization by 4/17. **Orders:** 4/14 1. Sit calmly with patient at least t.i.d. 2. Reinforce that most people have similar feelings in these circumstances. 3. Explore the specific problems associated with hospitalization. 4. Do not discourage crying if it occurs. ———————— S. Friedman, RN
Implementation (Documentation) 4/14	1115 Spent ½ hr talking. Shared that anxiety is a common feeling among patients. Asked to identify the most distressing aspect of this experience. States, "I don't have any health insurance." Asked if she would like to see a social worker to discuss a partial payment schedule. ———————— C. Skinner, SN
Evaluation (Documentation)	1115 Stated, "Oh yes. I didn't know that was possible. I'm so relieved. I thought I'd have to sell my car." No crying. Ate most of lunch. ———————— C. Skinner, SN

Expect to repeat information about the daily routine and names of staff and other patients. Anxiety may temporarily interfere with remembering.

Teaching Suggestions for Admitting and Discharging Patients From a Health-Care Agency

The following summary offers suggestions for teaching about admitting and discharging a patient from a hospital:

The patient should be taught about the hospital environment, his unit and room, hospital policies and procedures, and so on upon his admission to a hospital. This type of explaining should also be done when a patient is transferred within a hospital.

The patient should be well prepared for discharge through a planned teaching program, as described in this chapter. A program should include information about medications, treatments, and diet restrictions ordered for the patient and about any other factors influencing his health and well-being. Included in discharge planning should be instructions about when to call a physician if problems arise.

Applicable Nursing Diagnoses

Several psychosocial nursing diagnoses can apply to patients being admitted, transferred, referred, and discharged. Beginning students without any prior courses in psychology or psychosocial nursing may not yet have the knowledge to independently plan care for these problems:

- Altered Role Performance
- Altered Family Processes
- Impaired Adjustment
- Ineffective Family Coping: Disabled
- Ineffective Family Coping: Compromised
- Decisional Conflict
- Self-Esteem Disturbance
- Powerlessness

Nursing diagnoses that may be more within the level of competence for a beginning student include

- Anxiety
- Fear
- Social Isolation
- Altered Home Maintenance Management
- Altered Health Maintenance

Nursing Care Plan 11-1 shows an example of what the nurse may do for a patient with Anxiety. Anxiety is defined in the NANDA Taxonomy (1989) as "A vague uneasy feeling whose source is often nonspecific or unknown to the individual."

Bibliography

Anderson CA: Preparing patients for aeromedical transport. Journal of Emergency Nursing 13(4):229–231, 1987

Bishop JH, Klassen TM: Utilizing transfer agreements to create a continuum of care. Provider 15(11):27, 1989

Bodry E, Robins M, Forestier M: Diversional therapy . . . residents in a long-term care facility. Canadian Nurse 86(2):33–35, 1990

Boyd CR, Hungerpiller JC: Patient risk in prehospital transport: Air versus ground. Emergency Care Quarterly 5(4):48–55, 1990

Brent NJ: Referral by facsimile: New headache for home health care. Home Healthcare Nurse 7(6):4–5, 1989

Burns JJ, Fox A, Shelby IL: The survival of the community health nurse in a Medicare environment. Caring 6(4):80–83, 1987

Clews DL: Interhospital transport of the critically ill child. Holistic Nursing Practice 4(1):24–29, 1989

Cook MH: "First come, first served," admissions, key access issues. Provider 13(6):36, 38, 1987

Corkery E: Discharge planning and home health care: What every staff nurse should know. Orthopedic Nursing 8(6):18–27, 1989

Dewing J: What a relief . . . respite care. Nursing Times 86(8):43–45, 1990

Harris MD: The physician connection . . . physicians who refer patients for home care services. Home Healthcare Nurse 7(6):39–41, 1989

Johnson M, Maguire M: Give me a break: Benefits of a caregiver support service. Journal of Gerontological Nursing 15(11):22–26, 1989

LeSage J, Eicher J: Nursing home liaison program. Nursing Administration Quarterly 14(2):50–54, 1990

Loraine K, Grayson R: Plane truths: Flying with your patient. RN Magazine 53(1):40–43, 1990

Nolan MR: Addressing the needs of informal carers: A neglected area of nursing practice. J Adv Nurs 14(11):950–961, 1989

Paxton JM: Transport of the surgical neonate. Journal of Perinatal and Neonatal Nursing 3(3):43–49, 1989

Renna R: Caring, courtesy, understanding in critical care units . . . evaluating family/visitor perceptions. Nursing Management 18(8):78–79, 1987

Save time and improve your referrals. Colleague on Call 4(3):4, 1987

Saywell RM Jr, Woods JR, Holmes GL: Reducing the costs of patient transfers. J Nurs Adm 17(7/8):11–19, 1987

Taggert JS: Nursing home-based hospice programs meet community needs. Provider 15(10):58–60, 1989

Tompkins JM: Intrahospital transport of seriously ill or injured children. Pediatric Nursing 16(1):51–53, 1990

Welton JM: Going into business as a Medevac nurse. Am J Nurs 89(12):1639–1641, 1989

12

Promoting Rest and Safety Within the Patient's Environment

Define terms appearing in the glossary.

Describe a comfortable, attractive, and practical room for a patient in terms of space, furniture, personal-care items, decor, temperature, humidity, and ventilation.

List equipment ordinarily found in a patient's room and indicate how each type is used to fit the patient's needs.

Describe the steps in making an unoccupied and occupied bed.

Describe how a patient's privacy can be protected and ways to control noise and odors in a patient's room.

Describe methods to promote sensory stimulation.

List ten items to consider when helping to make a patient's environment safe and discuss common practices that ensure safety in each case.

Explain steps to take when an accident occurs.

List suggested measures for promoting a safe and comfortable environment in selected situations, as described in this chapter.

Summarize suggestions for instructing the patient.

Chapter Outline

Behavioral Objectives
Glossary
Introduction
The Environment
The Patient's Room
Furnishings in the Patient's Room
Modifying the Environment
Sensory Alteration
Ensuring the Patient's Safety
When Accidents Occur
Suggested Measures to Promote a Restful and Safe Environment in Selected Situations
Applicable Nursing Diagnoses
Teaching Suggestions to Promote a Restful and Safe Environment
Bibliography

Skill Procedures

Making an Unoccupied Bed
Making an Occupied Bed
Promoting Sensory Stimulation
Applying a Protective Restraint

Behavioral Objectives

When the content of this chapter has been mastered, the learner will be able to:

Glossary

Accident report A written report that describes an accident or error. Synonym for *incident report*.

Ambulatory Able to walk about, not confined to bed.

Asphyxiation Suffocation caused by lack of oxygen in the blood.

Cross-ventilation The movement of air that occurs as a result of opening windows that face each other on opposite walls of a room or building.

Environment All that surrounds and influences life and development.

Environmental psychologist A psychologist whose specialty is the study of how the environment affects behavior.

Humidity The amount of moisture in the air.

Incident report A written report that describes an accident or error. Synonym for *accident report*.

Protective restraints Devices that limit a person's movement to prevent harm.

Relative humidity The ratio between the amount of moisture in the air and the greatest amount of moisture the air could contain at the same temperature.

Rest A decreased state of activity that results in feeling refreshed.

Safety The protection from injury.

Sensory alteration Difficulty in processing information because of an excess or insufficient amount of stimuli.

Sensory deprivation A state in which a person receives less than optimal amounts of stimuli for well-being.

Sensory overload A state in which a person receives more than optimal stimuli for well-being.

Stimulus A change in the environment sufficient to cause a response. The plural of the word is *stimuli*.

Temperature The measurement of heat.

Ventilation Movement of air.

Introduction

Rest is a decreased state of activity that results in feeling refreshed. This state is in constant fluctuation. A variety of stimuli or emotions can cause a change that people vaguely identify as being tired. Examples of factors that can affect rest include an uncomfortable environment including furnishings, noise, odors, worry, and tension. Conditions that promote rest will be discussed in this chapter.

Safety is the protection from injury. The environment of a patient contains many potential hazards. This chapter also identifies specific hazards and accident prevention measures.

The Environment

The word *environment* refers to all of an individual's natural and man-made surroundings. The environment influences life and human development. When the environment is safe, clean, comfortable, and attractive, it can contribute to a sense of well-being.

The patient's room is the environment in which the nurse carries out the most personal kind of care. The room may be in a hospital, in the home, in a clinic—wherever the person receives care. A unit is an area in a hospital where patients with similar conditions are housed.

Many things in a patient's room or in a hospital unit cannot be changed by the nurse. However, sometimes the nurse can make modifications in the environment that do not involve major alterations. This chapter discusses nursing measures that help make the patient's environment more comfortable, safer, and more pleasant.

The Patient's Room

All individuals have a need to possess an area they can call their own. The characteristics of that area appear to vary among people. The city dweller may be content within a small efficiency apartment, whereas a farmer may feel a need for a barn and utility buildings on acres of property. Regardless of its characteristics, having and controlling a personal territory contributes to one's self-concept and self-esteem.

It has been observed that people will defend the area they have. Usually, the smaller the area, the more an individual will fight for it. Individuals often zealously claim and guard their seat on a park bench, for example.

The nurse should be aware of the importance of the patient's need for a personal area. Some may even refer to an assigned room as "my room." A person in a nursing home, for example, may feel offended if another sits in his usual chair for meals. Some occupy the same places at planned activities. The nurse shows respect for the patient's feelings by seeing to it that other patients, who may be confused, do not wander into another's room. The nurse should see to it that a person's personal items are not taken, lost, or damaged. What may seem as having little value to the nurse may be extremely valuable to the patient.

Walls and Floors

It is no longer the practice for health agencies to appear bare and sterile. Plain, white walls and imposing equipment are being replaced by more colorful furnishings within a functional decor. Floors and walls are more tastefully decorated. There is a new specialty within the field of psychology. An *environmental psychologist* is a specialist who studies how the environment affects behavior. Information is being accumulated on ways to alter a room and its furnishings to produce a particular mood or feeling. The use of color and design is being used in careful planning of a patient's environment.

Bright and stimulating colors are often annoying. Research indicates that various colors, such as blue and green, promote feelings of coolness and relaxation. These colors are being used to promote well-being in environments, like hospitals, that are associated with anxiety and tension. Most patients prefer a modest, simple decor. Many patients have been disturbed by wall coverings with large and distinct designs because they can create the illusion of faces and other objects. Pictures, bedspreads, and draperies may have the same effect if not selected carefully. Some patients feel dizzy when they look at floor or wall coverings with small designs, parallel lines, or tiny squares. Carpeting is now being used in areas within health agencies. This reduces noise and promotes a more homelike atmosphere.

When health agencies construct new patient care units, nurses are being consulted on their functional design as well as decor. Nurses may provide advice about equipping a patient's room for care in the home. It would be well to consider some of the points about walls and floors already discussed to promote the patient's comfort while still keeping the decorating pleasant.

Lighting

Good lighting, both natural and artificial, is important both to patients and to health workers. Light bulbs, shades, and lamps usually are easily adjusted so that good lighting is generally available. Many health agencies are now being built with large windows or sliding glass doors that can be shaded as needed. In addition to providing much more natural light, they make it pleasant for patients who enjoy looking or being outdoors.

Looking into light, seeing glare from artificial lights, and seeing light reflected from linens may be uncomfortable for patients and workers. In particular, older persons and those wearing glasses are bothered by glaring lights. Often moving furniture a bit and adjusting shades on lights will help to decrease glare.

Although light that brightens the entire room may be best for health workers, it may not be satisfactory for the patient when he wishes to read. A bedside lamp that is adjustable for brightness and for different angles is best.

Most persons prefer that a room be darkened when they rest and sleep. This can usually be accomplished by adjusting shades and draperies and by turning off artificial lights.

At night, a dim light is a valuable comfort and safety measure. Newer hospitals are installing night lights at the base of the floor and in hall areas. These lights illuminate the environment yet do not shine in the patient's eyes.

Humidity, Temperature, and Ventilation

A patient's comfort often depends on regulating environmental factors such as humidity, temperature, and ventilation. *Humidity* is the amount of moisture in the air. *Relative humidity* is the ratio between the amount of moisture in the air and the greatest amount of moisture the air could contain at the same temperature.

Temperature is the measurement of heat. Most people are comfortable in a room maintained in a temperature range of 20°C to 23°C (68°F to 74°F) and a relative humidity of 30% to 60%. Illness may influence the patient's comfort, and he may feel too warm or too cold even when the temperature and humidity are within average normal ranges.

Most health agencies and many homes have air-conditioning units that regulate temperature and humidity. In climates or buildings where humidity is very low, measures that add moisture to the air may be helpful. This may be done with the use of humidifiers or machines that produce steam or a fine mist of water.

Ventilation refers to the movement of air. A room with fresh air is comfortable, but a room with stale air is almost always uncomfortable. Air-conditioning units help keep the air fresh and clean. Windows may be used for ventilation when weather permits. Open windows that face each other but are located on opposite sides of a room or building promote cross-ventilation. *Cross-ventilation* is the movement of air in one opening and out the other. When ventilating rooms, take care to prevent drafts that could circulate microorganisms carried on air currents.

Furnishings in the Patient's Room

Manufacturers of hospital furnishings attempt to combine equipment that is both attractive and serves an utilitarian purpose. The items within a patient's room must be safe, durable, and comfortable.

The Bed

For the convenience of caregivers and patients, most health agencies have adjustable beds, which can be raised and lowered electrically or manually. The height of most beds is kept in a low position so that the patient can get in and out of the bed with less danger of falling.

The head, knees, and foot of the bed can be adjusted for comfort or to maintain a therapeutic position. Hospital beds can be rented or borrowed for patients who need home care. Mechanical beds designed for particular patient needs are discussed in Chapter 18.

The degree of rest is frequently related to the quality of the mattress. Other factors include the cleanliness and smoothness of the linen. Skill Procedure 12-1 describes a method for making an unoccupied bed. An unoccupied bed is made for patients who are ambulatory. An *ambulatory* patient is one who is able to walk and be out of bed. A guide for making an occupied bed can be found in Skill Procedure 12-2. The actions that are described for bedmaking promote good body mechanics and prevent the transmission of bacteria and dust. These practices contribute to the safety of both the nurse and the patient.

The Mattress

A good mattress adjusts to the shape of the body, yet supports it. A mattress that is too soft allows the body to sag and the patient may become uncomfortable and suffer backaches.

The covering of the mattress should be of good quality so that it will not tear or separate easily. Mattresses are not sterilized between patient use. Most health agencies use mattresses with a special waterproof coating. These mattresses can be washed after each patient use. A plastic drawsheet is unnecessary, although mattress pads are still used.

Pillows

Pillows may be filled with various materials and vary in comfort. Foam-rubber pillows are often used by persons who are allergic to kapok, feathers, and other commonly used materials. They are not easily molded, and, therefore, are often difficult to arrange in the most comfortable position for the patient. Also they tend to absorb and retain heat, causing the patient to perspire.

Most persons use pillows under the head for comfort. Nurses also find pillows helpful in aiding the patient to maintain a comfortable position in bed. This is discussed further in Chapter 18.

Pillows are generally not sterilized between patient uses, but it is general practice to protect them in some way. Hospital pillows are made from material that resists dirt and moisture; this is a great help in keeping them clean. Some require a separate cover to protect them. Plastic covers are commonly used. Their disadvantages include

(Text continues on page 223)

Skill Procedure 12-1. Making an Unoccupied Bed

Suggested Action	Reason for Action
Bring a laundry hamper and a clean chair to the bedside.	Having equipment on hand saves energy by avoiding trips to obtain necessary equipment.
Place an adjustable bed in the high position and lower the siderail.	Having the bed in the high position and the siderails down reduces musculoskeletal strain on the nurse.
Remove equipment attached to bed linens and check for personal items the patient may have dropped in the bed, such as a watch or dentures.	Equipment attached to the bed may be lost or ruined if it is accidentally sent to the laundry. It may be costly or impossible to replace lost or broken items.
Starting at the head of the bed, loosen all linen while moving around the bed.	Loosening linens helps prevent tugging and tearing. Moving around the bed while loosening linen reduces strain caused by reaching across the bed.
Remove pillowcases by slipping them off while the pillows lie on the bed.	Not lifting the pillows reduces drafts that may spread organisms and lessens strain on the nurse's arms.
Fold reusable linens, such as blankets, in place on the bed in fourths, and hang them over a clean chair.	Folding saves time and energy when reusable linen is replaced on the bed. Folding linens while they are on the bed reduces strain on the nurse's arms.
Snugly roll all the soiled linen inside the bottom sheet and place it directly into the laundry hamper. Do *not* place it on the floor or on furniture.	Rolling linens snugly and placing them directly into the hamper helps prevent the spread of organisms. The floor is heavily contaminated; soiled linen will further contaminate furniture.
Keep all soiled linen away from the front of the uniform.	The nurse must go from patient to patient. Organisms from soiled laundry may be transferred to the nurse's uniform and could spread disease to the nurse or other patients.
Wash hands thoroughly after stripping a bed and before making a clean bed.	Hands contain organisms from soiled laundry. Hand-washing reduces their transfer to the clean linen.
Bring necessary clean linens to the bedside.	Having linens on hand saves nursing time by preventing unnecessary trips to the linen storage area.
Place linens on a clean chair or on the overbed table in the same order in which they will be placed on the bed.	Having linens in the order in which they will be used saves nursing time.
Place the mattress pad on the bed so that, as it is unfolded, it will be in the proper place.	Opening linens by shaking them causes movement of air. Air currents can carry dust and organisms about the room. If linens were held with the arms extended, the nurse's arms would be strained.
Place the bottom sheet on the bed and unfold it.	Opening linens by shaking them causes air currents that may spread dust and organisms about the room.
Position the bottom sheet with its center fold in the center of the bed and the hem of the sheet even with the lower edge of the mattress. The seam should be on the underneath side.	Positioning the sheets in this manner allows for sufficient fabric to be tucked in at the top and sides of the mattress. Placing the seam underneath prevents the raised edge from irritating the skin of the patient.
Tuck the bottom sheet securely under the head of the mattress on one side of the bed, making a corner according to agency policy. A mitered corner is shown in Figure 12-1.	Having bottom linens free of wrinkles results in a comfortable bed. Making a mitered or square corner makes the bed look neat and prevents linen from becoming loose and wrinkled.
If a waterproof sheet is used, place it over the bottom sheet so that it will be under the patient's chest-to-knee area. Place the cotton drawsheet in the same manner over the waterproof drawsheet.	When a patient soils his bed, drawsheets can be changed without remaking the entire bed.

(continued)

Skill Procedure 12-1. Continued

Suggested Action	**Reason for Action**

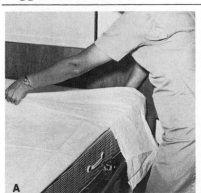 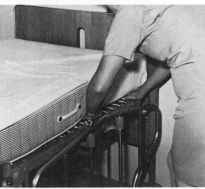 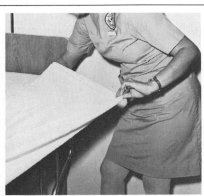

Figure 12-1 (*A*). To make a mitered corner, the nurse folds the sheet back on the bed and holds her right hand to form the corner. (*B*). The nurse tucks the bottom of the sheet, forming the corner under the mattress. (*C*). The nurse places a hand at the side of the mattress to hold the corner in place and with the other hand brings the sheet down over the corner. The nurse is then ready to tuck the entire length of the sheet under the mattress.

When pulling bottom sheets tightly, hold the hands with the palms downward so that pull is produced by the large muscles of the arms and shoulders. Bend the knees. Spread the feet as though to walk backward and rock back so that the weight of the body helps produce the force needed, as illustrated in Figure 12-2.

The longest and strongest muscles in the nurse's arms are at work in this position. Bending the knees and spreading the feet produce a wide base of support. Rocking backward uses the body's weight as a force. The nurse uses the body efficiently throughout these movements to reduce the effort of work.

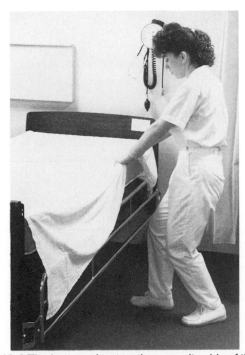

Figure 12-2 The bottom sheet on the opposite side of the bed is already tucked in securely. Note the position of the nurse as the sheet is pulled tightly before tucking it under the mattress. The nurse faces the work area. The feet are separated, and the knees are flexed. The sheet is grasped with the palms of the hands held downward.

(*continued*)

Skill Procedure 12-1. Continued

Suggested Action	Reason for Action
Tuck the linens from the bottom sheet, the waterproof sheet, and the drawsheet under the mattress. Move to the other side of the bed and do the same.	Making the bed on one side and then completing the other side saves time.
Place the top sheet on the bed with its center fold in the center of the bed and with the top of the sheet placed so that the hem is even with the head of the mattress.	Opening linens by shaking them spreads organisms and dust on air currents.
Make a toe pleat by making a small horizontal or vertical fold in the top sheet near the bottom of the bed, as shown in Figure 12-3, or slightly gather the linen before tucking it under the mattress. Place the blanket and the spread about 20 cm (8 in) from the top of the bed in the same manner as the top sheet.	Providing room for the patient's feet prevents top linens from forcing the patient's feet into an uncomfortable position.

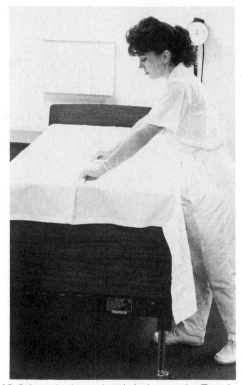

Figure 12-3 A vertical toe pleat is being made. For a horizontal toe pleat, the nurse would fold the top sheet so that the pleat would lie across the bottom of the bed rather than on the vertical plane.

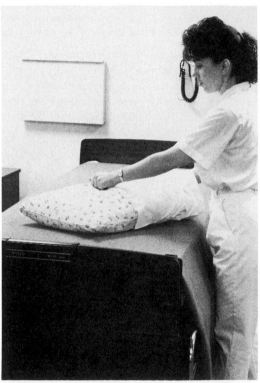

Figure 12-4 The nurse places protectors and cases on a pillow by gathering them first and then sliding them one at a time over the pillow, which rests on the bed.

Tuck top linens, blanket, and the spread securely at the foot of the mattress and make corners according to agency policy.	Securing bed linens without placing pressure on the patient's feet, results in a bed that is comfortable.
Turn the top of the sheet down over the spread and blanket.	Folding the sheet over the blanket and spread protects the patient's chin and face from irritation.
Place the pillow on the bed. Unfold the pillowcase in the same manner as that used for the other linen. Gather the pillowcase as you would gather hosiery, and slip the case over the pillow, as illustrated in Figure 12-4.	Opening linens by shaking them causes organisms and dust to be carried about on air currents. Covering the pillow while it rests on the bed reduces strain on the nurse's arms.

(continued)

Skill Procedure 12-1. Continued

Suggested Action	**Reason for Action**
Place the pillow at the head of the bed with the open end away from the door and the seam of the pillowcase toward the top of the bed.	The enclosed end of the pillow presents a neat and tidy view of the patient's room. The seam can create a source of pressure and discomfort as the patient lies in bed.
Fanfold or piefold the top linens, as illustrated in Figure 12-5, to the lower part of the bed.	Having linens folded to the bottom of the bed makes it more convenient for the patient to get into the bed.

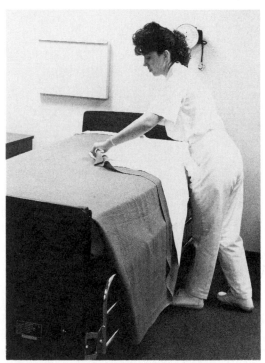

Figure 12-5 The nurse "piefolds" the top linen.

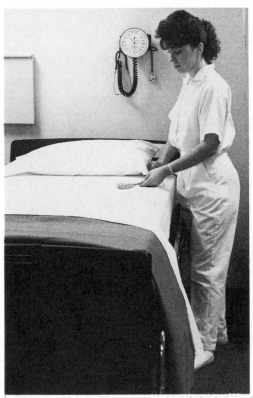

Figure 12-6 The nurse attaches the signal device to the bottom bed linen.

Secure the signal device on the bed according to agency policy, as shown in Figure 12-6.	Having the signal device handy for the patient makes it possible for him to call for assistance as necessary.
Adjust the bed to the low position.	Having the bed in the low position makes it easier and safer for the patient to get into bed.

being slippery and hot. The patient is always welcome to bring his own pillow from home if that would provide more comfort. The nurse should take care to identify and safeguard it from loss.

The Overbed Table

Overbed tables are conveniently used by patients for eating, reading, writing, and performing personal hygiene. They can also be used to support the patient in a forward-leaning position (Fig. 12-9). Health practitioners also find overbed tables convenient for holding equipment used for some procedures. Most overbed tables are designed so

that they can be lowered for the patient while he is in a chair. There is often a portion of the table that can be tilted and will support a book or newspaper. Some have mirrors that are convenient for the patient to use when combing hair, shaving, or applying makeup.

The Bedside Stand

A bedside stand is used for storing the patient's personal-care items. Although stands may vary among health agencies, certain features are handy for both patients and health personnel. The patient can handle the stand with greater ease when it is mounted on wheels. A drawer in the stand

Skill Procedure 12-2. Making an Occupied Bed

Suggested Action	Reason for Action
Elevate the height of the bed.	To avoid back strain, the patient should be at waist level to the nurse.
Cover the patient with a bath blanket and remove the top bed linen.	A bath blanket provides warmth and prevents exposure while the soiled linen is removed and the bed is remade.
Help the patient to the far side of the bed, where a siderail is in position. Loosen the bottom linens opposite the patient, roll them toward the patient, and tuck them as close to the patient as possible, as illustrated in Figure 12-7.	With the patient on the far side of the bed, the nurse is able to make half of the bed (bottom linens only). Rolling linen together with the cleaner side of the linens to the outside helps to prevent spreading organisms.

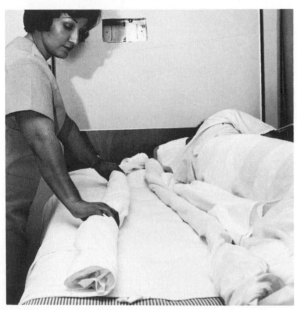

Figure 12-7 The nurse has the siderail in place so that the patient will not fall from the bed. The soiled linen is rolled close to the patient. The nurse has secured the bottom linen under the mattress and will roll all of it close to the soiled linen.

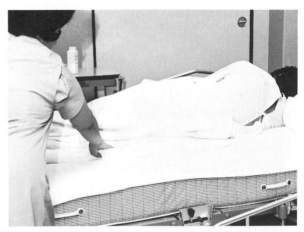

Figure 12-8 The far siderail is up. After assisting the patient over the rolls of clean and soiled linen and removing the soiled linen, the nurse pulls the clean linen toward her.

Place a clean bottom sheet on the bed. Unfold it in place. Tuck the sheet under the mattress securely on the side opposite the patient. Fanfold the sheet and place it near the rolled-up linen at the patient's back. Unfold the drawsheet in place and tuck it securely under the mattress. Place the siderail in position on the side where you are working.	Opening linens by shaking them causes drafts that could spread organisms. Having linens free of wrinkles results in a more comfortable bed.
Help the patient to roll over all linens to the clean side of the bed.	The nurse is now able to make the second half of the bed, bottom linens only.
Move to the opposite side of the bed and lower the siderail. Loosen soiled linens and continue to roll them together and place them in the hamper. Keep linens away from the uniform.	Avoiding stretching across the bed helps to prevent straining muscles. Keeping soiled linens rolled together and away from the uniform helps to prevent spreading organisms.
Pull the clean bottom sheet into place, as illustrated in Figure 12-8. Tuck it under the mattress. Do the same with the drawsheet. Be sure that linens are pulled and tucked firmly and securely.	Having linens free of wrinkles and well secured under the mattress results in a more comfortable bed.

(continued)

Skill Procedure 12-2. Continued

Suggested Action	Reason for Action
Assist the patient to the middle of the bed and onto his back. Place the top linens in place and make the remainder of the bed. Remove the bath blanket and fold it in place on the bed. Change pillow linens. Arrange the pillows comfortably for the patient. Put up the side-rails as indicated.	

Note: Some agencies recommend that both bottom and top linens be arranged before the patient is assisted to that side of the bed where bottom linen is clean. Follow agency procedure.

usually is used for the patient's personal possessions. The inside of the stand is used for the storage of items such as a washbasin, oral hygiene equipment, soap dish, bedpan, urinal, bath blanket, and so on. It is an important safety practice to keep the utensils used for elimination clean and separate from other items. This helps to control odors and the transmission of microorganisms present in stool.

Chairs

A straight chair with good arm and back support is comfortable for most patients. For very short patients, a footstool can be placed under the feet. Having chairs without arms available is desirable. For instance, these chairs are

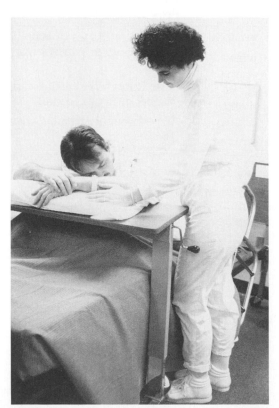

Figure 12-9 This patient is made comfortable by being supported on the overbed table in a forward-leaning position. The patient often welcomes this position after lying in bed.

more suitable when patients must be lifted out of bed and into chairs, because there are no arms to get in the way of those who are lifting.

Upholstered chairs are often very comfortable but are not practical for patients who find it difficult to raise themselves out of them. Elderly patients and those with limited movement usually find upholstered chairs difficult to use.

Personal-Care Supplies

The following items are basic supplies needed for giving personal care:

- Bedpan
- Drinking glass
- Emesis basin
- Mouthwash cup
- Soap dish
- Wash basin
- Water container
- Urinal.

Disposable personal-care items are in common use. Glass breaks easily; metal is noisy when handled; and enamel chips, making it hard to keep clean. Reusable items are cleaned and sterilized before being supplied to another patient as described in Chapter 16.

Most patients bring combs, brushes, shaving equipment, toothbrushes, and toothpaste with them when they are hospitalized. In some agencies, kits containing these items are available.

Diversional Items

Most health agencies have television sets and telephones for the use of patients. Although these items offer patients diversion and convenience, the nurse will wish to remember that they can also be hazardous in the room. Wiring on the floor, loose plugs, frayed cords, and television stands in doorways are some of the dangers they can present.

The patient may bring diversional items to health agencies when admitted, such as handicraft work and books. If a patient brings an electrical item, such as a tape player or radio, the same precautions mentioned above should be used. Also, the nurse should check agency policy concerning which types of electrical items are allowed.

Modifying the Environment

It is easy for health personnel who work each day in the same environment to be unaware of things that may be offensive to a patient. Some factors may be controlled, making the patient's stay in a health agency more comfortable.

Controlling Noise

Many patients complain of noises that often seem to be a part of every health agency. Much money and effort have gone into the design of buildings and into the use of carpeting, draperies, and acoustic ceilings to help reduce noise. Yet, many patients are disturbed by the hospital's noisy environment. Two of the most common complaints from patients are that staff allow telephones to ring and that they speak loudly when conversing on the phone. Patients and visitors find frivolous chatting and laughing by personnel difficult to accept and consider it an annoyance.

Controlling Odors

Illness tends to alter the sense of smell and may make mild odors that are usually pleasant become disagreeable. For example, the smell of food cooking is pleasant for a well person but may cause nausea in an ill person. There are various air deodorants on the market, but in general they seem to do little more than substitute one odor for another. However, they are frequently the only help when odors are hard to control and ventilation is insufficient. Removing soiled articles and opening privacy curtains may help to reduce odors in the patient's immediate area. The nurse should avoid using highly scented colognes or cosmetics. It is important for the nurse to be clean and free of offensive body odor.

Providing Privacy

Anyone who is being interviewed, examined, or cared for has the right to privacy. The nurse will want to remember that certain legal problems may develop when the patient's privacy is invaded, as Chapter 6 described. Patients also enjoy privacy when they have visitors. If a procedure, which may be embarrassing to the patient, cannot wait to be performed, visitors should be shown where they may wait until the care is finished. If the patient requests that a family member remain while the care is given, his wish should be respected. It is a thoughtful gesture to notify visitors or family, who have momentarily left a patient's room, when the care has been completed. Table 12-1 offers suggestions to help control noise and odors and provide privacy.

Table 12-1. Suggestions to Control Noise and Odors and Providing Privacy

Controlling Noise	Controlling Odors	Providing Privacy
Handle equipment as carefully as possible. Dropping articles and bumping things cause unpleasant noises.	Discard waste and refuse promptly.	Use cubicle drapes or screens when caring for patients who share rooms.
Handle dishes, silverware, and trays to prevent rattling them about.	Remove old flowers and stagnant water promptly.	Close doors when giving care to patients in private rooms.
Answer the telephone promptly and speak in a normal tone of voice.	Empty bedpans, urinals, and emesis basins promptly and clean them properly.	Drape patients carefully when giving care.
Avoid calling down corridors; go to people to whom you wish to speak.	Remove leftover food from rooms promptly.	Allow the patient privacy when using the bedpan or urinal, if it is safe to leave the patient.
Avoid laughing and social chatting in corridors and patient lounges.	Remember that patients find it offensive to receive care from nurses who are in need of deodorant, whose perfume is strong, or who have been smoking recently.	Knock before opening a closed door. Identify your presence outside the privacy curtains.
Limit reporting about patients to the nurses' station and conference rooms. In addition to causing noise, overheard conversations may be misinterpreted by patients.		Help visitors find the patients they wish to visit so that they do not enter a stranger's room.
Try to keep television sets and radios at a low volume. Remind patients courteously to keep the volume low. Have them use ear receivers if possible.		

Sensory Alteration

There may come a point at which environmental stimuli, or the lack of it, become harmful to a patient. A *stimulus* (plural is *stimuli*) is a change in the environment sufficient to cause a response. For example, an unexpected, loud noise is a stimulus that may cause a person to respond with fear. Stimuli are received through various senses (*i.e.,* sight, hearing, touch, smell, and taste).

When normal stimuli are absent or decreased, when their quality is poor, or when they are above normal in amount, well-being suffers. The person may experience a *sensory alteration*. This means a person is experiencing an excessive or insufficient stimulation, making it difficult to process information appropriately. Patients in hospitals and nursing homes are especially at risk for this. Patients typically show signs of loneliness and a variety of unusual states, such as fear and panic, depression, inability to concentrate, and boredom when sensory alteration is present.

Nurses use two additional terms when speaking of sensory alteration. *Sensory deprivation* is receiving less than optimal amounts of good-quality stimuli for the person's well-being. This includes monotonous or repetitive stimuli; the stimuli are present, but lack the variety to be noticed. *Sensory overload* means receiving more than optimal amounts of stimuli for well-being. Interestingly enough, the signs are similar when the patient suffers from either too many or too few stimuli over a period of time.

The most desirable amount of stimuli for well-being varies among people. For example, the noise in a crowded disco is tolerated well by some, while others find the noise intolerable. Also, the quiet and the slow pace of country living may be uncomfortable for the city dweller who is used to noise and bustle.

Knowledge of sensory alteration has implications for nursing. The actions described in Skill Procedure 12-3 suggest ways and reasons for promoting sensory stimulation in a health agency or the home. With experience, the nurse will find still other measures for helping to prevent sensory alteration. Efforts to adjust stimuli within a patient's environment are evidence of quality nursing care.

Ensuring the Patient's Safety

It will never be possible to prevent accidents completely. However, there are ways that injuries can be reduced. The nurse must take various safety precautions to limit the potential for accidents that may harm patients.

Signaling for Assistance

Health agencies use a signal system so that patients can call for assistance. A device, usually with a push button, is placed on the bed near the patient. It may be attached to the bed linen with a clasp. When the patient pushes the button, a light or bell signals the nurse. Some devices have an attachment that, when activated, sounds a loud buzzer, indicating that an emergency exists and help is needed immediately. Some health agencies use intercom systems for patients to communicate with the nurse. Signal devices are usually placed in bathrooms, lounge areas, and other places where patients gather.

It is very important to make certain that a signal device is convenient for the patient's use and that it is in working order. Nursing personnel must respond to the patient's signal promptly. Health practitioners can be held negligent when accidents occur because a patient cannot reach his signal device or does not know how to use it, or if the signal is ignored.

In the home, a bell placed at the patient's bedside can be used. Individuals with health problems who are at home should have a telephone within easy reach so that they can call for help if necessary. Some communities use the emergency assistance number, 911, which is easily remembered and can be dialed quickly. There are phones that dial specific numbers, such as the ambulance or fire department, automatically.

Identifying the Patient Accurately

It is important to check the patient's identification bracelet before giving nursing care, so that treatments and medications are not given to the wrong patient. As important as an identification bracelet is, the nurse should also ask an unfamiliar patient to state his name before giving care. A very ill, hard-of-hearing, or confused patient may respond even if the nurse calls him by the wrong name. Asking the patient to state his name is particularly important when caring for patients in clinics, nursing homes, and in home care, where identification bracelets may not be used. Legal problems may be very serious when health practitioners confuse one patient for another.

Using Restraints Safely

Protective restraints are devices that limit a person's movement to prevent harm. Movement is essential to life. Restricting movement can cause injury to the patient. The nurse who makes a decision to use a restraint also has some serious responsibilities to protect the well-being of the patient. Generally, if a patient becomes so restless or irrational that he may harm himself, other patients, or staff members, a temporary restraint may be necessary. Observe the following guidelines when applying restraints:

- Restrain someone only when there is no other means of preventing harm.
- Use the least restrictive type of restraint that will still protect the patient. Soft restraints, made from fabric like the one illustrated in Figure 12-10, are preferable to leather ones.
- Apply the restraint for the shortest amount of time

Skill Procedure 12-3. Promoting Sensory Stimulation

Suggested Action	Reason for Action
Move the bed to various places in the room. Rearrange the furniture and change the draperies occasionally. Use items such as pictures, flowers, and plants to vary what the patient sees.	Any stimulus becomes monotonous if it is not changed periodically.
Change the location of the patient so that he may look out windows that provide a change of scenery.	Changing the scenery and the activity in an area prevents boredom.
Encourage family members and friends to visit the patient as much as possible within the policies of the health agency.	A change in the faces and voices of people breaks monotony.
Encourage the patient to call relatives and friends when face-to-face visits are not possible. Some communities offer Dial-A-Friend services, which motivate shut-ins to make telephone contact.	The phone can be a substitute for personal visits. It helps stimulate individuals and provides a way to check on their safety.
Speak to the patient. Make conversation about what is happening in the world or community.	Giving explanations about nursing care is not enough in itself to prevent sensory alteration.
For the patient who is unconscious, tune and change radio stations and talk to the patient during the day.	An unconscious patient may still hear. Stimulating him through this sense may help the person gain consciousness.
Vary sounds as much as possible, especially when the patient must listen to the continuous sound of equipment.	Changing the position of equipment, even slightly, often changes its sound and adds some variety.
Encourage as much physical activity as permissible. Help the patient leave his room for visits to lounges or the lobby.	This increases the variety of stimulation a patient experiences.
Use touch appropriately and frequently. For example, give a backrub or hold the patient's hand.	Touch is a means for both communication and sensory stimulation.
Encourage the use of leisure-time activities. Provide reading and handicraft materials as alternatives to television and radio.	Using more than one sensory organ at a time, or varying its pattern of use, may divert the patient's interest to something new.
Be sure patients using eyeglasses or hearing aids have them available. Read to patients whose sight is limited or absent. Provide books, magazines, and calendars with large print for those with poor vision.	The nurse must make special efforts to compensate for those who have limitations of their sensory organs.
Help the patient to be aware of the time and date. Place a clock and a calendar in his room.	Patients who are not necessarily confused may lose track of the time and date if they lack the usual reminders.
Offer a variety of foods that provide different flavors, temperatures, and textures.	Varying the sensations associated with taste can provide another source of stimulation.
Relieve discomfort and sleeplessness as much as possible, using the nursing actions discussed in Chapter 10.	Prolonged pain and fatigue can contribute to an inability to interpret and respond to stimuli appropriately.

necessary. The vest restraint in Figure 12-11 may only be necessary while a patient is sitting in a wheelchair.

• Provide for as much movement as possible, even though the patient may need to be restrained. The waist restraint in Figure 12-12 protects the patient from falling or crawling out of bed, but still allows the patient to change his position independently.

• Restrain the fewest limbs or body parts possible. But,

if leg restraints are necessary, use wrist restraints also, as illustrated in Figure 12-13. If this is not done, the patient may remove the leg restraints or become accidentally hung by his heels in the restraints.

• Tie the restraint with a knot that is not likely to come loose, yet can be easily released by the nurse in an emergency. A half-bow knot, illustrated in Figure 12-14, meets these criteria.

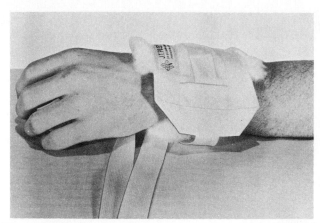

Figure 12-10 This type of restraint may be used for the ankle or wrist. It is soft and padded to prevent injury to the patient's skin. (Courtesy of the JT Posey Company, Arcadia, CA.)

- Fasten restraints in an area where the patient cannot reach the knot or buckle used to secure the restraint.
- Fasten restraints to the bed frame, which is more stable than the siderails.

Skill Procedure 12-4 describes suggested actions for applying a protective restraint.

Preventing Falls

Falls are among the most frequent causes of accidents for people of all ages. It has been estimated that three fourths of accidents in hospitals result from falls. Most falls are due to slipping, sliding, fainting, tripping or falling from a bed, wheelchair, toilet or commode. Display 12-1 identifies risk factors in accidental falls.

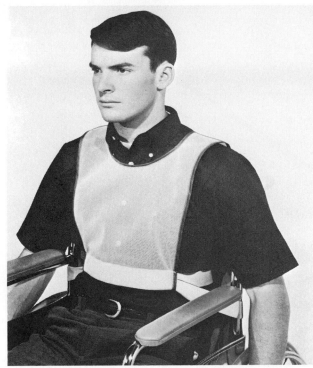

Figure 12-11 A restraining vest prevents the patient from leaving the wheelchair and helps support him. The waist belt on this restraint adjusts to fit the size of the patient without restricting his breathing. (Courtesy of the JT Posey Company, Arcadia, CA.)

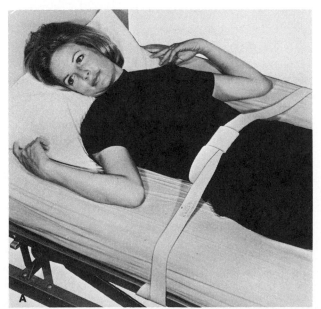 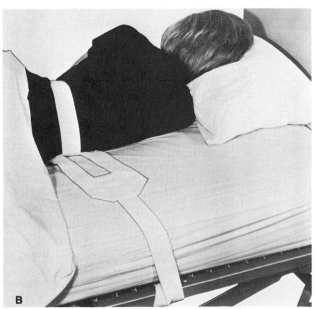

Figure 12-12 (*A*). This waist restraint is effective for keeping the patient in bed, while still allowing her to turn from side to side. (*B*). This safety roll belt allows freedom to roll but not to fall from the bed. (Courtesy of the JT Posey Company, Arcadia, CA.)

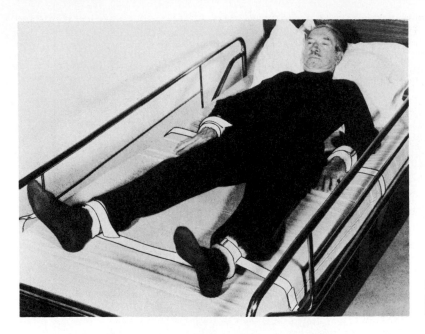

Figure 12-13 Limb restraints are applied to this patient's arms and legs. (Courtesy of the JT Posey Company, Arcadia, CA.)

Siderails on the bed help prevent patients from falling out of bed. Most health agencies have policies stating that siderails are to be up at all times except when care is being given. Patients sometimes ask that siderails be removed. Half or three-quarter siderails may be an acceptable alter-

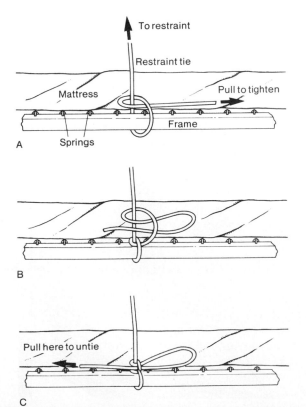

Figure 12-14 Follow this sequence for tying a half-bow knot. The knot will remain secure until the free end is pulled. It is a safe knot that can be quickly released.

native to the patient. An explanation of why the siderails are there will often result in gaining the patient's cooperation. If the patient continues to refuse to have the siderails raised on his bed, most health agencies require that he sign a release. However, obtaining a signed release does not relieve the nursing staff from maintaining the safety of the patient.

Sometimes visitors ask to have siderails down. They may say they will watch the patient. It should be remembered that the nurse, not the visitor, is responsible for the patient's safety. Therefore, extreme caution must be used before leaving siderails down.

Preventing Electrical Injuries

Health agencies and homes today contain a great variety of electrical equipment that can be extremely dangerous if used improperly. The danger of accidents from electrical shocks and from fires is always present unless precautions are taken.

Preventing Fires

Despite fire regulations and the use of fire-retardant material, hospital fires still occur. Figure 12-15 shows the causes of fires that occur in health-care facilities. Smoking accounts for the majority of fires in which there have been deaths, injuries, and property damage. Besides banning smoking for obvious health reasons, health agencies that have enacted no-smoking policies for patients, visitors, and staff may also reduce the incidence of fires.

One of the best ways to prevent deaths and injuries is to practice fire safety. Health agencies have regular fire drills so that all health workers know exactly what to do. When a fire occurs, the nurse should:

Skill Procedure 12-4. Applying a Protective Restraint

Suggested Action	Reason for Action
Assess the patient's behavior and his ability to co-operate.	Using a restraint is only justified if a patient presents potential harm to himself or others.
Obtain a written order from a physician for a restraint if the patient requires protection. A nurse should follow agency policy about the use of a restraint in an emergency.	Applying a restraint without just cause or a medical order could result in being sued for false imprisonment or battery. Consulting the doctor or a nursing supervisor helps substantiate that using a restraint is the most reasonable action to protect the patient.
Approach the patient slowly and calmly. Speak in a soft and controlled voice. Use the patient's name and make eye contact.	Some patients who need to be restrained are agitated and may become combative if they feel threatened.
Explain the reasons for needing the restraint. The patient should be reassured that use of the restraint will be discontinued when the possibility for harm no longer exists.	Even a confused patient may be able to understand some of the information. Since the nurse cannot evaluate the level of the patient's comprehension, an explanation is always in order.
Assess the skin and any other body part that will be affected by the restraint.	It is important to document any existing condition or subsequent alteration that may be related to the use of a restraint.
Protect any bony points or fragile skin that may be injured by a restraint.	The nurse has a responsibility to reduce or prevent unnecessary injury.
Position the patient comfortably and schedule position changes at least every 2 hours.	Complications due to immobility may develop if the patient's position is not changed at frequent intervals.
Apply the restraint following the guidelines already discussed. Make sure the restraint does not interfere with breathing or circulation.	The nurse must see that the device used to protect the patient does not itself become a source of harm.
Help the patient use a toilet, bedpan, or urinal at regular intervals. Feed a patient who must remain restrained at meals.	Restrained patients must depend on health personnel to take care of their basic needs.
Reassess the patient's ability to breathe and the circulation to the hands or feet as frequently as every 2 hours or as often as the agency's policy specifies.	The nurse is responsible for determining that the restraints are applied safely.
Objectively record a description of the patient's prior behavior and his physical and emotional response to the application of the restraint.	The record should show the reasons for the initial and continued use of a restraint.
Notify the patient's family that restraints have been necessary for the patient's protection.	The use of restraints is often misunderstood. Communication promotes understanding and cooperation.
Schedule, release, and document the removal of the restraints every 2 hours. Describe the condition of the skin, skin care, exercise of the restrained limbs, and the patient's behavior.	Restraints should only be used for the amount of time in which there is a potential for harm. The nurse is held accountable for preventing injuries that can be caused by the use of restraints.

- Evacuate the people in the room with the fire.
- Close the door to the room with the fire.
- Notify the switchboard using the proper code and location of the fire. Do not hang up until the operator repeats the information.
- Close all patient room doors and fire doors.
- Turn off oxygen in the vicinity of the fire. Use a manual resuscitation mask for patients who need continuous ventilation.

- Place moist towels or bath blankets at the threshold of doors where smoke is leaking.
- Use the appropriate fire extinguisher described in Table 12-2 if the fire is minor.

A shortened version of these steps may be remembered more easily using the term RACE. It comes recommended by the National Fire Protection Association. The letters

---

Display 12-1. Risk Factors for Accidental Falls

- Advancing age
- Impaired mobility
- Confusion
- Diarrhea or urinary frequency
- Impaired vision
- Sedating medication
- Postural hypotension
- Weakened state

---

stand for R—Rescue, A—Alarm, C—Confine (the fire), E—Extinguish.

When using a fire extinguisher, the nurse should:

- Free the extinguisher from its enclosure.
- Remove the pin that locks the handle.
- Aim the nozzle near the edge, not the center, of the fire.
- Move the nozzle from side to side.
- Avoid skin contact with the contents of the fire extinguisher.
- Return the extinguisher to the maintenance department for replacement or refilling.

Preventing Poisoning

Poisoning is a threat to the hospitalized patient because there are many poisonous substances in a hospital environment. Special precautions need to be observed, particularly in relation to various chemicals, such as those used for cleaning purposes. Safety associated with the administration of medications is discussed in Chapter 23.

Preventing Scalds and Burns

A hospital environment exposes some patients to the potential for scalds and burns. Equipment that provides heat as a therapeutic agent creates the possibility for hazards and injuries of this nature. Ill persons often become unable to handle items that they previously used with ease, such as hot coffee, tea, and soup. Many agencies have thermostats to regulate the temperature of hot water from taps. This precaution has helped reduce burns that have been caused when patients or personnel have carelessly used very hot water for baths and showers.

Preventing Drowning and Asphyxiation

Asphyxiation means suffocation because of lack of oxygen. Dangers of drowning and asphyxiation are relatively minimal among healthy persons, but they are a threat for many ill patients, especially those bathing in tubs without supervision.

Preventing the Spread of Infections

Chapters 16 and 17 discuss ways to prevent the spread of microorganisms. Observing practices presented in those chapters means a safer environment for everyone.

Table 12-3 offers more suggestions on helping to provide a safe environment for the patient as well as for health practitioners.

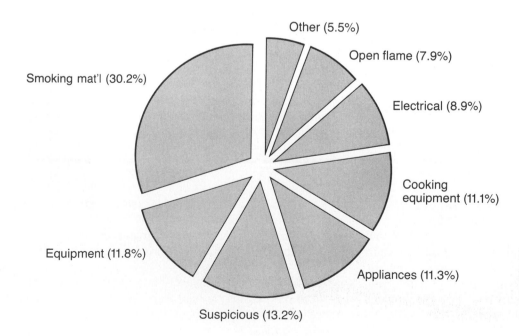

Other (5.5%)
Open flame (7.9%)
Electrical (8.9%)
Cooking equipment (11.1%)
Appliances (11.3%)
Suspicious (13.2%)
Equipment (11.8%)
Smoking mat'l (30.2%)

Figure 12-15 Smoking is the leading cause of fires in health-care facilities. Percentages are based on statistics prepared by the National Fire Protection Association, Quincy, MA 02269.

Table 12-2. Types of Fire Extinguishers

Type	Contents	Use
Class A	Water under pressure	Burning paper, wood, cloth
Class B	Carbon dioxide	Fires caused by gasoline, oil, paint, cooking fats, and other flammable liquids
Class C	Dry chemicals	Electrical fires
Class ABC (combination extinguisher)	Graphite	Fires of any kind

When Accidents Occur

Unfortunately, accidents occur despite efforts to prevent them. Human errors are sometimes made. In addition to possible harm to the patient, serious legal problems can be caused by accidents. Therefore, it is especially important to handle each accident with great care. The following steps are recommended when an accident occurs:

Check the patient's condition immediately. Note his condition and be ready to describe it accurately.

Call for help to assist you. For example, seek help in the event of a fall. Help is almost always necessary to move a patient so that injuries are not made worse.

Do *not* move a patient who has fallen until it is considered safe to do so. If a bone has been broken, moving the patient without proper support may cause further injury to bone and surrounding tissues.

Report the accident to the proper person promptly. Usually this is the supervising nurse, who will then notify the physician.

Comfort and reassure the patient. Explain that help is available and proper care will be taken. Indicate concern for the patient who is in discomfort. Experience has shown it is particularly important to maintain a helping nurse-patient relationship whenever an accident occurs. Feelings expressed by the patient, such as anger and fear, can be handled best when the

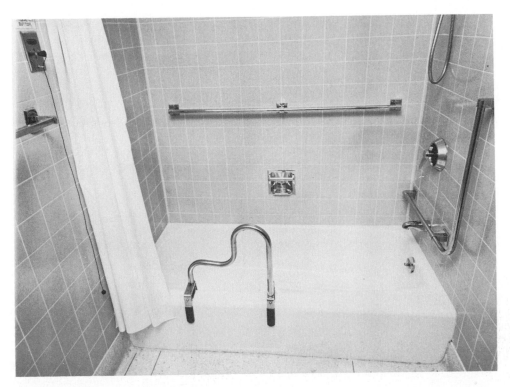

Figure 12-16 This photo illustrates several safety features. The support on the side of the tub helps the patient get in and out of the tub; several hand bars provide extra support; a mixer-type faucet controls water temperature; nonskid strips are affixed to the bottom of the tub; and a call cord is conveniently placed next to the tub.

Table 12-3. Dos and Don'ts for Providing a Safe Environment

Do	Don't
Helping to Prevent Falls Place adjustable beds in the low position when patients are getting in and out of bed. Use nonskid mats or strips in tubs and showers to prevent the patient from falling on slippery shower floors and bathtubs. Use tub and shower stools and sturdy handrails in bathrooms. Figure 12-16 illustrates several bathtub safety features. Have patients in wheelchairs use wide doorways, ramps, and elevators so that they are not tempted to try to walk stairs.	Do not use equipment and supplies for anything but their intended purposes. For example, chairs are dangerous step stools! Do not allow patients to use floppy, high-heeled, soft, or loose-fitting shoes when walking. The patient should wear good walking shoes with low heels to help prevent falling. Do not allow items such as books, magazines, handicrafts, shoes, and so on to be placed on floors and stairways. Litter on floors and stairways can easily cause tripping and falls. Do not leave spilled liquids on the floor. Mop or wipe up promptly. Also, see to it that signs are posted and warn patients and visitors when floors are wet and slippery after being scrubbed. Do not use throw rugs that slip easily or rugs that are torn or curled at the edges. Throw rugs are hazardous.
Helping to Prevent Electrical Injuries Use plugs and outlets with a ground when possible. These plugs have three prongs and will fit only into outlets with three-prong receivers. Remove a plug from a wall socket by grasping the plug. Pulling on the cord to remove the plug may damage both the plug and the wire. Use equipment for its intended purpose only. Using a hot plate, for example, is a dangerous way to warm a chilly room. Keep all electrical equipment in good working order and in good repair. Keep television sets, telephones, radios, hair dryers, and so on away from bathtubs and sinks.	Do not stand in water or wear wet shoes and then handle electrical equipment. Water conducts electricity. Do not kink cords. The fine electrical wires inside a cord may break. Do not use frayed or broken electrical cords or overload an electrical outlet. Overheating may occur and cause a fire. Do not use an appliance that overheats, produces a shock, or gives off an odor while being used. Never use faulty pieces of equipment. Test electrical equipment before use.
Helping to Prevent Fires Know where there are emergency exits. Know where fire extinguishers are kept and how to use them. Know the agency's policy and plan for fire and evacuation of patients. Remember that oxygen supports combustion. The smallest flame or a live cigarette can become a torch in the presence of concentrated oxygen. When a patient is receiving oxygen as part of his treatment, be sure the patient, his visitors, and his roommates know of the fire dangers. Post signs to show that oxygen is in use and that smoking is prohibited. Be sure smoking regulations are enforced. When patients and visitors are allowed to smoke, provide safe ashtrays, preferably ones from which a burning cigarette cannot fall. Many fires have started when wastebaskets were used for ashtrays.	Do not allow a confused, sleepy, or drugged patient to smoke unattended. Stay with the patient if he wants to smoke and take care of the cigarette for him when he has finished. Keeping cigarettes and matches out of his reach will prevent his using them when alone. Do not store materials saturated with solutions that could lead to spontaneous combustion unless they are in an airtight metal container. Certain cleaning solutions and acetone are offenders in this regard.

(continued)

Table 12-3. Continued

Do	Don't
Helping to Prevent Poisoning	Do not remove poisonous substances from their original containers and place them in another container. A poisonous substance may be mistaken for something entirely different because of the appearance of a container that ordinarily contains nonpoisonous contents. For example, poisonous cleaning solutions have been mistakenly drunk when the solution has been placed in a soft-drink bottle.
Be sure you know where emergency instructions on how to handle poisoning are posted in the health agency where you study or work. Having these instructions handy in the home is also important.	
Be sure that poisonous substances are conspicuously labeled.	
Put poisonous substances away immediately after use and store them where patients cannot get at them.	Do not place medications anyplace except where they are normally stored. Chapter 23 discusses further safety precautions when handling medications.
Helping to Prevent Scalds and Burns	Do not add hot water to a tub in which a patient is bathing without agitating it as you add the hot water. The patient may be burned by hot water that is not being mixed with the cooler water.
Place hot liquids, such as coffee and tea, in a place that is convenient for the patient. The nurse should plan to help a patient if he is unable to handle liquids safely on his own.	
Check the temperature of water being used by patients in tubs and showers. This is especially important if there is any doubt about whether the patient can safely regulate the temperature of water.	Do not use hot-water bags and heating pads without checking agency policy. Many agencies do not allow their use because of the danger of burning patients. Hot-water bags and heating pads are discussed further in Chapter 20.
Helping to Prevent Drowning and Asphyxiation	Do not leave a patient while he is in a bathtub if there is any danger of drowning.
When helping a patient eat, offer small bites of food and give him sufficient time between mouthfuls to chew food well. Offer fluids carefully also, especially if the patient must remain flat on his back or has trouble swallowing.	
	Do not leave a patient to feed himself if he requires help.
Use dentures for patients if available. Have food pureed or coarsely ground for those who lack teeth or can't chew.	Never "prop" a bottle for an infant and leave him unattended during feeding.
Place an unconscious patient on his side or abdomen.	

patient is helped to feel that personnel are sorry that the accident occurred, that care will be provided for him, and that prompt measures will be taken to prevent future accidents.

Do not offer explanations if you were not involved with the accident or without authorization to do so. It is best to consult a supervising nurse about explanations when an accident occurs.

Be *sure* to record exactly what happened in the patient's record after you have finished caring for the patient. The patient's record is discussed in Chapter 5.

After the patient is properly cared for and the physician has been notified, prepare an *incident* or *accident report*. All information related to the accident is entered on the form (Fig. 12-17), which is signed by those persons designated on the form.

These guidelines apply when any accident occurs within the health agency, regardless of the type (*e.g.,* errors in giving medication or a fall from a bed). Accident reports may be required even if visitors or personnel are injured. This form does not become part of the patient's permanent record; it is used to examine the circumstances surrounding the accident and prevent future accidents of a similar nature.

Suggested Measures to Promote a Comfortable and Safe Environment in Selected Situations

When the Patient Is an Infant or Child

Use mobiles over an infant's crib to add variety to the environment. Use objects that are safe for the infant who is able to grasp things in his hands.

Take into account that young infants respond best to colors with a high contrast, such as black and

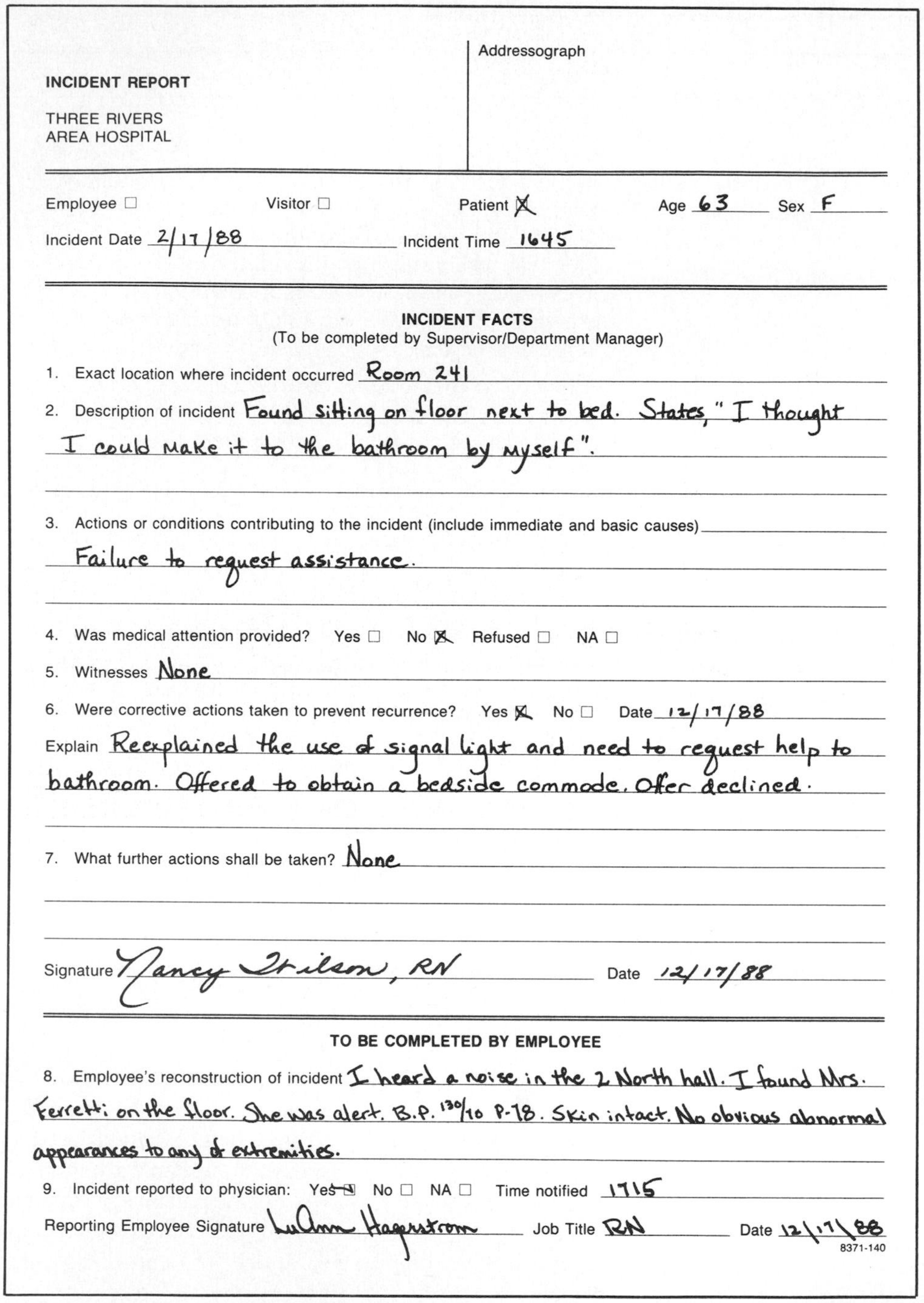

INCIDENT REPORT

THREE RIVERS
AREA HOSPITAL

Addressograph

Employee ☐   Visitor ☐   Patient ☒   Age _63_ Sex _F_

Incident Date _2/17/88_   Incident Time _1645_

INCIDENT FACTS
(To be completed by Supervisor/Department Manager)

1. Exact location where incident occurred _Room 241_

2. Description of incident _Found sitting on floor next to bed. States, "I thought I could make it to the bathroom by myself"._

3. Actions or conditions contributing to the incident (include immediate and basic causes) _Failure to request assistance._

4. Was medical attention provided?   Yes ☐   No ☒   Refused ☐   NA ☐

5. Witnesses _None_

6. Were corrective actions taken to prevent recurrence?   Yes ☒   No ☐   Date _12/17/88_

Explain _Reexplained the use of signal light and need to request help to bathroom. Offered to obtain a bedside commode. Offer declined._

7. What further actions shall be taken? _None_

Signature _Nancy Wilson, RN_   Date _12/17/88_

TO BE COMPLETED BY EMPLOYEE

8. Employee's reconstruction of incident _I heard a noise in the 2 North hall. I found Mrs. Ferretti on the floor. She was alert. B.P. 130/70 P-78. Skin intact. No obvious abnormal appearances to any of extremities._

9. Incident reported to physician: Yes ☒ No ☐ NA ☐   Time notified _1715_

Reporting Employee Signature _LuAnn Hagerstrom_   Job Title _RN_   Date _12/17/88_

8371-140

Figure 12-17 This is an example of an incident of accident report form. (Courtesy of Three Rivers Area Hospital, Three Rivers, MI.)

---

white. Older infants appear to prefer cool colors, such as blue and green. By the time they are toddlers, children like brilliant colors, such as red and yellow. These findings have resulted from studies that looked at the effects of environmental factors in stimulating development.

Keep small objects away from children, who frequently place them in their mouths and may choke. Examples include safety pins, marbles, small balls, and broken pieces from toys. Check stuffed animals for parts that may come off. For ex-

ample, the eyes on stuffed animals may be dangerous if they can be removed.

Fasten plastic sheeting *well* on a young child's bed. Keep plastic bags away from units housing children. Accidents from suffocation have occurred when a child's face has accidentally become covered with plastic material.

Keep crib sides up except when caring for an infant or young child. Keep a hand securely on a child when the siderails are lowered. Also, secure youngsters in highchairs to prevent their falling.

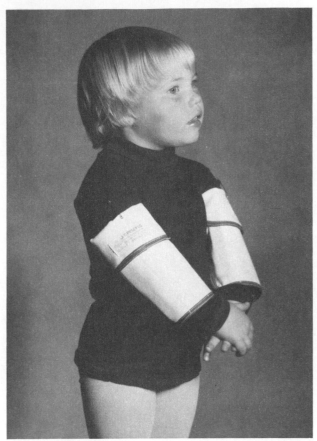

Figure 12-19 These elbow restraints have ties that may be fastened to the child's clothing. (Courtesy of the JT Posey Company, Arcadia, CA.)

Use restraints judiciously, as described earlier in this chapter. Various types are available for youngsters, such as a crib net, a bubble top, a control jacket, and a papoose or restraining board. Several additional ones are illustrated in Figures 12-18 through 12-20.

Explain to the child when he is old enough to understand, as well as to his parents, why restraints are needed.

Use safe and sturdy furniture and equipment for children. Be sure windows are well secured, electrical equipment is out of reach, and unused electrical outlets are covered. Serious shocks and even

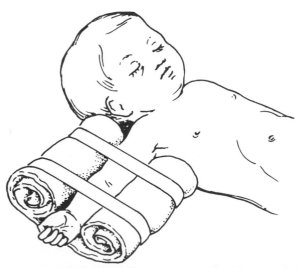

Figure 12-18 This sketch illustrates a method for restraining an infant's arm. The restraint is made with a diaper and secured with pieces of tape.

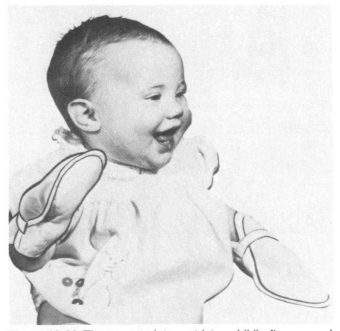

Figure 12-20 These restraints restrict a child's fingers and hands without restraining arm movements. They are particularly useful when a child scratches or picks. (Courtesy of the JT Posey Company, Arcadia, CA.)

NURSING CARE PLAN

12-1. High Risk for Trauma

Assessment

Subjective Data

States, "I'm afraid of falling. I've had some near misses at home since my last surgery. I get dizzy when I get to hurrying and my feet get all tangled up."

Objective Data

62-year-old man admitted for treatment of pneumonia. Difference of 20 mm of mercury in systolic pressure between lying and standing (135/85 lying; 115/80 standing). Fractured hip repaired following a fall during prior hospitalization for eye surgery. Wears eyeglasses at all times while awake. Has a walker but does not consistently use it. Takes a daily diuretic.

Diagnosis

High Risk for Trauma related to dizziness and impaired mobility.

Plan

Goal

The patient will ask for assistance when getting in and out of bed and will use his walker consistently while ambulating throughout hospitalization.

Orders: 7/5

1. Assess BP lying and standing daily @ 0800.
2. Use full siderails and keep the bed in low position.
3. Reinforce the need to use the call signal.
4. Assist to a sitting position until dizziness passes before standing.
5. Keep walker within reach at all times.
6. Help to put on nonskid slippers and glasses for ambulation. _____ B. JOYNER, RN

Implementation (Documentation)

7/6

0800   Full siderails up with bed in low position. BP 138/82 on R. arm while lying and 125/78 while sitting. Sat for 3 minutes on edge of bed. States, "I don't feel dizzy this morning. It usually hits me in the afternoon after my water pill kicks in." Helped with nonskid sneakers. _____ J. BUTLER, SN

Evaluation (Documentation)

0830   Tried to walk from bed to bathroom without using walker. Instructed to use the walker at all times. Location of call light in the bathroom identified. Said, "I hate having to depend on you." _____ J. BUTLER, SN

---

death have occurred when children have placed things, such as items made of metal, into an electrical outlet.

Know where every child is at all times. Children who play together in hospital rooms should be under adult supervision.

Group together children with similar degrees of illness. For example, grouping children who are convalescing from illness often provides them with good company for one another.

Keep the environment as flexible as possible so that children who are not acutely ill can be near friends and watch activity. These measures help prevent loneliness and sensory deprivation.

Never leave a child alone in a bathtub because of the danger of drowning.

Recommend gate guards or half-doors to close off the nursing work area, utility room, and medication room from curious children.

Remember that youngsters also have a need for their own personal area. Personal playthings are very important to a child. A place should be provided for playthings and none should ever be thrown away without consulting the child or his parents.

Expect that a child's room is not likely to be as tidy as an adult's room. Use large containers that will give the child easy access to toys and will provide ample storage space, thus promoting neatness.

When the Patient Is Helpless

Seek ways to provide a safe calling device for a helpless patient, such as one who is paralyzed. Several devices are available to help patients who cannot use a typical push button to call for assistance. One type has a plastic tube that is placed near the patient's mouth; when the patient puffs air into the tubing, the call system is activated. Another type has a switch in a large sponge and can be activated when slight pressure is made on it by any part of the body. Still another uses a highly sensitive touch plate.

Check a helpless patient at frequent intervals to be sure that he is not in danger.

When the Patient Is Elderly

Expect that the effects of being in a strange environment develop more quickly in an elderly person than in a young adult. The effects include confusion, disorientation, and anxiety. These observations illustrate the decreased ability of the elderly to adapt to change.

Take into account that older persons generally prefer a warmer room and usually are more sensitive to drafts than are young people.

In addition to a night light, provide an elderly patient with a flashlight, as indicated, to help orientation at night. Also, placing fluorescent tape at light switches and on doorknobs helps the patient orient himself to his environment.

Allow elderly persons to keep personal items close to them, even on their bed, if the items present no danger. Examples include eyeglasses, a purse, a sweater, or a blanket or pillow of their own. Familiar items close at hand help the elderly feel more secure and comfortable in a strange environment.

Be especially alert to sensory alteration among elderly persons. They tend to show the effects of sensory overload and sensory deprivation relatively quickly.

Teaching Suggestions to Promote a Comfortable and Safe Environment

The alert nurse will find many opportunities to teach patients how to prevent accidents. Safety measures apply to the home as well as to a health agency.

The nurse may teach by setting a good example. When care is given and the nurse expresses concern and interest in safety measures, patients will learn. Also, the patient is quick to realize when a nurse is not observing safety measures and will soon lose confidence.

The nurse has teaching opportunities when a family is preparing to set up a room for the home care of a patient. Safety and convenience are important, but so are the physical and psychological comforts an environment can offer when properly adapted to meet a person's needs.

Bibliography

Blakeslee JA: Speaking out: Untie the elderly. Am J Nurs 88(6):833–834, 1988

Burden B, Kishi D: Patient falls: Lowering the risk. Nursing 19(4):79, 1989

Collins HL: Who'd survive a fire on your unit. RN Magazine 51(7):32–36, 1988

Cushing M: Finding fault when patients fall. Am J Nurs 89(6):808–809, 1989

Daley I, Goldman L: A closer look at institutional accidents. Geriatr Nurs 8(2):64–67, 1987

Dallaire LB, Burke EV: A new program for reducing patient falls. Nursing 19(1):65, 1989

Easterling ML: Which of your patients is headed for a fall? RN Magazine 53(1):56–59, 1990

Garcia RM, Cruz M, Reed M: Relationship between falls and patient attempts to satisfy elimination needs. Nursing Management 19(7):80V–80X, 1988

Horrow JC: Electrical safety. Current Reviews in Respiratory and Critical Care 9(5):34–40, 1986

Huey FL: Price of no restraints. Geriatr Nurs 11(2):57, 1990

Jones WJ, Smith A: Preventing hospital incidents . . . what we can really do. Nursing Management 20(9):58–60, 1989

Kids and small objects: A dangerous combination. Patient Care 24(3):128, 131, 1989

Masters R, Mark SF: The use of restraints. Rehabilitation Nursing 15(1):22–25, 1990

Mohler G: Falls: Can they be prevented? Are restraints the only solution? Nursing Homes 36(4):24–26, 1987

Orey WJ: Is your fire prevention equipment really ready? Nursing Homes 36(2):28–32, 1987

Parsons MT, Levy J: Nursing process in injury prevention. Journal of Gerontological Nursing 13(7):36–40, 1987

Stutts AT: Fire: Critical issues. Nursing Homes 36(4):42–45, 1987

Tieaski L: Preventing falls. Journal of Practical Nursing 39(4):32–35, 1989

Ullman KV: Points to remember when fire strikes and life is a priority. Provider 12(10):51, 1986

Weinstein SA, Gantz NM, Pelletier C: Bacterial surface contamination of patients' linen: Isolation precautions versus standard care. Am J Infect Control 17(5):264–267, 1989

Weisiger KE: Making your patient safe at home. RN Magazine 50(2):59–60, 1987

Wheden MB, Shedd P: Prediction and prevention of patient falls. Image: The Journal of Nursing Scholarship 21(2):108–114, 1989

13

Obtaining Vital Signs

Chapter Outline

Behavioral Objectives
Glossary
Introduction
Body Temperature
The Pulse
Respirations
Blood Pressure
Frequency of Obtaining Vital Signs
Recording the Vital Signs
Suggested Measures to Obtain Vital Signs in Selected
    Situations
Applicable Nursing Diagnoses
Teaching Suggestions to Obtain Vital Signs
Bibliography

Skill Procedures

Cleaning a Glass Thermometer
Measuring Body Temperature Using a Glass
    Thermometer
Assessing Body Temperature Using an
    Electronic Thermometer
Assessing the Radial Pulse
Counting the Respiratory Rate
Measuring the Blood Pressure

Behavioral Objectives

When the content of this chapter has been mastered, the learner will be able to:

Define terms appearing in the glossary.
Summarize briefly how the body functions to maintain normal body temperature, pulse and respiratory rates, and blood pressure.
List factors that influence body temperature, pulse and respiratory rates, and blood pressure.
List average normal ranges for persons of various ages for body temperature, pulse and respiratory rates, blood pressures, and pulse pressure.
Describe characteristics of a normal and abnormal temperature, pulse, respirations, and blood pressure.
Describe how the vital signs are obtained, including obtaining body temperature using four different sites, pulse rate using six different sites, and blood pressure using two different sites.
Describe the following pieces of equipment and explain how each is used properly: a glass clinical thermometer, an electronic thermometer, a heat-sensitive thermometer, a tympanic thermometer, a sphygmomanometer, and a stethoscope.
Discuss the frequency with which vital signs are ordinarily obtained from hospitalized patients.
Demonstrate how to document vital signs on the patient's record.
Explain how to clean and disinfect a glass clinical thermometer.
List suggested measures for obtaining the vital signs in selected situations, as discussed in this chapter.
Summarize suggestions for instructing the patient.

Glossary

Apical pulse rate The number of heart beats that occur in one minute as heard over the apex of the heart with a stethoscope.
Apical-radial pulse rate The pulse rate obtained by two persons when one obtains the radial pulse rate while the other obtains the apical rate. Abbreviated A/R.
Apnea A period during which there is no breathing.
Arrhythmia An irregular pattern of heartbeats, and consequently an irregular pulse rhythm. Synonym for *dysrhythmia*.
Arteriosclerosis Loss of elasticity in arterial walls.
Atherosclerosis Narrowing of the inside of arteries due to deposits of fat.
Axilla Armpit.
Axillary temperature A measure of body heat obtained by placing a thermometer in the axilla.
Basal metabolic rate The minimum amount of energy

required to maintain body functions during periods of inactivity. Abbreviated BMR.

Blood pressure The force of blood within the arterial walls.

Bounding or full pulse A pulse that feels full and strong to the touch and is not particularly easy to obliterate with mild pressure.

Bradycardia A heart rate below 60 beats per minute in an adult.

Bradypnea A below-average or slow respiratory rate.

Cardinal signs Measurements of body temperature, pulse and respiratory rates, and blood pressure. Synonym for *vital signs*. Abbreviated VS, CS, or TPR and BP.

Celsius scale The original scale used in the centigrade thermometer.

Celsius thermometer An instrument having 0° for the temperature at which water freezes and 100° for the temperature at which water boils. Synonym for *centigrade thermometer*.

Centigrade thermometer An instrument having 0° for the temperature at which water freezes and 100° for the temperature at which water boils. Synonym for *Celsius thermometer*.

Cheyne-Stokes respirations A gradual increase and then gradual decrease in depth of respirations, followed by a period of apnea.

Constant fever A fever that continues, is consistently elevated, and fluctuates very little.

Crisis A rapid return of an elevated body temperature to normal.

Diaphragmatic respiration Respirations performed primarily by the diaphragm.

Diastole The time during which the heart muscle relaxes.

Diastolic pressure The least amount of pressure present in arteries when the heart muscle is in a state of relaxation.

Dyspnea Difficult and labored breathing.

Dysrhythmia An irregular pattern of heartbeats, and consequently an irregular pulse rhythm. Synonym for *arrhythmia*.

Exhalation The act of breathing out. Synonym for *expiration*.

Expiration The act of breathing out. Synonym for *exhalation*.

External respiration The process of exchanging oxygen and carbon dioxide between the lungs and the blood.

Fahrenheit thermometer An instrument having 32° for the temperature at which water freezes and 212° for the temperature at which water boils.

Febrile Having a fever.

Feeble, weak, or thready pulse Descriptions of abnormal pulse volume that require much effort to feel and are easy to obliterate with pressure.

Fever Above normal body temperature. Synonym for *pyrexia*.

Hypertension An abnormally high blood pressure.

Hyperthermia An abnormally high body temperature.

Hyperventilation Abnormally prolonged, rapid, and deep respirations.

Hypotension An abnormally low blood pressure.

Hypothermia A body temperature that is below the average normal range.

Hypoventilation A condition in which a reduced amount of air enters the lungs.

Inhalation The act of breathing in. Synonym for *inspiration*.

Inspiration The act of breathing in. Synonym for *inhalation*.

Intermittent fever A fever broken by periods of normal or subnormal temperature.

Intermittent pulse Periods of normal pulse rhythm broken by periods of irregular rhythm.

Internal respiration The process of exchanging oxygen and carbon dioxide between the blood and body cells. Synonym for *tissue respiration*.

Invasion The period when fever begins. Synonym for *onset*.

Korotkoff's sounds Sounds heard through a stethoscope while obtaining the blood pressure.

Lysis The gradual return of body temperature to normal.

Meniscus The curved surface at the top of a column of liquid in a tube.

Onset The period when fever begins. Synonym for *invasion*.

Oral temperature A measure of body heat obtained by placing the thermometer in the mouth under the tongue.

Orthopnea A condition in which breathing is easier when the patient is in a sitting or standing position.

Orthostatic hypotension A fall in blood pressure when a person assumes an upright position too quickly. Synonym for *postural hypotension*.

Palpitation Awareness of one's own heartbeat.

Peripheral pulses Those pulse sites, located distant from the heart, which can be assessed with relative ease.

Postural hypotension A fall in blood pressure when a person assumes an upright position too quickly. Synonym for *orthostatic hypotension*.

Premature contraction A pulsation that occurs sooner than has been the previous pattern.

Pulse A wave set up in the walls of the arteries with each beat of the heart.

Pulse deficit The difference between an apical and radial pulse rate.

Pulse pressure The difference between the systolic and the diastolic blood pressure.

Pulse rate The number of pulsations felt per minute.

Pulse rhythm The pattern of the pulsations and the pauses between them.

Pulse volume The quality of the pulsations felt.

Pyrexia Above-normal body temperature. Synonym for *fever*.

Radial pulse rate The pulse rate obtained by placing the fingertips on the radial artery at the wrist.

Rectal temperature A measure of body heat obtained by placing a thermometer in the rectum.

Remittent fever A fever that fluctuates several degrees but does not reach a normal temperature between fluctuations.

Respiration The act of breathing.

Sinus arrhythmia An irregular pulse rhythm characterized by slowing when an individual breathes out and accelerating upon breathing in.

Sphygmomanometer An instrument used to measure the pressure of blood within an artery.

Stertorous respirations A general term referring to noisy breathing

Stethoscope An instrument that carries sounds from the patient's body to the ear of the examiner.

Stridor A harsh, high-pitched sound heard on inspiration in the presence of an obstruction in larger airways, such as the larynx.

Systole The time during which the heart muscle contracts, causing blood to be pumped into the circulation.

Systolic pressure The maximum pressure exerted within arteries when the heart muscle contracts.

Tachycardia An abnormally rapid heart rate, between 100 to 150 beats per minute in an adult.

Tachypnea A respiratory rate that is more rapid than normal.

Thermometer An instrument used to measure the temperature of something; a clinical thermometer measures body temperature.

Thoracic respiration Respirations performed primarily by the intercostal and other thoracic muscles.

Tissue respiration The process of exchanging oxygen and carbon dioxide between the blood and body cells. Synonym for *internal respiration*.

Training effect Slowing of the heart rate, which results from regular, aerobic exercise.

Vital signs Measurements of body temperature, pulse and respiratory rates, and blood pressure. Synonym for *cardinal signs*. Abbreviated VS, CS, or TPR and BP.

Introduction

Changes in the way the body is functioning are often reflected in the body temperature, pulse and respiratory rates, and blood pressure. The body mechanisms that regulate them are very sensitive and respond quickly to changes in health. That is why they are frequently called *vital signs* or *cardinal signs*. They are commonly abbreviated VS, CS, or TPR and BP. Because vital signs serve as important indicators of the patient's condition, obtaining them is serious business—not just a routine task. The trend in the patient's vital signs should be analyzed each time they are taken by comparing the current measurements with those previously obtained.

Body Temperature

Body temperature normally remains within a fairly constant range as a result of a balance between heat production and heat loss. This process is regulated by a thermostatlike arrangement in the brain's hypothalamus. Heat is produced primarily by exercise and by the body's metabolism of food. Heat is lost from the body primarily through the skin, the lungs, and the body's waste products. When more heat is produced than is lost, the body's temperature will be above normal, or elevated. Conversely, when more heat is lost than produced, the body's temperature will be below normal, or subnormal. Figure 13-1 illustrates how heat loss and heat production determine the body's temperature.

The Clinical Thermometer

An instrument used to measure heat is a *thermometer*. A clinical thermometer is used to measure body heat. The thermometer is placed in the mouth to obtain an *oral temperature*. It is placed in the anal canal to obtain a *rectal temperature* and in the *axilla,* or armpit, to obtain an *axillary temperature*.

Body temperature is measured either in degrees of centigrade, abbreviated °C, or in degrees Fahrenheit, abbreviated °F. The *Celsius scale* was the original scale used in the centigrade thermometer. It was named after the man who devised it. Centigrade means a calibrated scale consisting of 100 equal parts. The *Celsius thermometer* or *centigrade thermometer* has a scale at which 0°C is the temperature at which water freezes and 100°C is the tem-

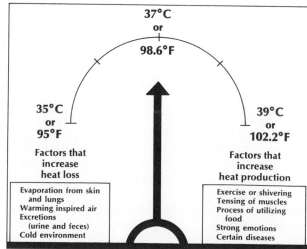

Figure 13-1 This illustrates the balance between factors that increase heat loss and factors that increase heat production.

Table 13-1. Equivalent Centigrade and Fahrenheit Temperatures*

Centigrade	Fahrenheit	Centigrade	Fahrenheit
34.0	93.2	38.5	101.3
35.0	95.0	39.0	102.2
36.0	96.8	40.0	104.0
36.5	97.7	41.0	105.8
37.0	98.6	42.0	107.6
37.5	99.5	43.0	109.4
38.0	100.4	44.0	111.2

*To convert centigrade to Fahrenheit, multiply by 9/5 and add 32. To change Fahrenheit to centigrade, subtract 32 and multiply by 5/9.

perature at which water boils. The Fahrenheit scale is used in the *Fahrenheit thermometer;* water freezes at 32°F and boils at 212°F. Table 13-1 gives comparable centigrade and Fahrenheit temperatures and explains how temperatures can be converted from one system to another.

The Glass Clinical Thermometer. The glass clinical thermometer most commonly used to measure body temperature contains mercury. It has two parts: the bulb and the stem. Mercury is a liquid metal and will expand when exposed to heat, causing it to rise in the stem of the thermometer. The stem is marked in degrees and in tenths of degrees. The range is from about 34°C or 93°F to about 42.2°C or 108°F. Fractions of a degree are recorded in even numbers, as 0.2, 0.4, 0.6, and 0.8. If the mercury appears to reach a bit more or less than an even tenth of a degree, it is usual practice to report the temperature to the nearest tenth. Figure 13-2 illustrates examples of glass clinical thermometers.

An oral thermometer has a long slender mercury bulb that provides a larger surface for contact with tissues under the tongue or in the axilla. A blunt-bulb thermometer is used to obtain a rectal temperature; the shape of the bulb helps prevent injury to or puncture of tissue when it is being inserted. Structurally, the design of the tip of an oral thermometer is weaker than the more uniformly shaped bulb of the rectal thermometer. Considering that an oral thermometer has a greater potential for breaking within the body cavity being measured, it is dangerous to use it for obtaining a rectal temperature.

When using a thermometer in the home or anywhere else, check to see whether it is oral or rectal. Some thermometers have this printed on them, but others do not.

Some authorities recommend that an oral thermometer be used for obtaining an axillary temperature. Others recommend a rectal thermometer. It is best to observe agency policy until there is general agreement about which thermometer is better for obtaining an axillary temperature.

The Electric, or Electronic, Thermometer. There are electric, or electronic, thermometers that measure body temperature in a matter of seconds. They have two temperature probes, one for oral and one for rectal use. Reports in the literature indicate that these thermometers are accurate and their use saves considerable nursing time. Figure 13-3 illustrates an electric thermometer.

Common Factors Influencing Body Temperature

A variety of factors normally influence body temperature.

Age. Newborns, infants, and young children normally have a slightly higher average temperature than that of adults. Elderly people tend to have a slightly lower-than-

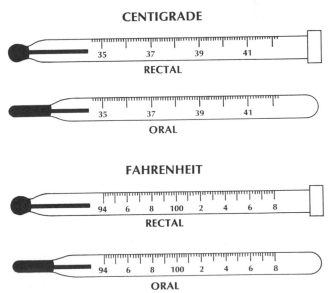

Figure 13-2 The two glass thermometers on the top use the centigrade scale to measure temperature; the two on the bottom use the Fahrenheit scale. Note the blunt bulbs on the rectal thermometers and the long thin bulbs on the oral thermometers.

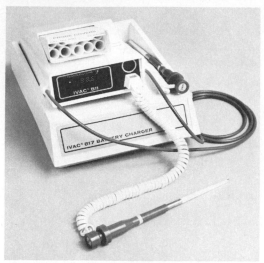

Figure 13-3 The upper portion of this electronic thermometer is portable. When not in use, its batteries are recharged electrically. Disposable probe covers are changed between each patient use. (Photograph courtesy of the IVAC Corporation, San Diego, CA.)

average adult temperature. The body temperatures of infants, young children, and the elderly are often influenced by environmental conditions. For example, the young and the elderly ordinarily require more clothing and bed covers than do young and middle-aged adults to maintain normal body temperature in a cool or cold environment.

Gender. Women demonstrate a slight rise in body temperature of about 0.6°C (1°F), rectally, when ovulating. This is most probably because of hormones that affect metabolism or tissue changes occurring in the body. The temperature returns to normal before menstruation.

Exercise and Activity. The minimum amount of energy required to maintain body functions during periods of inactivity is called the *basal metabolic rate* (BMR). Exercise and activity increase the need for energy. The body responds by increasing the metabolic rate. A byproduct of metabolism is heat production. Certain disease conditions, one being an overactive thyroid gland, can also increase the metabolic rate and, consequently, cause a rise in body temperature.

Time of Day. The vital signs normally fluctuate in circadian rhythm. For example, the body temperature is ordinarily about 0.6°C (1°F) lower in the early morning than in the late afternoon and early evening. This variation, which is considered normal, tends to be somewhat higher in infants and young children. An inversion of this cycle has been observed in persons who routinely work at night and sleep during the day.

Emotions. Persons having strong emotional experiences, such as fear and anger, are likely to have a higher

than average temperature. Conversely, persons experiencing apathy and depression are likely to have a lower than average body temperature.

Illness. A deviation from normal, either above or below normal, is often an indication of a disease process. An elevated temperature is commonly associated with infections and other disease conditions; a lower than average temperature is a characteristic of certain others. Elevated and subnormal temperatures are discussed later in this section.

Normal Body Temperature

The average normal temperatures for well adults in various body sites are as follows:

Temperature Scale	Oral Site	Rectal Site	Axillary Site
C	37.0°	37.5°	36.4°
F	98.6°	99.5°	97.6°

Elevated Body Temperature

An elevated body temperature is called *pyrexia,* or *fever.* A person with a fever is said to be *febrile. Hyperthermia* refers to an abnormally high body temperature.

The following are commonly associated with a fever:

- Pinkish, red (flushed) skin that is warm to touch
- Restlessness or, in others, excessive sleepiness
- Irritability
- Thirst
- Poor appetite
- Glassy eyes and a sensitivity to light
- Increased perspiration
- Headache
- Above-normal pulse and respiratory rates
- Disorientation and confusion (when the temperature is high)
- Convulsions in infants and children (when the temperature is high).

A patient is considered to be in danger when his temperature reaches beyond 41°C (105.8°F). An individual rarely survives when his temperature reaches 43°C (109.4°F).

The *invasion,* or *onset,* is the time when fever begins. It may begin suddenly or gradually. A chill with shivering usually occurs before rapid onset of fever. The skin is pale, due to constriction of small blood vessels in the skin, and the patient may state that he feels cold.

Fever and the manner in which it subsides may take a variety of courses. These courses are described and illustrated in Table 13-2. A fever that recurs following a period of normal body temperature may be a sign of relapse or complications; therefore, temperature should be reported promptly and will need continued frequent checking.

Table 13-2. Courses and Resolutions of Fever

Course or Resolution	Definition	Illustration
Constant fever	A fever that continues, is consistently elevated, and fluctuates very little.	
Remittent fever	A fever that fluctuates several degrees but does not reach a normal temperature between fluctuations.	
Intermittent fever	A fever broken by periods of normal or subnormal temperature.	
Crisis	A rapid return of an elevated body temperature to normal.	
Lysis	A gradual return of an elevated body temperature to normal.	

Subnormal Body Temperature

A body temperature below the average normal range is called *hypothermia.* The following are commonly associated with hypothermia:

- Pale, cool skin
- Listlessness
- Slow pulse and respiratory rates
- Decreased ability to solve problems
- Diminished ability to feel pain or other sensations.

Death usually occurs when the temperature falls below approximately 34°C (93.2°F). However, cases of survival have been reported when body temperature has fallen considerably lower. Sometimes the body temperature is lowered below normal for therapeutic purposes. There are some illnesses in which the patient typically has a subnormal temperature. Therefore, it is important to observe a patient just as closely when the body temperature falls below normal ranges as when it is elevated.

Selecting a Site for Obtaining Body Temperature

Health agency policy guides the nurse in selecting the site at which the body temperature is to be obtained. The oral site is ordinarily used for most persons, although the *axilla,* or armpit, is being recommended more often than it was in the past.

The axillary temperature is an accurate reflection of body temperature when it is obtained correctly. It may be the preferred site for a patient who has had oral surgery or facial injuries.

The following are advantages often cited for obtaining an axillary temperature:

- The axilla is readily accessible in most instances.
- It is a safe site to use.
- There is less danger of spreading microbes when compared with obtaining an oral or rectal temperature.
- Using the axillary site is less disturbing psychologically than using the rectal site for most patients.

For many years, it was believed that a rectal temperature was the most accurate reflection of the body's internal, or core, temperature. The exact placement of the thermometer, a lag in the rectal temperature when blood temperature changes, and the effect of stool in the rectum have been shown to influence the accuracy of a rectal temperature. Hence, the rectal site is probably no better than the oral or axillary route. Some persons are beginning to advocate that the rectal site be used only when the oral and axillary sites cannot be used. Tympanic thermometers described later in this chapter, are considered very accurate.

Further guidelines for selecting the site at which to obtain the body temperature in selected situations are given later in this chapter.

Keeping Clinical Thermometers Clean

Health personnel and health agencies are aware of a responsibility to protect patients from acquiring infections. Use of disposable or individual-use equipment is becoming common. One method adopted by some health agencies is to issue a glass clinical thermometer to each patient on admission. The same thermometer is used throughout the patient's time in the health agency. It is then sent home with him at the time of discharge. Each patient's thermometer is kept in a container at the bedside.

In some agencies, multiple glass thermometers are still issued from a central supply unit. The nurse is not expected to disinfect thermometers in most agencies. They are returned to the central supply unit to be cleaned for reuse. However, nurses should know how to clean and disinfect thermometers, especially when caring for patients in a clinic or office, in a school, or in a patient's home. If a nurse is unsure or questions the sanitary condition of a thermometer, or if there are no services for caring for thermometers between uses, the nurse should follow the suggested actions in Skill Procedure 13-1 for cleaning and disinfecting a glass clinical thermometer.

Thin, flexible, plastic sheaths shown in Figure 13-4 that cover a glass clinical thermometer are available. They are intended to maintain the cleanliness of one thermometer being used on multiple patients. The sheath is applied over the thermometer before insertion and disposed after one use. This decreases the spread of infections and the need for cleaning. However, it has been found that some brands of sheaths may perforate before or with use; other brands are very sturdy. Nurses and individuals who use protective coverings on thermometers should inspect them carefully. The product must be of sufficient quality to keep the thermometer clean in order to control the transmission of microorganisms from one patient to another. Any thermometer that is soiled must be cleaned and disinfected between uses.

Electronic thermometers are generally protected with hard, plastic, disposable probes. A separate probe is applied over the temperature sensor each time another patient's temperature is assessed. The probes can be attached and released without touching the area that is inserted in the patient. This method has also proven satisfactory in maintaining the cleanliness of thermometer equipment and preventing the spread of organisms.

Obtaining the Body Temperature

Skill Procedure 13-2 describes how to use a glass thermometer to obtain the body temperature when using the oral, rectal, and axillary sites. Skill Procedure 13-3 provides guidelines for using an electronic thermometer. As mentioned previously, the performance of all skills should begin and end with handwashing. Patients should always be prepared with proper explanations.

Skill Procedure 13-1. Cleaning a Glass Thermometer

Suggested Action	Reason for Action
Use a soft, clean tissue to wipe the thermometer.	Material on the thermometer interferes with disinfection. Soft material comes into close contact with all surfaces of the thermometer.
Hold the tissue at the stem part of the thermometer near the fingers and wipe down toward the bulb, using a firm twisting movement.	Cleaning from an area where there are few organisms to an area where there are numerous organisms minimizes the spread of organisms to cleaner areas. Friction helps loosen material on the thermometer.
Clean the thermometer with soap or detergent solution, again using friction.	A soap or detergent solution and friction loosen material on the thermometer.
Rinse the thermometer under cold, running water.	Cold water prevents breaking the thermometer. Rinsing helps remove material loosened by washing. Certain chemical solutions are not effective in the presence of soap—benzalkonium chloride is an example.
Dry the thermometer after rinsing it with water.	The strength of the chemical solution is decreased when water is added to the solution.
Place the thermometer in a chemical solution of the agency's choice for the prescribed length of time. Examples of solutions include glutaraldehyde (Cidex) or 90% alcohol.	Heat sufficient to kill organisms will ruin thermometers by causing the mercury to expand beyond the column within the thermometer. Chemical solutions must be used in a proper strength for the recommended time to be effective.
Rinse the thermometer with warm water after disinfecting it and store in a dry place.	Chemical solutions may irritate mucous membranes in the mouth or rectum and the skin in the axilla. Solutions may also have an objectionable taste and odor.
In home situations, it is generally considered safe to wash the thermometer well with soap or detergent and cool water, rinse it well, and then dry it with a clean tissue or cloth.	Family members often share the same types of organisms among themselves. Because these microbes are not strange to their bodies, simple cleansing, following infrequent use of the equipment, may be sufficient to prevent spreading infections.

Alternative Methods for Assessing Temperature

Several new types of thermometers are available. They range from very inexpensive disposable thermometers and limited-use skin devices to technologically advanced continuous monitors and a tympanic thermometer.

Disposable, Single-Use Thermometer. Disposable single-use thermometers are made from plastic strips.

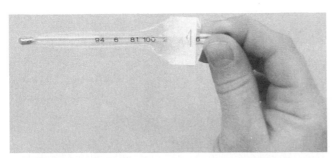

Figure 13-4 A glass thermometer can be covered with a disposable plastic sheath.

They register quickly, usually within 45 seconds. The degree of heat is indicated by a color change correlated with a number on the face of the strip. They are nonbreakable. The danger of cross-infection is eliminated because they are used only once.

Heat-Sensitive Patch or Tape. A temperature measuring patch or tape is commonly applied to the abdomen or forehead. It also changes color at different temperature ranges.

This type of assessment can be used with well infants born at term. Newborns usually are not capable of achieving a fever. In fact, a lower than normal body temperature is more common. Assessment is performed to determine if the infant needs some additional warming measure. Another application is for the layperson who does not have a glass thermometer or who cannot accurately use it. A patch or tape may be used to check a toddler or young child's temperature. It can help a parent, babysitter, or daycare teacher determine if the child needs to be seen by a health-

(Text continues on page 251)

Skill Procedure 13-2. Measuring Body Temperature Using a Glass Thermometer

Suggested Action	**Reason for Action**

Oral Method

Locate the type of thermometer used to measure temperatures in the particular health agency.	Some health agencies use glass clinical thermometers; some use flexible plastic sheaths to cover glass thermometers; some use electric thermometers with disposable probes.
Use a clean glove only in certain circumstances.	Saliva is not considered a body fluid that requires gloves as a barrier for human immune deficiency virus (HIV) unless it contains visible blood. The transmission of other nonbloodborne pathogens, such as pulmonary tuberculosis, can be reduced with the use of gloves.*
If the thermometer has been stored in a chemical solution, rinse it with water and wipe it dry with a firm twisting motion, using a clean, soft tissue.	A chemical solution may produce an objectionable taste or irritate mucous membranes. Soft tissue and a twisting motion help clean the entire surface of the thermometer.
Wipe from the bulb toward the fingers with each tissue.	Wiping from an area where there are few or no organisms to an area where organisms may be present minimizes the spread of organisms to cleaner areas.
Read the thermometer by holding it horizontally near eye level and turning it slowly between the fingers until the mercury line can be seen clearly, as illustrated in Figure 13-5.	Holding the thermometer near eye level makes reading it easier. Turning the thermometer will help to place the mercury line in a position where it can be read best.

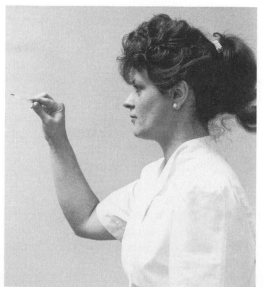

Figure 13-5 The nurse reads the thermometer by holding it near eye level and rotating it until the mercury line is clearly seen.

Grasp the stem of the thermometer firmly between the thumb and forefinger and, with a snapping wrist movement, shake the thermometer until the mercury is well into the bulb end below the lowest markings.	The mercury will not drop below the level of the previous temperature reading unless the thermometer is shaken forcefully.

(continued)

Skill Procedure 13-2. Continued

Suggested Action	**Reason for Action**

Oral Method

Cover the thermometer with a sheath, if that is agency policy.	Coverings promote sanitary conditions. They reduce the need to cleanse the thermometer between uses.
Place the mercury bulb of the thermometer under the patient's tongue and in the right or left posterior pocket at the base of the tongue.	When the bulb rests in a pocket where there is a rich supply of blood, and the mouth is closed, an accurate measurement of body temperature can be obtained.
Instruct the patient to hold the thermometer in place with his lips and to avoid biting it.	Room temperature is lower than body temperature. Unless the thermometer is enclosed within the mouth, the measurement may be inaccurate.
Leave a glass thermometer in place no less than 3 minutes if the patient is not feverish. If the temperature is borderline or elevated above normal, leave it in place for at least 5 minutes.	Allowing optimum placement time ensures accuracy. Optimum placement times are the recommendations from the most recent research conducted by Robinchaud–Ekstrand and Davies (1989).
Remove the thermometer and any plastic sheath that was used on the glass thermometer. Wipe it from the fingers down toward the bulb as shown in Figure 13-6, using a firm twisting motion. Discard tissues in a container for waste.	Mucus on the thermometer may make it difficult to read. Cleaning from an area where there are few organisms to an area where organisms may be abundant minimizes the spread of organisms to cleaner areas. Friction from the twisting motion helps to loosen matter.

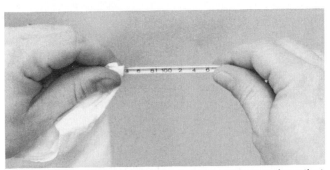

Figure 13-6 A tissue is used to remove oral secretions that could obscure the calibration marks on the thermometer.

Read the level at which the mercury expanded within the thermometer.	The calibrations on the glass thermometer indicate the patient's temperature.
Follow agency policy for handling the thermometer and record the patient's temperature.	Thermometers are generally kept in a certain location so that personnel may find them available when needed. Some nurses record the temperature directly on the patient's chart; others write it on a general sheet to be recorded later by a clerical assistant.

Rectal Method

Prepare the thermometer as suggested in the procedure for obtaining an oral temperature. Use a clean glove only in certain circumstances.	Feces is not considered a body fluid that requires gloves as a barrier for human immune deficiency virus (HIV) unless it contains visible blood. The transmission of other nonbloodborne pathogens, such as infectious diarrhea and Hepatitis A, can be reduced with the use of gloves.*

(continued)

Skill Procedure 13-2. Continued

Suggested Action	Reason for Action

Rectal Method

Suggested Action	Reason for Action
Place lubricant on a paper tissue and lubricate the lower tip over about a 2.5 cm (1 in) length.	Placing lubricant on a tissue prevents contaminating the lubricant supply. Lubricant reduces friction and helps to insert the thermometer, thereby minimizing irritation or injury of the mucous membrane in the anal canal.
Provide privacy around the bed.	The patient's body should be protected from the view of others.
With the patient on his side, fold back bed linens and separate the buttocks so that the anal opening is seen clearly.	If the thermometer is not placed directly into the anal opening, the bulb may injure tissue. Separating the buttocks well makes the anal opening easy to see.
While instructing the patient to breathe deeply, insert the thermometer about a distance of 3.5 cm (1½ in) in an adult. Do not use force to advance the thermometer.	Breathing deeply promotes relaxation of the round sphincter muscle in the anus and rectum. The thermometer may injure rectal tissue if force is applied.
Permit the buttocks to fall into place. Hold onto the thermometer. Leave a glass thermometer inserted 2 to 3 minutes.	Maintaining a hold on the thermometer will prevent it from being expelled before the temperature is recorded.
Remove the thermometer and wipe it as described earlier so that the numbers may be observed. Dispose of any sheaths or probe covers.	Fecal material and lubricant on the thermometer make it difficult to read.
Wipe away any excess lubricant or stool from the patient. Assist him to a comfortable position.	The patient is apt to feel soiled and uncomfortable if lubricant and residue of stool remain at the anus.
Care for equipment and record the temperature as agency policy directs.	Glass rectal thermometers are usually kept separate from oral thermometers to prevent accidentally mixing their use.

Axillary Method

Suggested Action	Reason for Action
Prepare the thermometer as suggested in the procedure for obtaining an oral temperature.	
Follow agency policy concerning whether to use a rectal or an oral thermometer.	Most often an oral thermometer is used for maximum contact with skin folds.
Place the bulb of the thermometer well into the axilla. Bring the patient's arm down close to his body and place the forearm over the chest toward the opposite shoulder, as illustrated in Figure 13-7. Stay with the patient so that the thermometer remains properly placed.	When the bulb rests against the superficial blood vessels in the axilla and skin surfaces are brought closely together to reduce air surrounding the bulb, an accurate measurement of body temperature can be obtained.
Leave the thermometer in place for at least 10 minutes, or longer.	Allowing sufficient time for the thermometer to reach its highest temperature results in an accurate measurement of body temperature.

(continued)

Skill Procedure 13-2. Continued

Suggested Action	**Reason for Action**

Axillary Method

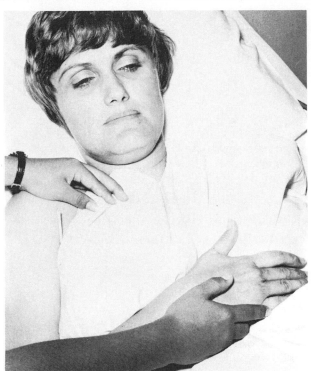

Figure 13-7 Note the position of the thermometer, well down into the axillary space. Bringing the patient's arm across her chest helps keep axillary tissue in good contact with the thermometer.

Follow agency policy regarding care of thermometer equipment and recording the patient's temperature.

---

*Update: Universal precautions for prevention of transmission of human immunodeficiency virus, hepatitis B, and other bloodborne pathogens in health-care settings. MMWR 37(24):378, 1988

---

care provider. Heat-sensitive tapes and patches can be reused several times. An example of a heat-sensing strip is shown in Figure 13-9.

Heat-sensitive patches or tapes are not as accurate as other assessment methods. They should be used clinically only when agency policy is being followed. If the results of the recording do not correlate with accompanying signs and symptoms, another more reliable assessment technique should be used.

Continuous-Monitoring Devices. Continuous-monitoring devices are used primarily in critical care areas. Probes may be inserted within the rectum or esophagus. They display continuous data on the patient's temperature. They are frequently used when a patient has

experienced extreme levels of hypo- or hyperthermia. Warming or cooling blankets are usually used at the same time. The assessment aids in evaluating the effectiveness of these devices.

Tympanic Thermometer. A noninvasive device to assess body temperature at the ear has been developed. A hand held probe is placed within the ear opening. It uses an infrared sensor to detect the temperature of the blood flowing through the eardrum. The blood that passes through this area is en route to the hypothalamus, the temperature-regulating center in the brain. For this reason, temperature assessed in this manner is said to be even more reliable than oral or rectal temperatures. The measured temperature is displayed on the screen of the elec-

Skill Procedure 13-3. Assessing Body Temperature using an Electronic Thermometer

Suggested Action	Reason for Action
Explain the procedure to the patient.	An explanation encourages cooperation and reduces apprehension.
Gather the following equipment: electronic unit, thermometer probe, probe cover, pencil or pen, paper or flow sheet. Lubricant and soft tissues will be needed if using a rectal route.	Organization contributes to efficient time management.
Use a clean glove only in certain circumstances.	Feces and saliva are not considered body fluids requiring gloves as a barrier for human immune deficiency virus (HIV) or hepatitis B virus (HBV) unless they contain visible blood. The transmission of other nonblood-borne pathogens, such as infectious diarrhea or pulmonary tuberculosis, can be reduced with the use of gloves.*
Wash your hands.	Handwashing deters the spread of microorganisms.
Remove the electronic unit from the charging area.	Charging maintains battery power for portable use.
Select the oral or rectal probe depending on which route is appropriate.	Probes should not be used interchangeably for oral and rectal assessment.
Attach a disposable cover over the probe.	Covering the probe prevents the transmission of organisms when the same equipment is used for several patients.
Place the covered probe beneath the tongue on the right or left side of the mouth.	Accuracy is improved with the thermometer placed on either side rather than under the middle of the tongue.
If using the rectal site, insert the lubricated rectal probe (using donned glove if needed) as described in Skill Procedure 13-2.	Positioning, lubrication, and insertion principles remain the same for an electronic thermometer as for one made of glass.
Hold the probe in place, as shown in Figure 13-8.	An unsupported probe tends to fall away from its location after insertion, making the measurement less reliable.

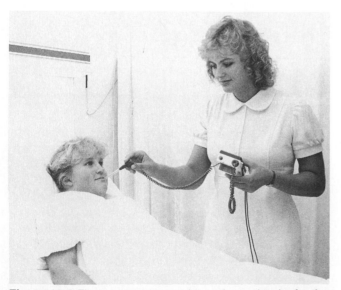

Figure 13-8 The nurse supports the probe and waits for the audible signal indicating that the patient's temperature has been measured.

(continued)

Skill Procedure 13-3. Continued

Suggested Action	Reason for Action
Maintain the thermometer probe in position until an audible sound occurs in 15–30 seconds.	A sound indicates that there are no further significant changes in the temperature.
Remove the probe from the patient's mouth or rectum. Note the numbers displayed on the electronic unit.	Leaving an electronic thermometer beyond the sound will not significantly change the accuracy of the reading.
Wipe lubricant from the rectum with soft tissues.	Removing lubricant and feces is a comfort and hygiene measure.
Release the probe cover while holding it over a lined receptacle, such as a wastebasket. If a glove was used, pull it off inside out.	This action prevents contact with surfaces that contain the patient's organisms.
Return the probe to its storage location within the electronic unit.	The probe is protected from becoming lost or broken if it is transported and stored together with the electronic unit.
Wash your hands.	Handwashing reduces the spread of microorganisms to other patients and to the nurse.
Report any abnormal findings to the appropriate person.	Additional action may be necessary based upon the validation and evaluation of the data.
Return the electronic unit, and reconnect it to a power source.	Equipment that is needed for other patients on a unit should be maintained for immediate use.
Record the temperature on the assessment, flow, or graphic sheet as indicated by agency policy.	The trend in recorded temperatures is used to identify nursing diagnoses, medical, and collaborative problems.

*Update: Universal precautions for prevention of transmission of human immunodeficiency virus, hepatitis B, and other bloodborne pathogens in health-care settings. MMWR 37(24):378, 1988

tronic unit. The use of a tympanic thermometer is demonstrated in Figure 13-10.

Research has shown this type of assessment to be very accurate. Time is saved in busy emergency rooms and other areas of the hospital because it can register body temperature in only 2 seconds. It is especially useful for critically ill patients, infants, and children because it can be used without rousing the patient, which interrupts sleep cycles. Toddlers are more likely to accept this route than a rectal one because it is noninvasive and quick. Infection rates are reduced because the ear does not contain mucous membrane and accompanying secretions.

The Pulse

Each time the heart beats, it forces blood into the aorta and then into smaller arteries. This causes the arterial walls to expand and distend. It produces a wave that can be felt as a light tap by the fingertips. This sensation is called the *pulse*.

Normal Pulse Rates

The *pulse rate* is the number of pulsations that occur in a minute. Normal pulse rates vary at different ages in life. Some common rates are listed in Table 13-3

Common Factors That Influence Pulse Rates. A variety of factors can influence pulse rate.

Age. Pulse rate varies with age. It is relatively rapid at birth and gradually diminishes from birth to adulthood. It tends to be increased above the average adult's pulse rate in old age. For example, the approximate average pulse rate of an adult is 80, but an elderly person may exhibit a pulse rate that tends to be higher than this.

Time of Day. As is true of body temperature, the pulse rate is lowest in the morning on awakening and increases later in the day.

Gender. On awakening in the morning, the pulse rate of the average man is approximately 60 to 65 beats per minute. The rate for women is slightly faster, by about 7 to 8 beats per minute, than for men.

Body Build. Tall, slender persons usually have a slower pulse rate than do short, stout persons.

Exercise and Activity. The pulse rate increases with exercise and activity. This reflects the heart's effort to increase blood circulation and oxygen distribution necessary for proper cell functioning. However, with regular aerobic exercise, a *training effect* can be observed. This means that the heart can adequately supply cells with

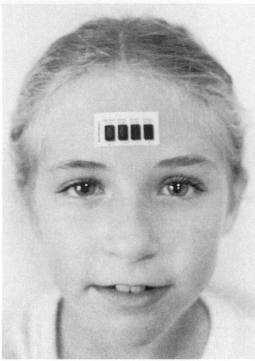

Figure 13-9 A self-adhesive thermometer has been applied to this child's forehead. Liquid crystals change color as the temperature changes. Although the calibration is not as precise as other thermometers, this method is easy to use for a quick assessment.

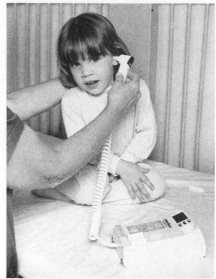

Figure 13-10 This child's temperature is being measured with a tympanic thermometer.

oxygenated blood with fewer beats. Those who are physically fit exhibit a slower pulse rate even during exercise.

Stress and Emotions. Stress increases the pulse rate. When a person is experiencing strong emotions, such as anger, fear, and excitement, the pulse quickens. Pain, which is stressful especially when it is moderate to severe, can trigger a faster heart rate.

Body Temperature. The body's need for energy is influenced by the body temperature. The body temperature may change due to illness, disease, or exposure to an environment that is either hot or cold. When body temperature is elevated the pulse rate increases to supply nutrients and oxygen to cells. When body temperature is low, cells have reduced requirements. The heart will not need to work as rapidly to meet the cells' needs; the pulse rate will be slower.

Blood Volume and Components. Excessive blood loss causes the pulse rate to increase. When there are decreased red blood cells or inadequate hemoglobin to distribute oxygen to cells, the heart rate accelerates in an effort to keep cells supplied.

Drugs. Certain drugs influence the heart rate. Some are intended to restore an abnormal rate to one that is normal. For example, digitalis preparations typically slow the heart rate. Sedatives slow the heart rate though they are given to promote rest. Caffeine and nicotine increase the heart rate.

Abnormally Rapid Pulse Rates

An abnormally rapid pulse rate is called *tachycardia*. An adult has tachycardia when the pulse rate is 100 to 150 beats per minute. The condition is usually a compensatory mechanism and occurs when there is a need to improve or increase blood circulation to the body's cells. Pulse rates can occur at rates higher than 150 beats per minute; very rapid heart rates may not oxygenate cells adequately. They may overwork the heart if sustained for very long.

The term *palpitation* means that the person is aware of his own pulse rate without having to feel for it over an artery. The pulse rate is ordinarily unduly rapid when palpitations are noted.

Abnormally Slow Pulse Rates

The term used to describe the pulse rate when it falls below 60 beats per minute in an adult is called *bradycardia*. A slow pulse rate during illness is less common than a rapid pulse rate, but, when present, bradycardia should be

Table 13-3. Normal Pulse Rates per Minute at Various Ages

Age	Approximate Range	Approximate Average
Newborn	120–160	140
1–12 months	80–140	120
1–2 years	80–130	110
3–6 years	75–120	100
7–12 years	75–110	95
Adolescence	60–100	80
Adulthood	60–100	80

reported promptly. The following are conditions in which bradycardia is likely to be present:

- In heart block, when the atria may beat at one rate while the ventricles beat at a slower rate.
- When the brain has increased pressure.
- In athletes whose heart muscles have become well developed and efficient.
- In patients who are developing a toxicity to the medication digitalis, or a medication that is similar in action.

The Rhythm of the Pulse

The *pulse rhythm* is the pattern of the pulsations and the pauses between them. The pulse rhythm is normally regular; that is, the beat and the pauses occur similarly throughout the time the pulse is being obtained.

An irregular pattern of heartbeats, and consequently an irregular pulse rhythm, is called an *arrhythmia*. It may also be called a *dysrhythmia*. Some common patterns of irregular rhythms include the following:

- One that slows when a person breathes out and speeds up when a person breathes in. This type is not considered dangerous and is often seen in some children and young adults. It is called a *sinus arrhythmia*.
- A pulsation that occurs sooner than the regular beats that have previously been noted. This is called a *premature contraction*. It is usually less intense than the regular beats. If several premature contractions occur in succession, or happen frequently in a minute, it could be a warning of a potentially dangerous situation.
- An *intermittent pulse* is one that has a period of normal rhythm broken by periods of irregular rhythms. It may be a serious sign, such as in certain heart diseases, or it may be a simple response to being upset or frightened.

Any arrhythmia should be reported promptly. More details about arrhythmias and their causes can be found in clinical textbooks.

The Volume of the Pulse

The *pulse volume* refers to the quality of the pulsations that are felt. The volume is usually related to the amount of blood pumped with each heartbeat. This amount usually remains fairly constant under normal conditions. Normal volume results in the ability to feel a pulsation easily and requires mild pressure on an artery with the fingertips to stop the feel of the pulse wave. These two characteristics are used to evaluate the volume or quality of the pulse. Some common abnormal observations in pulse volume include:

- A *feeble, weak, or thready pulse.* This term is used when the blood volume is small, making the pulse difficult to feel and, once felt, very easily stopped with pressure. A patient with a thready pulse usually also has a rapid pulse. A rapid, thready pulse is usually a serious sign and should be reported promptly.
- A *bounding* or *full* pulse. This occurs when a large blood volume produces a pronounced pulsation that is not easy to stop even with mild pressure.

Another way to describe the volume or quality of the pulse involves the use of numbers. This numbering system and its corresponding descriptions can be found in Table 13-4. It is best to follow agency policy when describing the volume of the pulse.

Selecting a Pulse Site

The rate, rhythm, and volume of the pulse may be assessed by compressing an artery against an underlying bone with the tips of the fingers. The arteries that are most often used are those located close to the skin surface. Most, but not all, are named for their adjacent bone. They include the tem-

Table 13-4. Identifying Pulse Volume

Number	Definition	Description
0	Absent pulse	No pulsation is felt despite extreme pressure.
1+	Thready pulse	Pulsation that is not easily felt. Slight pressure causes it to disappear.
2+	Weak pulse	Stronger than a thready pulse. Light pressure causes it to disappear.
3+	Normal pulse	Pulsation is easily felt. Moderate pressure causes it to disappear.
4+	Bounding pulse	The pulsation is strong and does not disappear with moderate pressure.

poral, carotid, brachial, radial, femoral, popliteal, dorsalis pedis, and posterior tibial arteries. They are collectively called *peripheral pulses* because they are distant from the heart. The locations of these sites are illustrated in Figure 13-11.

Usually the radial artery is the site commonly used for assessment. It is located on the inner (thumb) side of the wrist. Figures 13-12 and 13-13 show its location and the position of the fingertips during assessment using this site.

Obtaining the Radial Pulse Rate

The pulse rate obtained at the wrist is called the *radial pulse rate*. The actions described in Skill Procedure 13-4 describe the technique that may be used to obtain the radial pulse rate. The other characteristics of the pulse should also be assessed at the same time.

The Apical Pulse Rate

If the radial pulse is irregular or difficult to count, the apical pulse rate may be assessed. In the adult, the apical

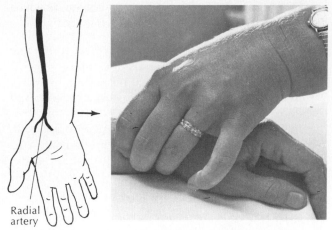

Figure 13-12 (*A*). The artist's sketch shows the location of the radial artery. (*B*). The nurse's fingertips and the patient's hand should be positioned as those in this photo when assessing the radial pulse.

pulse rate is counted by listening at the chest rather than feeling an artery. The heartbeats are best heard at the apex, or lower tip, of the heart as illustrated in Figure 13–14. The nurse places a stethoscope, described and illustrated later in this chapter, slightly below the level of the nipple on the chest to the left of the breastbone. The nurse listens for the "lub/dub" sound. These two sounds equal one pulsation that would be felt at a peripheral site. The rate should be counted for one minute. The rhythm may also be evaluated. The heart rate obtained in this manner is called the *apical pulse rate*.

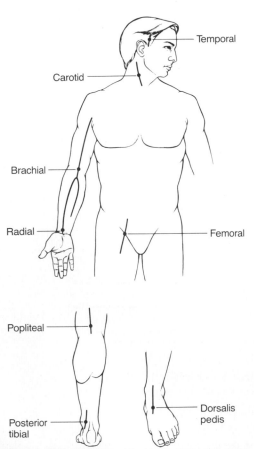

Figure 13-11 This diagram shows peripheral pulse sites. They may be used to assess the pulse characteristics of rate, rhythm, and volume. An absent, thready, or weak peripheral pulse may mean that there is an insufficient blood supply to that part of the body.

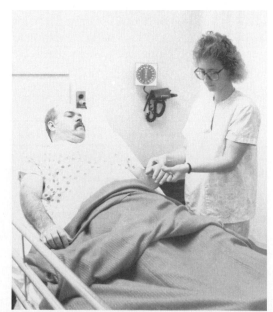

Figure 13-13 With the patient in a comfortable position, the nurse counts the patient's radial pulse. The temperature and respirations may also be obtained at the same time.

Skill Procedure 13-4. Assessing the Radial Pulse

Suggested Action	Reason for Action
Help the patient to a position of comfort. If he prefers lying down, have him rest his arm alongside his body with the wrist extended and the palm of the hand downward. The arm may rest on his abdomen if this is comfortable. If the patient prefers sitting, have him hold his forearm at about a 90° angle to his body and rest his arm on a support with the wrist extended and the palm of the hand downward. It is common to assess the pulse rate while the body temperature is being obtained. The nurse in Figure 13-13 is following this combination of actions.	These positions are usually comfortable for the patient and convenient for the nurse. An uncomfortable position for the patient may influence the heart rate.
Place the first, second, and third fingertips along the radial artery and press gently but firmly to compress the artery against the bone at the wrist. Rest the thumb on the back of the patient's wrist.	The fingertips are sensitive to touch and will feel the pulsation of the patient's radial artery. Using the thumb may result in feeling one's own pulse. This may result in an inaccurate assessment.
Gradually release the pressure while still feeling the pulsation. Note its rhythm and volume.	Too much pressure will shut off the pulse. If too little pressure is applied, the pulse will not be felt. The nurse should become aware of the feeling produced by the pulsation and the pattern of beats and pauses. The rate is not the only characteristic of the pulse that is assessed.
If the pulse is regular and feels normal, use a watch with a secondhand to count the number of pulsations felt for thirty seconds. Multiply this number by two to obtain the rate for one minute.	A watch with a sweep secondhand provides an accurate method for determining when a half minute has passed.
If the pulse is abnormal in any way, count the rate for a full minute. Repeat counting if necessary to determine an accurate rate and assessment of the rhythm and volume.	When the pulse is abnormal, a minimum of a full minute of counting is necessary to obtain a valid assessment of the rate, rhythm, and volume.
Use good judgment to gather more information about the pulse by assessing the pulse at other peripheral pulse sites or by listening to the heart beats at the apex of the heart.	Nurses who detect abnormalities in the pulse or observe other signs that indicate that the patient may have cardiovascular problems may order or obtain more data, which will help in identifying a nursing diagnosis or collaborative problem.
Record the pulse rate according to agency policy.	The rate of a pulse is often transferred and plotted on a graph. The characteristics of the rhythm and volume may be described in the patient's record.

The Apical-Radial Pulse Rate

Comparing the radial pulse rate with the apical heart rate may provide important information to health personnel. The rates should normally be equal, but for some patients they are not. Obtaining the *apical-radial pulse rate,* abbreviated A/R, requires two persons. One listens at the apex of the heart while the other feels the pulse at the patient's wrist. They use one watch placed conveniently between them, decide on a specific time to start counting, and count for a full minute. If a difference is noted in the two rates— and the rates have been counted accurately—the findings should be reported promptly. The difference between the apical and radial pulse rates is called the *pulse deficit.*

Figure 13-15 shows two nurses obtaining an apical-radial pulse rate.

Respirations

Respiration is the act of breathing. *Inhalation,* or *inspiration,* is the act of breathing in; *exhalation,* or *expiration,* is the act of breathing out. One act of respiration consists of one inhalation and one exhalation. Through the act of respiration, the body takes oxygen from the air and gets rid of carbon dioxide. The process of exchanging oxygen and carbon dioxide between the lungs and the blood is called *external respiration.* The process of exchanging oxygen and carbon dioxide between the blood and body cells is called *internal respiration* or *tissue respiration*.

The respiratory center in the medulla and specialized sensing tissue in the carotid arteries are very sensitive to the amount of carbon dioxide in the blood. These structures carry out a coordinated effort to adapt respirations to the body's needs without the person having to think about breathing. Nevertheless, breathing can be controlled voluntarily to a certain extent. For example, a person automatically controls his breathing when talking, singing, laughing, crying, eating, and so on. He can purposely take deep or shallow breaths. There are limitations, however, on how long a person can voluntarily hold his breath. When the body becomes desperate for oxygen and for getting rid of carbon dioxide, the person will have to breathe sooner or later. A new mother, not realizing this, may panic when her child has a temper tantrum and holds his breath. The child will eventually breathe whether he wants to or not.

Normally the lungs fill and empty through pressure changes from the contraction and relaxation of various muscles. Infants and young children use the diaphragm to a large extent. This is called *diaphragmatic respiration*. Adults primarily use their intercostal (between the ribs) muscles when breathing. Though the diaphragm is also used, this breathing is called *thoracic respiration*.

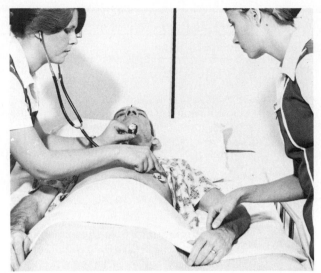

Figure 13-15 Obtaining an apical-radial pulse requires the simultaneous efforts of two nurses. Note that the patient's chest wall is exposed so that clothing does not interfere with hearing the apical pulse. It is best to warm the diaphragm of the stethoscope in the palm of the hand before placing it on the chest wall. A cold instrument placed on the patient could alter the pulse and respiratory rates.

Normal Respiratory Rates

Table 13-5 identifies normal respiratory rates for various ages; however, respiratory rates have been observed to vary considerably in well people. Factors that usually influence the pulse rate generally also affect the respiratory rate. The faster the pulse rate, the faster the respiratory rate, and vice versa. The relationship between the pulse and respiratory rates is fairly consistent in normal persons. The ratio is one respiration to approximately four or five heartbeats.

Abnormally Rapid Respiratory Rates

Above-average or rapid rate of respirations is called *tachypnea*. A rapid respiratory rate may be observed with an elevated temperature because the body is attempting to rid itself of excess heat. Also, the body's metabolic needs are increased at this time. Cells require more oxygen, thereby triggering increased respirations. Rapid respira-

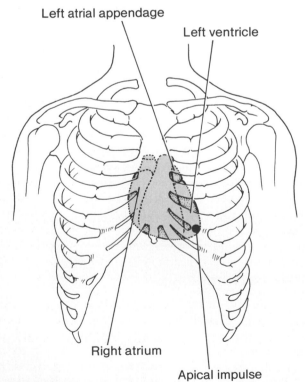

Figure 13-14 This sketch illustrates the location of the heart in the chest cavity and the area where the impulse for the apical pulse is normally found.

Left atrial appendage

Left ventricle

Right atrium

Apical impulse

Table 13-5. Normal Respiratory Rates at Various Ages

Age	Average Range
Newborn	30–80
Early childhood	20–40
Late childhood	15–25
Adulthood	
Male	14–18
Female	16–20

tions are common when diseases affect the cardiac and respiratory systems. *Hyperventilation* is a term that describes prolonged, rapid, and deep respirations. In an adult, a rate above 40 per minute in the absence of exercise is cause for alarm and should be reported promptly.

Abnormally Slow Respiratory Rates

A below-average or slow respiratory rate is called *bradypnea.* Certain drugs, such as morphine sulfate, will slow the respiratory rate. Slow respirations are also observed in the patient who has a brain tumor.

Hypoventilation is a term that describes a less than normal amount of air entering the lungs. This condition may occur when a person is taking shallow or slow breaths, or it may occur when an obstruction in the airway prevents a sufficient amount of air from reaching the lungs.

A respiratory rate of less than 8 per minute in an adult is cause for alarm and should be reported promptly.

Characteristics of Breathing

Breathing is normally automatic. Respirations are relatively noiseless and effortless. The amount of air exchanged with each respiration varies widely among different people. Athletes generally have an increased capacity to exchange oxygen and carbon dioxide with each respiration. The depth of respirations is referred to as shallow or deep, depending on whether the volume of air taken in is below or above average for that person. Periodically, each person automatically inhales deeply, filling the lungs with more air than inhaled with the usual respiration.

Certain terms are used to describe the nature and depth of respirations. *Apnea* refers to periods during which there is no breathing. This is a serious situation in which brain damage and death can occur if breathing or blood circulation is suppressed for more than 4 to 6 minutes. *Dyspnea* is difficult or labored breathing. Dyspneic patients usually appear to be anxious and worried as they experience the inefficient work of breathing. The nostrils flare (widen) as the patient fights to fill his lungs with air. Abdominal and neck muscles may be used to assist other muscles in the act of breathing. When observing the patient, it is important to note how much and what type of activity brings on dyspnea. For example, walking to the bathroom may bring on dyspnea in a patient who may not be distressed by sitting in a chair.

Some respiratory patterns have descriptive names. *Cheyne-Stokes respirations* refer to breathing that consists of a gradual increase in the depth of respirations followed by a gradual decrease in the depth of respirations, and then a period of apnea. Dyspnea is usually also present. The observation of Cheyne-Stokes respirations is a serious sign often occurring as death approaches.

Orthopnea is a characteristic in which breathing is facilitated by sitting up or standing. Dyspneic patients frequently find it easier to breathe in this manner. The sitting or standing position causes organs in the abdominal cavity to fall away from the diaphragm with gravity. This gives more room for the lungs in the chest cavity to expand, taking in more air with each breath.

Several terms are used to describe the nature of sounds that can be heard as a patient breathes. *Stertorous* breathing is a general term used to refer to noisy respirations. *Stridor* is a harsh, high-pitched sound that is heard on inspiration when there is a laryngeal obstruction. Infants and young children with croup often manifest stridor when breathing.

The nurse may listen to respirations with a stethoscope. The technique for assessing lung sounds is described in Chapter 14.

Assessing Respirations

The nurse frequently observes respirations. Not only is the rate important, but also the effort, pattern of breathing, and sounds associated with breathing are important. Skill Procedure 13-5 suggests techniques to use when obtaining the respiratory rate.

Blood Pressure

Blood is circulated through a loop involving the heart and blood vessels. *Blood pressure* is the force produced by the volume of blood pressure on the resisting walls of arteries. The arterial walls are normally elastic and expand as each new supply of blood is added to that which is already present.

Blood is pushed forward into the arteries during systole. *Systole* is the phase during which the heart works. It contracts and pumps blood out into the circulation. The pressure increases during this time. It is called the *systolic pressure.* The pressure is lower during *diastole,* the heart's resting phase. During that time the heart is filling with blood, which will be pumped out during the next systole. The pressure within the arteries that exists while the heart is at rest is called the *diastolic pressure.*

Blood pressure is commonly abbreviated BP. Its measurement is expressed as a fraction. The numerator is the systolic pressure and the denominator is the diastolic pressure. The pressure is expressed in millimeters of mercury, abbreviated mm Hg. Thus, a recording of 140/80 means the systolic blood pressure was measured at 140 mm Hg and the diastolic blood pressure was measured at 80 mm Hg.

Measuring the blood pressure helps to assess the efficiency of the circulatory system. The following are examples of information that blood-pressure findings directly reflect:

- Ability of the arteries to stretch and fill with blood
- Efficiency of the heart as a pump
- Volume of circulating blood.

Skill Procedure 13-5. Counting the Respiratory Rate

Suggested Action	**Reason for Action**
Observe the rise and fall of a patient's chest at a time when the patient is somewhat unaware of being watched. A convenient approach is to count the respirations while appearing to concentrate on counting the pulse.	Counting the respiratory rate while presumably still counting the pulse keeps the patient from becoming conscious of his breathing and possibly changing his respirations. Altering the characteristics of normal, automatic breathing may cause data to be inaccurate.
Note the placement of the sweep secondhand of a watch or clock. Count each rise and fall of the chest.	A complete respiration consists of one inspiration and one expiration.
If the respirations appear regular, even, and unlabored, count the number that occur for thirty seconds. The rate for one minute may be obtained by multiplying this number by two.	Sufficient time is necessary to observe the rate, depth, and other characteristics of the patient's respirations. Counting the respirations for 10 or 15 seconds does not provide sufficient data.
If the respirations are abnormal in any way, count them for a full minute and repeat if necessary for an accurate assessment.	A full minute of counting respirations and repeating the count if necessary allows time to collect and identify valid data.
Record information about the respirations according to agency policy.	Respiratory rates are often graphed in order to analyze any trends. Descriptions about other characteristics of the respirations are made in the patient's record.

Common Factors Influencing Blood Pressure

Various factors listed below influence blood pressure.

Age. Blood pressure rises with age. As individuals age, changes occur in the arteries. They lose their elasticity and become more rigid. This condition is called *arteriosclerosis.* Arteriosclerosis results in an even greater resistance to the heart's effort to fill arteries with blood. Arteries may also fill with deposits of fat, a condition called *atherosclerosis* that interferes with the amount of blood that can be contained within the arteries. Both conditions contribute to increasing blood pressure. The rate at which these conditions occur with aging depends on one's heredity and lifestyle habits such as diet and exercise. Normal blood pressure readings at various ages are listed later in this section of the chapter.

Time of Day. As is true of other vital signs, blood pressure tends to be lowest in the morning, on awakening, and highest later in the day and early evening.

Gender. Women usually have a lower blood pressure on the average than have men of the same age.

Exercise and Activity. Blood pressure rises during periods of exercise and activity. Regular exercise can result in maintaining the blood pressure within normal levels.

Emotions and Pain. Strong emotional experiences and pain tend to cause blood pressure to rise.

Miscellaneous Factors. As a rule, a person has a lower blood pressure when lying down than when sitting or standing, although the difference in most people may be insignificant. It has also been observed that blood pressure rises somewhat when the urinary bladder is full, when the legs are crossed, and when a person uses tobacco, drinks a caffeinated beverage, or is cold.

Normal Blood Pressure

Studies of healthy persons show that blood pressure can fluctuate within a wide range and still be normal. Because individual differences can be considerable, it is important to analyze the usual ranges and patterns of blood pressure measurements for a particular person. A rise or fall of 20 mm Hg to 30 mm Hg in a person's usual pressure is significant, even if it is well within the generally accepted range for normal. Table 13-6 offers a guide for average normal and upper limits of normal blood pressure measurements for various ages.

Abnormally High Blood Pressure

High blood pressure is called *hypertension.* It exists when the systolic pressure, or diastolic pressure, or both, is sustained at levels above the normal level for a person's age. Occasional elevation does not necessarily mean a person has hypertension. Data should be recorded and continue to be gathered to determine if a trend or pattern exists. Hypertension is not diagnosed until either of the following situations occurs.

- The average of two or more diastolic measurements on at least two different but subsequent visits exceeds the normal limit.

Table 13-6. Blood Pressures and Levels of Significant Hypertension for Children

Age	Normal* Systolic	Normal* Diastolic	Significant Systolic	Hypertension Diastolic
Newborn	<87 mm Hg	<68 mm Hg	>96 mm Hg	Undetermined
12 months	<105 mm Hg	<69 mm Hg	>112 mm Hg	>74 mm Hg
5 years	<109 mm Hg	<69 mm Hg	>116 mm Hg	>76 mm Hg
10 years	<117 mg Hg	<75 mm Hg	>126 mm Hg	>82 mm Hg
15 years	<129 mm Hg	<79 mm Hg	>136 mm Hg	>86 mm Hg
18 years	<136 mm Hg	<84 mm Hg	>142 mm Hg	>92 mm Hg

*Normal blood pressure is defined as systolic and diastolic blood pressures less than the 90th percentile for age and sex as calculated on male children used in averaged samples. Norms for females in these age groups average slighty less than those for males. The National Heart, Lung, and Blood Institute's Task Force on Blood Pressure Control in Children: Report of the Second Task Force on Blood Pressure Control in Children. Bethesda, Maryland, US Department of Health and Human Services, 1987.

- The average of multiple systolic measurements on two or more subsequent visits is consistently greater than the normal limit.

The 1988 Joint National Committee on Detection, Evaluation, and Treatment of High Blood Pressure considers a systolic pressure of 140 mm Hg or greater in adults 18 years or older, and a diastolic pressure of 90 mm Hg or greater, to be abnormally high. Other terms used to describe various adult blood pressure measurements can be found in Table 13-7. Not all health practitioners accept these figures and classification terms. The nurse is advised to check with the patient's physician when a question arises about whether hypertension may be present.

Some feel that an abnormally elevated diastolic reading is more indicative of a potentially dangerous condition than an abnormally elevated systolic reading. Certain recommendations concerning the evaluation and care of adult patients with blood pressure measurements at various levels are described in Table 13-8.

The following are examples of conditions commonly associated with hypertension:

- Obesity
- Arteriosclerosis and atherosclerosis
- Stroke
- Heart failure
- Kidney diseases.

Abnormally Low Blood Pressure

An abnormally low blood pressure is called *hypotension*. It exists when the blood pressure measurements are below the systolic normal values for the individual's corresponding age.

Having a consistently low pressure, 96/60 mm Hg for example, seems to cause no harm. In fact, low blood pressure is usually associated with efficient functioning of the heart and blood vessels. However, a low reading should be compared with the person's usual blood pressure to evaluate its significance.

The following are examples of common conditions with which hypotension may be observed:

- Changes in position, such as when a person rises to an upright position following periods of lying down or sitting. This is called *orthostatic hypotension* by some and *postural hypotension* by others.
- Shock due to blood loss or the inability of the heart to pump blood efficiently.

Table 13-7. Classification of Adult Blood Pressure Measurements

Blood Pressure (mm Hg)	Category*
Diastolic	
<85	Normal blood pressure
85 to 89	High normal blood pressure
90 to 104	Mild hypertension
105 to 114	Moderate hypertension
≥115	Severe hypertension
Systolic when DBP<90 mm Hg	
<140	Normal blood pressure
140 to 159	Borderline isolated systolic hypertension
≥160	Isolated systolic hypertension

*A classification of borderline isolated systolic hypertension (SBP 140–159 mm Hg) or isolated systolic hypertension (SBP ≥ 160 mm Hg) takes precedence over a classification of high normal blood pressure (DBP 85–89 mm Hg) when both occur in the same individual. A classification of high normal blood pressure (DBP 85–89 mm Hg) takes precedence over a classification of normal blood pressure (SBP < 140 mm Hg) when both occur in the same person.

Classification terms and measurements from the 1988 Joint National Committee Report on Detection, Evaluation, and Treatment of High Blood Pressure.

Table 13-8. Recommended Follow-Up for First-Occasion Elevated Blood Pressure Measurement

Blood Pressure (mm Hg)	Recommended Follow-Up*
Diastolic	
<85	Recheck within 2 years
85 to 89	Recheck within 1 year
90 to 104	Confirm promptly (not to exceed 2 months)
105 to 114	Evaluate or refer promptly to source of care (not to exceed 2 weeks)
≥115	Evaluate or refer immediately to a source of care
Systolic when DBP <90 mm Hg	
<140	Recheck within 2 years
140 to 199	Confirm promptly (not to exceed 2 months)
≥200	Evaluate or refer promptly to source of care (not to exceed 2 weeks)

*If recommendations for follow-up of DBP and SBP are different, the shorter recommended time period supersedes, and a referral supersedes a recheck recommendation.

Recommendations apply to adults age 18 or older as determined by the Joint National Committee Report on Detection, Evaluation, and Treatment of High Blood Pressure.

- Dilation of peripheral blood vessels, which may occur with severe allergic reactions or with drugs that are used to treat hypertension.

Checking for Postural Hypotension

Blood pressure falls in relation to position changes from lying to sitting or standing. The normal difference in systolic pressure tends to be no greater than 15 mm Hg lower than it was in a reclining position. The diastolic pressure may rise or fall 10 mm Hg from the lying pressure.

For most people the change in pressure is not noticeable. Internal pressure receptors make rapid adjustments to compensate for the changes in the distribution of blood volume. For some, however, the pressure drops much more dramatically. This phenomenon is called *postural hypotension*. It is also called *orthostatic hypotension*. Patients who have circulatory problems, dehydration, or those who take medications like diuretics or blood pressure medication are prone to postural hypotension.

A consequence of a sudden drop in blood pressure is dizziness and even fainting. It is always a safe practice to have a patient sit on the edge of the bed for a short time after lying down. Brace a patient while assisting him from a sitting to a standing position. Keep a chair close by.

The nurse may decide to assess a patient for the range in blood pressure changes from lying to upright positions. If so, the patient should be lying for at least three minutes. Repeat the measurement again after three minutes in a sitting or standing position. Any patient whose blood pressure varies more than 15 mm Hg should have special safety precautions identified on the nursing care plan. Always instruct the patient to seek assistance with position changes. The patient can be helped by instructing him to rise slowly after he has been lying or sitting.

Pulse Pressure

The difference between systolic and diastolic blood pressure measurements is called the *pulse pressure*. It is computed by subtracting the smaller figure from the larger. For example, when blood pressure is 126/88 mm Hg, pulse pressure is 38. A pulse pressure between 30 and 50 is considered to be in a normal range, with 40 being a healthy average.

Equipment Used to Obtain Blood Pressure

Blood pressure is usually measured with a sphygmomanometer and stethoscope, which will be described shortly. It is possible to palpate a blood pressure using only a sphygmomanometer. Only the systolic reading can be determined with this method. In critical care areas, the blood pressure can be monitored with a probe placed directly within the artery.

The Sphygmomanometer. A manometer is an instrument used to measure the pressure of a gas or liquid. A *sphygmomanometer* is used to measure the pressure of blood within an artery. It consists of a manometer and a cuff. The two types in common use are illustrated in Figure 13-16.

One type of sphygmomanometer uses a mercury gauge. A mercury gauge measures pressure with the use of liquid mercury within a column calibrated in millimeters. When using a sphygmomanometer with a mercury gauge, the manometer must be positioned vertically with the gauge at eye level. Before the blood pressure reading can be obtained, the mercury must be even with the 0 level at the base of the calibrated column. The surface of the column of mercury is slightly curved, like an inverted bowl. The curved shape is called the *meniscus*. The nurse notes the top of the meniscus while listening for certain sounds. If the meniscus is observed at a height above eye level, the pressure reading will appear higher than it really is. Conversely, if the meniscus is below eye level, the pressure reading will appear lower than it really is. Figure 13-17

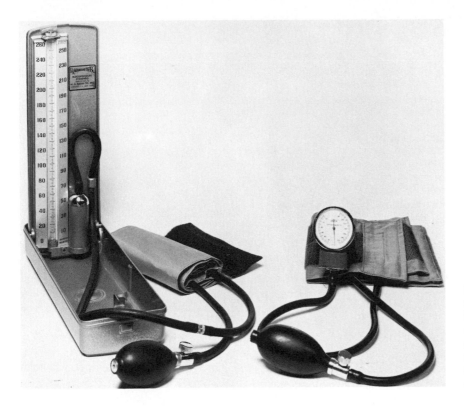

Figure 13-16 This photo shows a mercury manometer (*left*) and an aneroid manometer (*right*). One tube connects to the manometer; the other connects to the bulb. The screw above the bulb controls the air in and out of the bladder within the cuff. The cuffs on these two sphygmomanometers are self-securing.

illustrates the correct and incorrect observations of the meniscus.

The other type of sphygmomanometer uses an aneroid gauge. This type contains a needle that moves about a dial that is also calibrated in millimeters. The needle must be positioned initially at 0 to ensure an accurate recording. Either type of gauge, provided it is working properly and used correctly, can be used to measure blood pressure accurately. The readings obtained with one type of gauge are comparable to those obtained with the other.

The cuff contains an inflatable bladder, to which two tubes are attached. One is connected to the manometer, which registers the pressure. The other is attached to a bulb, which is used to inflate the bladder with air. A screw valve on the bulb allows the nurse to fill and empty the bladder of air. As the air escapes, the pressure is measured. Figure 13-18 illustrates the cuff and bladder.

The cuff should be of a size appropriate for the patient. A common guide is that the cuff width should be 40% of the circumference or 20% wider than the diameter of the arm or leg on which it will be applied. Figure 13-19 shows a quick way to determine the appropriateness of the cuff width. If the cuff is too wide, the blood pressure reading will be falsely low. If the cuff is too narrow, the blood pressure reading will be falsely high. The cuff should not cover more than two thirds of the length of the upper portion of the extremity after it is applied.

The bladder of the cuff should cover between 60% to

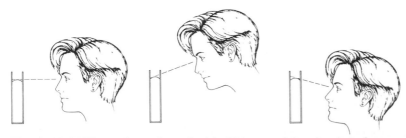

Figure 13-17 The surface of any liquid within a container tends to form a curve, called the meniscus. The curve may appear as an inverted bowl, as seen here. The meniscus of other liquids may appear cup-shaped. The sketch on the left illustrates the meniscus, and a reading made at eye level. The remaining sketches illustrate how blood pressure readings could vary when the eye is at different levels in relation to the meniscus.

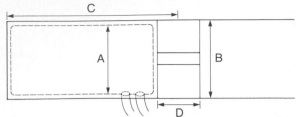

Figure 13-18 This drawing illustrates the bladder and cuff relationships of a sphygmomanometer. *A,* bladder width; *B,* cuff width; *C,* ideal arm circumference (A × 2.5); *D,* range of acceptable deviation from ideal arm circumference. Recommendations for Human Blood Pressure Determination by Sphygmomanometers. (© 1987, reprinted with permission of the American Heart Association.)

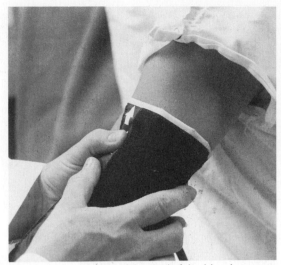

Figure 13-19 If the width of the end of the blood pressure cuff held lengthwise against the upper arm covers approximately 40% of the circumference of the arm, it is an appropriate size for the patient.

100% of the circumference of the extremity. Table 13-9 identifies the recommended bladder dimensions for blood pressure cuffs.

The Stethoscope. A *stethoscope* is an instrument that carries sounds from the body to the examiner's ears. The tip of the stethoscope magnifies sounds. Some stethoscopes have a cupped tip, called a bell; others have a flat disk tip, called a diaphragm; some have a tip that combines a bell and a diaphragm. The bell of the stethoscope is preferable when measuring blood pressure. The nurse obtains the blood pressure by noting the numbers on the gauge while listening for characteristic sounds. The parts of a stethoscope are shown in Figure 13-20.

If stethoscopes are used by various people, the eartips should be cleaned to avoid transferring organisms. Com-mon practice is to clean the tips with gauze or cotton balls dampened with alcohol. Individually owned stethoscopes also need cleaning to keep the eartips free of earwax and dirt. Lint and other debris allowed to collect in the tubing or behind the diaphragm will distort sound. Scrubbing stethoscopes regularly with a germicide is recommended.

Electronic Blood Pressure Meters. There are electronic blood pressure meters on the market that transform blood pressure measurements into audible sounds or a

Table 13-9. Recommended Bladder Dimensions for Blood Pressure Cuffs

Arm Circumference at Midpoint* (cm)	Cuff Name	Bladder Width (cm)	Bladder Length (cm)
5–7.5	Newborn	3	5
7.5–13	Infant	5	8
13–20	Child	8	13
24–32	Adult	13	24
32–42	Wide adult	17	32
42–50†	Thigh	20	42

*Midpoint of arm is defined as half the distance from acromion to olecranon. Use nonstretchable metal tape.

†In persons with very large limbs, indirect blood pressure should be measured in leg or forearm.

Reproduced with permission. Recommendations for Human Blood Pressure Determination by Sphygmomanometers, © American Heart Association, 1987.

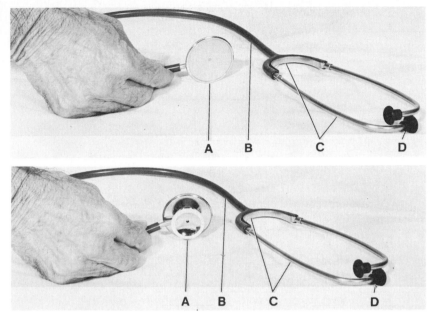

Figure 13-20 *A*. The chest piece on this stethoscope contains both a diaphragm (*top*) and a bell (*bottom*). The diaphragm is used for listening to high-pitched sounds. The bell is better for detecting low-pitched sounds. The bell is used when obtaining the blood pressure. *B*. The tubing may be rubber or plastic. Unnecessarily long tubing decreases good sound conduction. A length of about 50 cm (20 in) seems best. *C*. The brace and binaurals are the metal portions connecting the tubing and the chest piece. The binaurals should clear the examiner's face. The brace prevents the tubing from kinking. *D*. The eartips are rubber or plastic and should fit snugly but comfortably into the ears. The eartips should be placed so that they are directed downward and forward. If the eartips are not properly positioned in the ear canal, sound quality will be poor, and, in measuring the blood pressure, a falsely low systolic and falsely high diastolic pressure are likely to be obtained.

digital display of numbers, making a stethoscope unnecessary. They are helpful for patients who wish to obtain their own blood pressure. They also have been found useful by some to measure blood pressure on infants. Because of their delicate instrumentation, electronic machines should be recalibrated more than once each year. Patients using these devices for home use should also have their blood pressure checked periodically by health personnel.

Coin-Operated Sphygmomanometers.

Coin-operated blood pressure machines are most commonly located in drug and department stores and in shopping malls. The consumer is given directions for applying the cuff. Some of these sphygmomanometers supply a computer printout describing the blood pressure; others have a screen on which findings are displayed. Blood pressure recordings tend to vary as much as 5 to 10 mm Hg, usually on the higher side, when compared with standard sphygmomanometers. When calibrated accurately, errors tend to be related to improper cuff placement and noise in the environment.

Of concern to health practitioners is how well consumers using coin-operated sphygmomanometers understand and interpret findings and observe recommended follow-up care.

Korotkoff's Sounds

The nurse listens for a series of sounds when obtaining blood pressure. These sounds are called *Korotkoff's sounds*. Changes in sounds indicate the pressures that exist within the artery. These sounds are described in Table 13-10. Figure 13-21 is a diagram of the changes occurring in the brachial artery when Korotkoff's sounds are assessed.

The first sound heard in phase I represents the systolic pressure. It is recorded as the first number in the fraction. The diastolic pressure, the second number, is the level at which a change in the sound is first noted. Two figures are sometimes used to record the diastolic pressure. One is the first changed sound occurring in phase IV. The other is the last sound that can be heard, the beginning of phase V. An example of this type of recording would be BP 120/80/76. The number 76 indicates the point at which all sound disappeared. If sound is heard down to zero, this would be recorded as 120/80/0. If all sounds disappear when the diastolic pressure is noted, the blood pressure is recorded as 120/80/80.

Measuring Blood Pressure

Blood pressure can be measured directly or indirectly. Direct measurement involves inserting a cannula within an artery. The radial artery is most often used. Electronic equipment converts the pressure into a waveform. Some machines also indicate the numerical measurements of the systolic, diastolic, and mean arterial pressures on a digital screen.

Most blood pressure recordings are obtained indirectly. That is, they are determined by listening or palpating over an artery that lies superficially close to the skin. Skill Procedure 13-6 describes the standard technique to measure the indirect blood pressure on the arm.

Table 13-10. Korotkoff's Sounds

Phase	Description
I	This phase is characterized by the first appearance of faint but clear tapping sounds, which gradually increase in intensity. The first two consecutive tapping sounds represent the systolic pressure.
II	This phase is characterized by muffled or swishinglike sounds These sounds may temporarily disappear, especially in hypertensive persons. The disappearance of the sound during the latter part of phase I and during phase II is called the auscultatory gap and may cover a range of as much as 40 mm Hg. Failing to recognize this gap may cause serious errors in underestimating systolic pressure or overestimating diastolic pressure.
III	This phase is characterized by distinct and loud sounds as the blood flows relatively freely through an increasingly open artery.
IV	This phase is characterized by a distinct, abrupt muffling sound with a soft, blowing quality. The first of muffled sounds is considered to be diastolic pressure.
V	This is the last sound heard before a period of continuous silence. The second diastolic pressure reading is noted for adults when this occurs.

Obtaining a Blood Pressure at the Thigh. An indirect blood pressure may also be obtained on the thigh with a larger cuff than used on the arm. To perform this assessment, the patient lies on his abdomen or back and the cuff is applied. The bladder is positioned over the back side of the midthigh. The stethoscope is placed over the popliteal artery. The pulsation of this artery can be felt in back of the knee. The technique for measuring blood pressure remains the same as for the arm. The systolic pressure is usually a little higher when measured on the thigh than when measured on the arm. The diastolic pressure has been found to be about the same. Help the patient to a position of comfort after the blood pressure has been determined. Always document where the blood pressure was taken and indicate any alternative technique that was used.

Using Palpation to Determine Blood Pressure. Auscultating a blood pressure requires that the nurse listen for Korotkoff's sounds. Some circumstances may interfere with identifying the characteristic changes in these sounds. The nurse may have a hearing loss. A low pressure may make differentiating the phases of Korotkoff's sounds difficult.

The nurse may choose to palpate the blood pressure as an alternative. The technique is similar to the standard technique for measuring blood pressure using a stethoscope. The modifications include using the fingers over the brachial or popliteal artery throughout the assessment. After inflating the cuff 20 mm Hg to 30 mm Hg beyond arterial pulsation, the nurse gradually releases the pressure. The point at which the first pulsation is felt corresponds to the systolic pressure. The diastolic pressure cannot be measured using this technique. Palpations will continue to be felt as the air is released from the cuff's

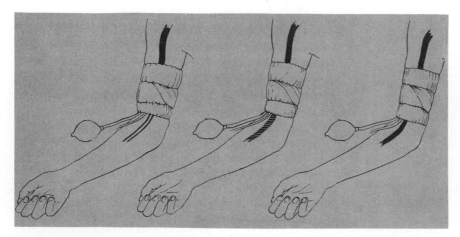

Figure 13-21 When the cuff has been inflated sufficiently, it will prevent the flow of blood into the forearm. No sound will be heard through the stethoscope at this time (*left*). When pressure in the cuff is reduced sufficiently for the blood to begin flowing through the brachial artery, the first sound is recorded as the systolic pressure (*center*). As the pressure in the cuff continues to be released, the muffled sound heard through the stethoscope is the diastolic pressure. At this time the blood flows freely through the brachial artery (*right*).

Skill Procedure 13-6. *Measuring the Blood Pressure*

Suggested Action	Reason for Action
Select a blood pressure cuff of an appropriate size for the patient.	A cuff that is too large or too small will produce a false reading.
Delay obtaining the blood pressure if the patient is emotionally upset, is in pain, or has just exercised, unless it is urgent to obtain the blood pressure.	Factors such as emotional upset, exercise, and pain will alter usual blood pressure readings.
Have the patient assume a comfortable lying or sitting position with the forearm supported at the level of the heart and the palm of the hand upward.	This described position places the brachial artery on the inner aspect of the elbow so that the bell of the stethoscope can rest on it easily.
Expose the area of the brachial artery by removing garments, or move a sleeve, if it is not too tight, above the area where the cuff will be placed.	Clothing over the artery interferes with the ability to hear sounds and may cause inaccurate blood pressure readings. Tight clothing on the arm causes congestion of blood and possibly inaccurate readings.
Center the inflatable area of the cuff over the brachial artery, approximately midway on the arm, so that the lower edge of the cuff is about 2.5 or 5 cm (1 to 2 in) above the inner aspect of the elbow. The tubing should extend from the edge of the cuff nearer the patient's elbow.	Pressure in the cuff applied directly to the artery will give the most accurate readings. If the cuff gets in the way of the diaphragm, readings are likely to be inaccurate. A cuff placed upside down with the tubing toward the patient's head will give a false reading in most instances.
Wrap the cuff around the arm smoothly and snugly, and fasten it securely or tuck the end of the cuff well under the preceding wrapping. Do not allow any clothing to interfere with the proper placement of the cuff.	A smooth cuff and snug wrapping produce equal pressure and help promote an accurate measurement. A cuff too loosely wrapped will result in an inaccurate reading.
Check that a mercury manometer is supported in a vertical position. The mercury must be within the 0 area with the gauge at eye level. If an aneroid gauge is used, the needle should be within the 0 mark.	Tilting a mercury manometer, inaccurate calibration, or improper height for reading the gauge can lead to errors in determining the pressure measurements.
Palpate the brachial pulse by pressing gently with the fingertips in the antecubital space.	The location of the pulse is the area that is likely to produce the most audible sounds during the assessment of the blood pressure.
Tighten the screw valve on the air pump.	The bladder within the cuff will not inflate with the valve open.
Inflate the cuff while continuing to palpate the artery. Note the point on the gauge where the pulse disappears.	To identify the first Korotkoff's sound accurately, the cuff must be inflated to a pressure above the point at which the pulse can no longer be felt.
Deflate the cuff and wait 15 seconds.	Allowing a brief pause before continuing allows the blood to enter and circulate through the arm.
Assume a position that is no more than 3 feet away from the gauge. The patient's position, the manner in which the cuff should be wrapped, the position of the manometer, and the nurse's position are illustrated in Figure 13-22.	A distance of more than about 3 feet can interfere with accurate readings of the numbers on the gauge.
Place the stethoscope earpieces in the ears properly.	The eartips should be directed downward and forward to fit the shape of the ear canal.
Place the bell of the stethoscope firmly but with as little pressure as possible over the artery where the pulse is felt. Do not allow the stethoscope to touch clothing or the cuff.	Having the bell directly over the artery makes more accurate readings possible. Having the bell firmly placed on the skin away from clothing and the cuff prevents missing sounds. Heavy pressure on the brachial artery distorts the shape of the artery and the sound of the pulse.

(continued)

Skill Procedure 13-6. Continued

Suggested Action	**Reason for Action**

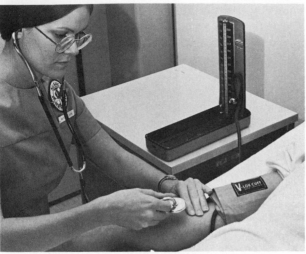

Figure 13-22 The nurse feels for pulsation over the artery and then places the bell of the stethoscope directly over the area. Note that the inflatable cuff is centered over the brachial artery slightly above the elbow and that the tubing leaves the cuff on the side nearest the patient's elbow.

Pump the pressure 30 mm Hg above the point at which the pulse disappeared.	Increasing the pressure above where the pulse disappeared ensures a period of time before hearing the first sound that corresponds with the systolic pressure. It prevents misinterpreting phase II sounds as phase I.
Loosen the screw on the valve. Slowly release the air at a rate of 2 to 4 mm Hg per second as the nurse is doing in Figure 13-23.	If air is released too slowly from the cuff, there will be congestion in the extremity, causing a false reading. If air is released too rapidly, sounds may not be accurately noted.

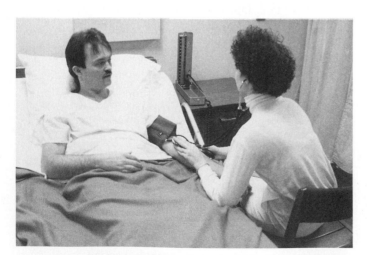

Figure 13-23 The nurse sits comfortably and keeps her eyes on the mercury manometer as she listens for the characteristic sounds associated with systolic and diastolic pressures.

(continued)

Skill Procedure 13-6. Continued

Suggested Action	Reason for Action
Note the point on the gauge at which there is an appearance of the first faint, but clear, sound, which slowly increases in intensity. Note this number as the systolic pressure.	Systolic pressure is the point at which the blood in the artery is first able to force its way through the vessel at a similar pressure exerted by the air bladder in the cuff. The first sound is phase I of Korotkoff sounds.
Read the pressure to the closest even number.	It is common practice to read blood pressure to the closest even number.
Do not reinflate the cuff once the air is being released to recheck the systolic pressure reading.	Reinflating the cuff while obtaining the blood pressure is uncomfortable for the patient and may cause an inaccurate reading. Reinflating the cuff causes congestion of blood in the lower arm, which lessens the loudness of Korotkoff's sounds.
Note the pressure at which the sound first becomes muffled. Also observe the point at which the last sound is heard. These may occur separately or at the same point.	The point at which the sound changes corresponds to phase IV of Korotkoff's sounds and is considered the first diastolic pressure reading. The point at which the last sound is heard is the beginning of phase V and is recorded in some agencies as the second diastolic pressure.
Allow the remaining air to escape quickly. Repeat any suspicious readings but wait at least 15 seconds between readings to allow normal circulation to return in the arm. Be sure to deflate the cuff completely between attempts to check the blood pressure.	False readings are likely to occur if there is congestion of blood in the arm while obtaining repeated readings.
If it is difficult to hear sounds when checking the blood pressure, raise the patient's arm over his head for 15 seconds just before rechecking the blood pressure.	Raising the arm over the head helps relieve congestion of blood in the arm, increases pressure differences, and makes the sounds louder and more distinct when blood enters the lower arm.
Inflate the cuff while the arm is elevated and then gently lower the arm while continuing to support it.	Supporting the arm while it is lowered prevents altering the pressure in the manometer by as much as 20 to 30 mm Hg.
Position the stethoscope and deflate the cuff at the usual rate while listening for Korotkoff's sounds.	The techniques used throughout the remaining assessment of blood pressure do not require any further modification.
Remove the cuff, clean and store the equipment.	Equipment that must be shared among personnel should be left in a manner ready for use.
Record the patient's position, the arm that was used to obtain the blood pressure, and the pressures that correspond to the systolic and diastolic readings.	Circumstances for assessing the blood pressure should be consistent for future comparisons.

bladder. When recording a blood pressure taken in this manner, it is important to indicate that it was assessed using palpation.

Assessing an Infant's Blood Pressure. Several techniques may be used to assess blood pressure in infants under the age of one. The nurse may choose to assess blood pressure using the infant's thigh, a doppler, or flush technique.

If the thigh is used, make sure that the cuff is an appropriate size. The thigh blood pressure is comparable to arm pressure under one year of age. The thigh systolic blood pressure tends to be higher thereafter.

Blood pressure may also be assessed using a doppler. A doppler is an instrument that converts the movement of blood into sound. A blood pressure cuff is positioned on the thigh. Conducting gel is applied over the popliteal artery. A transducer is substituted for the stethoscope. As air is released from the bladder of the cuff, the Korotkoff's sounds become audible. Use a capital D when charting the measurement, as in BP 86/40 D. This indicates that it was obtained by doppler technique.

If a thigh pressure is unobtainable or a doppler is unavailable, an infant's blood pressure can be assessed using the flush technique. This is best performed with the help of one other nurse. The principle of this technique is to reduce blood flow in the infant's hand or foot and observe the pressure at which flushing occurs when blood flow returns. The following steps are suggested.

- Apply a newborn or infant blood pressure cuff above the wrist or ankle.
- Raise the hand or foot to reduce blood volume within the extremity.
- Wrap the exposed hand or foot with an elastic bandage from the fingers or toes to the edge of the cuff as shown in Figure 13-24.
- Inflate the cuff to 120–140 mm Hg.
- Return the wrapped extremity to its natural position.
- Unwrap the bandage. The hand or foot should appear white.
- Release the air from the cuff at a rate of 2–3 mm Hg second.
- Ask the assistant to indicate when the extremity becomes pink or flushes.
- Note the corresponding pressure on the manometer.
- Record the pressure at which flushing occurred.

The flush pressure is comparable to the mean arterial pressure, that is, a pressure approximately between the systolic and diastolic pressures.

Frequency of Obtaining Vital Signs

Obtaining a patient's vital signs is part of most admission procedures. Health agency policies vary as to how often vital signs are obtained. For example, if a patient has a body temperature above normal, usual policy is that his vital signs are to be checked every four hours. For patients who have had surgery, most hospitals require that blood pressure be checked every 15 to 30 minutes until the patient is stable. Policies may require daily or even less frequent checking of vital signs for patients who are chronically or mentally ill. Blood pressure is often measured more frequently when a heart or blood vessel disease is present. All adults should have their blood pressure routinely checked at least every two years.

Regardless of the health agency's policy about the frequency of obtaining vital signs, the nurse must use judgment. Vital signs should be double-checked in the following circumstances:

- A change in the vital signs is noted and a trend is developing. For example, a gradual increase in the pulse rate is noted.
- Findings are very different from previous recordings. For example, a patient's vital signs may have been essentially normal and then an increase or decrease in one or all signs is noted.
- The vital signs are not in keeping with the patient's condition. The patient's condition suggests that his vital signs should be normal but they are elevated or decreased. Faulty equipment may be the cause. Reassess, using other equipment or sites for subsequent examinations.
- The vital signs could possibly be fraudulent. Occasionally, a patient may produce fraudulent vital signs, especially in relation to body temperature. Patients have been known to cause a thermometer to register falsely high readings by placing it on a light bulb or by rubbing it on bed clothing to create heat from friction. Conversely, they have been known to remove the thermometer before it registers properly. In these instances, the vital signs are not in keeping with the patient's condition. The nurse should remain with the patient while obtaining the vital signs when fraudulence is suspected.

Recording the Vital Signs

The manner in which vital signs are recorded depends on the health agency's policies. Different agencies use different forms and the nurse will use what is provided. Figure 13-25 is an example of a form used to record vital signs.

If anything unusual is observed while the nurse obtains the vital signs, it should be recorded and reported. Observations may be described in the patient's record. Many terms used to describe the vital signs were defined in this chapter. Although it is important to be familiar with these terms, it is recommended that a particular observation be described rather than labeled with a term. Doing so tends to avoid confusion. For example, the nurse would record that a patient is breathing very deeply rather than writing that the patient has hyperpnea.

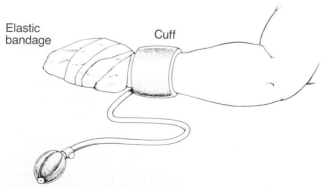

Elastic bandage   Cuff

Figure 13-24 The arterial blood within an infant's hand or foot is reduced by wrapping it from the fingers or toes and inflating the blood pressure cuff.

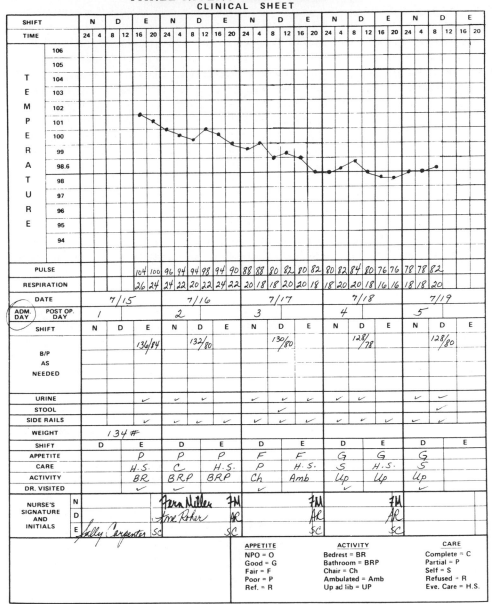

Figure 13-25 This graph illustrates how the vital signs are usually recorded. Plotting the figures on a graph helps to compare findings to determine any trends that may be occurring.

Suggested Measures to Obtain Vital Signs in Selected Situations

When the Patient Is an Infant or Child

Obtain infants' and young children's pulses and respiratory rates when they are quiet. It is best to obtain pulse and respiratory rates before obtaining the temperature because placing the thermometer often causes the youngster to cry.

Palpate an apical heart rate on children under 2 years of age for greatest accuracy. Obtaining the pulse rate at the radial artery is usually satisfactory after about 2 years of age. Palpating an apical rate is illustrated in Figure 13-26.

Observe an infant's or young child's abdomen to obtain the respiratory rate because respirations early in life are predominantly diaphragmatic.

Count the respiratory and pulse rates for a full minute when the patient is an infant or young child for greatest accuracy. A young child's pulse and respiratory rates normally tend to fluctuate more than an adult's rates.

Obtain the first temperature on a newborn rectally if this does not contradict agency policy. This tech-

Vital signs assessment is a part of every patient's care. The patient who requires frequent assessment or close monitoring of vital signs, however, may have nursing diagnoses such as
- High Risk for Infection
- High Risk for Altered Body Temperature
- Hypothermia
- Hyperthermia
- Ineffective Thermoregulation
- Fluid Volume Excess
- Fluid Volume Deficit
- Decreased Cardiac Output
- Impaired Gas Exchange
- Ineffective Breathing Pattern

Nursing Care Plan 13-1 describes approaches that can be used for a patient with hyperthermia. Hyperthermia is defined in the NANDA Taxonomy (1989) as, "A state in which an individual's body temperature is elevated above his/her normal range."

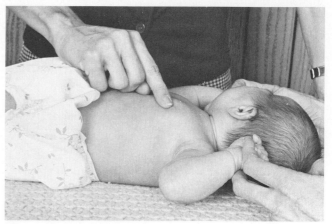

Figure 13-26 The index finger placed under the nipple and to the left of the sternum is the location for feeling an infant's apical pulse. The thin wall of an infant's chest makes this assessment possible. The apical pulse rate of an adult is obtained by listening to the heart.

Allowing an infant or young child to see, and possibly handle, the stethoscope before obtaining the blood pressure often helps decrease the youngster's fear of the equipment and procedure. The procedure should be explained to children old enough to understand.

When the Patient Cannot Cooperate

Obtain a rectal or axillary temperature from a patient who is subject to seizure activity or from patients who are unconscious, combative, irrational, or confused. A thermometer is likely to break in

nique helps assess whether the anus is patent. Do not force a thermometer if insertion is difficult.

Lubricate the bulb of a rectal thermometer *well* and insert the thermometer only slightly beyond the mercury bulb, about 1/2 to 1 1/2 inches, when obtaining a rectal temperature for an infant or child. The manner in which the thermometer is handled and inserted is important in preventing injury to rectal tissues.

Obtain an axillary temperature from infants and young children unless health agency policy indicates otherwise. Experienced nurses have found that obtaining an axillary temperature is safer and less disturbing to youngsters than is obtaining a rectal temperature. Also, studies have shown that there appears to be little, if any, difference between axillary and rectal temperatures obtained on infants and young children, especially when they are not seriously ill.

Hold an infant or young child in the arms while obtaining an axillary temperature, as the mother of the child in Figure 13-27 is doing. This technique is comforting for the youngster and promotes relaxation while obtaining the temperature.

Be *sure* the size of the blood pressure cuff is appropriate when obtaining blood pressure readings on infants and children.

Obtain blood pressure readings from children in a quiet room when they are not crying for most accurate readings.

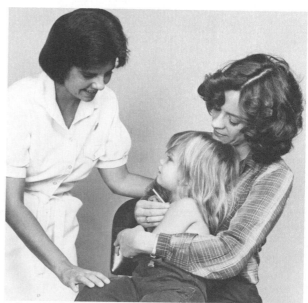

Figure 13-27 The nurse is teaching a mother how to obtain her youngster's axillary temperature. Note the correct placement of the thermometer.

NURSING CARE PLAN

13-1. Hyperthermia

Assessment

Subjective Data

Daughter states, "Mother insists on working in her garden in this heat. Luckily the neighbors saw her faint or who knows how long she would have lain there." Patient states, "I feel dizzy."

Objective Data

76-year-old woman. T—100.6 (o), P—104 thready and irregular, R-28, BP 106/52 in R. arm lying down. Skin is flushed, hot, and dry. Can identify daughter by name and relationship. Says this is summer, but cannot name the month or year. Knows she is in the hospital. Last meal and fluid consumed 6 hours ago. Not currently taking any type of medication.

Diagnosis

Hyperthermia related to overexertion in hot weather

Plan

Goal

The patient's body temperature will return to 98.6 ± 1° in 24 hours (1600 on 8/7).

Orders: 8/6

1. Assess vital signs $\overline{q}$ 4 h while awake on even hours.
2. Use only hospital gown while temp. is elevated.
3. Cover with just one cotton sheet while temp. is elevated.
4. Maintain bedrest and siderails.
5. Provide 1500 mL oral intake before bedtime. Likes lemonade, apple juice, and ginger ale.
6. Record I & O
7. When stable, instruct to:
   • wear a wide brimmed hat when outside
   • garden before 9 A.M. or after 7 P.M.
   • limit sun exposure to no more than 30 min
   • increase fluid intake on hot days
   • sit in front of fan after coming inside. —————————— S. EVANS, RN

Implementation (Documentation)
8/6

1800   T—100.4 (o), P—100 weak and irregular, R—20 $\overline{s}$ effort. BP 108/60 R. arm while lying down. Dress, undergarments, and stockings removed and given to daughter. Wearing hospital gown covered with top sheet. Bed is in low position with siderails up. Feels "dizzy" when head is elevated. BP 104/60 R. arm lying; BP 90/50 three minutes after assuming a sitting position. Bed rest maintained.
—————————— A. WHITE, LPN

Evaluation (Documentation)

2000   T—100 (o), P—96 full but irregular, R—20. BP 110/64 R. arm lying down. Skin is pink, dry, and cool. Drinking oral liquids. Urinating comparable amounts. Urine has changed from dark yellow to light yellow. Can identify current year correctly. No further dizziness experienced. Teaching postponed at this time.
—————————— A. WHITE, LPN

the patient's mouth if he cannot cooperate while an oral temperature is taken.

Locate the anal orifice digitally while using a lubricated finger cot or glove when the patient cannot be turned onto his side to obtain a rectal temperature. This technique avoids probing with the thermometer, which may injure local tissues. The technique also helps prevent placing the thermometer in a woman's vagina accidentally.

When the Patient's Activity or Emotional Status Is Likely to Influence the Vital Signs

Allow the patient to rest for a few minutes before obtaining the vital signs when he has been active or exercising. Activity and exercise tend to increase the pulse and respiratory rates and the blood pressure.

Except when necessary, avoid obtaining the vital signs when the patient is experiencing strong emotions, because they tend to increase vital signs. Examples of these emotions include fear, anger, and excitement.

Wait for 15 to 30 minutes before obtaining an oral temperature if the patient has recently had hot or cold fluids. This allows time for oral tissues to return to normal.

Wait about 5 minutes before obtaining an oral temperature if the patient has been smoking or has been chewing gum. This allows time for oral tissues to return to a normal temperature. One study showed that a patient's oral tissues had dropped to normal in about 3 minutes after chewing gum. It suggested that the exercise of oral muscles could falsely elevate a temperature taken during or immediately after chewing gum.

Delay obtaining an axillary temperature if the axilla has just been washed. The water and friction created by drying the skin may influence the temperature.

When the Patient Is Elderly

Count the pulse and respiratory rates of an elderly patient for a full minute for greatest accuracy. The rigidity of arterial walls that often occurs in the elderly results in a faster than normal pulse rate. The respiratory rate is often irregular due to certain chronic conditions frequently observed in the elderly.

Delay obtaining the vital signs unless necessary when the patient has been under stress or has been more active than usual. It has been observed that it may take as long as several hours for the vital signs to return to normal when an elderly patient has experienced psychological stress or more than usual exercise and activity.

When Certain Other Conditions Are Present

Avoid taking a rectal temperature from a woman in labor. The thermometer may injure the head of the infant passing through the birth canal.

Avoid obtaining a rectal temperature when the patient has had rectal surgery or has diarrhea. The thermometer is likely to injure tissue or increase the diarrhea.

Avoid obtaining an oral temperature when the patient breathes through his mouth. Examples of patients who usually are mouth breathers are those with respiratory tract diseases and obstructions in the nasal passages and those who have had oral or nasal surgery.

Observe agency policy about obtaining a rectal temperature when the patient has had a heart attack. It is thought by many that the thermometer may stimulate the vagus nerve causing the heart to slow to dangerous levels in some patients. However, one study to test this belief raised doubts and suggested that vagal stimulation may not be as harmful as once thought.

Obtain an axillary or rectal temperature from patients receiving oxygen by mask. The mask interferes with placing the thermometer in the mouth. Removing the mask may cause labored breathing due to a drop in the patient's oxygen level. The effect of oxygen therapy on oral temperatures has been studied in patients receiving oxygen by catheter or cannula. The conclusion was that the effect was so small that it probably had no significance for most clinical purposes.

Avoid obtaining an axillary temperature when the patient is in a state of shock. Blood circulation to the axillary area is likely to be poor and, as a result, the axillary temperature will be inaccurate. Shock is further discussed in Chapter 19.

Teaching Suggestions to Obtain Vital Signs

The following summary offers suggestions for patient teaching about obtaining the vital signs:

Nurses often teach home care patients or a family member how to obtain vital signs. The thermometer and equipment for obtaining the blood pressure are readily available in pharmacies and in medical supply stores.

Skill Procedures 13-1 through 13-6 can serve as guides when teaching patients or family members the techniques for obtaining vital signs and for cleaning a glass clinical thermometer.

Individuals who use sheaths to promote the cleanliness of an oral thermometer should be taught to inspect and evaluate the product carefully to determine its effectiveness.

The nurse should explain the normal findings for the vital signs and what abnormal findings constitute sufficient reason to contact a physician.

Bibliography

Baker NC, Cerone SB, Gaze N, Knapp TR: The effect of type of thermometer and length of time inserted on oral temperature measurements of afebrile subjects. Nurs Res 33(2):109–111, 1984

Bove PA, Owen L, Hekelman FP: Investigation of the methods used to teach blood pressure measurement techniques. Health Values 13(3):36–42, 1989

Brusch JL: Targeting the cause of unexplained fever. Emergency Medicine 21(5):108–110, 112–114, 119, 1989

Counselman FL: When fevers lead to seizures. Emerg Med Clin North Am 21(11):186–187, 190, 192, 1989

Haddock BJ, Merrow DL, Vincent PA: Comparisons of axillary and rectal temperatures in the preterm infant. Neonatal Network 6(5):67–71, 1988

Hahn LP, Folsom AR, Sprafka JM: Prevalance and accuracy of home sphygmomanometers in an urban population. Am J Public Health 77(11):1459–1461, 1987

Heinz J: Validation of sublingual temperatures in patients with nasogastric tubes. Heart & Lung: Journal of Critical Care 14(2):128–130, 1985

Henneman EA, Henneman PL: Intricacies of blood pressure measurement: Reexamining the rituals. Heart & Lung: Journal of Critical Care 18(3):263–273, 1989

Hon EH: Noninvasive blood pressure patterns. Journal of Perinatology 7(4):362–367, 1987

Howie JN: How and when should I respond to postop fever? Am J Nurs 89(7):984–986, 1989

Kunnel MT, O'Brien C, Munro BH: Comparisons of rectal, femoral, axillary, and skin-to-mattress temperatures in stable neonates. Nurs Res 37(3):162–164, 189, 1988

Martyn KK, Urbano MT, Hayes JS: Comparison of axillary, rectal and skin-based temperature assessment in preschoolers. Nurse Pract 13(4):31–32, 34–36, 1988

Mason DJ: Circadian rhythms of body temperature and activation and the well-being of older women. Nurs Res 37(5):276–281, 1988

Mauro AMP: Effects of bell versus diaphragm on indirect blood pressure measurement. Heart & Lung: Journal of Critical Care 17(5):489–494, 1988

Meier P: Bottle and breast feeding: Effects on transcutaneous oxygen pressure and temperature in preterm infants. Nurs Res 37(1):36–41, 1988

O'Brien EL: Clinical thermometry: In need of nursing research. Journal of Pediatric Nursing 3(3):207–208, 1988

Ogren JM: The inaccuracy of axillary temperatures measured with an electronic thermometer. Am J Dis Child 144(1):109–111, 1990

Pickering TG: Hypertension: Applications of ambulatory blood pressure monitoring. Consultant 29(1):115–116, 123–124, 1989

Preparing to take a patient's blood pressure. Nursing 19(6):65, 1989

Rebenson–Piano M, Holm K, Foreman MD, Kirchoff KT: An evaluation of two indirect methods of blood pressure measurement in ill patients. Nurs Res 38(1):42–45, 1989

Robichaud–Ekstrand S, Davies B: Comparison of electronic and glass thermometers: Length of time of insertion and type of breathing. The Canadian Journal of Nursing Research 21(1):61–73, 1989

Rudy SF: Measuring blood pressure: The vital sign. Emergency Medical Services 16(5):36, 38, 40–41, 1987

Sheehan MM: Blood pressure monitoring: Completing the picture . . . ambulatory blood pressure monitor. Nursing 20(4):79, 81, 1990

Taking accurate blood pressure readings. Nursing 18(4):32J, 32N, 1988

14

Performing Assessment Techniques

Chapter Outline

Behavioral Objectives
Glossary
Introduction
Gathering Information About the Patient
Purposes of Physical Assessment
Methods of Physical Assessment
Performing a Physical Assessment
Applicable Nursing Diagnoses
Suggested Measures to Assess the Patient's Health
   Status in Selected Situations
Teaching Suggestions to Assess the Patient's Health
   Status
Bibliography

Skill Procedures

Performing a Physical Assessment
Assessing Lung Sounds

Behavioral Objectives

When the content of this chapter has been mastered, the learner will be able to:

Define terms appearing in the glossary.
List information that is usually obtained in a health history.

Describe the steps for obtaining height and weight.
List examples of signs and symptoms.
List three purposes for assessing a patient's health status.
Identify four examination methods used during a physical assessment.
Describe the steps that a nurse follows when performing a physical assessment.
Describe the techniques used to assess each system of the body.
List several normal and abnormal findings that may be observed when examining a patient.
List suggested measures for assessing a patient's health status in selected situations, as described in this chapter.
Summarize suggestions for patient teaching offered in this chapter.

Glossary

Adventitious sounds Abnormal lung sounds.
Audiologist An individual who is a specialist in testing hearing.
Auscultation Listening to body sounds.
Constitutional sign or symptom A sign or symptom produced by the effect of a disease on the whole body. Synonym for *systemic sign* or *symptom*.
Crackles Intermittent, high-pitched, popping sounds heard in distant airways. Synonym for *rales*.
Cyanosis A bluish appearance to skin, nailbeds, and mucous membranes.
Distention Swelling or expansion of a part.
Ecchymosis The collection of blood in tissues, causing the skin to have a purplish color.
Edema Excessive fluid trapped in tissues.
Erythema A redness in areas of the skin.
Expectoration The act of expelling sputum from the throat or lungs through the mouth.
External hemorrhoid A vein that is stretched with blood and protrudes as a mass through the anus.
Fissure A groove or crack in the skin or mucous membrane.
Flush Reddish pink skin coloring, such as in a blush.
Fontanelle A soft spot between bones in the skull of a newborn.
Gurgles Continuous, low-pitched, bubbling sounds heard in larger airways. Synonym for *rhonchi*.
Health history Information about the patient's past and present health.
Inspection Purposeful observation.
Jaundice Yellow coloring of the skin.
Lesion An area of diseased tissue.
Local sign or symptom A sign or symptom limited to a particular part of the body.
Mental status Emotional mood and intellectual ability.

Mucoid Containing mucus.

Mucopurulent Containing mucus and pus.

Orientation The ability to identify time, place, and persons.

Otolaryngologist A physician who specializes in diagnosing and treating diseases of the ear, nose, and throat.

Otoscope An instrument used to examine the deep areas of the ear canal and eardrum.

Pallor A paleness of the skin.

Palpation Feeling or pressing on a part of the body.

Percussion Striking or tapping an area of the body.

Physical assessment The examination of the condition of the systems of the body.

Prodromal sign or symptom A sign or symptom appearing before the illness is obvious.

Purulent Containing pus.

Quadrant One fourth of a whole.

Rales Intermittent, high-pitched, popping sounds heard in distant airways. Synonym for *crackles*.

Rhonchi Continuous low-pitched, bubbling sounds heard in larger airways. Synonym for *gurgles*.

Rub A grating sound made as two dry tissue surfaces move over one another.

Sanguineous Containing blood.

Scar A mark left by the healing of a wound.

Sensory-perceptual status The appearance of sense organs, their state of functioning, and the ability of the mind to respond to stimuli.

Serosanguineous Containing serum and blood.

Serous Containing serum.

Serum The clear portion of blood.

Sign Observation or measurement made by an examiner.

Sputum Material expelled from the mouth by coughing or clearing the throat.

Symptom An observation that is felt and described by the patient.

Systemic sign or symptom A sign or symptom produced by the effect of a disease on the whole body. Synonym for *constitutional sign* or *symptom*.

Turgor The elasticity of skin.

Ulcer A craterlike open sore or lesion on the skin or mucous membrane.

Wheeze A whistling sound made as air moves through narrowed passages.

Wound A break in the skin.

Introduction

In Chapter 4, the components and principles of the nursing process were discussed. To review, the first step in the nursing process is assessment, or gathering information. One method of gathering information is to ask the patient questions about his health history. However, to gather information thoroughly, the nurse must perform a physical examination of the patient. That examination is referred to as a *physical assessment*. Though it is focused on the structures of the body, the nurse also takes the opportunity to gather information on the patient's mood, mental ability, and social interaction. This is in keeping with viewing man holistically, as discussed in Chapter 2.

This chapter discusses the information that a nurse usually obtains during assessment. It also describes the physical assessment techniques that are expected skills of a nurse generalist. Advanced physical assessment skills, which build on information given in this chapter, may be obtained by consulting specialty texts. The interpretation of abnormal findings is also excluded here; they are more appropriately discussed in clinical texts.

Gathering Information About the Patient

Though the nurse's responsibility for the depth of an assessment varies among health agencies and levels of practice, everyone should be familiar with its components. All nurses gather and record information that promotes the quality of a patient's plan for care.

Obtaining a Health History

Before examining each system of the body, the nurse gathers information that is unique to the patient. A *health history* summarizes the patient's past and present health. It generally includes the following information:

- Personal data, such as a patient's name, age, sex, marital status, and religion.
- The reason(s) for seeking health care at this time.
- The patient's description of his present state of health.
- The patient's past health problems, how they were treated, and the outcome.
- Information about the health of other family members, especially parents and grandparents.
- Information on lifestyle habits that affect health. This may include detrimental practices, such as the use of tobacco, alcohol, and other drugs. It may also include positive, preventive practices, such as monthly breast or testicular self-examination.

The physician also obtains a medical history. A medical history is usually obtained before admission to a hospital. If this has not been done, it is obtained shortly after admission. To avoid duplication, it is advantageous that the nurse be present when the physician obtains the medical history. Although the data gathered by the physician and the nurse are similar in content, the nurse uses the information differently.

Obtaining the Patient's Vital Signs

Obtaining vital signs is an example of one skill that assesses the cardiovascular and respiratory systems. However, because abnormal vital signs can reflect any number of problems related to other body systems, it is considered part of the general survey before any patient is examined. Obtaining vital signs is described in Chapter 13.

Obtaining the Patient's Height and Weight

It is common practice for the nurse to measure a patient's height and weight before the patient is examined. Although the patient may have weighed himself recently at home, it is best to weigh him again. This makes it possible to make comparisons while using the same scale. The patient's height is measured at the time of weighing. The following are recommended techniques to obtain a patient's height and weight:

- Check to see that the scale is calibrated at 0.
- Ask or assist the patient to remove his robe and shoes if he is wearing them.
- Place a paper towel on the scale before the patient stands on it in bare feet. This practice helps reduce patient contact with microbes that are spread through the use of hospital equipment by many patients.
- Assist the patient onto the scale.
- Slide the weights until the bar balances in the center of the scale, read the weight, and then write it down so the number is not forgotten.
- Ask the patient to stand straight in order to measure his height.
- Move the measuring bar down until it lightly touches the top of the patient's head, as the nurse in Figure 14-1 is doing.

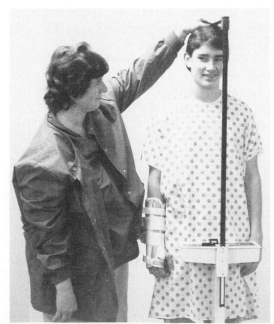

Figure 14-1 Before performing the physical assessment on each system of the body, the nurse obtains general information, such as the patient's height and weight.

- Note the height and write it down.
- Record the patient's weight and height on his record at the earliest appropriate time.

Measuring the patient's height and weight may be delayed temporarily if he is too ill. To make weighing easier for very ill patients, some agencies have portable or bed scales. The scale can be rolled to the patient's bedside, where he can be assisted or lifted onto it.

The nurse should be aware of signs or comments that suggest the patient is having recent, unexplained weight losses or gains, either of which may be an important diagnostic sign.

Noting Signs and Symptoms

While obtaining a health history or performing a physical assessment, the nurse notes signs and symptoms. Signs and symptoms are warnings the body gives when something is wrong. A *symptom* can only be felt and described by a patient. It is subjective in nature because it cannot be observed directly by another person. Pain and nausea are symptoms that can be felt and described only by the person who has them. A *sign* is something that can be seen by another person. It is objective in nature. A skin rash and swelling are examples of signs.

A *constitutional sign* or *symptom* is one that is produced by the effect of a disease on the whole body. Another term used by some nurses for this is *systemic sign* or *symptom*. Fever is a typical sign of most infectious diseases, such as a cold or chickenpox.

A *prodromal sign* or *symptom* is one that is noticed before an illness is obvious. A common prodromal symptom of flu is an aching sensation. A prodromal sign associated with measles is the appearance of white-centered spots inside the mouth.

A *local sign* or *symptom* is one limited to a particular part of the body. An example of a local sign associated with a sprained ankle would be swelling that is confined to the injured area; the local symptom would be the pain that is experienced in the ankle.

Examining the Patient

The role of the nurse when a patient is to be examined varies depending on the educational program or the health agency in which the nurse works. The general trend is that nurses are now taking increased responsibility in examining a patient, and some educational programs are preparing nurses accordingly. This component of the assessment phase within the nursing process is clearly stated in the ANA Standards for Nursing Practice.

Purposes of Physical Assessment

An examination of the patient serves several important purposes.

- It is an excellent way to evaluate an individual's current health status. It is a time when health practitioners can teach patients the importance of following healthful living habits.
- It helps to detect signs of early illness that can be treated more easily and effectively than long-standing illnesses.
- Findings of a physical assessment provide a database for identifying nursing diagnoses and collaborative problems.

Methods of Physical Assessment

Inspection, percussion, palpation, and auscultation are assessment methods that require the use of one or a combination of the nurse's senses. These techniques help the nurse gather information about the condition of the structures of the patient's body and the state of their functioning. Normal and abnormal findings are equally important.

Inspection

Inspection is purposeful observation. It is the most frequently used of the assessment methods. Using the term broadly, inspection refers to a technique in which the nurse uses many senses collectively to scan the patient. The information is interpreted rapidly to form an overall impression of the patient. Using the term more strictly, inspection refers to a technique in which the nurse simultaneously focuses vision and attention, looking for minute details. The nurse in Figure 14-2 is inspecting the mouth of a patient. With advanced instruction, some nurses learn to use instruments to inspect parts of the body that are potentially inaccessible to ordinary vision. For example, an ophthalmoscope is an instrument used to examine the inside of the eye.

Percussion

Percussion means striking or tapping a particular part of the body. The fingertips are most often used to cause a vibration of the tissue much like the drum-sticks on a drum. The effect of the tapping produces sounds. Mass produces a dull sound; empty or air-filled structures, like the lungs, generally produce a hollow sound. Any condition that changes the density of an organ or tissue, such as a tumor, collection of air, or fluid, will cause a change in the quality of the sound.

If percussion is performed correctly, the patient should not experience any discomfort. If pain is experienced it could mean that there is some injury or disease in that area.

Percussion is most often used to examine the lungs and abdomen. The nurse in Figure 14-3 is using percussion to assess the sounds produced in the abdomen. The area over the liver should sound differently from the area that contains only intestine because one is more dense than the other.

Palpation

Palpation uses the sense of touch to gather information. The examiner feels or presses on the body. The thyroid, breasts, and testes are types of glandular tissue that are often examined by palpation. The nurse should be able to gather data such as size, texture, temperature, movement of tissue, and associated discomfort when palpation is used as a method of assessment. It is important to compare structures when possible, such as the findings of one breast in relation to the other. The nurse in Figure 14-4 is examining the abdomen using the technique of palpation.

Patients can be taught to use some assessment methods. For example, the steps illustrated in Figure 14-5 provide simple instructions for using inspection and palpation to

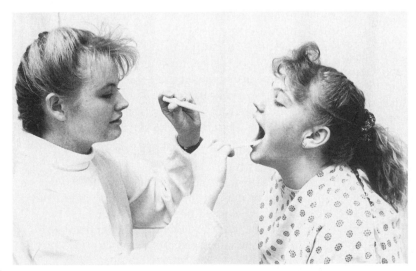

Figure 14-2 The nurse is using inspection to assess the patient's mouth, throat, and teeth.

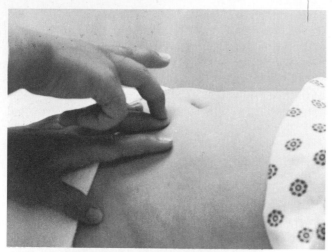

Figure 14-3 The nurse uses percussion to detect changes in the sounds in various abdominal areas.

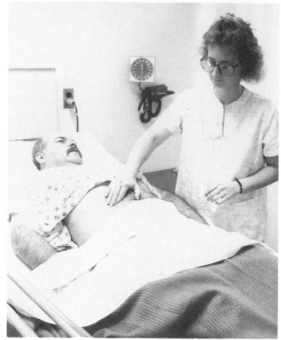

Figure 14-4 The nurse is palpating the patient's abdomen.

detect warning signs of breast cancer or other breast diseases. The nurse should instruct all women to perform self-breast examination. Men should also be instructed on using self-examination techniques to detect changes in the tissue of the testes.

Auscultation

Auscultation uses the sense of hearing. Some sounds, like a hoarse voice, may be heard with the nurse's ears. Others may require the use of a stethoscope to collect and amplify the sounds from structures deep within the body, such as the heart, lungs, and bowel. The nurse needs to practice this assessment technique to become proficient with its use. It is important to eliminate or reduce environmental noises while using auscultation. Figure 14-6 illustrates a nurse auscultating sounds within a patient's chest.

Performing a Physical Assessment

A beginning nurse should practice the techniques for performing various aspects of physical assessment. Table 14-1 lists assessment criteria that a competent nurse should be able to examine and interpret. Skill Procedure 14-1 describes the steps that the nurse may wish to follow when performing a physical assessment. The categories in Table 14-1 will be used as a framework in the next section to describe the techniques used to perform a particular area of assessment.

Assessing Sensory-Perceptual Status

Sensory-perceptual status is a complex combination of terms. It refers to examining the appearance of sense organs as well as their state of functioning. It also includes assessing the ability of the mind to interpret and respond appropriately to stimuli.

Examining a Patient's Mental Status. An arbitrary place to start a physical assessment is to evaluate the patient's mental status. *Mental status* most often implies the state of a person's mood and intellectual functioning. Nurses who specialize in mental health nursing will acquire advanced skills and terminology to assess the mental status of patients who require psychiatric treatment.

To assess mood, the nurse uses the technique of inspection. The nurse observes the patient's appearance, hygiene, speech, and behavior to determine how a patient may be feeling.

Terms such as anxious, frightened, and unconcerned are often used to describe the patient's mood. It is better to record the behavior the nurse observes. Some examples include: Muscles tense, jaw set, hands clenched, perspiring heavily; "Wearing soiled, wrinkled clothing, unbathed, sits and stares, does not respond to questions"; "Shouted obscenities at nurse. Threw a water pitcher at the wall."

The nurse also assesses the patient's intellectual functioning. The nurse uses direct questioning and active listening to assess the intellectual ability of patients. Some assessment techniques include the following:

- Adding simple numbers, like 3 + 5.
- Counting in groups of threes, such as 3, 6, 9, 12, 15.
- Requesting that the patient recall a series of numbers or words that the nurse verbally provides, such as duck, ring, soccer, bicycle, and church.
- Asking the patient to identify a common object, such as a watch, and explain its use.

1

In the shower:

Examine your breasts during bath or shower; hands glide easier over wet skin. Fingers flat, move gently over every part of each breast. Use right hand to examine left breast, left hand for right breast. Check for any lump, hard knot or thickening.

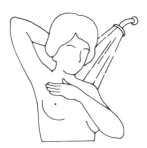

2

Before a mirror:

Inspect your breasts with arms at your sides. Next, raise your arms high overhead. Look for any changes in contour of each breast, a swelling, dimpling of skin or changes in the nipple.

Then, rest palms on hips and press

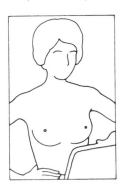

down firmly to flex your chest muscles. Left and right breast will not exactly match—few women's do.

Regular inspection shows what is normal for you and will give you confidence in your examination.

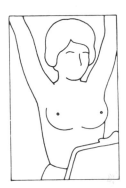

3

Lying down:

To examine your right breast, put a pillow or folded towel under your right shoulder. Place right hand behind your head—this distributes breast tissue more evenly on the chest. With left hand, fingers flat, press gently in small circular motions around an imaginary clock face. Begin at outermost top of your right

breast for 12 o'clock, then move to 1 o'clock, and so on around the circle back to 12. A ridge of firm tissue in the lower curve of each breast is normal. Then move in an inch, toward the nipple, keep circling to examine *every part of your breast,* including nipple. This requires at least three more circles. Now slowly repeat

procedure on your left breast with a pillow under your left shoulder and left hand behind head. Notice how your breast structure feels.

Finally, squeeze the nipple of each breast gently between thumb and index finger. Any discharge, clear or bloody, should be reported to your doctor immediately.

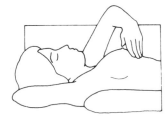

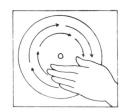

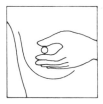

Figure 14-5 Following these steps, any woman can perform a breast self-examination. (Courtesy of the American Cancer Society.)

- Asking the patient to explain an abstract, but commonly used, figure of speech, such as, "That child is sharp as a tack."
- Asking the patient to explain a proverb, such as "Don't cry over spilled milk."
- Asking the patient to list several large cities in the United States.

These questions should be adjusted to the age or level of the patient's development. To be valid data, the errors should only be considered incorrect if they were within the person's expected intellectual capacity. For example, the nurse should not ask a 7-year-old child to multiply 2×4. More than one question should be asked to validate the response.

When recording the results of the intellectual assessment, it is helpful to quote what the patient actually answered. This is an example: "To the request 'Explain what it means if a boy is sharp as a tack,' the response was, 'The boy's head is pointed.'"

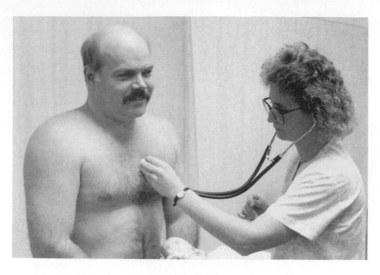

Figure 14-6 The nurse uses auscultation to listen to the patient's breath sounds.

Examining Vision and Eyes. Simple methods for assessing visual acuity, color perception, and the patient's field of vision were discussed in Chapter 2. For an accurate assessment of visual acuity, a Snellen chart or other eye- chart such as those shown in Figure 14-7 may be used. A complete eye exam is not generally performed on every patient who is hospitalized. The nurse may use these charts during school and employment screenings. The

Table 14-1. Physical Assessment by a Nurse Generalist

Physical System	Criteria	Physical System	Criteria
Sensory–perceptual	Mental status		Circulation (mucous membranes, nail beds)
	Vision and appearance of eyes	Neurological	Pupillary reactions
	Hearing		Orientation
	Touch		Level of consciousness
	Taste and smell		Grasp strength
Skin	Condition (color, turgor, character)	Gastrointestinal	Mouth, gums, teeth, and tongue (color, condition)
	Lesions		Gag reflex
	Edema		Bowel sounds
	Hair distribution		Presence of distention, impaction, hemorrhoids (external)
Respiratory	Rate, character		
	Breath sounds		
	Cough	Genitourinary	Lesions
Cardiovascular	Pulses (rate, quality, rhythm)		Presence of retention
	Apical Radial		Discharge (vaginal, urethral)
	Carotid Dorsalis pedis		Uterine response (pregnancy, postpartum)
	Brachial Posterior tibial	Musculoskeletal	Muscle tone, strength
	Femoral		Gait, stability
	Blood pressure		Range of motion

Carpenito L, Duespohl T: A Guide for Effective Clinical Instruction, 2nd ed, p 142. Rockville, Aspen, 1985. Reprinted with permission of Aspen Publishers, Inc., © 1985.

Skill Procedure 14-1. Performing a Physical Assessment

Suggested Action	**Reason for Action**
Assemble the equipment that will be needed to perform an examination. Some examples include: • stethoscope • sphygmomanometer • penlight • tongue blade • scales.	A physical assessment is time consuming. Having to search for equipment extends that time and tires the patient.
Introduce yourself to the patient and explain what is planned.	A nurse-patient relationship can be enhanced by setting the patient at ease and sharing information.
Give the patient an opportunity to use the bathroom or use a bedpan or urinal.	It is difficult to examine a patient when the urinary bladder is full or when the patient needs to have a bowel movement. Also, using the bathroom before an examination generally helps the patient feel more at ease.
Take the patient to an area that provides privacy; an examination room is preferred. If this is not possible, shut the door and pull the curtains within the patient's room.	A patient is likely to feel more comfortable being examined in an area where it is unlikely that there will be intrusions.
Wash hands before and at the completion of the examination.	Microbes are most often spread from dirty hands.
Follow agency policies about obtaining assistance with an examination.	Many agencies still require a woman to be present if a female patient is being examined by a man and, in some cases, vice versa. This is done for the legal protection of the examiner and the agency from charges that sexual assault was committed.
Make sure there is adequate natural or artificial lighting. The examination area should be comfortable in terms of temperature and ventilation.	Arranging the conditions of the environment promotes comfort during the examination
Assist the patient to put on an examining gown and provide a cover for other exposed areas.	A gown allows access to various parts of the body while still respecting the patient's modesty.
Explain that all information will be kept confidential and will only be used by health personnel to plan and carry out appropriate nursing care for the patient.	A patient is more likely to be candid in providing information if he feels the nurse is honest and sincere about protecting his rights.
Use techniques described previously in Skill Procedure 2-1 to promote effective communication.	The amount and depth of information obtained may depend on the skill with which the nurse communicates.
Be prepared to take notes, but try to avoid writing constantly.	The information must be accurately recorded on the hospital's record. The patient must feel that the nurse's priority of concern is for him as an individual, not the task.
Raise the bed or examination table to the nurse's waist level to avoid having to bend and stretch to reach the patient.	Good posture and body mechanics may be promoted by adjusting the height and position of the patient.
Take precautions that the patient will not fall off the table or bed.	The higher the patient is from the floor, the greater the potential for injury if a fall occurs.
Using the health agency's guide, begin to examine the patient. Explain each technique before it is performed.	Until a nurse develops practice, following a printed form will prevent omitting parts of the examination.

(continued)

Skill Procedure 14-1. Continued

Suggested Action	Reason for Action
Once the nurse is confident, the patient may be examined in any orderly fashion.	It is important to do a complete examination of the various systems of the body. The sequence through which the examination progresses is not important.
• From head to toe. • From an area further removed from the center of the body (distal) to one nearer the center of the body (proximal), such as from the toes to the hips. • From front (anterior) to back (posterior), such as the front of the chest wall and then the back of the chest wall. • From the middle of the body (medial) to the side of the body (lateral), such as from the eyes to the ears.	
Review the data that has been gathered to determine that it is complete.	The patient will be inconvenienced if parts of a physical assessment need to be rescheduled or repeated.
At the completion of the examination help the patient, if necessary, to dress.	The patient may prefer wearing his own personal bedclothes.
Assist the patient back to his room if the examination has been performed in another area.	Examination rooms may be needed for other patients.
Help the patient back into bed and adjust his position as he desires.	Concern for the patient's comfort should be expressed throughout his stay in a health agency.
Share a summary of the assessment findings with the patient, but avoid making medical interpretations of abnormalities that may have been revealed during the examination.	The patient has a right to information about his physical condition. The nurse and the patient will need to cooperatively determine which problems require attention and what measures are most suitable to the patient.
Make sure all equipment is cleaned or replaced.	The room should be ready for use for the next patient.
Record the assessment information on the appropriate form.	Data must be recorded accurately so that all health personnel may become aware of the patient's needs and problems.
Communicate any significant information to nursing or medical personnel.	Some findings may require immediate action.
Plan teaching sessions following the suggested actions in Skill Procedure 2–3.	The patient should be provided with information that will improve or maintain his health.

nurse working in an ophthalmologist's office may use these as a focus assessment when the patient is referred.

Most physical assessments include observations about the external structures and appearance of the eyes. Look at the pupils to determine if they are both round. Note any discoloration of the eyes or eyelids. Note other abnormal characteristics, such as swelling, crusting, tearing, or other secretions of the eyes, eyelashes, or eyelids.

Test extraocular movements. These are controlled by six pairs of muscles. Have the patient focus and track a finger or some other object like a pen without moving his head. Starting with the eyes centered, move the object side to side and diagonally from left to right and then right to left. The eyes should move symmetrically. These are called the six cardinal positions and are shown in Figure 14-8.

The nurse can assess the pupil's ability to change size while focusing on objects both near and far. This is called accommodation. Hold the finger or an object approximately 5 inches (12 cm) from the patient's nose. As the patient focuses on the object note if the pupils constrict. Constriction is a normal response. Ask the patient to look away from the object toward something more distant. The pupils should dilate.

The normal pupil response to light is discussed with neurologic assessment. However, the combined assessment of pupils is often abbreviated PERRLA, or pupils equally round and react to light and accommodation. If abnormal findings were noted this abbreviation would not be appropriate.

Assessing Hearing and the Ears. The characteristics and techniques for testing normal hearing were de-

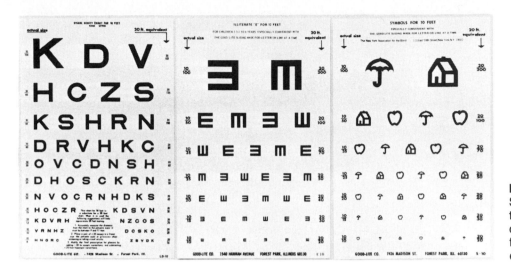

Figure 14-7 These are various Snellen charts used to test distant vision. The charts in the center and at far right are used for very young children and illiterate adults.

scribed in Chapter 7. If an individual responds poorly to the simple tests performed during the nurse's physical assessment, the patient may be referred to his physician or an *otolaryngologist,* a physician who specializes in diagnosing and treating diseases of the ears, nose, and throat. Another individual who is a specialist in testing hearing is an *audiologist.*

During a physical assessment, only the external ear is examined. The characteristics of the external ear can be assessed through visual inspection and palpation. The nurse may use the following techniques:

- Observe the appearance and feel of the skin areas behind and within the ear. Each ear should be compared with the other.
- Move the underlying cartilage about. The patient should not experience any discomfort.
- Shine a penlight into the ear canal to illuminate the area. To straighten the ear canal of a child, pull it down and back; on an adult, pull the ear up and back as

shown in Figure 14-9. Cerumen is commonly found within the ear canal. Any other type of drainage is abnormal, and its characteristics should be noted and reported. It is common for children to place objects in the ear, which then become fixed and difficult to remove. With advanced classes in assessment, some nurses learn to use an otoscope. An *otoscope* is a lighted instrument that facilitates deeper inspection of the ear canal and eardrum.

Assessing Touch, Taste, and Smell. To assess the senses of touch, taste, and smell the nurse may use various common objects. The nurse observes the accuracy with which the patient can identify substances or sensations produced by objects he cannot see. Note the following assessment techniques:

To Assess Touch:

- Instruct the patient to close both eyes throughout the examination.

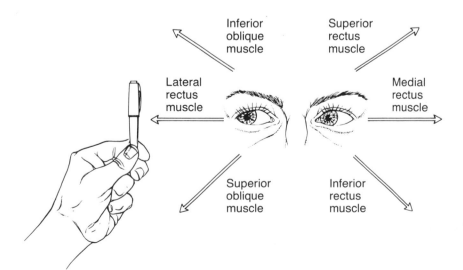

Figure 14-8 The nurse observes the ability of the patient to move his eyes in six different directions called the cardinal positions.

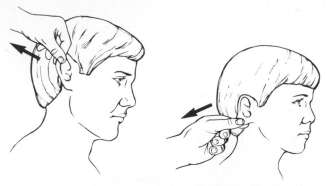

Adult: Pull ear superiorly   Children: Pull ear posteriorly
   and posteriorly   and inferiorly

Figure 14-9 The shape of the ear canal changes with growth. To allow better inspection, the nurse must position the ear differently for a child than for an adult.

- Touch the patient's skin on both sides of the body. Use a variety of objects that produce different sensations. The patient indicates if something is felt, and where.
- Opposite ends of an open safety pin may be used for assessing the patient's sense of touch. The patient identifies if the sensation is sharp or dull. An irregular pattern should be used to control for correct guessing.
- Drinking glasses containing warm and cold water can be applied to the skin on both sides of the body. The patient should correctly identify the temperature of the stimulus being used. Random patterns ensure more valid results.
- In some cases, a tuning fork may be struck and placed against a bony area, such as the wrist, to produce vibration.

To Assess Taste:
- Place small amounts of substances on the patient's tongue. Substances such as salt, sugar, and lemon should be readily identifiable. To assure valid responses the patient should rinse or sip water between substances.

To Assess Smell:
- Request that the patient alternately close off one nasal passage and smell a substance that gives off an easily identified odor. Examples include lemon, vanilla extract, coffee, peppermint, and rubbing alcohol. Several substances should be used to avoid inaccurate assumptions about results.

Assessing the Skin

The characteristics of healthy skin, mucous membranes, hair, and nails may be reviewed in Chapter 7. The nurse uses inspection and palpation to gather this information.

- Examine the entire surface of the body in one all-inclusive inspection, or note the condition of the skin as other structures are examined. For instance, while examining the eyes and ears, the condition of facial skin may be observed.
- Note the color of the skin. Though areas of the body may show slight variations, the color should be fairly even. Table 14-2 identifies terms that may be used to describe skin color.
- Feel the texture of the skin with the surface of the fingertips. The skin should feel soft except for areas of the palms and soles of the feet. A diseased area of skin is generally referred to as a *lesion*. There are many types of lesions. A *wound* is a break in the skin. An *ulcer* is a craterlike lesion on the skin or mucous membrane. A *scar* is a mark left by the healing of a wound or lesion. A *fissure* is a groove or crack in the skin or mucous membrane. The size, shape, depth, and location of a lesion should be noted. If drainage is present, it too is described as to amount and character. The amount is described as being scant, moderate, or profuse. Common terms for describing the appearance of drainage are as follows:
  Serous: Containing *serum,* or the clear portion of blood
  Sanguineous: Containing blood
  Serosanguineous: Containing blood and serum
  Mucoid: Containing mucus
  Purulent: Containing pus
  Mucopurulent: Containing mucus and pus
- Using the thumb and index finger, grasp and pull on the skin. This facilitates assessing skin *turgor,* or its elasticity. Normally the skin rebounds to its original appearance when released.
- Depress a finger into the skin over a bony area in the lower leg or top of the foot. If edema is present, an indentation remains. *Edema* is excess fluid that is trapped in the tissues. The skin may also appear taut, puffy, and shiny.
- Hair growth should be present in fine amounts over the body. Some patients may normally have excessive amounts.

Assessing the Respiratory System

Review the discussion on assessing the respiratory rate and character of breath sounds described in Chapter 13. Besides counting the respiratory rate and noting the pattern of breathing, the nurse may also assess the chest and respirations in the following ways:

- Observe the size and shape of the chest. Figure 14-10 shows some variations in chest contours.
- Observe that both sides of the chest rise and fall in synchrony with the respirations.
- Note the type and characteristics of any cough. A cough is described as nonproductive if no secretions from the respiratory tract are produced. If secretions can be raised, it is called a productive cough. Mucus is the watery secretion from mucous membranes.

Table 14-2. Common Color Variation of the Skin

Term	Description	Interpretation
Flush	A reddish pink coloring	A flush resembles a blush and is often seen when the temperature is elevated. The face and neck are affected more often than other parts of the body.
Erythema	A reddish coloring	When tissue is injured blood is sent to the area. This collection of blood is what contributes to characteristic redness of inflamed tissue.
Jaundice	A yellowish coloring	Jaundice is related to liver, gall bladder, and blood diseases. It involves all skin areas, but almost always the whites of the eyes are especially affected. Consuming excessive amounts of yellow vegetables can also discolor the skin and be confused as jaundice.
Pallor	Paleness	This is often associated with decreased numbers of red blood cells. In persons with dark skin, look for paleness of the oral mucous membranes, in the nail beds, and within the inner surface of the eyelids.
Ecchymosis	A purplish coloring	Ecchymotic areas, also called bruises, are usually the result of a collection of blood under the skin from blunt trauma.
Cyanosis	A bluish coloring	Cyanosis is associated with the lack of oxygen to the tissues. It can also be noted in the nail beds, lips, and mucous membranes.
Tan	A brown coloring	This may be associated with a person's ethnic origin. It may also occur with exposure to the sun or ultraviolet light. It may be seen in pregnant patients, where it is usually confined to the face and nipples.

Sputum, which consists of material expelled from the mouth by coughing or clearing the throat and which comes from the lower respiratory tract, is thicker than mucus. It may have a greenish yellow color when infection is present. *Expectoration* is a general term for the act of expelling secretions through the mouth.

Auscultating Lung Sounds. Listening to the lungs is a skill that requires frequent and repeated practice. Nurses should auscultate the lungs of classmates and family to acquire the ability to distinguish normal sounds from abnormal. Skill Procedure 14-2 describes the technique for assessing lung sounds.

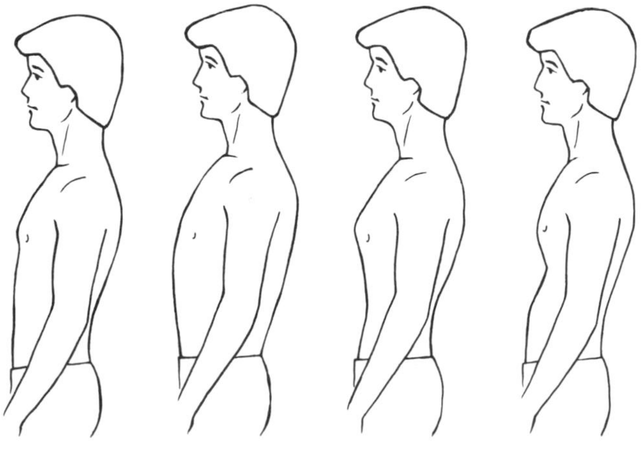

Normal Lung Sounds. Lung sounds are created by air moving in and out of air passageways. The airways vary in diameter as well as distance from the nose and mouth. The sounds, therefore, have different characteristics depending upon the location being auscultated.

The four types of normal lung sounds are tracheal, bronchial, bronchovesicular, and vesicular sounds. Tracheal sounds are heard, as the name implies, directly over the trachea. Because this airway is large and close to the mouth, the sound is loud and coarse. It is similar to wind blowing through a tunnel. Tracheal sounds are equal in length during inspiration and expiration separated by a short pause. Bronchial sounds are heard over the manubrium, the upper portion of the sternum. They are harsh and loud and are short on inspiration with a slight pause before a lengthier expiration. Bronchovesicular sounds are heard on either side of the center of the chest and back. These sounds are in the medium range. They are equal in length during inspiration and expiration with no noticeable pause. Vesicular sounds are soft, rustling sounds. They are heard in the periphery of all areas of the lungs. The inspirational sound is longer than the sound during expiration. There is no pause between the two. Figure 14-13 shows the locations of normal lung sounds.

Abnormal Lung Sounds. Abnormal lung sounds are also called *adventitious sounds.* They are heard in addition to normal lung sounds. Most abnormal lung sounds are

Figure 14-10 When inspecting the chest, the nurse may observe some of these common variations in contour. (*A*), normal chest; (*B*), barrel chest; (*C*), pigeon chest; and (*D*), funnel chest.

Skill Procedure 14-2. *Assessing Lung Sounds*

Suggested Action	Reason for Action
Wash hands.	Handwashing reduces the spread of microorganisms.
Explain the purpose and procedure for lung sound assessment.	Explanations promote cooperation and reduce apprehension.
Provide privacy.	The patient has the right to be protected from being seen by others.
Raise the bed to a high position.	A comfortable height for the nurse reduces back strain while conducting the examination.
Remove or loosen upper clothing.	Cloth rubbing on the stethoscope can interfere with an accurate assessment.
Reduce or eliminate environmental noise such as suction motors and humidifiers on oxygen equipment.	Controlling noise promotes optimum conditions for hearing lung sounds more distinctly.
Help the patient to a sitting position.	A sitting position allows the posterior, lateral, and anterior chest to be auscultated without changing positions.
Ask the patient not to talk.	Talking may interfere with the nurse's concentration and the ability to hear lung sounds clearly.
Warm the diaphragm of the stethoscope in the palm of the hand.	Metal can be cold and cause discomfort when applied to the skin. Body heat warms the metal by conduction.
Instruct the patient to breathe in and out through his mouth.	Breathing through the nose creates air turbulence that may distort lung sounds.
Apply the diaphragm to the upper back.	Lung sounds are best heard in the posterior. Heart sounds tend to obscure lung sounds on the anterior chest.
Listen during one complete respiration, e.g., inspiration and expiration, at each placement of the stethoscope.	Lung sounds may be identified by location, sound, rhythm, and occurrence during a respiratory cycle.
Wet chest and back hair or press more firmly if hair causes sound distortions.	Keeping hair flat with the surface of the skin increases the clarity of the lung sounds.
Move the diaphragm from side to side from the apices to the bases of the lungs as shown in Figure 14-11.	Abnormal sounds or an absence of sound may be localized. It is important that the assessment be thorough so as not to miss important data.

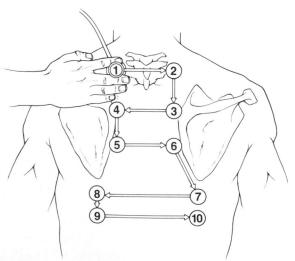

Figure 14-11 Lung sounds are compared by moving the stethoscope to a similar position on each side of the chest.

(*continued*)

Skill Procedure 14-2. Continued

Suggested Action	Reason for Action
Avoid placing the stethoscope over the scapulae or ribs.	Auscultating over bone reduces the ability to hear air as it moves throughout the lungs.
Auscultate the lateral and anterior chest similarly as shown in Figure 14-12.	All areas of the lung should be auscultated and compared bilaterally.

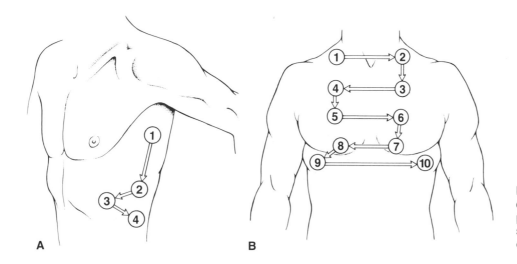

Figure 14-12 (*A*). Each side of the chest is auscultated and compared. (*B*). The anterior chest is systematically examined over each lung field.

Suggested Action	Reason for Action
Ask the patient to cough or breathe deeply if crackles or gurgles are heard.	Abnormal lung sounds that do not clear with coughing or deep breathing are more serious.
Reapply clothing and lower the patient's bed. Raise siderails that were lowered.	These actions restore comfort and safety.
Wash hands.	Handwashing reduces the spread of microorganisms.
Record normal and abnormal findings on the assessment sheet, narrative notes, or progress notes.	Documentation is one method of sharing information with colleagues. Trends can be identified by reviewing collected data.
Repeat assessments according to policy or the condition of the patient.	Auscultating lung sounds is especially important before and after suctioning and after inserting or repositioning an endotracheal tube.

caused by air moving through secretions or narrowed airways. They are generally divided into four categories: crackles, gurgles, wheezes, and rubs. Their names are somewhat descriptive of their sounds.

Crackles, also called *rales,* are intermittent, high-pitched, popping sounds heard in distant lung areas during inspiration. Some have compared the sound to a popular rice cereal as it becomes saturated with milk. Others suggest that rubbing strands of hair between the thumb and forefinger beside the ear simulates the sound of crackles. Crackles may be caused by the displacement of secretions that have accumulated in terminal bronchioles. This sound also has been attributed to air opening par-

tially collapsed alveoli. Crackles may clear with coughing, deep breathing, or a change in position.

Gurgles, also called *rhonchi,* are low-pitched, continuous, bubbling sounds heard in larger airways. They are more prominent during expiration. Incoming air moves mucus inward and bubbles through it during expiration. Some describe it as sounding like wet snoring. Gurgles will often clear with deep breathing or coughing. There are subcategories of crackles and gurgles. A physical assessment text is a good resource for a more detailed description.

A *wheeze* is a whistling or squeaky sound. It can be heard anywhere throughout the chest during inspiration

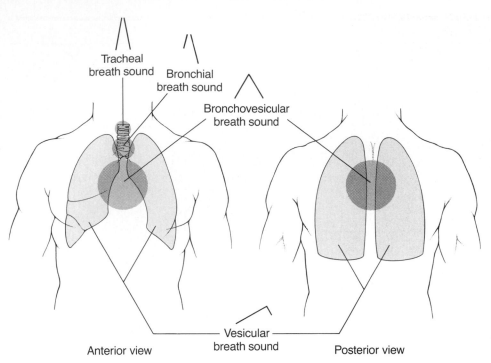

Tracheal breath sound

Bronchial breath sound

Bronchovesicular breath sound

Vesicular breath sound

Anterior view

Posterior view

Figure 14-13 The locations where normal lung sounds are heard. The marks above the labels illustrate the ratio of time during inspiration and expiration and the presence or absence of pauses between the two.

or expiration. Asthmatics usually wheeze on expiration. A wheeze occurs as air travels through a narrowed passage. Sometimes these sounds can be heard without even using a stethoscope. Coughing and deep breathing do not usually alter the wheeze.

A *rub* is the last category of abnormal lung sounds. It is a grating sound. The sound is created by two dry surfaces of tissue moving over one another. Ordinarily there is a thin film of fluid that helps membranes to glide noiselessly and smoothly across each other. When lung pleurae lose that fluid, the resulting friction causes a pleural rub. When a similar condition affects the heart, it is called a pericardial rub.

Assessing the Cardiovascular System

Many aspects of cardiovascular assessment have been discussed. Refer to Chapter 13 on obtaining and analyzing vital signs. The techniques for obtaining the patient's blood pressure and radial and peripheral pulses should be reviewed. The following actions are included when a nurse generalist assesses the cardiovascular system.

- Obtain the patient's blood pressure. On the basis of this finding, judge whether additional methods of blood pressure assessment are indicated. For example, the nurse may take blood pressure on both the right and left arm, or with the patient lying down and sitting up for comparisons. Data gathered must be valid to make accurate interpretations.
- Count the rate of the radial pulse; note its quality and rhythm.

- If there are any abnormal signs associated with the radial pulse, assess the apical pulse rate.
- Palpate the peripheral pulses on each side of the body. Observe the quality of the pulse at each location of the carotid, brachial, radial, femoral, posterior tibial, and dorsalis pedis pulse sites. The locations of these sites are illustrated in Chapter 13. If the peripheral pulses are difficult or impossible to palpate, assess blood flow using a Doppler probe. A Doppler is shown in Figure 14-14.
- Depress the nailbeds bilaterally on the thumbs and great toes. Note the rate of color return. It should be restored in less than 3 seconds. Compare the results of each two extremities.

Assessing Heart Sounds. While auscultating the anterior chest for lung sounds, the nurse has the opportunity to also assess heart sounds. No one knows exactly what causes heart sounds; they may be caused by the heart valves snapping closed at different times in the cardiac cycle. Four areas are auscultated because there are four heart valves. Some nurses use the words "Apple Pie To Make" to help them remember which valves are responsible for the sounds they are hearing. The first letter of each word stands for the following: A, aortic; P, pulmonic; T, tricuspid; and M, mitral. The locations where heart sounds from these valves are best heard are identified in Figure 14-15. The purpose for assessing heart sounds is to note their presence, count the heart rate, identify heart rhythm, and detect extra sounds that may be present in addition to normal ones.

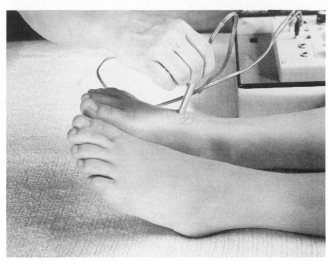

Figure 14-14 Conductive jelly is applied over the dorsalis pedis artery. The Doppler probe detects the movement of blood and amplifies its sound.

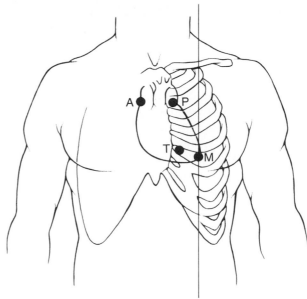

Figure 14-15 Though the auscultatory areas are not directly over the anatomical location of the heart valves, they are heard best in these locations.

Normal Heart Sounds. The two normal heart sounds are identified as S_1 and S_2. The first heart sound, S_1, correlates with the "lub" sound and S_2 correlates with "dub." The first sound is heard best with the bell of the stethoscope on the left side of the chest just below the nipple. This corresponds with the fifth intercostal space at the midclavicular line. This is exactly the same location described in Chapter 13 for counting the apical heart rate. Both normal heart sounds will be heard here, but the S_1 sound is louder and longer in this location. It can be identified positively by simultaneously palpating the carotid artery. A pulsation should be felt at the same time as the "lub" sound is heard.

This first heart sound is made by the combined closing of the tricuspid and mitral valves. Moving the stethoscope up one more rib space and toward the left border of the sternum, the tricuspid valve is more audible. The mitral and tricuspid valves close nearly, but not exactly, at the same time. A slight difference in the S_1 sound may be heard over the tricuspid area. If it is noted, it is called a split sound.

To auscultate for the S_2 sound, move the stethoscope to the second intercostal space to the right of the sternum. This is the best location for hearing the aortic valve. Now the "dub" sound should be louder. It is still shorter than "lub." The S_2 sound is made by the closing of the aortic and pulmonic valves nearly in unison. To hear the pulmonic valve and a possible splitting of the S_2 sound, move the stethoscope directly across to the opposite side of the sternum. Again, refer to Figure 14-15 for auscultating locations.

If the patient is obese or there is difficulty hearing the sounds, some modifications may help. One of the best actions is to move the heart closer to the chest wall. This can be done with the help of gravity by having the patient sit up and lean forward. Another position that may help is lying the patient flat and then turning him slightly to his left side.

Abnormal Heart Sounds. While listening and identifying normal heart sounds, the nurse may hear additional sounds. Children may normally have an extra heart sound that comes after the "dub" or S_2 sound called S_3. The sequence is S_1-S_2-S_3. An S_3 sound is abnormal in most adults. It is often heard in patients experiencing heart failure. Some say that when all three of these heart sounds are heard in sequence, their cadence sounds like the word "Ken-tuck-y."

An extra sound heard just before "lub," S_1, is identified as S_4. Its sequence in the cardiac cycle would be S_4-S_1-S_2. Some say this arrangement sounds like the word "Ten-ne-see."

Identifying abnormal heart sounds is a developed skill. If as a beginning student an unusual extra sound is heard, consult with another more experienced nurse or the physician. It could just be that a splitting of a normal sound is being heard, or it could be something much more significant.

Murmurs and a pericardial rub are also abnormal heart sounds that might be heard during auscultation. The description of murmurs is quite detailed. Interested students may wish to read more on the characteristics of murmurs in physical assessment or cardiology texts. Some excellent audiocassette tapes may also be available.

Assessing the Neurologic System

A complete examination of the nervous system is not a responsibility of a nurse generalist. A simplified physical assessment of this system can provide data indicating the need for a more extensive examination. A nurse generalist should evaluate pupillary reactions, orientation, level of consciousness, and strength of grasp. The neurological checklist is illustrated in Figure 14-16. Some patients require this assessment at frequent intervals to note significant changes. Note the scale for measuring pupil size. A standard for scoring the results of a neurological assessment has been developed. It is called the Glasgow Coma Scale. This standardization has helped to promote a common understanding of a patient's neurologic state among health personnel.

The following are techniques for assessing this system:

- Darken the room. Shine a penlight in the pupil of one eye. Repeat the action, testing the other pupil. Note the size and shape of each pupil and if they became smaller in response to the light. Observe if one pupil took longer to respond than the other. A dilated pupil that does not change should be reported immediately.

- Ask the patient to identify the date (day, month, year), his present location, and his name or names of family members. This is referred to as assessing the patient's *orientation.*

- Determine the patient's level of consciousness. If the patient is awake and responds appropriately to questions, no further testing of this component need be

---

Community Health Center of Branch County
Coldwater, MI 49036-2088 • Phone 517/278-7361

NEUROLOGICAL FLOW SHEET

PUPILS

2MM   4MM   6MM   8MM   10MM

R - REACTIVE   NR - NONREACTIVE
SR - REACT SLOWLY OR SLUGGISHLY

LEVEL OF CONSCIOUSNESS

GRADE I — ALERT, ORIENTED TO TIME, PLACE AND PERSON APPROPRIATE, OBEYS COMMANDS	**GRADE II** DROWSY, AROUSABLE, MAY BE CONFUSED, NOT COMPLETELY ORIENTED, MAY OR MAY NOT FOLLOW COMMANDS
GRADE III STUPOROUS, POOR RESPONSE TO VERBAL STIMULI, CONFUSED, INAPPROPRIATE, DOES NOT FOLLOW COMMANDS.	**GRADE IV** SEMICONSCIOUS, RESPONSE ONLY TO DEEP, PAINFUL STIMULI, MAY OR MAY NOT MOVE VOLUNTARILY.
GRADE V COMATOSE, NO RESPONSE TO PAIN, NO SPONTANEOUS RESPIRATIONS; COUGH AND CORNEAL REFLEXES ABSENT.	

DOCUMENTATION CODES — USING THE GLASGOW COMA SCALE

THE GLASGOW COMA SCALE PROVIDES A STANDARD REFERENCE FOR ASSESSING OR MONITORING A PATIENT WITH SUSPECTED OR CONFIRMED BRAIN INJURY. IT MEASURES THREE FACULTIES: RESPONSES TO STIMULI — **EYE OPENING, MOTOR RESPONSE**, AND **VERBAL RESPONSE** — AND ASSIGNS A NUMBER TO EACH OF THE POSSIBLE RESPONSES WITHIN THESE CATEGORIES. A SCORE OF THREE IS THE LOWEST AND 15 IS THE HIGHEST. A SCORE OF 7 OR LESS INDICATES COMA. THIS SCALE IS COMMONLY USED IN THE EMERGENCY DEPARTMENT OR AT THE SCENE OF AN ACCIDENT, AND FOR PERIODIC EVALUATION OF THE HOSPITALIZED PATIENT.

FACULTY MEASURED	GLASGOW COMA SCALE RESPONSE	SCORE
EYE OPENING	SPONTANEOUSLY	4
	TO VERBAL COMMAND	3
	TO PAIN	2
	NO RESPONSE	1
MOTOR RESPONSE	TO VERBAL COMMAND	6
	TO PAINFUL STIMULI - APPLY KNCUKLE TO STERNUM - OBSERVE ARMS:	
	LOCALIZED PAIN	5
	FLEXES AND WITHDRAWS	4
	ASSUMES DECORTICATE POSTURE	3
	ASSUMES DECEREBRATE POSTURE	2
	NO RESPONSE	1
VERBAL RESPONSE — AROUSE PATIENT WITH PAINFUL STIMULI, IF NECESSARY	ORIENTED AND CONVERSES	5
	DISORIENTED AND CONVERSES	4
	USES INAPPROPRIATE WORDS	3
	MAKES INCOMPREHENSIBLE SOUNDS	2
	NO RESPONSE	1
TOTAL — FROM 3 TO 15		

EXTREMITY — MOVEMENT

GRADE 2	MOVES VOLUNTARILY WITHOUT DIFFICULTY, REFLEXES NORMAL.
GRADE 1	WEAK, SLUGGISH, PARESIS.
GRADE 0	PARALYSIS, NO RESPONSE TO PAIN.

EXTREMITY — STRENGTH

S	STRONG
W	WEAK
A	ABSENT

DATE ▶

TIME	VITAL SIGNS				PUPILS — MM REACTION		LEVEL OF CONSC.	GLASGOW COMA SCALE	EXTREMITY MOVEMENT		STRENGTH		INTAKE			OUTPUT			MISC.
	T	BP	P	R	L	R			LEFT ARM	RIGHT ARM	LEFT LEG	RIGHT LEG	IV	PO	OTHER	URINE	NG	OTHER	

Figure 14-16 This neurological flowsheet is used by nurses to assess significant data about the nervous system. Points may be totaled to evaluate the patient's neurological status. (Courtesy of Community Health Center of Branch County, Coldwater, MI.)

made. If this is not the case, the nurse should progress through each of the following steps until there is a response. The patient's best response should be recorded. Perform the following techniques:

Observe if the patient responds to activity within the room.

If the patient continues to be unresponsive, say his name while touching him gently. Note if the patient awakens easily.

Shake the patient and call out his name more loudly. The nurse should use the first name as well as the patient's full name several times to stimulate a response.

Apply a painful stimulus, such as pinching the skin over the sternum. Note if the patient awakens, or attempts to pull away from the source of the pain, or if the patient shows some facial reaction.

- Ask the patient to grasp and squeeze the nurse's fingers. Observe the patient's ability to follow directions and the strength of the grasp. Compare each hand's strength with the other.
- Have the patient bend his knee and push as resistance to the movement is applied with the nurse's palm. Compare the response and strength of each leg.

Assessing the Gastrointestinal System

Various structures and areas associated with the gastrointestinal system are examined by nurse generalists. Basic assessments include the following:

- Request that a patient open his mouth and inspect the color and condition of the mucous membranes, gums, and tongue. A light and tongue depressor may be necessary for adequate inspection. Note the state of the patient's oral hygiene and condition of the teeth. Identify the use of dentures and bridges, or missing teeth.
- Using a tongue blade, press on the back of the tongue toward the oral pharynx to elicit the presence or absence of a gag reflex.
- Using a stethoscope, listen for bowel sounds in the four quadrants of the abdomen. A *quadrant* is one fourth of a whole. Figure 14-17 illustrates these four divisions. Bowel sounds are like "gurgles and growls." Normally bowel sounds are always present and active.
- Palpate the abdomen to assess its softness. If it feels hard, measure the abdominal girth with a tape measure for future comparisons. *Distention* is a swelling or expansion. Abdominal distention often occurs in illnesses of the intestinal tract and following abdominal surgery. The distention is usually caused by trapped gas that should normally be expelled through the anus. Tapping gently on the area will usually produce a hollow drumlike sound; if a mass is present, there will not be a hollow sound.
- If a patient cannot recall a recent bowel movement,

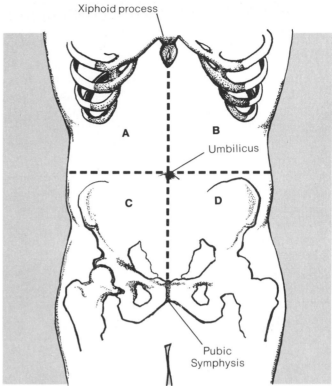

Figure 14-17 Quadrants of the abdomen: (*A*). The right upper quadrant (RUQ). (*B*). The left upper quadrant (LUQ). (*C*). The right lower quadrant (RLQ). (*D*). the left lower quadrant (LLQ).

insert a lubricated, gloved finger into the rectum. Feel for the presence and consistency of stool.
- Inspect the anus visually for the presence of hemorrhoids. *External hemorrhoids* are enlarged veins that appear as masses protruding from the anus.

Assessing the Genitourinary System

The genitourinary system assessment is combined because of its common location and also because it is a dual system in the male. Some common assessment techniques include the following:

- Apply gloves and examine the penis or labia. Retract the foreskin on an uncircumcised male and return it after inspection. The skin and mucous membrane should be intact, pink, and moist. No offensive odor or drainage should be present. Table 14-3 provides terms and descriptions of masses located anywhere on or within the body.
- Using the palm of the hand at the pubis, press downward to feel the crest of the bladder in the abdomen. An empty bladder should not be palpable.
- In much the same way as the bladder was palpated, the pregnant uterus (by the end of the third month) and the uterus of a woman who has just delivered a baby may be felt. The uterus is normally firm. Its level is described as being a certain number of fingers from the umbilicus.

Table 14-3. Characteristics of Abnormal Masses of the Body

Characteristic	Description
Mobility	Fixed—Does not move.
	Mobile—Can be moved with palpation.
Shape	Round—Resembles a ball.
	Tubular—Is elongated.
	Ovoid—Resembles an egg.
	Irregular—Has no definite shape.
Consistency	Edematous—Leaves indentation when palpated.
	Nodular—Feels bumpy to touch.
	Granular—Feels gritty to touch.
	Spongy—Feels soft to touch.
	Hard—Feels firm to touch.
Size	Measured in centimeters (1 cm = approximately ½ in).
Tenderness	Amount of discomfort when palpated—none, slight, moderate, or severe.

Assessing the Musculoskeletal System

The material in Chapter 9 may be used to supplement the following discussion about the assessment of the musculoskeletal system. The examination of the musculoskeletal system should include the following:

- Ask the patient to tighten and relax various muscles. Observe the patient's ability to accomplish this. Also feel the firmness of the contracted muscle.
- Request that the patient flex his arm and resist as the nurse attempts to straighten it. Evaluate the patient's strength in maintaining the flexed position.
- Instruct the patient to walk about the room. The patient should take each step first with the heel followed by the toe. Balance should be maintained. One arm should swing opposite the leg being advanced.
- Put the joints through range of motion (see Chapter 18). Note any restricted movement.

Table 14-4 summarizes the physical assessment of a patient as performed by a nurse generalist. It includes typical normal and abnormal findings. The nurse will acquire many more assessment skills as experience and knowledge are acquired. Only those techniques that beginning nurses would be expected to perform have been discussed in this chapter.

Table 14-4. Summary of Assessment Findings

Method	Normal findings	Abnormal findings
Mental Status/Mood		
Inspection	Expresses feelings of contentment and satisfaction with life. Shows evidence of coping with everyday living. Appropriate grooming and personal hygiene.	Moody, depressed, anxious, worried, angry. Poor grooming and hygiene. Restless or motionless. Inappropriate responses to events.
Mental Status/Intellectual Ability		
Inspection (in the sense of examining the answers to direct questions)	Has rational and coherent thought processes. Good attention span and memory.	Irrational, poor attention span and memory. Poor abstract thought. Unable to compute simple math.
Vision and the Eyes		
Inspection	Good visual ability with or without glasses or contact lenses. Appropriate color perception. No visual field loss. Eyes are bright. Pink mucous membranes. Eyes move equally in all directions.	Poor visual ability or blindness. Color blindness. Gaps in the field of vision. Dull or glossy eyes. Inflamed mucous membrane. Excessive tearing. Drainage from the eyes. Drooping eyelids.
Hearing and the Ears		
Inspection Palpation	Good hearing ability. Cerumen that is soft and easily removed. No drainage or discomfort. Skin that is intact, pink, warm, and slightly moist.	Limited hearing or deafness. Drainage. Soreness when the ear is moved. Dry cerumen that plugs the ear canal.

(continued)

Table 14-4. *Continued*

Method	Normal findings	Abnormal findings
Touch, Taste, Smell		
Inspection Palpation Percussion	Correct responses on both sides of the body to touch, texture, temperature, and vibration. Correct or very few incorrect responses to odors or flavors.	Absent, decreased, exaggerated, or unequal responses to the test substances.
Skin		
Inspection Palpation	Smooth, supple, and blemish free. Warm to the touch. No unusual color.	Blisters, wounds, lesions, rashes, swelling. Cool, edematous skin. Rough, dry, flaky skin.
Respiratory		
Inspection Palpation Auscultation	Symmetric chest. Clear breath sounds. Normal respiratory rate and rhythm. No cough.	Abnormal chest contour. Noisy breath sounds. Labored, slow, rapid, or irregular respirations. Cough, with or without raising sputum.
Cardiovascular		
Inspection Auscultation Palpation	Regular, strong heartbeats. Blood pressure within normal range for age. Palpable peripheral pulses. Immediate return of color to nailbeds.	Irregular heartbeats. Rates slower or more rapid than normal. Weak or absent peripheral pulses. Low or high blood pressure. Slow capillary filling in nailbeds.
Neurological		
Inspection Palpation	Pupils are equal and react to light. Oriented to person, place, and time. Alert and responds appropriately. Strong motor responses in all extremities.	Pupils sluggish or unequal. No response to light. Disoriented. Makes sounds that are not understandable. Weakness or paralysis in one or more extremities. No response to any stimuli.
Gastrointestinal		
Inspection Auscultation Palpation	Pink, moist mucous membranes. Regularly spaced teeth or well-fitting dentures or bridges. Rough-surfaced tongue. Gag reflex present. Soft abdomen with active bowel sounds present. No impaction or hemorrhoids.	Pale or dry mucous membranes. Diseased or missing teeth. Smooth, dry tongue. Absent gag reflex. Rigid abdomen. Diminished or absent bowel sounds. Hard, dry stool within the rectum. Hemorrhoids present.
Genitourinary		
Inspection Palpation	Intact skin and normal distribution of pubic hair. Pink, moist, mucous membranes. No lesions, drainage, or odors. Bladder nonpalpable. Firm uterus postdelivery located at or below the midline of the umbilicus.	Discharge from the penis or vagina. Lesions on the penis or vaginal mucosa. Distended bladder with dribbling of urine. Boggy, postpartum uterus located above the midline of the umbilicus.
Musculoskeletal		
Inspection Palpation	Firm, strong muscles. Good muscle control and coordination. Good posture and balance. Full range of motion in joints.	Muscle weakness, lack of control and coordination. Poor posture and balance. Limp or foot dragging during walking. Restricted range of motion.

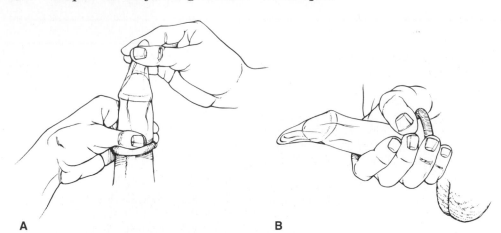

Figure 14-18 (*A*). When applying a condom, it should be rolled completely over the erect penis while pinching the space at the condom tip. This prevents forming an air bubble that could break and also provides a reservoir for semen. (*B*). The condom should be held at the base of the penis during its removal from the vagina.

Applicable Nursing Diagnoses

The nurse often has an opportunity to perform health teaching during a physical assessment. Some of the following nursing diagnoses may apply.
- Knowledge Deficit
- Noncompliance
- Decisional Conflict
- Altered Health Maintenance
- Health-Seeking Behaviors

Nursing Care Plan 14-1 is an example of actions to assist a person with the nursing diagnosis of Health-Seeking Behaviors. The definition for this according to the NANDA Taxonomy (1989) is, "A state in which an individual is actively seeking ways to alter personal health habits and/or the environment in order to move toward a higher level of health."

Suggested Measures to Assess the Patient's Health Status in Selected Situations

When the Patient Is an Infant or Child

An assessment of an infant's or child's health status is similar to that of an adult. However, rectal examinations may be deferred unless a disease condition is believed to be present.

Inspection of the external genitals should be done tactfully with a parent present.

Try to limit using restraints when examining an infant or child. Restraints tend to make matters worse if the child is crying or uncooperative. Often, a parent can provide helpful assistance by holding the child while the examination is conducted.

When a crying youngster is being examined, try to distract him with a toy or, for an infant, a pacifier.

Never leave a youngster alone on an examination table.

Plan to interview parents to obtain a health history for an infant or child. A record of immunizations is important.

Be sure to provide sufficient warmth when examining an infant or young child. Young children are likely to be irritable and to cry when they feel chilly.

Note the anterior and posterior fontanelles when examining the head of a newborn or infant. A *fontanelle* is a soft spot on the head lying between bones in the skull. The anterior fontanelle usually closes between 10 and 14 months of age but may close as late as 18 months of age. The small posterior fontanelle usually closes by 8 to 12 weeks of age.

Plan to measure the circumference of the chest and head when examining an infant. Measure the infant's length by placing him on a measuring board or on paper. Make a mark where the top of the head and the heel are located. Then measure the distance between the marks.

Check for cyanosis in an infant or young child on the palms of the hands and on the soles of the feet. These two areas often show signs of cyanosis before other parts of the body do.

Norms for vital signs differ for various age groups. Expect that infants and children will have more rapid heart and respiratory rates. The blood pressure will be lower than an average adult's blood pressure. The ranges for vital signs in infants and children can be found in Chapter 13.

NURSING CARE PLAN

14-1. Health-Seeking Behaviors

Assessment

Subjective Data

States, "I've been having sex with a lot of women. None of them have gotten pregnant and I haven't caught any diseases as far as I know. But, I don't want to take chances anymore."

Objective Data

19-year-old man scheduled for inguinal hernia repair as an outpatient in 3 days. Circumcised penis with bilaterally descended testicles. Slight bulge in R. inguinal area. No discharge from penis. Has vaginal sex at least four times a week. Currently has three sexual partners. Requests information on safe sex practices and use of condoms.

Diagnosis

Health-Seeking Behaviors: Preventing sexually transmitted diseases and pregnancy.

Plan

Goal

The patient will identify safe sex practices by 10/13 and use them during future sexual activities.

Orders: 10/10

1. Give assorted pamphlets and free condoms from Reproductive Control Clinic.
2. Emphasize the following safe sex practices:
   - Reduce sexual partners to one noninfected, faithful person.
   - Use a latex condom (Fig. 14-18) and nonoxynol-9 spermicide either over the tip of the condom or as a vaginal application.
   - Remove the condom-covered penis from the vagina before the penis becomes limp.
   - Do not have sexual contact again unless another condom is applied.
   - In the case that a condom breaks or leaks, urinate immediately and wash the penis with soap and water.
3. Give schedule of Reproductive Control Clinic hours. _____ B. VELASQUEZ, RN

Implementation (Documentation)

10/10   1300   Given the following pamphlets: "Choices" and "Understanding Safer Sex." Identified pages with illustrations for applying condoms. Given sample package of condoms. Clinic hours written on cover of pamphlets. Will discuss reading and use of condoms on return admission. _____ B. VELASQUEZ, RN

Evaluation (Documentation)

10/13   0630   Says he has read sex information pamphlets given during preadmission exam. Used one sample condom s̄ problems. Asked, "What can my girlfriend do if the condom breaks?" Advised immediate insertion of an applicator filled with foam spermicide. To reduce risks of sexually transmitted diseases, a female sex partner should urinate and also wash well with soap and water. Told to avoid douching as this may push infectious organisms higher into the uterus or Fallopian tubes. Plans to buy more condoms. Says "They're a lot cheaper than babies." _____ B. VELASQUEZ, RN

The chest wall of an infant is thin. Expect that the breath sounds may sound loud and harsh.

When the Patient Is an Adolescent

Be sure to obtain a health history from an adolescent in private. Adolescents are embarrassed relatively easily and are very aware of peer pressure. They respond more positively when their feelings are taken into account.

Recognize that adolescents want to participate in health decisions. They are not children and are eager to take beginning steps toward adulthood by learning to take responsibility for their health to the extent to which they are able and it is safe to do so.

Plan that health teaching can start during adolescence or when youngsters are old enough to comprehend and understand the relationships between their activities of daily living and their health.

When the Patient Is an Adult Female

Obtain a menstrual history that includes the age at which menstruation began, the regularity of the cycle, its length, and the first day of the last menstrual period.

Obtain an obstetrical history, including the number of pregnancies, live births, any multiple pregnancies, still births, and spontaneous abortions. Inquire about any elective terminations of pregnancy. Ask the patient to describe any problems associated with previous pregnancies, labors, and deliveries.

If the patient is pregnant, auscultate the fetal heart rate if the pregnancy is advanced enough for this to be audible.

When the Patient Is Elderly

Allow sufficient time to obtain a health history from an elderly patient. Be patient as the elderly person recalls the information from his past. Because of the lengthy span of years, it may take time for the patient to sequence the events and conditions affecting his health.

Try to let the elderly person set his own pace. Speak slowly, do not shout, do not interrupt him when he speaks, and take the time to listen. The elderly function best in an environment that is unhurried.

Never leave an elderly person alone on an examining table. Some may become confused or experience a disturbance in equilibrium. Falls from an examining table can be serious.

Expect physical changes that are in keeping with the patient's advanced years.

Teaching Suggestions for Assessing the Patient's Health Status

Suggestions for the instruction of patients were given several times in this chapter. They are summarized below.

The importance of having regular checkups should be included in a patient-teaching plan. It is especially important to help detect and treat illnesses in their early stages.

Health teaching should start no later than during adolescent years; many youngsters are able to understand the relationship between health and their activities of daily living.

Teaching the family of the patient is important also. Often, family members are excellent sources of support for promoting health and preventing illness. Teaching family members is essential when the patient is a child.

Examination of the breasts for tissue masses was described in Figure 14-5. Every woman should be taught how to examine her breasts and should be taught to do the examination at least once every month.

Adult males should be taught to examine the testicles for masses. The American Cancer Society has many pamphlets that may be used as teaching aids.

Bibliography

Bates B: A Guide to Physical Examination, 4th ed. Philadelphia, JB Lippincott, 1987

Bell I: Testicular self-examination. Nursing Times 86(9):38–40, 1990

Beyea S, Matzo M: Assessing elders using the functional health pattern assessment model. Nurse Educator 14(5):32–37, 1989

Brigdon P, Todd M: In search of the perfect assessment. Professional Nurse 5(4):181–184, 1990

Carlson K: Assessing a child's chest. RN Magazine 52(11):26–32, 1989

Ceilley RI, Goldberg GN, Prose NS: A guide to pediatric rashes. Patient Care 23(15):150–156, 159–160, 162–163, 1989

Champagne MT, Ashley ML: Use of a heart sound simulator in teaching cardiac auscultation. Focus on Critical Care 16(6): 448–456, 1989

Cohen KW, Byrne SM: The role of the nurse in assisting with eye examinations on premature infants. Neonatal Network 8(2): 31–35, 1989

Cramer JA, Wheel and RG: Pigmented lesions: A concise review. Patient Care 23(15):109–113, 116, 121–123, 1989

Crosby L, Parsons LC: Clinical neurologic assessment tool: Development and testing of an instrument to index neurologic status. Heart & Lung: Journal of Critical Care 18(2):121–129, 1989

Cuzzell JZ: Derm detective: Clues—bruised, torn skin. Am J Nurs 90(3):16, 18, 1990

Derdiarian AK: Effects of using systematic assessment instruments on patient and nurse satisfaction with nursing care. Oncology Nursing Forum 17(1):95–101, 1990

Frary T: Pediatric examination pearls. Journal of the American Academy of Physician Assistants 1(5):389–390, 1989

Gift AG: Clinical measurement of dyspnea. Dimensions of Critical Care Nursing 8(4):210–216, 1989

Goon JM, Berger DK: A model outreach program for health care screening. Journal of Pediatric Health Care 3(6):305–310, 1989

Jewell ML, Peters DA: An assessment guide for community health nurses. Home Healthcare Nurse 7(5):32–36, 1989

Kamenir S, Nahwegezhic R: Skin assessment: A tool for nursing staff. Perspectives 13(2):4–6, 1989

Killam PE: Orthopedic assessment of young children: Developmental variations. Nurse Practitioner 14(7):27–28, 30–32, 1989

Kittleson MJ: Assessing breathing patterns in first aid training. J Sch Health 60(2):67–68, 1990

Lindsey M: Abdominal assessment. Orthopaedic Nursing 8(4): 34–34, 1989

Lukes EN, Bratcher BP: Pre-employment physical examinations: Report of a pilot program. American Association of Occupational Health Nurses Journal 38(4):174–179, 1990

McCann J, Voris J, Simon M: Comparison of genital examination techniques in prepubertal girls. Pediatrics 85(2):182–187, 1990

McNaul J, Weisberg D, Hurley JF: What's going on in this child's chest? Respiratory Care 34(8):745–747, 1989

Ott MJ, Jackson PL: Precocious puberty: Identifying early sexual development. Nurse Practitioner 14(11):21, 14–18, 30, 1989

Rice EM: Geriatric assessment. Advancing Clinical Care 4(3):8–15, 1989

Schneiderman H, Garibaldi RA: Physical examination of HIV-infected patients: General appearance, vital signs, and skin part 1. Consultant 30(1):33–38, 41, 1990

Schneiderman H, Garibaldi RA: Physical examination of HIV-infected patients: Head and neck, eyes, mouth and throat, and lymph nodes part 2. Consultant 30(1):42–44, 47–48, 50–51, 1990

Schneiderman H, Garibaldi RA: Physical examination of HIV-infected patients: Respiratory and cardiovascular systems; abdomen and genitalia; neurologic examination part 3. Consultant 30(1):55–56, 61–63, 1990

Selby TL: RNs work to keep America healthy. American Nurse 22(2):3, 31, 1990

Tipton JH: A hospital-based approach to physical assessment. Journal of Nursing Staff Development 5(2):70–72, 1989

Toth M: Geriatric assessment teams: What they are and who they can help. Journal of Home Health Care Practice 2(1):1–8, 1989

Wilson D, Ratekin C: An introduction to using children's drawings as an assessment tool. Nurse Practitioner 15(3):23–24, 27, 30–32, 1990

Chapter Outline

Behavioral Objectives
Glossary
Introduction
Nursing Responsibilities When Special Procedures Are
    Performed
Advancements in Examinations and Tests
Interpreting Terms That Describe Tests
Examinations That Use X-Rays
Examinations of Electrical Impulses
Examinations That Detect Radiation
Examinations That Use Sound Waves
Examinations That Use Endoscopes
Examinations of Body Fluids
Suggested Measures to Assist With Examinations in
    Selected Situations
Applicable Nursing Diagnoses
Teaching Suggestions About Tests and Examinations
Bibliography

Skill Procedures

Assisting With an Examination
Using a Glucometer

Behavioral Objectives

When the content of this chapter has been mastered, the learner will be able to:

Define terms appearing in the glossary.

Describe the types of responsibilities a nurse assumes when assisting with patient examinations.

List common types of instruments, equipment, and supplies that are used during a physical examination.

Describe suggested nursing actions when assisting with an examination.

Interpret the word endings that pertain to tests and examinations.

Describe common examination procedures and give some indications for their use.

List suggested measures for assisting with examinations in selected situations, as described in this chapter.

Summarize suggestions for instruction of patients offered in this chapter.

Glossary

Allergy An unfavorable reaction to a substance to which the body is sensitive.

Amniocentesis The withdrawal of amniotic fluid from the pregnant uterus.

Angiography X-ray examination of blood vessels.

Biopsy The removal of a small specimen of tissue from the body for microscopic examination.

Bronchoscopy An examination that uses a bronchoscope to inspect the trachea and bronchi.

Cannula A hollow tube through which air or fluids may flow.

Cholecystogram An image of the gallbladder.

Cholecystography X-ray examination of the gallbladder and its ducts.

Computerized axial tomography An examination that uses narrow x-ray beams to view horizontal sections of a body part from various angles. Abbreviated CAT or CT.

Contrast medium A substance that makes hollow structures of the body more dense and, therefore, more distinct on an x-ray.

Cystoscopy An examination that uses a cystoscope to inspect the bladder and urethra.

Dorsal recumbent position The position in which a patient is on his back with his legs separated, the soles of his feet flat on the bed, and his knees bent.

Draping Covering a body part in such a manner that it does not interfere with the examination.

Echography An examination that produces images of structures through the use of ultrasound. Synonym for *ultrasonography.*

Electrocardiogram The image or paper strip showing waves produced during electrocardiography.

Electrocardiography An examination that produces an image of the electrical impulses produced by the contracting heart muscle. Abbreviated EKG or ECG.

Electrode A wire that connects the body, usually through contact with the skin, to a machine that records electrical impulses.

Electroencephalography An examination that records electrical impulses in the brain. Abbreviated EEG.

Electromyography An examination that records the electrical impulses produced by contracting skeletal muscle. Abbreviated EMG.

Endoscope An instrument used to view an internal part of the body.

Endoscopy An examination of a body part with an endoscope.

Erect position The normal standing position.

Fluoroscopy The study of body organs in motion with a fluoroscope. A fluoroscope uses roentgen rays to perform the examination.

Gastric analysis An examination of stomach secretions.

Genupectoral position The position in which a patient rests on his knees and chest. Synonym for *knee-chest position*.

Graft Living tissue that is relocated and substitutes for diseased tissue.

Head mirror A mirror worn on an examiner's head to direct light into an area.

Horizontal recumbent position The position in which a patient lies flat on his back with his legs together.

Intravenous pyelography X-ray examination of the urinary tract following the introduction of dye into a vein. Abbreviated IVP.

Invasive procedure An examination, test, or treatment in which the skin or parts of the body are entered.

Knee-chest position The position in which a patient rests on his knees and chest. Synonym for *genupectoral position*.

Lithotomy position A position that is similar to the dorsal recumbent position except that the feet are supported in stirrups.

Lumbar puncture A procedure for collecting body fluid by inserting a needle beneath the arachnoid layer of the meninges between the third and fourth or fourth and fifth lumbar vertebrae. Synonym for *spinal tap*.

Mammography X-ray examination of breast tissue.

Myelography X-ray examination of the spinal canal following the introduction of a dye into the subarachnoid space.

Ophthalmoscope An instrument used for examining the inside of the eye.

Otoscope An instrument used to observe the eardrum and external ear canal.

Pap test An examination of secretions from the female genital tract to determine whether cancer cells are present. Pap is from Papanicolaou, the name of the physician who devised the test.

Paracentesis The withdrawal of fluid from the abdominal cavity.

Proctoscopy An examination that uses a proctoscope to inspect the rectum.

Queckenstedt's test A test sometimes done during a lumbar puncture to determine if there is an obstruction to the flow of spinal fluid.

Radiation Energy that cannot be seen or felt.

Radionuclide A substance with an altered atomic structure that releases one or more types of radiation. Replaces the term radioisotope.

Radiopharmaceutical A radionuclide that has been prepared for administration to humans.

Retrograde pyelography X-ray examination of the ureters and kidneys following the introduction of dye directly into the ureters.

Roentgen rays Electromagnetic energy that passes through structures, producing an image on special film. Synonym for *x-rays*.

Roentgenogram The actual film image produced through roentgenography. Synonym for an *x-ray*.

Roentgenography A general term for all procedures that use x-rays to produce images of body structures.

Sigmoidoscopy An examination that uses a sigmoidoscope to inspect the lower colon.

Sims' position, right or left The position in which a patient lies on one or the other side of the body with the upper knee more bent than the other.

Specimen A sample of tissue, body fluid, secretions, or excretions.

Speculum An instrument used for opening a cavity so that it can be examined.

Spinal tap A procedure for collecting body fluid by inserting a needle beneath the arachnoid layer of the meninges between the third and fourth or fourth and fifth lumbar vertebrae. Synonym for *lumbar puncture*.

Stirrups Foot supports used when the patient is in the lithotomy position.

Suture Material used to close an incision.

Thoracentesis The withdrawal of fluid from the pleural cavity.

Tilt table A device that elevates or lowers the patient's body as he lies on it.

Tonometer An instrument used to measure pressure within the eye.

Transducer An instrument that picks up echoing sound waves.

Trocar An instrument used to pierce the skin and underlying tissue.

Tuning fork An instrument used to examine the patient's ability to hear or feel sensations.

Ultrasonography An examination that produces images of structures through the use of ultrasound. Synonym for *echography*.

Ultrasound Very high frequency, inaudible sound waves.

X-ray The actual film image produced through roentgenography. Synonym for *roentgenogram*.

X-rays Electromagnetic energy that passes through structures producing an image on special film. Synonym for *roentgen rays.*

Introduction

Many health personnel carry out examinations and special tests to obtain information about the patient. These are done to study how a patient's body is functioning and to locate disease processes. The nurse is often required to provide assistance by teaching and preparing the patient, supporting the patient physically and emotionally during an examination, assisting other health practitioners during an examination or test, and caring for the patient and equipment afterwards. This chapter gives a general overview of the nursing responsibilities when the nurse is not the primary examiner.

Descriptions of many common diagnostic tests are also discussed. Most of the tests described are not done routinely. They are performed only when the patient has a suspected health problem. However, a few, such as electrocardiography, may be used during routine, preventive examinations on people who are at potential risk for a certain disease.

An understanding of what is done during common procedures is important for the nurse to know. That information, and the reasons for which tests are usually performed, are necessary knowledge.

The nurse is responsible for carrying out test requirements. Policy and procedure manuals prepared by each health agency are available to the nurse. They describe the protocols that apply to individual tests. The usual preparation and aftercare of patients can be found in clinical or laboratory texts, which include nursing implications. Excellent examples are listed in this chapter's bibliography. These types of references are a valuable investment as a personal resource.

Nursing Responsibilities When Special Procedures Are Performed

The responsibilities of the nurse who assists with examinations and tests fall into several broad categories.

Understanding the Patient, His Illness, and His Plan of Care

Certain information is basic to understanding the measures used to restore an individual's health. Answers to questions such as the following will help a nurse apply general knowledge to the specifics of the individual:

- What is the patient's diagnosis?
- What is the probable cause of the patient's illness?

- How is the patient's illness interfering with normal body functions?
- How is the patient feeling physically and emotionally?
- How well is the patient responding to his present treatment?
- How does the examination or test fit into the plan for care?
- What does the patient know about his illness, tests, and treatment?
- What teaching possibilities exist?

Understanding the Procedure

To appropriately assist with an examination or test, the nurse must understand the nature of the procedure. Answers to questions such as the following will help provide the necessary information.

- What is the procedure and how is it defined?
- What are the purposes, or indications, for which the procedure is commonly used?
- What part of the body will be examined?
- Does the procedure require clean or sterile equipment?
- How shall the patient be positioned so that the procedure may be carried out efficiently, safely and comfortably?
- Will a specimen be obtained?
- What signs and symptoms will the patient experience?
- What measures can be used to prevent complications?
- What signs and symptoms indicate that the patient is not responding well to the procedure?
- What actions may be necessary if the patient develops complications?
- Where is emergency equipment kept?

Instructing the Patient

Ordinarily, the physician is responsible for explaining any *invasive procedure,* that is, one in which the skin or parts of the body are entered. These types of tests or examinations are often associated with potential health risks. The patient's signature on a special consent form is usually required. Informed consent was discussed in Chapter 6. The doctor must provide information to the patient from which he can decide to allow or refuse a procedure. It is recommended that each agency's policies be observed for obtaining a signed consent. Examples of procedures requiring consent include thoracentesis, paracentesis, and computerized axial tomography. These procedures are discussed later in the chapter.

Though the nurse does not hold the primary responsibility for providing information about tests and examinations, it often happens that the nurse must repeat explanations. An anxious patient may not grasp all the information the first time it is explained. There may be questions that come after the physician has left. The nurse should be sure that the patient understands the information. A thorough explanation will not eliminate all the stress a patient experiences, but it will reduce it. Stress can contribute to discomfort during an examination and may alter certain results.

No exact rules can be stated as to the best way to provide explanations to a patient. In general, the nurse is guided by the patient's questions, the requirements for the examination, the patient's condition, and each individual set of circumstances. Following the suggestions for teaching and providing emotional support, as discussed in Chapter 2, should lay a solid foundation for meeting the patient's needs.

Carrying Out Test Requirements

Many examinations and tests require special preparation of the patient in order to obtain accurate results. For example, some tests or examinations require that food or fluids be withheld, that the diet be modified, or that laxatives be administered before a test. The requirements for tests are usually located in a reference manual at each nursing unit. The nurse should refer to these written instructions each time a patient is undergoing a test rather than rely on memory. Special test preparations vary among health agencies. Nurses should follow the common practices at each place of employment.

After reviewing the special requirements, the nurse must provide directions to the patient, nursing staff, and other hospital departments affected by the test. All must cooperate so that the test can be carried out properly. If the nurse discovers that the preparations have not been carried out, it should be reported promptly. It may be necessary to cancel and reschedule the procedure in those instances.

Preparing Equipment and Supplies

The physician may wish to examine the patient from time to time. The nurse should have equipment and supplies ready for an examination. Items likely to be used are checked first to see that they are clean and in good working order. Most health agencies have a tray, basket, or cart for equipment ordinarily used during an examination. Although there are differences among agencies, items usually kept in readiness for a physical examination are described in Table 15-1. The equipment for a physical examination that is performed by a physician is much the same as that used by the nurse. Additional instruments may be used for a more extensive examination. Some commonly used instruments are illustrated in Figure 15-1.

Table 15-1. Common Examination Equipment and Supplies

Item	Description
Ophthalmoscope	An ophthalmoscope is an instrument used for examining the interior of the eye.
Otoscope	An otoscope is an instrument used for observing the eardrum and external ear canal.
Speculum	A speculum is an instrument used for opening a cavity so that it may be more easily examined. Nose and vaginal specula are those most commonly used.
Tonometer	A tonometer is an instrument used to measure the pressure within the eyeball. A mild anesthetic solution applied directly to the surface of the eye is used before placing a tonometer onto the eye's surface.
Head mirror	A head mirror is an instrument worn on the examiner's head to direct light into an area, such as into the throat.

The following items may also be used:

Sphygmomanometer	Stethoscope
Flashlight	Tongue depressors
Tape measure	Tuning forks
Skin pencil	Tissues and waste container
Sterile or clean gloves	Lubricant
Paper towels	Waste container for soiled instruments
Percussion hammer	Patient's gown
Material for draping	Lightweight blanket
Disposable pad	Pins, cotton, test tubes for hot and cold water, and various materials having different odors are included if a neurologic examination is to be done.
Containers and slides for specimens, as indicated	

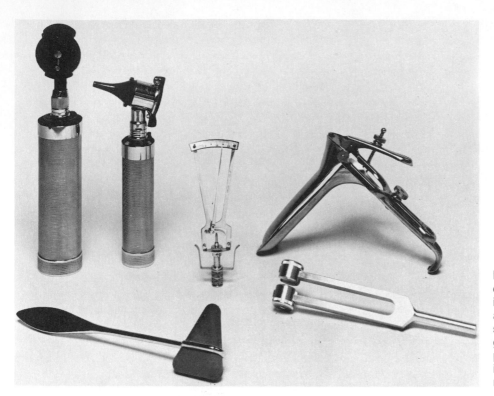

Figure 15-1 These instruments are often used during a physical examination. From top left to right are an ophthalmoscope, otoscope with speculum attached, tonometer, vaginal speculum. At lower left is a percussion hammer, and lower right is a tuning fork. Tuning forks are made in various sizes.

When special diagnostic examinations and tests are performed in the nursing unit, the nurse is usually responsible for obtaining the supplies and preparing the equipment prior to the procedure. The equipment and supplies will depend on the procedure and will vary among agencies. Some agencies have prepackaged trays with most, if not all, of the necessary items in readiness. While assembling and preparing materials, the nurse must maintain the cleanliness or sterility of the equipment. Practices that help to control microorganisms are discussed in Chapter 16.

Nurses giving patients daily care are not responsible for the equipment and supplies when an examination or test is carried out in another location, such as the x-ray department, the operating room, or a cardiac laboratory. Nor are nurses responsible for equipment or supplies when a special technician performs the procedure.

Preparing the Working Area

If the procedure is to be performed at the patient's bedside, the nurse will want to clear the area of unnecessary articles and provide privacy. Many nursing units contain an examination room that is clean, well-lighted, and stocked with frequently used equipment. If the patient is transported to such an area, the nurse will wish to explain that the reason is for the patient's comfort and convenience.

Any equipment and supplies that are needed should be arranged for easy access by the examiner. The functioning of instruments that require electric power, batteries, or lights should be checked prior to their use. This provides time to replace any nonfunctioning equipment or parts before the examination has begun.

Cleanliness or sterility of equipment should be maintained. The examination table should be covered with clean material, such as sheets or paper dispensed from a roll.

Preparing the Patient

Before an examination is performed, the nurse should check one more time that the required consent form is signed. Double-checking that test requirements have been fulfilled further prevents delays.

Just prior to the procedure, the nurse should provide the patient with the opportunity to care for his personal hygiene. Being clean promotes the patient's self-esteem and self-confidence in an unfamiliar situation.

In addition to the patient's hygiene measures, the nurse should observe the skin or site that will be examined. It may be necessary to cleanse it more thoroughly than just simply washing it. The area may even require shaving; this applies particularly to procedures where entry is made through the skin. The skin always contains microbes, some of which can cause disease if transferred to other tissues that the skin ordinarily protects. Antiseptics may also be used to reduce the numbers of organisms prior to entry through the skin.

The patient should be encouraged to use the bathroom or bedpan before the examination. While maintaining the privacy for elimination, the patient should be provided with a gown or other examination garments. These allow easy access to the various body areas, protect the patient from exposure, and avoid soiling personal clothing. Extra covers should be available if chilling occurs.

Positioning and Draping a Patient

The nurse is responsible for helping a patient to assume various positions and for draping a patient properly while he is examined. *Draping* is a term that refers to covering a body part in such a manner that it does not interfere with the examination. Draping avoids exposing the patient unnecessarily. Only those parts of the body being examined are exposed. Some agencies use disposable paper drapes. A bath blanket, drawsheet, or a bed sheet may also be used.

Positioning the patient facilitates the examination of specific body parts. With practice and knowledge of which area will be examined, the nurse can develop competence in positioning patients in an appropriate manner for any test or examination. Table 15-2 provides the names of common positions, describes the position, and identifies areas of the body that are usually examined in each position.

Table 15-2. Common Positions for Examinations and Tests

Description	Indications for Use
Erect Position	
The *erect position* is a normal standing position. The arms are held in a relaxed position at the sides of the body. The feet are 6 to 8 inches apart. The face should look straight ahead. The patient should wear a gown that opens in the back. Slippers may be worn.	This position is used to examine body contours, posture, balance, muscles, and extremities. When the patient walks, gait and muscle coordination can be observed.
Sitting Position	
The buttocks are firmly on the edge of the bed or at the foot of the examination table. The thighs are well supported. The knees should be bent and the feet should be positioned flat against the floor or a foot rest. A gown or paper vest may be used to cover the upper body; a bath blanket or paper sheet covers the waist and legs. This position is shown in Figure 15-2.	This position allows auscultation of the anterior, lateral, and posterior areas of the lungs. It facilitates inspection and palpation of the thyroid, breasts, and axillary areas. The reflexes in the elbows, wrists, knees, and ankles are easily examined in this position. Having the patient sit helps prevent back strain for the examiner while assessing the head and its related structures, such as the eyes, ears, nose, and throat.

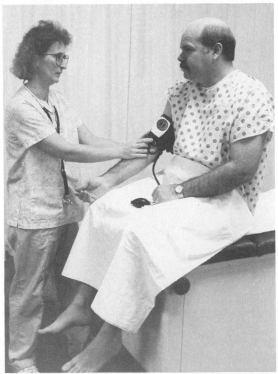

Figure 15-2 The nurse has instructed the patient to take this sitting position prior to his physical examination. The nurse has provided him with an examination gown and a drape. While waiting for the examiner, the nurse obtains the patient's vital signs.

(continued)

Table 15-2. Continued

Description	Indications for Use

Horizontal Recumbent Position

The *horizontal recumbent position* is one in which the patient lies flat on his back. The head is supported with a small pillow. The legs are together with the knees bent slightly to help relax the muscles in the abdomen. The patient is covered with a sheet and wears a gown. Areas of the drape may be folded back when a body part is examined.

This position may be used to examine the anterior parts of the body if the patient is too weak or uncomfortable in a sitting position. It is most commonly used to examine the heart, chest, and abdomen.

Dorsal Recumbent Position

The *dorsal recumbent position* is one in which a patient is on his back lying close to the edge, or center, of the bed or examination table. One pillow may be placed under the head. The legs are separated and the knees bent. The feet are flat against the surface on which the patient is lying. Figure 15-3 illustrates a dorsal recumbent position. A bath blanket is used to drape the patient. It is folded in such a way that the legs are covered, but a corner may be raised to expose the area between the legs as shown in Figure 15-4. A disposable pad may be placed under the patient's buttocks to avoid soiling bed linen.

The dorsal recumbent position is used most often to examine the rectum and vagina.

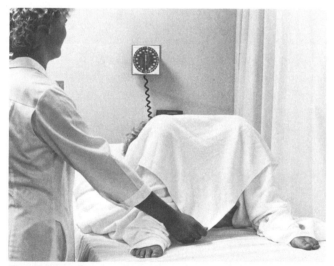

Figure 15-4 A bath blanket is used to drape a patient in a dorsal recumbent position. A corner of the rectangular drape is positioned at the head and between the feet, allowing the legs to be wrapped. When a procedure is about to be performed, the area covering the genitals is raised and placed over the abdomen.

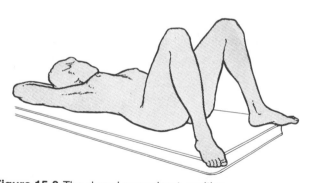

Figure 15-3 The dorsal recumbent position.

Lithotomy Position

The *lithotomy position* is similar to the dorsal recumbent position except that the feet are supported in stirrups. *Stirrups* are foot supports. In this position the patient's buttocks are brought to the edge of the end of the table. The draping is the same as for the dorsal recumbent position. An illustration of the lithotomy position can be seen in Figure 15-5.

The lithotomy position is used to examine the vagina with a speculum. It is also used when the internal female reproductive organs are palpated. Specimens from the cervix or vagina may be obtained in this position. It is also a position in which the rectum may be examined. Males or females undergoing inspection of the bladder with a cystoscope may be placed in a lithotomy position.

(continued)

Table 15-2. Continued

Description	**Indications for Use**

Lithotomy Position

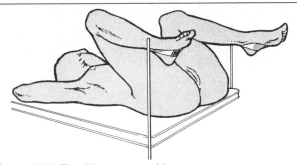

Figure 15-5 The lithotomy position.

Sims' Position

The *Sims' position* is a side-lying position. In the left Sims' position, the patient lies on his left side and rests his left arm behind his body. The right arm is forward with the elbow bent, and the arm rests on a pillow placed under the patient's head. The patient's body is slightly forward. The right knee is sharply bent; the left one is slightly bent. A left Sims' position is shown in Figure 15-6. A right Sims' position is the reverse of left Sims'. A disposable pad may be used under the buttocks. A bath blanket or paper sheet may be lifted at the hip to expose the area being examined.

The Sim's position is used to examine the external anus or examine the rectum internally with a lubricated, gloved finger. It is often a position used for nursing procedures such as administering an enema or inserting a rectal tube. These are discussed in Chapter 22. This position may be used in lieu of the lithotomy position when examining the vagina of a woman who has difficulty bending the knees or hips, as may be the case with arthritis.

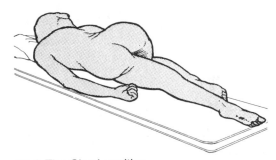

Figure 15-6 The Sims' position.

Knee-Chest or Genupectoral Position

The *knee-chest or genupectoral* position is one in which the patient rests on his knees and chest as illustrated in Figure 15-7. The head is turned to one side and may rest on a small pillow. A pillow may also be placed under the chest for added comfort. The arms are above the head, or they may be bent at the elbows and rest alongside the patient's head. The drape is placed so that the patient's back, buttocks, and thighs are covered. Only the area to be examined is exposed. It is a very difficult position for most patients, especially the elderly. Therefore, the nurse should not assist the patient into this position until the examiner is ready to begin. There are now examination tables with sectional parts that may facilitate maintaining this position without much patient effort.

This position is used when the internal condition of the bowel is examined with various endoscopes.

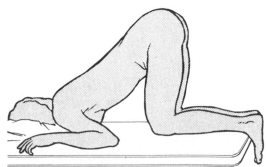

Figure 15-7 The knee-chest or genupectoral position.

Assisting With an Examination

During an examination, the nurse has responsibilities both to the patient and to the examiner. The doctor or technician may need help with handling equipment, directing lighting, and caring for specimens.

Specimens are samples of tissue, body fluids, secretions, or excretions. They may be sent to the laboratory following an examination. Each agency has its own policies concerning items such as the type of container for the specimen, how the specimen is to be preserved, and how the specimen is to be labeled. The nurse will wish to follow these policies so that test results are not inaccurate or delayed. Laboratory test results become a part of the patient's record. Figure 15-8 illustrates several examples of laboratory reports on specimens. The care of specimens, such as urine, stool, and sputum, are discussed later in this text.

The examiner may need equipment from the nurse. The nurse may also be required to hold drugs and injectable anesthetics. The nurse must check these labels carefully as described in Chapter 23. In addition, the container should be held in such a manner that the examiner can also read the label. These practices help to avoid errors and misunderstandings.

The nurse should always be aware of the patient's reactions during the examination. For example, the patient may be cold, perspiring, or in pain. The nurse may need to provide comfort measures and emotional support for the patient. Holding the patient's hand and offering words of encouragement may help the patient to withstand temporary discomfort. Assessments made by the nurse of the patient's physical condition may alert the physician to shorten or modify the examination in some manner.

Skill Procedure 15-1 is a summary of the nurse's responsibilities when assisting with an examination. For information about the responsibilities for preparing the patient and the aftercare associated with specific examinations, clinical texts that discuss the medical or surgical care of patients should be consulted.

Recording and Reporting Data

The agency's policies indicate what information to record and where it is recorded. Usually, the following items are included: the type of examination, the time the examina-

☐ COMPLETE U/A ☐ CATH ☐ VOIDED	Patient Height	Collection Started	Date to be Performed	Collected By
☐ STAT	Patient Weight	Collection Finished	Date Collected	Volume

ROOM, NAME, PAT. NO., PHY., BIRTHDATE, AGE, SEX

URINALYSIS

☐	COLOR Colorless Pale Yellow Dk Yellow Amber Red Orange
☐	CHARACTER Clear Slgt Hazy Hazy Cloudy Turbid Opaque
☐	pH 5.0 6.0 7.0 8.0 9.0
☐	PROTEIN 30 mg/dl 100 mg/dl 300 mg/dl Neg.Trace 1+ 2+ 3+
☐	GLUCOSE 0.1 g/dl .25 g/dl .5 g/dl 1. g/dl Neg. Trace 1+ 2+ 3+
☐	KETONES Neg. Trace 1+ 2+ 3+
☐	BILIRUBIN Neg. Trace 1+ 2+ 3+
☐	BLOOD Neg. Trace 1+ 2+ 3+
☐	UROBILINOGEN 0.1 1.0 2.0 4.0 8.0
☐	SPECIFIC GRAVITY 1.0______

☐ MICROSCOPIC
CASTS______/lpf
WBC /hpf
RBC /hpf
EPITHELIAL CELLS
Squamous______/hpf
Renal______/hpf
Transitional______/hpf
BACTERIA
CRYSTALS
MUCUS 1+ 2+ 3+ 4+
AMORPHOUS 1+ 2+ 3+ 4+
COMMENTS
TECH DATE TIME

☐	SODIUM		40-220 meg/24 hrs.
☐	POTASSIUM		25-120 meg/24 hrs.
☐	CHLORIDE		110-250 mg/24 hrs.
☐	CALCIUM		50-400 mg/24 hrs.
☐	PROTEIN		27-137 mg/24 hrs.
☐	AMYLASE		1-19 Iu/hr.
☐	CREAT. CLEARANCE		75-125 mL/min.
	Blood ______ mg	Urine______mg	

☐	PREGNANCY Tube Test	☐	PREGNANCY Slide Test
		☐	Stool for Occult Blood
☐	Stool for Polys	☐	Stool for pH
☐	Stool for Red Subst.	☐	Stool for O & P
☐		☐	

THREE RIVERS AREA HOSPITAL
214 SPRING STREET
THREE RIVERS, MICHIGAN 49093

7010-109 URINALYSIS/CHART COPY

SPECIMEN SOURCE	Date Collected	Time Collected	Collected By

☐ Throat Culture	☐ G.C. Culture	☐ Urine Culture	☐ Blood Culture	☐ Stool Culture
☐ Anaerobic Culture	☐ Other Please Specify		☐ MIC Requested	

PATIENT NAME, ROOM, BIRTHDATE, PATIENT NO., DR., AGE, SEX

☐ Gram______	PRELIMINARY REPORT:	FINAL REPORT:

ORGANISM	AMIKACIN	AMPICILLIN	CEFOTAXIME	CEFOXITIN	CEPHALOTHIN	CHLORAMPHENICOL	CLINDAMYCIN	ERYTHROMYCIN	GENTAMYCIN	METHACILLIN	NITROFURANTOIN	PENICILLIN	PIPERACILLIN	TETRACYCLINE	TRIMETH/SULFA	TICARCILLIN	TOBRAMYCIN	VANCOMYCIN						
1.																								
2.																								
3.																								

FORM NO.7010-139 TECH DATE TIME

THREE RIVERS AREA HOSPITAL
214 SPRING STREET
THREE RIVERS, MICHIGAN 49093

MICROBIOLOGY/CHART COPY

Figure 15-8 These are examples of forms used for laboratory reports. Each specimen has its own color-coded slip on which laboratory findings are entered. The forms contain a carbon copy, eliminating the need for duplicate copying. One copy is sent to the nursing unit, where it is attached to the patient's record.

Skill Procedure 15-1. Assisting With an Examination

Suggested Action	Reason for Action
Check to see that any required consent form has been signed and dated by the patient and a witness to the signature.	Lawsuits are possible when examinations, tests, and treatments are performed without the patient's informed consent.
Determine that all test requirements have been accomplished.	Incomplete or inadequate preparation for a test may result in its cancellation and need for rescheduling.
Inform the patient that the examination will occur shortly.	The patient may use the opportunity to complete personal hygiene, use the toilet or bedpan, and change to a clean examination gown.
Inquire if the patient has any questions about the examination.	Providing information can reduce anxiety.
Inspect the examination room. Determine if it is clean and contains the supplies and equipment that will be needed.	Ensuring the readiness of the work area and examination equipment prevents delays and inconvenience for the patient and the examiner.
Check the function of instruments. Arrange items that are likely to be used for the examination.	Nonfunctioning equipment can cause frustration and prolong the examination time as replacements are located.
Note that there is a supply of clean gowns, drapes, and protective pads.	It is just as important to have supplies available for the patient's use as they are for the doctor's use.
Complete any last-minute test requirements, such as cleansing or shaving the examination site.	Some measures are performed just prior to the examination.
Assist the patient in whatever manner is needed.	The patient may need help completing his hygiene, tying the gown, or donning a robe and slippers.
If the patient room is used for the examination, clear articles from the working area.	Clutter can result in disorganization and possible breakage of examination equipment.
Provide privacy around the bed or transport the patient to a private examination room.	The nurse must protect the patient from being observed and overheard during the examination.
Help the patient onto the examination table.	An examination table is generally higher than an average bed. The patient may need a step stool or a steady hand.
Assist the patient into a position that will facilitate the examination.	Various positions, previously discussed, provide the examiner access to the body part that will be examined.
Drape the patient and provide extra covers if he is chilled.	Examination gowns are lightweight. Though they cover the patient and allow access to the body, they do not provide much warmth.
Talk with the patient. Provide explanations for the actions that will take place.	Good communication techniques can help put the patient at ease.
Do not leave the patient alone.	Falls from an examination table can cause serious injury.
Introduce the patient to the examiner if they are unfamiliar with one another.	By extending social courtesy, the nurse can reduce the anxiety that comes from unfamiliarity.
Remain throughout the examination. This is especially important if the examiner and the patient are different sexes.	Having a third person present protects the examiner from accusations of impropriety.
Adjust the lighting to the specifications of the examiner.	Examinations requiring inspection are more accurately performed with adequate lighting.
Provide the examiner with instruments, supplies, and equipment as they are needed.	The examiner may be using sterile gloves and require the help of the nurse to keep them free of organisms.

(continued)

Skill Procedure 15-1. Continued

Suggested Action	Reason for Action
Be prepared to receive and label specimens that may be obtained.	Improperly contained specimens and lost or mislabeled forms can delay necessary and vital information about the patient's state of health.
Talk with and support the patient throughout the examination.	Attention and encouragement from the nurse may help the patient endure the experience.
After the procedure is completed, help the patient to a position of comfort.	Some examination positions are difficult to assume and maintain.
Clean the patient of any substances that caused soiling. Assist the patient with a clean gown.	The patient's comfort and hygiene should be restored.
Return the patient to his room, making sure that the signal is available if he requires further assistance.	The patient may wish to request additional comfort and care measures.
Check the patient for signs and symptoms related to the procedure at frequent intervals.	The nurse is accountable for the safety of the patient. Regular, frequent observations may detect desirable and undesirable outcomes.
Record information concerning the examination performed and the condition of the patient.	A record is kept, documenting the care of the patient while in the health agency.
Report significant information about the examination to others responsible for the patient's care.	Sharing information provides current data that contribute to changes in the patient's plan for care.
Restore the examination room to order. Return equipment to its proper location.	Facilities and equipment should always be ready for the next use.

tion was done, the name of the examiner, a description of what took place including any observations related to the patient's general condition. The person who performed the examination usually summarizes the findings on a different form than that used by the nurse.

If specimens were obtained, the nurse should describe their characteristics and note if they were sent for laboratory testing. The nature and amount of any drainage may also be described, using terms provided in Chapter 14.

In addition to the written account of the examination, the nurse should report significant information to other nursing team members. This may include that the examination has been completed, the patient's reactions during and immediately after the procedure, and any delayed reactions. When all the nursing team is kept aware of current events and changes in the patient's condition, the plan of care can be revised and kept up to date.

Caring for Equipment and Supplies

Local policy indicates the responsibilities of the assisting nurse in caring for used equipment and supplies. Everything that was used must be returned or replaced. Soiled, nondisposable equipment should be delivered to an area for cleaning, disinfection, or sterilization. Supplies for discard are placed in the proper receptacle to prevent the spread of disease-causing organisms. In some agencies, part or all of these responsibilities may be delegated to non-nursing personnel.

Advancements in Examinations and Tests

Technology now allows examination of internal areas of the body without major surgery. There are machines that can record electrical impulses, the deflection of sound waves, and the energy released from the radioactive substances. New tests on blood and other body fluids are constantly being developed. All these advances in testing and examinations have improved the ability to detect disease processes early. The remaining part of this chapter provides information about specific examinations and tests. The normal values and the significance of abnormal results can be found in laboratory texts.

Interpreting Terms That Describe Tests

The nurse can interpret many medical terms by learning the meaning of root words, prefixes, and suffixes. Words ending in "ography" are used with many names of tests. This suffix indicates a procedure in which an image is produced. For example, the word *cholecystography* combines the root word referring to the gallbladder, "cholecyst," with the suffix, "ography," to mean a procedure in which an image of the gallbladder is produced.

The actual image, or results of the test, is described by using a root word followed by the suffix, "ogram." The term *cholecystogram* refers to the image of the gallbladder, which may be held in the hand and examined. The word *electrocardiogram* refers to the visual image or paper strip showing waves produced during electrocardiography.

Words ending with "oscopy" describe examinations in which body structures are visualized with the aid of an instrument. For example, a *sigmoidoscopy* is an examination in which the sigmoid area of the colon is viewed by an examiner. Some instruments enhance the ability to see structures. They are described, using the word ending "scope." Most people are familiar with words like microscope and telescope. A sigmoidoscope is an instrument used to look at the sigmoid section of the colon. The terms otoscope and ophthalmoscope have already been used and defined in this text.

When a procedure involves puncturing a body cavity, the ending "centesis" is attached to a word. A *thoracentesis* is a puncture of the pleural cavity, which lies in the thorax. Procedures involving this type of action usually are done to collect body fluids. Sometimes the word *puncture* or *tap* is used in the name of these same types of procedures. For example, it is common that a nurse may assist with a bone marrow puncture or a spinal tap.

Learning root words for body structures, many of which come from Latin words, is a basic task for nurses. With this foundation and an understanding of the meanings of word endings, the nurse can interpret many technical terms. Only those referring to tests and examinations have been discussed here.

Examinations That Use X-Rays

Roentgenography is a general term referring to all procedures that use roentgen rays to produce images of body structures. *Roentgen rays* are also known as *x-rays*. They produce electromagnetic energy that passes through body structures leaving an image on special film. X-rays cannot be seen or felt. The actual film image that is produced is called a *roentgenogram,* but it is commonly known as an *x-ray. Fluoroscopy* is a technique that combines roentgen rays and a fluoroscope to visualize internal body structures in motion. It is performed at the same time that an x-ray is obtained.

When no other substance is used but the x-rays, it is called a plain film x-ray. X-ray examinations using plain film may be performed on almost any part of the body. For example, the chest, abdomen, teeth, sinuses, and bones may be studied. A plain film x-ray may be taken any time because there is no special preparation that is required before the procedure. No special care or observations are necessary following a plain film x-ray.

At times, details in the body cannot be visualized sufficiently through plain film x-ray examinations. Therefore, a contrast medium may be used. A *contrast medium* is a substance that fills a body organ or cavity and makes it appear more dense. This serves to make the shape of the structure more distinct when viewed on x-ray film. X-rays in which a contrast medium is used require special preparation of the patient. The nurse is responsible for the special preparation and aftercare of the patient following tests in which a contrast medium is used.

Some patients have adverse allergic reactions to certain contrast media (plural for medium). An *allergy* is an unfavorable reaction to a substance to which the body is sensitive. The reactions may be mild, causing signs and symptoms, such as nausea and vomiting, a skin rash, or itching. Others may have severe reactions such as shock, coma, and death. All patients should be asked if they have any allergies. When there is a history of allergies, this should be clearly indicated on the patient's record. Even if there is no history of allergies, the patient should be observed for allergic reactions to contrast media. Allergic reactions to contrast media substances, particularly those that contain dyes such as iodine, are relatively common.

There is a tendency now to be cautious about the number of x-rays that are taken. The energy that is used for imaging can cause cell changes when there is excessive or accumulated exposure.

Chest X-Rays

Description. A chest x-ray is a plain film x-ray that provides an image of the structures within the chest. Back, front, and side views are most commonly obtained. This is described as posterior and anterior (abbreviated PA) and lateral views of the chest.

Common Indications. Chest x-rays show the condition of the lungs, the ribs, the upper spine, and the size of the heart. They are useful, for example, in diagnosing pneumonia, broken ribs, and lung tumors.

Kidneys, Ureters, and Bladder (KUB), or Abdominal Plain Film

Description. A plain film of kidneys, ureters, and urinary bladder, abbreviated KUB, provides images of these three structures and also other soft tissues of the abdomen.

Common Indications. A KUB is used to help diagnose abnormalities in structures within the abdomen. Conditions such as enlarged kidneys or obstructions in the intestinal tract can be detected.

Upper Gastrointestinal X-Ray

Description. An upper gastrointestinal x-ray, sometimes called an upper GI, uses barium as a contrast medium to study the esophagus, stomach, and duodenum. Despite flavorings that are added to the barium, most people find them distasteful. The structures in the upper gastrointestinal tract may be studied in motion with fluoroscopy as the barium is swallowed. The patient may return to the x-ray department later to have further x-rays taken of the movement of the barium into the small intestine.

It is important that the patient be instructed that the characteristics of his stool will be assessed. The stool will appear white due to the presence of barium. If the barium is passed too slowly, it can thicken and obstruct the passage of normal stool. Laxatives are given to prevent this from occurring.

Common Indications. An upper GI x-ray is done commonly to help diagnose ulcers, tumors, or narrowing of the structures in the upper digestive system.

Lower Gastrointestinal X-Ray or Barium Enema

Description. A lower gastrointestinal x-ray may also be called a lower GI or a barium enema. This x-ray utilizes both air and barium, instilled as an enema, to enhance images of the lower intestine. Most patients find this examination tiring and embarrassing. Helping to reassure and support them is important.

To promote the emptying of barium from the lower bowel, laxatives are generally prescribed. Observation of the pattern and characteristics of the patient's bowel elimination is an important nursing responsibility associated with this test.

Common Indications. A lower GI is used to examine the position, contour, filling, and movement of barium within the colon. It is most often used to help diagnose growths within the bowel, obstructions, and other changes in the interior surface of the large intestine.

Cholecystography

Description. *Cholecystography* is an x-ray examination of the gallbladder and its ducts. A dye that serves as a contrast medium is given orally or, on occasion, the dye is introduced into a vein. The x-ray image is called a cholecystogram.

Patients undergoing cholecystography, and other tests of structures that lie behind the intestine, are required to receive laxatives and enemas in order that stool or gas not obscure the image that is being taken. This x-ray must often be repeated. Usually this is necessary when the bowel was not sufficiently cleansed or when there was insufficient concentration of the dye. The patient should always be offered an explanation so that he does not become alarmed and worried.

Common Indications. Cholecystography is most often used to determine the presence of stones and obstructions in the gallbladder or its system of ducts.

Intravenous Pyelography (IVP)

Description. *Intravenous pyelography,* abbreviated IVP, is an x-ray examination to study the urinary tract. A contrast medium that contains a dye is introduced into a vein during this procedure. The image that is produced is called an intravenous pyelogram.

The patient should be forewarned that the dye is likely to cause him to feel warm and to have a salty taste in his mouth. He may also experience nausea. These symptoms are not forms of an allergic reaction, but rather a common effect when the concentrated dye is instilled directly into the circulatory system.

Common Indications. An IVP is commonly used to help diagnose conditions that cause abnormal functioning of the urinary tract. It may help identify malformations, tumors, stones, cysts, and obstructions in the kidneys and ureters.

Retrograde Pyelography

Description. *Retrograde pyelography* is an x-ray examination of the urinary tract, similar to an IVP, except that the dye is introduced through small catheters. The catheters are threaded directly into the ureters with the use of an instrument called a cystoscope. The procedure using a cystoscope is discussed later in the chapter. The name *retrograde* is used because the dye is instilled in a direction opposite to the normal flow of urine.

Common Indications. This test is performed for the same reasons as an IVP. It is generally done when an IVP has not given sufficient results for diagnostic purposes. The IVP is more commonly performed because retrograde pyelography requires that the procedure be carried out in an operating room. A general or local anesthetic may be used.

Angiography

Description. *Angiography* is an x-ray examination of blood vessels. The blood vessels that supply the heart are those that are frequently examined. A contrast dye is used; it is introduced through a catheter that is inserted into a blood vessel.

Common Indications. An angiography is done to determine the location, extent, and degree to which blood vessels have narrowed. Narrowing interferes with the amount of blood that can reach cells delivering oxygen and other chemicals. Surgery may be done following an angiography. During surgery a graft is performed. A *graft* is living tissue that is relocated and substitutes for diseased tissue. In one type of surgery, a vein from the leg is removed and reattached so that it provides a bypass for blood around the narrowed blood vessel. The examination helps the surgeon know exactly where the graft must be placed before any incision is made. This test may also be performed after surgery to evaluate the success of the operation.

Myelography

Description. *Myelography* is an x-ray examination that uses contrast material to study the spinal canal. Water-soluble or oil-based contrast media may be used. It is instilled during a lumbar puncture that is described later in this chapter. The x-ray image that is obtained is called a myelogram.

The patient should be taught that a tilt-table is used during the examination. A *tilt-table* is a device that elevates or lowers the patient's body. This helps to move the contrast medium to various levels within the spinal canal.

Common Indications. Myelography is commonly used to detect spinal tumors, ruptured disks, and bony changes in the vertebrae.

Computerized Axial Tomography (CAT or CT)

Description. *Computerized axial tomography,* abbreviated CAT or CT, is a type of x-ray examination that views horizontal sections of the body from various angles. CAT involves the use of narrow x-ray beams, much more sensitive than ordinary x-rays. A contrast dye may be used in some instances. A computer makes mathematically calculated observations as the test is in progress. The CAT machine rotates about the motionless patient obtaining various views. Because a large area of the body is examined in layers, the name of this test may also be combined with the word *scan,* as in CAT scan. An example of a CAT scan is shown in Figure 15-9.

As a result of the high technology associated with the manufacturing and operation of this equipment, many small hospitals cannot afford to purchase one. Patients may be referred to larger hospitals for this specialized test.

Common Indications. Any part of the body may be examined by CAT. The most common uses include examinations of the head, chest, and abdomen. A CAT scan is useful in providing an image from which the size of normal and abnormal tissue can be evaluated.

Examinations of Electrical Impulses

Nerve activity produces electrical impulses. Machines have been developed that can record these electrical impulses. Analyzing the image of the electrical impulses can help identify normal and abnormal conditions. The electrical impulses produced by the heart, brain, and skeletal mus-

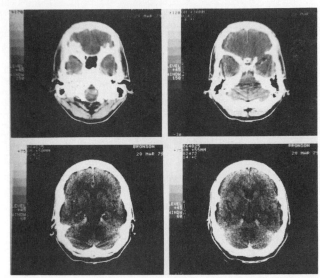

Figure 15-9 Progressive cross section images of the cranium using a CAT scan. The collective x-rays are evaluated to determine the size of soft and solid tissue structures.

cles are commonly examined. Wires, called *electrodes,* attached to the skin with suction and the help of a clear gel pick up the electrical impulses and transmit them to a machine. The machine converts the electrical energy into a visual image. The patient should be taught that although electrodes are connecting him to a machine, he will not receive any electrical shocks. Except for an awareness of the presence of electrodes, the patient usually does not experience any other sensations during the test. Most of these tests can be performed without any prior preparation.

Electrocardiography (EKG or ECG)

Description. *Electrocardiography* is an examination that records electrical impulses produced by the contracting heart muscle. It is abbreviated EKG or ECG. The recorded image of the electrical impulses, called an electrocardiogram, is illustrated in Figure 15-10.

Common Indications. EKG is used to assess the contraction of the heart muscle. The electrocardiogram can be interpreted to determine the heart rate, the rhythm, and evidence of heart damage, especially associated with a heart attack. This test may be performed to determine an individual's potential cardiac risk. Stress EKG was discussed in Chapter 9.

Electroencephalography (EEG)

Description. *Electroencephalography* is an examination that records an image of the electrical activity in the brain. It is abbreviated EEG. The recorded image is an

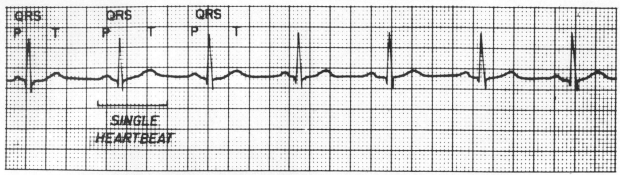

Figure 15-10 This is an example of an electrocardiogram. It illustrates normal heart functioning.

electroencephalogram. The patient's usual amount of sleep may be restricted before a scheduled examination. It is helpful to record the electrical impulses while the patient is awake and asleep. Natural sleep during the test is preferred to administering a drug to induce sleep.

The hair should be shampooed before the examination. This helps ensure that the electrodes, when applied to the head, remain in place. Natural oils on the scalp and hair may cause them to become loose. The hair will need to be rewashed following the test to remove the gel that was used to attach the electrodes.

Common Indications. EEG is used to help diagnose epilepsy, tumors, bleeding into the brain tissues, and various other diseases of the brain. The test is also used to determine if an unresponsive, comatose patient is brain dead.

Electromyography (EMG)

Description. *Electromyography* is an examination that records the electrical impulses produced by contracting skeletal muscle. It is abbreviated EMG. The record made of the electrical impulses is called an electromyogram.

There may be discomfort during this examination. Electrodes are inserted through the skin, which may cause slight pain. Uncomfortable sensations may also be felt when electrical stimulation is applied to muscles. This must be done to evaluate the ability of the muscle to respond. If the electrode makes contact with a nerve, an even greater amount of discomfort will occur. The patient should be asked to indicate when he feels pain so the examiner may make adjustments.

Common Indications. EMG is used to help identify and diagnose conditions that result in abnormal sensations, weakness, or paralysis. These may be due to nerve diseases or injuries. This technology is also being used in other ways. The electrical impulses from nerves are being harnessed to operate artificial limbs.

Examinations That Detect Radiation

Radiation is energy that cannot be seen or felt. The sun gives off radiation as well as heat and light. Types of radiation are identified as alpha, beta, and gamma. Gamma radiation is the most powerful of these. It can pass through objects and body tissue.

The atomic structure of some chemical elements, such as iodine, can be altered in such a way that it gives off radiation. It is then referred to as a *radionuclide.* This is a more current term replacing the traditional term *radioisotope.* Radionuclides prepared in forms that allow them to be administered to humans are called *radiopharmaceuticals.*

After a radionuclide is given, it will be circulated throughout the body. Some organs absorb only certain types of radionuclides. The organ that is targeted by the radionuclide emits radiation. A radionuclide is usually distributed fairly uniformly in normal tissues. It will be distributed unevenly, or be absent, in diseased tissues. A machine scans the organs and converts the energy into light. It is possible to produce an image in shades of black and white according to the amount of energy being released. Organs that are often studied for disease with radionuclides include the thyroid gland, liver, bones, and brain.

Tests using radionuclides are contraindicated for pregnant women or nursing mothers. The energy that is released can be harmful to the rapidly growing cells of an infant or fetus.

Thyroid Scan

Description. A thyroid scan is a type of examination in which a radionuclide is used. Radioactive iodine, identified as ^{131}I, is administered to the patient. It can be given either orally or injected into a vein. After allowing time for the thyroid to absorb the iodine, a scanner passes over the area of the patient's thyroid gland. The patient experiences no discomfort from the iodine or the machine.

Common Indications. A thyroid scan is done to evaluate the size, shape, and functioning of the thyroid gland. A normal thyroid gland absorbs the radioactive form of iodine evenly. The test is usually performed to diagnose a gland that is functioning excessively or insufficiently. These conditions will show alterations in the rate of absorption. Tumors may be identified by an uneven absorption within the gland. The shape or position of the gland may also be abnormal.

Examinations That Use Sound Waves

Ultrasonography is an examination that produces images of structures as they reflect or bounce back sound waves. This is similar to a bat or dolphin's echo location system. A synonym is *echography.* The sound produces waves of vibrations. They are of very high frequency, which neither can be felt nor heard by the human ear. This is the reason they are called *ultrasound* examinations. The various densities of body tissues reflect sound in different ways. Structures surrounded by fluid are the most readily examined by ultrasound.

A machine converts the deflected sound waves into a visual image. It can be viewed similarly to television. A recorded image is also obtained. It is called an ultrasonogram, sonogram, or echogram.

Ultrasonography is used to study the position, form, and functioning of various organs of the body. Ultrasonography can also be used to examine moving structures, such as the heart or a fetus.

Obstetric Sonogram (B Scan)

Description. The examination of a pregnant, or possibly pregnant, uterus using ultrasound is often called a B scan. This term refers to one of several methods for recording the echoing sound waves.

The pregnant uterus is especially easy to examine because the fetus is surrounded by fluid. A full bladder further enhances the transmission of sound waves. Fluid helps make the image of the structure within the fluid more distinct.

A gel is applied to the abdomen. The examiner moves a *transducer,* an instrument that picks up the echoing sound waves, over the abdomen while observing the image on a screen. The mother can also view her unborn child. Movement, if there is any, such as a beating heart or moving arms and legs, can also be observed. The sex of a fetus can sometimes be determined by the outline of its anatomy in the late stages of a pregnancy. A permanent image is made as a record of the test findings.

Common Indications. This test is often used to confirm that a pregnancy exists. It can also be used to determine the approximate age and growth of a developing fetus. Complications during pregnancy, such as an ill-located or attached placenta or fetal defects can be identified.

Examinations That Use Endoscopes

An *endoscope* is an instrument that can be inserted within the body. It is used for direct observation and inspection of internal body structures. The endoscope has a lighted mirror-lens system attached to a tube, which is sometimes flexible. *Endoscopy* is an examination of a body part with an endoscope. There are attachments for endoscopes that allow the examiner to obtain a biopsy. A *biopsy* is the removal of a small amount of tissue for microscopic examination.

Bronchoscopy

Description. A *bronchoscopy* is the direct inspection of the trachea and bronchi with a bronchoscope. It is generally carried out in an outpatient surgical department or in an operating room. The throat of the patient is anesthetized to prevent coughing and gagging as the scope is inserted. Food and fluids must be restricted until the patient can swallow and cough again. The nurse is held accountable for the safety of the patient who may have difficulty breathing due to swelling or aspirating secretions after this exam.

Common Indications. Bronchoscopy is used most commonly to help in the diagnosis of tumors, to remove foreign objects, to remove thick respiratory secretions, and to obtain specimens from the respiratory tract.

Proctoscopy and Sigmoidoscopy

Description. A *proctoscopy* and a *sigmoidoscopy* are examinations that allow direct inspection of the rectum and sigmoid colon with a proctoscope or sigmoidoscope. The patient will be placed in a knee-chest or Sims' position. There is no pain. The patient may experience some discomfort when the instrument is inserted its full distance. He may experience a strong urge to defecate.

Common Indications. A proctoscopy and a sigmoidoscopy are done most commonly to help in the diagnosis of inflammatory conditions of the bowel and to identify tumors in the rectum and sigmoid colon.

Cystoscopy

Description. A *cystoscopy* is an examination that permits direct viewing of the urethra, bladder, and openings to the ureters with a cystoscope. The patient will be placed in a lithotomy position for this examination. It is generally performed in an operating room, but the patient is usually awake. He is given a local anesthetic. General anesthetics may be given in special circumstances.

Common Indications. A cystoscope is used to examine urinary tract structures, to remove stones, to identify where a catheter should be threaded for retrograde pyelography, and to view and treat bladder tumors.

Examinations of Body Fluids

Some examinations of body fluids require that the physician collect the specimen at the bedside. Once the specimen has been obtained, it is sent to the laboratory for analysis. The nurse acts as an assistant to the physician. Prepackaged trays that contain most, if not all, of the necessary equipment are generally available. If they are not, the nurse should assemble supplies according to a prepared list. In some cases, as in tests on venous or arterial blood, the nurse coordinates the preparation and special care of the patient with laboratory personnel.

Some specimen testing on urine, gastric secretions, stool, and capillary blood may be performed by the nurse in the patient's bathroom, bedside, or utility room. These tests are usually repeated frequently and monitored for early, significant changes.

Several representative examples of procedures that are performed to collect and examine body fluids will be discussed. While assisting in procedures that require the help of a physician, the nurse also observes and supports the patient. If any unusual signs or symptoms are assessed, the nurse should inform the doctor in a manner that will not alarm the patient.

Gastric Analysis

Description. A *gastric analysis* is a procedure in which stomach secretions are obtained for examination. The gastric fluid is removed through a nasogastric tube to obtain the specimen. In Chapter 8, Skill Procedure 8-3 described the technique for inserting a nasogastric tube and can be reviewed again if necessary. Sometimes this test includes the administration of drugs known to stimulate the production of gastric acid to evaluate the stomach's response. The specimen is sent to the laboratory for examination.

A simpler form of examination may be performed by the nurse at the bedside. The gastric fluid is tested to determine its pH, the level of acidity or alkalinity. It only requires a bulb syringe and test strip if the patient has a nasogastric tube in place.

The nurse aspirates a small volume of fluid. A drop or two is applied to the test strip. The color change is compared with the chart on the test strip container. The color change correlates with a numerical value between 1 and 14. A number below 7 indicates acidity; alkaline fluids are above 7. Stomach secretions are normally between 1 and 3

unless the patient is receiving medications or has undergone other treatment to make them alkaline.

Another test performed by the nurse involves testing gastric fluid for blood. Blood may not be obvious with simple visual inspection. This is referred to as a hemoccult test. The prefix *hem* refers to blood and *occult* means hidden.

The nurse uses a liquid chemical reagent for this test. A sample of stomach fluid is applied to a permeable area of a cardboard slide. The chemical solution is dropped onto the specimen. After waiting 60 seconds, the nurse looks for a color change. If blood is present, the area turns blue. Detecting blood may indicate a need for treatment and perhaps further endoscopic or x-ray examinations.

Common Indications. Tests of this nature are generally performed to analyze the characteristics or effects of gastric acid present in the stomach. Excessively high acid levels are associated with gastritis and ulcers. Frequent monitoring may be done to evaluate the response of high-risk individuals to preventive treatment. However, absence of hydrochloric acid in the stomach or low levels also signify pathologic conditions.

Lumbar Puncture

Description. A *lumbar puncture* or *spinal tap* is a procedure that involves the insertion of a needle beneath the arachnoid layer of the meninges in the space between the third and fourth or fourth and fifth lumbar vertebrae. Cerebrospinal fluid is located in this space. It is collected and specimens are sent to the laboratory for microscopic examination. The spinal cord ends above this area so it cannot be injured. A local anesthetic is administered so that only sensations of pressure are experienced.

The patient is assisted to "curl up in a ball," as shown in Figure 15-11, or he is helped to assume a sitting position. This widens the space between the bony vertebrae so that the needle can be inserted easily. The nurse may need to help the patient maintain this position during the procedure.

Sometimes the nurse is asked to assist with *Queckenstedt's test* during a lumbar puncture. This is used to determine the presence or absence of an obstruction to the flow of cerebrospinal fluid. To perform this test, the nurse applies pressure with the hands to the patient's jugular veins in the neck. Or a blood pressure cuff is applied about the neck and inflated to 20 mm Hg. If there is no obstruction, the spinal fluid pressure will rise with compression and fall with its release. If an obstruction is present, the pressure will remain unaffected or require more than 20 seconds to become lowered.

Common Indications. This test may be performed for various reasons. It may be used to diagnose conditions that cause the intracranial pressure to be elevated, which

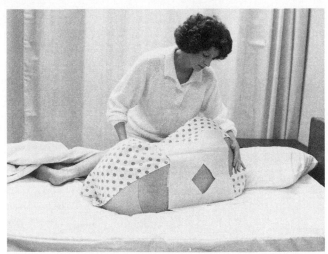

Figure 15-11 The patient is in position for a lumbar puncture. Note that his back is sharply arched as the nurse holds him at his knees and his shoulders. The sterile drape has been secured in place with adhesive strips. Helping the patient relax and having him take slow, deep breaths make holding the position easier for him. A small pillow is allowed under the head. Be sure the knees are not forced into the abdomen, which would affect spinal pressure.

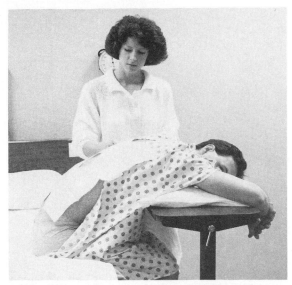

Figure 15-12 The patient rests over his bedside table in readiness for a thoracentesis. The nurse is securing the sterile drape with adhesive strips so that it cannot slip out of place over the working area. Some patients can rest over the back of a straight chair for a thoracentesis.

may occur with a brain or spinal cord tumor. A lumbar puncture may be used to lower the intracranial pressure by withdrawing some of the volume of fluid. Specimens of cerebrospinal fluid may be collected and sent to the laboratory to diagnose infections, like meningitis, and other diseases. A lumbar puncture may be performed in order to instill contrast medium when myelography is carried out. Finally, some conditions may be treated by instilling drugs directly into the spinal fluid after a similar amount of fluid has been withdrawn.

Thoracentesis

Description. A *thoracentesis* is a procedure during which the pleural cavity is entered and fluid is withdrawn. Normally fluid does not accumulate in the thorax. The patient is assisted into a sitting position, as shown in Figure 15-12. If the patient cannot sit, the nurse may have him lie on his unaffected side.

Common Indications. This test is performed to remove fluid or sometimes air from the pleural cavity. The fluid that is collected can be examined in the laboratory to determine if organisms are causing an infection. They may also be examined to help diagnose the presence of cancer. Removing accumulated fluid from the pleural cavity can be performed to ease a patient's labored respirations. This provides more room for the lungs to fill with air.

Paracentesis

Description. A *paracentesis* is a procedure that involves puncturing the skin and subsequently the abdomi-

nal cavity so that body fluid may be withdrawn. The patient is placed in a position shown in Figure 15-13. A local anesthetic is administered prior to using a piercing instrument called a *trocar*. A hollow sheath called a *cannula* surrounds the trocar. Once the trocar has been advanced to the depth desired, it is removed. Fluid drains through the cannula, tubing, and eventually into a drainage container. Large volumes of fluid can be expected.

It is important to have the patient urinate before the procedure. A full bladder could be accidentally punctured. The nurse may also obtain some evaluative assessments such as the patient's weight and the measurement of the abdomen. By repeating these assessments after the procedure, the nurse can collect objective information about its effectiveness.

Common Indications. This procedure is most commonly done to relieve pressure and dyspnea caused by the accumulation of excessive amounts of fluid. When this is done, the patient's ability to breathe may be improved because there will be more room for lung expansion. The patient, having had the weight from a large volume of fluid removed, should also be more comfortable. A sample of the fluid may be sent to the laboratory for microscopic examination.

Amniocentesis

Description. An *amniocentesis* is the withdrawal of amniotic fluid from the pregnant uterus. This test is preceded by an ultrasound of the abdomen to determine the location of the fetus and placenta. Following this the patient empties her bladder to reduce the possibility of

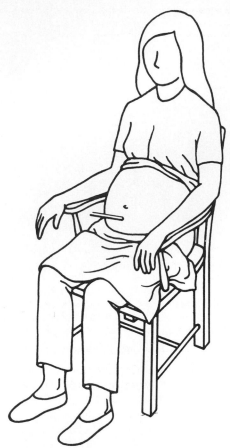

Figure 15-13 This sketch illustrates positioning for an abdominal paracentesis. Drainage occurs by gravity.

piercing it as the physician inserts a long thin needle through the abdomen. Fluid is aspirated through the needle for laboratory examination. The nurse monitors the patient's vital signs and the fetal heart rate before and after the test. It is also the nurse's responsibility to label the specimen properly and send it to the laboratory. The results of the test take three to five weeks.

Common Indications. This test is usually reserved for women at high risk for delivering an infant with genetic or congenital disorders such as spina bifida, Down's syndrome, and cystic fibrosis. The sex of the infant can also be determined with this test. Some choose not to know this information. In pregnancies where an early delivery is a necessity to ensure the health of the mother or the infant, it may be performed to evaluate fetal lung maturity, which indicates when the baby has the respiratory potential to survive outside the womb.

Capillary Blood Glucose

Description. This test involves pricking the finger with a spring-loaded lancet to obtain a drop of capillary blood. The blood is dropped onto a test strip. The level of glucose can be determined by visually comparing the color

changes on the strip with a color code chart. However, more exact levels are obtained when the test strip is inserted within a glucometer.

A glucometer is a machine that uses light reflectance to measure glucose. That is, it converts the amount of reflected light from the test strip into an equivalent blood sugar reading. The more light that is reflected, the lower the glucose level. This explains why it is critical to cover the test strip completely with blood and blot the excess in order to obtain accurate measurements.

Several companies manufacture glucometers. All are extremely accurate when used according to directions. Skill Procedure 15-2 provides general directions for using a glucometer.

Clinical Indications. Testing blood glucose is especially important in the care and treatment of diabetics. Their well-being is related to maintaining blood sugar within normal ranges. Monitoring helps to determine adjustments in diet, exercise, or medication throughout each day.

Capillary blood glucose may also be measured when nondiabetic patients receive high caloric tube or parenteral nutrition. These patients may require insulin temporarily to assist in metabolizing the carbohydrates found in these formulas.

Suggested Measures to Assist With Examinations in Selected Situations

When the Patient Is an Infant or Child

Tests and examinations performed on adults may also be performed on children. Test preparations and procedures may be adjusted in keeping with the child's body size or ability to cooperate.

Expect that the number of enemas or amount of laxatives are likely to be reduced when this is required prior to a test.

The use of laxatives or enemas should always be questioned if a child has abdominal pain or diarrhea.

The amount of time during which food and fluids are restricted before an examination may vary, depending on the physician's wishes.

Expect that the external jugular veins and femoral arteries are most likely to be used to obtain blood samples from an infant.

Expect that a sedative may be prescribed if a child has difficulty lying quietly during an examination.

Lead shielding, which protects the thyroid and genitals, should be provided for while undergoing dental x-rays.

Skill Procedure 15-2. Using a Glucometer

Suggested Action	Reason for Action
Assemble the following: lancet, lancet holder, test strips, glucometer, clean gloves, and a cotton ball or paper tissue depending on the blotting instructions of the manufacturer.	Gathering and organizing all necessary equipment promotes efficient time management.
Note the expiration date on the supply of test strips.	Outdated test strips may not produce accurate results.
Wash hands.	Handwashing reduces the transmission of microorganisms. Touching the pad of the test strip with unwashed hands can transfer substances that may alter the test results.
Turn on the machine. Test the machine's calibration using a control strip or solution provided by the manufacturer.	Reliability of the test results depends on the accuracy of the machine.
Explain the procedure to the patient.	Explanations decrease apprehension and promote cooperation.
Inspect the patient's fingers and thumbs for a non-traumatized area. The ear lobes and toes are acceptable alternates.	Repeated punctures in the same area can become painful.
Assemble the lancet within the spring-loaded holder.	Concealing the needle reduces the anticipation of pain.
Have the patient wash his hands thoroughly with soap and warm water and dry well.	Soap and friction clean the skin. Warm water dilates blood vessels, which facilitates obtaining an adequate drop of blood.
Avoid using alcohol as a skin antiseptic when performing this test.	Unless alcohol evaporates before the finger stick, it can alter the test results. Repeated use of alcohol dries the skin. Microorganisms can enter and remain in the cracks of dry skin.
Don clean gloves.	Gloves are worn as a universal precaution when the possibility of contact with blood exists.
Apply the lancet to the margin around the fingertip avoiding the central pad area as shown in Figure 15-14.	The center of the finger and thumbpads contain abundant sensory nerve endings. Puncturing this area increases the incidence of pain both during the test and later on.

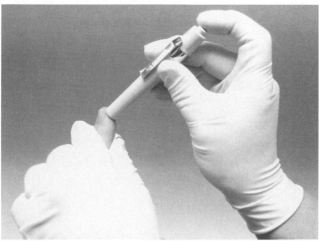

Figure 15-14 A puncture made with a lancet holder produces less trauma and pain than one made manually with just the lancet.

(continued)

Skill Procedure 15-2. Continued

Suggested Action	Reason for Action
Release the spring, causing the needle to pierce the skin.	The spring mechanism causes rapid penetration at a controlled depth. This produces an almost painless puncture.
Milk or squeeze the area to produce a large hanging drop of blood as shown in Figure 15-15.	Blood flow can be increased by stripping the blood toward the puncture area.
Touch the hanging drop of blood to the pad on the test strip. Make sure that the pad is completely covered.	The pad must be completely covered and saturated in order to produce accurate results. A thin film of blood does not penetrate the pad sufficiently.

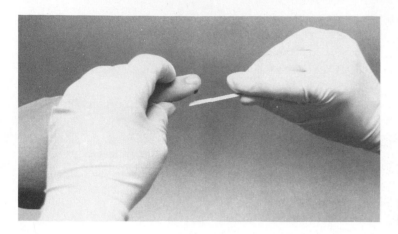

Figure 15-15 One drop of blood must be adequate enough to cover and saturate the test pad.

Press the start button on the glucometer to activate the timing of the test.	Accurate timing is critical to obtaining valid test results.
Place the test strip on a hard surface. Blot and reblot for 1 to 2 seconds when the machine beeps audibly.	Excess blood is removed through blotting. Some manufacturers recommend wiping with a cotton ball. Follow the manufacturer's directions.
Insert the blotted test strip immediately after blotting into the machine. Make sure that the pad faces the light window as shown in Figure 15-16. Shut the door to secure it in place.	The level of glucose is determined by the reflected light. Failure to close the door will allow light to enter and produce inaccurate results.

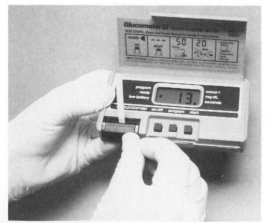

Figure 15-16 The test strip is inserted within the machine. When the timer reaches zero, the glucose level will be displayed.

(continued)

Skill Procedure 15-2. *Continued*

Suggested Action	Reason for Action
Note the number displayed on the screen of the glucometer at the end of the test.	Most glucometers display test results within approximately 1 to 2 minutes after the timer is activated.
Remove and compare the test strip with the color code chart on the container of test strips.	The color code is a visual method of checking the validity of the machine's results. The glucometer measurement and color code should be somewhat compatible. The glucometer is considered more exact.
Turn off the machine.	Glucometers operate by battery. The life of the battery is extended by turning the machine off when not in use.
Uncover the tip of the lancet holder exposing the needle tip. Press the sharp tip into its plastic cover, shown in Figure 15-17, remove the lancet, and dispose into a puncture-resistant container.	Gloves do not protect against punctures. Embedding the tip in plastic reduces the possibility of an accidental puncture while removing the lancet from its holder or during its disposal.

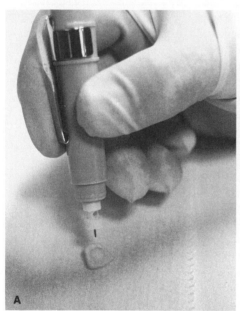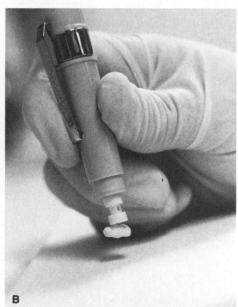

Figure 15-17 To avoid an accidental needle puncture with a used lancet, position it above the protective cap (*A*), and (*B*) pierce the cap with the sharp point.

Remove gloves and immediately wash hands.	Handwashing reduces the number of microorganisms on the hands.
Remove the equipment from the bedside if it does not belong to the patient.	Hospital equipment should be returned for the use of others.
Clean the light window with a clean, dry, lint-free cloth.	A dirty window interferes with detecting light reflection and distorts the test results.
Store the test strips in an area that is cool and dry.	Test strips can give false readings if stored in an area of high humidity or moisture, such as the bathroom. Their accuracy is best ensured at temperatures between 35° to 85°F (1.7° to 30°C).
Record the capillary blood glucose measurement on the patient's record.	A flow sheet helps to evaluate patterns and trends in blood sugar levels.
Verbally report abnormal blood sugar levels according to agency policy.	A normal premeal blood sugar is usually in the range of 80 to 120 mg. Additional treatment or testing may be necessary for values above and below this range.

Applicable Nursing Diagnoses

Patients undergoing tests and examinations may have these nursing diagnoses:

- Knowledge Deficit
- Anxiety
- Fear
- Impaired Adjustment
- Ineffective Family Coping
- Decisional Conflict
- Health-Seeking Behavior
- Powerlessness
- Spiritual Distress

Nursing Care Plan 15-1 is an example of the nursing process as it relates to the nursing diagnosis of Decisional Conflict. This diagnostic category has been defined in the NANDA taxonomy (1989) as, "The state of uncertainty about the course of action to be taken when choice among competing actions involves risk, loss, or challenge to personal life values."

Stroke and touch an infant or young child after a painful procedure. The warmth and touch offer reassurance and often console young children.

When the Patient Is Elderly

Expect that the elderly patient, especially one who is debilitated from illness, may not be able to tolerate having food and fluids withheld for long periods of time before certain examinations, such as an IVP.

Laxatives and enemas may exhaust some elderly patients. When there is a question, be sure to consult the physician. Be available to assist elderly patients with a bedpan or ambulating to the bathroom.

Elderly patients are often on daily medications for chronic conditions. The physician should be consulted about withholding medications when an elderly patient must remain fasting for a test or examination.

When the Patient Is Pregnant or Breast Feeding

Assume that any female who is sexually active and not using any form of birth control could be pregnant. X-rays should be delayed until the patient is questioned about the possibility of being pregnant.

Provide a lead apron to cover the chest and abdomen of any woman in reproductive years for whom x-rays are necessary.

Expect that examinations using x-rays or radio-

nuclides will not be used for women who are pregnant or breast feeding. Radiation may affect the cells of the rapidly growing fetus or infant.

Consult with a physician about omitting enemas and laxatives to prepare women in the advanced stages of pregnancy for tests and examinations.

Medications that are administered with tests or examinations may need to be withheld for the woman who is pregnant or breast feeding. Medications enter the bloodstream and breast milk and subsequently are distributed to the fetus or infant.

Teaching Suggestions About Tests and Examinations

Descriptions of what a patient may expect during a test or examination should be provided to all patients to prevent or relieve anxiety.

The patient should be instructed about test requirements or preparations. If the patient is going to be responsible for his own preparation, such as when a test is performed as an outpatient, the test instructions should be written. The patient should be given a phone number of a contact person if there are any questions.

Suggestions for the instruction of patients were given several times when describing specific examinations.

Women should be taught the importance of scheduling examinations that include a Papanicolaou's test, commonly called a *Pap test*. The test can be helpful in detecting cancer of the cervix during its early, still curable stages. It has been usual to recommend that regular Pap testing start at about 35 to 40 years of age. Some physicians perform this test at younger ages on women who take oral contraceptives. Some authorities state that after two negative Pap tests, done at 1-year intervals, a woman who is not at risk for cancer need have a Pap test only every 3 years.

Mammography, an examination of the breast tissue using x-rays, should be done as a baseline at about the age of 40. Mammographic examinations should be continued throughout the lifetime of an aging woman. This test can identify a cancerous lesion at least two years earlier than it can be felt. Women should consult with a physician about the frequency of these examinations. This often depends on risk factors obtained from a woman's health history.

Both men and women should have yearly proctoscopic and sigmoidoscopic examinations after the age of 40. Cancer of the colon and rectum oc-

NURSING CARE PLAN

15-1. Decisional Conflict

Assessment

Subjective Data

States, "I don't know what to do now that the amniocentesis shows that my baby will have cystic fibrosis. I know I can have an abortion, but I'm not sure I want to do that. I remember what it was like when my brother was always sick and then died. Why did this have to happen to me? I don't feel that any decision is possible right now."

Objective Data

28-year-old married woman who is 20 weeks pregnant. Date of last menstrual period: 7/2. Fetal heart rate is 140 in left lower quadrant. Says she has felt fetal movement. Had a younger brother who died at age 5 from cystic fibrosis. Sits with rigid posture almost immobile except wringing hands. Very little eye contact during interaction.

Diagnosis

Decisional Conflict related to birthing options of fetus with genetic disorder detected by amniocentesis.

Plan

Goal

The patient will make an informed choice concerning the outcome of the current pregnancy by the return office visit on 11/10.

Orders: 11/5

1. Ask to compose list of advantages and disadvantages to possible choices in writing before return on 11/10.
2. Encourage to discuss options with husband and other significant persons.
3. Offer referrals to the Cystic Fibrosis Foundation, pro-choice or right-to-life groups.
4. Support decision even if it is contrary to one's personal choice. _____ F. BROWN, RN

Implementation (Documentation)

11/5

1415   Shared that this decision is difficult—other women dealing with these same circumstances have also felt the same as she does. Reinforced that the choice is hers to make and also confident that she can make the one that is best for her. Asked to list any and all advantages and disadvantages in writing to help clarify options. Offered referral to supportive agenies. Asked for and was given the phone number of the Cystic Fibrosis Foundation. Encouraged to come with husband for sharing questions and concerns. _____ F. BROWN, RN

Evaluation (Documentation)

11/10

1300   Returned for office conference with husband. Contacted Cystic Fibrosis Foundation and attended a support group of parents. List of advantages and disadvantages completed by both patient and husband. Stated "The treatment of cystic fibrosis seems to have improved in the 20 years since my brother died. We talked it over and even if we had a normal baby, there's the risk it would die while we were alive. The people at the CF meeting made us feel like we're not alone." Scheduled next prenatal visit for 12/15. _____ F. BROWN, RN

cur with high frequency among men and women in the United States.

Men should understand the importance of an examination of the prostate gland. This is usually performed at the time of a physical examination. This gland undergoes changes, and may develop cancer, as men age. When the physician feels the outline of the prostate gland using a lubricated gloved finger inserted into the rectum, its size and texture may be assessed.

Bibliography

Barnie DC: Care planning in the endoscopy unit: Master care plan for the pre-endoscopy patient. Society of Gastrointestinal Assistants Journal 11(2):97–99, 1988

Barnie DC: Care planning in the GI endoscopy unit: Master care plan for the post procedure patient. Gastroenterology Nursing 11(4):266–267, 1989

Caine R: Essentials of monitoring the electrocardiogram. Nurs Clin North Am 22(1):77–87, 1987

Esposito N, Westgate P: Continuous EEG monitoring in the PICU. Journal of Pediatric Nursing 2(4):272–277, 1987

Gilden JL: Benefits from self-monitoring of blood glucose. Consultant 28(1):29–32, 34, 1988

Guthrie RA, Karem JH, Langer O: Self-monitoring of blood glucose. Patient Care 21(12):56–58, 60, 62, 1987

Harrison N, Smith B: Information wanted . . . what information should the relatives and friends of the patients be told? Nursing Times 86(6):46–48, 1990

Kenyon S: Making sense of obstetric ultrasound. Nursing Times 85(31):39–41, 1989

LaFontaine P: Alleviating patient's apprehensions and anxieties. Gastroenterology Nursing 11(4):256–257, 1989

Lopez EI: Prenatal diagnosis by ultrasound. Journal of Perinatal and Neonatal Nursing 2(4):34–42, 1989

Monroe D: Patient teaching for x-ray and other diagnostics. RN Magazine 52(12):36–40, 1989

Monroe D: Will your patient survive that trip to x-ray? RN Magazine 52(4):40–42, 44, 1989

Montana JA: Glucose meters. Journal of Pediatric Nursing 4(2):132–136, 1989

Nottingham A, Rambo A: Electrocardiographic phenomena in the transplanted human heart. Focus on Critical Care 13(6):41–46, 1976

Swartz M: Dealing with death in the endoscopy suite. Gastroenterology Nursing 11(4):242–244, 1989

Thompson J: Using medical radiation from the inside out. FDA Consumer 21(6):10–13, 1987

Thompson S: Ultrasonography: Intraoperative diagnoses of choledocholithiasis. American Association of Operating Room Nurses Journal 51(4):983–985, 1990

Thurlow JG: Informed consent: Every patient's right. Gastroenterology Nursing 12(2):132–134, 1989

Tomky D: A three-pronged approach to monitoring. RN Magazine 52(3):23–30, 1989

von Nostitz P: X-rays: What's safe? . . . how to lower your risks. Parents 62(4):209–212, 1987

Weck E: A primer on medical imaging part 2. FDA Consumer 23(4):12–15, 1989

Unit IV

Nursing Skills Related to Health Restoration

16

Controlling
Microorganisms

Chapter Outline

Behavioral Objectives
Glossary
Introduction
Characteristics of Microorganisms
Natural Body Defenses
Factors That Weaken Defenses
The Infectious Process Cycle
Description of Asepsis
Common Practices of Medical Asepsis
Methods of Disinfection and Sterilization
Principles of Surgical Asepsis
Common Practices Involving Surgical Asepsis
Applicable Nursing Diagnoses
Teaching Suggestions to Practice of Medical and
    Surgical Asepsis
Bibliography

Skill Procedures

Handwashing
Performing a Surgical Scrub
Using a Mask
Donning a Sterile Gown
Donning and Removing Sterile Gloves

Behavioral Objectives

When the content of this chapter has been mastered, the learner will be able to:

Define the terms appearing in the glossary.

Discuss the conditions that must usually be present to support the growth of microorganisms.

List examples of natural body defenses that protect individuals from acquiring infections.

List factors that increase the potential risk for acquiring infections.

Describe the cycle that explains how microorganisms are spread.

Explain the differences between surgical and medical asepsis.

Describe common nursing practices of medical asepsis; list examples from everyday living, personal grooming, and clinical practice.

Demonstrate proper handwashing; identify the actions that would be different when performing a surgical scrub.

Identify apparel that may be worn to prevent the spread of microorganisms between the patient and the nurse.

Describe the proper method for disposing of needles and sharp objects.

Discuss practices that should be followed when cleaning supplies and equipment.

Identify the difference between disinfection and sterilization.

List five factors that should be considered before selecting a method of disinfection or sterilization.

Identify four methods for destroying microorganisms with heat and four methods for destroying microorganisms with chemicals.

List principles that should be applied when carrying out sterile technique.

Demonstrate how to create a sterile field, add sterile items and liquids to a sterile field, handle transfer forceps kept in disinfectant, and don and remove sterile gloves.

Summarize the suggestions for instruction of patients that are offered in this chapter.

Glossary

Aerobic microorganism A microbe that requires free oxygen in order to exist.

Anaerobic microorganism A microbe that depends on an environment without oxygen for its survival.

Antibiotics A classification of drugs that have an anti-infective action.

Anti-infective agent A chemical that kills or suppresses the multiplication of microorganisms. Synonym for *antimicrobial agent.*

Antimicrobial agent A chemical that kills or suppresses the multiplication of microorganisms. Synonym for *anti-infective agent.*

Antiseptic A chemical used to prevent or inhibit the growth of microorganisms. In general, safe to use on living tissue. Synonym for *bacteriostatic agent.*

Asepsis The absence of infection.

Bacteriocide A chemical that kills microorganisms, but not necessarily spores. Synonym for *disinfectant* and *germicide.*

Bacteriostatic agent A chemical used to prevent or inhibit the growth of microorganisms. In general, safe to use on living tissue. Synonym for *antiseptic.*

Clean technique Practices that help confine and reduce the number of microorganisms. Synonym for *medical asepsis.*

Coagulation The thickening of a substance.

Concurrent disinfection Cleaning of a patient's contaminated supplies and equipment during the time he is in a health agency.

Contaminate To make something unclean or unsterile.

Disinfectant A chemical that kills microorganisms but not necessarily spores. Synonym for *bacteriocide* and *germicide.*

Disinfection A process by which pathogens, but not necessarily their spores, are destroyed.

Don To put on an article of clothing.

Germicide A chemical that kills microorganisms but not necessarily spores. Synonym for *bacteriocide* and *disinfectant.*

Host A person or animal on which or in which microorganisms live.

Medical asepsis Practices that help confine or reduce the number of microorganisms. Synonym for *clean technique.*

Microorganism A tiny living animal or plant, also called a microbe or organism, which can only be seen with a microscope.

Nonpathogen A harmless microorganism.

Nosocomial infection An infection acquired in a health agency.

Pathogen A microorganism that can cause an infection or a contagious disease.

Reservoir A place on which or in which microorganisms grow and reproduce.

Sepsis A state of infection.

Spore A microbe in an inactive state which allows it to survive extreme living conditions until more favorable ones exist.

Sterile field A work area that is free of all microorganisms.

Sterile technique Practices that render and keep objects and areas free of all microorganisms. Synonym for *surgical asepsis.*

Sterilization A process by which all microorganisms, including spores, are destroyed.

Surgical asepsis Practices that render and keep objects and areas free of all microorganisms. Synonym for *sterile technique.*

Susceptible host An animal or person who has the potential for acquiring an infection.

Terminal disinfection Final cleaning of a patient's contaminated equipment and supplies after he is discharged from a health agency.

Transfer forceps An instrument for handling supplies and equipment.

Vehicle of transmission The means by which organisms are carried about.

Introduction

Microorganisms, or what most people call germs, are everywhere though they cannot be seen without a microscope. They cover objects; they are in air, water, and on the surfaces of food. They are found on and within the body. Many are harmless; they are called *nonpathogens.* Those that cause infections or contagious diseases are called *pathogens.* The organism *Escherichia coli,* for example, is normally found in the intestinal tract where it does not cause disease. However, if it spreads to another part of the body, such as the urinary bladder, it is considered a pathogen because it may cause infection there. A *host* is a person or an animal on which or in which microorganisms live.

Some germs cause illnesses that are referred to as infections or infectious diseases. The human body has natural defenses that reduce the risk of acquiring infections. Still, all humans are affected from time to time. Sick persons are even more likely to acquire an infection because of weakened defenses.

A high priority in health care is to prevent disease, which includes infections, among individuals who are healthy and ill. Nurses do this by protecting an individual's natural body defenses and by safeguarding individuals who are at higher risk from pathogens. Health personnel do not wait until an infection develops; steps are taken to keep it from happening. The challenge to health personnel has been to carry out methods that prevent microorganisms from living, growing, and spreading. Techniques that are used to control organisms will be discussed in this chapter.

Characteristics of Microorganisms

A *microorganism* is a tiny living animal or plant. The word microorganism is often shortened to microbe or organism. Microorganisms include bacteria, viruses, fungi, yeasts, molds, rickettsia, and protozoa. Most nurses study the specific characteristics of each of these in microbiology courses.

All microorganisms are living substances and share some common characteristics. Certain conditions must be present to support life. They include:

Warmth. Microorganisms can survive at a wide range of temperatures. The normal temperature of the human body supports and promotes the growth of microorganisms.

Air. Most microorganisms require free oxygen to exist. These are called *aerobic microorganisms.* Those that survive without free oxygen are called *anaerobic microorganisms.* Some anaerobes are very dangerous because they grow rapidly in deep wounds where free oxygen is scarce, such as in nail punctures. The microorganism that causes tetanus (lockjaw) is one example.

Water and Nourishment. Microbes do not generally survive well in dry areas or places where nutrients are lacking. They depend on other sources, such as a human or animal, for water and food. Blood and the contents within cells can provide a continuous supply of the ingredients needed for the growth of organisms.

Darkness. Most microbes grow best in darkness and die when exposed to light.

Chemical Environment. An environment that is neither too acid nor alkaline is preferred by most microorganisms. Blood is relatively neutral and microbes often seek this as a medium to support their existence.

Following generations of reproduction, many microorganisms have gradually changed. They have been able to alter their structure or function to avoid becoming extinct. One example of an adaptive change is the ability to become spore forming. A *spore* is a microbe in an inactive state. During this state, a microbe changes its structure, usually by forming a thick outer cellular wall. This permits it to survive extremes of heat, cold, dryness, or lack of food. Spores can then develop into active microorganisms when conditions are more favorable for their growth.

Natural Body Defenses

The human body is equipped with various ways to protect itself. These methods are what allow humans to resist being overcome by microorganisms and to defend itself once they have become established in a part of the body. Table 16-1 is a summary of natural body defenses and the manner in which they provide protection.

Factors That Weaken Defenses

At times changes occur that weaken a person's normal defenses against microorganisms. An individual then becomes a *susceptible host,* one who is at risk of acquiring an

Table 16-1. Natural Body Defenses

Natural Defense	Effect on Microorganisms
Intact skin and mucous membranes	Unbroken surfaces of the skin and mucous membranes act as barriers that prevent the entry of organisms into the body.
Body hair	Hair that is present on or within areas of the body, such as the nose, trap and hold particles that contain microorganisms.
Body secretions, such as saliva, mucus, sebum, tears, perspiration, gastric enzymes, and urine	Body secretions contain chemical substances that weaken or destroy microbes.
Reflexes, such as sneezing, coughing, blinking, tearing, and vomiting	Reflex reactions occur spontaneously to expel microorganisms that enter a particular area of the body.
Physiological responses, such as the inflammatory response and the immune response	The body is capable of producing additional specialized cells and chemicals that are responsible for inhibiting the growth and spread of microorganisms.
Temperature regulation	By raising the body temperature above the normal range, many organisms can be destroyed or weakened by heat.
Cell repair and replacement	Manufacturing new cells that repair and replace those that are diseased, injured, or destroyed protects the body from further invasion of microorganisms.

infection. The following factors can result in reduced resistance to the entry of disease-causing organisms.

Poor Nutrition. The body depends on nutrients to grow, maintain, and repair healthy cells. Without proper nutrition, cells become weakened. Nutritional substances needed to produce body secretions and chemicals, examples of the body's natural defenses, can also be depleted.

Poor Personal Hygiene. The body traps microorganisms on the skin and hair, under nails, and in areas such as the mouth. Daily or more frequent hygiene removes microbes from those areas. Accumulation of trapped organisms provides the opportunity for their growth and multiplication.

Broken Skin or Mucous Membranes. Once the body's natural barriers have been broken, infectious microorganisms can invade more susceptible areas of the body. When cuts, incisions, or burns occur, individuals are at an increased risk for infection.

Age. Premature and newborn infants are at risk for infections because many of the natural defenses are not fully developed. The elderly are similarly at high risk because their defensive mechanisms are not always functioning at an optimum level.

Illness. When a disease disrupts normal functioning, the entire body is affected. Any reserves that would be ordinarily available to resist infection may be used up or reduced.

Certain Medical Treatments. Some useful forms of therapy, such as various drugs, may be prescribed for one illness yet reduce the body's ability to defend itself against infection. For instance, steroids, a type of hormone used to treat severe forms of arthritis, cancer, and transplant patients, may reduce the number of specialized cells that attack microorganisms.

The Infectious Process Cycle

Microorganisms move from place to place in a cycle. This is illustrated in Figure 16-1. If the cycle is broken anywhere, the organisms cannot grow, spread, and cause disease. Methods for controlling microorganisms are based on interrupting the cycle and thus preventing their spread. The focus of this chapter will be those practices that alter the *reservoir,* the place on which or in which organisms grow and reproduce, and practices that affect the vehicle of transmission. The *vehicle of transmission* is the means by which organisms are carried about. Additional techniques that interfere with the infectious process cycle will be discussed in Chapter 17 in relation to preventing the spread of contagious diseases.

Description of Asepsis

Health practitioners strive to eliminate pathogens. *Sepsis* means infection, and *asepsis* means the absence of infection. There are two methods used to reduce or eliminate the presence of microorganisms and thus prevent infections. These two methods are called surgical asepsis and medical asepsis.

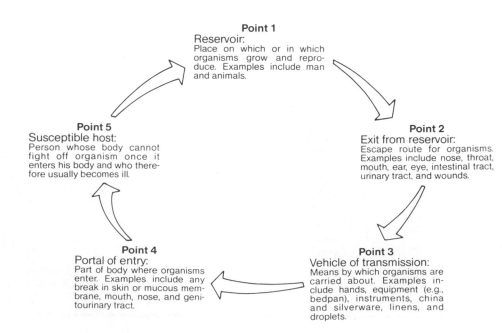

Point 1
Reservoir:
Place on which or in which organisms grow and reproduce. Examples include man and animals.

Point 5
Susceptible host:
Person whose body cannot fight off organism once it enters his body and who therefore usually becomes ill.

Point 2
Exit from reservoir:
Escape route for organisms. Examples include nose, throat, mouth, ear, eye, intestinal tract, urinary tract, and wounds.

Point 4
Portal of entry:
Part of body where organisms enter. Examples include any break in skin or mucous membrane, mouth, nose, and genitourinary tract.

Point 3
Vehicle of transmission:
Means by which organisms are carried about. Examples include hands, equipment (e.g., bedpan), instruments, china and silverware, linens, and droplets.

Figure 16-1 This sketch illustrates the infectious process cycle. Infections and infectious diseases are spread by starting from the reservoir (Point 1), and moving full circle to a susceptible host, (Point 5). Microorganisms can be controlled by using methods that interfere at any point within the cycle.

Surgical asepsis refers to the practices that eliminate the presence of all microorganisms, pathogens and non-pathogens as well as spores, from objects and working areas. A synonym for surgical asepsis is *sterile technique*. *Sterilization* refers to the process by which all microorganisms, including spores, are destroyed. Objects that are properly sterilized do not contain any living substances; they are sterile. Sterilization methods are discussed later in this chapter.

Medical asepsis is also called *clean technique*. It refers to practices that help confine or reduce the number of microorganisms, especially pathogens. Medical aseptic practices do not eliminate all organisms. Common practices of medical asepsis, such as handwashing, will be discussed.

To *contaminate* means to make something unclean or unsterile. In medical asepsis, clean areas and equipment are considered to be contaminated when they come in contact with something that harbors microbes. For example, the inside of a sink, the floor, and all items used by or for patients are considered reservoirs of microorganisms. The hands, which can be clean but never sterile, are considered contaminated after giving nursing care. In surgical asepsis, sterile areas and items are considered contami-nated if they have been touched by anything that is un-sterile.

The nurse must develop a strict conscience when carrying out and maintaining the principles of medical and surgical asepsis. If the nurse takes shortcuts in aseptic practices, possibly no one will be the wiser. However, the nurse's own health as well as that of patients is risked when there is a lack of concern for the spread of microorganisms.

Common Practices of Medical Asepsis

There are many times when medical asepsis is carried out in the course of everyday living and while giving patients nursing care. Examples of practices that promote cleanliness and reduce the spread of microorganisms are given in Display 16-1.

Using Antimicrobial Agents

Various types of antimicrobial agents are used in aseptic practices. An *antimicrobial agent* is a chemical that kills or

---

Display 16-1. Common Practices of Medical Asepsis

Examples in Grooming
Bathe and shower daily.
Use an antiperspirant to control underarm bacterial growth that causes body odor.
Change all clothing daily.
Shampoo hair regularly.
Style hair so it does not hang over food or a work surface.
Brush and floss teeth at least in the morning and evening.
Use only one's own hygiene items such as comb, washcloth, and toothbrush.

Examples in Everyday Living
Wash hands after using the toilet.
Wash hands before handling food.
Wash hands after having touched soiled items.
Dry hands with warm air or paper towels rather than cloth roller towels in public restrooms.
Cover the nose and mouth when coughing and sneezing.
Use disposable tissues rather than a cloth hand-kerchief.
Use disposable paper cups rather than a common glass in the bathroom.
Drink pasteurized milk.
Control pests such as rats, flies, and mosquitoes.
Follow serving regulations in restaurants that have salad bars and buffets.

Examples in Patient Care
Remain home when sick.
Wash hands before and after giving patient care.
Wash hands before and after handling equipment and supplies.
Wash hands before donning and after removing gloves.
Use liquid soap dispensers rather than bar soap.
Use faucets with knee or foot controls.
Dispose of body fluids, excrement, and secretions promptly.
Place wet or soiled patient-care items into a lined container.
Return used items to the dirty utility room.
Keep specimens covered until collection or testing is completed.
Clean stock equipment and supplies between each patient use.
Keep linens from touching the uniform.
Discard or clean any items that drop on the floor.
Unfold linen rather than shaking to avoid raising dust.
Wet mop and damp dust when cleaning patient units.
Clean the least soiled areas before those heavily soiled.

suppresses the multiplication of microorganisms. A synonym is *anti-infective agent*. Antimicrobial agents are used in the prevention and treatment of many kinds of infection.

Soaps and detergents can be considered antimicrobial agents. They are used for cleansing. By removing dirt, body oils, and debris, such as blood and secretions from skin or objects, the nurse also removes microbes that are present. Cleansing must be combined with some other sterilization method to completely remove all microorganisms and their spores from an object. Skin can never be completely free of microorganisms.

Antiseptics are chemical antimicrobial agents used to reduce the growth of microorganisms on living tissues. A synonym for an antiseptic is *bacteriostatic agent*. This category of anti-infective agents only prevents or inhibits the growth and reproduction of microorganisms. Bacteriostatic agents do not completely destroy all microbes; therefore, their use is not a form of sterilization. Examples of common antiseptics include iodine and hydrogen peroxide.

A *bacteriocide* is a substance that can destroy or kill microorganisms, but not necessarily spores. A *disinfectant* is a bacteriocidal substance. A synonym for bacteriocide and disinfectant is *germicide*. These antimicrobials are not intended for use on people. They are quite strong and would damage living tissue if used for the amount of time and strength necessary to destroy organisms. Though they render an object free of all active microbes, but not necessarily inactive spores, their use is not a form of sterilization. Examples of disinfectants include phenol, bichloride of mercury, and formaldehyde.

Antibiotics, such as penicillin, are examples of drugs that are anti-infective agents. Antibiotics have been lifesaving for many patients. However, they are only useful in reducing or destroying the growth of bacteria, one type of microorganism. Even so, not all bacteria are affected by all antibiotics. The physician must selectively match the type of bacteria with the appropriate antibiotic. Earlier indiscriminate use of antibiotics has been associated with causing adaptive changes among bacteria. Now some bacteria have changed in ways that allow them to resist the once effective action of many antibiotics.

Handwashing

Hands contain both resident and transient microorganisms. Resident microbes, as the name implies, are constantly present and not easily removed. Generally they are not pathogenic under most conditions. Transient microorganisms are deposited on the hands while touching contaminated sources. They are more pathogenic, but more easily removed during handwashing.

Handwashing is the single most effective way to prevent *nosocomial infections*. These are infections acquired after being admitted to a health agency. Improper, inefficient, or omitted handwashing is often the contributing factor in

these infections. Display 16-2 identifies situations when handwashing should be performed. Despite being warned about the importance of washing hands, carelessness still continues.

The importance of handwashing cannot be overemphasized. This text does not repeat this instruction every time a skill procedure is described; yet the nurse is expected to perform handwashing before and after care is given. There is an exception to this. When the hands are washed *after* giving care to one patient, and the nurse immediately provides care to another, the hands need not be washed a second time. Handwashing is a conscientious activity that shows a healthy respect for the potential hazards involved in spreading microorganisms.

Skill Procedure 16-1 describes the recommended actions for reducing the presence of organisms from the hands. The technique that is described is used when medical asepsis is practiced.

The handwashing procedure used prior to the activities in operating and delivery rooms is called a surgical scrub. Skill Procedure 16-2 describes the differences in the handwashing technique that should be followed when performing a surgical scrub.

Wearing a Uniform and Hospital Garments

On units where a uniform is worn, the nurse should follow aseptic principles. A clean uniform should be worn daily. Some prefer to wear a clean laboratory coat to reduce the spread of microorganisms onto or from the surface of clothing worn from home. An unprotected uniform should be changed after work and either laundered immediately or placed in a covered hamper. It is inconsiderate as well as potentially unsafe to expose others, such as one's family at home, or others in public places to microorganisms that are present on clothing worn while caring for patients.

Uniforms are not worn in all areas of a hospital. Atten-

Display 16-2. Handwashing Guidelines

Handwashing should be performed:
- When arriving and leaving work
- Before and after contact with each patient
- Before and after equipment is handled
- Before and after gloving
- Before and after specimens are collected
- Before preparing medications
- Before serving trays or feeding patients
- Before eating
- After toileting, haircombing, or other hygiene
- After cleaning a work area.

Skill Procedure 16-1. Handwashing

Suggested Action	Reason for Action
Remove or push the wrist watch up above the wrist. Wear only a plain wedding band.	A watch may become wet and damaged if it is not positioned out of the way. Grooves in watches, watchbands, or points in the stone settings of rings are reservoirs for microbes.
Approach the sink. Do not allow the uniform to touch the sink during the washing procedure.	The sink is considered contaminated. Uniforms may carry organisms from place to place.
Turn on the water. If hand-controlled knobs or levers are present use a clean paper towel when turning the water off.	Organisms accumulate on faucet controls. Touching them after the hands are clean leads to recontamination and the possibility of spreading microbes to oneself or others.
Regulate the temperature of the water so that it is comfortably warm.	Warm water makes better soap suds than cold. It also decreases the surface tension of body oils, which trap dirt and microorganisms. Hot water may dry and chap skin by removing oils from the skin.
Control the flow of water so that it does not splash from the sink.	Water splashed from the contaminated sink will spread organisms onto a uniform.
Wet the hands and suds them well as shown in Figure 16-2. Liquid soap is preferred; apply about a teaspoon.	Bacterial counts after washing are higher when less than 3 to 5 mL of liquid soap are used.

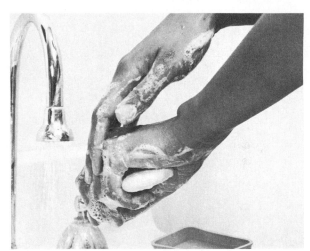

Figure 16-2 The nurse has regulated the temperature of the water and is wetting her hands.

Figure 16-3 The nurse scrubs well while continuing to hold the bar of soap in her hand.

Hold bar soap, as shown in Figure 16-3, until ready to rinse. If the bar is dropped, start the washing procedure again.	The soap is not considered clean until the outer layer is removed. Contact between the soap dish, the sink basin, or floor transfers microbes to the bar of soap.
With firm rubbing and circular motions, wash the palms and backs of the hands, each finger, the area between the fingers, and the knuckles.	Friction caused by firm rubbing and circular motions helps to loosen dirt and organisms. Dirt and organisms lodge between fingers and in skin crevices of knuckles, as well as on the palms and backs of the hands.
Wash the wrists and forearms. Wash up the forearms at least as high as contamination is likely to be present. Use firm rubbing and circular motions as illustrated in Figure 16-4.	Organisms may be present on the wrists and forearms as well as on the hands. In medical asepsis, the hands are considered to be more contaminated than other areas. Cleansing least contaminated areas (wrists and forearms), after the hands are clean, prevents spreading organisms from the hands to the forearms and wrists.

(continued)

Skill Procedure 16-1. *Continued*

Suggested Action	**Reason for Action**

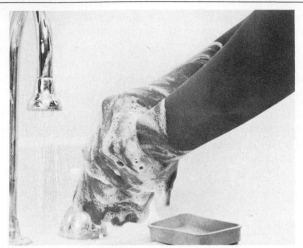

Figure 16-4 A thorough handwashing includes scrubbing the wrists. It also includes washing up the forearms to a distance at which contamination is considered present.

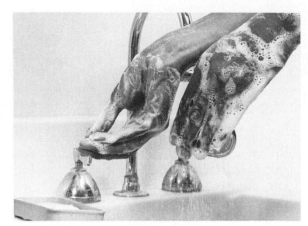

Figure 16-5 The nurse rinses the soap and replaces it without touching the soap dish, which is considered contaminated.

Wash the hands for at least 15 to 30 seconds before and after giving care if exposure to contamination is minimal. Use a 1- to 2-minute wash if exposure to contamination has been extensive. Use at least a 3- to 4-minute scrub if the hands are heavily contaminated, especially if contamination includes drainage from the body.	The amount of contamination on the hands determines the amount of time for washing the hands. For the safest precaution, it is best to overdo rather than underdo the washing.
Repeat the wetting, relathering, and washing procedure if the hands have been heavily contaminated.	When hands are heavily contaminated, second and third washings may be necessary to assure that all dirt and organisms have been removed.
After washing, rinse the bar of soap well under running water and drop the soap into the soap dish without touching the dish, as illustrated in Figure 16-5.	Accumulated dirt and organisms on unrinsed soap may be spread to the next user. The soap dish is considered contaminated.
Rinse the forearms, wrists, and hands, in that order, under running water.	Running water rinses dirt and organisms loosened with soap, water, and friction into the sink.
During the entire washing and rinsing procedure, keep the hands and forearms lower than the elbows so that water drips from the hands by gravity.	Water that holds dirt and microbes will drain away from the cleaner areas (forearms) to ones that are less clean (wrists and hands), and eventually into the sink.
Using as many paper towels as necessary, pat the forearms, wrists, and hands, respectively, to dry them well.	Drying the skin well prevents chapping. Drying more contaminated areas last prevents spreading remaining microbes to cleaner areas.
Apply lotion to the forearms, wrists, and hands.	Lotion helps to prevent chapping. Chapped skin is a reservoir for microorganisms that lodge and grow in roughened areas.

tion to asepsis is very important, especially on certain units. In the operating and recovery room, and obstetrical departments, it is expected that personnel change into an outer garment such as a scrub gown or suit. This reduces the microorganisms that individuals bring with them on clothing worn from home. Cover gowns worn over the

scrub attire are also used to maintain their cleanliness when leaving the unit for coffee or lunch breaks.

A plastic apron or cover gown should be worn during procedures where there may be soiling of the uniform with blood or body fluids. These items prevent saturation of the cloth fibers with subsequent penetration to the skin.

Skill Procedure 16-2. Performing a Surgical Scrub

Suggested Action	Reason for Action
Remove all fingernail polish if it has been applied.	Microbes can become lodged and inadequately removed from areas between the polish and nail.
Remove all jewelry including wristwatch.	Skin surfaces extending above the elbow will need to be scrubbed. Jewelry is a reservoir for organisms and should be removed and pinned to clothing or deposited in a safe place.
Apply a hair covering and mask.	Once the hands have been scrubbed, they can be recontaminated by touching other nonsterile items or parts of the body.
Turn on and regulate the water, using elbow, knee, or foot controls.	Controls that do not require hand regulation reduce the possibility for recontamination
Let the water flow over the skin while keeping the hands higher than the elbows.	In a surgical scrub, practices are used to keep the hands as free of microorganisms as possible. Wetting, scrubbing, rinsing, and draining should always be in a direction away from the hands.
Work up a lather and scrub the hands, using friction and circular motions as described for general handwashing.	An initial washing will remove a great deal of surface debris, but it is not sufficient for adequate cleanliness when surgical asepsis will be required.
Use an orange stick or similar nail cleaner for removing material beneath the fingernails, as shown in Figure 16-6.	Microorganisms can be trapped beneath nails. Washing loosens the debris so that it is more easily removed.

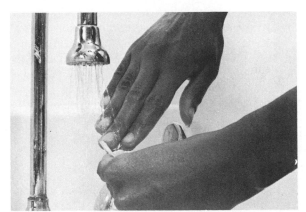

Figure 16-6 Organisms may be harbored under the nails. These areas are cleaned under running water by using a blunt orange stick or something similar.

Rinse in a direction from the fingertips to the elbows.	Sources of microorganisms flow away from the area that is to remain cleanest.
Relather the hands and use a soft brush to scrub all surfaces of the hands, then the wrists, and the forearms to just above the elbows. Scrub each hand separately. Follow the agency policy for the recommended time, which may be as long as 10 minutes.	Using a hand brush and extending the period of scrubbing time promote a high degree of cleanliness. The skin can never be sterile. Frequent use of surgical soaps has been shown to retard the growth of microorganisms. Some agencies have adopted policies in which subsequent scrubbing times may be reduced.
Rinse in a direction from the fingers to the elbows.	Water should flow away from the cleanest area, the hands.

(continued)

Skill Procedure 16-2. Continued

Suggested Action	Reason for Action
While keeping the hands higher than the elbows, dry each hand with a sterile towel. Use a different towel for each hand. Move the towel from the hand toward the elbow when drying.	Wet areas of the towel should never be brought back to dry cleaner areas. A second towel maintains the same degree of cleanliness for both hands.
Without touching any clothing being worn or letting the hands fall below the level of the waist, apply a sterile gown and gloves.	Unsterile clothing and areas below the waist are sources of organisms that could recontaminate freshly scrubbed hands.

Using Hair and Shoe Covers

Hair and shoe covers are generally used only during surgical procedures or when a baby is delivered. They control the spread of pathogens that may be present on loose, falling hair or present on shoes. When hair covers are worn, they should cover all the hair on the head. Shoe covers should cover the shoes as well as the open ends of the pant legs.

Using Clean Examination Gloves

Examination gloves can be used in situations that do not require sterility. Their purpose is to provide a barrier between the hands and substances that are likely to contain pathogens. Vinyl or latex gloves are equally protective in preventing contact with organisms in blood or body fluids as long as they remain intact. The use of gloves does not replace the need for handwashing before and after their use.

Gloves are worn only once. They must be changed between each patient contact. There is no special technique for the application of clean gloves. However, when removing soiled gloves, they should be pulled off the hands so they are turned inside out. This encloses the grossly contaminated surface within the gloves. Soiled gloves are then disposed in a lined and covered receptacle.

Using a Mask

A mask protects the patient and the nurse from airborne pathogens. Nasal and oral droplets contain pathogens carried on tiny beads of moisture. The mask prevents the patient from spreading pathogens to the nurse and vice versa. Dust and air currents are also filtered by the mask.

Most masks used today are disposable. They are kept in a dispensing box. The mask is applied after donning a hair cover, if that is required, and before performing a surgical scrub, which was discussed previously in this chapter.

The mask must cover both the nose and the mouth. It should be worn only once. While in place, the mask should not be touched. It should never be lowered onto the chest and then replaced over the face. A new mask should be obtained.

Moisture makes masks ineffective. The actual length of time a mask can be worn is questionable because it is affected by individual variables. It is best to change the mask when it becomes noticeably damp with repeated exhalation or perspiration. Skill Procedure 16-3 explains how to apply and remove a mask.

Wearing Protective Eyewear

Protective eyewear should be worn when there is a possibility that body fluid containing blood will splash into the eyes, mouth, or nose. If only goggles are available, their use should be combined with a mask. Some hospitals supply a multipurpose face shield, such as the one in Figure 16-9. It covers all areas where bloodborne organisms could enter through mucous membranes of the face. If protective eyewear is not worn, and blood or any other body fluid known to transmit pathogens contacts the eyes, flush and rinse the eyes with normal saline. Tap water can be substituted. The priority is to remove as much of the contaminated substance as soon as possible.

Disposing of Needles and Sharp Objects

Intact skin is the best barrier against infection. However, there is always the potential to receive punctures and cuts because nurses handle needles, scalpels, and other sharp objects. Because of the frequency of these accidents and their potential for transmitting bloodborne infections, nurses should never recap, bend, or break needles. The entire syringe or other sharp object must be deposited in a puncture-resistant container, such as the one shown in Figure 16-10. These containers are best located as close to the bedside as possible. They may be placed on the wall, a counter, or shelf.

If a cut or puncture occurs, the hands should be washed vigorously and bleeding promoted. The incident must be reported immediately to the infection control nurse, employee health department, or to emergency room personnel depending upon agency policy. The patient and employee can be tested for antibodies against bloodborne pathogens. Emergency preventive treatment can be insti-

Skill Procedure 16-3. Using a Mask

Suggested Action	**Reason for Action**
Don required cover garments, such as a hospital supplied scrub gown or suit, hair or shoe covers.	The mask is applied after the hair cover because it will be changed more frequently. It is donned just before preparation for a procedure to limit the accumulation of moisture.
Obtain a mask and determine its upper edge.	The upper edge must fit well over the bridge of the nose to prevent the possible spread of pathogens.
Position the mask so it covers the nose and mouth.	A mask should prevent the exit and entrance of large airborne particles through the nose and mouth.
If eyeglasses are worn, the frames should rest on top of the upper edge of the mask.	This prevents the lenses from becoming cloudy and obscuring vision when warm breath and body heat mixes with a cooler environmental temperature.
Tie the upper strings first above the ears at the back of the head.	The front of the mask must not touch the chest, which collects respiratory and oral secretions from breathing, talking, laughing, sneezing, and coughing.
Tie the lower strings snugly at the back of the neck, shown in Figure 16-7.	This encloses the mouth and nose, reducing the space where microbes could enter or leave.

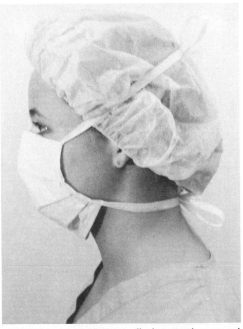

Figure 16-7 This nurse has applied a mask over a hair cap.

Do not touch the outer surface of the mask once it is secured.	Organisms can be transferred onto or from the hands through moisture within the mask.
Remove the mask by first untying the bottom strings.	Unfastening the bottom strings prevents the mask from falling by gravity onto the front of the gown or clothing.
Hold onto the upper strings as they are untied.	This frees the mask but prevents dropping it.
Touch only the strings, as shown in Figure 16-8, while discarding the mask into a lined container.	The mask is moist and contains a concentrated amount of organisms. Avoiding hand contact with the front of the mask reduces the spread of pathogens.

(continued)

Skill Procedure 16-3. Continued

Suggested Action	**Reason for Action**

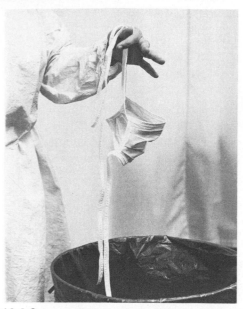

Figure 16-8 Once applied, the front of the mask should not be touched. Holding the soiled mask only by the ties, the nurse discards it. The length of time permissible to wear one mask is debatable. It should probably not be worn more than 20 to 30 minutes, provided it remains dry.

Wash hands.	Handwashing removes a large proportion of transient microbes transferred by touching the hair during the process of untying the mask.

tuted in the case of hepatitis. Its effectiveness, however, decreases if not initiated within 48 hours.

Cleaning Supplies and Equipment

Most health agencies now use disposable equipment. Disposables are used only once and then discarded. Most hospitals have central supply units where nonnursing personnel clean, disinfect, or sterilize reusable equipment and keep it in good working order. This department also dispenses disposable equipment and supplies according to patient needs. The use of central supply units and disposable equipment has helped reduce the spread of microorganisms in health agencies and the work required of nurses.

Nurses may still be responsible for cleaning some equipment and work areas. Duties concerning disinfection and sterilization vary. Occasionally, the nurse may have this responsibility when caring for patients in their homes. The nurse may need to teach individuals how to control the spread of microorganisms from equipment and supplies used at home.

The following guidelines describe safe and effective practices of medical asepsis when soap or detergent and water are used to clean supplies and equipment:

Wear waterproof gloves if items are heavily contaminated or if the skin is broken.

Disassemble and rinse reusable equipment as soon as possible after use, especially when time does not permit a thorough cleaning immediately. This prevents parts from becoming locked together.

Rinse items *first* under cool, running water. Hot water causes many substances to *coagulate* (that is, to thicken or congeal), making them difficult to remove.

Rinse reusable catheters and rectal tubes immediately after use to remove lubricant or body excretions. Leave them to soak if a thorough cleaning is not possible immediately. Force sudsy water through them for thorough cleaning.

Use hot water and soap or a detergent for cleaning purposes. Hot water and soap or detergent break up

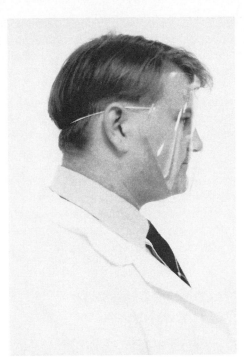

Figure 16-9 Wearing a face shield is an alternative to donning a mask and goggles.

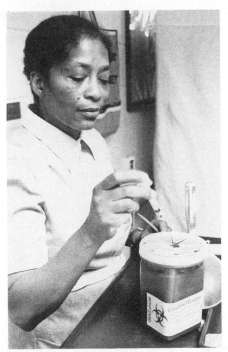

Figure 16-10 This nurse deposits a used, uncapped syringe into a puncture-resistant container. The container is on a movable medication cart that is located just outside the patient's room.

dirt and body secretions into tiny particles that can be more easily rinsed off with water.

A sponge or cloth may be used to create friction that helps loosen dirt and organisms from the surfaces of objects.

Use a brush with stiff bristles to loosen dirt as necessary. A brush is a necessity for cleaning small grooves and joints in instruments.

Use abrasive cleaners for removing stubborn stains, as on a washbasin or emesis basin.

Force sudsy water through the hollow channels of instruments to loosen dirt. Alcohol or ether may also be used and will help to break up oily substances.

Rinse items well under running water after cleaning with soap or detergent and water. This will rinse loosened dirt and organisms into the sink.

Dry equipment well to prevent rusting.

Treat gloves, brushes, sponges, cleaning cloths, and water used for cleaning as reservoirs for microorganisms. Clean or discard them accordingly.

Avoid splashing or spilling water on yourself or on the floor or other equipment during the entire procedure.

Consider hands heavily contaminated after cleaning equipment. Even when wearing gloves during cleaning, the nurse should perform handwashing as described earlier in this chapter.

For most purposes, thorough laundering of linen is sufficiently safe for cleaning. For linen used by individuals with contagious diseases, special precautions are neces-

sary within health agencies. These precautions are discussed in Chapter 17.

Certain items cannot be washed without being ruined. These include instruments used for taking blood pressure and for examining the eyes and the ears. Follow agency policy concerning the handling of such pieces of equipment. Wipe them with a small cloth or a cotton ball dampened with a disinfectant.

Completing Terminal Disinfection

The care given to cleaning contaminated supplies and equipment throughout the time a person is a patient in a health agency is called *concurrent disinfection*. When the patient is discharged, the room, bed, and furnishings are cleansed a final time to prepare them for reuse by another patient. This is called *terminal disinfection*. The housekeeping department is usually responsible for terminal disinfection. After the cleaning has been completed, the bed is made and the room is prepared to receive another patient, as described in Chapter 11.

Preparing for Disinfection or Sterilization

When supplies and equipment are clean, they are ready for disinfection or sterilization. *Disinfection* is a process by which pathogens, but not necessarily spores, are destroyed; sterilization destroys all microorganisms and spores. The nurse may be required to use good judgment when preparing reusable equipment for disinfection or sterilization. The following factors affect the nurse's choice of methods.

The Type of Microorganism. Some microorganisms are easier to destroy than others. However, it is rare that anyone can be certain what microorganisms are present. The safest practice is to overdo rather than underdo whatever method is available. Shortening the required time or reducing the chemical strength, temperature, or pressure is unwise.

The Number of Microorganisms. The greater the number of organisms, the longer it will take to destroy all of them. The number can be reduced by scrupulous cleaning prior to disinfection or sterilization. When organisms are protected under layers of grease, oil, blood, and pus, removing microorganisms becomes more difficult. Therefore, any method of disinfection or sterilization becomes potentially less effective and unreliable in their presence.

The Type of Contaminated Equipment. Some items cannot be exposed to all methods of disinfection or sterilization. Heat or chemicals may affect the composition of the equipment or sensitive gauges. Equipment with small grooves or openings, such as forceps or needles, requires thorough cleansing and exposure of all surfaces to destroy microorganisms.

The Eventual Reuse of the Equipment. Items used for certain procedures must be sterile, not just disinfected. All equipment used during operations must be sterile, for example.

The Aseptic Methods Available. Though some methods for disinfection or sterilization may be quicker or cheaper, they may not all be available for use. The nurse may have to use an alternative, yet reliable, method for controlling microorganisms.

Methods of Disinfection and Sterilization

Each agency may have various types of equipment and standards for destroying microorganisms. Table 16-2 is a list of various ways in which the growth of microorganisms can be checked. Some are more effective and feasible than

Table 16-2. Methods for Suppressing Growth of Organisms

Method	Examples	Explanation
Excessive heat	Boiling Free-flowing steam Steam under pressure Dry heat Pasteurization	Temperatures that exceed those at which microbes can survive will destroy organisms. Most of these techniques require special equipment that measures heat and pressure. The heat must be constantly maintained for a specific period of time.
Releasing oxygen	Hydrogen peroxide Hyperbaric oxygen chamber	Use of the oxygen can destroy anaerobic organisms. Hydrogen peroxide releases bubbles of free oxygen when instilled into a wound. Hyperbaric chambers deliver oxygen under pressures that exceed that in the atmosphere.
Exposure to light	Sunning Ultraviolet light	Light reduces microbial growth because most organisms prefer darkness.
Drying	Airing Hot-air oven Sunning	Eliminating water by using air, heat, or light can combine to interfere with the growth of microorganisms.
Cleaning	Handwashing Scrubbing Friction Soaking Rinsing	Removing dirt, body oil, blood, and other secretions can reduce the ability of microorganisms to grow.
Chemicals	Soaps Detergents Antiseptics Disinfectants Antibiotics Ethylene oxide gas	Chemicals work in a variety of ways to create a harmful environment that interferes with the ability of organisms to live, grow, and multiply.

others. The following is a discussion of the sterilization and disinfection methods that are more often used.

Destroying Microbes With Heat

The most common methods in which heat is used include boiling, free-flowing steam, dry heat, and steam under pressure. Microbes are destroyed when the heat exceeds that at which microbes can live. The higher the temperature, the quicker the microorganisms will die.

All organisms do not die instantly. To be sure that no microbes have survived, the heat is sustained at a particular temperature for a specified length of time. It is important to follow the established infection control policies because the standards for reliability vary with the method that is used.

Boiling Water. Placing equipment in boiling water for a period of time is a common method for destroying microorganisms with heat. Boiling water does not kill spores or other organisms that are particularly difficult to destroy unless items are boiled for a long time. Objects should be boiled at 100°C or 212°F for 15 minutes. The time may need to be lengthened in areas above sea level. Water begins boiling at lower temperatures at higher altitudes. Thus it may not reach the appropriate level of heat to destroy microbes. Use of boiling water is a convenient way to disinfect and sterilize items in the home.

Free-Flowing Steam. In order to destroy all microorganisms and spores, free-flowing steam has the same temperature and time requirement as the boiling water method. It is not a practical method of sterilization for all types of equipment. It is difficult to expose all surfaces of equipment to the steam.

Dry Heat. Dry heat, or hot air sterilization, uses equipment similar to a home baking oven. It is a good way to sterilize sharp instruments and reusable syringes because moist heat damages cutting edges and the ground surfaces of glass. Dry heat prevents rusting of objects that are not made of stainless steel.

Steam Under Pressure. Moist heat under pressure provides effective sterilization. In fact, this is the most dependable method for destroying all forms of organisms and spores. The autoclave is the type of pressure steam sterilizer that most health agencies use. The pressure makes it possible to achieve much hotter temperatures than the boiling point of water or free-flowing steam.

Pressure cookers used in many homes operate just as autoclaves do. Foods cooked in them are prepared more quickly than if prepared in an uncovered pot because of the higher temperature developed in the cooker. Pressure cookers may be used for sterilizing equipment in the home. Articles are placed on a rack above the level of water in the cooker.

Destroying Microbes With Chemicals

Chemicals used for disinfection or sterilization may be in the form of liquids or gases. Chemical liquids are commonly used as disinfectants. Studies have shown that chemical sterilization is difficult to accomplish. Some authorities believe that chemical solutions and gases are not safe or effective for sterilization. Generally, chemical gas is used as a sterilization method only when items are likely to be damaged by other methods or when a better method is not available.

Ethylene Oxide Gas. Items to be sterilized in this manner are exposed to the gas vapors in a chamber for a prescribed period of time. This method is used for certain types of equipment that may become damaged by heat or moisture. One positive advantage to ethylene oxide gas is that it can penetrate through outer wrappers quite well.

Ethyl Alcohol. Objects may be soaked in a 70% solution for 10 to 20 minutes. This is not considered a reliable sterilization method; its action should be regarded more as that of a disinfectant.

Phenol. One of the first disinfectants ever used was phenol. All others are compared with its effectiveness. It is used in a 2% to 5% solution. A newer disinfectant, hexachlorophene, is a derivative of phenol.

Bichloride of Mercury. Heavy metals, such as mercury, silver, and copper, are known to be bacteriostatic or bacteriocidal depending on the concentration of the chemical solution. Mercury is bacteriocidal when in a 1:1000 strength solution. However, it is corrosive to metals and highly toxic if accidentally consumed. Merthiolate and mercurochrome are antiseptics that contain mercury. These are less irritating and toxic than bichloride of mercury and therefore can be used on living tissue.

Principles of Surgical Asepsis

Surgical asepsis is based on the underlying principle that equipment and areas that are free of microorganisms must be protected from contamination. The practices that are involved in sterile technique are used whenever invasive procedures are performed. Sterile technique is used when surgery is performed, when inserting various types of equipment, such as catheters, when dressing wounds or incisions, when administering injections, and so on. These procedures increase the possibility of introducing organisms into the body, causing infection and disease.

For the sake of safety, sterile equipment is sometimes used even when it is not absolutely necessary. For example, the gastrointestinal tract and vagina are not considered areas that require surgical asepsis, since they already contain many nonpathogens; however, equipment inserted into these areas is usually initially supplied in a sterile condition. Table 16-3 lists principles that promote surgical asepsis.

Common Practices Involving Surgical Asepsis

There are many occasions in which the nurse will need to apply the principles of surgical asepsis. The following are some common practices that are often components of various nursing skills, which are discussed later in this text.

Creating a Sterile Field

A *sterile field* is a work area that is free of microorganisms. The inner surface of a wrapper that holds sterilized equipment is often used as a sterile field much like a tablecloth would be used. It acts as a sterile surface for resting sterile equipment or supplies. The nurse must open the sterile package in such a way as to keep the inside of the wrapper and its contents sterile. This may be done by performing the following steps, which are also illustrated in Figure 16-11.

- Position the wrapped package so that the outermost triangular edge can be moved away from the nurse shown in Figure 16-11A.
- The sides of the wrapper may be unfolded by touching the areas that will become the underneath surface

Table 16-3. Principles of Surgical Asepsis

Principle	Explanation
Items of questionable sterility should never be used.	It is better to err on the side of safety than to take a chance and have the patient acquire an infection
An item that has been disinfected only is not considered sterile.	Disinfection generally does not destroy spores.
The contents of any tampered or unwrapped package should not be used for a sterile procedure.	Any break in the integrity of a sterile package can contaminate the contents.
Refrain from using any sterile item after its expiration date.	Manufacturers base expiration dates upon the range of potential safe use of their product.
A sterile object should be opened by unfolding the wrapper on the far side of the package first and the nearest side last.	The risk of contamination is increased by reaching over a sterile area.
Opened wrappers are considered sterile to within 1 inch of the edge. The sterile margin of a peeled package is its inner edge.	The margins of any opened sterile item are the most likely to become contaminated.
A sterile object becomes contaminated when touched by anything unsterile.	Even clean surfaces contain microorganisms. Sterile objects may only touch other sterile objects.
A wet wrapper causes contamination.	Moisture causes wicking of microorganisms upward from the surface underneath.
An open sterile field and its contents become contaminated the longer they are unused.	Microbes can be deposited on previously sterile surfaces by air currents, dust, and lint.
Any unattended sterile field is considered contaminated.	Sterility cannot be ensured without continuous observation.
Coughing and sneezing or excessive talking over a sterile field cause contamination.	Microorganisms are present in the spray of oral and nasal droplets. They can fall onto sterile areas causing contamination.
Reaching across a sterile area causes contamination.	Accidental contact or depositing lint or dust transmits microorganisms.
Sterile objects must be maintained above waist level.	Areas below the waist are not within critical view. This poses the potential for undetected contamination.
Turning one's back on a sterile field must be avoided.	Without visual observation, it is difficult to determine if contact has occurred between unsterile and sterile objects.

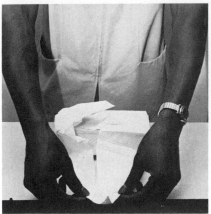 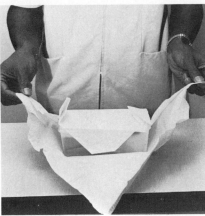 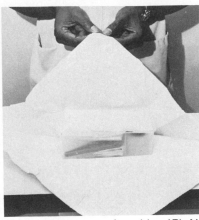

Figure 16-11 (*A*). The nurse opens a sterile package by unfolding the topmost part of the wrapper *away* from him. (*B*). Next, the nurse opens the second layer of the wrapper to the sides of the package. (*C*). As the last step, the nurse opens the final layer of the wrapper *toward* himself.

of the sterile field as the nurse is doing in Figure 16-11*B*.

- The final triangular fold can be pulled in the direction of the body as in Figure 16-11*C*. Opening the package in this manner avoids the possibility of touching a sterile field with the nurse's uniform and avoids having to reach across a sterile field.

Adding Sterile Items to the Sterile Field

There are times when sterile procedures will require supplies or equipment that may not be included in the wrapped package. The nurse will need to add items to the sterile field one at a time. There are several techniques that the nurse may find necessary to use.

Using Supplies Sterilized by the Health Agency. Equipment that has come packaged and sterilized from a health agency's central supply department can be opened similarly to the manner in which a sterile field is created. The nurse maintains a good hold of the sterile contents as each corner of the wrapper is unfolded. The corners are held so that they do not hang loosely. When the sterile contents have been exposed, the nurse can place the uncontaminated contents onto the sterile field and discard the wrapper. The nurse in Figure 16-12 is preparing to place a sterile basin on a sterile field using this described technique.

Opening Commercially Sterilized Supplies. Some supplies, such as gauze dressings, come packaged by medical supply companies. These packages usually have two loose flaps that extend above the sealed edges. By separating the flaps as the nurse is doing in Figure 16-13, the sterile contents can be dropped onto the sterile field without any contamination occurring. Using individually

wrapped sterile items for a single use has reduced the spread of microorganisms from supplies and equipment.

Pouring Sterile Solutions. When a sterile solution is needed, it can be added after the sterile equipment has been prepared. Common sterile solutions may be available in a variety of volumes. Choose the minimum amount that most likely will be needed. In the operating room any unused solution is discarded. Opening a large volume of sterile solution unnecessarily increases the cost to the patient.

When an opened solution will be used again in the immediate future, the inside of the cap should never come in contact with an unsterile surface. Hold the cap with the fingers so it faces downward similar to its position on the container. If holding is not possible, place it so the outside of the cap rests on a clean surface. These practices keep the inside of the cap from touching anything that is unsterile.

After a sterile solution has been opened and recapped, all subsequent uses should be preceded by pouring and discarding a small amount of the contents over the rim as the nurse in Figure 16-14 is doing. This practice is called "lipping." It washes any airborne contaminants from the mouth and rim of the container.

While pouring the nurse applies various principles of asepsis to avoid contaminating the opened supplies. The container is held above and in front of the nurse taking care not to touch unsterile to sterile surfaces. In addition, as shown in Figure 16-15, the height of the solution container prevents liquid from splashing onto the cloth sterile field.

Using Transfer Forceps. A *transfer forceps* is an instrument used to pick up and move sterile supplies. It is used commonly to add sterile items to a sterile field. The availability of single items in sterile wrappers is now reducing the necessity for using transfer forceps. If needed, a

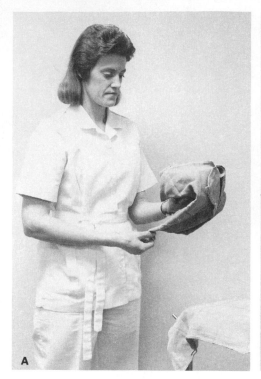
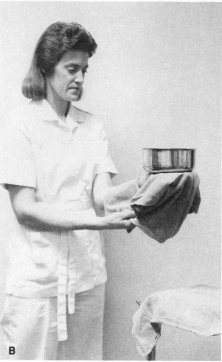

Figure 16-12 (*A*). While using one hand to support and hold a wrapped package, the nurse opens the outer flap in a direction away from the front of the uniform. (*B*). As each corner is subsequently unfolded, the nurse grasps the flaps to prevent them from touching the sterile field. The sterile contents of the unwrapped package can then be placed on the sterile field and the wrapper can be discarded.

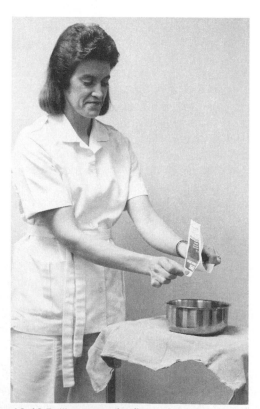

Figure 16-13 Pulling apart the flaps of sealed supplies opens the package in such a way that the contents are not contaminated.

package containing sterile transfer forceps is opened and used during the procedure. It is then discarded, if disposable, or resterilized after its use.

Transfer forceps, such as the ones shown in Figure 16-16, were kept stored in a container of disinfectant. They were used over and over by multiple individuals. This practice is now obsolete. Transfer forceps used in this manner are now considered suspect to contamination, because it is impossible to determine reliably the aseptic technique of all people who used the forceps. Furthermore, the disinfectant solutions in which these common-use transfer forceps were stored was subject to evaporation and deterioration unless replaced on a scheduled basis.

Donning a Sterile Gown

A sterile gown is used to protect the patient and sterile equipment from microorganisms that collect on the nurse's uniform. Sterile gowns are required during surgery and delivery of infants. They may be used during other sterile procedures.

Sterile gowns are made of cloth. They are sterilized after each use. Before wrapping a gown for sterilization, it is folded so that the nurse can touch the inside surface of the gown during the process of donning it. The nurse receives help in donning a sterile gown because reaching around to fasten the back would contaminate the sleeves. Skill

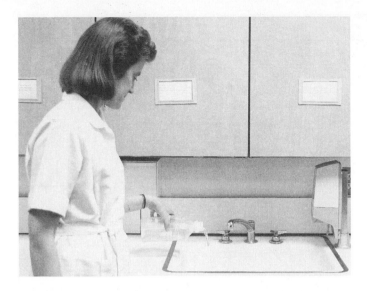

Figure 16-14 The nurse wastes a small amount of sterile solution by pouring it out of its container and into a sink. This carries away organisms that may be present on the outer rim.

Procedure 16-4 describes the technique for donning a sterile gown.

Donning and Removing Sterile Gloves

To *don* means to put on an article of wear. For certain procedures the nurse dons sterile gloves. When applied correctly, sterile gloves may be safely used to handle sterile equipment and supplies without contaminating these objects. They may be used to prevent transferring microbes, which are always present on the hands, to patients. Sterile gloves are included in some packages of supplies. They may also be packaged separately in glove wrappers. Skill Procedure 16-5 describes how to don sterile gloves and remove them.

Nonsterile gloves may be used as a barrier that protects the nurse from contact with grossly contaminated material. In this case, the gloves do not require any special technique for their application. However, nonsterile gloves should be removed following the techniques described in Skill Procedure 16-5.

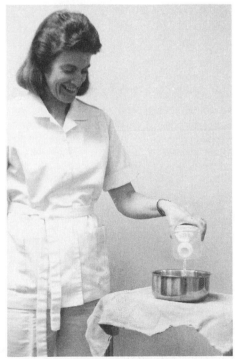

Figure 16-15 When adding sterile solution, the nurse holds the bottle close to the basin, pouring carefully so that it will not splash and wet the sterile field.

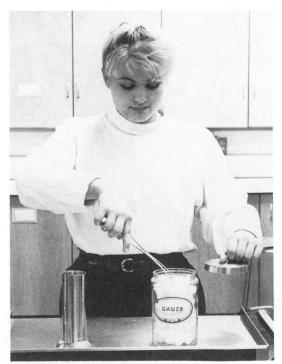

Figure 16-16 This nurse uses transfer forceps.

Skill Procedure 16-4. Donning a Sterile Gown

Suggested Action	Reason for Action
Apply a mask and hair cover.	These items should be applied before performing a surgical scrub so the hands are not contaminated from organisms that are present on the facial skin and hair.
Perform a surgical scrub.	A surgical scrub is the more effective handwashing technique for removing organisms from the hands, wrists, and forearms.
Pick up the sterile gown at the neck area.	Before sterilizing, gowns are wrapped so they can be touched on the inside, keeping the outer side sterile.
Hold the folded gown away from the front of clothing and other unsterile areas.	The gown could accidentally become contaminated by touching the uniform or other contaminated items.
Allow the gown to unfold while suspending it high enough that it will not come in contact with the floor as shown in Figure 16-17.	The floor is a reservoir of dirt and pathogens. Contact between a sterile gown and the floor causes contamination.

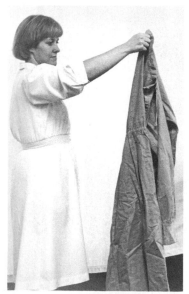

Figure 16-17 To prevent contaminating a sterile gown, it is picked up and held at the inner neck area, allowing the gown to unfold. The part being touched by the nurse will become the surface that eventually touches her uniform. The outside surface of the gown will remain free of organisms.

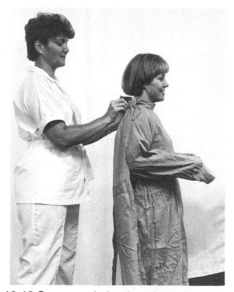

Figure 16-18 One nurse helps the other adjust a sterile gown. The assisting nurse touches only the inside of the sleeves and shoulder area of the gown. The fasteners will be contaminated once they are closed by the assistant. However, this area will not be touched during any sterile procedure.

Insert an arm into each sleeve without touching the sterile outer surface of the gown.	The side of the gown next to clothing is considered clean, but not sterile. The outside of the gown must remain free of microorganisms.
Have an assistant, like the one in Figure 16-18, pull the inside of the sleeves to expose the hands and adjust the fit of the gown.	Another person can help to adjust the fit by touching the clean surface. This prevents the wearer from accidentally touching skin, hair, or clothing that contains organisms.
Secure the gown in place by letting the assistant fasten the neck and waist closed.	Fastening the gown prevents it from opening and exposing a contaminated area.
Consider only the front of the gown from the chest to the waist, and the sleeves from above the elbow to the cuff, as sterile.	All other areas of the gown are considered unsterile because they are either unobserved, touch body surfaces, or can become moist from perspiration.

(continued)

Skill Procedure 16-4. Continued

Suggested Action	Reason for Action
Consider the cuff areas of a gown sterile only after they are covered with sterile gloves.	The cuff, while yet ungloved, is considered unsterile because a portion is in contact with the hand during donning.
Proceed with applying sterile gloves.	Situations that require the use of a sterile gown usually also require the application of sterile gloves.

Skill Procedure 16-5. Donning and Removing Sterile Gloves

Suggested Action	Reason for Action
Thoroughly wash the hands, following the techniques described for medical asepsis or a surgical scrub.	The hands can never be sterile, but the number of microorganisms can be reduced by conscientious handwashing.
Dry the hands well.	Wet hands interfere with glove application.
Select a package of gloves of the appropriate size.	Gloves that are too small will be difficult to don and may be easily contaminated. Gloves that are too large may be cumbersome to use.
Place the wrapped gloves on a work area that is at or just above waist level.	Sterile objects and equipment should not be positioned below the waist where contamination is likely to occur.
Open the wrapper containing the gloves without touching the inner surface. Paper wrappers may be peeled apart; cloth wrappers may be opened, using the technique described for creating a sterile field.	The inside of the wrapper and certain areas of the gloves must remain untouched or they will become contaminated.
Expose and identify the right and left gloves. They should appear similar to diagram A in Figure 16-19.	Gloves that are mismatched or are in reverse positions may prove awkward to apply and become contaminated.
Make sure that the cuff of each glove is folded down as represented by the shaded areas throughout the diagrams that are used as illustrations.	The side of the cuff that will eventually face the skin surface of the gloved hands is the only part that can be touched by bare hands as the gloves are applied.
Using the thumb and fingers of the nondominant hand, pick up the glove that will cover the dominant hand. Touch only the folded edge of the cuff, as shown in diagram B of Figure 16-19.	The outer surface of the glove must remain untouched to remain sterile.
Pull and stretch the glove while inserting the dominant hand. Do not allow any of the outside surface of the glove to touch the skin of either hand, the uniform, or other unsterile areas.	The sterile surface of gloves becomes contaminated when it comes in contact with skin or any other unsterile items.
Touching only the edge of the glove, as shown in diagram C of Figure 16-19, unfold the cuff.	The unfolded edge now exposes the maximum sterile surface of the gloves.
Insert the gloved hand beneath the folded cuff of the remaining glove, as shown in diagram D of Figure 16-19.	As long as sterile areas touch other sterile areas, no contamination occurs.
Using the gloved hand to pull and stretch, insert the hand, as illustrated in diagram E of Figure 16-19. Care must be taken that the gloved thumb, fingers, and hand do not touch the skin of the ungloved hand.	Sterile objects become contaminated with organisms when contact is made with unsterile areas.

(continued)

Skill Procedure 16-5. Continued

Suggested Action	**Reason for Action**

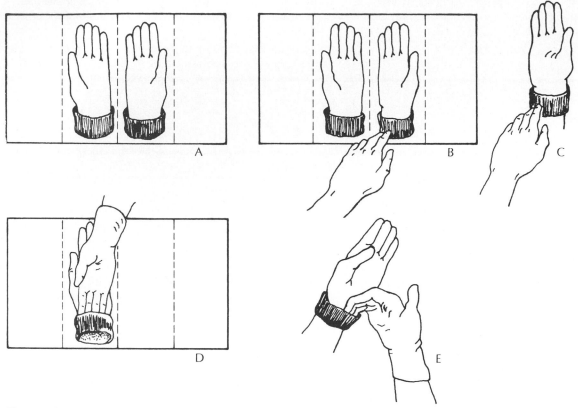

Figure 16-19 This illustrates the correct way of putting on sterile gloves. The shaded portion of the gloves may be touched by a bare hand but not by any part of a gloved hand.

Touching only the sterile surfaces of the gloves, pull and stretch them until they fit smoothly and firmly over all the fingers and surfaces of the hands.

Maintain gloved hands above the level of the waist.

To remove the gloves, grasp and stretch the area covering the wrist, as shown in photograph A of Figure 16-20.

Pull the glove, turning it inside out as illustrated in photograph B of Figure 16-20.

Reach under the cuff of the remaining glove. While touching only its inner surface, stretch it so that it too may be turned inside out as the nurse is doing in photograph C of Figure 16-20.

Discard the gloves according to agency policy. Disposable gloves can be deposited in a lined, covered trash container in a utility room for soiled equipment. Reusable gloves must be cleaned and disinfected before resterilization.

Sometimes wrinkles or air pockets form as gloves are being applied. These conditions can be corrected once the gloves are on both hands.

Lowering or dropping the hands to the sides creates the potential for contamination.

Following their use, the gloves are considered more contaminated than the bare hands. They should be removed so that additional organisms are not transferred to the hands.

Microorganisms from the patient are now enclosed within the inverted glove.

Neither ungloved hand should contact the contaminated surface of the gloves. This technique controls the spread of microorganisms to the nurse.

Medical asepsis includes proper disposal, cleansing, and disinfection to control the spread of microbes. Disposable gloves and other equipment are generally incinerated to destroy microbes with heat.

(continued)

Skill Procedure 16-5. Continued

Suggested Action	Reason for Action

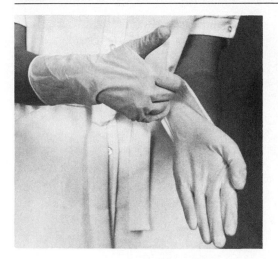

A

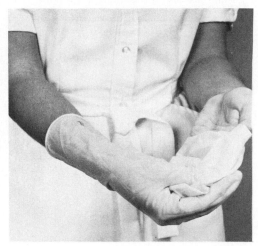

B

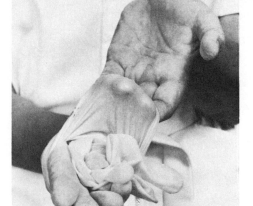

C

Figure 16-20 (*A*). The nurse grasps the first glove she will remove without touching her skin or the inside (clean surface) of the contaminated gloves. (*B*). The nurse pulls off the first glove, turning it inside out with the other gloved hand. (*C*). Next, the second glove is removed while touching only the inside (clean surface) of the glove. The nurse pulls the second glove off by turning it inside out also. Both gloves now enclose the contaminated areas; the clean surfaces are on the outside. The gloves are ready to be discarded.

Perform thorough handwashing immediately.	Organisms remaining on the hands before putting on gloves multiply rapidly in the warm, moist environment inside the gloves.

NURSING CARE PLAN

16-1. Knowledge Deficit

Assessment	**Subjective Data**

States, "The school nurse sent this note home saying there's been a case of hepatitis in my daughter's fifth-grade class. Isn't that what drug users get? Should I keep my daughter home from school? What will prevent her from catching it?" Patient is not experiencing any anorexia or tenderness in right upper quadrant.

Objective Data

11-year-old girl presently in the fifth grade. Public health department confirms one case of hepatitis A at this school. TPR is currently normal. Liver is not palpable. Denies nausea or diarrhea. Sclera of OU are white. Freshly voided urine is light yellow and tests negative for bilirubin with a chemstrip and Ictotest tablet. Will receive gamma globulin injection today.

Diagnosis

Knowledge Deficit: Cause and prevention of hepatitis A related to unfamiliarity with infectious diseases.

Plan

Goal

The child will satisfactorily return a demonstration of handwashing and mother will list at least three signs and symptoms of hepatitis at the end of this office visit.

Orders: 11/17

1. Explain that hepatitis A is spread primarily from stool of an infected person to the mouth of a susceptible individual.
2. Provide the following information and ask mother to recall at least three signs and symptoms:
   a. Hepatitis B is usually associated with IV drug use and contaminated blood.
   b. The incubation period of hepatitis A is 25 to 30 days.
   c. Handwashing is an excellent preventive measure and should be performed before eating and after each use of the toilet; staying home from school is not necessary.
   d. Signs and symptoms include low-grade fever, reduced activity, loss of appetite, nausea, abdominal pain, dark urine, light colored stool, and yellowing of the skin and white portion of the eyes.
3. Demonstrate handwashing and observe return demonstration emphasizing the following:
   a. Turn handles of school faucet on using a paper towel and let water run.
   b. Wet hands and lather with liquid soap from a hand-pump dispenser.
   c. Rub lathered hands for at least 30 seconds to 1 minute.
   d. Rinse, letting water flow from wrists to fingers.
   e. Dry hands with paper towel.
   f. Use a paper towel to turn faucet handle off. ————————— A. JOHANSON, RN

Implementation (Documentation)

11/7   1630   Differentiated between hepatitis A and B. States, "I'm so relieved that this case isn't caused by sharing drug needles." Provided with additional information on hepatitis as identified in care plan. Handwashing demonstration given. ————
——————————————————————————————— A. JOHANSON, RN

Evaluation (Documentation)

1645   Mother recalled the following signs and symptoms: fever, loss of appetite, nausea, and yellowing of eyes and skin. Child performed handwashing procedure as demonstrated. Given immune serum globulin injection in L. vastus lateralis muscle. ————————————————— A. JOHANSON, RN

Applicable Nursing Diagnoses

Everyone is susceptible to infections if contagious sources among individuals, equipment, and the environment are not controlled. Some nursing diagnoses that may apply for those especially at risk include

- High Risk for Infection
- Impaired Skin Integrity
- Bathing/Hygiene Self-Care Deficit
- Dressing/Grooming Self-Care Deficit
- Toileting Self-Care Deficit
- Altered Protection (accepted for testing since the publication of the 1989 NANDA taxonomy)
- Knowledge Deficit

Nursing Care Plan 16-1 has been developed to illustrate aseptic practices within a teaching plan for the diagnosis of Knowledge Deficit. The NANDA taxonomy presently does not contain a definition for this diagnostic category. It is still being developed. This definition from Carpenito (1989) therefore is being substituted: Knowledge Deficit is "the state in which an individual or group experiences a deficiency in cognitive knowledge or psychomotor skills regarding the condition or treatment plan." The orders in the sample care plan are specific to helping eliminate a particular contagious condition and preventing its spread and recurrence.

Teaching Suggestions to Practice Medical and Surgical Asepsis

The nurse may have many opportunities to teach patients practices and facts about medical and surgical asepsis.

It is important to teach patients common practices of medical asepsis that relate to everyday living. Many patients recognize the importance of common practices such as washing the hands after using the bathroom and before handling food, but some do not. By observing patients, the nurse may identify areas where instruction would be helpful in controlling the spread of microorganisms. Teaching can then be directed toward areas where it is most appropriately needed.

Soap or detergents and water remain among the best cleaning agents available, but patients may be confused about their differences. Both soap and detergents break up dirt into tiny particles that can be rinsed off more easily with water. Detergents have several advantages over soap. For example, they may be used in hard water and in cold water with better results than with soap. Studies have shown that soaps are about equal to each other in ability to clean. Soaps containing fragrances may be pleasant to use but appear to be no better for cleaning than plain green or odorless soap.

Some soaps and detergents contain agents that help destroy microorganisms but not necessarily their spores. However, studies have found that some of these agents can be harmful to humans. Therefore, many potentially harmful ones are available only with a physician's prescription. They may be used within high-risk areas of a hospital, such as the operating and delivery rooms.

The patient who gives himself care at home needs guidance in the proper way to handle sterile equipment and supplies and in how to sterilize reusable items. Teaching how to clean items properly is important also. Using boiling water at home is generally satisfactory. However, for the greatest safety, using disposable equipment should be recommended when practical.

The nurse acts as a model by observing sound practices of asepsis when giving care. This is a form of teaching also. Patients are generally quick to notice when questionable practices are used. The nurse who has not been attentive to personal grooming quickly loses credibility.

Bibliography

Bonnett KA: How to prevent needle sticks. Journal of Practical Nursing 38(2):33–35, 1988

Carpenito LJ: Nursing Diagnosis: Application to Clinical Practice, 3rd ed. Philadelphia, JB Lippincott, 1989

Crow S: Calling in sick: How to decide. Nursing 20(3):62–64, 1990

DeCrosta T: Nosocomial infections: Every patient is a target. Fighting the problem part 2. NursingLife 6(6):44–47, 1986

Ferwerda HE: Getting on top of infection control problems. Am J Nurs 89(9):1191, 1989

Ford CD: Disposal of sharps: Implications and control. Journal of Intravenous Nursing 13(1):42–47, 1990

Gidley C: Now, wash your hands! Nursing Times 83(29):40–42, 1987

Gundler C: AORN recommended practices format: Use of transfer forceps and splash basins. AORN J 46(2):320, 322, 1987

Hussain M: Hospital infection and its prevention. Point of View 26(3):9, 1989

Jones MA: Scrubbing with caution. Point of View 26(3):8, 1989

Larson E: Handwashing: It's essential—even when you use gloves. Am J Nurs 89(7):934–939, 1989

Mailhot CB, Slezak LG, Copp G: Cover gowns: Researching their effectiveness. AORN J 46(3):482–483, 486, 488, 1987

Manza RJ, Oesting HH: Handwashing: Re-examining the ritual. The Journal of Practical Nursing 37(3):14–15, 1987

McFarlane A: Why do we forget to remember handwashing? Professional Nurse 5(5):250, 252, 1990

Patterson P: Must that dropped package be discarded? OR Manager 6(4):1, 4, 6, 1990

Pottinger J, Burns S, Manske C: Bacterial carriage by artificial versus natural nails. Am J Infect Control 17(6):340–344, 1989

Proposed recommended practices: Surgical scrubs. AORN J 51(1):226, 228, 230, 1990

Recommended practices: Basic aseptic technique. AORN J 54(3):784, 786, 788–789, 1987

Recommended practices: Sterilization and disinfection. AORN J 54(2):440, 442, 44, 1987

Reybrouck G: Handwashing and hand disinfection. J Hosp Infect 8(1):5–23, 1986

Rohe J, Gelfant BB: The demise of aseptic technic. Point of View 26(1):17, 1989

Roth MK, Land GK: How to prevent infection in a home care patient. RN Magazine (9):61–62, 64, 66–67, 69–70, 1987

Sheehan A: Needle point . . . syringe/needle exchange schemes. Nursing Times 85(1):46, 1989

Stringer B, Walker M: Hepatitis. Canadian Nurse 85(8):38–40, 1989

Study reveals high prevalence of chapped hands, dermatitis. Hospital Infection Control 16(7):94, 1989

17

Preventing the Spread of Communicable Diseases

Chapter Outline

Behavioral Objectives
Glossary
Introduction
Progress Toward Infection Control
Limiting the Transmission of Pathogens
Types of Infection Control Practices
Common Transmission Barriers
Confining the Patient and Equipping the Room
Wearing Isolation Garments
Disposing of Contaminated Linen, Equipment, and
    Supplies
Handling Excretions and Secretions
Additional Infection Control Practices
Psychological Implications of Communicable Disease
    Control
Applicable Nursing Diagnoses
Suggested Measures to Control Communicable Diseases
    in Selected Situations
Teaching Suggestions to Control Communicable
    Diseases
Bibliography

Skill Procedures

Removing Isolation Garments (Gown, Gloves,
    and Mask)
Collecting and Transporting a Urine Specimen

Behavioral Objectives

When the content of this chapter has been mastered, the learner will be able to:

Define the terms appearing in the glossary.
List two explanations for the progress in controlling communicable diseases.
List seven factors that continue to contribute to the spread of communicable diseases.
List the routes by which microorganisms are most often transmitted. Give examples of each route.
List two general approaches for preventing microbes from spreading.
Identify two methods for infection control recommended by the Centers for Disease Control.
Name one type of isolation technique that is used but is no longer recommended by the Centers for Disease Control.
List seven groups of infection control practices included in category isolation.
Identify and explain how transmission barriers are used for infection control.
Demonstrate the recommended techniques for donning and removing gowns, masks, and gloves when caring for a patient with a contagious disease.
Demonstrate double-bagging technique.
Describe infection control techniques for using a watch, removing books, signing a document, and transporting a patient.
Discuss the psychological needs of a patient who requires infection control practices.
Identify factors related to controlling communicable diseases in young children and patients in intensive care areas.
Summarize suggestions for instruction of patients that are offered in this chapter.

Glossary

AFB isolation Infection control practices used to prevent the spread of the organism that causes tuberculosis.
Airborne transmission A route by which pathogens are transferred from an infected person to another on air currents containing suspended dust particles or residue of evaporated droplets.
Blood/body fluid precautions Infection control practices used to prevent the transmission of pathogens present in the blood or serum of an infected person.
Category isolation Several groups of infection control practices designed to limit the transmission of a variety of pathogens spread by a common route.
Communicable disease A disease that can be easily spread to others. Synonym for *contagious disease*.

Contact isolation Infection control practices that prevent the spread of highly contagious pathogens by direct or indirect contact.

Contagious disease A disease that can easily spread to others. Synonym for *communicable disease.*

Direct contact The route of transmission in which microorganisms are transferred when one is with or touching an infected person.

Disease-specific isolation A set of infection control practices unique to each communicable disease and its pathogen.

Double-bagging technique An infection control practice that involves placing a bag of contaminated items into another clean bag held by someone outside an isolation room.

Drainage/secretion precautions Infection control practices used when there is a possibility, though slight, for transmitting pathogens during direct or indirect contact.

Droplet transmission A route of transmission spread by particles of moisture released from the nose or mouth of an infected person.

Enteric precautions Infection control practices that limit the spread of pathogens present in the feces, or stool, of infected persons.

Indirect contact A route of transmission in which pathogens on contaminated objects are transferred to a susceptible host.

Infection control techniques Practices that prevent the transmission of pathogens from one host to another. Synonym for *isolation techniques.*

Infectious period The time when pathogens exit from an infected host.

Isolation techniques Practices that prevent the transmission of pathogens from one host to another. Synonym for *infection control techniques.*

Protective isolation Infection control practices used to prevent a highly susceptible person from acquiring an infection. Synonym for *reverse isolation.*

Respiratory isolation Infection control practices that limit the spread of organisms in the air or on droplets.

Reverse isolation Infection control practices used to prevent a highly susceptible, noncontagious person from acquiring an infection. Synonym for *protective isolation.*

Strict isolation Infection control practices used to prevent the spread of highly contagious diseases that are transmitted by more than one route. It may also be used when the pathogen is unknown.

Transmission barrier A garment or technique that blocks the transfer of pathogens from one person, place, or object to another.

Universal precautions Preventive practices that protect health-care workers from acquiring bloodborne viruses from unidentified, infected persons.

Vaccine A substance given to susceptible individuals to promote the body's natural defense against a specific contagious disease.

Vector An insect or animal that spreads pathogens.

Introduction

Communicable diseases are also called *contagious diseases* because they spread easily to others. These diseases are caused by pathogens. Practices called *isolation techniques* or *infection control techniques* are used to prevent the transmission of pathogens from one host to another.

Understanding the infectious process cycle, previously illustrated in Figure 16-1, is a foundation for the principles of infection control. Isolation techniques confine the reservoir of pathogens, block the vehicle or route of their transmission, interfere with the portal of entry, and protect susceptible hosts. The nurse should be familiar with the terms and practices of medical and surgical asepsis discussed in Chapter 16 before proceeding with the study of the skills associated with preventing the spread of communicable diseases found in this chapter.

Progress Toward Infection Control

At one time, contagious diseases were the leading cause of death. Today, many communicable diseases in the United States have been controlled or eliminated. Examples of two such diseases are poliomyelitis and smallpox.

There are several reasons for this accomplishment. One of the main factors has been the production and use of vaccines. *Vaccines* are substances given to individuals to promote the body's defenses against contagious diseases. Vaccines are given to infants, children, and susceptible individuals according to a routine schedule or immediate need.

The discovery and use of various types of drugs, such as antibiotics, have helped prevent the spread of communicable diseases. While many people still become ill with contagious diseases, drugs often help bring the infection under control more rapidly. Their use reduces the *infectious period,* the time when pathogens exit from their reservoir. The drugs make it possible to shorten the time during which infection control techniques are necessary.

Despite these advances, contagious diseases have not disappeared. Some predict that there will be an increase in communicable diseases in the future. This prediction is made on the basis that our society contains growing numbers of susceptible individuals. Among these are premature infants who would not have previously survived, an increase in the population of aging individuals, more and more recipients of transplanted organs who must take drugs that suppress the body's natural defenses, and a rising incidence of people acquiring AIDS (Acquired Immune Deficiency Syndrome) who also cannot resist pathogens.

Other facts that explain the continued occurrence and spread of contagious diseases include the following:

Some individuals are indifferent to the seriousness of communicable diseases and neglect acquiring vaccinations for themselves and their children.

Vaccinations are refused by some on the basis of religious beliefs.

Some organisms have developed methods to resist antibiotic drugs and remain a potential threat to health.

More young children are being cared for in preschool and day-care centers. One ill child can easily infect others.

Not all states require compulsory vaccination for school-age children.

Legal and illegal immigrants enter this country already sick or susceptible to contagious diseases.

Some individuals move frequently and do not maintain close medical care or accurate records.

Therefore, despite past accomplishments, nurses can expect the use of nursing skills to prevent spread of contagious diseases to be a continued challenge. These special infection control techniques are described in this chapter.

Limiting the Transmission of Pathogens

Microorganisms are transmitted by various routes. It is important to be aware of these routes because they form the bases for several kinds of techniques used to control the spread of communicable diseases. The routes of transmission are described in Table 17-1.

Isolation techniques limit the spread of contagious diseases in two general ways. One method protects other individuals in the general environment from the pathogens that are released from an infected person. This concept is illustrated in Figure 17-1. The other method, shown in Figure 17-2, protects a highly susceptible individual from microorganisms in the general environment.

Types of Infection Control Practices

Each health agency adopts its own infection control policies and practices. The procedures generally follow the recommendations from the Centers for Disease Control (CDC). This is a federal agency that studies pathogens, outbreaks of contagious diseases, and methods used to control them. Any health agency may modify the CDC recommendations. When modifications are made, they tend to be even more conservative than the CDC recommendations. Since isolation techniques may vary among

Table 17-1. Routes of Transmission

Route	Explanation
Contact Route—The Transmission of Communicable Pathogens by Touching the Microorganisms	
Direct contact	A nurse or others may acquire a communicable disease by being with or touching an infected person.
Indirect contact	Pathogens that remain on the surfaces of objects can spread diseases when they are touched and then enter a susceptible host. Common objects include bed linens, clothing, eating utensils, instruments, soiled tissues, and dressings.
Droplet spread	Moist material released when an infected person sneezes, coughs, talks, or laughs is considered contact spread because of the close association necessary between the infected person and the susceptible host. Droplets do not travel very far.
Vehicle Route—The Transmission of Communicable Pathogens Through Various Media	
Contaminated food, water, drugs, blood	When pathogens or their spores remain within food, water, drugs such as ointments, and blood they can be spread by being transferred through a portal of entry in the susceptible host.
Airborne	As air currents are created by walking, changing linen, sweeping, dusting, fans, open windows, and so forth, pathogens suspended on dust particles or residue of evaporated droplets can be transferred into a portal of entry.
Vectorborne	Insects and animals may carry pathogens from an infected person or contaminated water, food, or objects to a portal of entry in a susceptible host. Mosquitoes, flies, ticks, rats, and so on are are examples of vectors.

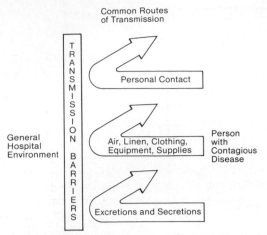

Figure 17-1 Following disease-specific or category isolation guidelines, transmission barriers can be used to prevent pathogens from being transferred from the infected person to the general hospital environment.

health agencies, nurses are advised to identify the principles underlying the practices rather than be concerned about their differences.

In the most recent guidelines from the CDC in 1983, two general types of isolation practices were recommended. They are category isolation and disease-specific isolation. Health agencies may choose to follow either of the two.

Another type of isolation practice is protective or reverse isolation. The CDC no longer recommends this type of isolation technique, but many hospitals continue to implement its use.

Regardless of the type of isolation practice that a health agency chooses to follow, the infection control practices that are required with its use are generally posted on the patient's door. Most instruction cards come in different colors and are located at eye level so all who enter the

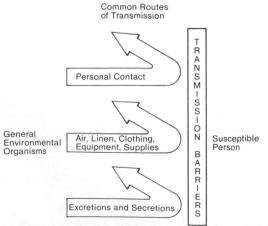

Figure 17-2 In protective, or reverse, isolation the susceptible person is protected from microorganisms. Transmission barriers are used to keep pathogens from the patient with weakened defenses.

room are made aware of the necessary precautions. An example of an isolation instruction card is illustrated in Figure 17-3.

Disease-Specific Isolation

Disease-specific isolation is a set of practices that limits the spread of a pathogen that causes a contagious disease. For instance, there are infection control practices that are designed specifically to prevent the spread of the meningococcus that causes one form of meningitis. The infection control practices would be different for this pathogen than those for controlling the spread of chickenpox, though each can be spread by respiratory secretions.

Infection control practices for each contagious disease can be as varied as there are kinds of pathogens. Most involve some combination of the skills necessary for carrying out the practices associated with category isolation. Therefore, a duplication of the discussion will be avoided. The skills described in this chapter can be utilized regardless of the type of infection control practice the health agency chooses to select.

Category Isolation

Category isolation includes a group of different isolation technique classifications. Each one utilizes practices that limit the transmission of a variety of pathogens spread by a common route, for instance, through blood, or stool, or body secretions, and so on. Category isolation groups include strict isolation, contact isolation, respiratory isolation, AFB (acid-fast bacillus) isolation, enteric precautions, drainage/secretion precautions, and blood/body fluid precautions.

Strict Isolation. *Strict isolation* is the most restrictive precautionary type of category isolation. It requires the use of the maximum number of infection control techniques. This type of isolation practice is used to prevent the spread of highly contagious diseases that can be transmitted by several routes, such as body secretions, contaminated articles, air, and so on. It may also be used when a contagious disease is suspected, but the pathogen has not been identified. Once identified, the type of category isolation practice may be changed.

Contact Isolation. When pathogens are transferred from an infected person immediately to a susceptible host, the route of transmission is by *direct contact.* When pathogens are transferred from contaminated articles used by an infected person, the route of transmission is by *indirect contact. Contact isolation* may be used if pathogens are almost certain to be spread by touching the patient or articles used by him. The infection control techniques that the nurse uses will depend on the type of care being administered.

Strict Isolation

Visitors—Report to Nurses' Station Before Entering Room

1. Masks are indicated for all persons entering room.
2. Gowns are indicated for all persons entering room.
3. Gloves are indicated for all persons entering room.
4. HANDS MUST BE WASHED AFTER TOUCHING THE PATIENT OR POTENTIALLY CONTAMINATED ARTICLES AND BEFORE TAKING CARE OF ANOTHER PATIENT.
5. Articles contaminated with infective material should be discarded or bagged and labeled before being sent for decontamination and reprocessing.

Figure 17-3 Instructions describing the precautions that must be practiced for each group of category isolation or disease-specific isolation are printed on a card and displayed on the door of the isolation room. This card is an example of strict isolation precautions, a type of category isolation.

Respiratory Isolation. *Respiratory isolation* prevents the spread of pathogens from droplet or airborne transmission. *Droplet transmission* refers to the drops of moisture released from the nose or mouth of an infected person when he coughs, sneezes, laughs, or talks. *Airborne transmission* is the transfer of pathogens from an infected person on suspended dust particles or on residue of evaporated droplets moved about on currents of air.

Enteric Precautions. Measures used to prevent the transmission of pathogens present in feces, or stool, are called *enteric precautions*. There may be only a few times during daily care that the possibility for transmission by this route would occur. The necessity to use enteric precautions need only be implemented on those specific occasions.

AFB Isolation. The pathogen that causes tuberculosis is an acid-fast bacillus (AFB). Practices used to prevent spreading this particular pathogen are, therefore, called *AFB isolation*.

Drainage/Secretion Precautions. *Drainage/secretion precautions* require that special infection control measures be used only when items or body areas containing pathogens from drainage will be handled. This type of isolation technique is used when the chance for spreading pathogens is slight, yet possible. This method contrasts with contact isolation practices in which there is strong likelihood for transmitting highly contagious organisms.

Blood/Body Fluid Precautions. *Blood/body fluid precautions* are used when a disease is spread through pathogens present in the blood or serumlike fluid of infected individuals. The disease is not spread by any other route. Special precautions are only necessary if the nurse or other susceptible individuals may be in contact with this vehicle of transmission.

Table 17-2 summarizes each of the types of category isolation and describes the infection control practices associated with them.

Universal Precautions

The transmission of bloodborne infections, especially AIDS caused by the human immunodeficiency virus (HIV) is a concern for all health-care workers. Anyone who is known to be infected with a bloodborne virus should be cared for following blood and body fluid precautions. However, there is a growing number of patients about whom that information is not known. Therefore, the Centers for Disease Control recommends using "Universal Blood and Body Fluid Precautions," also called "Universal Precautions." These recommendations are listed in Display 17-1.

Universal precautions are preventive practices that protect health-care workers from acquiring bloodborne viruses from unidentified, infected persons. This includes not only HIV, but also the virus that causes hepatitis B, and others.

The current list of body fluids with the potential for containing these infectious viruses includes blood and any body fluid containing visible blood, semen, vaginal secretions, cerebrospinal fluid, pleural fluid, peritoneal fluid, pericardial fluid, and amniotic fluid. Unless they contain blood, the following are not considered a vehicle of transmission: stool, nasal secretions, sputum, perspiration, tears, and vomitus. This does not preclude the ability for some of these substances to potentially transmit other diseases such as hepatitis A or tuberculosis. Other infection control and aseptic measures should be implemented if the patient is suspected of having a contagious disease transmitted by another route.

Protective Isolation

Protective isolation is used to prevent a highly susceptible, noncontagious person from acquiring an infection. Since

(Text continues on page 361)

Table 17-2. Category Isolation Practices

Technique	Purpose	Specifications	Examples of Diseases Requiring Technique
Strict isolation	To prevent transmission of highly communicable diseases spread by contact and airborne routes.	Private room necessary; door must be kept closed. Gowns must be worn by all persons entering room. Masks must be worn by all persons entering room. Hands must be washed on entering and leaving room. Gloves must be worn by all persons entering room. Articles must be discarded or must be double-bagged before being sent to other departments for disinfection/sterilization.	Chickenpox Diphtheria Smallpox
Respiratory isolation	To prevent transmission of organisms by droplets coughed, sneezed, or breathed into environment and by freshly contaminated articles.	Private room necessary; door must be kept closed. Gown not necessary. Masks must be worn by those coming close to the patient. Gloves not necessary. Articles must be discarded or must be double-bagged before being sent to other departments for disinfection or sterilization. Hands must be washed on entering and leaving room. Persons susceptible to specific disease should be excluded from patient area; if contact is necessary, susceptibles must wear masks.	Mumps Meningococcal meningitis Pertussis (whooping cough) Rubeola (measles) Rubella (German measles)
Enteric precautions	To prevent transmission of organisms through direct or indirect contact with infected feces.	Private room necessary for children or any patient who cannot be relied upon to practice good handwashing. Gown must be worn if soiling is possible. Mask not necessary. Hands must be washed on entering and leaving room.	Cholera Hepatitis, type A Typhoid fever

(continued)

Table 17-2. Continued

Technique	Purpose	Specifications	Examples of Diseases Requiring Technique
		Gloves must be worn by all persons having direct contact with patient or with articles contaminated with fecal material.	
		Articles must be disinfected or discarded; special precautions necessary for articles contaminated with urine and feces.	
Contact isolation	To prevent transmission of organisms that are highly contagious by direct or indirect contact, but do not require all the precautions of strict isolation.	Private room is necessary.	Impetigo
		Patients infected with the same organism may share a room.	Acute respiratory infections, such as bronchitis and influenza, in infants and children
		Masks are not necessary unless close contact will occur.	Rabies
		Gowns are necessary only if there is the potential for soiling.	Wound and burn infections that are draining and not covered, especially those caused by *Staphylococcus aureus* or group A streptococcus
		Gloves are necessary only if infective material will be touched.	
		Hands must be washed before and after care.	
		Articles must be discarded or double-bagged before being sent to other departments for disinfection/sterilization.	
AFB isolation (acid-fast bacilli)	To prevent transmission of the organism causing tuberculosis from droplets coughed, sneezed, or breathed into the air as well as present on contaminated articles.	Private room necessary with special ventilation.	Pulmonary tuberculosis that is active or strongly suspected in adult patients
		Gowns are not necessary unless clothing may be contaminated by droplets.	The secretions of young children and infants with this disease may contain few organisms in comparison with adults; for this reason, hospitals may choose not to place these patients in AFB isolation.
		Masks need only be worn if the patient currently has a cough or cannot be relied on to cover mouth.	
		Gloves are not necessary.	
		Hands must be washed on entering and leaving room.	
		Articles contaminated with secretions should be discarded, disinfected, or double-bagged before being sent to other departments.	

(continued)

Table 17-2. Continued

Technique	Purpose	Specifications	Examples of Diseases Requiring Technique
Drainage/secretion precautions	To prevent the remote, yet possible, transmission of organisms by contact with infected wounds, body secretions, and heavily contaminated articles.	A private room is usually not necessary. Gowns need only be worn if clothing is likely to be soiled by drainage or secretions. Masks are necessary if there is a danger of being splashed. Gloves need only be worn if touching drainage or soiled articles is likely. Hands must be washed before and after care. Articles contaminated with drainage or secretions must be discarded or double-bagged before being sent to other departments.	Minor or limited infected burns Minor or limited wound or skin infections Conjunctivitis
Blood/body fluid precautions	To prevent transmission of organisms by contact with blood or fluids that are likely to contain pathogens.	Private room is necessary for children or any adult who cannot be relied on to practice good handwashing. Gowns are necessary only if soiling with blood or body fluids is likely. Masks are necessary if there is a danger of being splashed. Gloves are necessary only if blood or body fluid will be touched. Hands must be washed immediately when there is contact with blood or body fluid and before caring for other patients. Avoid needle punctures; notify appropriate individuals if self-injury occurs. Articles contaminated with blood or body fluid must be discarded or double-bagged before being sent to other departments. Diluted sodium hypochlorite solution should be used promptly to clean up blood spills.	Acquired immune deficiency syndrome (AIDS) Hepatitis, type B Malaria

---

Display 17-1. Universal Precautions

Wear gloves when there is a possibility for hand contact with blood or any body fluid considered a potential source of bloodborne viruses.
Wear gloves when caring for a patient with nonintact skin or mucous membranes.
Avoid direct patient care and handling soiled equipment if one's own skin is not intact.
Wash hands immediately after removing gloves.
Wear any or all of the following additional protective garments when there is a possibility of being splashed with blood or body fluids: gown or plastic apron, goggles, mask.
Wash hands thoroughly and immediately with soap and water if contact with blood or body fluid occurs.
Dispose of uncapped needles, syringes, or sharp objects in a puncture-resistant container.
Use disposable ventilation devices rather than mouth-to-mouth breathing for pulmonary resuscitation.

---

this type of isolation utilizes techniques that are carried out in the opposite manner of other infection control practices, it is often called *reverse isolation*. Though infections may be acquired in a health agency, some patients are especially in danger. These individuals have weakened defenses. They are likely to die as a result of an infection

that most individuals would have little difficulty overcoming. Examples of individuals who need special protection are those with extensive burns, patients with leukemia, individuals receiving drugs, or radiation therapy that suppress the immune system.

The CDC has recently stopped recommending protective isolation. Research has shown that the patients for whom this type of technique has been used are susceptible even to organisms on and within themselves. Conscientious medical asepsis, such as handwashing, has proven to be just as effective in preventing infections in individuals with reduced natural defenses. However, many health agencies have chosen to continue implementing this type of infection control practice. Table 17-3 summarizes the infection control practices that are carried out for protective isolation.

Common Transmission Barriers

All isolation techniques utilize a combination of aseptic practices and the use of transmission barriers. A *transmission barrier* is a garment or technique that blocks the transfer of pathogens from one person, place, or object to another. Common transmission barriers that interfere with spreading pathogens include:

* Locating a patient and equipping the room to confine or restrict pathogens within that one area.
* Using gloves, masks, gowns, and occasionally hair and

Table 17-3. Techniques to Protect Individuals with Reduced Defenses

Technique	Purpose	Specifications	Examples of Diseases Requiring Technique
Protective or reverse isolation	To prevent contact between potentially pathogenic organisms and uninfected person who has seriously impaired resistance; patient is being protected from contamination	Private room necessary; door must be kept closed Gown must be worn by all persons entering room Mask must be worn by all persons entering room Hands must be washed on entering and leaving room Gloves must be worn by all persons having direct contact with patient Articles must be sterile or disinfected Cap and shoe covers are worn in some cases	Certain cases of leukemia Patients with extensive burns Transplant patients

shoe covers to prevent spreading microorganisms through direct and indirect contact.

- Caring for linen and, equipment such as bedpans, urinals, and eating utensils in such a way that pathogens are not transferred to others.
- Using infection control techniques to keep pathogens found within reservoirs of the patient's excretions and secretions from spreading.

Depending on the type of designated isolation technique, all or only some of these transmission barriers may be used.

Confining the Patient and Equipping the Room

Some organisms are able to remain alive and are capable of producing a disease even when separated from the infected person. The nurse needs to understand how to provide and maintain transmission barriers for organisms that can spread through the room environment.

Preparing an Isolation Room

To control the spread of most communicable diseases in a health agency, the patient is placed in a private room. In this way, no other patient is in direct contact with the infected or susceptible person as the case may be. On rare occasions, when more than one patient has the same contagious disease, a room may be shared. In epidemics, an entire unit may be separated from others rather than separating each individual patient.

It is preferred that the isolation room have a private bathroom with running water. This also aids in blocking the transmission of organisms that may be spread by transporting feces or urine, or by ineffective handwashing.

The room being used should have an instruction card posted on the door. The door of the room should remain closed. This provides a barrier to organisms and facilitates reading the sign. It is important that all personnel and visitors are informed of the need to follow the special precautions listed on the sign. The nurse may be called on to explain the purpose of isolation and to teach visitors special infection control techniques.

The room used for an isolation patient should be further designed so that when the door is opened, slight negative pressure or exhaust fans in the room prevent organisms from being pulled into adjoining areas on air currents. The opposite direction of air flow is desired when protective or reverse isolation is used. Slight positive pressure will carry organisms away rather than into the patient's room environment when the door is opened.

Each day, housekeeping personnel should clean the room of an isolation patient. The isolation room should be cleaned last since the cleaning equipment cannot be re-used in other patient's rooms. The room should be damp mopped to prevent the spread of pathogens on air currents. The mop head, if not disposable, can be deposited with the soiled linen. The mop handle can be wiped with a disinfectant. Solutions used for cleaning can be flushed down the toilet in most cases.

Stocking Isolation Room Equipment

The isolation room contains essentially the same equipment as any other hospital room with a few modifications. Equipment that would ordinarily be shared among non-contagious patients, such as a sphygmomanometer, should be left in the patient's room whenever possible for his exclusive use. This prevents the added task of cleaning and disinfecting it each time it must be used for another patient.

The patient should have his own thermometer. Disposable thermometers are preferred. If a glass thermometer is used, it should be left at the patient's bedside in a container of disinfectant. Cleaning the glass thermometer before placing it in the disinfectant and changing the disinfectant regularly are common techniques of medical asepsis. Electronic thermometers are not recommended. They are difficult to clean thoroughly in order to make them safe for the next patient.

Certain items should be placed within the room for concurrent disinfection. Concurrent disinfection refers to the ongoing daily cleaning or disposal of used equipment and supplies. Items such as a container for soiled laundry, lined waste containers for burnable trash, lined receptacles for items that require disinfection and sterilization, and liquid soap dispensers are examples of equipment that are needed if they are not presently located in each room. Figure 17-4 shows a nurse placing contaminated linen into a supported laundry bag.

Wearing Isolation Garments

Garments act as physical barriers for preventing the transfer of pathogens onto a nurse's uniform, a visitor's street clothing, or skin. Still, handwashing cannot be ignored. Inadequately washed hands transmit more microorganisms than any other vehicle. Therefore, *handwashing is the single most important means of preventing the spread of microorganisms*. The hands should be washed before and after contact with each patient. Handwashing should also be done when touching articles or sources containing the patient's secretions or excretions. Handwashing should be done even following those occasions when gloves are worn. The technique for handwashing may be reviewed in Chapter 16.

Five garments may be worn to prevent spreading organisms by contact. These garments include gowns, masks, gloves, and sometimes hair and shoe covers. In some

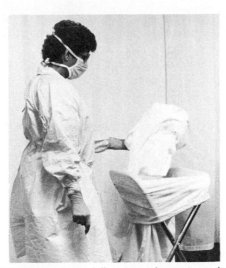

Figure 17-4 Contaminated linen, equipment, and supplies must be kept temporarily within a patient's room. This nurse places contaminated linen into a laundry container. The nurse avoids shaking the linen, which may create air currents and spread pathogens in that manner.

cases, only one type of garment may be required, depending on the pathogen's route of transmission.

Using a Gown

The use of a gown is the most efficient method of protecting the uniform and clothing of care givers or visitors from contamination with pathogens. Many variations of gowns exist, but all have the following common characteristics:

- Gowns open in the back to protect the front of the individual. This is the area most likely to be in contact with the patient.
- Gowns intended for use in isolation have close-fitting wristlets to help avoid contaminating the skin of the forearms.
- Fasteners are located on isolation gowns at the neck and waist to keep the gown securely closed, covering all the wearer's clothing.

Any gown in need of repair, such as one with torn areas or missing fasteners, should not be used.

When wearing a gown is necessary, it is worn only once and then discarded. Discarded cloth gowns may be placed within the patient's laundry hamper, removed with the soiled linen, washed, and then used again. Disposable paper gowns are placed in a waste container and eventually burned following removal from the patient's room.

No special procedure needs to be followed in putting on a clean gown when disease-specific category isolation are carried out. However, when protecting the patient who is at high risk for acquiring an infection, the nurse must don a sterile gown. This helps to reduce the potential for transmitting organisms within the environment and present in and on the nurse to the patient. Refer to Skill Procedure 16-4 for suggested actions for donning a sterile gown.

Using a Mask

Various isolation techniques require the use of masks when diseases can be spread by droplets or the airborne route. Clean masks should be stored with other isolation garments and clean supplies located outside the patient's room. Some health agencies have designed isolation units with anterooms. Cupboards within the anteroom contain frequently used supplies. This avoids cluttering the hallway.

The mask should be applied before entering the patient's room. If a nursing cap is worn, the nurse may remove it and leave it outside the room. Removing the nursing cap facilitates mask application and avoids possible contamination of the cap while giving patient care. Allow the patient to see the nurse's face before donning the mask. This is a thoughtful gesture. It helps keep the patient oriented and prevents feelings of alienation while being separated from contact with others. For the sequence used to remove a mask following the completion of patient care, refer to Skill Procedure 17-1.

Using Gloves

Gloves are required when a disease is highly contagious by direct contact. The gloves only need to be clean, not sterile. The nurse in Figure 17-5 is wearing the garments required for strict isolation. They include a gown, mask, and gloves.

Gloves are worn only once. However, they may need to be changed during patient care. The order in which gloves are removed with other strict isolation garments can be found in Skill Procedure 17-1.

Gloves are not a total and complete barrier to microorganisms. Leakage occurs approximately 2% of the time (Korniewicz, 1989). The percentage increases with the stress of their use. Handwashing should be repeated immediately after gloves are removed.

Removal of Isolation Garments

There is a recommended sequence for removal of isolation garments. This sequence prevents contamination of the nurse when leaving the isolation room before caring for others. The suggested actions described in Skill Procedure 17-1 are based on a situation in which wearing a gown, mask, and gloves is required. These garments are required for strict isolation.

The principle for removing isolation garments involves

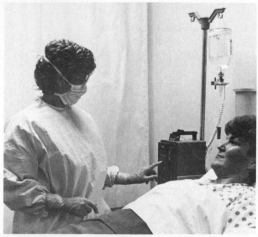

Figure 17-5 The nurse is wearing typical strict isolation garments. The gown, in this case a paper disposable type, is properly fastened. Note that to avoid steaming of eye-glasses, the frames rest over the upper part of the mask. Some prefer to tape the edge of the mask to the skin over the bridge of the nose to further prevent slipping and steaming of the glasses.

making contact between two contaminated surfaces or two clean surfaces. Garments of greater contamination are removed first while preserving the clean uniform underneath. With this principle as a guide, modifications for removing other combinations of required garments can be applied.

Disposing of Contaminated Linen, Equipment, and Supplies

Various receptacles placed within the patient's room are used to hold and collect contaminated items. As soiled waste and other articles accumulate, they are removed. A double-bagging technique may be used. A *double-bagging technique* involves placing bags containing contaminated articles into a second bag held by someone outside the room. The nurses in Figure 17-8 are double-bagging contaminated items.

The Centers for Disease Control (CDC) is now relaxing its recommendation concerning double-bagging. Its revised position is that a single bag probably provides adequate protection as long as it is strong enough to resist puncturing and care is taken to avoid touching the outside of the bag with articles that are placed within (CDC Guidelines for Isolation Precautions in Hospitals, 1983). When either of these two criteria cannot be met, double-bagging is still appropriate. Even when linen is contaminated with blood or body fluids, double-bagging is unnecessary as long as the bags that are used prevent leakage (American Hospital Association, 1988). One study (Maki, Alvarado,

Hassemer, 1986) at the University of Wisconsin Hospital and Clinics found that a single 2-mil polyethylene bag did not produce significantly greater surface contamination than that found on the outside of doubled bags.

All hospital personnel, including those in the dietary, laundry, and housekeeping departments should be following universal precautions as they perform their work-related responsibilities. Despite these findings, some hospitals may continue to require double-bagging. Existing policies should be followed.

Disposing of Burnable Trash

A lined wastebasket or other receptacle is used to collect items that can be destroyed by burning. Items such as old newspapers, unwanted magazines, dressing, tissues, disposable syringes, and food that cannot be flushed in the toilet may be placed in the container. Moist items such as food, soiled dressings, or wet tissues should be wrapped before depositing to prevent the spread of pathogens by vectors. A *vector* is an insect, such as a fly, or an animal that spreads pathogens. The bag and the contents are destroyed by incineration. The heat also kills the pathogens on the contaminated articles.

Caring for Nonburnable Items

Most health agencies currently use disposable equipment that may be burned. Reusable items may be collected separately in the room, bagged, and then sterilized by gas or steam under pressure. Contaminated needles are collected in a specially marked container in the room to prevent accidental needle punctures.

Disposable basins, bedpans, and urinals are best used for patients with contagious diseases. When that is not the case, stainless steel equipment may be rinsed with cold water, washed with soap and water, bagged, and sterilized before reuse.

Some health agencies use disposable eating utensils for isolated patients. They may be bagged with other burnable trash. Personnel caring for dietary equipment wear gloves. Most health agencies use dishwashers, which leave eating utensils free of pathogens. If this is not the case, the rinsed and prewashed dishes should be boiled for at least 20 to 30 minutes before reuse.

Handling Excretions and Secretions

Organisms can escape from the patient through body excretions and secretions. Urine, feces, respiratory, oral, vaginal, penile, and wound drainage may require special infection control practices.

Skill Procedure 17-1. Removing Isolation Garments (Gown, Gloves, and Mask)

Suggested Action	Reason for Action
Before removing the gloves, untie or unfasten the waist closure, which is located in the front of the gown.	The front of the gown receives the most contact with the patient. It, along with the gloves, is considered one of the most contaminated areas of isolation garments. Touching two highly contaminated areas will not add further to the contamination.
Remove gloves and place them in the proper container. Care should be taken to avoid touching the outer surface of the gloves with bare hands, as is illustrated in Figure 17-6.	Gloves that have had direct contact with the patient contain large numbers of pathogens. They should be removed before using the hands to touch or remove other isolation garments.

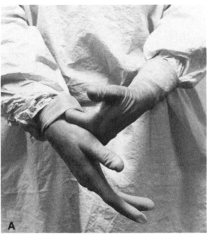 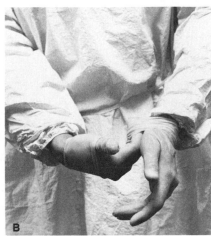 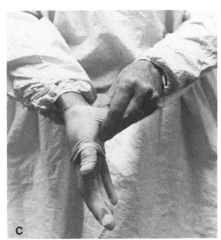

Figure 17-6 This series of steps shows a method of glove removal that prevents contamination of the nurse's hands. (*A*). The first glove is stretched and pulled down to form a cuff exposing the inner surface of the glove. (*B*). Before completely removing the first glove, the nurse takes off the second glove by pulling it inside out without touching the bare hand. (*C*). Touching only the inside of the contaminated glove, the bare hand is used to pull the remaining glove inside out. The removed gloves are discarded in the appropriate container.

Wash the hands, following medical aseptic practices described in Chapter 16, if there was any contact with the gown or outside of the gloves.	Handwashing is the best technique to remove any pathogens that may have possibly been transferred. Handwashing is appropriate at any time during the removal of isolation garments if contamination occurs.
Remove the mask, following the suggested actions in Skill Procedure 16-3. Discard it in the disposable trash or laundry container.	The mask ties are considered clean, since they are well above the waist and front of the body. There is no danger of contamination in touching the ties with clean hands.
Untie or unfasten the neck closure of the isolation gown.	The back of the gown is considered one of the least contaminated areas of isolation garments. Use clean hands to unfasten the gown for removal.
Remove the gown but avoid touching the front of it. Some people insert their fingers at the shoulder as illustrated in Figure 17-7. Others slide a finger under the cuff and pull the sleeve down.	Touching the front of the gown would transfer organisms to the nurse's clean hands. If the nurse uses the last suggested method to pull off the sleeves, it should be noted that the cuff area had been covered by gloves and is essentially clean. If gloves were not worn, the first method should be used or the hands should be washed again.

(continued)

Skill Procedure 17-1. Continued

Suggested Action   **Reason for Action**

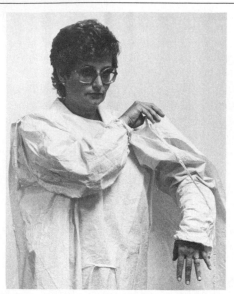

Figure 17-7 Touching clean hands on the inside of an isolation gown facilitates its removal without contaminating the hands.

Suggested Action	Reason for Action
Fold the outside of the gown to the inside, holding it away from the uniform. Roll up the gown and discard it in the trash container, if disposable, or place it in the linen hamper, if it is cloth.	Folding the contaminated surface to the inside prevents touching the surface, which contains pathogens.
Wash the hands again.	Handwashing before leaving removes organisms that may have possibly been transferred during garment removal.
Using a clean paper towel to protect the bare hand, open the isolation door.	The door knob is a reservoir of pathogens within the patient's room. The clean paper towel acts as a transmission barrier between the pathogens and the clean hands.
Discard the paper towel into the wastebasket inside the patient's room.	Once the paper towel has touched the door knob, it is contaminated. It should not be carried out of the room.
Pick up one's watch if it had been placed on a clean surface earlier. This is discussed later in the chapter.	Since the watch is on a clean surface and the nurse's hands are clean, the watch may be handled without contacting any pathogens.
Leave the room, taking care not to touch anything. Go directly to a utility room and wash the hands one final time.	A final handwashing removes organisms that may have been transferred by undetected contact with contaminated objects. It is always safer to overdo rather than underdo any practice that controls the spread of organisms.

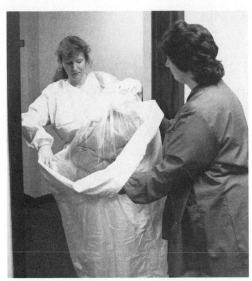

Figure 17-8 The nurse wearing a gown puts a bag of contaminated items into a second bag, the outside of which is kept clean. Note that the nurse holding the second bag has folded back a cuff. This helps prevent contamination of the outside of the second bag and her own hands as she receives contaminated items.

Disposal of Urine and Feces

Except in a few rural areas, waste water treatment systems are capable of destroying pathogens in urine and feces. Thus, these wastes may be discarded into the toilet. When the sewage system is inadequate for the destruction of organisms, the urine and feces may need to be treated with a disinfectant before disposal. Local policies should be observed in these instances.

The nurse should always follow general medical asepsis principles discussed in Chapter 16 when handling containers that hold urine and feces. Handwashing is always required. Safe practice for cleaning the bedpan or urinal requires that it be emptied, rinsed thoroughly with cold water, and washed with a solution of water, soap, detergent, or disinfectant.

Tissues and other paper or gauze items contaminated by wound, nose, mouth, vaginal, or penile drainage need to be deposited in a separate bag before they are added to the trash. They are removed along with other burnable items.

Removing Specimens

Specimens may need to be collected for laboratory analysis. Laboratory technicians are required to follow the same isolation precautions as nursing personnel and visitors.

When the nurse sends a specimen to the laboratory from a patient in isolation, the outside of the container should be protected from contamination. Skill Procedure 17-2 describes how to collect and remove a urine speci-

men from an isolation room without contaminating it. A container that has come in contact with a potential reservoir of the infecting pathogen should be bagged and labeled on the outside of the bag. Laboratory personnel follow universal precautions when handling all blood and body fluid specimens collected from patients.

Contact With Blood

The Occupational Safety & Health Administration has issued an interim mandate for hepatitis-B vaccination before completing its final report on protection standards involving infectious wastes. Employers are now required to provide free immunizations for health-care workers who are exposed to blood and body fluids once or more per month.

Hepatitis B is only one of several diseases that can be spread by blood. Regardless of having received the vaccine, whenever there is a possibility for contact with blood or body fluids, gloves should be worn.

Gloves will not prevent the transmission of HIV, hepatitis C, and other bloodborne pathogens if gloves are punctured. Therefore, nurses must be careful to avoid accidental punctures. Most health-care agencies have now equipped all patient rooms with puncture resistant containers such as the one in Figure 17-10. The nurse should deposit all sharp and blood-contaminated objects immediately within the container. Blood spills should be cleaned wearing gloves and using a 1:10 dilution of household bleach.

All laundry personnel handling soiled linen from the operating room or other patient-care areas should use gloves and gowns or aprons. The linen is washed in hot water that is at least 160°F (71°C) for 25 minutes. At temperatures lower than this, special low-temperature washing chemicals are added.

Additional Infection Control Practices

Additional techniques may be used to limit the spread of pathogens in unusual situations. These practices may be required on infrequent occasions, but the nurse should be aware of the suggested actions to follow.

Using a Watch

The need for a wristwatch is not always necessary. Many hospital rooms have a wall clock with a sweeping second hand. If a wall clock is unavailable and isolation garments would interfere with the ability of the nurse to read a watch, it can be protected from contamination by placing it within a transparent plastic bag. Before leaving the room, the nurse can open the bag, allow the watch to fall onto a clean surface, wash hands, and pick up the watch when leaving the room.

Skill Procedure 17-2. Collecting and Transporting a Urine Specimen

Suggested Action	Reason for Action
Obtain the appropriate specimen container.	In this case an unsterile specimen container for a routine urinalysis is used.
Leave the lid cover for the specimen container outside the patient's room on the supply cart.	The lid is not necessary in the room and could possibly be contaminated in the removal of the specimen from the room.
Place the specimen container on a clean paper towel.	Paper towels are usually stacked in a dispenser in such a way as to avoid any contact with pathogens. Each towel dispensed is considered clean. By going directly to the towel dispenser without touching the patient or other objects in the isolation room, the nurse's hands are still considered clean.
Prepare the patient to void in a bedpan or urinal.	The urine must be transferred into the specimen container.
Pour the urine from the urinal or a pitcher into the specimen container as shown in Figure 17-9. The outside of the specimen container must not be touched by the nurse's hands or the container that holds the urine.	Touching the specimen container with any source of pathogens will cause contamination to occur.

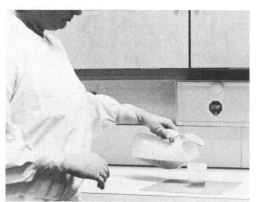

Figure 17-9 Before touching anything in the patient's room, the nurse removes a clean paper towel from its dispenser. The clean urine specimen container is then placed on the paper towel. The clean surface of the container is touching the clean surface of the paper towel. The nurse pours the urine into the specimen container, taking care not to touch the urinal or the urine to the outside of the specimen container. If this occurs, the specimen must be removed by double-bagging.

Clean the bedpan or urinal and replace it in the bedside unit.	All care of the patient and equipment must be completed before removing the specimen.
Remove the isolation garments according to the sequence described in Skill Procedure 17-1.	The nurse must be free of the patient's pathogens before picking up the clean specimen container and leaving the room.
Pick up the specimen container with one clean hand. Use a paper towel to open the door, and leave the room.	Because the specimen container has not been in contact with any contaminated objects, it may be removed without double-bagging.
Place the lid, which was left outside the room, on the specimen container and attach the laboratory identification slip.	The lid has remained clean because it was not taken into the patient's room.
Send the specimen to the laboratory as soon as possible.	Once specimens have been obtained, they should not remain on the nursing unit, where they may be spilled or misplaced or may deteriorate.

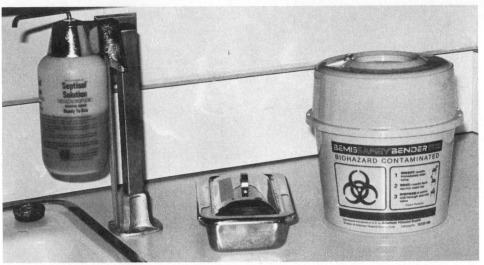

Figure 17-10 The container on the right has been placed near the sink in an isolation room. It is used to collect contaminated needles and other sharp objects.

Transporting Patients

Patients in isolation may need to be transported from their rooms to other departments. For example, a patient may need to be taken to the x-ray department. During the time of transport, it is necessary to use practices that will prevent the spread of pathogens from the patient to other individuals and to the wheelchair or stretcher.

Coordination between departments within the health agency is important. The department to which an isolation patient is to be transported should be made aware that the patient has a communicable disease. Unnecessary waiting in an area used by others may also increase the risk of spreading pathogens.

The nurse may use certain precautions for transporting a patient with a communicable disease. The surface of the wheelchair or stretcher should be protected from patient contact by a clean sheet or bath blanket. A second one should cover as much of the patient's body as possible during transport. The linen acts as a transmission barrier to pathogens from the patient to the transport vehicle and the environment. Figure 17-11 shows a patient with a communicable disease being taken to another area of the hospital. Any hospital personnel having direct contact with the patient should don and remove garments similar to those used in patient care.

When returning the patient to the isolation room, the nurse can deposit the soiled linen in the linen hamper within the patient's room. The nurse should take care to touch only the surface that has not been in direct contact with the patient's body. Some agencies also spray or wash the transport vehicle with disinfectant before reuse by another patient.

Removing Reading Material

For the patient in strict isolation who feels well enough to read, newspapers, magazines, and books can provide welcome diversion. As was already mentioned, unwanted newspapers and magazines can be removed with the

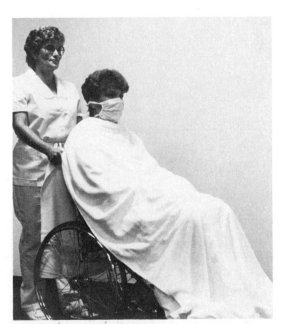

Figure 17-11 The wheelchair used for transporting an isolation patient is protected from contact with the patient by lining it with a clean bath blanket. A similar one covers the patient. This patient's communicable disease can be spread by droplets; therefore, the patient is required to wear a mask during the time outside the isolation room.

bagged, burnable trash. The patient may want to keep hardcover books, a prayer book, or a Bible. If the pathogen can be spread in this manner, two options exist. The surface of the book can be wiped with a disinfectant. If this is unacceptable, the book can be placed in a paper bag and gas sterilized.

Signing Documents

Occasionally patients with communicable diseases are required to sign documents such as consent forms, business correspondence, and legal papers. These items often represent a negligible vehicle for transmitting pathogens, since they are only in the patient's environment for a brief period of time. Nevertheless, a clean paper towel is used as a transmission barrier between the document and the overbed table. After the patient has read the document, another paper towel is placed in the area where the patient's hand will rest during signing. Figure 17-12 shows how a document is protected. After the patient has signed, the nurse may pick up the document with clean hands and leave the room. The paper has not been contaminated and no sterilization is required.

Psychological Implications of Communicable Disease Control

Regardless of the isolation technique that is used, one need for patient care remains a priority: attention to the psychological effects of isolation.

Understanding the Patient's Feelings

Experienced nurses have found that patients requiring infection control measures often feel feared by others. They, themselves, are generally frightened of the disease, since special precautions are required for their care. They feel "unclean" because everyone must wash their hands so frequently and be careful of handling contaminated articles. They feel alone and neglected because they cannot leave the room; visitors sometimes stay away. Particular effort needs to be made to demonstrate that the microorganisms, not the isolated patient, are unwanted.

When the patient resents the isolation precautions, the nurse needs to show acceptance of the patient as a person and allow him time for expressing his feelings. The nurse understands the holistic concept that emotions can influence the patient's recovery.

Providing Human Contacts

Loneliness is often a problem for the patient in isolation because the patient is usually deprived of his usual contact with others. Studies have shown that extensive isolation of the patient from others can be very traumatic. The goal, therefore, is to minimize this situation as much as is safely possible. While precautions are being used, it is important to plan frequent contact with the patient. Visitors should be encouraged to come whenever and as often as the agency's policies and the patient's condition permit. The nurse should emphasize that as long as the precautions are followed, they are not likely to acquire the disease.

Providing Sensory Stimulation

Being isolated from others and prevented from participating in activities outside the isolation room can easily lead to sensory deprivation and depression. The nurse must use preventive measures to help the patient experience a variety of sensory stimulation. Suggestions for providing sensory stimulation were discussed in Chapter 12.

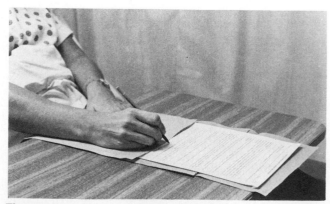

Figure 17-12 Clean paper towels protect a document from contact with the overbed table as well as from contact with the patient's hand during signing.

Applicable Nursing Diagnoses

Some of the nursing diagnoses that may apply when caring for a patient in isolation or one who is very susceptible to pathogens include the following:

- High Risk for Infection
- Altered Protection (accepted for testing since the publication of the 1989 NANDA taxonomy)
- Impaired Skin Integrity
- Social Isolation
- Ineffective Coping
- Diversional Activity Deficit
- Powerlessness
- Fear

Nursing Care Plan 17-1 applies the nursing process to a patient with the nursing diagnosis of High Risk for Infection. This diagnostic category is defined in the NANDA taxonomy (1989) as, "The state in which an individual is at risk for being invaded by pathogenic organisms."

NURSING CARE PLAN

17-1. High Risk for Infection

Assessment	**Subjective Data**
	States, "I get sick so easily when I'm taking these antirejection drugs. Seems like every time I turn around I've caught a cold, the flu, or get pneumonia. The slightest cut gets infected."
	Objective Data
	23-year-old man received a second kidney transplant four days ago following rejection of cadaver kidney implanted five years ago. Temperature 98° F. Present white blood count is 3,000. Has been receiving hemodialysis through arteriovenous cannula in L. arm three times a week for the past month. Receiving Prednisone and Imuran.
Diagnosis	High Risk for Infection related to immunosuppression secondary to antirejection drug therapy.
Plan	**Goal**
	The patient will remain free from infection throughout his hospitalization.
	Orders: 5/11
	1. Follow protective infection control policies.
	2. Assign staff who are free of infectious symptoms.
	3. Restrict visitors to wife and instruct on aseptic techniques.
	4. Assess vital signs, including temperature $\bar{q}$ 4 h.
	5. Inspect site of arteriovenous cannula for redness, swelling, discomfort, and drainage $\bar{q}$ day.
	6. Change vascular dressing and all invasive vascular lines $\bar{q}$ day. Use betadine followed by alcohol as a skin prep. Apply Neosporin ointment to insertion site. Cover with transparent dressing.
	7. Provide oral care p.c. & HS followed by prescribed antifungal oral suspension. Instruct to position half of the solution on one side of the mouth and retain as long as possible before swallowing. Repeat on opposite side with remaining solution. ———————————————————————G. LOPEZ, RN
Implementation (Documentation)	
5/11	1630 T—98 ^{4}(o), P—88, R—20, BP 148/98 R. arm while sitting. Currently in protective isolation. Wife instructed on handwashing, gowning, mask and glove technique. Returned demonstration satisfactorily. ————————————W. HILL, LPN
Evaluation (Documentation)	
	1945 TPR remain normal—see graphic sheet. Arteriovenous site is not red and shows no evidence of swelling or drainage. No pain noted. Blood flowing through dialysis cannula. No streaks or separation of plasma from cells observed. Mouth care given according to written nursing orders. No white patches seen on oral mucous membranes. ———————————————————————W. HILL, LPN

Suggested Measures to Control Communicable Diseases in Selected Situations

When the Patient Is an Infant or Child

Infants and children represent a group of individuals that are at high risk for acquiring contagious disease. Young children often play in close contact with one another for long periods of time. Handwashing is often infrequent and inadequate. They share eating utensils and food. They may not cover their mouth while coughing and sneezing. For these reasons, as well as others, they acquire communicable diseases at a higher frequency than other age groups. Prevention and care for them is often a special challenge.

Newborns who have a contagious disease require special care. Some health agencies separate a sick infant from healthy infants in a nursery. However, if there is adequate personnel, opportunity for thorough handwashing, and sufficient space between newborns, a private room for the infant may not be necessary.

Until the source of an infection in a nursery is identified, groups of infants born within the same 24- to 48-hour period may be kept in a single nursery. Personnel assigned to care for these infants should remain constant. The room is then cleaned thoroughly when all the infants have been discharged.

Children with the same contagious disease may be placed in a room together. Nurses must observe them closely, since young patients cannot always be relied on to remain within the isolated area.

When the Patient Is in an Intensive Care Unit

Patients in intensive care units are at higher risk for acquiring an infection because they require more invasive equipment while in a weakened condition. Furthermore, these patients are grouped closely together. In an emergency, personnel may be required to move quickly and frequently from patient to patient without time for handwashing.

The optimum precaution would be to place the intensive care patient with a communicable disease in a private room. When this is not possible, the isolation area may be marked off by cubicle curtains or tape on the floor. Instructional cards are posted nearby. Conscientious handwashing continues to be one of the most critical precautions for limiting communicable diseases.

Teaching Suggestions to Control Communicable Diseases

The following are teaching suggestions that may be carried out while providing care for the patient in isolation.

The patient and his family need to have an accurate understanding of the disease and of how to carry out the required precautions.

Family members may need much help in understanding why the patient may be depressed and how to cope with it.

Health agency staff should review the practices involved in isolation technique frequently. Patients are quick to observe differences in the practices of personnel. This can cause confusion and even mistrust in the quality of care.

Bibliography

American Hospital Association: Management of HIV Infection in the Hospital, 3rd ed. Chicago, 1988

Becker L, Lagomarsino W: Isolation guidelines for perinatal patients: Creating a new protocol. Matern Child Nurs J 12(6):400–404, 1987

Campbell B: Using universal precautions in infection control. Hospital Trustee 13(1):16–18, 1989

Centers for Disease Control: Guidelines for prevention of transmission of human immunodeficiency virus and hepatitis B virus to health-care and public safety workers. MMWR 38(6S):3–37, 1989

Centers for Disease Control: Recommendations for prevention of human immunodeficiency virus (HIV) transmission in health-care settings. MMWR 36(2S):3S–18S, 1987

Centers for Disease Control: Update: Universal precautions for prevention of transmission of human immunodeficiency virus, hepatitis B virus, and other bloodborne pathogens in health-care settings. MMWR 37(24):377–388, 1988

Controversies in care: New OSHA rules under fire from all angles. Am J Nurs 90(1):18, 22, 1990

Craft K: Do you really know how to handle sharps? RN Magazine 53(8):33–35, 1990

Dickerson M: Protecting yourself from AIDS: Infection control measures. Critical Care Nurse 9(10):26–28, 1989

Garner JS, Simmons BP: Centers for Disease Control: Guidelines for isolation precautions in hospitals. Infect Control 4(Suppl):245–325, 1983

Goldrick BA: Effectiveness of an infection control programmed unit of instruction in nursing education. Am J Infect Control 15(1):16–19, 1987

Gruca JAK: A systems look at infection control. Nursing Management 18(3):50–51, 1987

Kim MM, Mindorff C, Patrick ML: Isolation usage in a pediatric hospital. Infect Control 8(5):195–199, 1987

Korniewicz D: Leakage of virus through stressed vinyl and latex examination gloves. Fifth International Conference on AIDS; Montreal, June 1989

Jackson MM, Lynch P: Education of the adult learner: A practical approach for the infection control practitioner. Am J Infect Control 14(6):257–271, 32A–35A, 1986

Jackson MM, Lynch P, McPherson DC: Why not treat all body substances as infectious? Am J Nurs 87(9):1137–1139, 1987

Larson E: Change and infection control. Am J Infect Control 14(6): 246–249, 1986

Maki DG, Alvarado C, Hassemer C: Double-bagging of items from isolation rooms is unnecessary as an infection control measure: A comparative study of surface contamination with single and double-bagging. Infect Control 7(11):535–537, 1986

Moeller KI, Swartzendruber EJ: Suppressing the risks of bone marrow suppression. Nursing 17(3):52–54, 1987

New guidelines for preventing transmission of the A.I.D.S. virus. Nursing 17(11):22, 24, 1987

Preventing infections transmitted by contact. Nursing 18(3):112, 1988

Radany MH, Perry S, McCallum: Is it safe to reuse disposables? Am J Nurs 87(1):35–38, 1987

Schweizer RT, Allen B, Ruddell C: Infection control and the transplant patient. Asepsis 11(1):2–13, 1989

Taylor L, Josse E: Nursing aid: Developing infection control. Nursing Times 84(49):32, 1986

The CDC guidelines. The Journal of Practical Nursing 38(2): 26–31, 1988

Tribulski JA: The true odds of getting AIDS from a patient. RN Magazine 51(5):64, 67–68, 70, 1988

Wells R: Who's at risk? Nursing Times 83(45):16–17, 1987

18

Caring for the Inactive Patient

Chapter Outline

Behavioral Objectives
Glossary
Introduction
Dangers of Inactivity
Helping to Prevent Disuse Syndrome
Using Positioning Devices
Using Protective Bed Devices
Using Specialty Beds
Turning and Moving the Patient
Positioning the Patient Confined to Bed
Transferring the Patient
Maintaining Joint Mobility
Preparing the Patient for Walking
Suggested Measures to Prevent Inactivity in Selected
   Situations
Applicable Nursing Diagnoses
Teaching Suggestions to Prevent Inactivity
Bibliography

Skill Procedures

Turning the Patient
Moving the Patient Up in Bed
Positioning the Patient
Transferring the Patient To and From a Stretcher
Moving the Patient To and From a Chair
Performing Range-of-Motion Exercises

Behavioral Objectives

When the content of this chapter has been mastered, the learner will be able to:

Define the terms appearing in the glossary.
Describe at least ten signs or symptoms associated with the disuse syndrome.
List 10 positioning devices used for the safety and comfort of inactive patients confined to bed and explain the purpose of each.
List five pressure-relieving devices and an indication for the use of each one.
Demonstrate how to turn and move patients safely.
Demonstrate how to position a patient on his back, side, and abdomen, and in a sitting position.
Identify the purpose and demonstrate range-of-motion exercises.
Describe four exercises that help prepare a patient to walk.
Demonstrate how to transfer a patient to a stretcher and chair and back to bed again.
Identify the manner in which a cane and walker should be used.
Describe ways in which a patient is prepared for crutch walking.
Describe or demonstrate four basic gaits for crutch walking.
List suggested measures to prevent inactivity in selected situations, as described in this chapter.
Summarize the suggestions for instruction of patients that are offered in this chapter.

Glossary

Abduction The act of moving a body part away from the center of the body.
Active exercise An exercise performed by a person without assistance from others.
Adduction The act of moving a body part toward the center of the body.
Alignment Being positioned in a straight line.
Atelectasis An incomplete expansion or collapse of a portion of lung tissue.
Atony Decreased muscle tonus.
Atrophy The wasting away of body tissue.
Axillary crutches Crutches that fit under the upper arms into the axillae.
Canadian crutches Crutches that fit the forearms by means of frames or metal cuffs. Synonym for *Lofstrand crutches.*
Circumduction Movement in a circular direction.
Constipation A condition in which stool becomes dry and difficult to pass.

Contracture A fixed decrease in a joint's range of motion.

Dangling The position in which a person is sitting on the edge of the bed with his legs and feet over the side of the bed.

Decubitus ulcer Breakdown of skin as a result of prolonged pressure over a bony prominence. Synonym for *pressure sore.*

Disuse syndrome The collective signs and symptoms that develop as a result of inactivity.

Dorsiflexion Movement of the foot at the ankle so that the toes point toward the kneecap.

Embolism A sudden blockage of an artery by a blood clot.

Embolus A clot that moves within circulating blood. Plural is emboli.

Extension The act of straightening or increasing an angle that brings parts into or toward a straight line.

External rotation The act of turning outward.

Fecal impaction A condition in which stool becomes so dry that it cannot be passed.

Fecal incontinence The inability to control bowel elimination.

Feces The product of intestinal elimination, also called stool.

Flexion The act of moving so that the angle between adjoining parts is reduced; bending.

Foot drop A common condition associated with inactivity in which the foot cannot assume a position of dorsiflexion.

Fowler's position A sitting position.

Gluteal setting Isometric exercises in which the muscles of the buttocks are alternately tensed and then relaxed.

Hyperextension A position in which the angle between adjoining parts is made larger than its normal or average range.

Hypostatic pneumonia An inflammation of the lungs due to decreased ventilation and retained secretions.

Internal rotation The act of turning inward.

Lateral position A position in which a person lies on his side.

Lofstrand crutches Crutches that fit the forearms by means of frames or metal cuffs. Synonym for *Canadian crutches.*

Neutral position A joint's normal position of alignment.

Passive exercise An exercise in which one person moves the body parts of another person.

Phlebitis An inflammation of a vein.

Plantarflexion Movement of the foot so that the toes point in a direction away from the head.

Platform crutches Crutches on which the patient's forearm is supported.

Pressure sore Breakdown of skin as a result of prolonged pressure over a bony prominence. Synonym for *decubitus ulcer.*

Prone position A position in which a person lies on his abdomen.

Quadriceps setting Isometric exercises in which the muscles in the front of the thigh are alternately tensed and relaxed.

Rotation The act of turning.

Spasticity A sudden, continuous, and involuntary muscle contraction.

Supine position A position in which a person lies on his back.

Syndrome A group of signs and symptoms that occur together.

Thrombophlebitis Inflammation of a vein accompanied by a thrombus.

Thrombus A stationary blood clot. Plural is thrombi.

Tonus The normal, slight, continuous contraction of muscles.

Transfer To move a person from one place to another.

Trapeze A triangular piece of metal hung by a chain over the head of a bed.

Urinary incontinence The inability to control urination.

Valsalva's maneuver Forced exhalation against a closed glottis.

Introduction

Research has shown that activity is essential for health. Inactive patients require movement and exercise. This chapter describes how to turn, move, position, exercise, and promote mobility to prevent complications associated with inactivity.

Dangers of Inactivity

Some patients are so inactive that their health deteriorates. Multiple complications can and do occur among individuals whose activity and movement are limited. These complications are grouped together under the term *disuse syndrome*. The word *syndrome* means a set of signs and symptoms that occur together. The disuse syndrome refers to the collective signs and symptoms that develop as a result of inactivity. These signs and symptoms occur in many systems of the body, not just in the musculoskeletal system.

It has been demonstrated that a person needs only about 2 hours of activity in every 24 hours to prevent many problems associated with the disuse syndrome. The dangers of inactivity illustrate the importance of a nursing care plan that includes activity and exercise for the patient. The following discussion deals with the effects associated with the disuse syndrome.

The Muscular System

Muscular weakness develops quickly with inactivity. When inactivity is prolonged, muscle weakness may become so severe that the effects are more damaging than the original illness.

Tonus refers to the normal, slight, continuous contraction of muscles. Decreased muscle tonus, called *atony*, develops with inactivity. In time, there is the development of *atrophy*, which is the wasting away of muscle cells.

Most patients experience backaches after being in bed for several days. Poor posture in bed and a soft mattress most frequently are responsible for backaches. These backaches are caused by the stretching of back muscles and failure to support them properly in bed.

The Skeletal System

One problem associated with the disuse syndrome is osteoporosis, which was also discussed in Chapter 8. This condition is characterized by loss of minerals, especially calcium, from the bones. The result is that the bones become less dense. When this condition occurs, the bones are brittle, fracture easily, and often become deformed. The calcium leaves the bone and is eliminated through the urinary tract. This predisposes the inactive patient to kidney stone formation.

Poor alignment also affects structures of the skeletal system. *Alignment* refers to positioning the body in a straight line. Allowing joints to remain bent and stationary for long periods of time can limit their range of motion.

Inactivity may eventually lead to a *contracture*, which is the decrease in a joint's range of motion due to the shortening of a muscle, disuse of a joint, or improper positioning. A joint can become fixed within a matter of days unless preventive measures are used. Patients often refer to a contracture as a "locked" or "frozen" joint.

Ordinarily the foot can easily be moved from a position of plantarflexion to dorsiflexion. *Dorsiflexion,* shown in Figure 18-1, means the foot is in a position in which the toes point upward. It is important to position the feet of an inactive person in dorsiflexion. This is the joint position that is necessary for walking. In a normal standing position, the foot is at a right angle to the leg, with the toes pointing straight forward. When a person takes a step the heel strikes the floor, followed by the toes.

Plantarflexion, also shown in Figure 18-1, means the foot is in a position that allows the toes to point downward. When the patient is in bed on his back, the foot tends to assume the position of plantarflexion. If this position is maintained for a period of time, a condition known as foot drop occurs. *Foot drop* is a type of contracture that results from prolonged plantarflexion, lack of movement of the ankle joint, and shortening of muscles at the back of the calf. This condition makes walking difficult or impossible since the heel and foot cannot be placed flat on the floor. In order to prevent permanent disuse, the foot must be kept in dorsiflexion and exercised.

The Cardiovascular System

Normally, when muscles contract during activity, they squeeze veins, helping to move blood back to the heart.

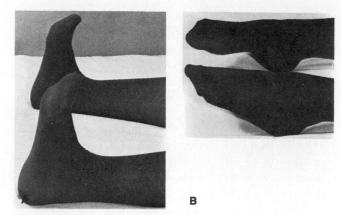

Figure 18-1 The feet in (*A*) dorsiflexion and (*B*) plantarflexion, which can lead to foot drop.

Lack of activity reduces this circulatory assistance. It contributes to sluggish circulation which allows blood to pool in the veins. This can lead to several circulatory complications.

The flow of blood may be so slowed in the lower legs that a clot forms. A *thrombus* is a stationary blood clot. It frequently causes a slowing or block in the flow of blood through a blood vessel. A thrombus is often accompanied by an inflammation of the vein in the area in which it is located. The suffix "itis" refers to the presence of an inflammation. When combined with the root word for vein, "phleb," it forms the word phlebitis. *Phlebitis* is an inflammation of a vein. A *thrombophlebitis* is a condition in which a thrombus lies within an inflamed vein.

An embolus can develop from a thrombus. An *embolus* is a blood clot that is no longer stationary, but moves within circulating blood. The sudden blockage of an artery or vein with a blood clot is called an *embolism.* If the thrombus or embolus lodges in a blood vessel supplying a vital organ, like the arteries that supply the heart muscle, the lungs, or the brain, the life of the patient could be in danger. If the blockage is not promptly relieved, the embolism may prove fatal. Periodic movement, especially of the lower extremities, can reduce the risk of cardiovascular complications.

The Respiratory System

Inactivity and poor posture cause a decrease in the movement of the thorax and a loss in tonus of the muscles of respiration. As a result, the exchange of oxygen and carbon dioxide is diminished. The normal chemical balance of the blood may be placed in jeopardy.

Inactivity causes a pooling of respiratory secretions. The patient tends to lose the ability to raise and expectorate them. This predisposes the patient to respiratory infections and a poor exchange of oxygen and carbon dioxide. *Hypostatic pneumonia* is a condition associated with inactivity that results from retained secretions.

Still another possible result of inactivity and poor posture is *atelectasis,* which is an incomplete expansion or collapse of small areas of lung tissue. Secretions that block air passageways predispose the patient to the condition.

The Urinary System

A reduction in the passage of urine, urinary tract infections, and urinary stone formation are the most common urinary complications that result from inactivity. There are many reasons that explain why an inactive person is predisposed to these complications.

Pressure from the accumulation of urine within the bladder signals a person that he should urinate. When a person is in a reclining position, the amount of pressure on sensitive muscles is reduced. The bladder continues to fill. As urine remains in the bladder, organisms can grow and multiply, leading to an infection. Substances normally dissolved in urine can crystallize as urine is retained for longer periods of time within the bladder. The crystals eventually form stones if the urine is not kept dilute and frequently passed. As the muscles that control urination are used less, their tone decreases. *Urinary incontinence,* the inability to control urination, may develop as a further complication.

The Gastrointestinal Tract

Anorexia is often associated with inactivity. When the patient is eating poorly, ensuring that he has a well-balanced and nourishing diet becomes a problem.

The movement of food in the gastrointestinal tract and proper intestinal elimination also become problems with inactivity. Gravity acts along with abdominal muscle movement to propel food and stool through the intestinal tract. Gravity is more effective in a standing position. As stool remains in the intestinal tract for long periods of time, more and more water is absorbed from the stool. The stool becomes dry and difficult to pass. This is known as *constipation.* It is a common symptom associated with the disuse syndrome.

Feces is another word for stool. A *fecal impaction* is a further complication of constipation. This is a condition in which the stool becomes so dried that it cannot be passed. Removing a fecal impaction is discussed further in Chapter 22. When an inactive person acquires a fecal impaction, liquid stool from above the hardened mass is sometimes released around the dry feces. It may seem that the patient is experiencing *fecal incontinence,* the inability to control bowel elimination, or has diarrhea; the actual problem may be just the opposite.

The Integumentary System

The skin's response to inactivity is ordinarily easy to see and occurs rapidly. A *decubitus ulcer,* also called a *pressure sore,* is a condition in which areas of skin are actually destroyed as a result of diminished blood supply caused by pressure from an inactive person's body weight. This is a common problem that occurs when a person sits or lies in the same position for prolonged periods of time. The formation of a decubitus ulcer is even more likely to occur when the patient is also incontinent of urine or stool. When that is the case, pressure plus the moisture and organic substances in the waste products of elimination contribute to the breakdown of skin. The prevention and care of a pressure sore is discussed in greater detail in Chapter 20.

Changes in Metabolism

The metabolic rate decreases when patients are inactive because the body requires less energy to function. Body temperature is lowered; there is a decrease in hormonal secretions. In fact, most of the body's processes are carried out at a reduced capacity.

Sleep Pattern Disturbance

Sometimes inactive individuals sleep as a result of boredom rather than to compensate for fatigue. Frequent naps change the cycles of REM and NREM sleep.

Psychosocial Changes

It is normal to be up and about, to work, to exercise, and to enjoy outlets for recreation and diversion. When a patient cannot participate in these normal activities, his mental attitude and motivation generally suffer. Feeling depressed is common. The person often loses interest in carrying out activities of daily living. Anger may occur as a result of feeling dependent on others.

Inactive persons may become more self-centered, since their "world" is confined to the immediate environment around themselves. They may appear impatient and demanding to others whose lives include varied activities.

Helping to Prevent Disuse Syndrome

When a patient is inactive, the nurse must carry out measures that prevent the disuse syndrome. This may involve performing passive exercises. *Passive exercise* is an exercise in which one person moves the body parts of another. Some patients may have to be encouraged to do active exercises. *Active exercise* is an exercise performed by a person without assistance from others.

Policies about exercise and activity vary. A physician's order may be necessary in some situations. In others, the primary nurse or nursing team leader takes responsibility for writing nursing orders for the patient's activity and exercise. It is recommended that the nurse follow orders on the nursing care plan and consult the supervising nurse if there are any questions.

It is self-defeating to both the patient and the nurse to write unrealistic orders for activity. A more practical approach is to evaluate the patient's present abilities and maintain them. The nurse can then consult with the patient about mutually agreed upon goals and methods for increasing levels of activity and exercise.

Several of the following nursing approaches can be used to avoid the dangers of limited activity that accompanies most illnesses:

- Teach the patient the importance of activity. This should include explaining that activity and exercise are a part of quality care.
- Encourage and supervise active exercises as much as is possible and safe for the patient. The nurse can build on the patient's abilities and encourage efforts he can take on his own.
- Carry out passive exercises as indicated and gradually help the patient move toward active exercising.
- Change the helpless patient's position every 1 to 2 hours and use different positions to promote comfort, variety, and exercise.
- Remain supportive when the patient seems uninterested, fearful, or opposed to activity and exercise.

The remainder of the chapter discusses various devices and nursing measures that are commonly used to prevent the disuse syndrome through positioning, exercise, and mobility.

Using Positioning Devices

Some patients' activity and exercise may be limited to moving within a bed. The nurse may be required to use many skills for positioning, musculoskeletal support, movement, and exercise that some patients are independently unable to carry out.

It is just as important for the body to be in good alignment and posture when lying down as it is when standing or sitting. There are many devices that help to maintain good body alignment in bed and to prevent discomfort or pressure. It should be remembered that any position, no matter how comfortable or anatomically correct, must be changed frequently.

Adjustable Bed

The adjustable bed was described in Chapter 12. In the high position, this bed is helpful for the nurse when giving care. When it is in the low position, it enables the patient to get in and out of bed with greater ease. Raising the head of the bed helps the bedridden patient see and look about without twisting and bending his neck. Also, he is in a nearly vertical position without the effort of standing, which helps make more effective use of gravity and prepares him for the day when standing and walking will begin.

Mattress

For a mattress to be comfortable and supportive, it must be firm but have sufficient give to permit good body align-

ment. A nonsupportive mattress promotes an unnatural curvature of the spine.

Bed Board

If the mattress does not provide sufficient support, a bed board may help to keep the patient in better alignment. Bed boards usually are made of plywood or some other firm material. The size varies with the needs of the situation. If sections of the bed such as the head and foot can be raised, it may be necessary to have the board divided and held together with hinges. For home use, full bed boards can be purchased or they can be made from sheets of plywood.

Pillows

The primary purposes of pillows are to provide support and elevation of a body part. Small pillows are ideal for support or elevation of the head, extremities, shoulders, or incisional wounds. Specially designed, heavy pillows are useful to elevate the upper part of the body when an adjustable bed is not available as, for example, in the home.

Turning Sheet

Most healthy individuals reposition themselves several times an hour, even during sleep. Many ill or injured patients are inactive. This may be due to weakness, loss of consciousness, sedation, or pain. The nurse assumes the responsibility of turning a patient who is inactive. Methods for turning and moving a patient are described later.

A turning sheet is a helpful positioning device. It is used to prevent friction while a helpless patient is moved, lifted, and tilted from side to side. The sheet can also be used to help transfer a patient from the bed onto a stretcher.

A draw sheet or a separate flat sheet folded in quarters can be used as a turning sheet. The sheet extends from the upper back to the upper thighs. Nurses on each side of the bed roll the sheet closely to the patient's body. Each grasps the rolled sheet tightly. Working as a team they slide and roll the patient into an alternate position. Care must be taken to keep the sheet dry and free of wrinkles.

Sandbags

Sandbags are used when an extremity needs firm support. They can be used to keep the foot or leg from turning outward. When sandbags are properly filled, they are not hard or rigid, but rather pliable. They can be shaped to fit body contours. To promote proper alignment and positioning, sandbags can be placed along the outer surface of the leg from the hip to the knee or ankle. They should be placed so that they do not create pressure on bony prominences. They should be covered with absorbent material, such as a sheet or bath blanket, to avoid accumulation of moisture next to the skin. These precautions help prevent the development of a decubitus ulcer. Sandbags are available in various sizes.

Trochanter Rolls

Trochanter rolls prevent the legs from turning outward. They received their name from anatomical landmarks of the femur. The femur is the long, large bone in the thigh. The trochanters are bony ridges at the head of the femur near the hip. The top of the femur and the depression into which it fits within the pelvis form the ball and socket joint of the hip. This type of joint permits the leg to be moved in multiple directions, one of which is outward rotation. Placing a positioning device at the trochanter helps to keep the leg from rotating outward. Trochanter rolls are illustrated in Figure 18-2. They can be made and used in the following manner:

- Fold a sheet lengthwise in half or in thirds and place it under the patient so that it extends from the hips to about the knees.
- Place a rolled-up bath blanket or two bath towels under each end of the sheet that extends on either side of the patient. If the roll is too short, the leg will have very little support.
- Roll the sheet around the blanket so that the end of the roll is underneath. In this way, it cannot unroll itself and the weight of the patient will hold it securely. The patient will be lying on a section of linen that has a large roll on either side of him so that his legs cannot turn outward.
- Fix the rolls close to the patient and firmly against the hips and thigh on each side.

Hand Rolls

The most important hand function to preserve is the ability to grasp and pick up objects. If positioning of the hands is overlooked, they will become so contracted that they may no longer be useful. To maintain their function, the thumb is held away from the hand slightly and at a moderate angle to the fingers. A rolled washcloth or a ball secured in the hand can be used to maintain this position. There are several commercial hand supports available, like the one in Figure 18-3. They are especially helpful if the patient needs hand and thumb support for extended periods of time.

Positioning should always be accompanied by periodic movement and exercise. Positioning the hands alone will not prevent contractures from forming, but if they occur, the thumb and fingers will still be in a position for some use.

Footboard and Foot Splints

Footboards and foot splints are used primarily to keep the feet in the normal walking position. This position prevents foot drop, which is illustrated in Figure 18-4. The board is placed between the foot of the bedstead and the mattress. If the patient is short and cannot reach the board, a foot splint can be used. The splint may be an improvised sturdy box or wooden block padded with linen. On some commercial foot-boards, there are supports that hold the foot in dorsiflexion as well as prevent outward rotation of the foot and lower leg. Another type fastens to the sides of the mattress with a clamp. It can then be placed on the mattress in the appropriate position for the patient. A foot splint is illustrated in Figure 18-5. Some nurses have found that having the patient wear ankle-high tennis shoes in bed will also help prevent foot drop. The shoes must be removed regularly, and proper foot care should be given.

If a foot splint or footboard is not readily available, a temporary foot support can be made with a pillow and large sheet. The pillow is rolled in the sheet, and the ends

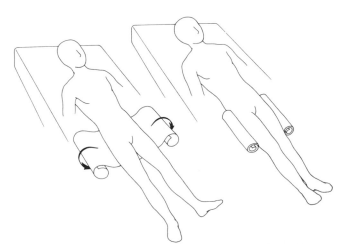

Figure 18-2 These two sketches illustrate how trochanter rolls are used to support the patient's hips so that the legs do not rotate outwardly.

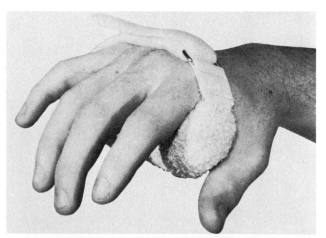

Figure 18-3 This is an example of a palm grip that helps prevent contractures of the fingers and thumb. (Courtesy of the JT Posey Corporation, Arcadia, CA.)

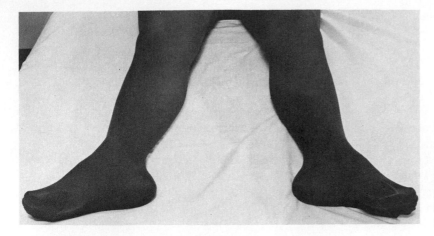

Figure 18-4 This is a typical position of the legs and feet when they are not properly supported in bed. The toes point downward and the legs rotate outward.

of the sheet are twisted before being tucked under the mattress. The tucked ends should be placed under the mattress at an angle toward the head of the bed to help keep the pillow in place. A pillow support does not provide the firmness of a board or splint and, therefore, should eventually be replaced as soon as possible with something more sturdy.

Foot splints such as the ones shown in Figure 18-6 are also used to prevent foot drop. A foot splint allows more variety of body positioning while still maintaining the foot in a neutral position.

Trapeze

A *trapeze* is a triangular piece of metal hung by a chain over the head of the bed. The patient grasps a trapeze and can then move himself about in bed. Unless arm movement or lifting is undesirable, a trapeze is an excellent device to help and encourage a bedridden patient to be active. A trapeze is illustrated in Figure 18-7.

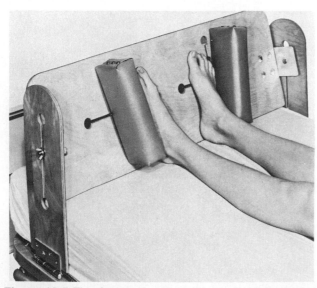

Figure 18-5 This foot support can be fastened at any level along the side of the mattress. Special supports help prevent the feet and legs from rotating outward. (Courtesy of the JT Posey Company, Arcadia, CA.)

Using Protective Bed Devices

Several other items assist the patient with independent activity. Some protect the inactive patient from harm or complications.

Siderails

Siderails are a valuable self-help device to aid patients in changing their own position, moving about, and exercising while in bed. For example, with siderails in place, the patient can safely turn himself from side to side and sit up in bed. These activities help patients maintain or regain muscle strength and joint flexibility after periods of time when they have had to lie in bed.

Mattress Overlays

The skin of anyone confined to bed is predisposed to break down. Several items can be placed over a standard hospital mattress that aid in the prevention or early treatment of impaired skin due to pressure.

Pressure is greatest over an area where a bony prominence is in contact with a hard surface. There is not much resilience. The blood vessels are easily compressed to the point that blood flow is occluded. Tissue then dies and the skin no longer remains healthy and intact.

Foam Mattress. Several types of foam mattresses are available. They are made from latex or polyethylene and covered with a sheet. Many are convoluted or made with a series of elevations and depressions so as to resemble an egg crate. Others are waffle cut and are much thicker. The density of the foam and the manner in which the foam is formed determines the degree of pressure reduction formed. Egg-crate foam mattresses provide minimal pressure reduction and are often used for comfort only. Thicker waffle-shaped foams offer much greater pressure reduction and can be used to prevent skin breakdown.

Foam acts almost like a layer of subcutaneous tissue. It conforms to the patient's body shape and acts like a cushion. It redistributes the pressure over a greater area, thus reducing the effect on one or a few specific parts of the

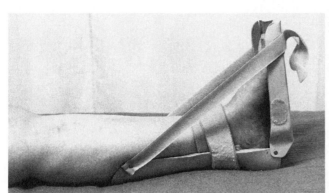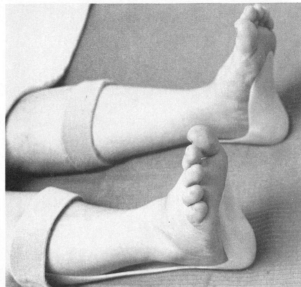

Figure 18-6 These are two different types of foot splints that are applied directly to the patient.

body. Foam contains channels and cells filled with air. This allows some evaporation of moisture and escape of heat, which also reduces the potential for skin breakdown.

Gel and foam cushions also have been used in a similar way. When placed in a wheelchair, they prevent the "hammock effect." This refers to the posterior and lateral compression concentrated on the coccyx and hips that occurs when sitting in a vinyl sling.

Static Air Mattress. A static air pressure mattress is one that is filled with a fixed volume of air. It is similar in appearance to those used at the beach or for camping. It suspends the patient on a buoyant surface and distributes the pressure on the underlying tissue. There is much less possibility for evaporation of moisture than with foam because of the nonabsorbent quality of plastic. Sharp objects can damage the integrity of the mattress. If the mattress becomes underinflated so that the patient is no longer lifted off the bed, its effectiveness as a pressure-relieving device is lost.

Alternating Air Mattress. An alternating air mattress is similar to one that is static with one exception. Every other channel inflates as the one next to it deflates. The process is then reversed. Through the wave-like redistribution of air, pressure over bony prominences is cyclically changed. This process allows improvement of blood flow with enough frequency to keep the tissue supplied with oxygen.

It is important that the tubing connecting the mattress to its motor-driven compressor does not become kinked. Some patients are disturbed by the noise.

Water Mattress. Water is another buoyant substance. A mattress filled with sufficient volume of water not only

supports the body weight but equalizes the pressure per square inch over the body surface. This effect is maintained regardless of any shift in a patient's body position. Many claim that sleeping in a water bed produces beneficial emotional and physical effects. Some say that the rocking motion produces a feeling of tranquility.

Water mattresses weigh a great deal. The structure of the floor and the frame of the bed must ensure that the weight can be supported. Puncturing leads to damage. Filling and

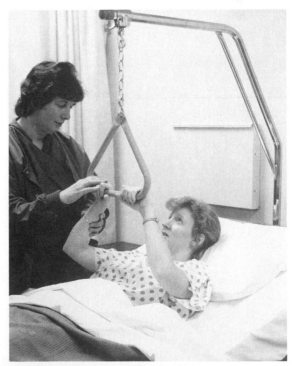

Figure 18-7 The nurse explains how the patient can lift herself and move about in bed by using the trapeze.

emptying, though only done once, are nevertheless time consuming.

Cradle

Tight linen over the toes can contribute to foot drop. Recall that a toe pleat or fold in the top sheet is used to avoid this. A high footboard may also be used to help keep the bed linen off the patient's feet or legs. A cradle is a frame that is usually made of metal and constructed so that it can be secured to the mattress. It forms a shell over the patient's lower legs. It is often used for patients with burns, painful joint disease, and fractures of the leg.

Using Specialty Beds

A variety of specialty beds can be used to relieve pressure as well as prevent other problems associated with inactivity and immobility. Specialty beds provide modified mattresses and frames with more functions than a standard hospital bed, even one with a mattress overlay.

Specialty beds are costly. Their use is billed separately. Therefore, the condition of the patient should justify the selection of a specialty bed. Table 18-1 identifies the indications when particular types of beds may be considered.

Current medical equipment manufacturers are working to redesign a more therapeutic mattress for hospital beds so that the need for specialty beds will be reduced. This is undoubtedly to prepare for the possibility that Medicare and other insurance carriers will eliminate or reduce payments billed for their use.

Low-Air-Loss Bed

A low-air-loss bed, shown in Figure 18-8, is one that contains inflated air sacs within its mattress. It maintains capillary pressure well below pressure that could interfere with blood flow. The bed can be adjusted to a variety of positions, such as sitting, and flat with the head lower or higher than the feet. Regardless of the changes in position, the mattress selectively responds by redistributing the air to maintain low pressure to all skin areas.

Air-Fluidized Bed

This air-fluidized bed, shown in Figure 18-9, contains a collection of tiny beads within a mattress cover. The beads

Table 18-1. Pressure-Relieving Devices

Device	Examples	Indications for Use
Foam mattress or gel cushion	Egg crate Geo-Matt® Spencegel® pad	Intact skin and minimal risk for breakdown Changes in position occur spontaneously or require minimal assistance
Static air, alternating air, or water mattress	TENDER™ Cloud Sof-Care® Pulsair® Lotus	At some risk for skin breakdown OR The skin has a superficial or single deep break but pressure is easily relieved
Oscillating support bed	Roto Rest® Tilt and Turn Paragon 9000	Need for prolonged bedrest with immobilization At high risk for systemic effects of immobility, such as pneumonia and skin breakdown
Low-air-loss bed	KinAir® FLEXICAIR® Mediscus	Combination of the following: Impaired skin Risk factors for further skin breakdown continue to exist Altering positions is limited, less than adequate, or impossible Requires assistance for frequent transfers from bed
Air-fluidized bed	CLINITRON® FluidAir®	Combination of the following: Impaired skin Risk factors for further skin breakdown continue to exist Altering positions is limited, less than adequate, or impossible Seldom transferred from bed
Circular bed	CircOlectric®	Current or high-risk for skin breakdown due to multiple trauma especially if it involves the head, neck, or spine Burns that require frequent dressing changes or topical applications

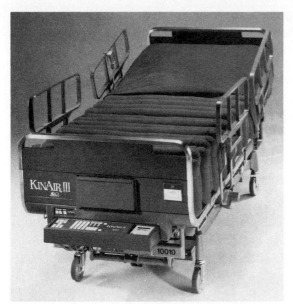

Figure 18-8 This is an example of a low-air-loss bed. (Courtesy of Kinetic Concepts, Inc., San Antonio, TX.)

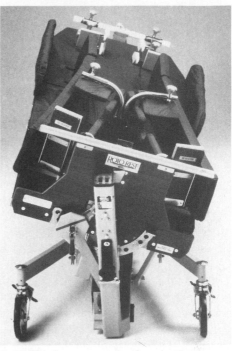

Figure 18-10 This is an example of an oscillating support bed. (Courtesy of Kinetic Concepts, Inc., San Antonio, TX.)

are blown upward on warm air. When suspended, the dry beads take on the characteristics of fluid. The patient literally floats on the lifted beads. Excretions and secretions drain away from the body and through the beads. This prevents skin irritation and maceration from moisture. The pressure-relieving effects of this type of bed have been shown to speed the healing of severely impaired tissue.

An air-fluidized bed is better allocated for a patient who is difficult to transfer in and out of bed and is, therefore, likely to remain in bed for long periods of time. Fluid balance may become a patient-care problem because of accelerated evaporation caused by the warm, blowing air. Puncturing or tearing the mattress is also a potential problem affecting function.

Oscillating Support Bed

Oscillation is the swinging between two extremes of an arc. Fans that oscillate turn on a fixed base circulating air in various directions. An oscillating bed is based on the same principle. It relieves skin pressure by continuously rocking the patient slowly from side to side in a 124° arc as shown in Figure 18-10. Foam-covered supports applied to the head, arms, and legs prevent sliding and shearing of skin.

Oscillation also helps to mobilize respiratory secretions and reduce pulmonary complications. The bed moves the patient over 300 times per day (Bennett–Canclini, 1985), a

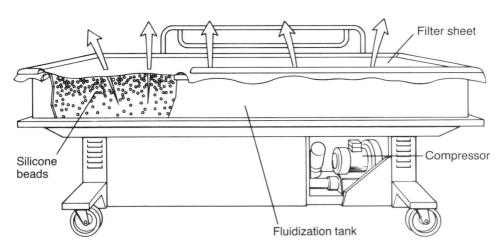

Filter sheet

Silicone beads

Compressor

Fluidization tank

Figure 18-9 Air blows through silicone beads on an air-fluidized bed. This reduces pressure on the capillaries, which helps maintain blood flow.

record that would be difficult to match even with continuous nursing care. Compartments within the bed can be removed temporarily to facilitate assessment and care of the posterior body.

Circular Bed

A circular bed has the capacity to rotate the patient in a full 360° circle. However, the rotation is not continuous, as it is with an oscillating bed. The circular bed, shown in Figure 18-11, supports the patient on a 6- or 7-foot anterior or posterior platform suspended across the diameter of the frame. While in motion, the patient is sandwiched between the two.

This bed allows the patient to remain passively immobilized during a position change. Because the bed mechanically rotates the patient, there is less strain on the nurse. Patients with extensive burns experience less pain with repositioning. Turning facilitates access to the patient from all aspects for nursing care. Instructed patients can learn how to operate the bed in order to make minor adjustments in their own position. This promotes a sense of control among otherwise dependent patients.

Turning and Moving the Patient

Before learning to position a patient, the nurse must learn skills for turning and moving a patient. These skills are important to prevent injury to the nurse and the patient. Many of the principles of body mechanics are related to

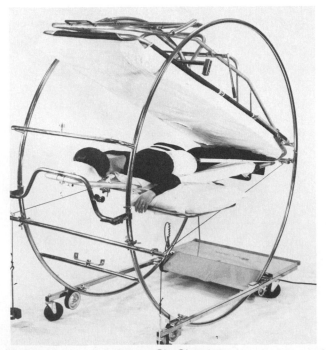

Figure 18-11 In this photo, a CircOlectric bed has been turned so that the patient rests in the prone position. (Courtesy of the Stryker Corporation, Kalamazoo, MI.)

the techniques for turning and moving an individual whose weight may equal or exceed that of the nurse. Skill Procedures 18-1 and 18-2 describe and illustrate the suggested actions when the patient requires turning and moving.

Positioning the Patient Confined to Bed

The proper positioning of the patient in bed is essential to promote comfort and provide for proper body alignment. Changing positions in bed may be the only exercise some patients get. An inactive patient's position should be changed at least every two hours. It should be done more frequently if any signs or symptoms of the disuse syndrome have been assessed. When the position of the patient is changed, it presents a good opportunity for providing skin care. Techniques for skin care are described in Chapter 20.

The Supine Position

The *supine position* is one in which the person lies on his back. There are two primary concerns when using the supine position. One concern is pressure on the back of the body where pressure sores commonly develop, especially in the area at the end of the spine. The second is toe pressure from linens, which, when combined with gravity, forces the feet into the foot-drop position.

The Lateral Position

A *lateral position* is one in which an individual lies on his side. Foot drop is of less concern in this position because the feet are not being pulled down by gravity as they are when the patient lies on his back. However, there is concern when using this position if the upper shoulder and arm are allowed to rotate forward and fall out of alignment. This tends to interfere with proper breathing.

The Prone Position

A *prone position* is one in which an individual lies on his abdomen. Lying on the abdomen is a comfortable and relaxing position for many patients. It is a helpful alternative for the person with pressure sores. The position also provides for good drainage from bronchioles, stretches the trunk and extremities, and keeps the hips in an extended position. However, the prone position is often contraindicated when the patient has respiratory distress or heart disease, since it interferes with chest expansion. It may be uncomfortable for patients with recent abdominal surgery or those with back pain.

Fowler's Position

Fowler's position is a sitting position. With the head of the bed elevated 45 to 60°, it is referred to as a semi-Fowler's

(Text continues on page 395)

Skill Procedure 18-1. Turning the Patient

Suggested Action	**Reason for Action**

Turning the Patient From His Back Onto His Side

Turning the Patient Toward the Nurse
Raise the bed to the high position.

The nurse needs to maintain adequate balance and prepare to center the weight over the widest base of support.

Have the patient flex his knees and place his arms across his chest.

This positioning helps prevent the patient from rolling back, partially prepares him for lying on his side, and prevents him from rolling onto his arm.

Place one hand on the patient's shoulder and one on the hip on the far side.

The heaviest part of the body is centered in the pelvis. Using the arms and hands in this way will help move the patient most efficiently by distributing the weight more evenly.

Spread the feet, flex the knees, place one foot behind the other, and while rocking backward, gently roll the patient, as illustrated in Figure 18-12.

This provides a wide base of support for balance. It makes use of the longest and strongest muscles. Rocking provides a momentum and uses the nurse's own body weight to reduce the effort required to move the patient.

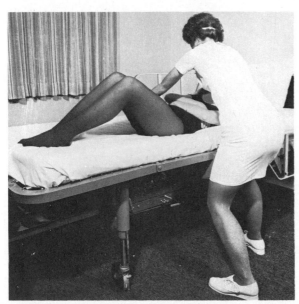

Figure 18-12 Notice the nurse's position as she prepares to rock backward while turning the model from her back to her side.

Raise the siderails on the working side and move to the other side of the bed.

Having siderails in place prevents the patient from rolling out of bed.

Turning the Patient Away From the Nurse
Raise the bed to the high position.

The nurse needs to maintain adequate balance and distribute the weight over the widest base of support.

Place a hand under the patient's shoulders, spread the feet, flex the knees, place one foot behind the other, and, while rocking backward, gently pull the patient to the middle of the bed.

This position creates momentum and uses the nurse's body weight to assist with moving the heaviest parts of the patient while distributing the bulk of the mass over the widest base of support.

OR

(continued)

Skill Procedure 18-1. Continued

Suggested Action	Reason for Action

Turning the Patient From His Back Onto His Side

Stand at the patient's shoulder area. While using the same foot positions, place the arms under the patient's shoulders and move the shoulders to the center of the bed. Move parallel to the patient's hips. Use the same actions to move the hips.

To prevent a personal injury, an alternative technique may be used if the nurse is slight, the patient is extremely heavy, or cannot help in any way. It involves moving portions of the patient's body in separate actions. This dual maneuver is shown in Figure 18-13.

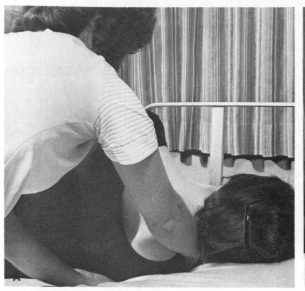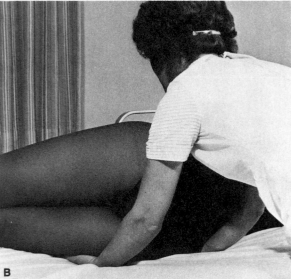

Figure 18-13 The lightweight patient can be moved to the center of the bed in one maneuver. For most adults, it is best to move the shoulders first (*A*) and then the hips (*B*).

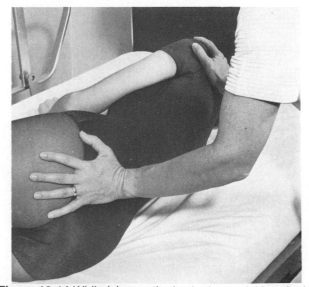

Figure 18-14 While lying on the back, the model is asked to flex her knees. The nurse then gently pushes the model at the hip and shoulder areas to roll her away from the nurse.

(continued)

Skill Procedure 18-1. Continued

Suggested Action	Reason for Action

Turning the Patient From His Back Onto His Side

Continue to spread the feet and flex the knees. The nurse can roll the patient away by pushing at the shoulder and hip areas of the patient, as shown in Figure 18-14.	Lowering the nurse's center of gravity, distributing weight over a wide base, and using the longest and strongest muscles facilitate moving a patient while avoiding personal injury. Rolling requires less effort than lifting because it avoids overcoming gravity.

Turning the Patient From His Back Onto His Abdomen

Turning the Patient Toward the Nurse

Place the patient's arm nearest the nurse under his buttock with the palm up. Bring the far leg over the leg nearest the nurse, and turn the patient's face away from the nurse, as illustrated in Figure 18-15.	This position secures the patient's arm and leg so that he does not injure or roll onto them and prevents him from turning onto his face.
Grasp the patient's far hand and hip. The nurse's feet should be spread, the knees flexed, and one foot should be behind the other. Gently pull on the arm while rolling the hips toward the nurse, turning the patient onto his abdomen, as shown in Figure 18-16.	This positioning will roll the heaviest parts of the patient's body comfortably. The nurse's positioning gives stability by providing a wide base of support and lowering the center of gravity. The body weight of the nurse is used to assist the nurse's arms while rolling the patient.
Move the patient to the center of the bed.	Centering the patient provides sufficient area to position the head, arms, and legs properly.

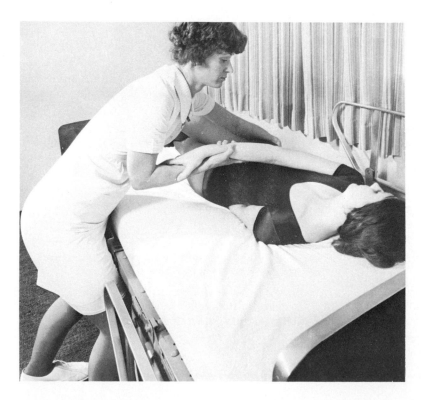

Figure 18-15 The nurse grasps the model's far hand and hip and prepares to rock backward to turn the patient from the back-lying to the face-lying position.

(continued)

Skill Procedure 18-1. *Continued*

Suggested Action	Reason for Action

Turning the Patient From His Back Onto His Abdomen

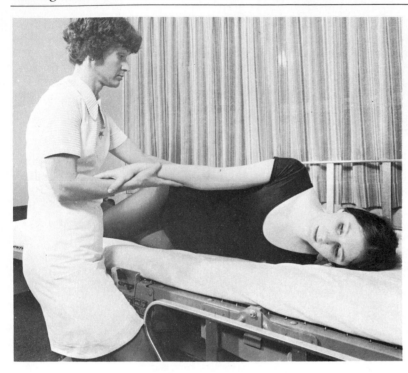

Figure 18-16 As the nurse rocks backward, she brings the model from her back to her abdomen while gently pulling on the far arm and hip to roll the model toward her.

Turning the Patient Away From the Nurse

Raise the siderails on the opposite side of the bed.

The raised siderail will prevent the patient from accidentally rolling out of bed.

Stand on the side of the bed with the lowered siderails and move the patient toward the nurse.

Bringing the patient toward the nurse avoids stretching and allows room to accommodate the patient's body after it is turned.

Place the patient's arm that is most distant from the nurse under the buttock, with the palm up. Bring the near leg over the far leg, and turn the patient's head toward the nurse, as illustrated in Figure 18-17.

This positioning helps prevent the patient from rolling onto his face and arm and secures his leg for comfortable rolling.

Place one arm under the patient's upper leg with an elbow at the level of the patient's buttock. Place the other arm under the patient's shoulders with a hand on his lower shoulder.

This positioning will help move the heaviest parts of the patient's body comfortably.

The feet of the nurse should be spread, and the knees should be flexed.

This positioning gives stability by providing a wide base of support and balance.

Pull by straightening the arms. This will gently roll the patient onto his abdomen, as illustrated in Figure 18-18. With this maneuver, the patient is centered on the bed.

The strongest muscles in the arms are used to roll the heaviest parts of the patient's body. Pulling, pushing, and rolling use less effort than lifting.

(continued)

Skill Procedure 18-1. Continued

Suggested Action	Reason for Action

Turning the Patient From His Back Onto His Abdomen

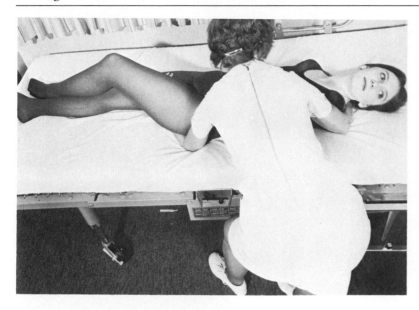

Figure 18-17 The nurse prepares to roll the model from her back to her abdomen. The model will roll away from the nurse.

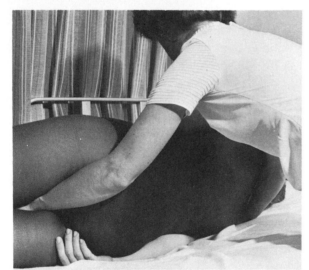

Figure 18-18 The nurse straightens her arms and the model rolls from her back to her abdomen.

Turning the Patient From His Abdomen Onto His Back

First Technique

Place the patient's hand that is most distant from the nurse under the thigh on the same side. Cross his near leg over his far leg, and turn the patient's face toward the nurse.

This positioning secures the patient's arm and leg so that he does not injure or roll on them and prevents him from turning onto his face.

Grasp the patient's far hand by reaching under the patient. Place the other hand on the patient's uppermost hip, as illustrated in Figure 18-19.

This positioning will prepare the nurse for pulling and rolling the patient.

(continued)

Skill Procedure 18-1. Continued

Suggested Action	Reason for Action

Turning the Patient From His Abdomen Onto His Back

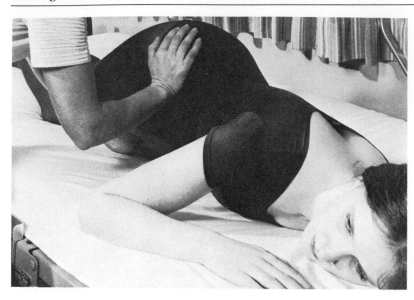

Figure 18-19 The nurse grasps the model's far hand and prepares to push on the near hip to have the model roll from her abdomen to her back.

Spread the feet and flex both knees.

This positioning gives stability by providing a wide base of support and balance.

Pull the patient's hand while pushing on his hip and gently roll him away onto his back, as illustrated in Figure 18-20.

This motion uses the strong muscles of the arms to roll the heaviest parts of the patient's body. Pulling and rolling require less effort than lifting.

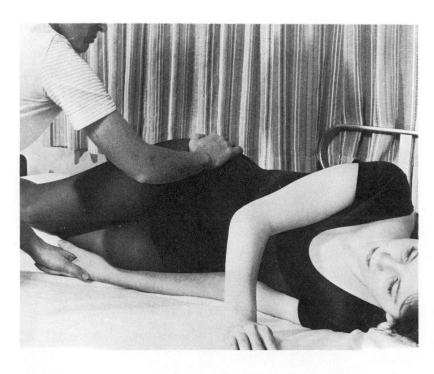

Figure 18-20 The nurse pulls on the model's far hand and pushes on the near hip as the model rolls from her abdomen to her back.

(continued)

Skill Procedure 18-1. Continued

Suggested Action	Reason for Action

Turning the Patient From His Abdomen Onto His Back

Second Technique

Place the patient's far hand under his far thigh, cross his near leg over his far leg, and turn the patient's face in the direction of the nurse. One arm of the nurse should be inserted between the patient's legs to a level where the elbow is even with the patient's knee. The nurse's hand should be on the patient's thigh. The other arm is placed under the patient's chest with that hand on his far shoulder.

This positioning secures the patient's arm and leg so that he does not injure or roll on them and prevents him from turning on his face. This positioning will prepare the nurse to pull and roll the patient.

Spread the feet and flex the knees.

This positioning gives stability by providing a wide base of support and balance.

Pull, using both arms, and use the momentum gently to roll the patient onto his back.

This motion uses the strong muscles of the arms to roll the heaviest parts of the patient's body. Pulling and rolling require less effort than lifting.

Turning the Heavy Patient Onto His Back, Using Two Nurses

One nurse should stand at the patient's head with one arm under the patient's upper chest with the hand on the far shoulder. The patient's face should be turned toward the nurse.

This technique uses two people, each of whom moves an area that involves the heaviest parts of the patient's body.

The second nurse should place the patient's hand at his side with the palm up. One arm is inserted between the legs of the patient grasping the hand of the patient. The second hand is placed on the near hip. The positions of the two nurses prior to turning can be seen in Figure 18-21.

The second nurse will be helping to move the lower area of the body as the first nurse moves the upper body. The patient is positioned in such a way that injury will not occur during rolling.

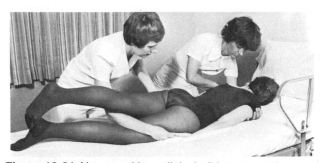

Figure 18-21 Nurses with a slight build may need to work together to turn a patient who is heavy. Each nurse is in the proper position to turn the patient.

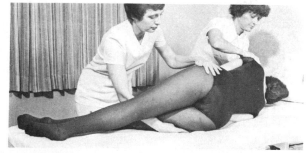

Figure 18-22 Two nurses share the work of turning a patient from the abdomen onto the back.

The nurse at the upper area of the body pulls on the lower shoulder while pushing on the upper one. The second nurse pulls the patient's hand and pushes on the patient's hip. Figure 18-22 shows the patient being gently turned from the abdomen onto his back.

The opposing movements serve to roll the patient onto his back. Pulling, pushing, and rolling require less effort than lifting.

Skill Procedure 18-2. Moving the Patient Up in Bed

Suggested Action	Reason for Action

One-Person Technique When the Patient Can Assist

First Technique

Remove the pillows from under the patient's head and place one against the headboard.

Have the patient flex his knees and place one arm under the patient's shoulders and the other under his hips, as illustrated in Figure 18-23.

The pillow at the head of the bed prevents having the patient accidentally hit the headboard as he is moved.

The patient flexes his knees so that he can assist by pushing with the strong muscles of his legs. The nurse uses the strong muscles of the arms to move the heaviest part of the patient's body comfortably.

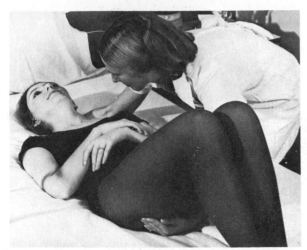

Figure 18-23 The nurse hugs the model by grasping her under the buttocks and shoulder to move her up in bed. Notice that a pillow protects the headboard.

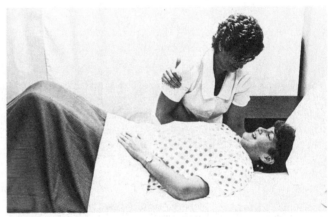

Figure 18-24 The nurse and the patient lock arms so that each can share in the work of moving upward in bed. The knees of the patient are flexed to help push as the nurse pulls the patient's upper body.

Assume a position of hugging the patient.

Spread the feet, flex the knees, and rock toward the head of the bed while the patient pushes with his feet.

It is easier to move a heavy object when it is close to one's center of gravity.

Such positioning and motion give the nurse stability by providing a wide base of support and balance. Rocking creates momentum that combines with the nurse's body weight to assist the muscles of the upper arms to move the patient up in bed.

Second Technique

Repeat positioning the pillow and flexing the patient's knees as described previously.

The nurse should stand facing the head of the bed. The patient and the nurse should lock arms. This is done when the nurse grasps the patient's shoulder while the patient grasps the nurse's upper arm. The nurse's opposite arm should be placed under the patient's shoulder, supporting the head and neck as shown in Figure 18-24.

Spread the feet by placing one foot in front of the other, and flex the knees.

Care must be taken to avoid injuring the head of the patient. The patient will use the strong muscles of his legs to help move his body.

Locking arms doubles the arm strength for moving. Using mutual strength and the strong muscles in the patient's lower legs eases movement.

Placing one foot in front of the other forms a wide base of support and balance. Flexing the knees helps use the strongest muscles of the legs more efficiently.

(continued)

Skill Procedure 18-2. Continued

Suggested Action	Reason for Action

One-Person Technique When the Patient Can Assist

Rock back and forth, putting weight on one foot and then on the other while counting 1, 2, 3. Explain to the patient that on the count of three, which will coincide with the forward rocking motion, the patient should push with his legs as the nurse pulls the locked arm.

Momentum, using strong muscles, and coordinated effort help move the weight of the patient up in bed with the least amount of effort.

Two-Person Technique

When the Nurses Slide the Patient
Protect the headboard with a pillow, as described previously.

Have the nurses, who are facing each other on opposite sides of the bed between the patient's hips and shoulders, join hands under the widest part of the patient's shoulders and hips.

This positioning facilitates moving the heaviest parts of the patient's body comfortably and provides for the best use of the nurses' arm muscles.

The nurses should spread their feet, flex their knees, and lean close to the patient by locking hands with each other under the patient's buttocks and shoulders, as illustrated in Figure 18-25.

This positioning provides a wide base of support and balance and moves the weight of the patient into the nurse's center of gravity.

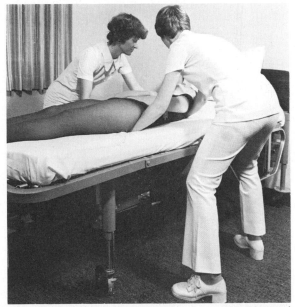

Figure 18-25 These nurses are properly positioned to rock as they move the model up in bed.

Rock in unison toward the head of the bed. Upon a previously agreed signal, move the patient up in bed. The patient may even assist by flexing his knees and pushing when the signal is given.

Momentum, and using the coordinated strength of each person's muscles, will help move the weight of a patient with ease. Rocking, pushing, and pulling require less effort than lifting.

(continued)

Skill Procedure 18-2. Continued

Suggested Action	Reason for Action

Two-Person Technique

When the Nurses Slide the Patient, Using a Drawsheet
Protect the headboard with a pillow, as explained previously.

Place a drawsheet under the patient so that it extends from the patient's head to below his buttocks and roll the sides of the sheet up close to each side of the patient's body.

The sheet will act as a sling to help carry and slide the patient up in bed.

Have the nurses, who are facing the foot of the bed on opposite sides near the patient's chest and waist, take a firm grip of the rolled drawsheet on each side, as illustrated in Figure 18-26.

This positioning prepares the nurses to use their arm muscles and the weight of their bodies to slide the patient, using the drawsheet.

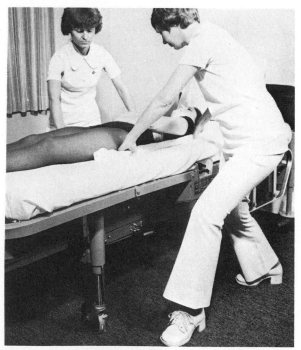

Figure 18-26 The nurses grasp the rolled drawsheet and rock to move the model up in bed.

Have the nurses spread their feet, place the leg nearest the bed behind them, flex their knees, and rock backward. Upon reaching a given signal that coincides with a backward motion, the nurses slide the patient up in the bed.

Such positioning and motion give the nurses stability by providing a wide base of support and balance. They use their own weight, momentum, and the strongest muscles in the arms and legs to slide the patient. Sliding requires less effort than lifting.

At the completion of the rocking motion, each nurse has the elbow nearest the patient on the mattress.

If the technique has been performed correctly, the elbow will rest on the mattress to counteract the shift in the center of gravity.

This same procedure can be performed with the nurses facing the head of the bed.

Some nurses prefer to observe the face of the patient and the progress of the movement toward the head of the bed. However, the work seems easier when the backward rock is used, perhaps because different combinations of muscles are used.

position; a 90° elevation is a high Fowler's position. This position is especially helpful for patients with dyspnea. It causes abdominal organs to drop away from the diaphragm, relieving pressure on the chest cavity. This allows the lungs and heart to fill efficiently. It also makes eating, conversing, and looking about easier than from a lying position.

Skill Procedure 18-3 illustrates and describes how to position a patient properly in the supine, lateral, prone, and Fowler's positions.

Transferring the Patient

In this chapter, the word *transfer* refers to moving a patient from place to place. For example, the patient is transferred when he is moved from a bed to a chair and back to bed, or to and from a stretcher. The patient assists in an active transfer; transfer done entirely by others or by mechanical means is a passive transfer.

Basic Guidelines When Transferring the Patient

Certain techniques are used when transferring a patient to help prevent injury to the patient as well as to the nurse. The following are basic recommended guidelines:

Know the patient's diagnosis, capabilities, weaknesses, and any movement he is not allowed. For example, patients who have had surgery on bones or joints may not be permitted full weight bearing or certain movements.

Put on braces and other devices a patient may use before getting him out of bed.

Plan exactly what will be done while transferring a patient so that the appropriate techniques will be used. Without planning, the nurse or the patient may be injured.

Explain what will be done to the patient. Then, use his ability to assist as much as possible to reduce the work.

Remove obstacles that may make transferring more difficult. For example, furniture such as chairs, bedside tables, and overbed tables should not be in the way.

Elevate the patient's bed as necessary so that the work is being done at a safe and comfortable level.

Lock the wheels of the bed, wheelchair, or stretcher so that they cannot slide about as the patient is moved.

Observe sound principles of body mechanics so that muscles are not strained and injured. It is a good idea to review these principles in Chapter 9 before transferring a patient.

Be sure to keep the patient in proper alignment during transfer procedures so that the patient is also protected from strain and muscle injury.

Support the patient's body, especially near the joints.

Avoid grabbing and holding an extremity by the muscles, which will injure tissues and often put unnecessary strain on joints.

Avoid causing friction on the patient's skin. Roll or push the patient when possible rather than pull him across bed linens. Friction can be reduced by sprinkling powder or cornstarch on the patient's skin and linens.

Use smooth rather than jerky movements when transferring the patient. Jerky motion tends to put extra strain on muscles and joints and is uncomfortable for the patient.

Use mechanical devices when they are available for transferring patients. Many health agencies have them and some persons also have these devices in their homes. Thoroughly understand how the device operates; be sure the patient is properly secured and is informed of what will occur. Patients who do not understand or are afraid may not be able to cooperate and may suffer injury as a result.

Be realistic about how much you can safely do without injury. Two small-statured women cannot safely lift and carry a patient weighing 250 pounds without straining their muscles.

Transferring the Patient To and From a Stretcher

Considerable care must be taken to prevent injuring the patient and the nurse when transferring a patient to and from a stretcher. If he is unconscious or helpless, the extremities and the head must be supported especially well.

The most convenient way to move a patient is to place a sheet under him and then pull carefully on the sheet to slide the patient from one surface to another such as from a bed to a stretcher and from a stretcher back to bed. When the patient must be lifted and carried, a three-carrier lift is recommended. It is described and illustrated in Skill Procedure 18-4.

Transferring the Patient from a Bed to a Chair and Back to Bed

A correct sitting position was described in Chapter 9. The chair in which a patient sits should make it possible for him to maintain good posture. Figure 18-34 illustrates ways in which necessary adjustments may be made when the chair does not accommodate a patient well.

In general, upholstered chairs should be avoided. The patient tends to sink into an upholstered chair, making it difficult for him to maintain good posture and to get into and out of it.

When the Patient Can Assist With the Transfer. If a patient can assist and stand while he is being transferred from a bed to a chair or wheelchair, the following techniques are used:

(Text continues on page 399)

Skill Procedure 18-3. Positioning the Patient

Suggested Action	Reason for Action
The Supine Position	
Remove all pillows and positioning devices used in the current position.	Positioning devices interfere with the movement of the patient.
Move the patient to the center of the bed.	Centering the patient provides sufficient area to properly position the head, arms, and legs.
Place a *small* pillow under the upper shoulders, neck, and head so that the head and neck are held in proper alignment.	The position of the head should appear similar to one if the patient were standing. The chin should not be pressed into the neck, nor should the head tilt backward.
Bring the arms out to the side, bend the elbows, and place the forearms on pillows so the palms face downward.	Slight flexion and pronation of the joints in the upper extremity promote comfort.
Place handrolls in the patient's hands, if necessary.	Handrolls help maintain the position for potential use of the fingers and thumb.
Elevate the wrist above the level of the elbows, and the elbows above the shoulder. This may be accomplished by compressing the pillow more at one end, or by overlapping two pillows.	Elevation helps drain blood from the distal areas of the body back to the heart.
Place a *small* roll just above the patient's knees, *not* directly under them. The knees should be bent only 5° to 10°.	Hyperextension of the knees must be avoided. Slight flexion is preferred. If the roll is placed under the knees or if they are bent more than 10°, the pressure may slow circulation through blood vessels or cause pressure and damage to nerves in the area.
Use a footboard to hold the patient's feet at right angles to his lower legs.	Maintaining the feet in a position of dorsiflexion will help to prevent foot drop.
Place sandbags or trochanter rolls alongside the hips and thighs. Figure 18-27 shows a patient who has been placed in a supine position.	Trochanter rolls help prevent permanent external rotation, which can also interfere with the ability to walk normally.

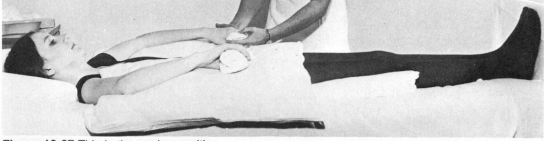

Figure 18-27 This is the supine position.

Suggested Action	Reason for Action
Arrange top linens, using a toe pleat, or spread them over a high footboard or cradle.	Relieving pressure on the toes helps to prevent footdrop.
The Lateral Position	
Remove all pillows and positioning devices used in the current position.	Positioning devices interfere with the movement of the patient.
Center and move the patient to the outer side of the bed.	There must be room for the arms and legs, which will extend from the midline of the body when using this position.

(continued)

Skill Procedure 18-3. Continued

Suggested Action	Reason for Action

The Lateral Position

Place a *small* pillow under the patient's head and neck.

This prevents rotation of the neck, which may lead to a contracture or, at the very least, some discomfort.

Place the arm on the side on which the patient is lying straight out from his body; bend the elbow about 90° so that it is resting alongside the pillow at the patient's head. This may be observed in Figure 18-28, which shows a person in a lateral position.

The patient should not lie on his arm. This can interfere with circulation. Pressure on nerves may cause the hand to feel tingly and numb. It can cause discomfort from the pressure of body weight.

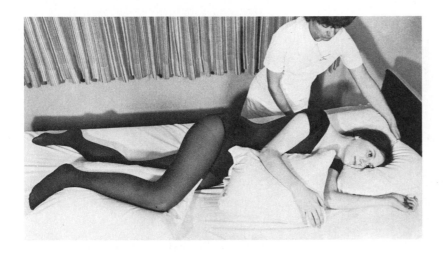

Figure 18-28 The model has been properly placed in a lateral position.

Place a pillow under the uppermost arm.

The pillow holds the arm in such a way as to promote circulation.

Use handrolls, if needed.

If the patient does not move one or both hands, handrolls may help prevent permanent loss of finger and thumb function.

Slightly bend the knee on the side on which the patient is lying.

Sligh· flexion promotes comfort for the patient.

Bring the top leg forward and slightly bend that knee also. Place pillows under the thigh, leg, and foot.

Supporting the upper leg in this manner prevents it from falling onto the bed and causing internal rotation and adduction of the femur.

Pull the hip on which the patient is lying slightly backward.

The hip is stabilized with this movement, thus preventing the patient from rolling forward.

Cover the patient with linen and blankets as desired.

The pressure and weight from linen is less likely to contribute to foot drop in this position than in others.

The Prone Position

Remove all pillows and positioning devices used in the current position.

Positioning devices interfere with the movement of the patient.

Move the patient down in bed so that when he is turned, his feet can be positioned over the edge of the mattress or be supported on pillows just high enough to keep the toes from touching the bed.

A prone position can contribute to foot drop unless the feet are positioned correctly. If a pillow is used, the knees should not be bent more than a few degrees to avoid contributing to a knee flexion contracture.

(continued)

Skill Procedure 18-3. Continued

Suggested Action	Reason for Action

The Prone Position

Place the arms at the side of the body or with the elbows flexed about 90°.

This prevents the patient from lying on his arms, which would interfere with comfort and circulation.

Use handrolls as indicated.

Handrolls help maintain functional use of the fingers and thumb.

Place a very *small* pillow under the patient's head if he wishes, or the head may rest directly on the mattress. The person in Figure 18-29 has been properly placed in a prone position.

A pillow supports the head and prevents flexion of the neck.

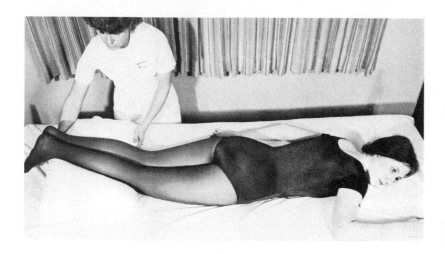

Figure 18-29 The nurse has placed this model in a prone position.

Slip a small pillow into the space at the lower end of the ribs and the upper abdomen if the patient is thin.

This type of support prevents hyperextension of the back and facilitates breathing.

Fowler's Position

Remove all pillows and positioning devices used in the current position.

Positioning devices interfere with the movement of the patient.

Center the patient on his back so that when the head is elevated, the break in the bed will be at the hips.

The back should be straight. Flexion at any point in the spine will cause discomfort from poor alignment and interfere with ventilation.

Raise the head of the bed to the desired height.

The height of elevation may be adjusted according to the physician's order, the comfort of the patient, or the activity the patient may perform.

Allow the patient's head to rest against the mattress, or support it with a small pillow.

The neck should not be flexed or hyperextended.

Support the forearms on pillows so that they are elevated sufficiently to prevent a pull on the patient's shoulders.

Pulling on the shoulders contributes to stress on the joint and discomfort.

Support the hands on pillows so that they are in line with the forearms and slightly elevated in relation to the elbows.

This positioning prevents a contracture at the wrist and promotes circulation through the hands.

(continued)

Skill Procedure 18-3. Continued

Suggested Action	Reason for Action

Fowler's Position

Use handrolls if the patient is extremely inactive.	Handrolls help to maintain the fingers and thumb in a functional position.
Elevate the knees for brief periods only. Figure 18-30 shows a person being placed in Fowler's position.	Flexion of the knees promotes comfort, but it may slow the circulation of blood from the legs and put pressure on nerves. Patients who have had blood clots or who are at risk for developing them should never have the bed gatched at the knees. Prolonged flexion of the knees can cause contractures that interfere with standing and walking.

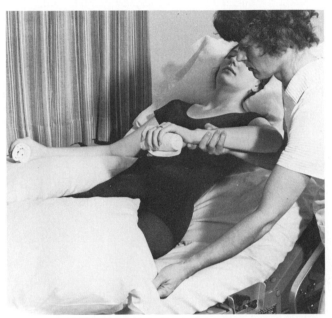

Figure 18-30 The model is in Fowler's position. Notice that the break in the bed is at the hips so that the back is in proper alignment.

Support the feet at right angles to the lower legs using pillows, and footboard, or a foot splint.	Keeping the foot in a position of dorsiflexion will prevent foot drop.

Use equipment with firm and stable surfaces. If the mattress is soft and the patient sinks into it, place a bedboard under it before transferring the patient to a chair or wheelchair.

Take the patient's condition into account. For example, if the patient is weaker on one side of his body than on the other, or if he has a leg or arm that is weaker than the other, transfer him to his stronger side. This means placing a chair or wheelchair alongside the bed on the patient's stronger side.

Make the distance for transferring as short as possible. Place the chair or wheelchair parallel to and near to the head of the bed. Be sure the wheels of a wheelchair are locked and the foot supports are in the up position.

Place short bedrails in the up position so that the patient can grasp a rail to sit up in bed and steady himself as he moves. This is illustrated in Figure 18-35.

Stand on the side of the bed on which the patient will be moving. Do not reach across the bed to assist the patient. Help the patient to a sitting position.

Allow the patient to sit a few seconds until you are sure he is not feeling faint.

Pivot the patient a quarter of a turn by supporting his shoulders and legs.

Dress the patient appropriately, as he sits at the side of the bed. If he is going to walk, help him put on shoes and stockings. Hard-soled and well-fitting shoes will give him more support than will loose, floppy slippers.

Place the bed in the low position.

(Text continues on page 402)

Skill Procedure 18-4. Transferring the Patient To and From a Stretcher

Suggested Action	Reason for Action

From a Bed to a Stretcher

Place the stretcher at a right angle to the foot of the bed with the brakes locked.

This places the stretcher out of the way when the carriers pivot from the bed, yet close enough so that the patient will only need to be lifted and carried a short distance.

Arrange the carriers according to height, with the tallest person at the patient's head.

The tallest person usually has the longest arm grasp, making it easier to support the patient's head and chest.

Stand facing the patient while sliding arms under him. The arms of the middle carrier are placed under the patient's waist and buttocks. One arm of the carrier at the head is under the patient's head, neck, and shoulder area and the other arm is directly against the middle carrier's arm at the bottom of the patient's chest. The carrier at the patient's feet has one arm against the middle carrier's lower arm and the other arm under the patient's legs and ankles, as shown in Figure 18-31.

The greatest weight is in the middle of the body. Having the middle carrier's armspread smaller than that of the others and supported by the other two carriers helps prevent strain on this person.

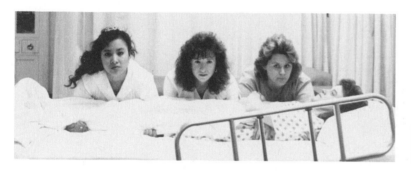

Figure 18-31 The patient has been moved to the edge of the bed and the carriers are positioned to lift her.

Slide the arms under the patient as far as possible and slide the patient to the edge of the bed.

Moving the patient near to the carriers at the edge of the bed helps position the mass of the patient within the nurses' center of gravity. This makes it easier and safer to lift the patient.

Spread the feet and flex the knees.

This position provides a wide base of support and balance. It prepares for using the leg muscles more effectively.

Place the arms further underneath the patient and log-roll him onto the chests of all three carriers at the same time the patient is being lifted from the bed. During logrolling, the patient's head should turn with his shoulders. Figure 18-32 illustrates the position of the carriers and patient when he is lifted from the bed.

Rolling reduces the effort of lifting. Keeping the patient's head and shoulders straight places the back in correct alignment.

Pivot and move to the stretcher. On signal, bend the knees, as the body of each carrier is lowered with that of the patient, as shown in Figure 18-33.

This maneuver reduces the strain on the back muscles of the carriers while letting the large leg and arm muscles do the work of lowering the patient.

Secure additional persons if the patient is extremely heavy, has a large cast, or in some other way presents special problems.

Nurses are responsible for the safety of the patient and will be held accountable should an injury occur.

(continued)

Skill Procedure 18-4. Continued

Suggested Action	Reason for Action

From a Bed to a Stretcher

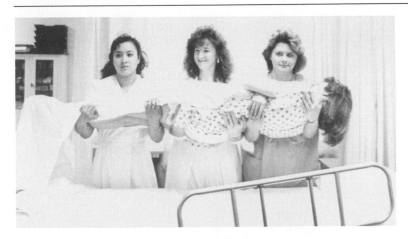

Figure 18-32 The patient has been logrolled onto the chests of the three carriers. Notice that the patient's head and back are straight and in proper alignment.

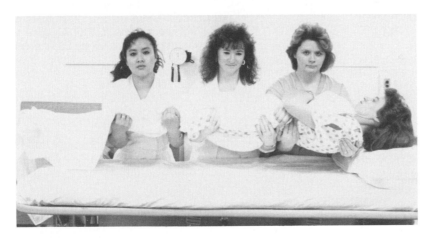

Figure 18-33 On signal, the patient is gently lowered onto the stretcher.

From a Stretcher to a Bed

Suggested Action	Reason for Action
Lift and move the patient from the stretcher, as was described when transferring him from the bed to the stretcher.	The same techniques are applicable in either situation.
Place the patient on the bed but near the edge when carrying him from the stretcher.	Trying to place the patient in the middle of the bed after carrying him from the stretcher causes strain on the backs of the carriers. Also, the patient is likely to be dropped onto the bed if an attempt is made to place him in the middle of the bed.
Have one carrier support the patient at the edge of the bed.	One person supports the patient so that he will not fall into the bed.
Have the other carriers go to the opposite side of the bed and place their arms underneath the patient in preparation for sliding him to the center of the bed.	Sliding the patient to the middle of the bed requires less energy than lifting the patient.
Measures should be taken to reduce friction during sliding.	Friction can injure the patient's skin.
At a given signal, the carriers should use one of the techniques described earlier for moving or sliding the patient up in bed.	Cooperative efforts by all carriers reduce the possibility of straining back muscles or acquiring other injuries.

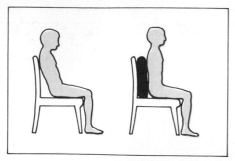

If the chair is too deep, place a pillow or cushion at the patient's back.

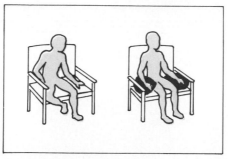

If the chair is too wide and the patient tends to lean to one side, place a cushion or pillow on each side.

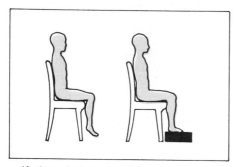

If the chair is too high, support the patient's feet to promote good posture and relieve pressure on the back of the knees.

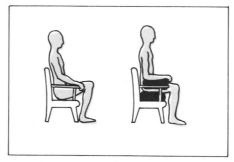

If the chair is too low, place a cushion on the seat and, if necessary, pad the arms of the chair.

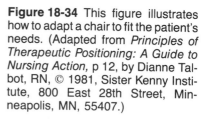

Figure 18-34 This figure illustrates how to adapt a chair to fit the patient's needs. (Adapted from *Principles of Therapeutic Positioning: A Guide to Nursing Action,* p 12, by Dianne Talbot, RN, © 1981, Sister Kenny Institute, 800 East 28th Street, Minneapolis, MN, 55407.)

Face the patient, spread the feet to provide a wide base of support and balance, put one foot forward between the patient's feet, and flex the knees to provide stability and the most effective use of the strong leg muscles. The patient puts his hands on the nurse's shoulders, while he is held in the axillary areas. Grasping the patient on his chest wall is uncomfortable and

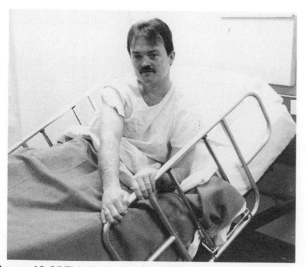

Figure 18-35 This illustrates how a patient can use siderails to help move in bed.

restricts breathing. Helping the patient out of bed is illustrated in Figure 18-36.

As the patient's upper body is supported, ask the patient to lift himself from the bed.

Maintain a wide base of support while pivoting with the patient so that his back is toward the chair.

Bend the knees and keep the back straight as the patient is lowered into the chair or wheelchair, as illustrated in Figure 18-37. Have the patient assist by holding onto armrests on the chair or wheelchair if they are available as he is being lowered into it.

Sometimes a patient may end up sitting too far from the back of a wheelchair. An easy way to move him back is to place a folded towel in the wheelchair before placing the patient in it. Have one end of the towel hanging out the back of the wheelchair and the rest of it on the seat. Once the patient is seated, it becomes relatively easy to move the patient back by standing behind the wheelchair, bracing the feet, and pulling on the towel from the back of the chair. This technique avoids friction on the patient's skin and requires less energy than lifting him back into the chair. The same techniques are used, but in reverse order, when transferring the patient from a chair back to bed.

When the Patient Cannot Assist With the Transfer. If a patient cannot stand before he sits in a chair, it is

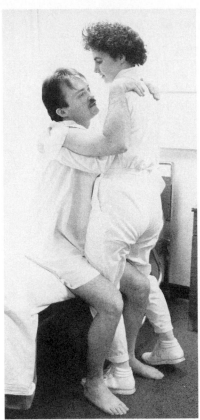

Figure 18-36 The nurse assists the patient out of bed. Notice the placement of the nurse's and patient's hands. Some nurses prefer to lock arms to assist the patient to a standing position.

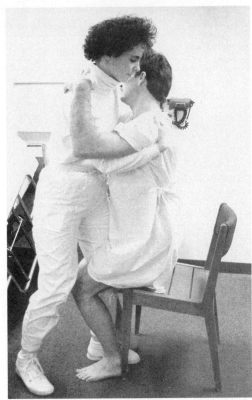

Figure 18-37 After helping the patient to his feet, the nurse assists him into a chair. A chair with arms would provide another means for the patient to help support and guide himself into the chair.

best to have two persons lift the patient from the bed into a chair. However, one person can do so unless the patient is simply too heavy for one nurse to handle. The single-person technique is handy for home use and in situations when only one person is available. It is described in Skill Procedure 18-5.

Some agencies have a mechanical, hydraulic lift, such as the one in Figure 18-40. It is used for transferring heavy or helpless patients. Slings are placed under the thighs and upper back while the patient is in bed. Chains are hooked through the eyelets in the slings. The patient is then lifted and transported to a wheelchair, toilet, car seat, or back to bed, and lowered into place. When used correctly a mechanical lifter is safe and helps prevent injuries among personnel.

Maintaining Joint Mobility

Each joint in the body has a range of motion, abbreviated ROM. That is, it has the capacity to move in certain directions. The direction of movement differs at various joints and depends on the shape and structure of the bones forming the joint. For example, the joint at the shoulder allows movement of the arm in a complete circle; it is a ball and socket joint. The joint at the elbow moves like a hinge. The amount of movement, or the joint's range, can be measured.

An active patient generally uses all his joints in the process of performing activities of daily living. However, an inactive patient may be unable to perform a variety of activities. The joints eventually sustain reduced range of motion and can become totally nonfunctional. In addition to changing the patient's positions in bed, the nurse ensures that the inactive patient's joints remain flexible.

A good exercise for the inactive patient is to move each joint through its full ROM by purposefully exercising each one to the extent its structure allows. ROM exercises may be carried out by the patient as active exercises or by the nurse as passive exercises. The patient may do some of them on his own while the nurse assists with others.

Basic Guidelines Using ROM Exercises

The following are basic guidelines when the patient is helped to put joints through ROM:

Know the patient's diagnosis and why ROM exercises are to be used. This knowledge helps the nurse in determining what exercises are needed and which ones may be contraindicated.

Skill Procedure 18-5. Moving the Patient To and From a Chair

Suggested Action	Reason for Action
Place a chair parallel with and against a point near the patient's buttocks.	Having a chair as close as possible decreases the distance to which he must be moved.
Place arms under the patient's head and shoulders and slide the upper portion of the patient's body to the edge of the bed. Move the lower portion of the patient's body by pulling with arms placed under the waist and beneath the buttocks. A rocking motion created by placing one foot in front of the other with the knees bent will help to move the weight of the patient.	Positioning the patient near the edge will reduce the energy required for transferring the patient. The more lifting that must be done, the more strain on the nurse's muscles.
Place arms well under the patient's axillary areas from the rear. The patient's head and shoulders may rest on the nurse.	Supporting the upper portion of the patient's body increases the mass over the nurse's own center of gravity where there is more support.
Move to the back of the chair while pulling the patient into the chair. Lean against the back of the chair to keep it from moving and to provide a base for support. Rock back while pulling the patient into the chair. This is illustrated in Figure 18-38.	Pulling and sliding require less effort than lifting. Rocking creates momentum that supplements the effort of the strong muscles in the nurse's arms and legs that are used to move the patient.

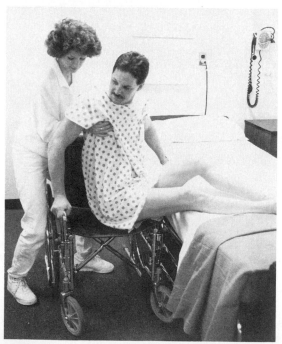

Figure 18-38 With the chair near the bed and while supporting the patient from the back, the nurse gently moves the helpless patient onto the chair. The nurse has a wide base of support, bends her knees, and rocks back as the patient slides to the chair.

Flex knees, grasp the chair near the seat, rock back, and pull the chair with the patient away from the bed until the patient's feet are on the edge of the bed.	Sliding the chair that supports the weight of the patient reduces the effort for the nurse.
Bend from the knees rather than from the waist while supporting and lowering the patient's legs and feet to the floor.	When the knees are flexed to lower the body, rather than bending from the waist, the nurse uses the musculoskeletal system more effectively and avoids personal injury.

(continued)

Skill Procedure 18-5. *Continued*

Suggested Action	**Reason for Action**
To move the patient back into the bed, slide the chair directly alongside the bed with the patient facing the foot of the bed.	Sliding the chair with the patient on it requires less energy than lifting. If the floor has a polished surface, the chair may be slid on a small rug or cloths.
Flex the knees and pivot the patient's legs onto the edge of the bed.	Using the strong muscles of the legs rather than weaker muscles of the back helps reduce strain on the nurse.
Go behind the chair, grasp the patient in the axillary areas from the rear, and roll him onto the bed, as illustrated in Figure 18-39. Have a wide base of support and rock to move the patient onto the bed.	Rolling rather than lifting the patient, having a wide base of support, and rocking reduce the strain on muscles.

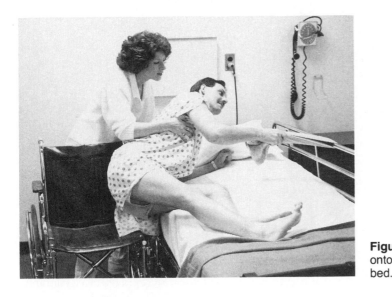

Figure 18-39 The nurse places the patient's feet and legs onto the bed first as she rolls him off the chair and onto the bed.

Slide the chair away using a foot. The nurse's body should be braced against the bed to prevent the patient from falling out of bed.	The nurse must clear away objects that interfere with controlling and supporting the patient.
Help the patient into a position of comfort, such as on his side, back, or abdomen.	A patient's position should be changed frequently. A Fowler's position is too similar to the position of the patient in a chair. Pressure should be relieved from the buttocks and heels. The hips should be extended after being flexed for a period of time.

Teach the patient what exercise is being undertaken, why, and how it will be done. Using a show-and-tell technique is recommended. A patient at ease and relaxed about exercising can more actively take part in it.	To conserve energy and to avoid strain and injury, use good body mechanics when placing a patient through ROM exercises.
Use ROM exercises twice a day and do the exercises regularly to maintain or increase joint flexibility. Each exercise is carried out two to five times. Many exercises can be carried out when the patient is being bathed. Routine tasks, such as eating, dressing, bathing, and writing also help to put certain joints through full ROM and should be encouraged.	Avoid overexertion and using exercises to the point at which the patient experiences fatigue. The purpose of moving the joints is not to exhaust or tax the patient. Certain exercises may need to be delayed until the patient's condition allows, such as those that require a standing position.
	Follow a pattern to avoid omitting any joint of the body. Begin at the head and move progressively down the body or vice versa.

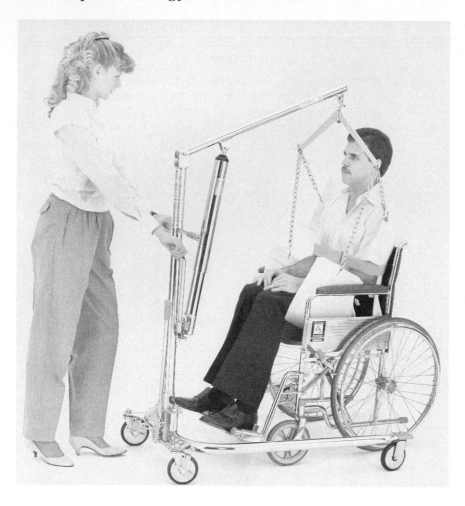

Figure 18-40 Many patients rent or purchase a hydraulic lift. With the aid of this equipment, the patient can be much more mobile than before. (Courtesy of Ted Hoyer & Company, Oshkosh, WI.)

Start gradually and work slowly. All movements should be smooth and rhythmic. Irregular, jerky movements are uncomfortable for the patient.

Support the joint being exercised. Use a firm but comfortable grip when holding the patient's joints. This technique gives the patient a feeling of adequate support. Grasping muscles or tendons is likely to cause injury or discomfort.

Move each joint until there is resistance but not pain. Movements should not be forceful. Uncomfortable reactions should be reported and exercises halted until further instructions are obtained. Excessive stretching of joints may lead to injuries and even bleeding into joints. When the patient cannot speak, watch for nonverbal signs, such as facial expressions, to judge discomfort.

Place each joint in its *neutral position,* that is, it's normal position of alignment, when beginning and finishing each exercise.

Stop ROM exercises if *spasticity,* which is sudden, continuous, and involuntary muscle contraction, occurs. Gentle pressure on an extremity tends to cause the muscle to relax. Moving a joint more slowly often helps prevent spasticity.

When moving extremities, keep friction to a minimum to avoid injuring the skin. Some agencies use powder boards to assist when exercising the legs. The boards are made of smooth material, such as fiberboard, and sprinkled with powder to reduce friction.

Expect that the patient's respiratory and heart rates may increase within the upper limits of normal during ROM exercise, which is good. These rates should return to the resting rate within a few minutes. Otherwise, the exercises are probably too strenuous for the patient.

Use passive exercises as necessary. When the patient is able to do for himself, encourage active exercises to move joints through their range of motion. Family members can be taught to perform ROM with patients. Exercises should continue at home after a period of hospitalization if the individual continues to be inactive.

Skill Procedure 18-6 describes and illustrates the actions that should be carried out when performing ROM exercises.

(Text continues on page 416)

Skill Procedure 18-6. Performing Range-of-Motion Exercises

Suggested Action	**Reason for Action**
Place one hand beneath the neck of the patient and the other on the patient's forehead, as the nurse in Figure 18-41 is doing. Lift the neck while the forehead is gently pushed down.	Joints must be supported during ROM. This action moves the joints of the cervical spine in a position of hyperextension. *Hyperextension* is a position in which the angle between adjoining parts is made larger than its normal or average range, or more than 180°.

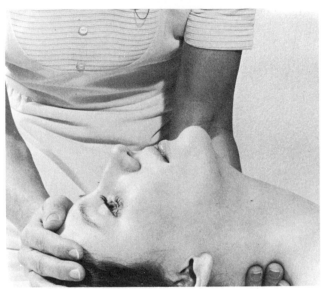

Figure 18-41 Hyperextension of the neck.

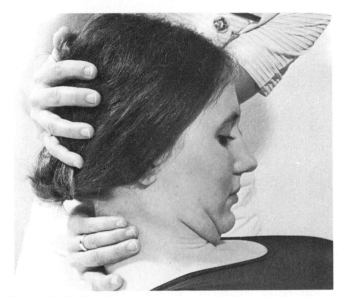

Figure 18-42 Flexion of the neck.

Repeat each joint exercise between two and five times at least twice a day.	Repeated and frequent exercise of joints helps to maintain and restore a joint's flexibility.
Place one hand under the neck and one under the back of the head, as shown in Figure 18-42. Move the head so the chin is in the direction of the chest.	This action puts the joints of the cervical spine into a position of flexion. *Flexion* is the act of moving or bending so that the angle between adjoining parts is reduced.
Place a hand on either side of the head and turn the head from side to side, as the nurse in Figure 18-43 is doing.	This action puts the joints of the cervical spine through rotation. *Rotation* is the act of turning.

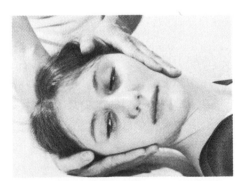

Figure 18-43 Rotation of the neck.

(*continued*)

Skill Procedure 18-6. Continued

Suggested Action	**Reason for Action**
Grasp and support the elbow and wrist of either arm. Bring the arm straight up and over the head to across the back of the head as far as possible, as shown in Figure 18-44.	The inactive patient usually maintains this joint in a position of extension. *Extension* is a position that brings parts into or toward a straight line. The action described moves the joint of the shoulder to a position of flexion.

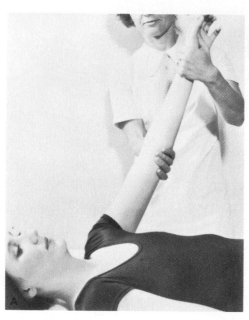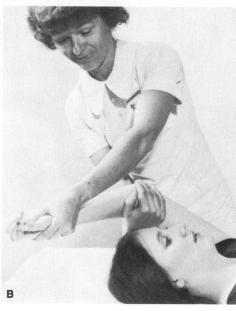

Figure 18-44 (*A*). Extension of the shoulder. (*B*). Flexion of the shoulder.

When the patient is on his abdomen or is able to sit, the arm can be moved beyond its neutral position toward the back, as shown in Figure 18-45.	This action moves the shoulder to a position of hyperextension.

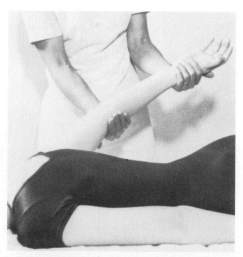

Figure 18-45 Hyperextension of the shoulder.

(continued)

Skill Procedure 18-6. Continued

Suggested Action	Reason for Action
With the patient on his back, stabilize the elbow and move the forearm first to a position in which the hand is above the head and then brought down to the side. Follow the direction of the arrows in Figure 18-46.	This movement puts the shoulder through external and then internal rotation. *External rotation* is the act of turning outward; *internal rotation* is the act of turning inward.

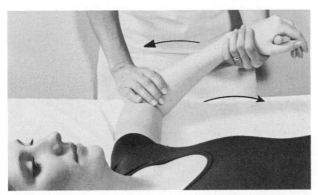

Figure 18-46 The shoulder is in external rotation when moved toward the head. It is in internal rotation when moved toward the feet.

If the patient is able to stand or sit on the edge of the bed, support the elbow and wrist while moving the shoulder joint in a full circle, as illustrated in Figure 18-47.	This exercise moves the shoulder through circumduction. *Circumduction* is circular movement. Confinement in a bed generally prevents this exercise from being performed.

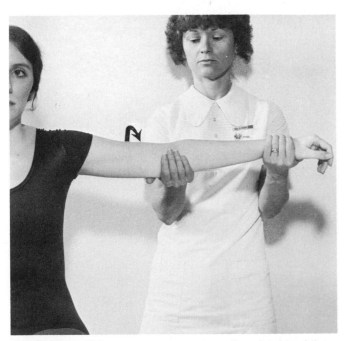

Figure 18-47 This movement exercises the shoulder joint through circumduction.

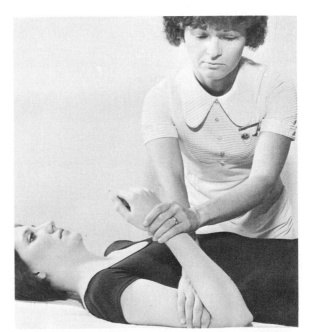

Figure 18-48 Moving the forearm toward the head produces flexion of the elbow joint.

Bring the arm so it rests in neutral position at the side of the body. Stabilize the arm above the elbow and bend the forearm toward the head as shown in Figure 18-48.	This position puts the elbow joint into a position of flexion.

(*continued*)

Skill Procedure 18-6. Continued

Suggested Action	**Reason for Action**

Return the arm to neutral position. Support the wrist and elbow and bring the arm outward from the body and then across the chest, as is being done in Figure 18-49.

These movements exercise the elbow and shoulder joints, facilitating first abduction and then adduction. *Abduction* is movement away from the body; *adduction* is movement toward the center of the body.

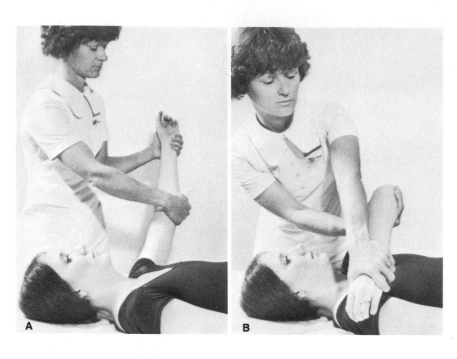

Figure 18-49 (*A*). The arm is brought out to the side into a position of abduction. (*B*). The arm is then brought across the chest to a position of adduction.

Prepare to exercise the wrist and fingers by supporting the joint at the hand and at the lower forearm. The bed can be used to support the arm.

Support of the joint prevents injury and promotes control during exercise.

With the hand held straight, bend the wrist first toward the inner forearm and then toward the outer forearm, as the nurse is doing in Figure 18-50.

This action moves the wrist from a position of extension, flexion, and then hyperextension.

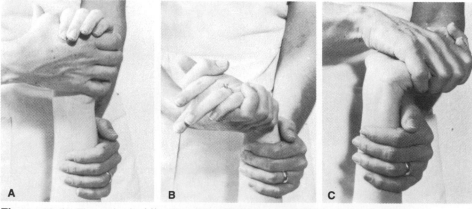

Figure 18-50 The wrist is (*A*) extended, (*B*) flexed, and (*C*) hyperextended.

(*continued*)

Skill Procedure 18-6. Continued

Suggested Action	**Reason for Action**

While stabilizing the forearm, move the hand in a twisting movement first in one direction and then in the other, as the nurse in Figure 18-51 is doing.

This action moves the wrist through external and internal rotation.

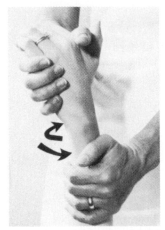

Figure 18-51 Turning the wrist moves the joint through rotation.

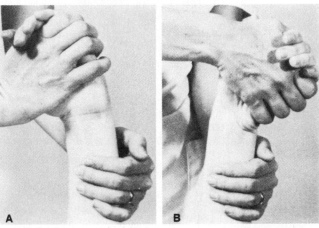

Figure 18-52 (*A*). Bending the wrist away from the body produces abduction. (*B*). Bending the wrist toward the body produces adduction.

Bend the thumb side of the hand toward the wrist and then away from the wrist, as is shown in Figure 18-52.

This moves the wrist through abduction and then adduction.

Support the wrist and bend the thumb and fingers into the palm of the hand as shown in Figure 18-53. This should be followed by straightening all the fingers and the thumb.

This exercise places the joints of the fingers in a position of flexion followed by extension. An inactive patient may eventually acquire a permanent flexion contracture. ROM exercise that promotes extension helps maintain flexibility of the fingers.

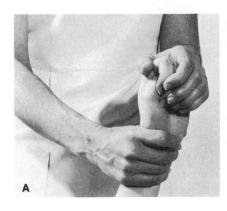

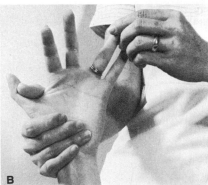

Figure 18-53 (*A*). The joints of the fingers are flexed by bending them. (*B*). The fingers are extended by straightening them.

Turn each finger and thumb, as illustrated in Figure 18-54.

Turning exercises the joints of the fingers and thumb through rotation.

(continued)

Skill Procedure 18-6. Continued

Suggested Action	Reason for Action

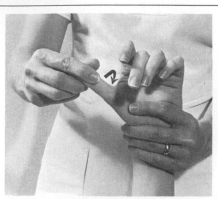

Figure 18-54 Exercising the thumb and then each finger by moving them in a twisting motion puts the joints through rotation.

With the patient flat in bed, support the knee and ankle while moving the leg out to the side and then back toward the center of the body, as the nurse in Figure 18-55 is doing.

This position moves the leg into positions first of abduction and then adduction. The hip joint of an inactive patient is usually frequently moved from flexion to extension when his position is changed from a lateral and Fowler's position to a prone and supine position.

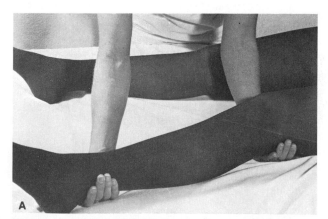 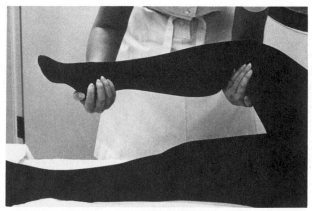

Figure 18-55 (*A*). Hip abduction occurs when the leg is moved away from the center of the body. (*B*). Bringing the leg across and toward the midline of the body produces adduction of the hip.

Support the knee and ankle and turn the leg outward, as shown in Figure 18-56, then inward.

This exercise alternates the position of the hip from external rotation to internal rotation.

With the patient on his abdomen, lift the leg backward, shown in Figure 18-57, as far as is comfortable while supporting the knee and ankle.

This exercise moves the hip joint to a position of hyperextension.

When the patient is able to stand, have the patient transfer his weight to one leg, lift the opposite leg, and turn it in a circular motion as shown in Figure 18-58.

This exercise moves the hip joint through circumduction.

With the patient lying in a supine position, place one hand beneath the knee and one under the ankle. Bend the knee in the direction of the head. These actions are shown in Figure 18-59.

When the knee is straight, the joint is in extension; when the knee is bent, the joint is in flexion. Sitting and gatching the knees place the knees in flexion. Positions of flexion should be alternated frequently with periods of extension.

(continued)

Skill Procedure 18-6. Continued

Suggested Action	Reason for Action

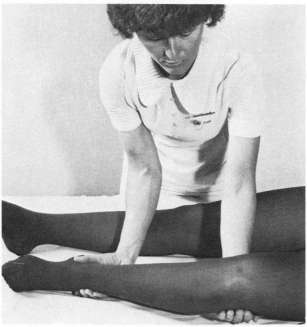

Figure 18-56 Turning the leg outward produces external rotation of the hip.

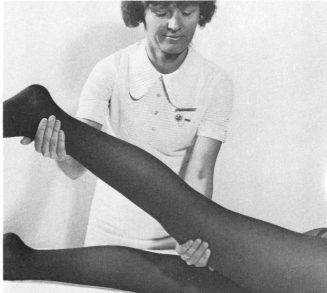

Figure 18-57 While the model lies on her abdomen, her leg is brought up as far as is comfortable to produce hyperextension of the hip.

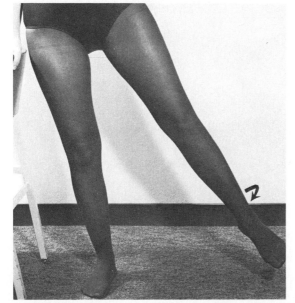

Figure 18-58 The model stands to demonstrate a method for maintaining joint mobility of the hip by moving it in a circular pattern called circumduction.

Prepare to exercise the ankle by using one hand to support the heel and the other to support the lower leg, leaving the ankle free to move.

Grasping the muscle of the calf can cause discomfort or injury to the patient.

(continued)

Skill Procedure 18-6. Continued

Suggested Action	**Reason for Action**

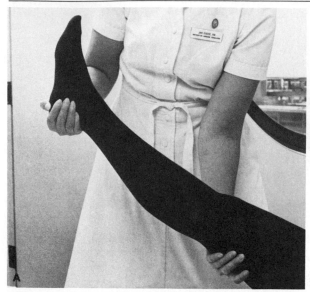 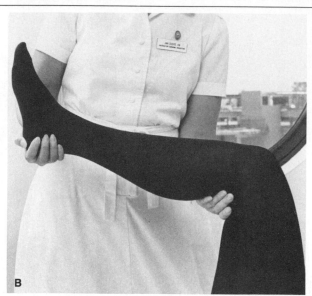

Figure 18-59 (*A*). The leg is brought off the bed with the knee in a position of extension. (*B*). Bending the knee places the knee and hip joints in a position of flexion.

Pull as through stretching the heel so that the toes point in the direction of the head. Follow this by stretching the foot so that the toes point downward, as shown in Figure 18-60.	This exercise alternates dorsiflexion with plantarflexion. Positioning and exercising the ankle to maintain dorsiflexion can help maintain an inactive person's ability to eventually stand and walk.

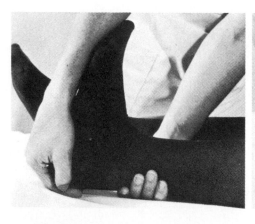 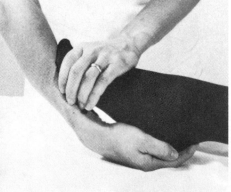

Figure 18-60 (*A*). The foot is brought up into a position of dorsiflexion. (*B*). The foot is then brought down to a position of plantarflexion.

Support the ankle and turn the foot to the middle of the body and then to the outside of the body, shown in Figure 18-61.	This exercise alternately moves the ankle from internal to external rotation.
Let the bed support the foot. Hold the foot at the arch area, bend and then straighten the toes, as the nurse in Figure 18-62 is doing.	This movement causes the joints of the toes to become flexed and then extended.
To exercise the remaining areas of the spine, help the patient assume a curled-up position while sitting, as shown in Figure 18-63.	Bending the spine causes the joints to be placed in a position of flexion.

(continued)

Skill Procedure 18-6. Continued

Suggested Action	Reason for Action

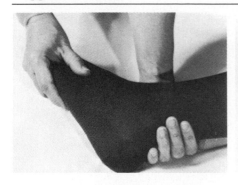 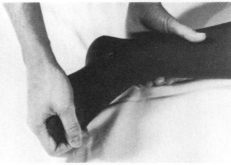

Figure 18-61 (*A*). The ankle is rotated in an inward direction. (*B*). The ankle is rotated in an outward direction.

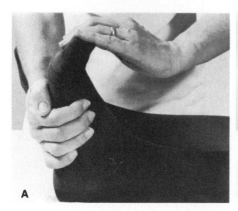 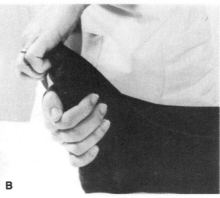

A **B**

Figure 18-62 (*A*). The joints of the toes are straightened to a point of hyperextension. (*B*). Bending them produces flexion.

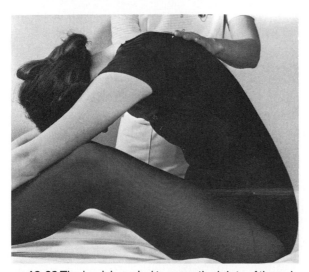

Figure 18-63 The back is curled to move the joints of the spine into a position of flexion. This movement could also be achieved with the patient lying on her side.

(*continued*)

Skill Procedure 18-6. Continued

Suggested Action	Reason for Action
With the patient lying on his abdomen, help him to arch his back by bringing the shoulders off the bed, as the person is doing in Figure 18-64.	With the back straight, the spine is in a position of extension. Arching changes the position of the spinal joints to hyperextension.

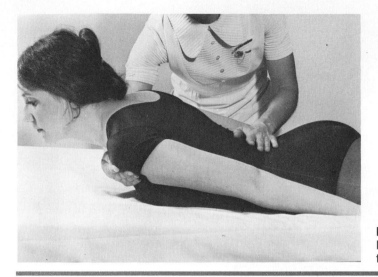

Figure 18-64 By bringing the shoulders off the bed while lying on the abdomen, this model demonstrates hyperextension of the joints of the spine.

Preparing the Patient for Walking

When patients are confined to bed for short periods of time, preparing them for increased activity may be simply a matter of assisting them out of bed and helping them to walk. However, some patients may require special preparation, especially those who have been in bed for long periods of time. In addition to the positioning and joint movements, certain other exercises and activities will help prepare the musculoskeletal system for weightbearing and activity.

Assisting With Isometric Exercises

Isometric exercises were discussed in Chapter 9. They are exercises that involve contracting and relaxing muscle groups with little, if any, movement. Patients who perform these exercises must be taught to avoid using them with a closed glottis. The glottis is closed when one tries to stifle a sneeze or cough or when one grunts with a strain. Forcing exhalation against a closed glottis is called *Valsalva's maneuver.* Avoiding Valsalva's maneuver is especially important for patients with heart diseases. Straining against a closed glottis tends to raise blood pressure and can cause the heartbeat to become irregular. When performing isometric exercises, the patient should understand that the muscle contraction should be followed by muscle relaxation every few seconds. Patients tend to misunderstand

and think they should keep the muscles in a contracted state for long periods of time. This tires and strains muscles rather than exercises them.

Quadriceps Setting. *Quadriceps setting,* sometimes shortened to quad setting, is an isometric exercise in which the muscles on the front of the thigh are alternately tensed and relaxed. These muscles are some of the strongest of the leg muscles. Their tone must be maintained so the inactive patient can eventually stand and support his body weight. They also help in moving the leg during walking. They are exercised as follows:

1. Have the patient contract the quadriceps femoris muscles by pulling the kneecaps toward the hips. The patient will feel that he is pushing his knee down into the mattress and pulling his foot upward.
2. Contract the muscles for several seconds and then relax them for an equal amount of time.
3. Count slowly to four with each contraction and relaxation to establish a rhythm.
4. Contract and relax the muscles two to three times each hour but not to the point of fatigue.

Gluteal Setting. The muscles in the buttocks are also important for body support and movement. To perform gluteal setting exercises, the patient pinches the buttocks together and then relaxes. The guidelines for performing gluteal setting are the same as those for quad setting. Strengthening these muscles helps prepare the patient for walking as well as for climbing stairs.

Assisting With Push-Ups

Push-ups strengthen muscles of the shoulders and arms. These muscles are important for holding onto a chair as the patient begins to walk again. Also, they are needed for patients who must learn to walk with crutches or with a cane. Push-ups are done as follows:

Have the patient sit up in bed. The patient then lifts his hips off the bed by pushing down with his hands on the mattress. If the mattress is soft, a block or books are placed on the bed under the patient's hands.

Another technique requires that the patient lie on his abdomen and place his hands near his body at approximately shoulder level, palms down on the mattress, with the elbows sharply flexed. He then straightens his elbows while lifting his head and shoulders off the bed, as illustrated in Figure 18-65.

Push-ups can be done when a patient sits in an armchair. He places his hands on the arms of the chair and then raises his body out of the seat. Push-ups are usually done three or four times each day.

Using a Tilt Table

Some patients may have been inactive and confined to bed for so long that they need to gradually become used to being in an upright position. They may faint or remain too weak to support their body weight. A tilt table is a device that looks very much like a stretcher with a foot piece. The patient is transferred and secured to the tilt table. The entire body of the patient is progressively raised to a standing position. Eventually, when the patient can tolerate being upright, he may be assisted with walking.

Assisting the Patient to Dangle

Another exercise that helps prepare the patient for being out of bed is referred to as *dangling*. The patient is placed on the side of his bed with his feet on the floor or on a

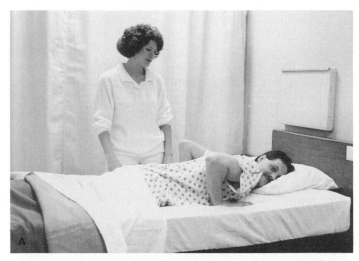

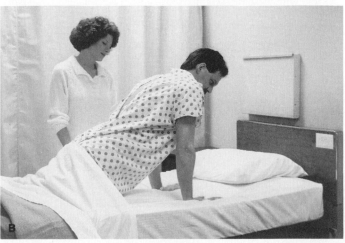

Figure 18-65 (*A*). The patient is in position to begin push-ups. (*B*). He lifts himself off the bed as he straightens his elbows, then lowers himself by flexing his elbows to return to his original position.

footstool, as shown in Figure 18-66. The exercise is carried out as follows:

1. Place the patient in Fowler's position for a few minutes to accustom him to the sitting position. This reduces the possibility for injury should he feel faint from a drop in blood pressure.
2. Stand at the side of the bed and assist the patient to the edge of the bed.
3. Place the bed in low position.
4. Pivot the patient a quarter of a turn by supporting his shoulders and legs. Swing the patient's legs over the side of the bed. The patient may wish to place his hands on the nurse's shoulders for support.
5. Rest the patient's feet on the floor.
6. Remain with the patient and be ready to put him into a lying position if he feels faint or if his pulse rate is significantly affected by dangling.

Assisting the Patient to Walk

Despite strengthening exercises, some patients may still need progressive assistance to eventually take steps independently. There are several possible devices and techniques that provide support and assistance with walking.

Parallel Bars. Some health agencies have parallel bars that help a patient begin to walk. The patient grasps a

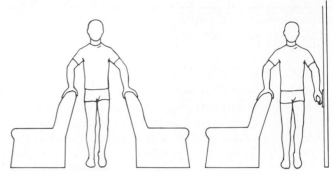

Figure 18-67 This sketch illustrates how a patient can use two sturdy chairs, or a chair and a doorknob, for support as he prepares to walk.

bar on either side of him and starts to walk as he supports himself on the bars. When parallel bars are not available, almost any two *stable* pieces of furniture can be used. Examples include the backs of two heavy chairs, the footboards of two beds, or a hall rail and a chair. Figure 18-67 illustrates this technique, using two sturdy chairs and a chair and doorknob.

Walking Belts. A walking belt is helpful for some patients. One is illustrated in Figure 18-68. The patient has the security of support until he feels ready to walk on his own. The nurse can anticipate if the patient is losing his balance and prevent injuries from an uncontrolled fall.

Walking With a Nurse. The nurse should walk alongside the patient who is just beginning to ambulate,

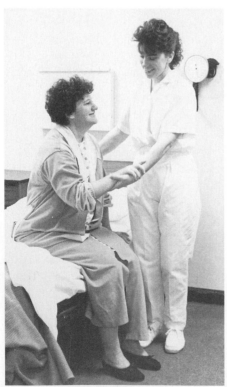

Figure 18-66 The patient dangles in preparation for getting out of bed. The bed is in the low position to allow the patient's feet to rest on the floor. The nurse remains ready in case the patient should feel weak or faint.

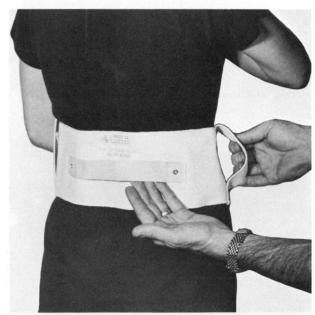

Figure 18-68 This is an example of a walking belt. Handles on the sides and in the back give firm grips for the person assisting the patient. (Courtesy of the JT Posey Company, Arcadia, CA.)

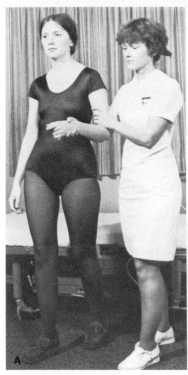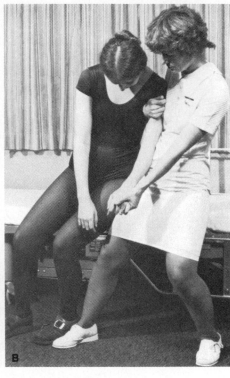

Figure 18-69 (*A*). Note that the nurse walks hand-in-hand with the model. (*B*). When the model slumps to fall the nurse slips her arm into the model's axillary area, puts her foot that is nearer to the model out to one side to provide a wide base of support, and supports the model on her hip until help arrives.

keeping an arm under his in an arm-in-arm manner. If the patient begins to feel faint, the nurse can quickly slide an arm up and into the patient's axillary area. By placing one foot out to the side to form a wide base of support, the patient can then rest on the nurse's hip until additional help arrives to assist. This is illustrated in Figure 18-69.

Using Aids for Ambulation

Several devices may be used for support and safety. These may be used temporarily or permanently to assist with ambulation.

Canes. Canes may be used to help a patient walk. One type is a straight walking stick with a rubber cap on the end to help prevent the cane from sliding along the floor. A cane should be placed about 10 cm (4 in) to the side of the foot. It should be held in the hand on the uninvolved side. If the nurse helps the patient, support and assistance should be provided on the involved side. The patient should assume an erect position when walking with a cane. Leaning over a cane results in poor body posture.

Another type of cane, the quadripod or "quad" cane, has four legs, which give extra support for the patient. A patient may use one cane or two, depending on the amount of support he needs.

Walkers. A walker is one of the most stable forms of ambulatory aids. It is used by patients who require considerable support and assistance with balance. Patients who are learning to walk again after prolonged periods in bed or following hip surgery often use a walker. The patient should hold onto the handgrips at the side of the walker. The elbows should be flexed about 30° with the feet about 15 cm to 20 cm (6 in to 8 in) apart, for a wide base of support while walking. To maintain good posture, the patient should hold himself straight and look ahead, not at the floor. Figure 18-70 illustrates a patient using a walker.

Crutches. Crutches require considerable physical strength and balance to use. There are many safety hazards involved with their use. For this reason most elderly or inactive patients are supplied with a walker rather than crutches.

Types of Crutches. Axillary crutches fit under the arm into the axillary area. Most patients learn to use this type of crutch in the beginning of ambulation and when the use of crutches is a temporary measure.

There are crutches with no axillary support. One type is called *Lofstrand* or *Canadian crutches.* They are illustrated in Figure 18-71. This type of crutch has a frame or metal cuff that extends beyond the handgrip. These crutches are generally used by well-experienced patients who need permanent assistance with walking.

Another type of crutch is called the *platform crutch.* This type of crutch is designed to support the forearms. It is especially useful for patients unable to bear weight with their hands and wrists. Many patients with arthritis use them. As Figure 18-72 illustrates, the patient's weight is distributed over the entire forearm.

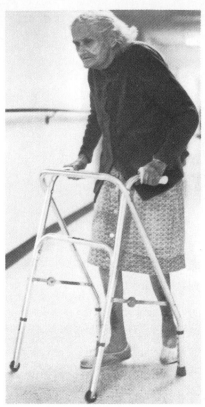

Figure 18-70 This elderly lady stoops over somewhat when she walks, perhaps as a result of osteoporosis. However, she is using her walker properly.

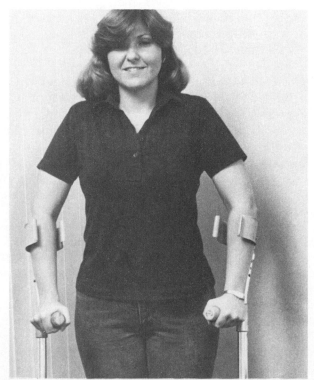

Figure 18-71 Lofstrand or Canadian crutches have bands to fit around the forearms to help keep them in place.

Measuring the Patient for Axillary Crutches. There are two common methods for measuring a patient for axillary crutches. With the patient in bed on his back and wearing shoes, the nurse measures the distance from the fold at the axillary area to the feet and adds 5 cm (2 in). Using the second method, measure the distance from the fold at the axillary area to a point 15 cm to 20 cm (6 to 8 in) away from the patient's heel. The measurement of crutch length includes the axillary pads and crutch tips. The handgrips are adjusted so that with the patient standing, the elbows are slightly bent (about 30°) and the wrists are bent backward (hyperextended) slightly. There should be room for two fingers in the space between the top of the axillary bar of the crutch and the fold of the axilla when the patient stands. Safety rubber suction tips on the ends of crutches prevent slipping. It is important to be sure the tips are clean and not worn.

Preparing for Crutch Walking. Several exercises help a patient prepare for crutch walking. Pushups help strengthen the arm and shoulder muscles. The muscles in the hand can be strengthened by squeezing a ball 50 times or more a day. Handgrips can be purchased that are also used for this purpose.

The following recommended steps help a patient prepare for using axillary crutches:

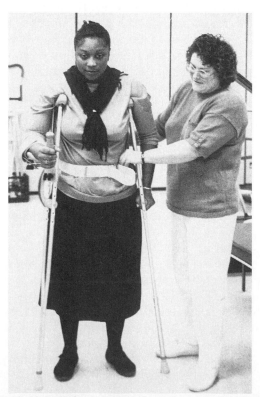

Figure 18-72 A platform crutch allows the patient to distribute weight bearing on the forearm. This patient wears a type of walking belt. The person assisting the patient holds onto the belt to offer support and security until the patient has mastered the skill of walking with crutches.

1. Assist the patient into a chair that is close to a wall when he is ready to get out of bed.
2. Help the patient stand against the wall with the crutches placed in his hands.
3. Have the patient sway from side to side on his crutches while standing slightly away from the wall. This helps the hands and arms become used to weight bearing.
4. Have the patient lean against the wall and pick up one crutch to about 15 cm (6 in) from the floor and then place it back down on the floor. He should do the same with the other crutch and repeat this exercise several times. It helps the patient learn how to manage his crutches. He is ready to start to walk after he has shown that he can handle his crutches with ease and comfort.
5. Have the patient assume a posture with the crutches that allows the line of gravity to go through a wide base of support. The crutches should be placed about 10 cm to 20 cm (4 to 8 in) in front and about the same distance to the side of the feet, forming a triangle for good balance.
6. Teach the patient he is to support himself on the crutches with his arms and hands. If he supports himself by placing his weight on the axillary area, he may irritate the skin. Also, the weight tends to cut off circulation and places pressure on nerves to the arms and hands, which may result in permanent paralysis.
7. Cover the place where the patient rests his hands

with adhesive or moleskin if the patient's hands tend to slip on the hand supports.

Crutch-Walking Gaits. In many agencies, a physical therapist teaches the patient how to use crutches. However, it is important for the nurse to observe that the patient uses his crutches properly. The nurse is often required to provide assistance after the initial teaching has been done. Also, the nurse may be responsible for teaching patients how to use crutches in the home.

Table 18-2 describes several basic crutch-walking gaits. Some use the term *point* in their name. Point refers to the number of supports being used during ambulation. For instance, during a two-point gait a crutch and one leg represent the support that is utilized as one leg and the other crutch are picked up and moved forward; in a three-point gait, two crutches and one leg act as supports, and so on.

Using Recreation for Exercise

The concept of exercise need not be limited to dull routines that many find tedious and boring. Patients can be encouraged to move about while enjoying leisure-time activities.

Arts and crafts can often be a rewarding use of leisure time. Activities such as painting, clay modeling, knitting, and using a saw or sander in woodworking are examples of recreation that exercises the fingers, hands, wrists, elbows, and shoulders. Family members are often eager to provide materials that the patient will enjoy while gaining therapeutic benefits.

Table 18-2. Common Crutch-Walking Gaits

Gait	Condition for Use	Method for Use
Two-point gait	The patient must be able to bear some weight on each leg.	The patient bears weight on both feet. The right crutch and left foot are moved forward. Then, the left crutch and the right foot move forward. It resembles a normal walking pattern.
Three-point gait	Weight-bearing is allowed on one leg. The other foot cannot bear weight or can bear only limited weight.	Both crutches and the leg that cannot bear weight move forward and then the foot permitted to bear weight comes through. The crutches are brought forward immediately and the pattern is repeated. The gait is illustrated in 18-73.
Four-point gait	Weight-bearing must be permitted on both feet; however, those using this gait may need to move slower because they lack balance, are weak, or have limited ability to move.	Only one point is moved forward at a time in a sequence like this: left crutch, right foot, right crutch, left foot. Some may progress from this gait to a two-point gait as their condition improves. The patient in 18-74 is using a four-point gait.

(continued)

Table 18-2. Continued

Gait	Condition for Use	Method for Use

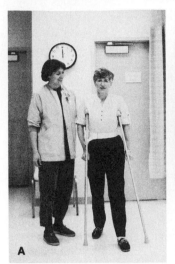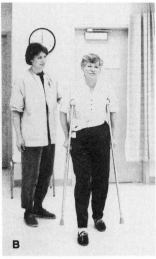

Figure 18-73 (*A*). When using the three-point gait, one foot (in this case the patient's right foot) is permitted to bear weight. The patient is placing both crutches and her left foot, which can bear only limited weight, forward. (*B*). After shifting her weight from her right foot to her crutches and to the foot with limited weight-bearing ability, she then brings her right foot through and in front of her to receive her weight.

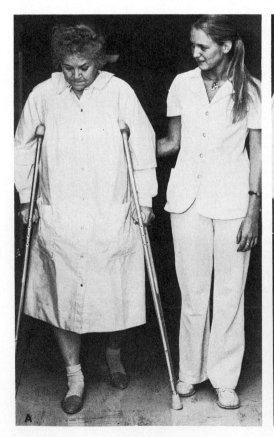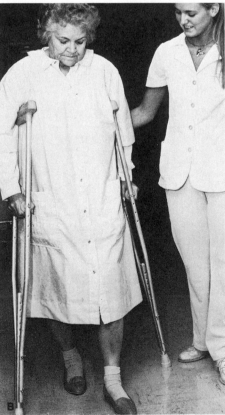

Figure 18-74 This patient is using the four-point gait for crutch walking with axillary crutches. (*A*). The left crutch is placed forward first, and the patient moves her right foot forward in position to receive weight. (*B*). The right crutch is then placed forward, and the patient's left foot is brought forward in position to receive weight.

(*continued*)

Table 18-2. Continued

Gait	Condition for Use	Method for Use
Swing-through and swing-to gait	In this gait, one or both legs are involved. Usually, a patient using this gait has leg braces. The gait produces rapid movement, but it does not resemble normal walking.	The crutches are advanced together. The body weight is shifted from the legs to the hand grips. The legs are swung either slightly beyond the crutch tips or just parallel with them. The person in 18-75 is using a swing-through gait.

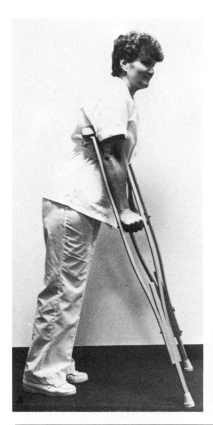
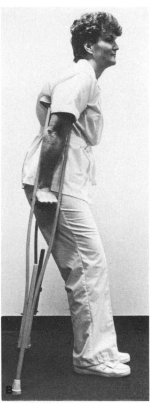

Figure 18-75 The nurse demonstrates a swing-through gait as it would be done by a person with involvement of both legs. (*A*). Both crutches are brought forward. (*B*). After shifting the body weight to the handgrips, the nurse swings her legs forward through the space between the crutches. Some patients, for instance those with a leg cast, use this gait while supporting their weight on one leg.

Suggested Measures to Prevent Inactivity in Selected Situations

When the Patient Is an Infant or Child

Most infants and children enjoy bathing and the freedom for movement it allows. Use water play as a means of promoting activity and exercise.

Mobiles hung above an infant's bed can be a source of sensory stimulation and can provide motivation for hand activity.

Soft foam action toys such as footballs, basketballs, and frisbies can be used safely inside to promote large muscle movement among children.

Many songs for children can be used along with actions to provide an enjoyable means for exercise.

Pet therapy can help children exercise by providing an opportunity for stroking, walking, and playing with an animal.

Children may enjoy riding stationary bicycles as a means of indoor activity.

Using scissors to cut out colorful pictures from magazines or used greeting cards can provide a pleasurable activity as well as hand exercise. Children often enjoy pasting the cut-out pictures into a scrapbook.

Periodically assess the measurement of a child's ambulatory aid, such as canes and crutches, so that they remain appropriate for the growth of the child.

Inspect the rubber tips of crutches or other ambulatory devices. The tips should be replaced if they

NURSING CARE PLAN

18-1. Unilateral Neglect

Assessment	**Subjective Data** States, "Somebody's arm and leg are in my bed." **Objective Data** 76-year-old man previously treated for hypertension. Admitted now for a stroke. Left side of face droops. Unable to smile or show teeth completely when asked. Tongue deviates from midline. Not able to see objects placed on L. side of body. Does not eat food on left side of plate and tray. No movement of L. upper or lower extremities. No response to touch or pain stimuli on L. side. Cannot differentiate between warm or cold on the left, but can do so on right.
Diagnosis	Unilateral neglect related to unawareness of objects in L. visual field secondary to stroke.
Plan	**Goal** The patient will identify his own L. arm and leg and assist with bathing, exercising, and dressing the L. side of his body by 4/21. **Orders:** 4/19 1. Each shift, show the patient three objects held on the R. side of the patient's visual field. 2. Locate the same three objects on the L. side of the bed, wall, or room and instruct the patient to turn his head and identify where each is located. 3. Have the patient locate and touch his left arm and leg. 4. Instruct the patient to bathe his left arm in the A.M. and follow with inserting sleeve over left hand and arm; on remaining shifts have patient grasp his left arm and perform range of motion of shoulder, elbow, wrist, and fingers. _ S. LABADIE, RN
Implementation (Documentation) 4/19	1745 While standing on R. side of bed, patient was shown a pen, flashlight, and watch. Flashlight placed by left hand, watch buckled to left siderail, and pen placed on top sheet. Instructed to turn head to the left and identify relocated items, L. arm, and L. leg. ————————————————— J. PERRY, LPN
Evaluation (Documentation)	1800 Able to scan left side and correctly identify objects and body parts. Able to grasp left hand and extend arm over head. Right elbow flexed and extended; arm adducted. Pronation, supination of hand, flexion and hyperextension of R. wrist and fingers performed by patient five times each. Assisted with abduction of arm and circumduction of shoulder. ——————————— J. PERRY, LPN

are worn. They must be cleaned to remove dust and dirt that build up.

When the Patient Is Elderly

Consider the disuse syndrome as a serious threat to the elderly and work conscientiously to help prevent it.

Balance periods of activity with periods of rest. The elderly often have arthritis. Expect that it will take the patient some extra time in the morning before he can gradually resume activity.

Elderly patients may enjoy the stimulation and activity associated with playing board games and card games.

Puzzles with large-sized pieces can be used as a means of solitary activity.

Remove any objects that may present an obstacle or hazard to the use of a walker or cane so that further injury is avoided. Common problems are

Applicable Nursing Diagnoses

Many nursing diagnoses may apply to the care of inactive patients, including the following:
- Impaired Physical Mobility
- Constipation
- Urinary Retention
- Altered Tissue Perfusion
- Ineffective Airway Clearance
- High Risk for Disuse Syndrome
- Unilateral Neglect
- Impaired Skin Integrity
- Impaired Tissue Integrity
- Sleep Pattern Disturbance
- Bathing/Hygiene Self-Care Deficit
- Hopelessness

Nursing Care Plan 18-1 illustrates the steps in the nursing process for a patient with Unilateral Neglect. This diagnostic category is described as, "A state in which an individual is perceptually unaware of and inattentive to one side of the body" in the NANDA taxonomy (1989).

throw rugs, electrical cords, chair legs, and water on the floor.

Teaching Suggestions to Prevent Inactivity

Suggestions for preventing and counteracting inactivity have been described in this chapter. They are summarized below:

Few people are aware of the dangers of inactivity. Most seem to believe that complete bedrest during illness is essential to regain health and they are reluctant to return to activity. Bedrest is often very important for patients, but without some planned activity the patient is likely to develop serious complications. Therefore, it becomes important for the nurse to teach patients the many dangers of inactivity and to gain their cooperation to return to activity as soon as possible.

It is important to explain what is going to be done, and why, when transferring patients and when performing exercises. When patients have this information, accidents are less likely to occur.

Most patients assume a "coffin position," which is similar to the supine position, unless properly taught the benefits of other positions in bed. Teaching the patient the benefits of changing positions in bed is important, especially when this may be among the few activities allowed.

It is important to use necessary precautions when transferring patients and when helping them walk—and to teach why precautions are necessary.

Patients often do not recognize their limitations or the state of weakness that follows a period of inactivity. Accidents are likely to occur when teaching has been inadequate. Although certain patients need to be encouraged to engage in activity and exercise, others may tend to take on more than is safe.

Patients need repetitive teaching about the use of crutches, canes, and walkers. Using these devices improperly can lead to accidents and injury.

Bibliography

Beaver MJ: Mediscus low air-loss beds and the prevention of decubitus ulcers. Critical Care Nurse 6(5):32–33, 36–39, 1986

Belanus AR, Paradiso C, Konzelmann NM, Roosma MC: Helping yourself and your patients when working with Clinitron therapy. Rehabilitation Nursing 10(1):29–30, 1985

Benison B, Hogstel MO: Aging and movement therapy: Essential interventions for the immobile elderly. Journal of Gerontological Nursing 12(12):8–16, 1986

Bennett–Canclini S: The kinetic treatment table: A new approach to bed rest. Orthopaedic Nursing 4(2):61–70, 1985

Bristow JV, Goldfarb EH, Green M: Clinitron therapy: Is it effective? Geriatr Nurs 8(3):120, 124, 1987

Conine TA, Choi AK, Lim R: The user-friendliness of protective support surfaces in prevention of pressure sores. Rehabilitation Nursing 14(5):261–263, 1989

Cuzzell J, Willey T: Pressure relief perennials. Am J Nurs 87(9): 1157–1160, 1987

Fink MP, Helsmoortel CM, Stein KL, Lee PC, Cohn SM: The efficacy of an oscillating bed in the prevention of lower respiratory tract infection in critically ill victims of blunt trauma. Chest 97(1):132–137, 1990

Fischer AA, Goldberg L, Lyles BD Jr: Mobilizing the sedentary patient. Patient Care 21(4):14–17, 20–21, 27–28, 1987

Hahn K: Left vs. right: What a difference the side makes in stroke. Nursing 17(9):44–47, 1987

Kunkler CE: The nursing-therapy connection: Bedside treatment. Orthopaedic Nursing 6(4):37–40, 1987

Livesley B: Airwaves take the pressure. Nursing Times 82(32):67–68, 71, 1986

Lucke K, Jarlsberg J: How is the air-fluidized bed best used? Am J Nurs 85(12):1338, 1340, 1985

Maklebust J: Pressure ulcers: Etiology and prevention. Nurs Clin North Am 22(2):359–377, 1987

Mandzak–McCarron K, Drayton–Hargrove S: Ambulation aids. Rehabilitation Nursing 12(3):139–141, 1987

Munro BH, Brown L, Heitman BB: Pressure ulcers: One bed or another? Geriatr Nurs 10(4):190–192, 1989

Passarella P, Gee Z: Starting right after stroke . . . Bobath principles. Am J Nurs 87(6):802–208, 1987

Peletier G, Poppe SR, Twomey JA: Controlled air suspension: An advantage in burn care. J Burn Care Rehabil 8(6):558–560, 1987

Pires M: What's it like to be a rehabilitation clinical nurse specialist. NursingLife 7(3):18–19, 1987

Sanchez DG, Bussey B, Petorak M: How air-fluidized beds revolutionize skin care. RN Magazine 46(6):46–48, 1983

Wahlquist G: The family in rehabilitation. Rehabilation Nursing 12(2):62, 1987

Willey T: High-tech beds and mattress overlays: A decision guide. Am J Nurs 89(9):1142–1145, 1989

19

Caring for the Patient Undergoing Surgery

Chapter Outline

Behavioral Objectives
Glossary
Introduction
Types of Surgery
Locations for Surgery
Types of Anesthesia
Identifying Surgical Risk Factors
Informing the Patient
Predonating Blood
Providing Psychological Support
Caring for the Patient Before Surgery
Resuming Care After Surgery
Laser Surgery
Suggested Measures When Giving Preoperative and
    Postoperative Care in Selected Situations
Applicable Nursing Diagnoses
Teaching Suggestions Related to a Surgical Experience
Bibliography

Skill Procedures

Teaching Deep-Breathing Exercises
Teaching the Patient to Cough
Teaching Leg Exercises
Using Antiembolism Stockings
Preparing the Patient for Surgery
Caring for the Postoperative Patient

Behavioral Objectives

When the content of this chapter has been mastered, the learner will be able to:

Define the terms appearing in the glossary.

List at least five reported benefits that occur when patients are well taught and prepared for surgery.

Discuss at least two reasons for predonating blood before surgery.

Design a plan of care for the preparation of a patient who is to have surgery, including psychological care.

Demonstrate teaching deep-breathing, coughing, and leg exercises.

Measure and correctly apply antiembolism stockings.

Discuss methods for preoperatively preparing the surgical site.

Describe the actions that are generally included in the immediate preparation of a patient for surgery.

Describe the postoperative care after receiving a patient from the recovery room.

List ten usual types of postoperative orders.

List 18 to 20 possible postoperative discomforts and complications, indicate typical signs and symptoms, and describe nursing measures to prevent and to help overcome them.

Discuss several ways in which the nurse can help the family of a surgical patient and the benefits of such efforts.

List five advantages of laser surgery.

Identify three safety hazards and special precautions associated with laser surgery.

Summarize suggestions offered in this chapter for teaching the surgical patient and his family.

Glossary

Ambulatory surgery Surgical procedures performed on patients who enter and leave the hospital all on the same day. Synonym for *outpatient surgery*.

Anesthesia The loss of sensation.

Anticoagulant A medication that inhibits or delays blood clotting.

Autologous transfusion The administration of one's own blood.

Dehiscence The separation of layers of a wound.

Depilatory cream A substance used to remove hair.

Directed donor A blood donor selected by the patient.

Evisceration The separation of a wound with exposure of body organs.

General anesthesia The use of an anesthetic agent that eliminates all sensation as well as consciousness.

Hiccups Intermittent spasms of the diaphragm. Synonym for *singultus*.

Incentive spirometry A method for measuring a patient's respiratory efforts.

Laser Light energy that can incise tissue, coagulate blood, and vaporize tissue.

Local anesthesia The use of an anesthetic agent that eliminates sensation in the area of a procedure but does not alter consciousness.

Microabrasion Scraping away of skin not usually visible with ordinary vision.

Nebulizer A device that converts a liquid into a fine mist.

Operating room The area in which a surgical procedure is performed.

Outpatient surgery Surgical procedures performed on patients who enter and leave the hospital all on the same day. Synonym for *ambulatory surgery.*

Parotitis An inflammation of the parotid glands. When the condition occurs postoperatively, it is frequently called surgical mumps.

Plume Smoke produced as a consequence of vaporizing tissue with a laser.

Pneumonitis An inflammation of the lungs.

Reacting room The area in which a patient is closely observed after surgery until his condition is stable. Synonym for *recovery room.*

Receiving room The area in which a patient waits immediately prior to surgery.

Recovery room The area in which a patient is closely observed after surgery until his condition is stable. Synonym for *reacting room.*

Regional anesthesia Loss of sensation in a large area of the body without affecting consciousness.

Shock The reaction of the body to inadequate circulation. Hypovolemic shock occurs with the loss of blood volume.

Singultus Intermittent spasms of the diaphragm. Synonym for *hiccups.*

Surgery Procedures that involve entering tissue and removing or reconstructing structures that are diseased, injured, or malformed.

Topical anesthesia A type of local anesthetic applied to the surface of mucous membranes.

Trendelenburg position The position in which the head is lower than the feet.

Introduction

Some illnesses or conditions can be treated through surgery. *Surgery* involves entering tissue and removing or reconstructing structures that are diseased, injured, or malformed. This chapter discusses basic care of the surgical patient. It includes care that, in general, applies to all surgical patients, regardless of diagnosis or type of surgery. Clinical textbooks more appropriately discuss specific disorders that require particular kinds of surgery.

Types of Surgery

Surgical procedures are classified according to the urgency with which they must be carried out. They are described in Table 19-1. Nursing care of the patient is frequently influenced by the type of surgery a patient is having. For example, providing psychological support, physical care, and teaching is affected by the time available with the patient prior to surgery. Emergency surgery requires split-second coordination and attention to priorities. Elective surgery allows a more relaxed pace with time to attend to details. Regardless of the type of surgery, the nurse must be competent in performing the skills required for preoperative and postoperative care.

Locations for Surgery

Surgery can be done in various locations. Traditionally, surgery has been performed in special areas within hospitals. The surgical units generally include a *receiving room,* where the patient waits immediately prior to surgery; one or more *operating rooms,* where surgery is performed;

Table 19-1. Types of Surgery According to Their Urgency

Type	Description	Example
Optional	Surgery is performed at the request of the patient.	Surgery for cosmetic purposes
Elective	Surgery is planned at the convenience of the patient. Failure to have the surgery does not result in catastrophe.	Surgery for the removal of a superficial cyst
Required	Surgery is necessary and should be done relatively promptly.	Surgery for the removal of a cataract
Urgent	Surgery is required promptly, within a day or two if at all possible.	Surgery for the removal of a malignant tumor
Emergency	Surgery is required immediately for survival.	Surgery to relieve an intestinal obstruction

and a *recovery* or *reacting room,* where the patient is closely observed after surgery. Until recently, most surgical patients were admitted to the hospital the day before surgery and were prepared to spend a period of time there during recovery.

Now there is a trend to perform more and more *ambulatory* or *outpatient surgery.* This type of surgery is performed in hospitals, but it allows the patient to come to and leave the health care agency the same day that the surgery takes place. This type of surgery is generally reserved for those patients who are in an optimum state of health and whose outcome is expected to remain uneventful. Some advantages and disadvantages of outpatient surgery are listed in Table 19-2.

Some surgical procedures are performed in a doctor's office. These are usually types of procedures that do not present any exceptional risks for the patient. They also do not require much anesthesia. *Anesthesia* is the loss of sensation.

Types of Anesthesia

The types of drugs that produce anesthesia are intended to eliminate the uncomfortable sensations associated with an invasive procedure. The type of anesthetic agent that is used is based on several factors:

- The location and extent of the surgical procedure
- The potential for experiencing pain or other discomfort with the procedure
- The patient's current state of health
- The level of the patient's anxiety
- The personal feelings of the patient about certain types of anesthesia.

Following consideration of these factors, the patient may receive general, regional, local, or topical anesthesia. *General anesthesia* eliminates all sensation and produces loss of consciousness. It can be administered by the inhalation of gases or by injection of drugs into the circulatory system. *Regional anesthesia* produces loss of feeling in a large area of the body, such as the pelvis and lower extremities, by instilling an anesthetic agent into the spinal canal. The patient remains alert with regional anesthesia. *Local anesthesia* eliminates sensation in the immediate area of the procedure without altering the patient's state of consciousness. Local anesthesia may be achieved by injecting an anesthetic agent into and around the tissue where the procedure will be performed. *Topical anesthesia* is a type of local anesthesia applied to the surface of mucous membranes and eliminates discomfort for a relatively short period of time.

Identifying Surgical Risk Factors

Each patient who will undergo surgery should be evaluated for potential risks. The nurse shares the responsibility for assessing factors that pose a hazard for the patient undergoing surgery. Experience has shown that certain risk factors increase the possibility that complications will occur. The number and type of risk factors influence the preoperative preparation, the type of anesthetic, and postoperative care of surgical patients. Some risk factors may be so great that surgery may be postponed.

Some risk factors and complications that may result are listed in Table 19-3. Old age, obesity, and chronic diseases, such as diabetes mellitus, are common surgical risk factors that are discussed in more detail at the end of the chapter. In addition to the conditions listed, the nurse should report any abnormal vital signs and laboratory test results. Specific complications associated with surgery are discussed later in this chapter.

Informing the Patient

A patient is usually told about the need for surgery by his own physician. This often happens before the patient is admitted to the hospital. In some instances, the patient

Table 19-2. Evaluation of Outpatient Surgery

Advantages	Disadvantages
Lowers the surgical costs due to the reduced use of hospital services	Reduces the time for establishing a nurse-patient relationship
Reduces the time spent away from home, school, or place of employment	Requires intensive preoperative teaching in a short amount of time
Interferes less with the individual's usual daily routine	Reduces the opportunity for reinforcement of teaching and for answering questions
Provides the potential for more rest and sleep before and after surgery	Allows for fewer delays in assessing and preparing a patient once he arrives for surgery
Allows more opportunity for family contact and support	Requires that care of the patient following discharge be carried out by unskilled individuals

Table 19-3. Surgical Risk Factors

Condition	Complication	Explanation
Old age	Delayed healing, disuse syndrome	The elderly patient may have decreased body functions that prolong cell growth and repair. Inactivity may lead to many complications.
Dehydration	Reduced circulation, reduced urine output, blood clots	When the water volume of blood is low, cells may not receive adequate chemicals or oxygen. Blood that is thick is more apt to clot.
Inadequate nutrition	Poor healing, skin breakdown	Without appropriate nutrients, cell maintenance, growth, and repair cannot take place.
Cigarette smoking or use of other tobacco products	Pneumonia, atelectasis, poor circulation, blood clots	Smoking causes an increase in mucous production that can plug air passages or lead to an inflammation in the lungs. Nicotine constricts blood vessels, slowing the movement of blood.
Obesity	Poor healing, hypostatic pneumonia	Fatty tissue has a reduced blood supply. This interferes with the delivery of oxygen, nutrients, and other chemicals needed for tissue repair. An overweight person generally moves less and breathes less deeply.
Use of certain drugs, such as anticoagulants, aspirin, oral contraceptives, steroids	Bleeding, clotting, slowed healing, reduced response against infection	Anticoagulants, including aspirin, can interfere with clotting. Oral contraceptives increase the tendency to clot. Steroids alter the ability to heal and fight infection due to their anti-inflammatory action.
Substance abuse or dependence, such as alcohol	Withdrawal symptoms, altered reaction to anesthetic agents	Reduction in the usual amount of an addicting substance may cause dangerous symptoms.
Psychological fear	Emotional stress, tensed muscles, elevated blood pressure, rapid heart rate	Stimulation of the sympathetic nervous system accelerates many body functions. Tense muscles and an overly excited state of consciousness may interfere with achieving the desired state of anesthesia.

may be admitted for diagnostic studies and then learn that surgery is advised. The physician must inform the patient of the risks and benefits of surgery, the likely outcome if surgery is not performed, and alternative methods of treatment other than surgery. These are components of informed consent that were discussed previously in Chapter 6. Obtaining written consent will be discussed again later in this chapter. The patient is always entitled to obtain second opinions before making a decision.

Predonating Blood

Surgery, except in a few circumstances, means there will be blood loss. For some, blood loss requires blood replacement. Many currently fear the rare but potential consequences of blood transfusions. Although blood is tested, the risk of contracting AIDS and hepatitis still exists. There is also the risk of a transfusion reaction. The blood banking system is not perfect.

For these reasons, more and more people are choosing

to predonate their own blood. Receiving one's own blood is called an *autologous transfusion*. It can be accomplished in two different ways. One way is to begin donating a unit of blood weekly up to within one week of the scheduled date of surgery. This process can be started six weeks before surgery since blood can only be safely stored for 42 days. On rare occasions blood can be donated every three days. Regardless of the frequency, no blood will be accepted if the donor's iron stores (hemoglobin) become depleted. A hemoglobin below 11 g disqualifies the donor. Blood can be frozen longer, up to three years. However, arrangements for long-term storage must usually be made through private blood-banking firms. This option, obviously, is more costly.

Another way to receive an autologous transfusion involves recycling the patient's blood that is suctioned during an operation. Bloody drainage is collected and the red blood cells are filtered out, washed, and replaced in the form of a transfusion to the patient.

Some individuals are preselecting their own donors from among relatives and friends. They are called *directed donors*. A directed donor must have the same blood type of the recipient or a compatible type. Otherwise, the donated blood becomes part of the general blood bank supply. The hospital must also agree to store and reserve the directed donor's blood for the future surgery patient. Some feel that receiving blood from directed donors is not much safer than the blood from unidentified donors.

Criteria for autologous and directed donations differ among regions and, in some cases, hospitals. Table 19-4 is a list of guidelines that are common among various centers around the United States.

Providing Psychological Support

Keeping in mind holistic concepts, the nurse understands that a patient's emotional state can affect his physical condition. Because fear and stress create potential risk factors

---

Table 19-4. Autologous and Directed Blood Donor Guidelines

Common Features

Collected in blood centers, mobiles, hospitals
Require 72 hours from collection to delivery
Require donor appointment
Will be tested under routine protocol

Autologous Donation	**Directed Donation**
Donor must weigh 95 pounds.	Donor must weigh 110 pounds.
Donor must be at least 14 years old.	Donor must be at least 17 years old.
Exceptions made in medical history.	Must meet volunteer donor medical history criteria.
Requires physician order.	Patient's physician must be informed of directed donation.
Used only for transfusion to donor.	May be transfused to others if not needed by intended patient.
Blood type does not need to be known at time of donation.	Donors should know blood type of patient.
Units that test positive for disease (other than HIV) will be issued.	Units that test positive for HIV or hepatitis will not be used.
Donation frequency may be greater than one unit every 56 days; iron therapy may be necessary and is ordered by physician.	May donate one unit every 56 days.
Additional fee to hospital or recipient may be charged for holding blood on reserve.	Additional fees may be charged to the recipient, the donor, or hospital.

Information used with permission of Great Lakes Region, American Red Cross, 1990.

for the surgical patient, the nurse has an important responsibility for providing psychological support for the patient.

The need for psychological support will vary greatly among patients. For example, the patient's age, diagnosis, cultural and educational background, family responsibilities, and occupation are typical factors that affect the need and approaches for psychological support.

By putting oneself in the patient's position, a nurse can begin to help patients cope with upcoming surgery. Answering certain questions such as the following can provide a beginning:

- How would I feel if I were about to have the type of surgery this patient is to have?
- What would frighten me most about the surgical experience?
- Who would I most like to be with me?
- What would I like the nurse to do to help me through this experience?

Psychological stress is usually based on a fear of the unknown. Therefore, another way to provide emotional support is by anticipating common concerns of the patient. Then, by providing information and instructions, the patient's stress level may be reduced. Experience has shown that the following questions are most frequently asked by patients about to have surgery:

- What is the surgical procedure and why is it being done?
- Will I lose control of my body functions while I am unconscious?
- How long will I be in the operating and recovery rooms?
- When may I see my family after surgery?
- Will I have pain when I wake up?
- Will I know where I am?
- Will I be sick from the anesthesia?
- Will I have tubes in me when I wake up?
- Will I need a blood transfusion?
- What can I eat and drink after surgery?
- What kind of incision will I have? How long will it take to heal?
- Will I be disfigured? Can I lead a normal life?
- How long will it take before I can return home, go to work, or go to school?

This list of questions is by no means complete; some patients may ask still other questions. On the other hand, not every patient will be interested in answers to every question listed. However, these questions may help to guide the nurse in being alert to areas in which the patient may have concerns.

Psychological support not only involves providing information. It includes observing and taking the time to listen to the patient and others who are concerned about the patient. It is usually of no help simply to say that everything will be all right and that there is no cause for worry. The helpful nurse will be available to provide an opportunity for individuals to talk about their problems and express feelings. In this manner, the nurse can often determine whether the patient wishes to see some other support person, such as his minister, priest, or rabbi, before surgery. Steps can be taken to arrange a visit if this has not already been done.

Emotional care continues during the postoperative period in a manner similar to that in preoperative care. The nurse should be alert to feelings and worries that patients may not be able to express specifically. For example, the patient may ask, "How am I doing?" when he really means, "Do you think I'll make it?" The nurse may need to interpret the patient's underlying question and explain what is happening to the extent to which individuals are interested or able to understand.

Caring for the Patient Before Surgery

Experienced nurses have found that the better patients are taught and prepared for surgery, the fewer postoperative problems or complications that occur. When compared with patients who have had little or no preparation during their preoperative care, studies have noted the following:

- Well-prepared patients understand more about the surgery they are to have.
- They feel more in control of the actions and consequences affecting their care.
- They experience less postoperative pain and anxiety.
- They are better motivated for self-care.
- They require less time in the hospital.
- Their recuperative period is shortened.

These findings certainly indicate the advantages in preparing patients for their surgical experiences.

Most often, teaching is done on an individual basis. However, when an opportunity for teaching a group of preoperative patients exists, the nurse is encouraged to use this method. Very often, patients offer each other emotional support and find that sharing experiences with others makes the surgical experience less frightening.

Nurses have also learned that it is very helpful to include close family members in preoperative teaching. This is especially important when a patient may be unable to understand all the nurse's teaching or when the patient will be going home the same day of surgery. Most relatives are eager to be informed, cooperative, and helpful.

The discussion that follows includes information that could be included in the preparation of patients undergoing surgery. Any preoperative teaching should be documented on the patient's chart as it is carried out. This provides a record of what teaching has been done and what still needs to be completed.

Promoting Activity and Exercise

Inactivity poses a hazard for the surgical patient. Postoperative patients tend to want to move about as little as possible. They are often fearful of pain and of opening an incision. If patients are allowed to function in this manner, postoperative complications, including some associated with the disuse syndrome, are very likely to develop.

The nurse should explain to the preoperative patient that postoperatively he will be helped to move and turn, to change his position frequently, to dangle, and even to walk soon after surgery. Most surgical patients are helped out of bed the same day of their operation. Skills for promoting movement and mobility are described in Chapter 18.

Preventing Respiratory Complications

Many factors increase the risk of respiratory complications even for the patient who is reasonably healthy and active before surgery. As mentioned previously, inactivity interferes with adequate ventilation. Refraining from food and water tends to thicken respiratory secretions. Inhaled anesthetics are combined with oxygen, which has a drying effect on mucous membranes. The nurse has an opportunity preoperatively to teach the patient measures that will counteract these effects in order to prevent or restore respiratory function.

Performing Deep-Breathing Exercises. Normally, individuals yawn, sigh, or take deep breaths automatically every 5 to 10 minutes to keep the small air passageways of the lungs open. Those who receive general anesthesia are dependent on the person administering the anesthetic to provide occasional deep breaths. The reduction of automatic deep breathing, inactivity during surgery, and a tendency to breathe less deeply after surgery to avoid pain combine to predispose the surgical patient to respiratory complications. Less than optimal ventilation may be accompanied by the collection of thickened secretions within the respiratory tract. Deep-breathing and, in some cases, coughing are important measures to prevent the possibility of hypostatic pneumonia and atelectasis.

Deep breathing exercises consist of helping a patient to use diaphragmatic and pursed-lip breathing. This helps open small air passageways and to inflate the lungs fully with air. Skill Procedure 19-1 describes and illustrates the actions that the nurse can teach the patient in order to improve ventilation.

Skill Procedure 19-1. Teaching Deep-Breathing Exercises

Suggested Action	Reason for Action
Place the patient in a sitting position, if that is possible.	A sitting position lowers the abdominal organs away from the diaphragm so that the lungs have the maximum amount of room for expansion. A sitting position may not be allowed following all surgical procedures.
Place a pillow between the lower back and the bed or have the patient sit 2 to 4 inches from the back of a chair.	Having the back away from the bed or chair further allows room for full expansion of the lungs.
Flex the knees if the patient has an abdominal incision.	Flexion creates less tension on abdominal muscles and therefore less discomfort when the chest expands.
Help the patient relax.	Tense muscles interfere with full lung expansion.
Explain that the pattern for deep-breathing should be repeated three or four times with a few seconds of rest between each inspiration.	To compensate for the period of inactivity during surgery and restricted ventilation afterwards, deep breathing must be performed several times when it is actively practiced.
Emphasize that the breathing should be done *slowly*.	Rapid breathing causes hyperventilation. It does not allow enough time to exhale carbon dioxide, which can lead to dizziness, lightheadedness, weakness, tingling around the mouth and fingertips, and even fainting.
Have the patient place his hands on his abdomen, as the nurse is demonstrating in Figure 19-1.	Practicing with the patient helps reinforce the correct movements for diaphragmatic breathing.
Instruct the patient to take a deep breath while counting to about five or seven, with a second for each count, making the abdomen swell to become larger.	This type of breathing moves the diaphragm downward, increasing the area of the thorax and elevates the lower ribs to allow the greatest amount of room for the lungs to expand.

(continued)

Skill Procedure 19-1. Continued

Suggested Action	**Reason for Action**

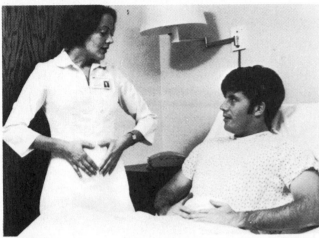

Figure 19-1 The nurse teaches the patient to make his abdomen larger as he takes a deep breath through his mouth. He holds his breath to the count of three before exhaling.

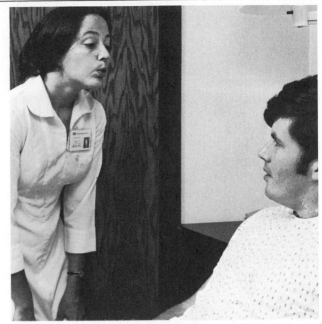

Figure 19-2 The nurse demonstrates exhaling through pursed lips.

Follow local custom for explaining the process for inhalation. In some agencies, the patient is instructed to inhale through his mouth or nose.

Have the patient hold his breath to the count of three to four after inhaling deeply.

Instruct the patient to exhale slowly through pursed lips to the count of 12 to 15 or, if he cannot exhale for that long, for as long as it took him to inhale. The patient in Figure 19-2 is being shown how to exhale.

Have the patient compress his abdomen toward the spine while exhaling or bend slightly forward.

Practice the deep-breathing exercise several times until the patient can perform it correctly.

Explain that postoperatively he should plan to breathe deeply every 1 to 2 hours while he is awake. These exercises should continue for the first 2 to 3 postoperative days, or possibly longer if he has respiratory problems.

Inhaling through the nose prevents gulping and swallowing air, which can lead to discomfort if the stomach and intestines fill with air.

Retaining a high volume of air opens and fills air passages throughout the lungs and helps prevent bronchioles and alveoli from narrowing or collapsing.

Exhaling slowly through pursed lips increases the air pressure within the alveoli more than during quiet expiration, opens air passageways, and helps to maximize the exhalation of carbon dioxide.

Rather than passively releasing air, this movement increases intraabdominal pressure, which moves the diaphragm upward to empty the lungs of a higher volume of expired air.

Patients should be competent at performing this before surgery. Pain and anxiety after surgery limit the patient's attention and may interfere with the ability to learn.

To achieve the goal of preventing respiratory complications, this exercise must be performed at frequent intervals until the patient breathes well and normal breath sounds are heard throughout the lungs.

Using Incentive Spirometry. Some patients may have difficulty understanding and carrying out the instructions for deep breathing. Others, such as smokers or individuals with chronic respiratory diseases, who are at higher risk for developing respiratory complications, may require additional assistance. A method other than deep breathing may be needed to ensure that the patient is adequately inflating the lungs.

Incentive spirometry is a method for measuring the patient's respiratory efforts. One type of incentive spirometer is illustrated in Figure 19-3. Depending on the type used, each provides a signal that can be seen or heard. Reaching the signal acts as an inducement for inhaling with maximal effort. Some equipment can be set at a certain level for inhalation, usually 500 mL. The depth of inhalation can be increased as the patient learns to inhale more deeply.

Some spirometers contain a nebulizer. A *nebulizer* is a device that converts a liquid into a fine mist. Water or liquid medications can be inhaled through this attachment. The nebulizer helps liquefy respiratory secretions so that they do not become thick and plug respiratory passageways.

The use of this equipment is best taught preoperatively according to the manufacturer's instructions. It is commonly used for about five days postoperatively, ten times during each waking hour. It is recommended that the patient take up to five normal breaths between each deep breath on an incentive spirometer. Sessions of deep breathing should be avoided immediately after meals because of the danger of causing nausea.

Most patients quickly learn to use an incentive spirometer so that they can carry out the procedure without a nurse in attendance. However, the nurse should monitor a patient from time to time to note that the spirometer is used properly. Such monitoring also demonstrates the nurse's interest, which, in turn, tends to motivate the patient to use incentive spirometry as prescribed.

Raising Secretions. Cilia, hairlike structures that line the respiratory tract, move secretions to the upper airways. Coughing is an automatic method for clearing airways of secretions. Deep breathing alone may provide enough stimulus to produce a natural cough. Encouraging patients to drink adequate amounts of fluid will help keep the secretions thinned so they are more easily raised.

It is generally agreed that, unless moist secretions can be heard in the lungs, forced coughing should not be routinely performed postoperatively. The forced exhalation created by coughing tends to collapse small airways and alveoli, doing more harm than good. Patients undergoing some types of surgery, such as that on the eye or brain, or those having had a hernia repaired, should not cough unless specifically ordered to do so. Coughing is dangerous for these patients because it increases pressure in the operative area. However, these surgical patients may perform deep-breathing exercises.

For those patients who have noisy respirations or wet lung sounds, coughing should be performed to help raise and expectorate the accumulated secretions. Skill Procedure 19-2 describes the technique for teaching a patient how to cough properly.

Avoiding Thrombi and Emboli

Inactivity and gravity cause blood to pool and settle in lower areas of the body. Blood tends to become thickened due to the restriction of fluid and food prior to surgery. The surgical patient should avoid positions that tend to keep blood trapped in the lower extremities. Such things as sitting for a prolonged period of time should not be allowed. Placing pillows directly beneath the knees or gatching the bed can interfere with blood flow, leading to the formation of clots. Measures can be used during the postoperative period to prevent circulatory complications. The nurse can explain their use preoperatively.

Performing Leg Exercises. The temporarily inactive surgical patient can perform leg exercises to promote circulation and help prevent the formation of blood clots. Alternate contraction and relaxation of muscles create a pulselike effect on vein walls that helps move blood toward the heart. Recommended techniques for leg exercises are described in Skill Procedure 19-3.

Wearing Antiembolism Stockings. To help prevent thrombi formation, antiembolism stockings are often or-

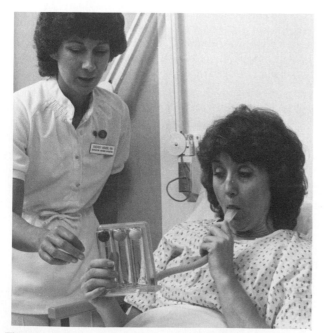

Figure 19-3 The goal when using this spirometer is to raise the three balls during inhalation.

Skill Procedure 19-2. Teaching the Patient to Cough

Suggested Action	**Reason for Action**
Position the patient in a sitting position, unless contraindicated, with the patient leaning slightly forward. A side-lying position may be used by those who may not sit.	A sitting position lowers abdominal organs away from the diaphragm so that the lungs have the maximum amount of room for expansion. A sitting position may not be allowed for all surgical patients. Leaning forward increases intrathoracic pressure, promoting raising of secretions.
Splint the abdomen if that is where the operative site will be. This can be done with applied hand pressure, with a folded towel or pillow, or with a bath blanket about the middle of the body, as shown in Figure 19-4.	Applying pressure supports the area of an abdominal incision. The patient will feel less discomfort with a splinted incision and will likely produce a more effective cough.

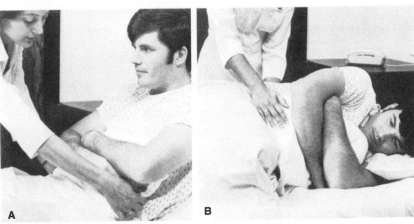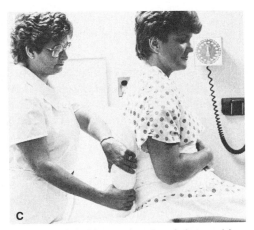

Figure 19-4 (*A*). A rolled towel can be used as a splint over a wound when the patient coughs. (*B*). The patient can bring up his knees while lying on his side and put pressure on a pillow against an incision for support when coughing. (*C*). This nurse has wrapped a bath blanket around the patient's chest and abdomen. When the blanket is rolled to support the incision snugly, the patient is encouraged to cough.

Have the patient inhale deeply and then have him give two or three hacking coughs as he exhales. The mouth should be open with the tongue out for best results, as illustrated in Figure 19-5.	Hard coughing should be avoided because it may injure the tissues in the respiratory tract.

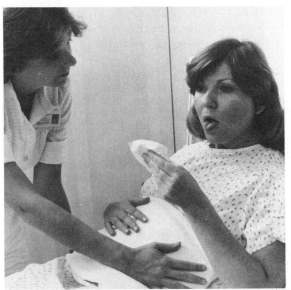

Figure 19-5 The patient is producing a hacking cough with tongue extended, raising secretions from the respiratory tract.

(continued)

Skill Procedure 19-2. Continued

Suggested Action	Reason for Action
Follow the coughing effort with a deep breath and then with another cough if secretions are still present.	Deep breathing following coughing helps inflate collapsed lung tissues.
Explain that the patient should expectorate raised secretions into a tissue.	The pressure created by coughing should move secretions to a higher area, where they can be expelled.
Have the patient dispose of the tissue in a waste container.	Secretions may contain pathogens that could be spread if touched by others.
Listen postoperatively for the presence of secretions after the patient coughs.	Normal breath sounds should sound like air moving in and out of passageways. When secretions accumulate, the nurse may not hear any sounds in an area or they will sound like wheezes, crackles, or gurgles as the patient breathes in and out.

dered for patients with limited activity. The stockings are manufactured by several companies. They come in thigh length or knee length in various sizes. Some stockings fit either leg; others are designed for right or left. Their elastic woven fiber acts to support the walls and valves of veins much as a girdle supports abdominal muscles. The support of the vein wall prevents it from stretching and distending with blood. As blood is pumped from the lower areas of the legs upward, the stockings help the valves close. Closed valves prevent blood that has been moved forward toward the heart from falling back into the lower legs and feet.

In addition to inactive and bedridden patients, people with vein disorders or circulatory disturbances, those who spend a great deal of time on their feet, and pregnant women often find elastic stockings helpful to prevent edema and improve circulation in the legs. Skill Procedure 19-4 describes and illustrates the actions for applying and using antiembolism stockings.

Obtaining Written Consent

The importance of having a consent form signed preoperatively was discussed in Chapter 6. It is a nursing responsibility to check that one has been obtained before proceeding with preparing a patient for surgery. A consent form for a surgical procedure is illustrated in Figure 19-10.

Preparing the Surgical Site

Hair and skin harbor organisms. For this reason, the skin at and around the site of the surgery is specially prepared preoperatively. The skin cannot be sterilized, but measures can be taken to reduce the chances of introducing organisms into the operative site.

Cleansing the Skin. An area of skin much larger than the immediate area around the incision is ordinarily prepared before surgery. This precaution further reduces the chances of infection.

Some agencies permit the patient to participate in preparing his skin by showering or scrubbing with a specified type of soap for a certain period of time. Usually the nurse is required to scrub the surgical site.

Removing Hair. Recent studies have shown controversy about the traditional approach used to prepare the surgical site. This included shaving the body in a wide area surrounding the eventual incision. Examples are shown in Figure 19-11. Shaving is done to remove microorganisms

Skill Procedure 19-3. Teaching Leg Exercises

Suggested Action	Reason for Action
Position the patient on his back with the head of the bed slightly elevated.	Leg exercises require that the patient flex the knee and toes, which is most easily performed in a supine position. Raising the head helps the patient observe foot movements and relaxes the abdominal muscles.
Instruct the patient, as the nurse is doing in Figure 19-6, to alternately dorsiflex and plantarflex his feet followed by moving each foot in clockwise and then counterclockwise circles.	Movement of the feet helps to move blood, pooled there by inactivity and gravity, out of the most distant areas of the legs.

(continued)

Suggested Action

Reason for Action

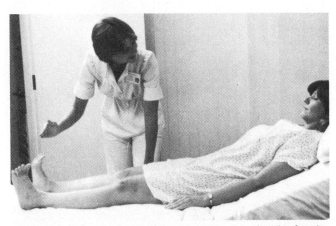

Figure 19-6 The patient is being taught to exercise the feet by performing alternate dorsiflexion and plantarflexion followed by moving the toes in circles. This begins to circulate blood that has pooled in the lowest areas of the legs back to the heart.

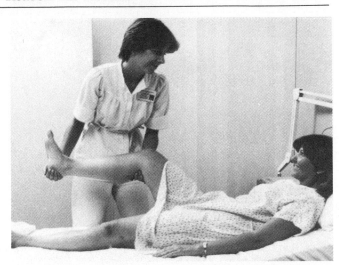

Figure 19-7 The patient is taught to bend her knee. The nurse provides assistance if the patient cannot independently perform the exercise.

Request that the patient bend one knee and then the other, sliding each as far up the mattress as possible and then back again. Or, the nurse can assist the patient with this movement, as shown in Figure 19-7.

Have the patient straighten and then raise each leg alternately as high off the bed as comfort will allow and return it to the bed, as illustrated in Figure 19-8.

Actively using the muscles of the thigh to flex and extend the knee creates a pumping action that moves blood back to the heart.

Elevation assists gravity to move blood in the direction of the heart.

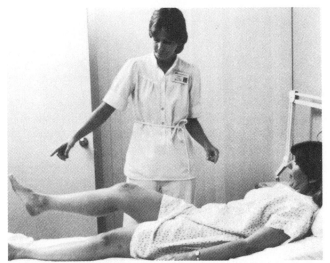

Figure 19-8 The patient extends her knee as she allows her leg to drop slowly back onto the bed. Each leg is exercised in this manner.

Inform the patient that leg exercises should be performed five times each and repeated when awake every 2 hours postoperatively until resuming ambulation and normal activity.

Until a reasonable level of activity is resumed, leg exercises must be performed as a substitute for ambulation.

Suggested Action	Reason for Action
Measure the patient's leg from the flat of the heel to the bend of the knee, and the calf circumference. For thigh-high stockings, measure the length to mid-thigh; in addition to the calf measurement, also measure thigh circumference.	Determining a patient's size is important for achieving the purpose of the stocking. Improperly fitting stockings are uncomfortable and will do little good and may even do harm.
Plan to apply stockings in the morning before the patient is out of bed or after elevating the feet for at least 15 minutes.	Before the feet are lowered, there is a minimal amount of pooled blood in the lower legs and feet. Elevation helps gravity move blood toward the heart.
Clean and dry the feet. Apply cornstarch or talcum powder if desired.	Hygiene provides an opportunity for assessment. Powder helps reduce friction when the stockings are applied.
Take care not to massage the legs during hygiene.	Massaging may break a clot loose, if it is present, and cause it to circulate in the body.
Apply the stocking using either of two methods. Turn the stocking inside out and insert the toes. Or, gather the stocking down from the top, insert the foot, and thread the leg through the stocking. Both methods are shown in Figure 19-9.	Though elastic, these stockings do not have a wide range of stretch. Applying the stockings in graduated amounts helps ease their application and prevents forming uncomfortable wrinkles.

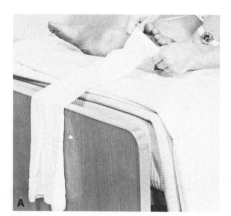 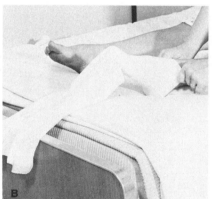 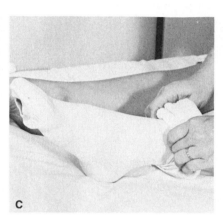

Figure 19-9 (*A*). This type of antiembolism stocking is turned inside out to the foot. (*B*). The inverted stocking is then put on the foot and properly positioned over the heel. (*C*). This stocking has been gathered and is pulled the length of the leg. The opening, which should cover the toes, is somewhat larger to allow for extra room and comfort.

Check the position of the patient's heel in the stocking.	An improperly positioned heel area may interfere with wearing slippers and walking or cause discomfort.
Stretch the toe area of the stockings and mold the toes and forefoot into good alignment if the stockings do not have a toe opening.	Pressure and poor alignment of the toes should be relieved so that circulation, the condition of the skin, or movement are not restricted.
Smooth the stocking wrinkles.	Folds and wrinkles can cut off circulation and cause enough pressure to break down skin.
Remove the stockings and assess the patient's comfort, temperature, and signs of swelling at least twice a day or on each shift.	Damage to skin and problems with circulation can develop quickly. Frequent observation aids detection and correction of problems early.
Wash soiled stockings at least every three days or more often if necessary.	Laundering clothing is an example of personal hygiene.
Dry the stockings on a flat surface.	Drying on a flat surface prevents altering the shape and size of stockings due to stretching.
Immediately replace soiled stockings with a clean pair.	Removing stockings for an extended period of time defeats their purpose.

```
              THREE RIVERS AREA HOSPITAL
              THREE RIVERS, MICHIGAN   49093

              AUTHORIZATION FOR MEDICAL
                       AND/OR
                  SURGICAL TREATMENT
```

                                                                    a.m.

                    Date *July 18*   19**88**   Time **2:30** (**p.m.**)

I, the undersigned, a patient in Three Rivers Area Hospital, hereby authorize

Dr. *Robert Morrison, M.D.*   (and whomever he may designate as his assistant)

to administer such treatment as is necessary, and to perform the following operation

Exploratory Laparotomy and Appendectomy   .

                    (Name of operation and/or procedure)

and such additional operations or procedures as are considered therapeutically

necessary on the basis of findings during the course of said operation, with the

following exception, **None**   .

I also consent to the administration of such anesthetics as are necessary, with

the exception of **None**   .

                    (None, spinal anesthesia, or other)

I hereby certify that I have read and fully understand the above AUTHORIZATION

FOR MEDICAL and/or SURGICAL TREATMENT, the reasons why the above named surgery is

considered necessary, its advantages and possible complications, if any, as well as

possible alternative modes of treatments, which were explained to me by

Dr. **Morrison**   .

I also certify that no guarantee or assurance has been made as to the results

that may be obtained.

Gary Holmes   *Judi Ebbert, RN*
  (Patient or nearest relative)   (Witness)

_____
    (Relationship)

I hereby certify that I have explained to **Gary Holmes**

(a patient at Three Rivers Area Hospital), the reasons why the above named surgery

is considered necessary, its advantages and possible complications, if any, as well

as possible alternative modes of treatment.

Robert Morrison, M.D.   *7-18-88*
  (Surgeon signature)   (Date)

7181-102

Figure 19-10 This consent form has been signed by the patient to grant permission for surgery. (Courtesy of Three Rivers Area Hospital, Three Rivers, MI.)

attached to the hair. The theory is valid. However, it has been found that a razor causes microabrasions. A *microabrasion* is a scraping away of skin that cannot be seen with normal visual inspection. This skin is ordinarily a barrier against pathogens. When skin is abraded, it allows an entry site for microorganisms. Microbes tend to grow even more vigorously in the plasma-rich environment of the impaired skin. Their growth compounds during the time between shaving and the actual surgery.

Some surgeons are eliminating hair removal completely before surgery. They are relying on appropriate cleansing of the skin to reduce the numbers and types of skin pathogens. Limited research on statistically small numbers of patients have shown no significant differences in infection rates among those patients left unshaved versus any other type of hair removal.

If hair needs to be removed, it is being restricted to the area of the incision and a narrow margin where tape may

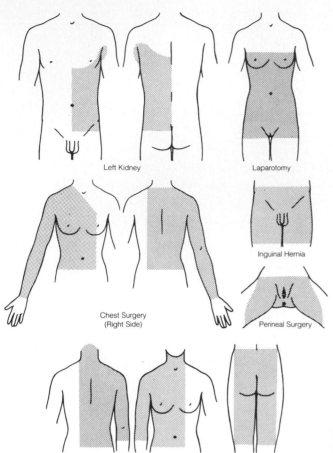

Left Kidney   Laparotomy

Chest Surgery
(Right Side)   Inguinal Hernia

Perineal Surgery

Breast Surgery (Right Side)   Rectal Surgery

Figure 19-11 These sketches illustrate the areas of skin that may be shaved preoperatively for various types of surgery. Follow the physician's order or local policy, which may differ regarding preparation of the surgical site.

be applied. Hair clipping is now being substituted for shaving in more and more instances. Those surgeons who request shaving postpone hair removal until just before the procedure. It is performed while the patient is in the operative holding area.

Some use a depilatory cream as an alternative method for hair removal. A *depilatory* chemically separates the hair at the skin surface. Many who use this method say that the cream is messy, it takes more time than any other method for hair removal, and causes skin irritation among some sensitive patients.

Covering the Prepared Surgical Area. In some instances, the surgeon may order that sterile dressings be applied to the scrubbed or shaved skin. This is likely to be the case when surgery involving the musculoskeletal system is done. The following aseptic practices should be followed when covering is required:

- Create a sterile field and add the following sterile items: basin, water, gauze squares, rolls of gauze, and sterile towels.

- Don sterile gloves.
- Rinse and dry the cleansed or shaven area with sterile gauze as the nurse in Figure 19-12 is doing.
- Wrap the dried area with rolls of gauze, as shown in Figure 19-13.
- Cover the wrapped gauze with sterile towels, as illustrated in Figure 19-14. The area should be wrapped snugly but not so tightly that it causes discomfort or endangers proper circulation.
- Secure the dressings, as in Figure 19-15.

Carrying Out the Preoperative Routine

Most agencies follow similar routines for the basic physical preparation of the preoperative patient. Skill Procedure 19-5 provides a sequence of care that is most commonly performed before a patient's surgery. Not all the actions will be required for all patients. Any omission of a commonly practiced preoperative routine should be questioned. There could have been an oversight on the part of the nurse, attending physician, or other hospital person-

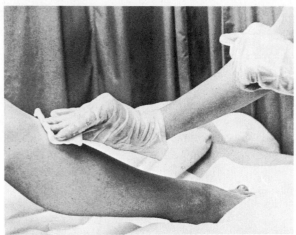

Figure 19-12 The nurse has donned sterile gloves and rinses soap from the skin with sterile gauze and sterile water.

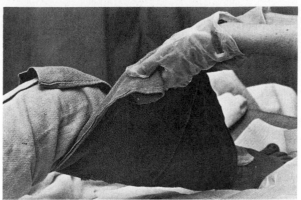

Figure 19-14 Sterile towels are then used to cover the dressings on the patient's leg.

nel. Appropriate steps may be taken to rectify the situation to avoid delaying the surgery.

Judgment is required in emergency situations. The preoperative preparation of the patient is adapted to meet the patient's needs in the best possible manner while still conserving time.

Completing a Preoperative Checklist. Most health agencies have a checklist to guide the nurse's actions while preparing the preoperative patient for surgery. The checklist is a summary of priority actions that must be completed before an operation can begin. Having all the information on one sheet of paper eliminates searching through the patient's chart to determine that they have been carried out. Before the patient leaves the preoperative unit, the nurse responsible for his care and an individual who works in the operating room review the checklist. If any areas of the checklist are incomplete, the patient remains on the nursing unit until clarification takes place. An example of a preoperative checklist is illustrated in Figure 19-17

Resuming Care After Surgery

Most health agencies have recovery rooms where patients remain until they are conscious and their condition stabilizes. Nurses working in recovery rooms have special training in the immediate care of the postoperative patient. Their role is not discussed here.

Preparing a Patient's Room

While the patient is in the operating and recovery room, the nurse prepares an unoccupied bed, as described in Chapter 12. The top linen is folded to the side or bottom of the bed until the patient is transferred from the stretcher. Absorbent pads may be placed over the drawsheet to protect bottom linens from soilage. Equipment and supplies that are likely to be needed are available. They will include items such as blood pressure equipment, extra tissue wipes, an emesis basin, and a pole for hanging intravenous fluid. The nursing unit will be informed by the recovery room nurse if other items, such as suction or oxygen equipment, will be needed.

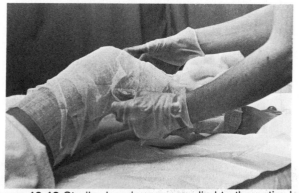

Figure 19-13 Sterile dressings are applied to the entire leg.

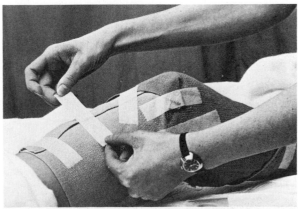

Figure 19-15 The nurse completes the procedure by securing the sterile dressings to prevent them from slipping out of place. Notice how strips of tape are used along the long axis of the leg to hold the two sterile towels together.

Skill Procedure 19-5. Preparing the Patient for Surgery

Suggested Action	**Reason for Action**

Early Before Surgery

Determine that a physical examination, laboratory tests, and special examinations have been ordered and completed.	Knowledge of the patient's condition is important to help prevent complications, correct abnormalities, and reduce surgical risks.
Assess the health status of the patient.	Being aware of each individual's problems is the basis for the preparation and planning of patient care.
Obtain a signed consent for surgery.	Legal implications are serious when surgery is performed without proper consent.
Assess vital signs on admission and again periodically before surgery. Report abnormal vital signs promptly.	Abnormal vital signs may indicate conditions that increase the surgical risks. Surgery may need to be postponed or canceled if they are not within normal ranges.
Provide a light meal or restrict to nothing by mouth.	A nonactive and empty gastrointestinal tract prevents aspiration of undigested food if vomiting occurs. It reduces postoperative nausea and abdominal distention.
Carry out the physician's orders for special measures to promote bowel elimination.	An empty bowel reduces postoperative abdominal distention and constipation.
Prepare the surgical site acording to the policies of the health agency.	A clean operative area reduces chances of introducing organisms into the operative field.

Nearing the Time of Surgery

Provide for mouth care and a partial or complete bath as time permits.	Early scheduling of surgery may shorten the time available for complete bathing in the morning.
Care for valuables, such as jewelry, a watch, or money the day of surgery. If the patient objects to removing a ring, it can be secured in place with adhesive tape or with a strip of gauze, as shown in Figure 19-16, unless there is danger of burning with electrical equipment.	Lost or damaged valuables may result in serious legal problems. Observe agency policy on how to safeguard valuables.

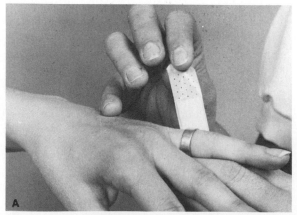 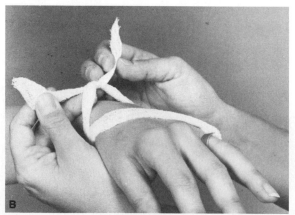

Figure 19-16 (*A*). A plastic bandage strip can be used to secure a ring in place when a patient does not wish to remove it. The gauze section of the strip is placed over a stone when one is present in the ring. (*B*). Another way to secure a ring is to use bandaging gauze to tie the ring in place.

(continued)

Skill Procedure 19-5. Continued

Suggested Action	Reason for Action
Nearing the Time of Surgery	
Remove prostheses, such as artificial limbs and eyes. Follow agency policy regarding the removal of dentures and bridgework. Store prostheses properly and safely according to agency policy.	Prostheses may be lost or accidentally damaged during surgery. Dental appliances may become dislodged or chipped, and cause choking during surgery.
Remove glasses, contact lenses, wigs, false eyelashes, and cosmetics such as lipstick, nail polish, and rouge.	Glasses and other items may become lost or damaged. Contact lenses may damage the eyes. Cosmetics interfere with the assessment of skin, lips, and nailbeds.
Assist the patient to dress in surgical wearing apparel, such as a hospital gown and hair covering. Antiembolism stockings are applied preoperatively in some agencies.	Hospital garments are used for convenience and to prevent soiling or damage to personal garments. Caps prevent the transmission of organisms on loose strands of hair. Stockings reduce the formation of thrombi due to inactivity during surgery.
Remove hairpins, clips, and combs. Rubber bands may be used to secure hair in place.	Sharp hair devices may accidentally injure the scalp.
Provide an opportunity for bowel and bladder elimination shortly before surgery.	A full bladder or bowel may cause discomfort or interfere with the surgical procedure.
Verify that the patient is wearing an identification bracelet.	Misidentification of surgical patients can lead to serious physical injury and legal problems.
Check the patient's history of allergies and administer preoperative medications at the time specified.	A sedative, usually a narcotic, is given to help the patient into a relaxed state. A drug to dry mouth secretions may also be given to minimize the danger of aspiration.
Explain to the patient that he will feel drowsy and thirsty depending on the medications that have been administered.	Informing the patient about the action of drugs will reduce the anxiety and fear of the unexpected.
Raise all siderails, attach the signal cord, and advise the patient to remain in bed.	It is unsafe for the patient to ambulate after receiving preoperative medications, since they may cause the patient to feel dizzy and fall.
Complete all charting and the preoperative checklist.	Personnel in the operating and recovery rooms will need the patient's completed record.
Assist with transferring the patient from the bed onto a stretcher. Explain the need for any belts and the continued use of siderails.	A medicated patient may have difficulty moving onto a stretcher. Belts and siderails are used so that the patient does not fall off the stretcher.
Direct the family or friends to the surgical waiting area.	The surgeon or other personnel may come to this area to communicate personally with the family.

Receiving the Patient

When the patient returns from the recovery room, the nurse should be prepared to continue making frequent and appropriate assessments of his condition. Skill Procedure 19-6 describes the actions that are commonly carried out during the immediate postoperative period on the nursing unit.

Planning Postoperative Care

The patient's postoperative care is guided by written nursing and medical orders. Many health agencies follow previously adopted standards for care. The plan for care is designed to include measures for preventing postoperative complications and discomforts and treating them when they occur. The following are general types of measures included in postoperative orders:

- The frequency with which vital signs are to be checked once they have stabilized.
- The type, amount, and rate at which intravenous fluid therapy is to be administered.
- The concentration and method for administering oxygen.

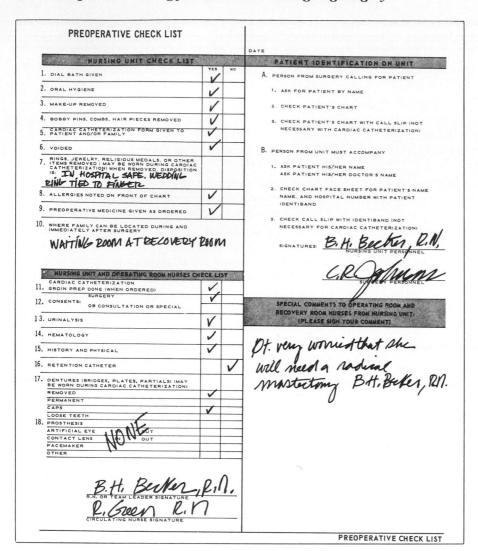

PREOPERATIVE CHECK LIST

DATE

NURSING UNIT CHECK LIST

	YES	NO
1. DIAL BATH GIVEN	✓	
2. ORAL HYGIENE	✓	
3. MAKE-UP REMOVED	✓	
4. BOBBY PINS, COMBS, HAIR PIECES REMOVED	✓	
5. CARDIAC CATHETERIZATION FORM GIVEN TO PATIENT AND/OR FAMILY	✓	
6. VOIDED	✓	
7. RINGS, JEWELRY, RELIGIOUS MEDALS, OR OTHER ITEMS REMOVED (MAY BE WORN DURING CARDIAC CATHETERIZATION) WHEN REMOVED, DISPOSITION IS: IN HOSPITAL SAFE, WEDDING RING TIED TO FINGER		
8. ALLERGIES NOTED ON FRONT OF CHART	✓	
9. PREOPERATIVE MEDICINE GIVEN AS ORDERED	✓	
10. WHERE FAMILY CAN BE LOCATED DURING AND IMMEDIATELY AFTER SURGERY WAITING ROOM AT RECOVERY ROOM		

NURSING UNIT AND OPERATING ROOM NURSES CHECK LIST

	YES	NO
11. CARDIAC CATHETERIZATION GROIN PREP DONE (WHEN ORDERED)	✓	
12. CONSENTS: SURGERY	✓	
OB CONSULTATION OR SPECIAL		
13. URINALYSIS	✓	
14. HEMATOLOGY	✓	
15. HISTORY AND PHYSICAL	✓	
16. RETENTION CATHETER		✓
17. DENTURES (BRIDGES, PLATES, PARTIALS) (MAY BE WORN DURING CARDIAC CATHETERIZATION)		
REMOVED	✓	
PERMANENT		
CAPS	✓	
LOOSE TEETH		
18. PROSTHESIS		
ARTIFICIAL EYE OUT	NONE	
CONTACT LENS OUT		
PACEMAKER		
OTHER		

B. H. Becker, R.N.
R.N. OR TEAM LEADER SIGNATURE
R. Green R.N
CIRCULATING NURSE SIGNATURE

PATIENT IDENTIFICATION ON UNIT

A. PERSON FROM SURGERY CALLING FOR PATIENT

  1. ASK FOR PATIENT BY NAME

  2. CHECK PATIENT'S CHART

  3. CHECK PATIENT'S CHART WITH CALL SLIP (NOT NECESSARY WITH CARDIAC CATHETERIZATION)

B. PERSON FROM UNIT MUST ACCOMPANY

  1. ASK PATIENT HIS/HER NAME
    ASK PATIENT HIS/HER DOCTOR'S NAME

  2. CHECK CHART FACE SHEET FOR PATIENT'S NAME, NAME, AND HOSPITAL NUMBER WITH PATIENT IDENTIBAND

  3. CHECK CALL SLIP WITH IDENTIBAND (NOT NECESSARY FOR CARDIAC CATHETERIZATION)

SIGNATURES: *B. H. Becker, R.N.*
      NURSING UNIT PERSONNEL

C.R. Johnson
      SURGERY PERSONNEL

SPECIAL COMMENTS TO OPERATING ROOM AND RECOVERY ROOM NURSES FROM NURSING UNIT: (PLEASE SIGN YOUR COMMENT)

Pt. very worried that she will need a radical mastectomy B.H. Becker, R.N.

PREOPERATIVE CHECK LIST

Figure 19-17 An example of a preoperative checklist. The nurse responsible for the patient's care signs when a listed action has been completed. These checks and double checks help to avoid errors and to assure that the patient has been properly readied for surgery.

- Medications to be given following surgery. Ordinarily, orders include drugs to control pain and sleeplessness.
- The type of food and fluids that the patient may have. Typically, the patient initially has ice chips and sips of water. If the patient tolerates this well, clear fluids and finally a soft diet may be ordered. Food and fluids are restricted if the patient has gastric or intestinal suctioning.
- The recording of fluid intake and output.
- Care for the wound.
- The frequency for turning and positioning.
- The time when dangling and ambulation should be started.
- Laboratory examinations to be done.

Detecting Postoperative Complications

The nurse must be alert for changes that indicate complications may be occurring. Some signs and symptoms indicate a life-threatening situation, while others may only be minor discomforts. Table 19-5 is a list of common problems that may occur during the postoperative period and their implications for nursing care.

Assisting the Family of a Surgical Patient

Keep in mind that relatives, too, are fearful and worried about the patient. To ease their anxiety, they should be given information about what to expect when the patient returns from surgery.

The nurse should be sure to explain the agency's visitation policies to family members. Most agencies allow close family members to be with the patient before he goes to surgery. They also generally allow family members generous visiting privileges during the immediate postoperative period.

Family members appreciate knowing where they may wait and how long the patient is expected to be in the operating and recovery rooms. It is better not to predict specific times. Delays sometimes occur, causing relatives

Skill Procedure 19-6. Caring for the Postoperative Patient

Suggested Action	Reason for Action
Verify the identify of the patient by checking his wristband.	Misidentification of the patient can lead to serious errors. An identification bracelet is more reliable than verbal responses.
Transfer intravenous fluid bottles, equipment used for oxygen, drainage tubes, and containers to the hospital bed.	Stretching or pulling tubing may cause discomfort or dislocation unless there is sufficient slack to allow for the distance during transfer.
Assist with moving the patient from the stretcher to the bed.	A patient who is drowsy, in pain, or who has not fully regained feeling in his legs will not be able to provide much help during transfer.
Place the patient on his side when possible, or if he must be on his back, turn his head to one side. Keep the patient who has had spinal anesthesia flat.	A side-lying position or turning the head to one side prevents secretions from draining into air passageways. A flat position for a patient who has had spinal anesthesia helps prevent headaches.
Cover the patient with extra blankets if he seems to be chilled.	Operating and recovery rooms are usually air-conditioned. Blood loss and a lowered room temperature can lower the patient's body temperature.
Raise the siderails and fasten the signal cord within the patient's reach.	The patient should not attempt to get out of bed. Siderails and the signal cord provide a means for ensuring the safety of the patient.
Obtain a brief report from the person in charge of transporting the patient, if this was not provided earlier on the phone.	To provide continuity of care, the nurse who assumes responsibility for the patient should be aware of anything unusual that may have occurred in the operating or recovery room.
Check the patient's vital signs. A typical routine is to check them every 15 minutes until stable. Frequent checking, as often as every 5 to 10 minutes, is indicated if the patient's condition is not stable.	A change in vital signs may be one of the earliest indications that a complication is occurring.
Note the color of the patient's skin especially around the mouth and nailbeds.	Blood loss and poor ventilation can be detected by pale or cyanotic color in these areas.
Allow an oral airway to remain in place if one is present.	An airway keeps upper air passages open. The patient will expel an oral airway when reflexes in his throat return to normal.
Check the patient's dressings. Report if there is a large amount of bright red bleeding. Feel under the patient's body, along the side, and the bottom linen.	Dressings absorb blood. An unusual amount of bright red blood may indicate that hemorrhage is occurring. Gravity may influence the direction of drainage so that instead of saturating the dressings, the blood flows down the side or under the patient.
Check the patient's postoperative orders for instructions about specific settings for oxygen, suction, and so on.	The nurse is responsible for carrying out any orders that affect the patient's immediate care.
Observe the site of an IV. Count the rate at which intravenous fluid is infusing.	Intravenous fluid is used to supplement oral fluids and nourishment. The type and rate of infusion must provide appropriate amounts of fluid.
Assess the patient's level of consciousness. Help the patient become oriented by telling him that his surgery is over and that he is back in his room.	General anesthesia alters consciousness. The patient may still be sleepy but easily aroused. Though he may not communicate, he may understand what he hears.
Instruct the patient to take several deep breaths and move his feet and legs as soon as he is able to cooperate.	Preoperative instructions should be implemented as soon as possible to avoid respiratory and circulatory complications.

(continued)

Skill Procedure 19-6. *Continued*

Suggested Action	Reason for Action
Provide mouth care using specially prepared swabs, or wet a washcloth or gauze to moisten the patient's lips and tongue.	The patient recovering from anesthesia may be disturbed by thirst, yet not be alert enough to swallow safely.
Administer pain-relieving medication as soon as the patient's condition safely permits.	Pain-relieving medication can cause drowsiness, decrease respirations, and lower other vital signs. This may tend to interfere with the accurate assessment of the patient's reovery from anesthesia.
Assess the patient's bladder for distention. Offer the use of a bedpan when the patient feels the need to urinate. Measure the amount voided. Notify the physician if more than 8 hours have passed since the patient's last voiding.	An accurate record of the patient's fluid balance must be kept after surgery. Additional measures may be needed if the patient is not able to void.
Communicate with the patient's relatives about his condition and the plans for nursing care.	The family is naturally concerned. Without explanations, they may misjudge the patient's condition or the priorities for care.

unnecessary worry. Also, the nurse will wish to tell the family where meals and snacks are available while they wait and where they can make telephone calls. The family support system is an important part of every patient's care. Both the patient and his family benefit when a nurse takes this into account and wisely uses the family's support for the patient.

Laser Surgery

Laser stands for light amplification by the stimulated emission of radiation. The principle of laser technology involves converting one source of energy, usually electrical, into light energy. The concept is attributed to Albert Einstein in the early 1900s. The first prototype was built in 1960 and used therapeutically to treat eye problems.

Stimulation involves a solid, gas, or liquid medium. Substances such as carbon dioxide, argon, and neodymium–yttrium aluminum garnet (Nd:Yag) are the types commonly used in surgical procedures. All substances, including the ones used in lasers, are composed of atoms in motion. Stimulating the atoms causes them to increase their activity or energy state. The laser machine contains the energy. The focused energy can then be released toward a confined area of tissue.

The tissue absorbs the light energy converting it to heat. By controlling the power, time, and direction of the energy, the laser beam can be used to incise tissue, coagulate bleeding vessels, and vaporize tissue.

The thrust to reduce health-care costs and days spent recovering from surgery is making laser surgery more popular. This technology is becoming more available in doctors' offices as well as in ambulatory and in-patient surgery departments. It is being used as an alternative to conventional surgical procedures such as removing gallbladders, hemorrhoids, and tonsils. Nurses are finding their surgical roles expanding in this area. Along with the traditional nursing responsibilities for preoperative teaching, intraoperative support, and providing postoperative discharge instructions, operating room nurses are pretesting and troubleshooting laser machines. They are enforcing laser safety precautions. They are even assisting with the mechanical operation of the machine. Nurses are taking courses and training others who will be using the equipment; certification in this area will no doubt be available soon.

Benefits of Laser Surgery

Besides cost-effectiveness, several other benefits are associated with laser surgery:

- Reduced need for anesthesia
- Smaller incisions
- Minimal blood loss
- Reduced swelling around the incision
- Less pain following the procedure
- Decreased incidence of wound infection
- Reduced scarring
- Less time recuperating.

Lasers are also being used in conjunction with flexible endoscopes. This allows the surgeon to destroy diseased tissue, relieve obstructions, and control bleeding internally without making any incision at all.

Laser technology is being used in a new form of cancer treatment. It is called photodynamic therapy (PDT). PDT involves the administration of a dye intravenously. When

(Text continues on page 451)

Table 19-5. Common Postoperative Problems

Discomfort/Complication	Implications for Nursing

Cardiovascular Problems

Hemorrhage and Shock

Shock is the body's reaction to inadequate circulation. Clinical texts describe various types of shock. Hypovolemic shock is discussed here and occurs postoperatively when blood volume is lost due to hemorrhage. It constitutes an emergency situation.

- Observe for signs and symptoms of hemorrhage and shock, which include excessive blood on dressings; a rapid, thready pulse; a drop in blood pressure; pale, cold, clammy skin; rapid respirations; low body temperature; restlessness and anxiety; and finally listlessness and unconsciousness. The patient will die if remedial action is not taken.
- Check vital signs frequently and report adverse changes promptly.
- Check dressings frequently for signs of excessive bleeding. Be sure to check under the patient for bloody drainage.
- Be prepared to place the patient in shock in the *Trendelenburg position,* in which the head is lower than the feet, as illustrated in Figure 19-18. This positioning encourages blood to flow from the extremities to vital body organs. The position is *not* used for patients who have had spinal anesthesia or brain surgery. Some agencies require a physician's order before patients can be placed in this position.

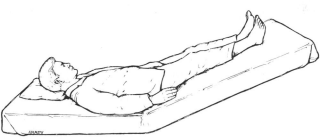

Figure 19-18 This sketch illustrates the Trendelenburg position. The lower extremities are elevated at an angle of about 20 degrees, the knees are straight, the trunk is horizontal, and the head is slightly elevated. (Brunner LS, Suddarth DS: Textbook of Medical-Surgical Nursing, 6th ed, p 366. Philadelphia, JB Lippincott, 1988)

- Place an extra covering on the patient for warmth. *Do not* overheat the patient. This would cause blood to be diverted from vital organs to the skin.
- Be prepared to administer prescribed emergency drugs, intravenous infusions, a blood transfusion, and oxygen.
- Put manual pressure on a bleeding area, if possible, to try to stop the bleeding. The patient may need to be returned to the operating room if the bleeding does not stop.

Thrombophlebitis

Thrombophlebitis occurs as a result of various factors, singly or in combination: injury to veins, dehydration, and slowed circulation after surgery. Thrombophlebitis usually develops between 7 and 10 days after surgery.

- Observe for signs of thrombophlebitis, which include pain or cramping in the calf, painful swelling of the leg. Body temperature may be elevated.
- Use measures to help prevent thrombophlebitis, which include keeping the patient well hydrated, using leg exercises, and early ambulation.
- Avoid anything that may decrease circulation to the legs, such as gatching the knees.

(continued)

Table 19-5. *Continued*

Discomfort/Complication	Implications for Nursing
Cardiovascular Problems	
	• Avoid massaging the legs and use antiembolism stockings as prescribed.
	• When thrombophlebitis develops, be prepared to restrict the patient's activity. Administer a prescribed *anticoagulant,* which is a drug that inhibits or delays blood clotting.
	• Expect that hot, moist packs may be ordered to be placed on the affected leg.
Respiratory Problems	
Atelectasis Atelectasis is the most common postoperative respiratory complication. It is often accompanied by *pneumonitis,* which is an inflammation of the lungs. Atelectasis is caused by a mucous plug that closes off small respiratory passages.	• Observe for signs and symptoms of atelectasis, which include dyspnea, and decreased breath sounds. Fever is often present with pneumonia. • Use measures to encourage ventilation, especially deep-breathing exercises, incentive spirometry, coughing when secretions are present, and early ambulation. • Oxygen therapy may be necessary.
Pulmonary Embolism A pulmonary embolism is most often caused by a blood clot that has dislodged from its original site. It is often preceded by deep-vein thrombophlebitis.	• Observe for signs and symptoms of pulmonary embolism, which include coughing, bloody sputum, a sharp pain in the chest, cyanosis, extreme anxiety, dyspnea, and a rapid and irregular pulse rate. • Use preventive measures such as early ambulation, exercise, and activity, antiembolism stockings, and encouragement of a liberal fluid intake. • Be prepared to administer prescribed oxygen therapy, analgesics, bedrest, and anticoagulants when a pulmonary embolism has occurred.
Hiccups *Hiccups* are intermittent spasms of the diaphragm. A synonym is *singultus.*	• If possible, remove the cause of hiccups, such as gastric or abdominal distention and irritation from drainage tubes in the upper gastrointestinal tract. • When the cause cannot be eliminated, the following measures often relieve hiccups: Have the patient rebreathe in and out of a paper bag. Have the patient hold his breath while swallowing water. • Be prepared to administer a prescribed medication, such as chlorpromazine hydrochloride (Thorazine), if hiccups persist.
Respiratory Infections Respiratory infections include bronchitis, lobar pneumonia, bronchopneumonia, and pleurisy.	• Observe for signs and symptoms of various respiratory infections; these include fever, expectorations of purulent sputum, cough, elevated pulse and respiratory rates, flushed skin, dyspnea, and pain with inspirations. • Use preventive measures to improve respiratory functioning; these include deep-breathing exercises, coughing, incentive spirometry, early ambulation, and activity as prescribed. • Encourage fluid intake. • Be prepared to administer prepared antibiotics and oxygen therapy when an infection is present.
Airway Obstruction	• Observe for signs and symptoms of blocked respiratory passages; these include cyanosis, noisy and difficult respiration, or lack of respirations. • Use suction to remove secretions and debris that may be blocking air passages.

(continued)

Table 19-5. *Continued*

Discomfort/Complication	Implications for Nursing
Respiratory Problems	
	• Open the patient's airway by tilting his forehead and lifting the chin. • Be prepared to use an oral airway to facilitate breathing. • Expect that an endotracheal tube or a tracheostomy may be needed when other measures fail to open respiratory passages.
Gastrointestinal Problems	
Nausea and Vomiting Nausea and vomiting occur in many postoperative patients. They often result from an accumulation of stomach contents before peristalsis returns and from handling the intestine during surgery.	• Offer fluids and food only as ordered. Intravenous infusions are ordinarily used during the early postoperative period. • Use measures described in Chapter 8 to help prevent and relieve nausea and vomiting. • Support and splint the surgical wound when the patient retches and vomits.
Thirst Thirst is the result of preoperative medications used to decrease secretions, fluid loss during surgery, and preoperative fluid restrictions.	• Provide mouth care with commercially prepared swabs. • Moisten the lips and tongue with a clean wet washcloth or gauze square. • Offer ice chips or sips of fluid, if permitted. Hot tea with lemon juice is often useful. • Use measures described in Chapter 25 for the care of patients with limited fluid intake.
Parotitis *Parotitis* is inflammation of the parotid glands. It is often called surgical mumps. Poor oral hygiene predisposes a patient to parotitis.	• Observe for signs and symptoms of parotitis; these include pain, swelling, and redness in the area of the parotid glands. • Use measures described in Chapter 7 to assure good oral hygiene.
Abdominal Distention Abdominal distention generally results from inactivity of the gastrointestinal tract due to medications, anesthesia, handling of internal organs during surgery, the patient's inactivity, and changes in fluid and food intake.	• Observe for signs and symptoms of abdominal distention; these include a swollen abdomen and abdominal pain. • Keep the patient NPO postoperatively until bowel sounds are heard. • Use measures described in Chapter 22 for the prevention and relief of abdominal distention. • Encourage exercise and activity to the extent permitted.
Constipation Constipation may be due to reduced fluid and food intake and inactivity.	• Observe the patient for signs and symptoms of constipation, as described in Chapter 18. • Begin postoperative exercise and activity as soon as permitted after surgery. • Use measures described in Chapter 22 to relieve and prevent constipation.
Urinary-Tract Problems	
Retention, Retention with Overflow, and Urinary-Tract Infections These complications occur most often among patients having surgery	• Observe for signs and symptoms of retention, retention with overflow, and infection in the urinary tract, as described in Chapter 21.

(continued)

Table 19-5. Continued

Discomfort/Complication	Implications for Nursing
on the anus, vagina, or lower abdomen. Infections are common when the patient must be catheterized or has an indwelling catheter.	• Use measures described in Chapter 21 to help prevent and relieve retention, retention with overflow, and urinary-tract infections. • Use measures described in Chapter 21 when catheterizing a patient and when caring for a patient with an indwelling catheter.

Pain and Sleeplessness

Pain is almost always present at the site of surgery. Sleeplessness is common postoperatively, especially when pain is present.	• Observe the patient for signs and symptoms of pain and sleeplessness, as described in Chapter 10. • Administer prescribed medications to relieve pain and sleeplessness, as indicated. • Use measures described in Chapter 10 to promote comfort, rest, and sleep. • Carefully check dosages of narcotics prescribed to control pain postoperatively.

Problems Related to the Skin and Mucous Membranes

Dehiscence *Dehiscence* means that layers of the wound separate. Dehiscence may involve only top layers or it may include all layers of the wound. It usually occurs about 1 week after surgery. *Evisceration* is present when internal organs are exposed and escape from the wound.	• Observe for signs and symptoms of dehiscence, which include a separation of the wound. When evisceration occurs, the patient is likely to say that "something gave way" and is likely to be very anxious. • Handle evisceration as an emergency and be prepared to return the patient to the operating room. • When evisceration occurs, cover exposed organs with sterile gauze moistened with warm sterile normal saline. Do *not* try to replace organs. • Use measures described in Chapter 20 to care for the wound and to help prevent dehiscence. When the patient coughs, be sure the wound is well supported.
Wound Infection A wound infection may be localized or it may affect the patient systemically.	• Observe for signs and symptoms of a wound infection; these include fever, rapid pulse and respiratory rates, general malaise, discomfort, swelling in the area, and redness. An elevated temperature occurring after 72 hours postoperatively suggests a wound infection. • Use measures described in Chapter 20 to care for the surgical wound.
Decubitus ulcers and symptoms of poor personal hygiene	• Observe measures to promote personal hygiene described in Chapter 7 and to prevent and care for decubitus ulcers as described in Chapter 20.

Musculoskeletal Problems

General muscle weakness and contractures are likely to occur if efforts to prevent them are not taken.	• Observe for signs and symptoms of musculoskeletal weakness, as described in Chapter 18. • Use measures described in Chapter 18 to prevent musculoskeletal problems by using exercise and activity for the patient to the extent permitted.

(continued)

Table 19-5. Continued

Discomfort/Complication	Implications for Nursing
Nutritional Problems	
Fluid imbalances and malnutrition may result when efforts to prevent them are not taken.	• Observe for signs and symptoms of fluid imbalances and malnturition, as described in Chapters 8 and 25. • Expect that intravenous therapy, certain medications, and a nourishing diet will be used to help prevent fluid imbalances and malnutrition.
Hypothermia	
Hypothermia decreases the availability of oxygen for cells due to slowed circulation. It can also cause a slow or irregular heartbeat. A body temperature below 35.6°C (96°F) is typical of hypothermia.	• Observe for signs of hypothermia; these include a low body temperature, shivering, and skin that is cold to touch. • Apply blankets to the patient to prevent and correct hypothermia. • Expose the patient as little as possible when assessing him postoperatively. • Consider pain as a possible cause of hypothermia and use measures to overcome it. • Be prepared to administer warm, humidified oxygen when hypothermia is present.
Disturbances in Psychological Status	
Disorientation is likely to occur as a result of sensory alterations and the use of analgesics. Emotional distress may occur as a result of alterations in body image.	• When caring for the patient postoperatively, observe for signs of disorientation. Also observe for signs of emotional distress in the patient's behavior and communication patterns. • Use measures described in Chapter 12 to prevent and overcome sensory alterations. • Be prepared to listen to the patient so that he can express his concerns. • Use measures described in Chapter 2 to develop and maintain a helping nurse-patient relationship.

body cells absorb the dye, they become sensitive to light. Tumor cells are destroyed when the malignant tissue is bombarded with light from an argon tunable dye laser. Patients undergoing this form of treatment must be instructed on methods for preventing exposure to sun and bright artificial light for up to six weeks.

Laser Safety

Several unique precautions for laser use apply to staff and patients. A chief concern is eye protection. The doors of laser rooms should be posted with signs warning of their use. Everyone, including the patient, is required to wear eyeglasses or goggles depending upon the type of laser being used. Prescription glasses with side shields, but not contact lenses, may be adequate in some cases. Special goggles with filters may be required for others. The awake patient should be provided with similar eye protection. The anesthetized patient's eyes can be taped closed. For procedures involving the face, anesthetic drops are instilled and lead coverings placed on the eyes. Even the patient's teeth may need to be covered with plastic or rubber mouth guards.

Because heat is produced, fire and electrical safety are paramount. Volatile substances such as alcohol and acetone are not used around lasers. Muscle relaxants are used as an alternative to anesthetic gases. Even methane gas produced in the intestine can be potentially explosive. It has been attributed to causing one laser death. Use of polyvinyl chloride airways are contraindicated. Before enough information was available, accidents occurred because polyvinyl chloride ignited and burned. Surgical instruments are sometimes coated black to avoid absorption of any scattered beam. Jewelry can reflect and deflect laser light. Consequently, no metal jewelry can be worn.

Another concern is the health hazards that involve plume. *Plume* is the smoke produced as a consequence of vaporizing tissue with a laser. It contains carbon, water, and intact cells. It is accompanied by an offensive odor.

Smoke evacuators are used at the operative site. Their effectiveness varies with the type of laser and evacuator equipment.

The smell, nausea, and burning and watering of eyes, though uncomfortable, are not hazardous; however, the potential inhalation of airborne cells and viruses is dangerous. A conventional surgical mask, even doubled, is not sufficient in filtering substances that measure less than 0.30 microns. Viruses can be as small as 0.12 microns. Thus it is possible, but not yet proven, that the HIV virus could be transmitted by inhaling laser plume. Manufacturers are developing more effective filters for smoke evacuators. Not all hospitals have budgeted funds for replacement or conversion of their present smoke evacuators. Additional research needs to determine the biohazards of laser plume and the most effective means of preventing its inhalation.

Suggested Measures When Giving Preoperative and Postoperative Care in Selected Situations

When the Patient Is an Infant or Child

Remember that a properly signed consent form is as important for an infant or child as for an adult. Parents or guardians must sign consent forms for minors.

Carefully check the child preoperatively for signs of a skin rash, fever, and an upper respiratory infection. Children are more likely than adults to have an upper respiratory infection or a communicable disease. The onset is often rapid. Unless an emergency exists, surgery needs to be postponed if an infection is present.

Take into account that an infant or child receives most of his emotional support from his parents. Therefore, the parents should be taught about the surgical experience, as described in this chapter, so that they can anticipate what will happen and be in a position to support their children through the experience. Parents are being allowed to accompany their child in some hospitals during the induction of anesthesia and also as the child awakens in the recovery room.

During the preoperative period, work at developing a friendly and trusting relationship with a child having surgery. The child will then be ready to trust the nurse who provides postoperative care.

Just as for an adult, teach a child about the surgical experience, equipment likely to be used, and the experience of pain at a level the child understands. Some hospitals include tours in advance of outpatient surgery. With this teaching, the child

---

> ### Applicable Nursing Diagnoses
>
> Patients undergoing surgery are likely to have nursing diagnoses such as:
> * Knowledge Deficit
> * Fear
> * Pain
> * Impaired Skin Integrity
> * High Risk for Infection
> * High Risk for Fluid Volume Deficit
> * Ineffective Breathing Pattern
> * Ineffective Airway Clearance
> * Body Image Disturbance
>
> Nursing Care Plan 19-1 has been developed to show nursing orders that may help in the resolution of Body Image Disturbance. NANDA defines this category in its 1989 taxonomy as, "Disruption in the way one perceives one's body image."

---

will enjoy benefits similar to those of an adult who has been properly taught preoperatively.

Assure a child that he will not be left alone. Encourage him to talk about his fears as much as he is able. Tell him it is all right to cry, answer his questions, and correct the misconceptions most children have of surgery.

Allow the child to take his own stuffed animal, doll, or familiar blanket with him to the operating room as a form of emotional support. Communication among personnel will generally provide for its safekeeping during surgery and replacement with the child in the recovery room.

Use visual aids to explain a surgical procedure to the extent that a child can understand the procedure. Drawings, x-ray films, and pictures are helpful. Use of a doll as a substitute for a patient has been successful for role-playing with many youngsters.

Modify methods to encourage deep breathing. Balloons, party horns, or pinwheel toys may be used.

When the Patient Has Diabetes Mellitus

Preoperatively, help work toward good control of a patient's diabetes. Surgical risks are lessened when the patient's disease is under control.

Be prepared to make adjustments in the patient's insulin dosage. A longer-acting dose may be prescribed the night before, or a somewhat smaller dose than usual may be ordered in the morning by injection or by intravenous drip. Postoperatively, insulin dosages are generally regulated according to periodic blood testing for glucose levels.

Expect that it may be likely that wound healing will

NURSING CARE PLAN

19-1. Body Image Disturbance

Assessment

Subjective Data

States, "I hate myself for agreeing to this operation. This 'thing' fills up, it bulges, and smells. No one will ever want to come near me again."

Objective Data

31-year-old woman with prior history of ulcerative colitis admitted four days ago for colectomy with ileostomy. Asks that room freshener be sprayed frequently. Applies perfume heavily. Positions herself more than 5 feet from visitors.

Diagnosis

Body Image Disturbance related to fear of rejection based on altered elimination.

Plan

Goal

The patient will demonstrate acceptance and less self-consciousness about ostomy by interacting with a visitor within 3 feet by 10/9.

Orders: 10/5

1. Spend at least 15 minutes with patient midmorning, midafternoon, and early evening without performing direct care to communicate acceptance. During interaction:
   a. Sit within 3 feet to show by example that closeness is not a problem.
   b. Empathize with the patient; agree that this change is difficult to accept.
   c. Offer to contact another person with an ostomy through the United Ostomy Association to share mutual feelings and experiences while still in the hospital.
   d. Offer referral to an enterostomal nurse therapist for suggestions on odor-control techniques.
2. During ostomy teaching sessions and care of the stoma, implement the following:
   a. Avoid facial expressions that may communicate disgust or repulsion with the care of the ileostomy.
   b. Use terminology such as "your stoma" (avoiding any depersonalized or pet names) to promote the concept that the stoma is not a separate entity but rather part of her natural body.
   c. Avoid using gloves when performing direct care to convey that personal contact is not a problem. ———————————————— N. Nunn, RN

Implementation (Documentation)

10/5

1330 Interacted socially for approx. 15 min. Sat within 3 feet. Patient moved her own chair away to provide more distance. Reinforced that adjusting to an ostomy is difficult. Explained the purpose of the United Ostomy Association and gave booklet, "So You Have ... Or Will Have An Ostomy." Offered to contact another person with an ostomy or the enterostomal therapist. ——————— G. Orsini, LPN

Evaluation (Documentation)

10/6

1030 Demonstrated stoma care without the use of gloves. Used the term "your ostomy" and "your appliance" during teaching session. Pt. used the term "Mt. Vesuvius" when referring to stoma. Page mark noted in ostomy booklet indicating that reading has begun. States "I don't know if talking with someone else will help. Not everyone has friends like mine." ——————— G. Orsini, LPN

be delayed in patients with diabetes. Wound dehiscence is also more likely, especially if the patient is obese.

When the Patient Is Obese

Expect that the care of an obese postoperative patient is likely to be more difficult than for a patient who is of average weight. Much of this is due to inactivity.

Be especially careful to use nursing measures meticulously to promote respiratory functioning. The obese person tends not to move about and takes shallow breaths. Therefore, special efforts are required to help prevent respiratory complications.

Observe the patient carefully for wound dehiscence and poor wound healing because of the reduced blood supply to fatty tissue. Delay in wound closure increases the risk for postoperative wound infections.

When the Patient Is Elderly

Expect that many elderly persons suffer from poor nutrition. Most elderly persons require a diet high in protein before and after surgery.

Anticipate that elderly patients suffering with chronic diseases are more likely to experience postoperative complications. Chronic diseases especially likely to predispose a patient to postoperative complications include anemia, diabetes mellitus, and various respiratory and cardiovascular diseases.

Administer medications with caution, since most elderly persons do not metabolize or excrete medications as well as do younger adults. Therefore preoperative and postoperative medications are ordinarily prescribed in smaller than average doses. Use noninvasive measures described in Chapter 10 to help control pain and sleeplessness. This practice reduces the dangers of adverse medication reactions.

Monitor the vital signs, urinary output, and laboratory findings carefully when the surgical patient is elderly. With advancing age, the patient is more susceptible to shock and other postoperative complications.

Anticipate the need to help elderly persons become oriented postoperatively. They are more likely to be disoriented in a strange environment.

Expect slower wound healing in most elderly persons due to less-than-adequate nutrition and poorer circulation to tissue.

Take into account that the elderly have diminished physical reserves. This explains why their organ functions slowly return to normal after surgical intervention. Therefore, meticulous preoperative and postoperative care are especially important to help prevent postoperative complications.

Teaching Suggestions Related to a Surgical Experience

Many teaching suggestions for the care of the surgical patient preoperatively and postoperatively were given in this chapter. Although teaching must be geared to meet each patient's needs, the following additional teaching suggestions are appropriate in most situations:

Many patients will not have used a bedpan or urinal before hospitalization for surgery. It is helpful to show the patient a bedpan or urinal and demonstrate its use preoperatively. Understanding this alternative method for elimination may be helpful in reducing or eliminating postoperative urine retention or constipation.

Patients are generally fearful of tubes. They accept them better and are more cooperative when they are taught why they are used. Commonly used tubes include urinary catheters, intravenous lines, and drainage tubes at the site of the incision. Patients should also be prepared if oxygen and suctioning equipment will be used postoperatively.

Checking vital signs and dressings may seem routine to a nurse. However, many patients are disturbed and fear their condition is poor when a nurse is checking frequently. If the patient understands that he will be checked frequently, it relieves unnecessary postoperative anxiety.

The fear of pain and sleeplessness often contributes to anxiety. Therefore, the patient should be taught that measures will be used to keep him as comfortable as possible. Explaining that he will be consulted postoperatively about pain and sleeplessness and measures to relieve them is especially reassuring for most patients.

The purposes of not being allowed to eat or drink for a period of time postoperatively should be explained. Most patients are interested in knowing how nutritional and fluid needs are met when they are not eating and drinking normally.

Explanations and the purposes for measures provided before and after surgery should always be offered before carrying them out.

Teaching postoperatively should also include instructions on whatever the patient needs to learn about self-care for when he goes home.

Family members of patients are very often of critical importance. As this chapter points out, it is important that they, too, are taught so that they are able to support the patient in the best way possible.

Bibliography

Ball KA: Controlling smoke evacuation and odor during laser surgery. Today's OR Nurse 8(12):4–10, 1986

Ball KA: Laser safety. Today's OR Nurse 8(10):10–14, 1986

Birdsall C, Carpenter K, Considine R: How is autotransfusion done? Am J Nurs 88(1):108, 110–111, 1988

Brazen L: OR experiences are for student nurses . . . operating room scene. Today's OR Nurse 11(2):18–23, 35–37, 1989

Butler S: Current trends in autologous transfusion. RN Magazine 52(11):44–55, 1989

Cunningham JD: "What have I done?": The issue of informed consent. Rehabilitation Nursing 14(4):202–203, 1989

Dexeus R: Atelectasis/pneumonia: Prevention for the abdominal surgical patient. Dimensions in Oncology Nursing 3(4):26–28, 1990

Ewing G: The nursing preparation of stoma patients for self-care. J Adv Nurs 14(5):411–420, 1989

Gawron CL: Body image changes in the patient requiring ostomy revision. Journal of Enterostomal Therapy 16(5):199–200, 1989

Harrison EM: Clinical aspects of a laser program. Journal of Urological Nursing 7(3):466–468, 1988

Johnson J: New light on lasers. Nursing Times 85(33):28, 30–33, 1989

Kuroc E: Photodynamic therapy: The nurse's role. Laser Nursing 1(2):8–10, 1986–1987

Lehr PS: Surgical lasers: How they work, current applications. AORN J 50(5):972–877, 1989

Love C: Deep vein thrombosis: Threat to recovery part 1. Nursing Times 86(5):40–43, 1990

McConnell E: Identifying Mrs. Frohne's postoperative complication. Nursing 19(6):72–74, 1989

Ogilvie L: Hospitalization of children for surgery: The parents' view. Children's Health Care 19(1):49–56, 1990

Patterson P: Hair clipping superior to preoperative shave. Today's OR Nurse 12(3):37, 1990

Payman BC, Dampier SE, Hawthorne PJ: Postoperative temperature and infection in patients undergoing general surgery. J Adv Nurs 14(3):198–202, 1989

Phillips A: Are blood transfusions really safe? Nursing 17(6):63–64, 1987

Proposed recommended practices: Laser safety in the operating room. AORN J 49(3):284, 286–287, 290, 1989

Scuderi J, Olsen GN: Respiratory therapy in the management of postoperative complications. Respiratory Care 34(4):281–291, 1989

Swindale JE: The nurse's role in giving pre-operative information to reduce anxiety in patients admitted to hospital for elective minor surgery. J Adv Nurs 14(11):899–905, 1989

Tovar MK, Cassmeyer VL: Touch: The beneficial effects for the surgical patient. Association of Operating Room Nurses Journal 49(5):1356–61, 1989

Trauger P: Rules easing on directed donations to blood banks. Today's OR Nurse 11(5):43, 1989

What happens next? . . . Preoperative education booklet. Today's OR Nurse 11(8):16–17, 1989

20

Promoting Tissue Healing

Chapter Outline

Behavioral Objectives
Glossary
Introduction
Types of Wounds
The Body's Reaction to Injury
Promoting Skin Integrity
Caring for a Wound
Performing an Irrigation
Caring for a Wound With a Drain
Packing a Wound
Applying Wet to Dry Dressings
Securing a Dressing
Removing Sutures and Staples
Using Bandages and Binders
Understanding the Use of Heat and Cold
Applicable Nursing Diagnoses
Suggested Measures to Promote Tissue Healing in
    Selected Situations
Teaching Suggestions to Promote Tissue Healing
Bibliography

Skill Procedures

Preventing Pressure Sores
Changing an Occlusive Dressing
Changing a Gauze Dressing
Irrigating a Wound
Irrigating an Eye
Irrigating an Ear
Administering a Douche
Applying Bandages and Binders
Applying a Compress

Behavioral Objectives

When the content of this chapter has been mastered, the learner will be able to:

Define the terms appearing in the glossary.

Discuss how the body reacts to injury and how healing occurs.

List and describe at least five types of wounds.

Describe factors that predispose a patient to the development of a pressure sore. Discuss susceptible patients, common locations, and how a pressure sore is best prevented and treated.

List five reasons for leaving a wound undressed and five purposes of a dressing.

Demonstrate how to change a dressing on a clean, open wound and how to secure it.

Describe how to care for a drain, pack a wound, and remove sutures and staples.

Demonstrate how to irrigate a wound, the eye, the ear, and the vagina.

List five purposes of bandages and binders and recommended actions when applying them.

Demonstrate the application of a roller bandage using each of six basic turns.

Discuss six factors that affect applications of heat and cold and list common purposes for using such applications.

Describe how to use the following hot and cold applications: ice and hot water bags, alcohol and cool water baths, hypothermia blankets, electric heating pads and K-pads, sitz baths, hot soaks and packs, light cradles and heat lamps.

Demonstrate the application of cold or hot compresses.

List suggested measures for promoting tissue healing in selected situations, as described in this chapter.

Summarize suggestions for the instruction of patients offered in this chapter.

Glossary

Abscess A collection of pus or a foreign body surrounded by tissue.

Bandage Material applied in a manner to cover a part of the body.

Binder A type of bandage designed to cover or support a large body part, such as the abdomen or chest.

Circular turn A technique for wrapping a roller bandage in which one turn completely overlaps another.

Closed wound Injured tissue without a break in skin or mucous membrane.

Compress Local application of moisture.

Debridement A method of cleaning a wound of debris.

Douche A vaginal irrigation.

Dressing A protective covering placed over a wound.

Figure-of-eight turn A technique for wrapping a roller bandage in the manner of the number 8.

First intention A type of wound healing in which the edges are directly next to one another. Synonym for *primary intention*.

Four-tailed binder A type of cover that supports the chin.

Granulation tissue An area of repaired cells that appears pinkish red from an increased blood supply.

Hyperthermia A high body temperature.

Hypothermia A low body temperature.

Inflammation The naturally occurring defensive response of the body to injury.

Insulator A substance that is a poor conductor.

Irrigation A procedure that involves instilling solution into an area of the body.

Malaise Loss of energy.

Open wound Injured tissue in which there is a break in the skin or mucous membrane.

Recurrent turn A technique for wrapping a roller bandage by layering the bandage back and forth over a rounded surface.

Regeneration A process in which destroyed cells are replaced with identical cells.

Resolution A type of healing process in which damaged cells are able to recover.

Roller bandage A continuous strip of material wound on itself to form a roll.

Scar formation A process in which destroyed cells are replaced by connective tissue.

Scultetus binder A binder with many tails.

Second intention A type of wound healing in which widely separated edges must heal inward toward the center.

Shearing force Damaging effect to skin that occurs when compressed layers of tissue move upon each other.

Sitz bath A method for applying moist heat in which the patient is placed in a tub with enough water to cover his hips.

Soak Placing part of the body in water or in a medicated solution.

Spica turn An adaptation of the figure-of-eight wrap in which all turns overlap and cross each other, forming a sharp angle.

Spiral-reverse turn A wrapping technique in which the spiral is reversed halfway through each turn.

Spiral turn A wrapping technique in which one turn partly overlaps the previous one.

Staples Wide metal clips used to hold a wound together.

Straight binder A rectangular piece of material that is long enough to encircle the body.

Sutures Materials used to join the edges of tissue together.

T-binder A binder shaped like the letter *T*.

Third intention A type of wound healing in which temporarily separated wound edges are eventually brought together at a later time.

Trauma A general term for injury.

Wound Injured skin or soft tissues of the body.

Introduction

Everyone acquires a wound at one time or another. A *wound* is damaged skin or soft tissues of the body. It occurs as a result of *trauma,* a general term referring to an injury. Some examples of trauma include physical injury, such as cuts, blows, or even poor circulation to tissue, strong chemicals, and excessive heat or cold.

The body has remarkable ability to recover when tissue is injured. This chapter will discuss several methods through which the body repairs wounds. It will also describe nursing actions that can be taken to prevent wounds from occurring and actions that support the healing processes of the body.

In most health agencies, measures described in this chapter require a physician's order. In others, some of them may not. The nurse should observe the policies of the agency where care is given.

Types of Wounds

In general, there are two types of wounds, open and closed. An *open wound* means there is a break in the skin or mucous membrane. Such a wound may be caused by an accident, or it may be an intentional wound, such as that made by a surgeon. A *closed wound* has no break in skin or mucous membrane. Table 20-1 provides a list and descriptions of various types of open and closed wounds.

The Body's Reaction to Injury

Regardless of the type of wound, the body immediately reacts to the injury. First, the body produces an inflammation and later implements one of several mechanisms for tissue healing.

The Inflammatory Response

An *inflammation* is a naturally occurring defensive response of the body to injury. Its purpose is to limit tissue damage, remove injured cells and debris, and prepare the wound for permanent repair. Several activities occur during an inflammation before the wound can actually heal. The sequence of these activities gives the characteristic local signs and symptoms associated with an inflammation:

Table 20-1. Types of Wounds

Open Wounds	Description
Incision	A clean separation of skin and tissue with smooth, even edges
Laceration	A separation of skin and tissue in which the edges are torn and irregular
Abrasion	A wound in which the surface layers of skin are scraped away
Avulsion	Stripping away of large areas of skin and underlying tissue, leaving cartilage and bone exposed
Ulceration	A shallow area in which skin or mucous membrane is missing
Puncture	An opening of skin, underlying tissue, or mucous membrane caused by a narrow, sharp, pointed object

Closed Wounds	Description
Contusion	Injury to soft tissue underlying the skin from the force of contact with a hard object; sometimes called a bruise

swelling, pain, decreased function, redness, and warmth. Systemic signs and symptoms also occur; they include *malaise,* a general loss of energy, and a slightly elevated temperature.

Events associated with the inflammatory response occur in the following sequence:

1. The injured cells release chemical substances. These chemicals alter cell membranes and allow fluid from within the cells to pour out into the surrounding tissue. This causes swelling and congestion, which limit movement and function. Consequently, injuring substances are prevented from traveling to other parts of the body and causing further injury. Another chemical, released at the same time, causes the sensation of pain to be transmitted along nerve cells. Finally, chemicals cause blood vessels to dilate, producing the redness and warmth associated with inflamed tissue.

2. White blood cells are drawn to the injured area and begin to engulf dead cells and debris. Neutrophils, the body's largest number of white cells, appear first. They encircle the injured area and begin to consume small particles. Monocytes, which migrate somewhat later, are able to remove larger-sized debris in the area of injury. Any substances that escape these cells travel to the lymph system and are destroyed there.

3. Once the area has been cleaned, cells called fibroblasts and a substance called collagen fill the injured area. These two act as building blocks and "glue" to temporarily repair the area that was damaged. They are the components in a scab.

4. The body begins to send new projections of capill-

aries into the area to supply replacement cells with oxygen and nutrients. This produces pinkish red tissue, called *granulation tissue,* that is gradually replaced by skin and scar tissue. The supply of blood through these capillaries will eventually diminish and the area will appear similar in color to the surrounding tissue.

Healing Mechanisms

Wound healing involves the body's efforts to restore the structure and function of cells in the injured area. This is done either by the recovery of injured cells, a process called *resolution;* by replacement of damaged cells with identical new ones, called *regeneration;* or by the production of a nonfunctioning substitute for the destroyed cells, a process called *scar formation.* Cells that can no longer be duplicated when injured are replaced with scar tissue. A scar consists of connective tissue that is strong but does not have the elasticity or capacity to function like the cell it replaces. The aim is to minimize the amount of scar tissue and thereby preserve the appearance and the function of the injured tissue. The type of healing and the time required for permanent repair depends on the extent of injury and the type of tissue involved.

There are three mechanisms by which wounds heal. They are called healing by first intention, second intention, and third intention. Each is illustrated in Figure 20-1. The distance between the edges of a wound determines the area of scar tissue.

First Intention Healing. *First intention* healing, also called *primary intention,* occurs when wound edges are

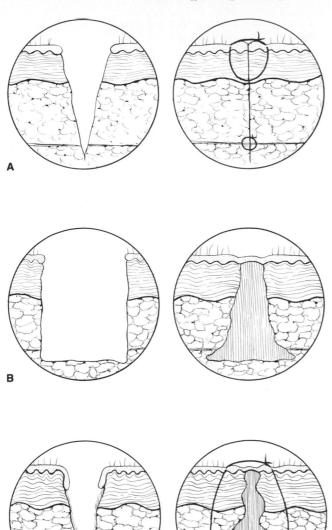

A

B

C

Figure 20-1 (*A*). Smoothly separated wound edges are held together with suture facilitating first intention healing. This is the optimum method of healing because it ensures minimal scar formation. (*B*). Second intention healing requires that the body produce material to fill the area between separated wound edges. Healing takes place slowly from the wound margin toward the center. (*C*). Third intention healing shows delayed closure, early formation of granulation tissue around the margin of the edges, and then the use of suture to join the wound edges together.

directly next to one another. There is only a narrow space that must be filled with replacement tissue. Only a small scar results. Closing a wound with sutures or material that produces a similar effect, such as butterfly strips, steri-strips, or staples, facilitates healing by first intention.

Second Intention Healing. Healing by *second intention* involves replacing damaged cells between wound edges that are relatively far apart. This occurs when the edges of the wound cannot be stretched to achieve closure. In some cases the rate of second intention healing is slowed by the presence of drainage from an infection, a blood clot, or debris that fills the space between the wound edges. Granulation tissue extends from the edges of the wound toward the center. This tissue is easily dislodged. Therefore, the nurse must take care to avoid reinjuring the healing wound.

Third Intention Healing. *Third intention* healing involves a wound with widely separated edges that are later brought together with some type of closure material. The wound is usually one that is fairly deep and likely to contain accumulating fluid. In some cases, the surgeon may intentionally place a drain or pack gauze into the wound to provide for drainage. This keeps the edges of the wound temporarily apart. Once the drain or gauze is removed, the edges of the wound can be closed and the healing completed. The amount of scar tissue that develops with third intention healing is similar to the end result of second intention healing.

Factors Affecting Healing

If the injury is overwhelming and the body is unable to cope with it, death occurs. When this is not the case, several factors, mentioned below, affect the outcome of healing.

The Extent of Injury. The more tissue that is damaged, the greater the demand on the body's reparative processes. It will take longer for healing to take place as the limited supplies of the body must be replenished to meet the continued demands. The ability to close an open wound greatly affects the rate of healing and prevention of complications. It may be necessary to use skin grafts to close a wound when the skin covering a large area has been destroyed.

The Blood Supply to the Area. An adequate blood supply is necessary for healing. Healing is delayed when oxygen, nutrients, and specialized cells cannot be delivered to the injured area. The tissue of an obese person heals more slowly; individuals with poor circulation, such as the elderly, take longer to heal. The nurse must assess the injured area frequently to determine that edema, tight bandaging, or positioning do not interfere with an adequate blood supply.

The Type of Injured Tissue. Skin and mucous membranes close and heal fairly quickly, sometimes in a day's time. Deeper structures take longer to repair. Surgeons account for this by using different types of suture material for joining various layers of tissue. Sutures that hold muscle layers together are designed to dissolve at a slow rate.

Some damaged cells, such as heart muscle and nerve tissue, never regenerate. Healing is prolonged and less than satisfactory as the dead cells are removed and replaced by scar tissue.

The Presence of Debris. Drainage, dead or damaged tissue cells, embedded fragments of bone, metal, glass, or other substances can act as foreign bodies and interfere with good tissue healing. Cleaning an area of this sort of material is referred to as *debridement.* The physician, but sometimes a nurse, performs debridement. The nurse is usually responsible for the initial cleansing of a wound and wound irrigation.

The Presence of Infection. Because the patient's primary protective barrier is weakened when skin and mucous membranes are opened, the need for preventing microorganisms from entering the body becomes especially important. Careful handwashing before caring for the wound probably is the single most effective method of preventing infections. Although it is not possible to sterilize the skin, practices of surgical asepsis are used when caring for an open wound. Precautions are also taken for persons with closed wounds because of the lowered resistance of the damaged tissue to infection.

When an infection is present, a collection of white blood cells and dead pathogens collects within a wound. This material is called pus. Until the body absorbs it, or it drains from the wound, healing will be delayed. An *abscess* occurs when the body walls off a collection of pus and healing occurs around it. Treatment of an abscess varies, but healing will not completely take place until it is removed. In some cases a surgical procedure to open and drain the abscess may be performed. Local application of heat and immobilization of the part may also be used.

The Health of the Patient. The promotion of high-level wellness helps the body deal with trauma. Adequate rest, relief from emotional tensions, a nourishing diet, and adequate fluid intake are particularly important for healing. As mentioned in Chapter 19, individuals with chronic diseases, such as diabetes mellitus, or those with conditions or medications affecting the immune system will have a reduced capacity for healing.

Promoting Skin Integrity

Intact skin is a barrier against microorganisms. It also helps to retain fluids and proteins within cells and tissues. A pressure sore is an area where skin has been injured; there may be eventual destruction of underlying tissue as well. The terms pressure sore, decubitus ulcer, and pressure ulcer are used interchangeably. Nurses are wiser to channel their energies into preserving skin integrity than to be faced with the need for aggressively treating a pressure sore.

Understanding the Causes of Pressure Sores

The primary cause of a pressure sore is unrelieved compression of capillaries that supply blood to the skin and its underlying tissue. The mechanism for destruction is as follows. The body weight compresses the tissue and blood vessels against a hard surface. As a result, the cells supplied through the vascular network lack oxygen and a means of carrying away waste products of metabolism. Cells eventually die if these conditions are prolonged and unrelieved.

Pressure above 32 mm Hg occludes blood flow. Body cells can tolerate increased pressure, but tolerance is affected by the amount and duration of the pressure. In other words, high pressure over a short amount of time has been shown to be as detrimental as lower amounts of pressure for longer time.

Inactive or immobilized patients are at highest risk for skin breakdown. For example, pressure on bony prominences from sitting on a hard surface has been measured at from 5 to 15 times higher than that which will occlude capillary blood flow. Lying on an innerspring mattress produces over twice the occlusive pressure. Active individuals self-adjust their body weight to relieve pressure at frequent intervals. The nurse needs to implement frequent position changes and pressure-relieving techniques for patients who cannot independently shift their own weight.

Friction to the skin and shearing forces also contribute to altering the integrity of skin. Friction causes abrasions to the skin. *Shearing force* is the damaging effect that occurs when compressed layers of tissue move upon each other. This tends to tear and separate the attachment between the epidermal and dermal layers of the skin. For example, a patient who is partially sitting up in bed will experience shearing forces when his skin sticks to the sheet. Tissues underlying the skin move downward with his body weight. This may also occur in the patient who sits in a chair but slides down while his skin sticks to his clothing and the back of the chair.

Wrinkles in linen and various types of debris in a bed or on a chair, such as crumbs, irritate and damage skin so that a pressure sore is likely to develop. Other contributing factors include fecal and urinary incontinence, inadequate nutrition and poor hydration.

Pressure sores most often develop on areas of the body where there is excess pressure on bony prominences. Figure 20-2 illustrates common areas where pressure sores tend to develop. They also frequently occur over the heels, the ankles, elbows, and even over the ears.

Recognizing the Signs of a Pressure Sore

The earliest sign of excessive pressure is a pale appearance to the skin over a bony area of the body. The pallor is due to poor blood circulation in the area. This is followed by

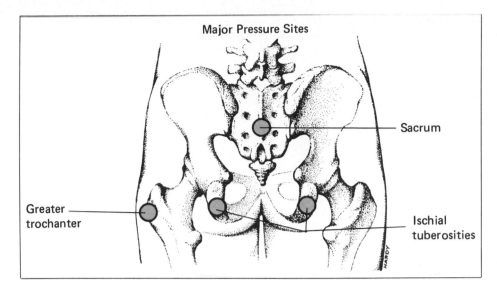

Major Pressure Sites

Sacrum

Greater
trochanter

Ischial
tuberosities

Figure 20-2 Sites at which about 75% of all pressure sores occur. Other bony prominences include the areas at the heels, the elbows, the ankles, the knees, and the back of the head. (Brunner LS, Suddarth DS: The Lippincott Manual of Nursing Practice, 4th ed, p 60. Philadelphia, JB Lippincott, 1986)

reddened skin as the body oversupplies the area with blood to improve the effect caused by diminished circulation. Unless the circulation is improved promptly, the area will become dark and cyanotic. As cells die, the skin breaks down, forming an open ulcer.

Pressure sores may be classified according to stages, depending on the assessed characteristics of the skin. Table 20-2 lists the stages of pressure sores, illustrates each stage, and describes the characteristics of each classification.

Identifying Individuals at Risk for Developing Pressure Sores

Any patient, regardless of diagnosis, who is not moving about is at risk for developing a pressure sore. Other candidates are patients who are eating poorly, have a low hemoglobin, have lost a great deal of weight, or are very thin. There is also a high risk for others who are unable to control urination and bowel movements, have draining wounds, or are feverish and perspire freely. Totally or partially paralyzed patients and those who are in casts and require immobilization need careful watching. The bedridden patient is especially susceptible, but patients in chairs and wheelchairs also develop decubitus ulcers. Table 20-3 provides an assessment guide for predicting individuals who are at risk for developing pressure sores. Using this guide, the nurse may develop nursing orders using measures designed to prevent the occurrence of pressure sores in susceptible individuals.

Preventing Skin Breakdown

There are many interventions that help prevent pressure sore formation. Some recommended techniques are provided in Skill Procedure 20-1.

Treating Pressure Sores

Preventive measures described in Skill Procedure 20-1 should continue if a pressure sore develops. However, additional actions must be taken to restore the skin's integrity. The approaches that are appropriate are different, depending on whether the pressure sore is a closed wound, as in Stages I and II, or has extended to an open wound, as in Stages III and IV.

One of the principal differences involves whether to keep the area of the pressure sore moist or dry. During the prevention and treatment of a closed pressure sore, the focus is on keeping the area dry; the reverse is true when treating an open pressure sure. When the surface of the skin is broken, the nurse must maintain a moist environment. Moisture promotes the movement of epidermal cells to the surface of the wound, causing it to seal over and heal. A dry, crusted area retards this process. Many health care personnel are now using occlusive dressings, such as Op-Site®, Tegaderm®, and DuoDERM®, over open pressure sores. These prevent tissue fluid from evaporating away from the area of skin breakdown. Suggestions for applying occlusive dressings are provided later in this chapter.

Other measures, including the use of enzyme ointments, debridement techniques, and direct application of oxygen, are being used to promote healing of late-stage pressure sores. They have been reported to be effective for at least some patients. The selection of methods depends on local policy. Nursing orders should clearly direct the schedule and techniques that should be followed. By far the best approach is to prevent the formation of pressure sores with good nursing care initially.

Table 20-2. Classification of Pressure Sores

Classification	Appearance	Description
Stage I	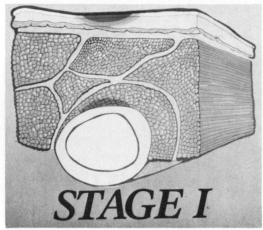 **Figure 20-3** First-stage pressure sore.	The chief sign associated with the first stage is redness. The skin does not return to normal color, even when the pressure is relieved.
Stage II	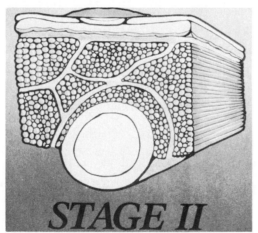 **Figure 20-4** Second-stage pressure sore.	Redness persists, usually accompanied by blistering or a shallow break in the skin.
Stage III	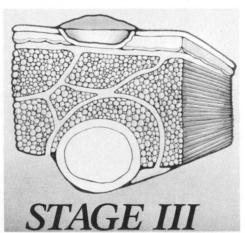 **Figure 20-5** Third-stage pressure sore.	The break in the skin becomes deeper, extending to subcutaneous tissue.

(continued)

Table 20-2. *Continued*

Classification	Appearance	Description
Stage IV	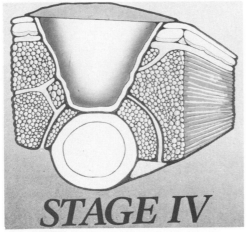	The ulcer involves loss of all skin layers exposing muscle and bone.

Figure 20-6 Fourth-stage pressure sore.

Illustrations courtesy of Evonne Fowler, clinical nurse specialist in gerontology, Los Angeles Harbor College, Wilmington, CA.

Caring for a Wound

The tissues of open and closed wounds are more susceptible to further injury than is healthy, intact tissue. Prevention of additional injury and the promotion of healing are two principal goals of wound care.

The Undressed Wound

Closed wounds are left undressed. Some open wounds are left undressed if the wound has sealed itself and can be protected from injury and irritation. This is true even of wounds that have been surgically created and sutured. There may be occasions when a wound is left undressed for most of the day and then covered at bedtime. Many small cuts and abrasions are handled in this manner.

These are common reasons for leaving wounds undressed:

- Friction and irritation of the dressing may injure skin tissues.
- Exposure to air helps keep the wound dry. A wet dressing may pull organisms into the wound like a wick or blotter.
- A dark, warm, moist area under the dressing is the type of environment that promotes the growth of microorganisms.
- A dressing may interfere with circulation to the part, causing a delay in healing.

The Dressed Wound

A protective covering over a wound is called a *dressing*. A dressing is applied to:

- Keep a wound clean and restrict entry of organisms
- Absorb drainage
- Control bleeding
- Protect the healing area from additional injury
- Hold antiseptic medication next to the wound
- Protect an area that may be sensitive to environment temperature changes
- Cover an area of disfigurement.

Types of Dressings

Several types of dressings may be used to cover a wound. The challenge is to match the characteristics of the dressing with the requirements for the individual wound.

Gauze Dressings. Dressings made of woven cloth fibers have been the traditional form of wound cover. Gauze dressings come in many forms such as squares, rolls, and tubes. They are highly absorbent and are valuable during initial wound care because they are porous and collect a large volume of drainage. Though inexpensive initially, their cost increases when saturation makes frequent replacement necessary.

Eventually, as bleeding diminishes, the gauze may adhere to the wound causing trauma to healing tissue during removal. Fibers can become embedded in the wound. To avoid tissue injury, gauze strips impregnated with vaseline may be used. Another type moistened with iodine has some bacteriostatic action.

Gauze dressings interfere with wound assessment. Inspection can only be accomplished by removing the dress-

(Text continues on page 467)

Table 20-3. Determining Patients at Risk for Pressure Sores*

Mental Status	Continence	Mobility	Activity	Nutrition	Circulation	Temperature	Medications
4							
Alert	Continent	Fully mobile	Ambulatory	Good	Immediate capillary refill	98°–99° F. (36.6°–37.2° C)	No analgesics, tranquilizers, or steroids
3							
Apathetic	Incontinent of urine (without catheter)	Slightly limited	Walks with assistance	Fair	Delayed capillary refill	99°–100° F. (37.2°–37.7° C)	One of the above
2							
Confused	Incontinent of feces	Very limited	Confined to wheelchair	Poor	Mild edema	100°–101° F. (37.7°–38.3° C)	Two of the above
1							
Stuporous or comatose	Incontinent of urine and feces	Immobile	Bedridden	Cachectic	Moderate to severe edema	>101° F. (>38.3° C)	All of the above

*Evaluate patients for each of the above categories, then assign appropriate score. Patients with a score of 16 or less on this assessment scale are at significant risk for developing pressure sores.

From Shannon ML: Five famous fallacies about pressure sores. Nursing84(14):34–41. Reprinted with permission from the October Issue of Nursing 84, Copyright 1984 by Springhouse Corporation. All rights reserved.

Skill Procedure 20-1. Preventing Pressure Sores

Suggested Action	Reason for Action
Change the patient's position *often,* as frequently as every hour or two, for a patient at risk for bedsores.	Changing the patient's position helps relieve pressure and restore circulation.
Use the supine position as infrequently as possible	The back-lying position causes pressure to many vulnerable areas on the body.
Tilt the body obliquely at a 30° angle. Use pillows to support the body in this position.	An oblique position is the ideal position to avoid pressure over bony prominences on the posterior and lateral sides of the body.
Keep the skin dry and clean.	Dampness and uncleanliness predispose the patient to skin breakdown.
For skin that is frequently wet or subjected to shearing forces, use a protective skin barrier such as Newskin® Spray or a plasticized coating such as Bard Barrier Film® and Incontinent Spray.	These products contain chemicals that take on the form and function of a second layer of skin. They help to keep the natural skin intact.
Use skin cleansers that do not destroy the natural acid condition of the skin.	Bathing with alkaline soaps destroys the ability of the skin to retard the growth of bacteria and fungi.
Rinse off soap, detergent, or skin cleansers well with water.	Residues left on the skin can be irritating and predispose the patient to skin breakdown.
Avoid using waterproof materials on the patient's bed.	Waterproof materials tend to cause the patient to perspire and to prevent evaporation of water. They also retain urine next to the skin of incontinent patients. Moisture on the skin predisposes the patient to skin breakdown.
A sheepskin is no longer being advocated for preventing pressure sores.	Synthetic sheepskins tend to become stiff and hard after washing. The hide backing on natural sheepskins will not allow urine to drain away from an incontinent patient.
Avoid massaging reddened areas. Gentle massage over bony prominences is recommended *before* any redness is apparent.	Once a pressure sore is forming, massage may cause separation of skin layers. Massage of healthy tissue promotes circulation to the area.
Protect areas especially prone to friction, shearing forces, and pressure, such as the heels and elbows. Figure 20-7 shows a heel protector.	Special protective devices reduce friction and provide a cushioning effect to body areas subject to skin breakdown.
Use a bridging technique like the one illustrated in Figure 20-8 to protect the tissue over bony areas.	Relieving counter-pressure from a hard surface can improve the circulation of blood to an area prone to skin breakdown.
Avoid using a mattress that is so hard that it causes pressure on parts of the body. A water mattress, as illustrated in Figure 20-9, shows how pressure is distributed on the mattress. Other types of pressure-relieving mattresses, or specialty beds are also available.	The even distribution of the patient's weight, at the same time as the counter-pressure from the mattress is reduced, helps improve circulation and prevent injury to skin.
Use only one sheet and avoid tightly tucked linen covering a pressure-relieving mattress.	Re-creating a rigid surface defeats the purpose of the mattress.
Use smaller pressure-relieving pads, like the one shown in Figure 20-10, for those times when the patient is sitting in a chair.	Sitting increases the weight and pressure on bony areas in the buttocks greater than that when lying down. A portable small pad relieves pressure during inactive time spent out of bed.
Change a patient's sitting position frequently. Try not to raise the head of the bed more than 30°.	Pressure and shearing forces increase in proportion to the head elevation of the patient.

(continued)

Skill Procedure 20-1. Continued

Suggested Action	**Reason for Action**

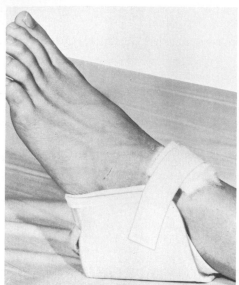

Figure 20-7 This device protects the heel from friction when moving across the bed linen and mattress. Other pressure-relieving measures are recommended in addition to the use of this type of product. (Courtesy of the JT Posey Company, Arcadia, CA.)

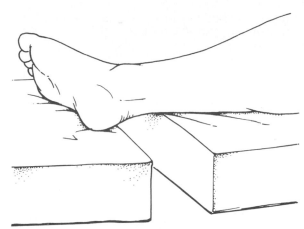

Figure 20-8 The sketch illustrates a way to create a bridging effect by supporting the leg and foot. This positioning technique prevents pressure on the ankle and bottom of the heel.

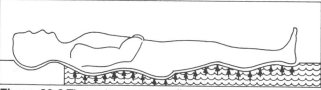

Figure 20-9 The water mattress allows for even distribution of the patient's weight, thereby reducing areas of pressure. It can be used for the prevention of decubitus ulcers and as an aid in healing them.

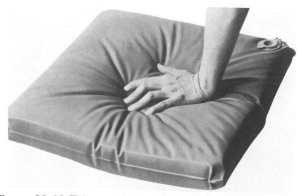

Figure 20-10 This example of a flotation gel pad illustrates how weight can be distributed to relieve pressure areas. This type is especially handy for patients who are allowed to sit in a chair or a wheelchair. (Courtesy of the JT Posey Company, Arcadia, CA.)

Use cornstarch if the patient's skin sticks to the bed, chair, or bedpan.

Lift or use a turning sheet rather than slide the patient when he is moved.

Avoid using doughnuts and air-inflated rings, or use them only with the greatest of care and for very short periods of time.

Friction and shearing force have a damaging effect on skin. Cornstarch absorbs moisture and reduces trauma to skin.

Reducing friction can promote and maintain skin integrity.

Rings may relieve pressure over an area but they restrict circulation where the body part rests on the ring, causing more problems than they solve.

(continued)

Skill Procedure 20-1. Continued

Suggested Action	Reason for Action
Keep bed linens and clothing dry, clean, and free of wrinkles.	Wrinkles, soilage, and moisture irritate the skin and predispose the patient to skin breakdown.
Do everything possible to help keep the patient in the best possible physical condition. This includes seeing that he eats a nutritious diet, takes plenty of fluids, has sufficient rest, and gets as much exercise as possible.	Healthy, well-nourished, hydrated patients are less prone to injury and deterioration.

ing. Though periodic dressing changes are necessary with any type of covering, gauze dressings are usually changed more frequently than other kinds. Therefore patients are more apt to experience more overall discomfort with repeated removals and reapplication.

Gauze dressings are usually secured with tape. Some patients are hypersensitive to adhesives and care must be taken to use hypoallergenic tapes. Roller bandages may also be used to secure gauze dressings.

Transparent Dressings. Transparent dressings, known by trade names such as Op-Site® and Tegaderm® shown in Figure 20-11, offer several advantages over gauze dressings. One feature is that they are clear. This permits wound assessment without removing the dressing. When a transparent dressing is used, only the thin, single layer is applied over the wound. It can be pressed to conform to the surface of the skin. This is preferred by most patients over bulky layers of gauze. Transparent dressings are self-adhesive and under most circumstances do not require additional tape. Ordinarily this type of dressing does not need changing for two to seven days.

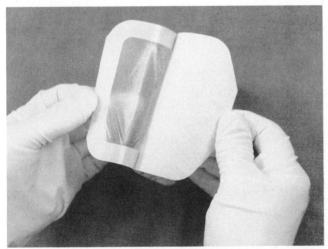

Figure 20-11 The backing is being removed from this occlusive dressing to reveal a transparent window. The framed edge makes handling easier. It is removed after the adhesive side is pressed over the wound.

Perhaps the best feature of transparent dressings is their selective permeability. That is, they let some substances into the wound area and keep others out. Oxygen and moisture vapor can move through the dressing toward the wound. They keep the wound moist. A moist wound undergoes accelerated healing. New cells first form at the wound margin. They extend toward the center at a more rapid rate in a moist environment. In addition, transparent dressings keep bacteria and liquids such as urine, stool, or drainage out of a second adjacent wound. This keeps the wound clean and reduces secondary skin irritation and infection.

Unfortunately, transparent dressings are not absorbent. As wound drainage accumulates, it has a tendency to loosen the dressing. Once the dressing is no longer intact, many of its original purposes are defeated. Manufacturers have recently designed a pouch dressing made of transparent material. The pouch collects the drainage. The volume within the pouch is reduced through evaporation, which extends the longevity of the original dressing.

Hydrocolloid Dressings. Hydrocolloid dressings such as DuoDERM® and Tegabsorb® are also waterproof and, like transparent dressings, promote a moist healing environment. They are ideal for covering wounds such as the one in Figure 20-12 that must heal by second intention. They are preferred for a wound that produces a lot of drainage. The underside of the dressing reacts with moisture in the wound to form a gel-like substance. The gel maintains the integrity of the dressing longer than the transparent type by preventing leaking and loss of adhesion.

Unless the dressing becomes loose or there are supporting signs of infection, it can remain undisturbed for up to seven days. Thus, healing and comfort are promoted in the absence of mechanical trauma from removal and reapplication of a dressing.

Unlike transparent dressings, hydrocolloid dressings keep air from reaching the wound. Reports in the literature by Hunt and colleagues (1981) and Galub (1983) indicate that a lack of oxygen acts as a stimulus for capillary growth.

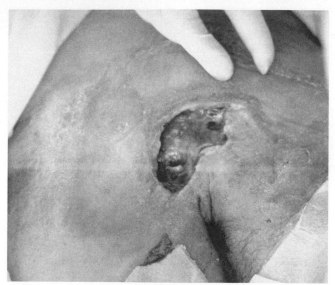

Figure 20-12 This patient has developed a Stage IV pressure sore in the sacral area. (Courtesy of E.R. Squibb & Sons, Inc., Princeton, NJ.)

Skill Procedure 20-2 describes the technique for applying an occlusive dressing such as the transparent and hydrocolloid types.

Preparing a Patient for a Dressing Change

A patient's outlook and self-esteem improves when he is included in planning for dressing changes. Mutual cooperation makes the patient a partner in his care. The patient and the nurse should discuss where, when, and how the dressing will be changed. If changing a dressing is likely to be a painful experience, the nurse should give the patient a prescribed medication about 15 to 30 minutes before a dressing change to reduce discomfort.

Dressings may be changed in a treatment room or in an operating room in some agencies. In most cases, dressings are changed while the patient is in bed. Some agencies have dressing carts that are wheeled from one patient to another. However, to help prevent cross-infection, the preferred method is to have individual dressing trays that

---

Skill Procedure 20-2. Changing an Occlusive Dressing

Suggested Action	**Reason for Action**
Wash hands.	Handwashing reduces the spread of microorganisms.
Assemble the following: clean and sterile gloves, waterproof container for refuse, dressing, gauze squares, tape is optional. Refer to Skill Procedure 20-4 if the wound will require irrigation.	Organizing supplies and equipment facilitates effective time management.
Choose dressing size that will extend approximately 2 in beyond the wound edge.	Attachment to an adequate area of healthy tissue reduces the possibility it will loosen as fluid collects underneath.
Don clean gloves.	Gloves act as a barrier against direct contact with drainage that contains blood, serum, and microorganisms.
Press on the skin at the margin of the dressing with one hand while using the fingers on the other hand to peel the edge away from the skin.	This approach helps to avoid tearing fragile skin that could be pulled away with the dressing.
Ease the dressing from all edges toward the center of the wound.	The wound heals toward the center; pulling toward the wound edge could reinjure healing tissue.
Remove the clean gloves turning them inside out enclosing the soiled dressing inside.	Enclosing the removed dressing within the soiled gloves contains pathogens.
Dispose of the gloves and dressing within a waterproof receptacle.	A waterproof receptacle prevents potential leakage and spread of pathogens.
Wash hands and don sterile gloves.	Hands are rewashed to remove microbes that multiply on gloved hands.
Irrigate or cleanse the wound as indicated.	Debris interferes with healing.
Pat the skin dry with gauze squares where the dressing will cover intact skin.	The adhesive on the dressing will not adhere to wet or oily skin.
Peel the paper backing exposing the adhesive surface as shown in Figure 20-13.	The backing maintains the sterility of the surface that will be in contact with the skin.

(continued)

Skill Procedure 20-2. Continued

Suggested Action	Reason for Action

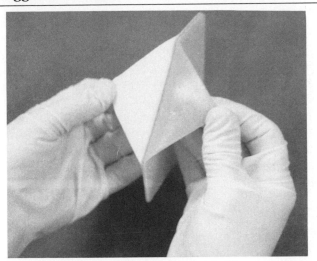

Figure 20-13 The backing is being peeled from this hydrocolloid dressing.

Center the dressing over the wound and press it in place.

Pressing rather than stretching the dressing avoids creating a shearing force on intact skin.

Smooth the peeled area of dressing from the center outward until it adheres to healthy skin.

Smoothing outward helps to avoid wrinkles in the dressing or air bubbles beneath it.

Press the dressing down within folds of the skin as the nurse in Figure 20-14 is doing.

Following body folds helps to avoid forming a gap that would permit leaking or evaporation of the moist environment.

Tape the edges with hypoallergenic tape, shown in Figure 20-15, if the patient is able to take a shower, tub bath, or receives hydrotherapy.

Tape acts as a secondary reinforcement against potential loosening.

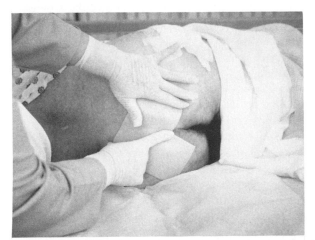

Figure 20-14 The nurse has trimmed an occlusive dressing to cover a sacral pressure sore. To avoid air leaks, the dressing is pressed so it covers the area within folds of skin. (Courtesy of E.R. Squibb & Sons, Inc., Princeton, NJ.)

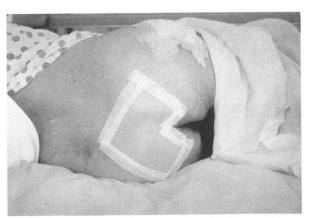

Figure 20-15 Though hydrocolloid dressings are self-adhesive, the tape has been used here to prevent loosening of the dressing as the gel builds underneath. (Courtesy of E.R. Squibb & Sons, Inc., Princeton, NJ.)

(continued)

Skill Procedure 20-2. Continued

Suggested Action	Reason for Action
Remove gloves and immediately wash hands.	Handwashing removes organisms that grow and multiply on gloved hands.
Date the dressing.	A date serves as a handy reminder for the next dressing change.
Make the patient comfortable in a position that avoids pressure on the dressed wound.	Pressure that exceeds 32 mm Hg occludes capillary blood flow.
Return or dispose of soiled equipment in the dirty utility room.	Keeping soiled items separate from clean is a medical aseptic practice to prevent the spread of pathogens.
Chart the appearance of the wound, the technique for cleansing or irrigation, and description of the dressing.	The description of the wound aids in evaluating the response of the patient to the implemented plan of care.

contain the equipment and supplies necessary for each patient. Commercially prepared, sterilized, and individually packaged supplies selected according to the patient's needs are used.

It is best to avoid changing a dressing immediately before or after a meal because of the effect it may have on the patient's appetite or digestion. A considerate nurse will schedule a dressing change other than during visiting hours. The patient will feel more in control of the events surrounding his care if the nurse considers his wishes as long as the choice does not create a potential hazard to his care.

The patient should receive explanations about the steps that will be followed when changing his dressing. In some instances, patients do not wish to look while their wounds are dressed. This is particularly true for patients whose wounds involve changes in their appearance or body functions, such as when an extremity has been amputated or a breast has been removed. The nurse can make positive statements, such as "There's less drainage today," as a verbal progress report. Patience and empathy will have a more positive effect on the nurse-patient relationship than coercion or shaming.

Organizing Equipment and Supplies for a Dressing Change

The following equipment and supplies are suggested for a dressing change on a clean open wound:

- A sterile cloth or paper on which to set up a working field. This can be the wrapper that covers a sterile dressing kit or an instrument set.
- Forceps or a clean glove to handle soiled dressing materials.
- Sterile forceps and a pair of sterile gloves with which to apply sterile dressing materials.
- A sterile cup in which to place antiseptic solution or commercially prepared sterile antiseptic swabs.

- A special solvent if a spray-on adhesive preparation was used to secure the previous dressing.
- Sterile normal saline if the dressing tends to stick to the wound.
- A waterproof bag to receive soiled dressings and wet cleansing materials.
- Dressings of various sizes and amounts depending on the size and condition of the wound.
- Tape for securing the dressing. Many patients are allergic to adhesive tape. Micropore tape, or paper tape, is less damaging to skin when it is removed. Also, few individuals seem to experience skin reactions with its use.

Skill Procedure 20-3 describes how to use this equipment and supplies when changing a dressing on a clean open wound. Practices of surgical asepsis are required to prevent introduction of organisms into the wound.

Performing an Irrigation

Wounds and other cavities of the body sometimes require an irrigation. An *irrigation* is a procedure that involves instilling solution into an area of the body. Irrigations are generally performed to cleanse and remove drainage and debris. All irrigations will require a solution, an instillation device, and a basin to receive soiled irrigation solution as it drains away from the area.

Various types of solutions may be used. Some are identified in Table 20-4. The nurse should follow the physician's order or the agency's policy regarding the choice of irrigating solution. Warming the solution may produce some comfort for the patient and stimulate increased blood flow that will aid in healing.

The instillation device will often depend on the volume of solution that must be instilled. An asepto syringe, a bulb syringe, or even a commercial wound irrigating device

(Text continues on page 475)

Skill Procedure 20-3. Changing a Gauze Dressing

Suggested Action	Reason for Action
Provide privacy.	The patient has a right to expect that others will not be see the procedure.
Position the patient so that he is comfortable and so that the working height promotes the nurse's posture and body mechanics.	Comfort for the patient and convenience for the nurse make contamination of the area while working less likely.
Expose the area of the wound but cover the areas that do not require attention.	Unnecessary exposure can cause chilling and embarrassment.
Remove materials securing the dressing. If materials other than tape have been used to secure the dressing, loosen and place them away from the wound.	The soiled dressing must be removed and properly disposed in order to prepare the wound for cleansing and redressing.
Loosen the end of an adhesive strip and gently pull it with quick, short, strokes toward the wound. Pull the tape while holding it as nearly parallel to the skin as possible, as illustrated in Figure 20-16. When hair is present, pull the tape in the direction of hair growth, if possible.	Pulling adhesive tape toward the wound prevents separating wound edges in the process of repair. Short, quick strokes and pulling in the direction of hair growth help prevent discomfort for the patient.

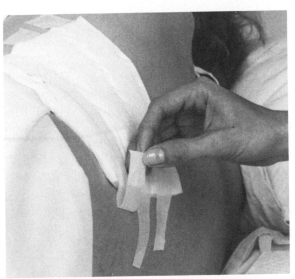

Figure 20-16 The nurse removes adhesive that is securing the patient's dressing. Notice that it is being pulled toward the wound and that the tape is held as nearly parallel to the patient's skin as possible.

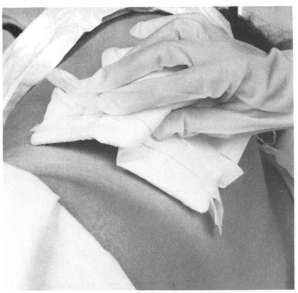

Figure 20-17 The nurse's gloved hand provides protection from organisms that may be present on the soiled dressing. Forceps may be used in place of a glove.

Lift off the dressing while touching only the outside area. If the dressing is soiled, use a forceps or gloved hand, as illustrated in Figure 20-17.	Microorganisms can be transferred by contact with the drainage on soiled dressings.
Discard the soiled dressings in a waterproof bag, as illustrated in Figure 20-18, for later disposal. Be careful not to touch the dressing materials to the outside of the bag.	Confining organisms within a waterproof bag acts as a transmission barrier controlling the spread of organisms to others.
Place used forceps on a paper towel away from the work area. If a disposable glove or forceps is used to remove the soiled dressing, it may also be placed in the waterproof container with the soiled dressing.	Equipment used to handle soiled dressings are contaminated and should not be placed near sterile materials. The material from which disposable items are made will melt and be destroyed when burned.

(continued)

Skill Procedure 20-3. Continued

Suggested Action	**Reason for Action**

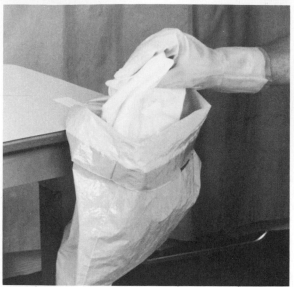

Figure 20-18 The soiled dressing and contaminated equipment and supplies are placed in a waxed bag.

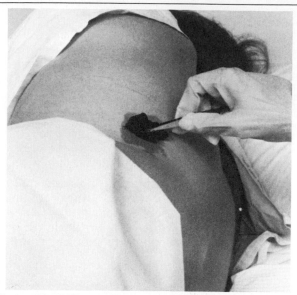

Figure 20-19 The wound is cleaned with a gathered gauze square moistened with povidone-iodine (Betadine).

Suggested Action	Reason for Action
If a dressing sticks to a wound, moisten it with sterile water or normal saline, unless contraindicated. Remove the dressing only when it is completely free.	Granulation tissue is easily dislodged by gauze that contains dried secretions. Moistening the dressing will liquefy the dried secretions, thereby reducing trauma and bleeding in the healing wound.
Wash hands before continuing to care for the wound.	Handwashing is one of the most important medical aseptic techniques to reduce the spread of pathogens.
Set up the sterile field on the overbed table or a similar, stable, convenient, work area.	Appropriate location of the sterile field will help prevent contamination of the equipment later.
Add all the equipment and supplies for the dressing change, including the antiseptic solution to the sterile field.	Poor organization wastes time. Having all necessary materials ready prevents having to seek assistance. Leaving to obtain the items would risk contaminating the sterile field.
Don sterile gloves.	To prevent contaminating items that will be placed in contact with an open wound, sterile gloves must be worn.
Gather the edges of a small gauze square containing no cotton filler with sterile forceps, as the nurse in Figure 20-19 has done.	Gathering permits absorption of a greater volume of antiseptic without dripping. Fibers from cotton-lined gauze squares tend to remain in the wound.
Using one gauze square or swab for each stroke, cleanse the wound and skin around it, following one of the three methods illustrated in Figure 20-20.	Moving away from the wound and using one swab for each stroke prevents bringing organisms present on the skin into the wound.
Dispose of the gauze squares or swabs with the other soiled material in the waterproof container. Take care not to touch the sterile forceps or glove to any contaminated or unsterile areas.	Placing a wet gauze or swab on a cloth or paper sterile field will pull organisms from the underneath surface, thereby contaminating that area.
Allow the antiseptic to dry well.	Dressings may become moist and pull organisms into the wound if excessive antiseptic remains on the skin. Tape may not securely hold the dressing in place if the skin is wet.

(continued)

Skill Procedure 20-3. *Continued*

Suggested Action	**Reason for Action**

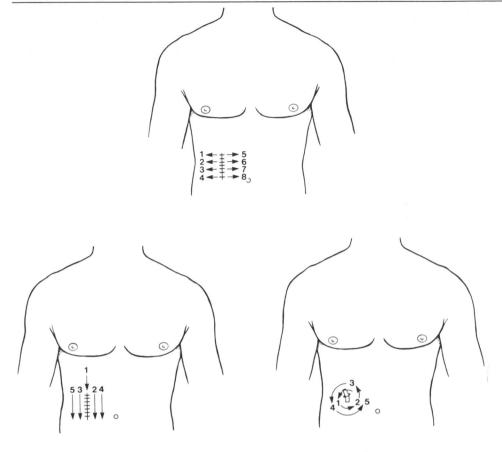

Figure 20-20 The nurse cleanses a wound from the incision, outward by following any of the numbered patterns shown in the illustration.

Look at the wound carefully. Assess the healing process and look for signs of infection, such as unusual drainage, puffiness, and tenderness.	The nurse is responsible for assessing the wound and recording the findings that are observed on the patient's record.
Cover the wound with sterile gauze dressings, as illustrated in Figure 20-21. Position the dressing with sterile forceps or gloved hands. The very outer surface of the last dressing may be considered clean rather than sterile.	Touching the wound surface with one's hands can transfer pathogens that may lead to a wound infection.
Consider the effect of gravity on the drainage. Use extra amounts of dressing materials on the lower sides of draining wounds.	Material from a wound will drain downward due to gravity. Applying extra material at the lower edges will help absorb drainage when the patient walks or lies in bed.
Secure the dressing with tape. Fold a portion of the end of the tape back over on itself.	Tape helps prevent the dressing from coming loose or changing position. Fashioning a tab promotes ease of tape removal and may reduce discomfort the next time the dressing is changed.
See the text for suggestions for other methods of securing dressings.	Some patients may be sensitive to tape or their wounds may require some additional reinforcement.
Dispose of the contaminated, soiled material. Care for used instruments according to agency policy.	Careless handling of equipment and supplies spreads organisms to others.

(continued)

Skill Procedure 20-3. *Continued*

Suggested Action	**Reason for Action**

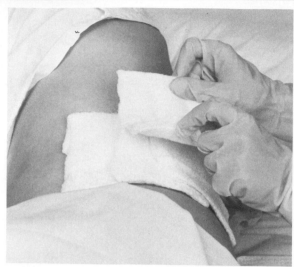

Figure 20-21 The nurse has removed soiled gloves and has donned a sterile pair. Layers of gauze squares and pads are placed over the wound to absorb the drainage. Excess dressing material should be avoided, since it may cause discomfort.

Suggested Action	Reason for Action
Record the care and appearance of the wound.	Careful documentation is important in validating the care provided and the progress of the patient's condition.

Table 20-4. *Solutions Used in Wound Care*

Type	**Use**	**Disadvantages**
Povidone-iodine (Betadine®)	Kills bacteria, spores, fungi, and viruses	Many patients are allergic to iodine Interferes with tissue granulation at strengths >1% Can elevate serum iodine levels by being absorbed from large wounds
Sodium hypochlorite (Dakin's solution)	Antimicrobial Debrides wounds	Inhibits blood clotting at the wound site Irritates skin around the wound
Hydrogen peroxide	Mechanically removes debris from wounds	Can dislodge clots that have formed Prolonged use could inhibit tissue granulation Can cause pockets of air to form, separating layers of tissue and delaying healing
Acetic Acid 1/8%	Inhibits organisms such as *Pseudomonas, Trichomonas,* and *Candida*	Irritates healthy skin surrounding the wound
Normal Saline and Ringer's Solution	Removes debris from wound without cell injury Rinses more toxic antiseptics from wound	No bacteriostatic or bacteriocidal action

Adapted from Thomason SS: Front-line antiseptics. Geriatr Nurs 10(5):235–236, 1989. Used with permission from American Journal of Nursing Company.

may be used. Some have found that the pulsating fluid from a Water-Pik® is an effective method to loosen wound debris. It usually requires two nurses, one to operate the device while the other suctions the fluid.

Any wound irrigation that is performed in a body area containing intact tissue will not necessarily need to follow principles of sterile technique. However, when an irrigation is required for an incision or other open wound, surgical asepsis should be followed. The drainage basin does not need to be sterile because it will receive solution contaminated with organisms and debris from the irrigated area. An emesis basin or round basin may be used. Universal precautions should be followed when an irrigation may produce a spray that would include blood or body fluids known to transmit bloodborne viruses.

A wound irrigation is usually carried out just before applying a new dressing. Skill Procedure 20-4 describes the suggested actions for performing a wound irrigation.

Irrigating Body Structures

Minor changes can be made in the technique used for irrigating a wound when other structures, such as the eye, ear, or vagina need to be cleansed. Variations usually involve differences in the position of the patient, volume, temperature, and types of solutions used.

Eye Irrigation. In an emergency—for example, when splashed with an irritating chemical—the objective is to act quickly. The longer the substance remains in the eye, the greater the seriousness of the injury. Blindness is a poten-

Skill Procedure 20-4. Irrigating a Wound

Suggested Action	Reason for Action
Wash hands.	Handwashing reduces the spread of microorganisms.
Assemble the following equipment: gloves, waterproof receptacle, absorbent pad, emesis basin, solution, basin, Asepto syringe, skin protectant such as zinc oxide or vaseline if an irritating solution will be used, gauze squares.	Collecting necessary items promotes organization and effective time management.
Add items needed for universal precautions such as goggles and mask or face shield, cover gown or apron.	During a wound irrigation, body fluid containing blood can splash the face or uniform.
Warm approximately 100 to 200 mL of irrigating solution to 90°–95°F (32.2°–35°C). This can be done by setting the container of solution in a basin or sink with warm water.	Tepid to warm temperatures promote comfort and reduce the potential for thermal injury to the tissue.
Explain the procedure to the patient and provide time for comfort measures such as using the bathroom.	An explanation reduces anxiety and promotes patient cooperation.
Provide privacy.	The patient has the right to be protected from being observed by others.
Position the patient so fluid will flow into the wound and drain away from the irrigated area. For an abdominal wound the usual position is supine or dorsal recumbent.	Irrigation and drainage are accomplished by gravity.
Protect the bed with an absorbent pad.	Time and effort are conserved by protecting the bed linen.
Loosen the tape on the dressing, don gloves, and remove the soiled dressing.	Gloves protect the hands from direct contact with drainage that may contain pathogens.
Deposit the dressing within a waterproof receptacle.	Containing soiled items is a medical aseptic practice that controls the spread of microorganisms.
Remove gloves turning them inside out, dispose, and wash hands immediately.	Handwashing removes microbes that grow and multiply in the warm, moist environment within gloves.
Prepare irrigation equipment.	Refer to the principles of asepsis discussed in Chapter 16.
Place a kidney or emesis basin with the curve conforming to the body contour below and to the side of the wound.	Keeping the basin close to the body helps reduce the amount of irrigant that may leak onto the absorbent pad.

(continued)

Skill Procedure 20-4. *Continued*

Suggested Action	Reason for Action
Don wearing apparel selected for universal precautions.	The nurse uses judgment in selecting apparel that will prevent direct contact with blood and body fluids.
Apply skin protectant such as zinc oxide or a petroleum-based ointment to the healthy tissue surrounding a wound if an irritating solution will be used.	Zinc oxide or petroleum-based ointment provide a moisture-proof barrier against irritating solutions such as sodium hypochlorite or acetic acid.
Without touching the wound itself or using a great deal of pressure, instill solution over or into the wound.	The flow of the solution mechanically loosens debris and moves it out of the area.
Tilt the patient toward the drainage basin and wait a short time for draining to be completed.	Gravity causes fluid to flow from a higher to lower level.
Dry any skin areas that may have become wet with solution or drainage.	Drying the patient shows concern for his comfort.
Remove skin protectant if an occlusive dressing will be applied.	Moisture and oily substances interfere with the ability of tape or an occlusive dressing to adhere to the skin.
Apply a fresh dressing over the wound.	A dressing acts as a barrier to microbes in the absence of intact skin.
Change any wet linen or patient clothing. Help to a position of comfort.	Wet linen and a strained position contribute to discomfort.
Remove gloves and other garments when there is no longer any potential for contact with bloody drainage or serum.	Gloves and other garments are a temporary barrier used while there is a potential for contact with blood and body fluids.
Wash hands immediately.	Organisms grow rapidly within the warm, moist conditions inside gloves.
Remove soiled equipment and care for it according to agency policy.	Disposing of soiled equipment aids in controlling the spread of microorganisms.
Record the condition of the wound and the procedure that was carried out.	The patient's chart is a record of his care and response to prescribed treatment.

tial consequence if treatment is delayed or inadequate. It is important to flush the eye immediately and continuously with water. Tap water from a faucet, water fountain, or showerhead is appropriate. It is likely that the eye will have to be held open, since the natural tendency is to squeeze the eyelids shut. Goggles should be worn when working with caustic liquids or substances that could be propelled into the eyes. Skill Procedure 20-5 describes the technique for irrigating an eye in nonemergency situations.

Ear Irrigation. It should always be determined that the tympanic membrane, the eardrum, is intact before irrigating the ear. If it is not, the solution can enter the middle ear, become trapped, and contribute to discomfort and growth of pathogens. In addition, it would be wise to perform a gross inspection if a foreign body is suspected. Children are notorious for putting small buttons and other objects in their mouth, nose, and ears. They often wedge and become irretrievable. If the item is a bean, pea, or similar dehydrated substance irrigation is contraindicated. The solution can cause the item to swell and become fixed

even more tightly. Solid objects may require removal with an instrument. An exception would be in the case of a live insect. The insect can be suffocated by instilling and briefly retaining water or oil within the auditory canal. The dead insect will usually pass out as the fluid drains from the ear. Skill Procedure 20-6 gives suggested actions for irrigating the ear to remove dried secretions or other debris.

Vaginal Irrigation. A vaginal irrigation is commonly called a *douche*. Douching is not recommended as a routine practice. The vagina contains helpful microbes called *Döoderlein bacilli*. They promote a weak acidic quality to natural vaginal secretions. The acidity creates a hostile environment for other organisms. Therefore, they actually help to prevent vaginal infections. Removing these helpful organisms through repeated douching reduces their numbers and beneficial effect.

Douching is also contraindicated within 24 to 48 hours of a vaginal exam involving a Pap test. Irrigation can remove abnormal cells that could otherwise be collected and identified in the vaginal secretions. Abnormal cervical

Skill Procedure 20-5. Irrigating an Eye

Suggested Action	Reason for Action
Wash hands.	Handwashing reduces the spread of microorganisms.
Assemble the following equipment: gloves if a local infection is present, towel, emesis basin, solution, basin, Asepto syringe, cotton balls or gauze squares, waterproof receptacle.	Universal precautions do not apply to eye drainage unless it is visibly contaminated with blood. Gloves act as a barrier against contact with other pathogens.
Warm 60 to 240 mL of irrigating solution to 98.6°F (37°C).	A solution that is near body temperature is soothing and not likely to cause thermal injury.
Explain the procedure to the patient and provide time for comfort measures such as using the bathroom.	An explanation reduces anxiety and promotes patient cooperation.
Provide privacy.	The patient has a right to be protected from being observed by others.
Place the patient in a sitting position with the affected eye tilted toward the side.	Gravity controls the direction in which fluid flows.
Protect the bed with an absorbent pad.	Time and effort are conserved by protecting the bed linen and patient's clothing.
Moisten a cotton ball or corner of gauze square and wipe the eye from the nose toward the ear if matter is visible on the lids or lashes.	Wiping away from the nasolacrimal duct reduces the potential for spreading infectious organisms to the nose and sinuses.
Discard each cotton ball into the waterproof receptacle after one wipe. Use a separate corner of the gauze square if additional strokes are needed.	Reuse of a soiled item replaces debris and organisms back into the cleansed area.
Position the emesis basin at the side of the face. An alert patient can assist.	The basin collects draining irrigant and prevents the discomfort of solution dripping onto the face or into the ear.
Separate the lids with the fingers of the nondominant hand.	Holding the lids apart controls the blinking reflex.
Fill the syringe and position it approximately 1 inch (2.5 cm) above the eye, as shown in Figure 20-22.	Holding the tip close to the eye aids in controlling the direction of the solution.

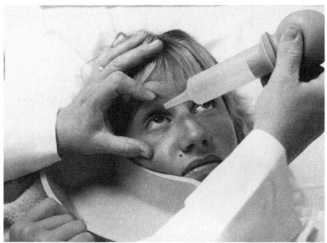

Figure 20-22 The nurse prepares to flush the eye with irrigating solution.

(continued)

Skill Procedure 20-5. Continued

Suggested Action	Reason for Action
Direct the flow onto the conjunctiva rather than the cornea.	The force of water on the cornea can cause discomfort and reflex blinking.
Have the patient close his eye periodically.	Periodic closure helps to circulate the solution over all areas of the eye.
Dry the face and any other areas that have become wet with irrigating solution.	Drying the patient shows concern for his comfort.
Change any wet clothing or bed linen and return the patient to a position of comfort.	Wet linen and a strained position contribute to discomfort.
Remove soiled equipment and care for it according to agency policy.	Caring for soiled equipment is an appropriate medical aseptic practice.
Wash hands.	Handwashing removes transient microorganisms.
Record the condition of the eye and the procedure that was carried out.	The patient's chart is a record of his care and response to prescribed treatment.

bleeding may also be obscured by douching before an exam.

Douching is not an effective method of birth control. By the time a douche could be administered, some sperm already would have entered the cervix and be inaccessible to removal by irrigation.

Vaginal irrigation is appropriate as a method of instilling an antiseptic solution to treat an existing infection, such as

the yeast, *Candida,* or the protozoan, *Trichomonas.* A mixture of 1 to 2 tablespoons of white vinegar (acetic acid) to a quart of water is often as effective as more expensive over-the-counter douching products. Some infections respond better to prescribed vaginal instillations of creams or dissolvable tablets. The best recommendation for itching, burning, or vaginal drainage is to be examined and follow the suggested treatment.

Skill Procedure 20-6. Irrigating an Ear

Suggested Action	Reason for Action
Wash hands.	Handwashing reduces the spread of microorganisms.
Assemble the following equipment: cotton-tipped applicator, waterproof receptacle, towel, emesis basin, solution, basin, Asepto syringe, glove and one or two cotton balls.	Collecting all necessary items at one time promotes organization and effective time management.
Warm up to 500 mL of solution to 98.6°F (37°C).	Warmer or cooler temperatures can cause nausea and dizziness when instilled in some patients.
Explain the procedure to the patient and provide time for comfort measures such as using the bathroom.	An explanation reduces anxiety and promotes patient cooperation.
Provide privacy.	The patient has a right to be protected from being observed by others.
Protect the shoulder and bed with a towel or an absorbent pad.	Time and effort are conserved by protecting the bed linen and patient's clothing.
Place the patient in a sitting position. Inspect the ear for dried secretions or accumulated drainage.	The ear is assessed more easily with the patient in a sitting position.
Moisten a cotton-tipped applicator in the irrigating solution and clean the pinna and outer area of the ear.	Cleansing is more effective after physically removing excessive debris. To avoid injury, the applicator should not be placed within the auditory canal.

(continued)

Skill Procedure 20-6. *Continued*

Suggested Action	Reason for Action
Discard the applicator after one stroke. Use a fresh applicator if additional removal is indicated.	Reuse of a soiled item redeposits debris back into a clean area.
Have the patient tilt his head so fluid will drain from his ear.	Gravity aids drainage.
Place a kidney or emesis basin below the ear. An alert patient can assist.	The basin collects draining irrigant and prevents the discomfort of solution dripping down the neck.
Straighten the ear canal of an adult by pulling the pinna upward and backward as shown in Figure 20-23. Pull the ear downward and backward for a young child.	Straightening the ear canal aids in filling the chamber to its maximum depth and volume. The angle of the canal changes with growth.

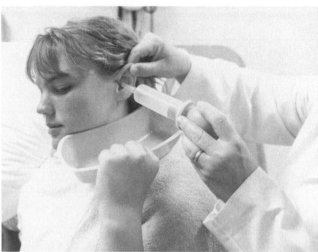

Figure 20-23 The nurse has straightened the ear canal before instilling the warm irrigating solution.

Fill the syringe and direct the flow toward the roof of the auditory canal, not toward the tympanic membrane. Do not close off the ear canal with the tip of the syringe.	Controlling the direction and volume of the solution prevents discomfort and possible perforation of the eardrum.
When the irrigation is finished, place a cotton ball loosely within the ear. Instruct the patient to lie on his side.	A cotton ball absorbs residual moisture and drainage from the ear.
Change any wet clothing or bed linen.	Replacing wet linen with dry demonstrates concern for the patient's comfort.
Remove soiled equipment and care for it according to agency policy.	Caring for soiled equipment is an appropriate medical aseptic practice.
Don a clean glove and remove the cotton ball after 15 minutes.	A glove acts as a barrier from direct contact with a source of pathogens.
Observe the drainage and enclose the cotton ball within the removed glove. Dispose of the glove and its contents in a waterproof receptacle.	Containing soiled articles helps control the spread of microorganisms.
Record the characteristics of the drainage and the condition of the ear, as well as the procedure that was performed.	The patient's chart is a record of his care and response to prescribed treatment.

Occasionally a douche is administered preoperatively before gynecologic surgery. Skill Procedure 20-7 identifies the suggested actions for irrigating the vagina.

Caring for a Wound With a Drain

Drains are hollow tubes through which liquid secretions from a wound are removed. At one time most drains were inserted directly into the wound. This has been found to delay healing and provide an entry site for pathogens. Now surgeons are inserting drains so that they exit from a separate location beside the wound. Some drains are su-

tured in place while others may be prevented from slipping beneath the skin by placing a safety pin or clip on the end extending from the wound.

Closed drains are being used more often in place of open drains. A closed drain is connected to a drainage receptacle, such as the one in Figure 20-24. A vacuum or suction machine causes a pulling action to remove drainage. The end of an open drain remains free. It relies on gravity to remove secretions that are then deposited into an absorbent dressing. Open drains are made from various materials. Some are flat flexible rubber tubes, such as a Penrose drain; some are silicone or plastic with one or more openings at the base for removing drainage.

Skill Procedure 20-7. Administering a Douche

Suggested Action	Reason for Action
Wash hands.	Handwashing reduces the spread of microorganisms.
Assemble the following equipment: cotton bath blanket, gloves, bedpan, irrigation bag and nozzle, absorbent bed pad, sanitary napkin.	Organizing supplies promotes efficient time management. Gloves should be used as a universal precaution against contact with vaginal secretions that may contain blood and bloodborne viruses.
Inspect the douche nozzle for burrs, chips, or cracks.	A damaged nozzle or one with a rough surface could injure tissue within the vagina.
Warm 1000 to 1500 mL of the prescribed solution to 100.5° to 110°F (40.5°–43.3°C).	The vagina can tolerate temperatures slightly warmer than body temperature.
Explain the procedure to the patient and provide time for comfort measures such as using the bathroom.	A full bladder can cause discomfort and interfere with filling the vagina with solution.
Provide privacy.	The patient has the right to be protected from being observed by others.
Place the patient in a dorsal recumbent position and cover with the cotton bath blanket.	The bath blanket will provide warmth and prevent exposure of the patient after top linen is removed.
Fanfold the top linen to the bottom of the bed and drape diagonal corners of the bath blanket about the legs.	The top linen must be removed in order to have adequate access to the vagina.
Place a bedpan beneath the patient.	The vagina has no sphincter. The bedpan will collect the draining solution.
Substitute lying in a bathtub as an alternative if the patient can self-administer the irrigating solution.	Sitting on the toilet or standing in the bathtub interferes with filling the distal areas of the vagina.
Elevate or suspend the container of solution 18 to 24 inches (45–60 cm) above the hips.	The higher the container, the faster and more forceful the flow. A rapid instillation is not likely to be retained long enough to achieve effective cleansing.
Empty the air from the tubing by letting some solution flow into the bedpan.	Instilled air occupies a portion of available space needed for solution. It may also cause discomfort from distention.
Allow some of the solution to flow over the vulva.	The patient should be consulted about the comfort of the warmed solution. The area to be irrigated may be even more sensitive than adjacent tissue.
Don gloves and separate the labia.	Gloves act as a barrier against bloodborne viruses and other organisms present in the vaginal cavity or secretions.

(continued)

Skill Procedure 20-7. Continued

Suggested Action	Reason for Action
Insert the nozzle downward and backward within the vagina.	To avoid injury the nozzle should follow the anatomical contour of the vagina.
Unclamp the tubing and gently rotate the nozzle as the fluid is instilled.	Rotation helps direct the solution to all areas of the vagina.
Have the patient contract the perineal muscles, as though trying to stop urination, and then relax them four or five times during the irrigation.	Contracting helps to fill and distend the folds of the vaginal mucous membrane. Relaxation allows drainage to take place.
Clamp the tubing, remove the nozzle, and elevate the head of the bed after the solution has been instilled.	Sitting will promote draining of the remaining irrigation solution.
Remove the bedpan and dry the perineum. Position a sanitary napkin in place.	A sanitary napkin will continue to collect and absorb any fluid that continues to leak from the vagina.
Remove the drape and replace the top bed linen.	The drape is no longer needed after the procedure is finished.
Empty the contents of the bedpan noting the characteristics of the drained solution	Assessment aids in evaluation of the implemented plan of care.
Clean and replace the bedpan and reusable equipment in the bedside stand.	Clean equipment can be reused for the same patient.
Remove gloves and dispose in a waterproof receptacle.	Containing soiled equipment is an appropriate medical aseptic practice.
Immediately wash hands.	Handwashing removes organisms that grow and multiply within gloves.
Document the procedure and pertinent assessments.	The patient's chart is a record of his care and response to the implemented plan of care.

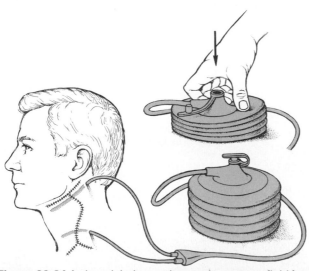

Figure 20-24 A closed drain may be used to remove fluid from a wound. The fluid travels through the catheters into a collector. This device facilitates wound drainage by creating a vacuum when it is flattened and sealed.

When caring for a drain, the nurse should do the following:

Assess the characteristics and amount of drainage. Drains can become kinked or plugged. If this happens, an abscess may develop within the wound or drainage may ooze from the insertion site.

Cleanse the area around a drain using separate equipment and gloves than those used to clean the wound. This avoids transferring organisms that may be present in one area but not in another.

Clean the skin around the drain, using the circular method described earlier. It may be helpful and may provide more comfort to the patient if the drain is elevated with several thicknesses of gauze squares while care is being provided. This avoids pulling on the drain from its point of attachment.

Shorten a drain by using forceps and a *gentle* twisting motion to pull the drain out for the prescribed distance. Cut off the excess length with sterile scissors. Replace the sterile safety pin or clip near the exposed end of the drain. Periodic shortening of a drain promotes healing from the base of a wound to the surface.

Remove a drain using the same techniques for shortening. The patient may be premedicated to reduce any potential discomfort. Refer to the discussion later in this chapter concerning removal of sutures, if the drain has been secured in this manner.

Encircle an open drain with a drain dressing. A drain dressing is a gauze or telfa square. It is precut on one side to the center of the dressing. To improvise a drain dressing from gauze squares, refer to Figure 20-25.

Packing a Wound

A draining wound, especially when it is deep and has pockets, may be packed. Packing materials help to soak up drainage and remove large debris from a wound that may not move freely through a drain. Long strips of gauze impregnated with iodoform, an antiseptic substance, may be used. The strip may be cut when the desired amount has filled the wound. The physician or the nurse generally changes the packing at the same time that the dressing is changed. This requires assembling additional supplies. The wound should be packed using sterile forceps or gloved hands. The packing should be inserted gently and with care to prevent injury to the wound or displacement of any granulation tissue that may be present. Packing promotes second or third intention healing.

Applying Wet to Dry Dressings

A technique for surface debridement of a wound involves applying a wet to dry dressing. The moist dressing keeps the area soft and traps the debris within the dressing as it slowly dries. The wet dressing is covered by a dry dressing to promote the comfort of the patient. When the dressing is changed, the trapped material is lifted from the wound.

If the dressing is not changed frequently, there is a risk that healing tissue may adhere to the dressing and be pulled away from the wound. Wet dressings, especially those that do not contain an antiseptic, may contribute to the growth of pathogens.

Securing a Dressing

Securing a dressing often requires ingenuity and resourcefulness. Factors such as the size of the wound, its location, and the amount and nature of the drainage, the frequency with which the dressing needs changing, and the activities of the patient should be taken into account.

The following recommendations describe basic techniques for securing a dressing:

Plan to use adhesive or paper tape for most dressings. These are available in various widths. The length is cut according to need. Elasticized tape permits more

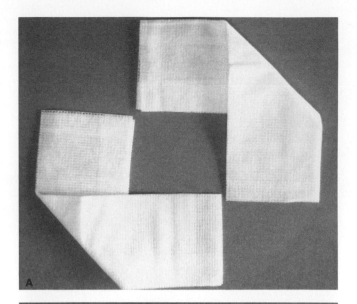

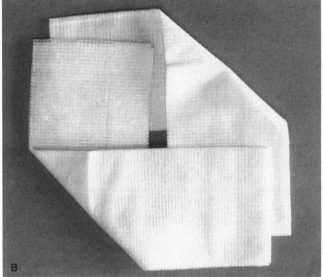

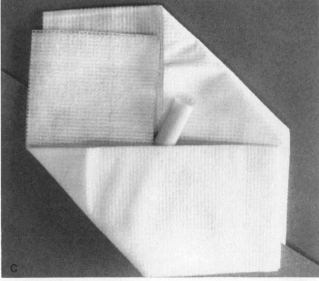

Figure 20-25 (*A*). Two gauze squares have been refolded forming right angles. (*B*). The two gauze strips are overlapped. (*C*). The drain protrudes through the center of the overlapped gauze.

movement of a body part without pull on adjacent tissues.

Consider clipping the area if tape must be applied over hairy areas. Try to avoid shaving because it can cause microabrasions and an entry site for organisms.

Remove adhesive remnants when applying new tape. The remains of adhesive may be removed with acetone, but it is very drying and irritating to the skin. A better technique is to apply an ointment, such as A and D ointment, to the adhesive remnants, allow them to "soak" for a few minutes, and then wipe the area gently with soft tissues.

Fold under each end of an adhesive strip, creating a tab, as illustrated in Figure 20-26. This technique helps in grasping the tape and lifting it off when it is to be removed.

Apply a protective coating on the skin before using tape when dressings must be changed frequently. This helps protect the skin from irritation. A preparation often used when skin is not irritated is compound tincture of benzoin. Another suitable preparation is collodion, which is treated plant cellulose in ether or alcohol. Other products, such as karaya paste or powder, or Skin Gel, used for protecting the skin around an ostomy, may also be used around some wounds.

Moisten adhesive with a little alcohol if the adhesive does not stick well to the skin. Alcohol dissolves the oils present on skin surfaces.

Try using liquid adhesive for securing a small dressing on a wound with little or no drainage. The edges of the outer piece of gauze are cut to fit over the wound, painted with liquid adhesive, and then glued to the skin.

Do not cover the entire surface of the dressing with tape. To do so does not permit the escape of heat and moisture from the skin. This predisposes the patient to skin irritation and destruction.

Observe the patient for sensitivity to adhesive. Investigate any complaint or discomfort associated with adhesive. Signs include redness, swelling, and blister formation. Various kinds of nonallergic tapes, such as those made of silk or paper, are available for a sensitive patient.

Use Montgomery straps for securing a dressing when it must be changed frequently. They do not require removal with each dressing change. They can be handmade or purchased commercially. The adhesive end of the strap is placed on the skin well away from the wound. The end of the strap near the wound remains free because the adhesive side has been turned back on itself, similar to a large tab. Gauze or cloth strips passed through eyelets are tied over the wound to secure the dressing. When the dressing is changed, the straps are untied and turned back to allow for wound care. The skin is protected appropriately before the straps are applied to the patient. These straps are illustrated in Figure 20-27.

Center the tape over the middle of the dressing. Press each end of the tape gently away from the direction of the wound. Keep the skin smooth; avoid bulging or bunching the tissue.

Secure a dressing so that it is snug enough to prevent the dressing from slipping. Loose-fitting dressings cause friction as the patient moves. Also, try to secure a dressing so that it fits a body contour for the patient's comfort.

Consider using a type of bandage or binder when adhesive is impractical. Bandages and binders are discussed later in the chapter.

Removing Sutures and Staples

Clean open wounds are held together with temporary materials to promote healing by first intention. Some methods of wound closure include butterfly tapes, steri-

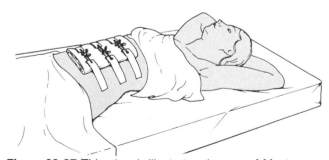

Figure 20-27 This sketch illustrates the use of Montgomery straps. Cut strips of adhesive, 5 cm to 7.5 cm (2 to 3 in) wide. Fold back one end of each strip onto itself for about 7.5 cm (3 in), sticky side to sticky side. Fold in half again, and cut a slit into the middle of the folded edge. When the strip is unfolded, there is an opening through which cotton twill or gauze is passed for tying the straps in place. The adhesive strips should be cut sufficiently long so that they extend about 15 cm (6 in) beyond the wound on each side. Montgomery straps can be used for 2 to 3 days and should then be replaced to help prevent excessive skin irritation.

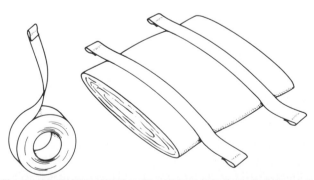

Figure 20-26 The sketches illustrate how to fold back the ends of adhesive strips. The technique helps in the removal of tape so that the ends can be easily grasped. The edges had been turned back for easy removal of tape from the patient who was shown earlier in Figure 20-16.

strips, sutures, and staples. Butterfly tapes and steri-strips are adhesive-backed materials applied to the skin surface.

Sutures are natural fibers, such as silk, or synthetic substances, such as nylon, that provide a union between open edges of a wound. Lay people refer to them as stitches. *Staples* are wide metal clips that also hold tissue together. Sutures and staples are inserted into the skin and underlying tissues. Staples have an advantage in that they are less likely to compress tissue if a wound swells. Staples do not encircle the wound; they merely form a bridge that holds the two sides together.

All wound closure material is intended to remain in place until the wound has healed sufficiently to prevent reopening. Depending on the location this may be a few days to as long as two weeks. The nurse may be directed by the physician to remove the sutures or staples. For individuals with slower healing, every other suture may be removed. This will be followed by removal of the other sutures a few days later. A weak incision may be held together with steri-strips after the sutures or staples are removed. The technique for removing sutures is illustrated in Figure 20-28. Staples are removed with a special instrument shown in Figure 20-29.

Using Bandages and Binders

A *bandage* is material that covers an injured body part. Usually, bandages are dispensed in rolls of various widths. A *binder* is a type of bandage. The term binder is generally used when the bandaging covers or supports a large body area, such as the abdomen, chest, or breast. Some texts use the terms synonymously, although in the strictest sense they do not have the same meaning.

Purposes of Bandages and Binders

Bandages and binders serve a variety of purposes:

- They can be used to hold dressings in place, especially when adhesive cannot be used or when a dressing is large.

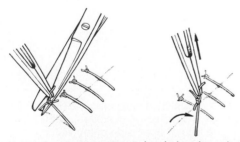

Figure 20-28 To remove sutures, begin by cleansing the incision line. Use a forceps to grasp and elevate the knot. Carefully insert the tip of the scissors just under the knot. If sutures seem to stick, moisten them with normal saline for a few minutes. If the patient is allowed to shower, schedule suture removal following personal hygiene. Cut the suture *below* the knot as close to the skin as possible. Pull the knot gently to remove the suture.

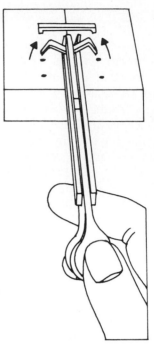

Removing staples

Figure 20-29 The staple remover is placed in the middle of the metal staple. Squeezing bends the bridge area and lifts the embedded teeth of the staple from the skin.

- They prevent tension on sutures when properly applied.
- They limit motion to promote healing.
- They are used to support a part of the body, protect an injured area, and prevent further injury.
- They provide comfort and a sense of security for the patient.

Fabrics for Bandages and Binders

Bandages and binders are made from various fabrics to achieve certain desired results. Table 20-5 describes each type of material and indicates the purposes for their use. An Ace bandage is commonly used in health agencies. It is made from elasticized material. An example of an Ace bandage is shown in Figure 20-30.

Selecting a Bandaging Technique

Most fabrics used for covering a body part are roller bandages. A *roller bandage* is a continuous strip of material wound on itself to form a cylinder or roll. These rolls are prepared in various widths and lengths. When applying a roller bandage, it is wrapped around a body part. The outer surface of the bandage is placed next to the patient's skin. When the bandage is begun, the end is held in place with one hand while the other hand passes the roll around the part. Once the bandage is anchored, the remainder of the roll is passed from hand to hand, with care being taken to exert equal tension with each turn. Unequal tension may interfere with proper circulation to the part. The terminal

Table 20-5. Comparison of Fabrics Used for Bandages and Binders

Fabric	Description	Uses
Gauze	Light, porous, soft, prepared in a roll or tube	Readily fits a body part. Promotes a cool feeling because it allows circulation of air.
Muslin, flannel, synthetic fabrics	Tightly woven, strong, firm	Useful when support and comfort are desired. Feels more like an article of clothing. Helps keep an area warm. Well suited for home use, since they may be washed and reused.
Elasticized materials	Strong, stretchable, molds well to body contours; some are self-adhering (*i.e.,* sticks to itself)	Provides firm support and immobilization. Can exert pressure to control bleeding and swelling.
Stockinet	Tubular, stretchable material in various widths or diameters	Encircles a body part, making it convenient for covering the head, chest, or length of an extremity. Applies a uniform amount of pressure. Remains in place better than a wrapped bandage. Simple and quick to use.

end of the bandage may be secured with adhesive, clamps, or with safety pins. None of these methods should be done in a way that produces pressure on the patient's skin or wound.

There are six basic turns used when applying roller bandages. The choice of turning technique depends on the shape of the body part. Some wrapping techniques may be used separately or in combination, depending on the purpose and the part being bandaged. Table 20-6 describes each turn, lists its purpose, and provides illustrations for its application.

Applying Bandages and Binders

The nurse should follow some basic guidelines when applying bandages and binders. Skill Procedure 20-8 describes suggested actions that can provide principles to follow when covering a body part.

Removing a Roller Bandage

If a roller bandage is not going to be reused, it is best to remove it by freeing the bandage material with bandage scissors. Cutting should be done on the side opposite the injury or wound, from one end to the other, so that the bandage can be opened its entire length. If the material is to be reused, it may be unwrapped and rewound by rolling the loosened end and passing it as a ball from one hand to the other. If an elastic roller bandage has become soiled, wash it and dry it on a flat surface. Hanging stretches the elastic fibers and decreases the usefulness of the bandage.

Applying Commonly Used Binders

Some commonly used binders include the T-binder, four-tailed binder, scultetus binder, and straight binder. A triangular binder, known as a sling, is discussed further in Chapter 26. The following is information concerning the application of binders that are frequently used in the care of patients.

Using a T-Binder. A *T-binder* looks like the letter T and is used for securing dressings on the perineum and in the groin. A single T-binder has a tail attached at right

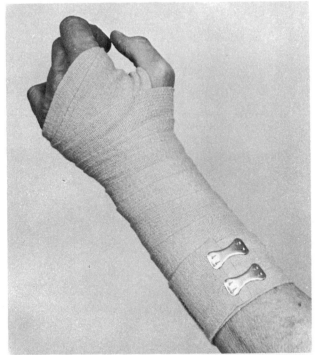

Figure 20-30 An Ace bandage has been applied to a patient's forearm to immobilize the wrist. This type is not self-adhering. The bandage is secured with clips that hold the end of the bandage in place.

(Text continues on page 488)

Table 20-6. Basic Wrapping Techniques for Roller Bandages

Description, Purpose, and Illustration

Circular turn: Hold the free end of the bandage with one hand and return to the exact point of starting without pulling so tightly as to create a tourniquet effect.

Purpose: To anchor and secure a bandage when it is started and ended.

Illustration:

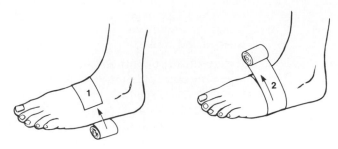

Figure 20-31 A circular turn is wrapped firmly but not tightly around the end of the foot. Note that bandaging is started at the side of the foot so that the end will not cause pressure over a bony area on the upper foot or create discomfort on the bottom of the foot when the patient walks.

Spiral turn: Partly overlap the previous turn. The overlapping varies from one half to three fourths of the width of the bandage, depending on the purpose of the bandage.

Purpose: To wrap a part that is cylindrical in shape, such as the fingers, arms, legs, chest, and abdomen.

Illustration:

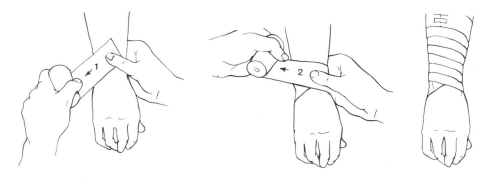

Figure 20-32 A roller bandage is applied using a spiral turn. Note that instead of an initial circular turn, the bandage was started obliquely to anchor it around the wrist.

Spiral-reverse turn: This is wrapped similarly to a spiral, the difference being that each layer is reversed halfway through the turn.

Purpose: To bandage a cone-shaped body part, such as the thigh or leg.

Illustration:

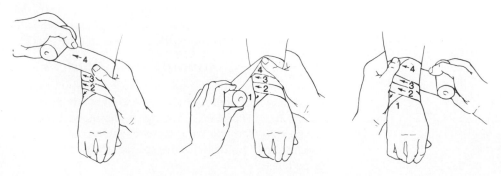

Figure 20-33 This is the procedure for making the spiral reverse turn with a roller bandage.

(continued)

Table 20-6. Continued

Description, Purpose, and Illustration

Figure-of-eight turn: This turn consists of oblique overlapping turns that alternately ascend and descend. Each turn crosses the one preceding it so that it resembles the number 8.

Purpose: To bandage around joints such as the knee, elbow, ankle, and wrist. This turn provides for a snug bandage, which in some cases is useful for immobilization.

Illustration:

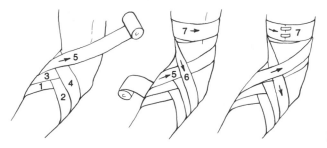

Figure 20-34 This illustrates the figure-of-eight turn.

Spica turn: The spica turn is an adaptation of the figure-of-eight wrap. The wrap consists of ascending and descending turns with each overlapping and crossing the other to form a sharp angle.

Purpose: To bandage the thumb, breast, shoulder, groin, or hip.

Illustration:

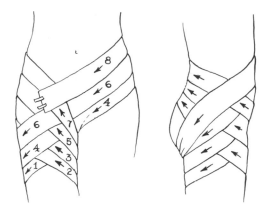

Figure 20-35 The numbers and arrows indicate the technique for wrapping a roller bandage in a spica.

Recurrent turn: In the recurrent turn, the roll is passed back and forth over the tip of the body part from one side to the other after the free end has been anchored. It is important to be sure that the tension on each turn is equal. Uneven overlapping of turns should be avoided. All skin should be covered to prevent swelling of exposed tissue. To hold the recurrent turns in place, the bandaging may be completed by using a figure-of-eight turn.

(continued)

Table 20-6. Continued

Description, Purpose, and Illustration

Purpose: To bandage rounded surfaces, such as the head or the stump of an amputated limb.

Illustration:

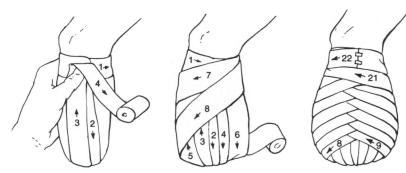

Figure 20-36 This illustrates the sequence for wrapping a roller bandage around a stump. A circular turn is followed by several recurrent turns. A circular turn should not be used to anchor a bandage on a stump if circulation will be compromised. The patient or an assistant can hold the recurrent turns securely. The bandaging can then be completed, using a figure-of-eight technique covering the length of the stump and the previous recurrent turns.

angles to a belt. A double T-binder has two tails attached to a belt. The single T-binder is used for females and the double T-binder for males. The belt is placed around the waist and secured with safety pins. The single or double tails are passed between the legs and pinned to the belt. T-binders are illustrated in Figure 20-37.

Using a Four-Tailed Binder. A *four-tailed binder* consists of a rectangular piece of material that has four tails, two on each side. An illustration of this type of binder can be seen in Figure 20-38. The rectangular area is placed into the hollow area beneath the lower lip. The first of two tails is tied in the back of the head. Care should be taken that the knot is positioned somewhat to the side so that it does not put pressure on the bones of the spine. The remaining tails are drawn up to the top of the head and secured with a knot.

Using a Scultetus Binder. A *scultetus binder* is the name given to a binder with many tails. Each tail is about 5 cm (2 in) wide, attached to the sides of a rectangular piece of flannel or muslin. Among other purposes, it may be used to support the wound of an obese patient to prevent dehiscence. When a scultetus binder is applied to the abdomen, the patient lies on his back and on the center of the binder. The nurse should be sure the binder is free of

wrinkles. The lower end of the binder is placed well down on the hips but not so low that it will interfere with the use of a bedpan or walking. The tails are brought out to either side to wrap around the lower part of the abdomen. A tail from each side is brought up and placed obliquely over the abdomen until all tails are in place. The last tails are fastened with safety pins. Figure 20-39 illustrates the application of a scultetus binder to the abdomen.

Using a Straight Binder. A *straight binder* is a rectangular piece of material, usually about 15 to 20 cm (6 to 8 in) wide and long enough to more than circle the body. This straight piece of fabric can be applied to the abdomen or chest. Sometimes a binder is applied to the breasts of a newly delivered mother to suppress the formation of milk. A breast binder is often equipped with shoulder straps so that it will not slip down on the trunk. When straight binders are used, they must be adjusted to fit the contours of the body. This is usually done by making small tucks in the binder. The tucks can be secured with safety pins.

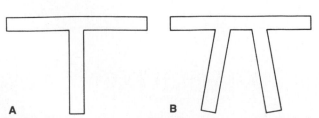

Figure 20-37 (*A*). A single T-binder. (*B*). A double T-binder.

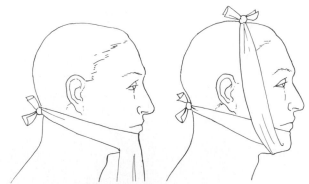

Figure 20-38 A four-tailed binder.

Skill Procedure 20-8. Applying Bandages and Binders

Suggested Action	Reason for Action
Observe principles of medical asepsis when applying bandages and binders.	Bandages and binders should be clean and dry. Handwashing controls the transfer of organisms.
Select a bandage or binder material according to the effect desired.	Some bandages or binders are meant only to hold a dressing in place, while others are intended to exert pressure, immobilize, and so on.
Avoid an unnecessarily thick or extensive bandage.	Heavy and extensive bandaging makes the area uncomfortably warm and cumbersome for the patient.
Choose the size of bandage or binder appropriate for covering the body part.	Covering the chest or thigh will require larger sized materials than that for a forearm or finger.
Support the part to be bandaged in normal anatomic alignment. Joints should be slightly flexed rather than extended or hyperextended.	Improper alignment contributes to healing in a position of deformity.
Use absorbent material to separate any two skin surfaces that touch one another, such as between fingers and toes, in the axillary area, under the breasts, in the folds of the groin or abdomen.	Padding absorbs moisture and reduces skin irritation or breakdown. It also promotes separate healing for surfaces that may each contain an open wound.
Pad bony prominences over which bandages and binders are placed. Hollows in the body contour may be filled with padding.	Padding cushions and distributes pressure equally over all skin surfaces. It promotes comfort and prevents skin breakdown.
Determine the appropriate technique for encircling a body part if a rolled bandage is being used.	Various turning techniques are used depending on the body part that is bandaged.
Begin at the lowest point of the body part and bandage in a direction toward the heart. The heel should not be left exposed when the foot or leg is bandaged.	Bandaging toward the heart helps prevent venous congestion and interference with circulation. Swelling is likely to be accentuated in the unbandaged area due to uneven compression on tissue and blood vessels.
Leave a small portion of an extremity, such as the fingertips or toes, exposed.	Exposing fingertips and toes on a bandaged extremity helps a nurse observe for signs of swelling and changes in circulation.
Apply a bandage or binder with sufficient pressure, using neither too little nor too much. Avoid applying a binder on the chest too snugly.	Sufficient pressure provides for adequate support and immobilization, and ensures that the bandage will stay in place. Too much pressure may interfere with circulation or respiration, and cause discomfort.
Unwind a roller bandage gradually and only as it is required.	This provides better control of the roll to keep equal tension throughout the area being covered.
Apply a bandage over a wet dressing or draining wound less tightly than usual.	If a wet dressing, saturated with secretions, dries, it is likely to shrink, causing more pressure than when it was originally applied.
Test the circulation in a bandaged extremity by applying pressure on the nailbeds. Compare with an unbandaged extremity if possible.	In normal circumstances, the area will blanch first and then return to its original color quickly when pressure on the nailbed is released. If the bandage is too tight, the blood may be trapped or it may not be able to leave and return very quickly.
Report any of the following signs promptly: coldness, numbness of the part, swelling, bluish or very red coloring, throbbing, tingling, or pain.	Prolonged poor circulation to an area can result in death of cells or slowed healing. Corrective action should be taken if signs of impaired circulation are present.
Place pins and clips used to secure the bandage or binder well away from a wound or tender and inflamed area. Also, place them so that they do not cause unnecessary pressure on a part of the body.	Pressure from pins and clips is uncomfortable, may interfere with circulation, and may cause injury to skin and nerve tissues.

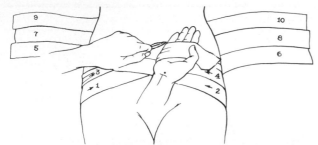

Figure 20-39 This illustrates the procedure for applying a scultetus binder.

Understanding the Use of Heat and Cold

Before applying heat or cold to the body, the nurse will wish to be familiar with certain facts to give safe care.

The Immediate Effect of Cold Applications. The immediate effect of cold applications is that blood vessels in the area constrict; that is, they become smaller. The opposite occurs when heat is applied. The reverse effect occurs with prolonged use of heat or cold. For example, eventual blood vessel constriction will occur with prolonged use of heat. Therefore, applications should not be left in place for long periods of time. The recommended durations for various heat and cold applications are provided when they are described later in this chapter.

Nerve Receptors for Heat and Cold in the Skin Adapt to Temperature. An important characteristic of heat and cold receptors is that they adjust readily if the stimulus is not extreme. For example, if the arm is placed in warm water, the sensation of warmth soon diminishes because of the adaptability of the heat receptors. The same phenomenon occurs if cool water is used. This is important to remember. Once the receptors adapt, the patient may become unaware of temperature extremes until tissue damage occurs. The patient usually is not familiar with this adaptability process and may request that the heat or cold be increased beyond the point of safety.

The Temperatures That the Skin Can Tolerate Vary Among Persons and on Different Parts of the Body. Some can tolerate very warm and cold applications more safely than others; young children, elderly, diabetic patients, and individuals with circulatory diseases have a low safety margin. Certain areas of the skin are also more tolerant of temperature than are others. Those parts of the body where the skin is thinner, for example the inner forearm, chest, and abdomen generally are more sensitive to temperature than exposed areas where the skin is often thicker. Therefore, it is important to apply warm and cold applications well within the generally known safe limits of temperature. In addition, the skin should be observed so that persons who are more sensitive to temperature will

not suffer tissue damage, even though applications have been applied within recommended temperature ranges.

Heat and Cold Are Transferred Directly From One Substance to Another by Conduction. A poor conductor is called an *insulator.* Water is a relatively good conductor of heat while air is a poorer conductor. Therefore, the skin will tolerate greater extremes of temperature if the heat or cold is dry rather than moist. For example, a moist hot compress should be applied at a lower temperature than a cloth-covered hot water bottle to prevent burning the skin. The air between the bag and the dry cloth that covers the hot water bottle acts as an insulator.

The Body Tolerates Greater Extremes in Temperature When the Duration of Exposure Is Short. When duration is lengthy, the temperature range that the body can tolerate safely is narrower. The area involved is also important. In general, the larger the area to which heat or cold is applied, the less tolerant is the skin to the extreme in temperature.

The Condition of the Patient Is an Important Factor to Consider When Heat and Cold Are Being Applied to the Body. Special care is indicated for patients who are debilitated or unconscious. Patients who have disturbances in circulation are more sensitive to injury from heat and cold. Broken skin areas are also more subject to tissue damage and less tolerant of heat and cold.

Common Uses of Cold Applications

Use good judgment when deciding to use hot or cold applications. Generally, using a cold application immediately following an injury is best to control swelling and pain. Later, the use of heat promotes comfort and improved circulation, which speeds healing.

Cold is most commonly used for the following clinical reasons:

- To limit the accumulation of fluid in body tissues (edema). If edema is already present, the application of cold acts to retard its relief because circulating blood in the area is at a minimum and excess fluid will not be reabsorbed efficiently.
- To control bleeding by constricting blood vessels.
- To relieve pain, such as at the site of a sprain.
- To produce an anesthetic effect. Cold may be used for this purpose for certain surgical procedures and for the relief of discomfort at the site of an injection.
- To reduce body temperature and the body's metabolic rate.

Common Uses of Heat Applications

Heat is most commonly used for the following clinical reasons:

- To promote circulation to an injured area and thereby hasten healing.

- To aid in removing debris from an infected or dirty wound.
- To relieve muscle spasms.
- To relieve pain by promoting muscle relaxation. Some individuals have learned that they have good relief from pain when they use warm applications. Others use cold applications. Still others may find that alternating between hot and cold applications works best for them. The reason for the difference is not clearly understood.
- To help overcome feelings of chilliness.
- To help raise body temperature when applied over a large area of the body.

Ensuring Safe Temperatures for Applications of Hot and Cold

No one optimum temperature can be stated for hot or cold applications. The selection of temperature depends on factors such as the duration of the application, the method of the application, the condition of the patient, and the condition and sensitivity of the skin. For short periods of time and for small areas, the maximum safe limits for hot or cold temperatures can be tolerated without discomfort or tissue damage. For longer periods, it is considered dangerous to expose skin to extreme temperatures except in rare life-threatening situations. These situations require constant monitoring. Table 20-7 provides the temperature ranges for various levels of hot or cold water.

Other special considerations should guide the safe temperature for applications of heat or cold. Very hot and cold temperatures should be avoided in an area of skin disease. They should also be avoided when patients have circulatory or heart disorders because of the danger of causing damage to tissues already in a state of distress.

Selecting a Method for Applying Cold

There are several ways that cold temperatures can be applied to the skin. Some of the more common methods are discussed below.

Using an Ice Bag. Rubber or plastic ice bags are frequently used for applying cold to an area. Ice collars are smaller than most ice bags and are used for the neck and other small areas.

An ice bag should be prepared as follows:

Fill an ice bag one-half to two-thirds full with ice chips or small cubes. This makes it easy to mold the bag to fit body contours. Also, small pieces of ice reduce the amount of air, which acts as an insulator in the bag.

Pour water over the cubes or chips to eliminate sharp edges and then remove the water from the bag.

Twist the top of the bag and cap it. This technique removes excess air from the bag.

Table 20-7. Temperature Ranges for Applications of Heat and Cold

Level of Heat	Temperature Range
Very hot	40.5°C to 46.1°C (105°F to 115°F)
Hot	36.6°C to 40.5°C (98°F to 105°F)
Warm and neutral	33.8°C to 36.6°C (93°F to 98°F)
Level of Cold	**Temperature Range**
Tepid	26.6°C to 33.8°C (80°F to 93°F)
Cool	18.3°C to 26.6°C (65°F to 80°F)
Cold	10°C to 18.3°C (50°F to 65°F)
Very cold	Below 10°C (Below 50°F)

Check for leaks in the bag and at the cap to prevent the patient from becoming wet should there be a flaw in the bag.

Cover the ice bag and place it on the patient. The cover provides for comfort for the patient and absorbs moisture that condenses on the outside of the bag. Many bags are made with a soft outer covering, making another covering unnecessary.

Allow the ice bag to remain in place no more than one-half to one hour and then remove it for approximately one hour. In this way, the tissues are able to react to the desired immediate effects of the cold. Signs of excessive cold include mottled skin and numbness in the area being treated.

Try using a rubber or plastic glove when a small area is involved. The ice is placed in the glove, excess air is removed, and the glove is tied shut securely. This type of ice bag has been found useful for patients who have had mouth or dental surgery.

Wrap an ice cube in gauze with one side of the cube exposed to massage an area. Use a small circular motion when massaging. This technique is useful for applying cold to a small area for a short period of time when an ice bag is unsuitable for a small area.

Place ice chips in a zip-lock plastic bag when a plastic bag is not available.

Commercially prepared cold packs are available. They retain a constant degree of cold for several hours. Figure 20-40 illustrates and describes one pack that can be used for either cold or hot applications.

Using Cold Compresses. *Compresses* are local applications of moisture. They may be either hot or cold depending on their desired purpose. They are applied similarly with the exception of the temperature of the solution. Skill Procedure 20-9 describes the suggested actions for applying compresses.

Providing a Cool Water or Alcohol Bath

There are times when a cool bath is recommended for reducing a patient's elevated temperature. Usually cool water is used, but 70% alcohol may be added to tepid water in severe circumstances. The alcohol should be diluted in twice its volume of water. The patient and the nurse may experience discomfort from the fumes if the bathing occurs in a small area. Tepid sponging, discussed in Chapter 7, should be used for children; using alcohol is not recommended.

Alcohol and cool water reduce body temperature through evaporation. The heat from the body is conducted to the moisture, which is then vaporized into the atmosphere. Alcohol evaporates at a lower temperature than does water. Therefore, when alcohol is added, it increases the speed of evaporation.

The recommended procedure for giving a cool water or alcohol bath is as follows:

Prepare plain water initially at a temperature of about 85°F (29.4°C). As the patient adjusts to this temperature, it can be lowered even further to about 65°F (18.3°C) by gradually adding ice chips to the water. The temperature for a mixture of alcohol and water should be between 85°F to 90°F (29.4°C–32.2°C). Alcohol and water do not require ice or further cooling of the solution.

Protect the patient's bed with waterproof material because the patient will be sponged while in bed.

Have the room comfortably warm so that the patient does not chill. Shivering tends to increase body temperature through the contraction of muscles in the skin. This defeats the purpose of the bath.

Prepare several ice bags and one hot water bottle. One ice bag is placed on the patient's head. Others are placed in the groin and axillary areas where blood vessels are close to the skin surface. The ice bags help to cool the patient further. The hot water bottle is placed at the patient's feet for comfort and to help prevent the patient from shivering.

Drape the patient properly to prevent shivering as various parts of the body are exposed for bathing.

Sponge the face and forehead, the neck, arms, and legs for 3 to 5 minutes, and the back for 10 minutes. Usually, the anterior of the chest and the abdomen are not sponged. Cover but do not dry each part as it is sponged. Move on from one part of the body to another and continue bathing for 25 to 30 minutes. If the bath is short in duration, the body does not adjust to the coolness; it then reacts to conserve heat, and the patient's temperature may go higher.

Check the patient's color and pulse during the bath. Discontinue bathing if the patient is reacting unfavorably.

Pat the patient dry after the bath is completed. The friction of rubbing him dry may increase body temperature.

Check the patient's body temperature about one-half hour after the bath to evaluate the effectiveness of the cool bath.

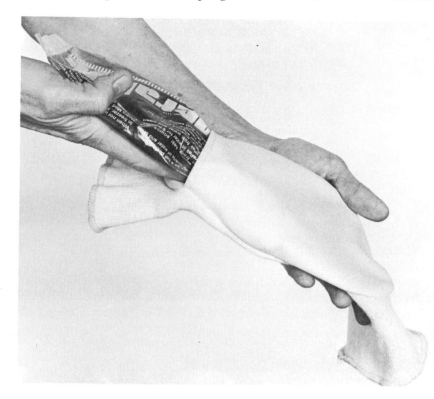

Figure 20-40 A hot and cold gel pack, which is prefilled and reusable, is being inserted into the pocket on a band. A gel pack can be stored in a freezer without the sleeve for cold applications. The gel remains malleable even when its temperature is below freezing. It can be dropped in hot water or heated in a microwave for hot applications. (Courtesy of Hydro-Med Products, Inc., Dallas, TX.)

Skill Procedure 20-9. Applying a Compress

Suggested Action	Reason for Action
Assemble equipment following appropriate principles of medical or surgical asepsis.	Medical asepsis is used most often, but sterile technique is practiced when there is an open wound.
Place an appropriate amount of solution over absorbent material, such as gauze or even a clean washcloth.	The texture and the thickness of the material used depend on the area to which the compress is applied.
Warm or cool the solution to the desired temperature within those considered in a safe range to achieve the desired purpose of the application.	Consider the duration of the application, the condition of the patient, the condition and sensitivity of the skin, and the area to be covered.
Explain and plan the procedure with the patient.	A patient can cooperate and feel more in control of his care when he can understand and is permitted to participate.
Place the patient in a position of comfort.	An uncomfortable position can lead to muscle strain if maintained for the duration of the compress.
Protect the bed linen with absorbent material.	Covering the linen and ensuring absorption will reduce the need to change all the bed linen.
Wring the compress material of excess liquid. Sterile forceps or gloves may be used for sterile compresses.	The compress should be moist but not dripping. Cold or hot saturated compresses can injure tissue, since water is a relatively good conductor.
Shake the compress once or twice quickly.	Incorporating air into the layers of compress material acts to trap air, keeping the compress at a rather constant temperature.
Allow some of the liquid to drop onto thinner skin near the area of the intended compress.	Thinner skin is generally more sensitive than other areas. If the temperature feels comfortable in this area, it will be easily tolerated in other areas.
Place the compress gently on the affected area.	Pressure or rapid change in surface temperature may cause discomfort.
Lift the compress after a few seconds to inspect the patient's skin.	Assessing the effect of the compress on the skin helps prevent subsequent injury.
Place a dry covering over the moist compress and enclose both in waterproof material. Some nurses prefer placing the dry cover on the outside and the waterproof material next to the wet compress.	The dry covering and waterproof cover will act as insulators and prevent rapid temperature change and moisture loss from the compress.
Mold and secure the coverings to fit the contours of the body surface.	Air is a poor conductor of heat or cold. When openings allow air movement, rapid changes in the original temperature decrease the effectiveness of the compress.
Remoisten the compress material frequently enough to maintain the temperature. Usually the patient can indicate when this should be done.	The temperature should be maintained within a fairly constant range within the duration of the compress.
Use warming or cooling devices, such as an ice bag or hot water bottle, over the compress material, if available.	Heat or cold may be conducted from one source to another and promote a constant temperature.
Continue applying the compress for approximately 15 to 20 minutes four or five times a day.	Prolonged applications of hot or cold may cause the reverse effect to tissue.
Provide comfort measures during and following treatment.	The patient may need to be warmed or cooled due to the effect of the compress, drafts, and exposure of the compress area.

(continued)

Skill Procedure 20-9. Continued

Suggested Action	Reason for Action
Remove the compress and dispose of the wet material according to agency policy. If compress material contains body secretions, bag them in a waterproof container and dispose of them properly.	Unsoiled wet compress material can be placed in a lined receptacle. Soiled compresses must be wrapped separately in a waterproof container for burning to avoid spreading organisms.
Dry the patient as necessary after completing the procedure.	Restoring the comfort of the patient is a considerate act.
Assess the effect of the compress on the skin as well as the patient's evaluation.	Changes in the plan of care are based on the responses of the patient to treatment measures.
Chart significant observations and any other pertinent information according to agency policy.	The patient's chart is a written record of the patient's care and progress.

Occasionally, a patient may be immersed in a tub of cold water to which a large volume of ice cubes has been added. This type of cold application, though primitive, could be used in the absence of any other sophisticated equipment. Its use would be reserved for treating severe heat stroke or other cases of life-threatening hyperthermia.

Using a Hypothermic Blanket. A low body temperature is referred to as *hypothermia*. Blankets and pads through which a thermostatically controlled solution is circulated are also used in many health agencies to produce hypothermia. Some are disposable and used for one patient only. The blanket is connected to an adapter for circulating cool solution. The patient should be covered with a bath blanket and one should be placed underneath his body above the cooling device. Some machines have been coated with a soft fabric on the cooling surface. The manufacturer's instructions and agency procedures should be observed because each type of equipment operates slightly differently.

It is important that the patient's temperature be checked frequently. Some machines constantly register the body temperature through a probe inserted within the rectum. The cooling device is removed when the patient's temperature is a couple degrees *above* the desired level. The body temperature will "drift," that is, it will continue to cool a bit more after the blanket is removed. Ice packs placed in the axillary areas and groin may be used simultaneously. Medication may also be ordered to depress the heat regulating center in the brain, thereby helping to lower body temperature.

Selecting a Method for Applying Heat

Various methods may be used for applying heat. The applications of heat must be treated just as cautiously as the applications of cold. When heat is applied, the patient will require monitoring. If a large area of the body is involved with the application of heat, it is best to determine the patient's temperature before and after the heat is removed

to determine any influence on body temperature. If the condition of the patient is poor or if he appears to be reacting unfavorably, monitoring all the vital signs is recommended.

Using Electrical Heating Pads. The electric heating pad is a popular means for applying dry heat. It is easy to use, provides constant and even heat, and is relatively safe when used on low settings. Careless handling may result in injury to the patient or the nurse as well as damage to the pad.

Because of possible injury, many health agencies have a policy that prohibits the use of heating pads. If the patient insists on using a heating pad, the health agency may require him to sign a release to free the hospital of responsibility.

Because heating pads are commonly used in the home and in some agencies, the nurse should be familiar with their proper use. The heating element of an electric pad consists of a web of wires that converts electric current into heat. Crushing or creasing the wires may impair proper functioning, and portions of the pad will overheat. Burns or a fire may result. Pins should be avoided for securing the pad because there is danger of electric shock if a pin touches the wires. Pads with waterproof coverings are preferred, but they should not be operated in a wet or moist condition because of the danger of short circuiting the heating element and consequently causing electric shock.

Heating pads for home use have a selector switch for controlling the heat. After the heat has been applied and a certain amount of adaptation of nerve endings in the skin has taken place, the patient often increases the heat. Many persons have been burned in this manner. Health agencies that use heating pads usually have preset pads, which cannot be reset to temperatures that may burn the patient.

Heating pads should be covered with flannel or similar material. This helps make the heat more comfortable for the patient and protects the skin. However, it is important not to cover the pad too heavily because heavy covering over an electric pad prevents adequate heat dissipation. The patient should not lie on a heating pad because heat will accumulate and may cause burns.

Applying a Hot Water Bottle. A hot water bottle is actually a flexible bag made of rubberlike material designed to hold water. Hot water bottles are commonly used to apply dry heat. Many health agencies do not allow the use of hot water bottles. Too often, they have been used carelessly and patients have been burned. However, they are commonly found in the home and the nurse should be familiar with their proper use.

The following are recommended techniques for the use of hot water bottles:

Prepare water that has been accurately checked with a thermometer. A safe temperature range for infants under 2 years of age, the elderly, the diabetic, and the unconscious patient is from 40.5°C to 43.3°C (105°F to 110°F). For older children and adults, the range is from 46.1°C to 51.6°C (115°F to 125°F). It is unsafe to fill a hot water bottle with water that has not been checked with a thermometer.

Fill the bag about two-thirds full to keep the bag easy to mold and as light in weight as possible.

Place the bag on a flat surface, allow water to come to the opening, and then cap the bag, or twist the unfilled portion of the bag and then cap it. These techniques expel excess air, which acts as a poor conductor of heat.

Check for leaks in the bag and at the cap.

Place a flannel cover on the bag and put the bag on the patient. The cover provides comfort and helps prevent burns because the cloth acts as an insulator. Many bags are made with a soft outer covering, making a second cover unnecessary.

Alternately remove and replace hot water bottles every hour or two to gain the most effectiveness from the heat, unless continuous heat is ordered. In the latter case, change the water in the bag at regular intervals to keep it as near to the optimum temperature as possible.

Teach the patient about the temperature of water in the bag. Many patients seem to think that the water is not hot enough. Unless the patient receives a proper warning, it is likely that the patient or a willing visitor may fill the bottle with extremely hot water from the tap.

Using a Hyperthermia Pad. *Hyperthermia* refers to a high body temperature. Commercial pads and blankets like those discussed for hypothermia can be used to raise body temperature. One type of pad is a K-Matic® pad, or K-Pad, which is used in some health agencies in place of hot water bottles. The pad has a tubular construction that is filled with water and then heated electrically. A thermostat on the pad automatically keeps the temperature of the water in the pad at a constant and correct temperature. The pad is filled about two thirds, excess air is removed, and the pad is then covered to help prevent burns before applying it to a patient. Figure 20-41 illustrates a K-Pad.

Giving a Sitz Bath. Patients are often seated in tubs filled with sufficient water to cover the hips as a means of applying tepid or hot water to the pelvic area. These baths are referred to as *sitz baths*. The legs and feet remain out of water. Special tubs and chairs are available that are designed so that the patient's buttocks fit into a rather deep seat, which is filled with water of the desired temperature. The reusable type requires careful cleaning and disinfection between uses. A disposable type is also available and is especially helpful in preventing cross-infections. A regular bathtub may be used but is not as satisfactory because the heat is also applied to the legs. This alters the effect desired in the pelvic region.

The following are recommended techniques to observe when giving a sitz bath:

Prepare water for a sitz bath at 43.3°C (110°F) if the purpose is to apply heat to the area. Use water of about 33.8°C to 38.8°C (98°F to 102°F) if the purpose is to produce relaxation or to promote healing in a wound by cleansing it of discharge and dead tissues.

Place the patient in the tub and cover his back, shoulders, and lower legs with a cotton blanket. This prevents the patient from feeling chilly during the procedure.

Be sure the patient's legs, which are placed over the edge of a sitz tub, are comfortable. The short patient may need a towel placed over the edge of the tub and his feet placed on a stool so there is no excess pressure in the area behind the knees.

Place cold compresses or an ice bag on the patient's head if he desires this for general comfort.

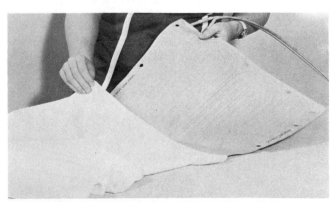

Figure 20-41 K-Pads, which come in various sizes, are used for heat application.

Place a towel in the patient's lumbar region if the tub feels uncomfortable against the patient's back. Twenty to thirty minutes may feel like a very long time if one's body is not comfortable or in good alignment.

Allow the patient to remain in the tub for 20 to 30 minutes to receive maximum benefit from the bath.

Check the temperature of the water during a sitz bath several times so that it is as constant as possible. While adding hot water to the tub, be sure to agitate it in order not to burn the patient.

Assess the patient's pulse rate and look for signs or symptoms of weakness. The movement of large quantities of blood to the pelvic region may cause the patient to faint. Do not leave the patient alone unless you are absolutely *sure* it is safe to do so and then be certain a call bell is within easy reach for the patient.

Cover the patient well and encourage him to stay out of drafts after the bath so that he does not become chilled.

Encourage the patient to rest for a short time after the bath until normal circulation returns. This will help him avoid feelings of faintness.

Preparing Soaks. Placing part of the body in water or a medicated solution is referred to as a *soak*. If a soak is prescribed for a large wound, such as one that covers an entire arm or lower leg or even an area of the torso, a compromise with sterile technique may be necessary. The vessel into which the body area is placed is sterilized before use if possible. If this is not possible, the vessel should be scrupulously cleaned. A Styrofoam chest serves as a good vessel at home and helps keep the solution at the ordered temperature. Tap water may be used for soaks because it is generally accepted as free from pathogens.

During the treatment, which is usually 15 to 20 minutes per soak, the temperature should be kept as constant as possible. This may be done by discarding some of the fluid every 5 minutes or so and replacing it with solution at a higher temperature. However, care must be taken to avoid burning the patient. When hot solution is added, the nurse quickly stirs or otherwise mixes it into the cooler solution to prevent discomfort or tissue damage.

The recommended procedure for a soak is as follows:

Prepare the water or ordered solution at a temperature of 40.5°C to 43.3°C (105°F to 110°F) unless ordered otherwise. This temperature provides heat sufficient for therapeutic purposes. Place the water or solution in an appropriate vessel.

Place the part to be soaked in a comfortable position and in good body alignment in the vessel. For example, an arm basin placed on top of the bedside stand may cause the patient's shoulder to be out of alignment. It may also cause pressure on the back of the patient's

arm. Also, a hand basin may be situated to cause wrist fatigue if care is not taken.

Look for pressure areas after the part is in the soak and offer additional support with towels or pads to prevent tissue injury.

Continue the soak for the prescribed time, usually 15 to 20 minutes.

Check the temperature of the water regularly so that the temperature is kept as constant as possible. Remove some of the cool water and add hot water as necessary. Agitate the hot water as more is added so that the patient will not be burned.

Remove the part after the soak is completed, dry it well, and cover it in the manner ordered.

Applying Hot Moist Packs. The application of several layers of hot moist cloths to a relatively large body area is referred to as a pack. Packs differ from soaks primarily in two ways: the duration of the application is usually longer than that of soaks, and the initial application of heat is generally more intense. Packs are usually applied at temperatures as hot as the patient can tolerate them. Because of their potential to injure the patient, a pack should never be used on an unresponsive patient or one who cannot perceive heat when applied to the skin. The nurse is responsible to assess frequently and remove the pack if there is any likelihood that it is producing thermal injury.

A commercially available hot pack is shown in Figure 20-42. This type is submerged in boiling water. It is then enclosed within the core of several turkish towels that are

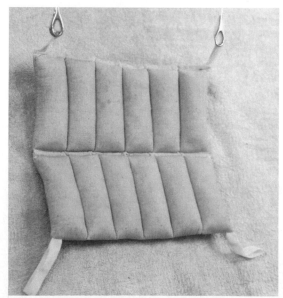

Figure 20-42 Tissue forceps are used to lift this commercial hot pack onto towels. It will subsequently be wrapped over and over again within the towels so there are multiple layers between the hot core and the patient's skin.

overlapped around it. The steam penetrates the towels. The pack is applied to the affected part. Many individuals with low-back pain or other conditions causing muscle pain purchase these types of packs for self-use. The manufacturer recommends that this type of pack be stored in a sealable plastic bag before it dries out. If not being used for long periods of time the sealed pack can be stored in the freezer compartment of a refrigerator.

Using Other Miscellaneous Methods of Applying Heat.

A cradle with an electric light bulb enclosed in a metal frame is sometimes used to apply dry heat to extremities. It is a good way, for example, to help circulation in an extremity, to provide general warmth for the patient, and to help dry a cast. The bulb should be 25 watts and placed no closer to the patient than 45 to 60 cm (18 to 24 in).

Heat lamps with bulbs no more powerful than 60 watts can be used to apply dry heat. They should be placed no closer than 45 to 60 cm (18 to 24 in) from the patient and for no longer than 15 to 20 minutes at a time. However, the patient should be checked every 5 minutes. The desired effect from a heat lamp is to have the skin become warm and pink. Redness and discomfort are signs that the patient is receiving a burn.

Ultraviolet and infrared lamps can also be used to apply dry heat. Diathermy, which produces heat in tissues by the use of high-frequency currents, may be used. Generally, trained workers are responsible for using diathermy, ultraviolet, and infrared lamps, but the nurse will wish to observe the patient's reactions to these types of heat applications.

Applicable Nursing Diagnoses

Patients who have problems with tissue healing are likely to have nursing diagnoses from the following list:
- Impaired Skin Integrity
- Impaired Tissue Integrity
- Altered Tissue Perfusion
- High Risk for Infection
- High Risk for Injury
- Impaired Physical Mobility
- Pain

Nursing Care Plan 20-1 was developed for a patient diagnosed with Impaired Tissue Integrity. NANDA defines this diagnostic category in its 1989 taxonomy as, "A state in which an individual experiences damage to mucous membrane, corneal, integumentary, or subcutaneous tissue."

Suggested Measures to Promote Tissue Healing in Selected Situations

When the Patient Is an Infant or Child

Plan to promote general well-being when a child sustains trauma, especially if it involves a large area. Infants and children do not tolerate injury as well as adults. Be sure the patient receives proper nourishment, sufficient fluid intake, rest and sleep, and emotional support to promote healing.

Take into account that infants and children do not tolerate applications of heat and cold as well as adults do. Be *sure* that the temperatures of applications are within normal safe ranges. Check the child skin and general physical reaction to heat and cold applications frequently. Heating pads are not recommended for infants and children because of the danger of burning. Hot water bottles and ice bags should never be placed directly on the skin without proper protection of the bag and skin.

To hold an ice collar in place on a child, put the collar in a piece of stockinet.

In an emergency, recommend that a parent use a bag of frozen vegetables, such as peas or corn, as a method of applying cold. It molds easily to body contours and will not drip as much as melting ice cubes when becoming warm.

Be sure to assess a child frequently while giving a cool bath. Note signs of chilliness, poor skin color, and changes in the pulse rate. Discontinue the procedure if unfavorable reactions occur.

When the Patient Is Unconscious

Be especially careful when applying hot and cold application to an unconscious patient. His circulation is usually poor and he is unable to report symptoms of discomfort and tissue injury. Hot water bottles and heating pads should *never* be placed directly on the patient's skin without adequate coverings. Many authorities recommend not using heating pads or hot water bottles for unconscious patients because of the danger of burning.

When the Patient Is Elderly

Plan to give the best possible nursing care to promote general well-being when tissue trauma is present. Elderly persons do not tolerate injury or heal as well as younger adults. Physical reserves wane with the years. Be sure the patient receives proper nourishment, sufficient fluid intake, rest and sleep, and emotional support to promote healing.

NURSING CARE PLAN

20-1. Impaired Tissue Integrity

Assessment

Subjective Data
States, "I have no feeling below my upper back and chest."

Objective Data
18-year-old man with spinal cord injury at the C-7 (7th cervical vertebrae) level two years ago following an auto accident in which he was not wearing a seat belt and was thrown from the car. Admitted for treatment of a pressure sore over the coccyx that has not responded to home treatment. The skin over the coccyx is open and measures 2 in × 3 in × ½ in. Approximately 2 in of intact skin around the sore remain red and warm even after pressure is relieved. Tissue within the ulcer is gray with a yellow base. Elbows and heels are reddened but skin is intact. Wears an external catheter. Bowel elimination is regulated with the use of a suppository q̄ 2 days.

Diagnosis

Impaired Tissue Integrity: Stage III pressure sore over coccyx and Stage I over bilateral heels and elbows related to unrelieved pressure secondary to immobility.

Plan

Goal
The coccygeal pressure sore will develop a ⅛ in margin of granulation tissue around the circumference of the wound by 8/30. The elbows and heels will blanch with pressure relief by 8/18.

Orders: 8/15
1. Reposition q̄ 2 hours until an air-fluidized bed can be obtained.
2. Avoid the supine and Fowler's position as much as possible.
3. After bathing spray heels and elbows with Bard Barrier Film®.
4. Until results of wound culture are obtained, care for the open wound as follows:
   • Mix Shur Clens® with water and cleanse wound
   • Rinse with normal saline
   • Pack the wound loosely with a continuous strip of gauze moistened with normal saline
   • Cover with an ABD pad
   • Repeat above routine q̄ 4 h as the packing becomes dry.
5. If wound culture is negative for pathogens:
   • Eliminate wet to dry dressing
   • Clean, dry, and cover wound with Op-Site® and leave in place for 5 days.
   • If drainage collects, pierce Op-Site® and aspirate fluid from underneath. Seal opened area with a small reinforcement of Op-Site® over punctured area.
6. Measure open pressure sore q̄ 3 days (8/18, 8/21, etc.) during day shift.   R. ROSEN, RN

Implementation (Documentation)
8/16

1700	Turned q̄ 2 h alternating side to side using a 30° lateral position with slight elevation of the upper body. ———————————————————— A. FOX, LPN	
1900	Transferred from hospital bed to Clinitron® Bed. Explained principle for use and discontinuation of turning schedule. ———————————————— A. FOX, LPN	
2000	Dressing and packing removed. Wound cleansed with Shur Clens® and rinsed with saline. Repacked with saline-moistened gauze and covered with ABD secured with paper tape. ———————————————————— A. FOX, LPN	

Evaluation (Documentation)

2045   Removed packing contains white debris. Tissue within wound looks pink with slight bleeding. Wet to dry dressing drying more rapidly with Clinitron® bed therapy. Will change in 3 h and evaluate again. Evidence of skin coating on elbows and heels. These areas still appear red over bony prominences. States, "I really like this bed, I wasn't sleeping much at night with all that turning going on." Advised that fluid intake must be increased to compensate for increased evaporation from skin due to blowing air from bed. Placed on I & O. — A. FOX, LPN

As individuals age, they lose body fat underlying the skin. This, combined with a tendency to have drier skin, and inactivity predispose the elderly to decubitus ulcers.

Check bedridden elderly persons frequently for early signs of skin breakdown. They ordinarily have a decreased sense of pressure on the skin, as well as of pain, heat, and cold. Plan preventive measures described previously in this chapter for anyone at high risk for developing pressure sores.

Be especially careful to apply heat and cold applications with care to prevent tissue damage. Be sure the temperatures of heat and cold are within the normal safe range and inspect the patient's general response to therapy frequently.

Teaching Suggestions to Promote Tissue Healing

Suggestions for teaching patients who have had tissue injury are summarized below.

Patients with tissue injuries are often not hospitalized when the injury is relatively small; if hospitalized, they may be discharged before wounds are healed. Therefore, they or family members need to be taught how to care for the wound and signs indicating complications, such as profuse or foul-smelling drainage, puffiness, and tenderness in the area of the wound.

Teaching patients about the normal characteristics of the body's reaction to injury and how to care for an open wound helps them to overcome commonly held fears about the strength of wound healing and wound closure techniques.

Patients being taught how to give themselves a douche at home should be instructed to lie in a bathtub. Administering a douche while sitting on a toilet will not result in a thorough cleansing since the solution will not come in contact with all the tissue within the vagina. This occurs because there are no muscles to retain the solution; therefore, solution will flow out by gravity before reaching the upper levels of the vaginal canal.

Bibliography

Arnell I: Aggressive and successful prevention of skin breakdown. Today's OR Nurse 10(10):10–14, 37–39, 1988

Barnes SH: Patient/family education for the patient with a pressure necrosis. Nurs Clin North Am 22(2):463–474, 1987

Boykin A, Winland–Brown J: Pressure sores: Nursing management. Journal of Gerontological Nursing 12(12):17–21, 1986

Chagares R, Jackson BS: Sitting easy: How six pressure-relieving devices stack up. Am J Nurs 87(2):191–193, 1987

Conforti C: Pressure sores: Dressed for successful healing. Nursing 19(3):58–61, 1989

Cooper DM: Optimizing wound healing: A practice within nursing's domain. Nurs Clin North Am 25(1):165–180, 1990

Fowler EM: Equipment and products used in management and treatment of pressure ulcers. Nurs Clin North Am 22(2):449–461, 1987

Galub J: Wound dressing technology revives old concept: Don't expose wound to air. Nursing Homes 32(5):32–35, 1983

Gosnell DJ: Assessment and evaluation of pressure sores. Nurs Clin North Am 22(2):399–416, 1987

Hunt TK, Knighton DR, Silver IA: Regulation of wound healing angiogenesis: Effect of oxygen concentration. Surgery 90:266–270, 1981

Jeter KF, Tintle T: Principles of wound cleansing and wound care. Journal of Home Health Care Practice 1(1):43–47, 1988

Jones PL, Millman A: Wound healing and the aged patient. Nurs Clin North Am 25(1):263–278, 1990

Kundin JI: A new way to size up a wound. Am J Nurs 89(2):206–207, 1989

LaFoy J, Geden EA: Postepisiotomy pain: Warm versus cold sitz bath. Journal of Obstetrical and Gynecologic Nursing 18(5):399–403, 1989

Lindsey B: Cold and heat application in musculo-skeletal injury. Journal of Emergency Nursing 16(1):54–57, 1990

Maklebust J: Pressure ulcers: Etiology and prevention. Nurs Clin North Am 22(2):359–377, 1987

Messner R: The prevention of pressure sores. Journal of Practical Nursing 37(1):16–17, 1987

Morison MJ: Wound cleansing—which solution? Professional Nurse 4(5):220–222, 224–225, 1989

Nightingale K: Making sense of . . . wound drainage. Nursing Times 85(27):40–42, 1989

O'Hara MM: Leeching: A modern use for an ancient remedy. Am J Nurs 88(12):1656–1658, 1988

Reese JL: Nursing interventions for wound healing in plastic and reconstructive surgery. Nurs Clin North Am 25(1):223–234, 1990

Trelstad A, Osmundson D: Water Piks: Wound cleansing alternative. Plastic Surgical Nursing 9(3):117–119, 1989

Wooding–Scott M, Montgomery BA, Coleman D: No wound is too big for resourceful nurses. RN Magazine 51(12):22–25, 1988

21

Promoting Urine Elimination

Chapter Outline

Behavioral Objectives
Glossary
Introduction
Understanding Urinary Structures and Function
Factors That Influence Urinary Elimination
Assessing Urinary Function
Toileting the Patient
Managing Incontinence
Using an External Catheter
Using Intermittent Straight Catheterization
Using Urethral Catheterization
Eliminating Urine From a Surgical Opening
Obtaining Urine Specimens
Performing Common Urine Tests
Suggested Measures to Promote Urinary Elimination in
    Selected Situations
Applicable Nursing Diagnoses
Teaching Suggestions to Promote Urinary Elimination
Bibliography

Skill Procedures

Placing and Removing a Bedpan
Managing Incontinence
Applying an External Catheter
Inserting an Indwelling Catheter in the Female Patient
Inserting an Indwelling Catheter in the Male Patient
Managing an Indwelling Catheter
Irrigating an Indwelling Catheter Using an Open
    System
Using a Three-Way Catheter for Irrigation
Collecting a Clean-Catch Midstream Specimen

Behavioral Objectives

When the content of this chapter has been mastered, the learner will be able to:

Define terms appearing in the glossary.

Explain how urine is formed and eliminated.

List and discuss at least six alterations in normal patterns of urinary elimination.

Describe normal and some abnormal characteristics of urine.

Describe how to toilet a patient. Include using the bathroom, a commode, bedpan, and urinal.

List nursing measures commonly used when caring for patients with urinary incontinence and urinary retention.

List several reasons for catheterization.

Demonstrate how to catheterize female and male patients.

Outline a teaching program for helping a patient to learn intermittent self-catheterization.

Identify the potential hazards of using an external catheter and nursing measures to avoid them.

Describe at least 12 to 24 management techniques for a patient with an indwelling catheter.

List at least eight nursing measures for a patient with a urinary diversion.

Describe how to collect urine specimens using the following methods: voiding, clean-catch midstream, 24-hour collection, straight catheter, indwelling catheter, and urinary stoma.

Explain how to test a urine specimen for sugar and acetone, and explain how to determine the specific gravity of urine.

List suggested measures for promoting elimination from the urinary bladder in selected situations, as described in this chapter.

Summarize suggestions for the instruction of patients offered in this chapter.

Glossary

Albuminuria The presence of albumin in urine. Synonym for *proteinuria*.

Anuria The lack of urine production.

Appliance A collecting bag that is placed over a stoma.

Burning The feeling of warmth and local irritation when voiding.

Catheter A tube for instilling or removing fluids.

Catheterization The act of introducing a hollow tube into a body structure.

Clean-catch midstream specimen A voided urine specimen collected under conditions of thorough cleanliness after the first 30 mL of urine are voided.

Commode A chair with an opening in the seat under which a receptacle is placed to collect urine and stool.

Condom A device used by males for birth control.

Credé's maneuver The application of light pressure over the lower abdomen that aids in releasing urine.

Cutaneous triggering Stimulating skin to promote voiding.

Cystometrogram A test that measures the capacity of the bladder.

Diuresis The excessive production and excretion of urine. Synonym for *polyuria*.

Dysuria Difficulty in voiding.

External catheter A device for collecting urine that fits over the outside of the penis.

Frequency Voiding at frequent intervals.

Glycosuria The presence of sugar in urine.

Hematuria The presence of blood in urine.

Indwelling catheter A catheter placed in the bladder and secured in place. Synonym for *retention catheter*.

Kegel exercises Perineal exercises that help strengthen muscles that control voiding.

Lumen Space within a tube.

Meatus The external opening of a canal in a body structure.

Micturation The act of emptying the urinary bladder. Synonym for *urination* and *voiding*.

Nocturia The need to urinate during the night.

Oliguria The production and excretion of scant amounts of urine.

Overflow The involuntary escape of urine associated with an extremely full bladder.

Polyuria The excessive production and excretion of urine. Synonym for *diuresis*.

Port An opening in a piece of equipment.

Proteinuria The presence of albumin in urine. Synonym for *albuminuria*.

Pyuria The presence of pus in urine.

Residual urine Urine remaining in the bladder immediately after voiding.

Retention catheter A catheter placed in the bladder and secured in place. Synonym for *indwelling catheter*.

Second voided specimen A term describing a urine sample collected one-half hour after a patient has emptied his bladder.

Specific gravity The weight of a liquid substance compared with the weight of water.

Stoma An artificial opening in the body formed with natural tissue.

Straight catheter A catheter that is immediately withdrawn following its use.

Stress incontinence The escape of urine from the bladder during times of increased abdominal pressure.

Urgency A strong feeling that urine must be eliminated.

Urinalysis A laboratory study of urine.

Urinary incontinence The inability to retain urine in the bladder.

Urinary diversion Procedure in which the ureters are surgically implanted elsewhere.

Urinary retention A condition in which urine is not being excreted from the bladder.

Urinary suppression A condition in which the kidneys are not forming urine.

Urination The act of emptying the urinary bladder. Synonym for *micturation* and *voiding*.

Urine Waste released from the urinary system.

Urinometer An instrument for measuring the specific gravity of urine.

Voiding The act of emptying the urinary bladder. Synonym for *micturation* and *urination*.

Introduction

Elimination of excess water and wastes is a basic need for all forms of life. The urinary system eliminates excess fluid and toxic substances in a waste solution called *urine*. This is one of the chief mechanisms by which the health of an individual is maintained. When this function becomes impaired, it can be life threatening.

In this chapter the process of urinary elimination is briefly reviewed. Methods for assessing urinary function and promotion of urinary elimination are also discussed. The chapter describes skills that the nurse may be required to use when the usual methods of elimination are temporarily or permanently altered.

Understanding Urinary Structures and Function

The urinary tract is one of several routes from which wastes are excreted from the body. Other routes include the large intestine, lungs, and skin. The urinary system consists of structures that produce urine, collect urine, and transport it from the body.

The Kidneys and Ureters

The kidneys perform the major responsibility for maintaining the balance of water and other chemicals in blood and cells. The blood delivers these substances to microscopic structures called nephrons in the kidneys. The nephrons selectively remove excess water and substances for which the body has no need, thus forming urine. Urine is transported from the kidneys through the ureters to the urinary bladder. As long as this selective process takes place, the fluid and chemical content of the body remains relatively constant.

The Urinary Bladder

The bladder is a structure that temporarily collects and holds urine. It is made up of several layers of smooth muscle tissue. At the base of the bladder, a round ring of muscle tissue forms the internal sphincter, which guards the opening between the urinary bladder and the urethra.

As the volume of urine increases, the bladder expands and pressure increases within it. When the pressure becomes sufficient to stimulate stretch receptors located in the bladder wall, the desire to empty the bladder becomes noticeable. Usually this occurs in adults when about 150 to 250 mL of urine collect in the bladder.

The Urethra

The urethra is the final passageway for urine. In men, the urethra is a structure that also functions as a passageway for sperm. The male urethra is about 14 to 16.5 cm (5½ to 6½ in) in length. The female urethra is 4 to 6.5 cm (1½ to 2½ in long). It serves no reproductive function in the female.

Another sphincter, this one called the external sphincter, is located in the urethra. It is under voluntary control; that is, one can contract and relax this muscle at will. When the sphincter is contracted, urine is held within the bladder. Upon relaxation of the external sphincter, urine is released.

The Urinary Meatus

The word *meatus* refers to an external opening of a canal in the body. The opening at the end of the urethra in both the male and female is called the urinary meatus. This is the terminal structure of the urinary system and the only part that can be seen with the eyes. *Urination,* the process of emptying the bladder, takes place when urine flows out of the meatus. Synonyms for urination are *voiding* and *micturation.*

Factors That Influence Urinary Elimination

A variety of factors influences the amount, content, and characteristics of urine or its elimination:

- The amount of urine normally produced varies with fluid intake. The greater the amount of fluid intake, the larger will be the amount of urine, and vice versa. If large amounts of fluid are being excreted by the skin, lungs, or intestine, the amount formed by the kidneys will decrease.
- The content and characteristics of urine are related to the individual's dietary intake and the chemical com-

position of body fluids. These conditions are in a constant state of fluctuation; yet, the kidneys maintain a relatively stable balance of all the constituents within blood and cells.
- The frequency of voiding depends on the amount of urine being produced. Since fluid intake is reduced during the night, less urine will be formed. Most healthy adults do not void during sleeping hours.
- The intervals at which individuals void generally is determined by habit. Everyone learns to respond to the impulse of a filling bladder on an individual basis. Some respond earlier than others to the urge to void. The intervals are insignificant as long as the overall total amount voided is adequate.
- Increased abdominal pressure—such as that which occurs during pregnancy and with coughing, sneezing, and lifting heavy objects—can increase the urge to void and even force urine through the external sphincter and meatus. This is known as *stress incontinence.*
- Under certain conditions, it may be difficult to relax muscles sufficiently to void. For example, this may occur when a urine specimen is needed. It may also happen when a person is embarrassed or shy about using a bedpan or having to urinate in a public restroom.
- Women find it easier to void in a semi-sitting or sitting position than in the back-lying position. For the bedridden female patient, elevating the head of the bed and flexing the knees are helpful. If allowed, the patient may be assisted to a commode or to the bathroom. Men find it easier to void when standing, and this position is preferred when the male patient's condition permits.

Assessing Urinary Function

The nurse uses assessment techniques to evaluate all the systems of the body. The process of assessment can be reviewed in Chapter 4, and the specific techniques for physical assessment of the genitourinary system can be found in Chapter 14. The nurse can obtain a broad base of information when recording the patient's health history and assessing his patterns of elimination. The nurse adds to the assessment by using examination techniques such as inspection, palpation, and percussion.

Identifying Abnormal Urinary Patterns

Certain terms pertain to the signs and symptoms associated with abnormal urinary patterns. The nurse should become familiar with the definitions that follow.

Urinary suppression indicates that the kidneys are not forming urine. *Anuria* refers to the absence of urine. If the kidneys are not producing urine, the bladder will remain empty. *Oliguria* is the production of a small volume of urine, usually less than 500 mL of urine in 24 hours when an oral intake has been adequate and no other excessive amount of fluid has been lost. The prolonged inability to produce urine can eventually lead to death.

The nurse must use assessment techniques to determine why there is a reduction in urinary elimination. It could be due to suppression or urinary retention. *Urinary retention* means that urine is being produced but is not being emptied from the bladder. This should be suspected when a patient is consuming normal amounts of liquids and the bladder feels distended when palpated. The patient may even feel a desire to void, but only eliminates small amounts.

Residual urine is urine retained in the bladder immediately after voiding. In the case of urinary retention, the volume may be as high as 100 to 150 mL. Urine that is retained in the bladder can support the growth of organisms leading to an infection. Dissolved substances, such as calcium, can precipitate while dwelling in the retained urine and form bladder stones.

The urge to void is usually experienced when there are approximately 150 to 250 mL of urine in the bladder. A normal daytime pattern for an adult is to urinate every 4 to 6 hours. When an individual experiences a need to void more often than this, it is referred to as *frequency*. A strong feeling that urine must be eliminated is called *urgency*. The person with urinary retention often experiences frequency and urgency.

Frequency and urgency are also symptoms that are associated with a lower urinary tract infection. An additional symptom is *dysuria*. Dysuria refers to difficult or uncomfortable voiding. *Burning* is the feeling of warmth and local irritation while urine is being passed.

Polyuria means producing an excessive amount of urine. *Diuresis* is a synonym. Ordinarily, the amount of fluid that is consumed is nearly matched by the amount of urine eliminated. Certain fluids act as natural diuretics and cause a temporary increase in the production of urine and the frequency of urination; examples include coffee, tea, and cocoa. Alcohol inhibits the production of antidiuretic hormone (ADH), which explains the increased urination while drinking and the dry mouth and other symptoms of fluid depletion experienced later. These substances also irritate the bladder and increase the perceived urge to urinate. *Nocturia* is present when individuals are repeatedly awakened during the night with the urge to void.

Urinary incontinence is the inability to control the release of urine from the bladder. The six recognized types of incontinence are stress, urge, reflex, functional, overflow, and total incontinence. They are differentiated in Table 21-1. The treatment of incontinence is complex because there are so many variations and etiologies. It is even possible for one individual to have multiple types of incontinence. Diagnosing the particular manner in which there is involuntary loss of urine is instrumental in helping patients to manage or regain control of urinary elimination. Figure 21-1 shows an example of a log that can be used for recording data.

Examining Urine

Data about the functioning status of the urinary system may be obtained by collecting and examining urine. The nurse routinely assesses the color, amount, clarity, and odor of urine. Table 21-2 is a summary of the normal characteristics of urine. Reviewing the results of laboratory tests performed on urine also can contribute assessment data. The techniques for collecting and performing specific urine tests are discussed later in this chapter.

Identifying Abnormal Characteristics of Urine

Various terms are used to describe abnormalities in the contents of urine. These terms are formed by combining a common suffix referring to urine and a prefix that specifies a substance. Some of these terms include the following:

Hematuria refers to urine that contains blood. When blood is present in large enough quantities, the urine becomes reddish brown in color; smaller amounts may make the urine appear smoky. The nurse must assess carefully to determine that the blood is coming from the urinary tract rather than from the rectum, or from the vagina of a menstruating female.

Pyuria is pus in the urine. The urine appears cloudy. Normal urine, when it stands and cools, may also become cloudy. The two should not be confused.

Albuminuria means that there is albumin in the urine. Albumin is a type of protein found in plasma. For this reason, the term *proteinuria* is sometimes used as a synonym. The nephrons should not permit albumin to filter through into urine. The presence of albumin may be an early indication of impaired kidney function.

Glycosuria refers to glucose, a type of sugar, in the urine. Glucose should be reabsorbed into the blood stream. When the amount of sugar in the blood exceeds the nephrons' ability to return it to the circulation, glucose is deposited in the urine. This may occur on occasions after an individual eats foods that contain a great deal of sugar. It may even be associated with a period of emotional stress when the body requires a surge of glucose for additional energy. However, sustained glucose in the urine is one of the most common symptoms of diabetes mellitus.

Toileting the Patient

Some patients may need assistance with toileting. Illness sometimes affects patients' strength and ability to eliminate independently. The nurse may promote urinary elimination or help the patient with the use of a toilet, commode, bedpan, or urinal.

Table 21-1. Types of Incontinence

Type	Description	Example	Common Causes
Stress	The loss of small amounts of urine during situations when intraabdominal pressure rises	Dribbling is associated with sneezing, coughing, lifting, laughing, or rising from a bed or chair	Loss of perineal and sphincter muscle tone secondary to childbirth, menopausal atrophy, prolapsed uterus, or obesity
Urge	The need to void is perceived frequently with short-lived ability to sustain control of the flow	Voiding commences when there is a delay in accessing a restroom	Bladder irritation secondary to infection; loss of bladder tone due to recent continuous drainage with an indwelling catheter
Reflex	Spontaneous loss of urine when the bladder is stretched with urine, but without prior perception of a need to void	Automatic release of urine that cannot be controlled by the individual	Damage to motor and sensory tracts in the lower spinal cord secondary to trauma, tumor, or other neurological conditions
Functional	Control over urination is lost due to inaccessibility of a toilet or a compromised ability to use one	Voiding occurs while attempting to overcome barriers such as doorways, transferring from a wheelchair, manipulating clothing, acquiring assistance, or making needs known	Impaired mobility, impaired cognition, physical restraints, inability to communicate
Total	Loss of urine without any identifiable pattern or warning	A person passes urine without any ability or effort to control	Altered consciousness secondary to a head injury, loss of sphincter tone secondary to prostatectomy, anatomic leak through a urethral/vaginal fistula
Overflow	Urine leaks because the bladder is not completely emptied and remains distended with retained urine	The person voids small amounts frequently or a catheter drains a small volume and urine dribbles or leaks from the urethra	Overstretched bladder or weakened muscle tone secondary to obstruction of the urethra by debris within a catheter, an enlarged prostate, constipated stool, or postoperative bladder spasms

Promoting Urinary Elimination

The following nursing measures should be followed when the patient needs assistance with urination.

- Provide privacy. Voiding may not occur if the patient is tense or worried about being observed or interrupted.
- Help females to assume a sitting position. Sitting is the natural position women assume for elimination.
- Assist males to stand in front of a toilet or stand at the bedside when using a urinal. Standing is the natural position men assume when urinating.
- Maintain an adequate intake of oral fluids. The urge to urinate depends on the pressure exerted against stretch receptors as the bladder fills.
- Use the power of imagery and suggestion to help

patients initiate voiding. This may be done by running water from a tap within hearing distance of the patient. Placing the patient's hand in warm water or running water over the perineum may also be tried.

Assisting the Patient to a Bathroom

Some patients are able to use the toilet in a bathroom for elimination. The nurse's responsibilities depend on the patient's condition but, in general, include the following:

- Help the patient walk to the bathroom and stay with the patient if necessary. After being in bed, the patient is often weak and may faint.
- If it is safe to leave the patient alone in the bathroom, be sure that the bathroom door is unlocked and a signal device is handy.

BLADDER RECORD

TIME INTERVAL	Column 1 URINATED IN TOILET	Column 2 LEAKING ACCIDENT	Column 3 LARGE ACCIDENT	Column 4 FLUID (OZ)	Column 5 REASON
6–8 A.M.					
8–10 A.M.					
10 A.M.–12 P.M.					
12–2 P.M.					
2–4 P.M.					
4–6 P.M.					
6–8 P.M.					
8–10 P.M.					
10 P.M.–12 A.M.					
OVERNIGHT					

Number of pads used today: _____

Comments: _____

Figure 21-1 This bladder record is an assessment tool to diagnose types of incontinence. Column 1 — Place a check next to the time urination occurred in the toilet, commode, bedpan, or urinal. Column 2 — Place a check next to the time there was accidental leakage. Column 3 — Place a check next to the time there was a large accident. Column 4 — Record fluid intake. Column 5 — Note any reason for the accident (for example, upon coughing or lifting something heavy). (Adapted from Jakouac-Smith, DA: Continence restoration in the homebound patient. Nurs Clin North Am 23(1):207–218, 1988)

- Wait close by, ready to provide the patient with assistance.
- Help the patient clean the perineum of any residue from elimination if that is necessary.
- Observe the characteristics of the urine or stool before flushing the toilet.
- Provide the patient the opportunity for handwashing before leaving the bathroom.
- Help the patient back to bed, leaving him clean and comfortable.
- Make the necessary notations on the patient's record.

Using a Commode

A *commode,* is a chair with an opening in the seat under which a receptable is placed. It is sometimes used for elimination at the bedside. This may be necessary when the patient is weak or when walking to a bathroom is contraindicated. The patient can be helped from bed in the same manner as assisting a patient from a bed to a chair, described in Chapter 18. Some commodes are equipped with wheels, which allow the patient to be taken to the bathroom for more privacy during elimination. If that is the case, the opening in the seat can be positioned over the toilet. Characteristics of the urine should be noted before flushing.

Using a Bedpan

A bedpan can be used either for the elimination of urine or stool. Bedpans are made from stainless steel or plastic. One type, called a fracture pan, is more flat on the end that fits toward the back of the buttocks. It is used for individuals who cannot sit or elevate their hips. Skill Procedure 21-1 describes how to place and remove a bedpan.

Using a Urinal

A urinal is a container for collecting urine. Because of anatomical differences, it is easier for females to use a bedpan for urination. However, there are specially designed urinals that may be used by females under certain circumstances. In addition to the actions regarding privacy, hygiene, and disposal of wastes described for using a bedpan, the following actions may be helpful when a male patient uses a urinal:

- To avoid wet linen, make sure that the urinal is empty before handing it to the patient or placing it in position.
- Warm the outside of a metal urinal in the same way that a steel bedpan is warmed, by running warm water over its surface.
- To assist a patient who cannot place the urinal himself, instruct the patient to spread his legs a short distance.

Table 21-2. Characteristics of Normal Urine in Healthy Adults

Item	Description
Amount	Approximately 1000–1500 mL of urine in each 24-hour period. The average is about 1200 mL.
Color	Golden yellow to amber. If the urine is concentrated, such as early in the morning or after a period of little fluid intake, the color will be darker. It will be lighter if the urine is dilute.
Clarity	Clear. Urine may turn cloudy on standing, owing to normal phosphate precipitation.
Odor	Faintly aromatic. Some foods, such as asparagus, and certain drugs cause a pungent odor.
Specific gravity	1.005 to 1.025. A wider range has been noted in some healthy adults.
Acidity	Average pH of 6 for persons on a standard diet. A range of 4.6 to 8 is normal. Vegetarians excrete slightly alkaline urine. A high-protein diet increases the acidity of urine. Certain drugs influence the acidity/alkalinity of urine.
Protein	Negative.
Glucose	Negative. Glucose may be found in the urine if the person has eaten concentrated sweets, such as candy.
Ketone bodies	Negative.
Sediment	Negative for red blood cells. Negative for white blood cells. Occasional epithelial cells. Occasional hyaline casts.

- Hold the handle of the urinal and direct it at an angle between the patient's legs so that the bottom rests on the bed.
- Lift the penis and place it well within the inside of the urinal.

Managing Incontinence

Urinary incontinence may be either permanent or temporary, depending on its cause. It is a problem faced by many elderly persons. Family members often need the nurse's help on ways to deal with incontinence in the home. The best approach is to assist with bladder retraining. This may not be possible or realistic for all incontinent patients. When total rehabilitation is not an option, other nursing skills may be implemented. These may include measures that help to reduce the frequency or limit the consequences of incontinence.

Assisting With Bladder Retraining

For some patients, a bladder retraining program may be useful. However, to start this type of plan when there is little or no possibility of achieving results can be emotionally damaging to the patient. It can also affect the morale of the nursing team. Even if the program of retraining is likely to succeed, the patient must be helped to understand that it will be a slow process and that the gains may be slight and very gradual. It will require the combined effort and dedication of all the nursing team as well as the patient and his family.

The following is a list of suggestions that may be developed into a more specific plan for bladder retraining:

- Assess for any regularities or patterns in the patient's periods of dryness versus incontinence. Success is more likely if the nurse can adapt measures that correspond to the filling and emptying of the patient's bladder.
- Set realistic goals with the patient. The nurse may find that the patient desires so badly to regain control of his bladder that he sets unrealistic and self-defeating goals. The nurse may have to help keep expectations within reason. Setting very limited, specific, short-range goals may promote more positive results.
- Plan a schedule with the patient for attempts to void. This schedule should correlate with the patient's

Skill Procedure 21-1. Placing and Removing a Bedpan

Suggested Action	Reason for Action
Bring the bedpan, toilet tissues, and equipment for the patient to wash and dry his hands.	Having equipment on hand saves time by avoiding unnecessary trips to the storage area.
Warm the bedpan by rinsing it with warm water if the bedpan is made of metal.	A cold bedpan feels uncomfortable and may make it difficult for the patient to void.
Close the patient's room door and pull the privacy curtains around the patient's bed.	The patient's right to privacy should be respected. Most are especially embarrassed about being observed during elimination.
Spread a layer of cornstarch over the surface that contacts the body if the patient is prone to skin breakdown.	Cornstarch absorbs moisture and reduces friction and shearing forces.
Place an adjustable bed in high position.	Having the bed in high position promotes the nurse's good use of body mechanics.
Place the bedpan on the chair next to the bed or on the foot of the bed while preparing to position the patient.	To avoid spreading organisms, the bedpan should be placed in an area that is somewhat distant from clean articles.
Raise the top linen enough to determine the location of the patient's hips and buttocks.	This prevents unnecessary exposure while still allowing the nurse to place the bedpan.
Instruct the patient to bend his knees and press his weight downward on his heels.	Elevating the hips provides clearance for placing the bedpan.
Help the patient lift his buttocks by placing one hand under his lower back.	The nurse uses less energy when the patient can assist.
Slip the bedpan into place beneath the buttocks, as illustrated in Figure 21-2.	Proper placement ensures that soiling will not occur during elimination.

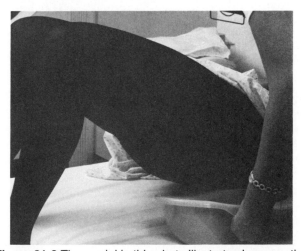

Figure 21-2 The model in this photo illustrates how a patient can help raise himself onto a bedpan. One hand of the nurse is placed under the patient's lower back to help lift, and the other hand slips the bedpan under the patient.

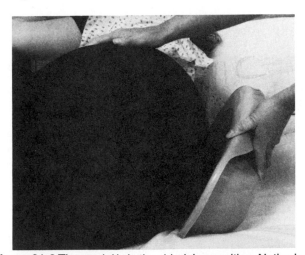

Figure 21-3 The model is in the side-lying position. Notice how the bedpan is tucked under the patient. The nurse then rolls the patient onto the bedpan.

If the patient is entirely helpless, two people may be required to place the patient on a bedpan.	Sharing the work reduces the possibility of injury when turning and positioning a helpless patient.
Place the helpless patient on his side while positioning the bedpan against the buttocks.	Turning a patient to the side takes less effort than lifting.
Roll the patient onto the bedpan, as shown in Figure 21-3.	Rolling takes less energy when positioning a patient.

(continued)

Skill Procedure 21-1. Continued

Suggested Action	Reason for Action
Look to see that the patient's buttocks rest on the rounded shelf of the bedpan, as is the case in Figure 21-4.	The weight of the patient should be supported, yet should allow sufficient room for elimination.

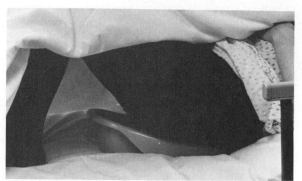

Figure 21-4 The bedpan is properly placed. The patient is sitting in such a way that soiling should not occur.

Suggested Action	Reason for Action
Raise the head of the bed slightly, if permitted.	This position generally makes it easier for the patient to eliminate and avoids strain on the patient's back.
Leave the signal device and toilet tissue within easy reach of the patient.	Falls can be prevented when the patient does not have to reach for items he needs.
Leave the patient if it is safe to do so. Raise the siderails before leaving.	Attending patients and using siderails help prevent falls or other accidents.
Return promptly to assist the patient with toileting hygiene.	Patients find sitting on a bedpan uncomfortable. Prolonged pressure can lead to skin breakdown.
Remove the bedpan in the same manner in which it was offered.	Proper lifting or turning helps prevent injury.
Place the patient on his side if he is not capable of removing residue that remains from elimination.	Cleaning the patient prevents offensive odors and skin irritation.
Wrap the hand with toilet tissue. Use one stroke from the pubic area toward the anal area. Discard the tissue and use more until the patient is clean. Spread the buttocks to clean the anal area.	Care must be taken to prevent introducing organisms into the urinary meatus. A principle of medical asepsis includes cleaning from an area that is less soiled to one that is more heavily soiled.
Place soiled toilet tissue into the bedpan unless a specimen is required.	Toilet tissue mixed with a specimen makes laboratory examination more difficult. Tissue used for wastes contains organisms and should be disposed of properly.
Help the patient to a position of comfort and offer the patient supplies to wash and dry his hands, assisting him as necessary.	Handwashing is one of the most effective methods of controlling the spread of organisms.
Assess the characteristics of elimination; collect a specimen; measure the urine if necessary.	The products of elimination may provide data that will aid in a medical or nursing diagnosis.
Do not discard contents of a bedpan if urine or stool appears abnormal in any way. Obtain a sample of the contents from the bedpan in a sealed container.	Disposing of abnormal urine or stool prevents having it analyzed by the laboratory.
Record information according to agency policy.	It is important to keep accurate records.

(continued)

Skill Procedure 21-1. Continued

Suggested Action	Reason for Action
Empty the contents of the bedpan into the patient's toilet or flushable hopper in a dirty utility room.	Sanitary measures include disposal of urine and stool into a sewage treatment system.
Clean the bedpan and replace it in an area that is located separately from clean articles or possessions used by the patient.	Keeping items used for elimination separate from cleaner items helps prevent the spread of organisms.
Wash hands before performing any other nursing tasks.	Conscientious handwashing prevents the spread of organisms by health personnel.

assessed voiding patterns. For example, if it is noted that a frequent wetting time is 10:30 A.M., voiding could be attempted at 10:00 A.M. If night incontinence is a problem, awaken the patient and have him void. If no pattern is apparent, develop a schedule that meets the needs of the patient. An opportunity for voiding should be made at least every 2 to 3 waking hours. It can be extended or shortened to correspond with a patient's periods of continence.

- Discourage strict limitation of liquid intake. The patient should have adequate amounts of fluids to keep urine diluted and prevent fluid imbalance. Also, when the patient's bladder is kept reasonably full, he is more apt to be successful when attempting to void.
- Everyone involved in the patient's care must be aware of the developed schedule and conscientiously carry it out. Unless everyone is dedicated to the plan, enthusiasm will be lost as goals remain unachieved.
- Teach the patient to take note of any sensation that precedes voiding. Examples include chilliness, perspiring, muscular twitching, and restlessness. Males may experience a spontaneous erection triggered by a full bladder. It is important that the patient recognize these signs and use them as indications for voiding.
- Encourage a relaxed atmosphere and as nearly normal circumstances for elimination. A toilet or a commode is preferable. However, simulating the positions for elimination can be done using a bedpan or urinal.
- Suggest that the patient bend forward in a slow, rhythmic manner. This increases abdominal pressure on the bladder. The nurse may also suggest that the patient use *Credé's maneuver.* This involves applying light pressure with the hands over the bladder.
- Experiment with the success of other measures that may stimulate urination, such as listening to running water or placing a hand in a basin of water. Whatever helps to accomplish a small goal can encourage individuals to persevere with the plan.

Selective Continence Techniques

The type of technique used to restore the patient's continence must be carefully matched with the type of incontinence and its etiology. Table 21-3 identifies methods that

are associated with greater success. Some are elaborated upon further in the following discussion.

Strengthening Pelvic Floor Muscles

Strengthening pelvic floor muscles is one method to control some types of incontinence. It is especially helpful for stress incontinence and may extend the time needed for control in urge incontinence.

The pelvic floor muscle exercises, also called *Kegel exercises,* increase the tone of the pubococcygeus muscles. They form a ring around the vagina and anus. These muscles are used to voluntarily hold back urine, intestinal gas, or the passage of stool. The patient can be taught to perform these exercises by instructing him to

- Tighten the internal muscles (not the stomach, legs, or buttocks) for 10 seconds.
- Relax the muscles for the same amount of time.
- Repeat contraction and relaxation 10 to 25 times during one exercise period.
- Perform the exercise routine 3 to 4 times a day.

The isometric exercises can be supplemented by actually stopping the urinary stream several times during voiding. This practice can be performed at each elimination throughout the day. Improvement should be noticed within two weeks of consistent exercising. Increased control will become even more obvious after a month of continued repetition of the exercise program.

Using Cutaneous Triggering Mechanisms

Cutaneous triggering may be useful for some incontinent paralyzed patients. This technique promotes voiding by manually stimulating certain skin areas. Before implementing this technique, the nurse should determine whether a voiding reflex is present.

A voiding reflex is present if the anal sphincter tightens as a thermometer is inserted or responds similarly to other tactile stimulation in the genital area. Patients who experience reflex incontinence can learn to stimulate the release of urine although they cannot voluntarily initiate or curtail it. The most successful approach involves tapping the suprapubic area.

Table 21-3. Nursing Approaches for Incontinence

Type of Incontinence	Nursing Approach
Stress incontinence	Pelvic floor muscle strengthening Weight reduction
Urge incontinence	Maintain fluid intake of at least 2000 mL/day Omit bladder irritants, such as caffeine or alcohol Administer diuretics in the morning
Functional incontinence	Modify clothing Facilitate access to a toilet, commode, or urinal Assist to a toilet according to a preplanned schedule
Reflex incontinence	Cutaneous triggering Straight intermittent catheterization
Total incontinence	Absorbent undergarments External catheter Indwelling catheter
Overflow incontinence	Hydration Adequate bowel elimination Maintain patency of catheter Perform Credé's maneuver

The following actions can be performed by the nurse and eventually taught to the patient.

- Palpate the bladder for distention every 2 to 3 hours.
- Position the patient on a bedpan, toilet, or in a 45° sitting position with a urinal in place.
- Tap repeatedly over the bladder wall as many as 50 times for approximately 5 seconds.
- Move to an adjacent area and repeat unless voiding commences.

Other alternatives may be attempted if tapping is unsuccessful. The penis or the skin of the inner thigh may be stroked, the pubic hairs can be pulled, a thermometer or gloved finger can be inserted within the rectum, or the inguinal area of the abdomen can be massaged lightly. It may take longer stimulation, perhaps several minutes, with these substituted forms to trigger urination. A pause lasting at least 1 minute should be observed before switching to another mechanism for stimulation.

Once a successful triggering mechanism is discovered, it should be used with each subsequent attempt to stimulate voiding. Depending on the level of spinal injury some patients can be taught to bear down using their abdominal muscles once voiding has commenced. This may aid in further emptying the bladder.

Performing Credé's Maneuver

Patients who experience urinary retention and overflow incontinence may be helped by performing Credé's maneuver. This technique facilitates bladder emptying by increasing intraabdominal pressure above urethral pressure, thus allowing urine to be expelled.

Credé's maneuver is performed by placing the palmar surfaces of the hands below the navel, as shown in Figure 21-5, or one hand can be placed on top of the other. The hands press inward and downward over the bladder. Bending forward at the hips while seated on a toilet or bedpan can also augment the Credé's maneuver. This method is not advised for patients with reflex incontinence because the external sphincter may remain contracted despite increased pressure.

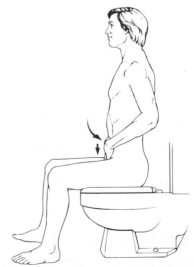

Figure 21-5 Credé's maneuver involves pressing inward and downward on the abdomen just below the navel.

Keeping the Incontinent Patient Dry

Incontinence is a source of embarrassment for most individuals. For many, it represents a loss of control similar to infancy. In addition to the physical care of incontinent patients, nurses must be particularly dedicated to maintaining the individual's dignity. Skill Procedure 21-2 and the discussion that follows provide suggestions that may reduce the effects of involuntary urination.

Using an External Catheter

Leaking urine can be collected with an *external catheter*. This is a device that fits over the outside of the penis. Examples of external catheters are illustrated in Figure 21-6. Because of the differences in male and female anat-

omy, external catheters are more effective when used for males. The external catheter can be attached to a leg bag while the patient is mobile. While in bed, the catheter is connected to a gravity drainage bag.

Applying an External Catheter

When an external catheter is used, certain problems may occur. First, and perhaps the most hazardous, is that the appliance may be applied too tightly and may restrict blood flow to the skin and tissues of the penis. Second, moisture accumulates beneath the appliance and can lead to breakdown of the skin that covers the penis. Third, the catheter may not fit well or for some other reason may allow urine to leak. If applied properly and checked frequently, these problems can be avoided. Skill Procedure

---

Skill Procedure 21-2. Managing Incontinence

Suggested Action	Reason for Action
Explain to the patient that efforts will be made to help him.	Incontinence is a difficult problem psychologically and physically. The patient's morale and cooperation can be strengthened when he knows others support him.
Help the patient restore normal functioning if there is a possibility for success.	Urinary incontinence should not be a condition to which every patient becomes resigned.
Encourage the patient to establish a routine for attempting to void.	A routine may be all that is needed to help restore function for some patients.
Take chronically ill and elderly patients to a bathroom or offer a bedpan or urinal every 2 to 3 hours.	Providing frequent opportunities to void may decrease the accidental loss of urinary control.
Use hygienic measures to keep the incontinent patient dry, clean, and comfortable.	Accumulated urine forms ammonia, which can cause strong odors. Lying on wet linens can quickly irritate skin, leading to its subsequent breakdown.
Teach the patient Kegel exercises when possible. These exercises consist of contracting the muscles, simulating or actually halting urination.	*Kegel exercises* are perineal exercises that help strengthen muscles that control voiding. The patient should repeat at least 10 to 25 contractions as often as 3 to 4 times daily.
For a male, apply an external catheter that covers the outside of the penis.	Helping the patient remain dry improves a patient's sense of dignity. External catheters have not been found to be effective for incontinent women.
Use absorbent pads and waterproof undergarments for male or female patients.	Disposable briefs have been reported to function effectively and allow the patient freedom of movement without obvious soiling.
Keep a urinal in place if the incontinent patient is a bedridden male. Protect the skin from contact with the urinal by covering it with terrycloth wristbands, or a similar material.	Covering a urinal that is kept in place with terry cloth helps prevent irritation and chafing in the genital area, absorbs perspiration, and prevents the urinal from slipping out of place.
Obtain a physician's order for inserting an indwelling catheter, as a last resort.	Because of the high risk for infection, an indwelling catheter should only be used as a temporary measure or when the patient's psychological or physical comfort is at stake.
Demonstrate tact and understanding. Provide opportunities for the patient to express his feelings and concerns.	Discouragement and depression can be relieved by sharing the burden with an empathetic listener.

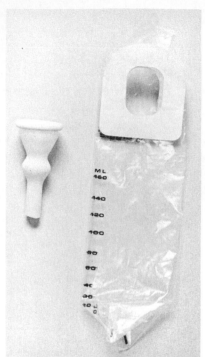

Figure 21-6 External urinary devices, such as these, permit collection of urine from males. The device on the right is used for pediatric patients.

21-3 describes the application and care involved when using an external catheter.

Constructing a Condom Catheter

A *condom* is a device used by males for birth control. It fits over the penis and collects semen, fluid that contains sperm. For the individual who may wish to avoid paying the price of a commercially manufactured external cathe-

ter, a homemade version using a condom is simple to make. These steps should be followed:

- Insert a flexible drainage tube within the condom.
- Secure the closed end of the condom and the tip of the drainage tube together. This can be done using dental floss, a rubber band, or similar material.
- Perforate the tip of the condom to provide an opening through which urine can drain. This does not have to be large; a hole made with a safety pin will do.
- Reverse the direction of the condom so that the connection is now inside, leaving just the drainage tube extending from the closed end of the condom.
- Wrap the area of the connection once again to make sure it will not come apart.
- The condom catheter is now ready for application.

Using Intermittent Straight Catheterization

For the patient who tends to have urinary retention or reflex incontinence that does not respond to cutaneous triggering, intermittent straight catheterization may be the best approach. Intermittent catheterization has an advantage in that the catheter is not left in place. It is removed once the bladder has been drained of urine. This procedure may need to be repeated several times during each day. However, the incidence of infection and other complications is less than with indwelling catheters.

Some patients can be taught to self-catheterize. When done in the home, the patient uses clean technique rather than the strict aseptic technique used in the hospital. Patients tend to resist the organisms in their own home environments much more effectively than those that are harbored in health-care agencies.

Skill Procedure 21-3. Applying an External Catheter

Suggested Action	**Reason for Action**
Explain the procedure to the patient.	Explanations reduce anxiety and promote patient cooperation.
Assemble the following: soap, water, towel, condom catheter, drainage tubing, collection device. Optional: disposable gloves and an additional adhesive strip or Velcro strap.	Organization promotes efficient time management.
Provide privacy.	The patient has the right to be protected from being seen by others during his care.
Place the patient in a supine position and cover him with a cotton bath blanket.	Lying on his back places the patient in the best position for care. The bath blanket provides warmth and maintains a sense of modesty.
Wash hands.	Handwashing reduces the spread of microorganisms.

(continued)

Skill Procedure 21-3. Continued

Suggested Action	Reason for Action
Don disposable gloves if desired.	Semen, though not likely to be present during this procedure, is a source for the transmission of HIV. It has not been implicated in work-related contact between patients and health-care workers.
Wash, rinse, and dry the penis well.	The integrity of the skin is maintained with appropriate hygiene.
Wind the adhesive strip in an upward spiral about the penis as shown in Figure 21-7.	A circular application could produce a tourniquet effect and constrict blood flow to the penis.

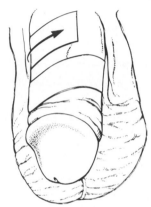

Figure 21-7 A spiral wrap is less likely to interfere with blood supply.

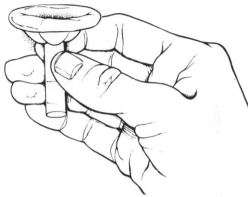

Figure 21-8 The condom catheter can be controlled better if it is rolled to its base.

Roll the condom on itself toward the drainage end of the catheter shown in Figure 21-8.	The easiest way to apply the catheter is to unroll it.
Hold approximately 1–2 in (2.5–5 cm) of the balloon portion as shown in Figure 21-9 and unroll the remainder over the penis.	Leaving a space below the urethra prevents direct contact with the catheter and possible irritation to the meatus.

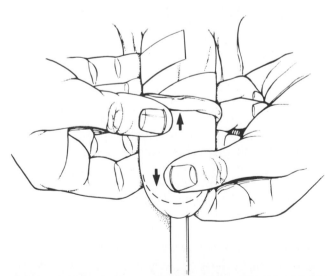

Figure 21-9 The condom catheter is pressed as it is unrolled over the penis so it remains in contact with the adhesive spiral.

(continued)

Skill Procedure 21-3. *Continued*

Suggested Action	**Reason for Action**
If necessary, secure the upper end of the unrolled catheter with a second elasticized adhesive strip or a Velcro strap, but not so tight as to interfere with circulation.	A second method for holding the catheter in place may be needed to ensure that it will not come loose.
Connect the drainage tip to tubing and a collection device such as a leg bag or gravity drainage bag.	A leg bag conceals the fact that a catheter is used. When the patient reclines, it should be replaced with a gravity drainage bag.
Maintain the penis in a downward position.	Urine drains by gravity.
Inspect the penis at least every two hours for circulatory problems due to swelling or tight adhesive.	Tissue respiration depends on adequate blood circulation.
Check that the space left at the tip of the catheter has not twisted.	A twisted catheter obstructs the flow of urine.
Empty the leg bag periodically as it fills with urine.	A full leg bag can become heavy and leak.
Remove and change the catheter daily or more frequently if it becomes loose or too tight.	A clean catheter should be applied following daily hygiene.
Wash the external catheter and leg bag with mild soap and water. Rinse the equipment with a 1:7 solution of vinegar and water.	External catheters and leg bags can be reused as long as they remain intact.
Remove the external catheter and substitute a waterproof garment at night if the flow of urine is difficult to maintain.	There are greater consequences from an obstructed flow of urine than from accumulation within an absorbent bedpad or undergarment.

Using Urethral Catheterization

A *catheter* is a hollow tube for instilling and removing fluids. *Catheterization* of the urinary bladder is the introduction of a catheter through the urethra into the bladder for removing urine.

The dangers of introducing a catheter into the bladder are injury and infection. An object forced through a narrowing, an irregularity, or a curve can cause injury to mucous membranes. Microorganisms can enter the bladder by being pushed in as the catheter is inserted. The procedure of catheterization is used as infrequently as possible due to the hazards involved in their use. Only when the benefits outweigh the risks should the nurse propose insertion of a catheter. The nurse should also advocate for its early removal.

Indications for Catheterization

There are several common reasons for catheterizing a patient.

- Occasionally, a patient is catheterized to obtain a urine specimen entirely free of contamination. However, collecting a voided, clean-catch midstream specimen is now replacing the need to obtain a specimen by catheterization. This method will be discussed later in the chapter.
- A catheter is inserted before some types of abdominal or vaginal surgery to keep the bladder empty of urine. This permits the surgeon a better view and palpation of internal tissue. It also prevents accidentally injuring a full bladder with surgical instruments.
- Catheterization sometimes becomes necessary when, for whatever reason, a patient cannot void and nursing measures to induce voiding have failed.
- Catheterization is used when the amount of residual urine left in the bladder after voiding must be measured or to differentiate suppression from retention.
- Catheterization may be used to remove urine from a greatly distended bladder.
- Catheterization may be used as a last resort to control incontinence. This should only take place if the patient has an open wound or his skin shows signs of breakdown. Frequent hygiene and changing linen present fewer risks than those that are potentially possible with the use of a catheter.
- A catheter may be inserted to monitor and accurately assess the fluid loss and replacement on critically ill patients.

Types of Urethral Catheters

There are many types of catheters that are manufactured for instilling or removing fluid from various parts of the body. Urethral catheters are intended to be inserted through the urinary meatus and progress up the urethra into the bladder. These catheters are manufactured in various diameters that correspond with the size of the meatus. For adults, sizes 14, 16, and 18 are generally used; the higher numbers indicate larger diameters.

A *straight catheter* is intended to be inserted and withdrawn immediately following its use. An *indwelling catheter* is placed in the bladder and secured there for a period of time. It is sometimes called a *retention catheter*. A drainage tube and collection device must be connected to this type of catheter.

The most commonly used indwelling catheter is called a Foley catheter. It has a balloon that can be inflated after the catheter is in place. The balloon prevents the catheter from slipping out of the bladder. An indwelling catheter is illustrated in Figure 21-10.

Although there are several types of indwelling catheters, the principles on which they operate are similar. The catheter has a double or triple lumen. A *lumen* is a space within a tube; in a catheter, it refers to the separate channels within the same tube. One lumen provides a passage for fluid that inflates the balloon. This portion of the catheter may be self-sealing or require a separate clamp. A second lumen is the channel through which the urine drains. A third lumen, available on some catheters, is made specifically for instilling irrigation fluid.

Preparing for Catheterization

Sets are now available that contain the required equipment needed for catheterization. They are packaged in a manner that ensures that the equipment is sterile. Once the contents of a catheterization set have been used, the set may be thrown away. Sets include the catheter, a drape, a

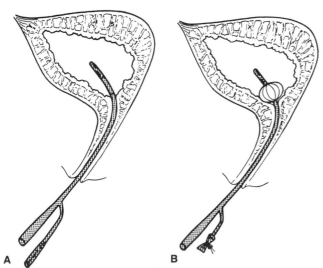

Figure 21-10 (*A*). A straight catheter does not have an additional lumen leading to a balloon. It is used one time to drain the bladder and removed immediately afterwards. (*B*). An indwelling catheter has a balloon that is inflated to prevent the catheter from slipping from the urinary bladder.

receptacle to receive urine, cleaning materials, a lubricant, a specimen container, and sterile gloves.

The preparation of a patient includes explaining that usually there is a sensation of pressure rather than pain when the catheter is inserted. Do not dismiss any report of pain, however, since introducing a catheter in swollen or injured tissue may cause discomfort.

Inserting a Catheter

The technique for inserting a catheter is described in Skill Procedures 21-4 and 21-5. The procedure can be used when either a straight or indwelling catheter is inserted. The main difference involves testing and inflating the balloon, which would not be done with a straight catheter.

Connecting a Closed Drainage System

An indwelling catheter is attached to a receptacle that collects urine. It is positioned lower than the bladder so that drainage occurs by gravity. A closed drainage system, as illustrated in Figure 21-23, is most commonly used. Urine follows a continuous sterile passageway from the bladder to the collecting container.

To ensure that the urine moves directly into the container, it must not become trapped within the tubing. The length of tubing from the bed to the collection bag cannot contain loops. Gravity controls the movement of fluid downward, not upward. If the tubing loops, fluid will be trapped and interfere with the continuous flow of urine. Some nurses use a plastic clip or safety pin to fasten the drainage tubing to the bed linen. This keeps the tubing hanging in a vertical line into the collection bag. When moving the patient or changing linen, these devices should be unfastened to avoid causing the patient discomfort or displacement of the catheter.

The tubing is generally long enough to give the patient freedom to move about. However, it is important that the drainage tube does not become compressed by the weight of the patient's body. Placing it over the top of the patient's thigh is an acceptable practice. Care must be taken that the siderails or other parts of the bed do not obstruct the flow of urine.

The drainage bag should never be positioned higher than the bladder. The urine that has been collecting for a period of time could then flow back into the bladder, possibly carrying organisms with it. Occasionally, a patient must be transported in a wheelchair. It may be difficult to position the collection system and the tubing lower than the bladder. It is better in that situation to apply a clamp between the catheter and the bag until it is possible to reattach the drainage system to the bed. Before doing so, check to make sure that clamping the catheter for a brief period of time will not cause injury to the patient. For some patients, the catheter should never be clamped.

Many closed drainage systems have graduated markings

(Text continues on page 524)

Skill Procedure 21-4. Inserting an Indwelling Catheter in the Female Patient

Suggested Action	**Reason for Action**
Explain the procedure to the patient.	An explanation reduces anxiety and promotes cooperation.
Gather the following equipment: catheterization kit, additional light source if needed, and a cotton bath blanket.	Organization promotes efficient time management.
Raise the bed to a high position.	Back strain and fatigue are reduced when the nurse does not bend from the waist while performing the procedure.
Position an additional lamp at the foot of the bed if the lighting in the room is not adequate or ask an assistant to hold a flashlight.	The nurse needs adequate light to identify the urinary meatus.
Pull the privacy curtains around the bed.	The patient has a right to be protected from the view of others during care.
Position the female in a dorsal recumbent position with the knees flexed and the feet about 2 ft. apart, as shown in Figure 21-11.	This is the optimal position for access to the urinary meatus during female catheterization.

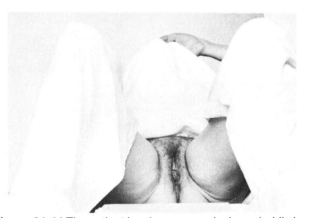

Figure 21-11 The patient has been properly draped while in a dorsal recumbent position, which is most often used.

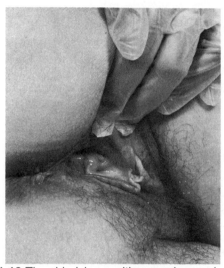

Figure 21-12 The side-lying position may be used when unusual circumstances prevent placing a female patient in a dorsal recumbent position. The photo illustrates that this position allows for good visualization of the meatus and surrounding area.

If the dorsal recumbent position causes pain or is difficult to assume for other reasons, place the patient on her side with the upper leg slighted hyperextended as shown in Figure 21-12. A Sims' position is another possible alternative.	Abduction of the legs may cause discomfort for some patients; alternate positions provide visualization and access to the female urethra.
Cover the patient with a bath blanket and fold the top linen to the foot of the bed.	Covering the patient shows concern for modesty.
Drape the bath blanket so that the abdomen and each leg is covered separately. Refer to Figure 15-4 in Chapter 15.	Appropriate draping provides warmth and access to the patient without exposing the entire lower body.
If the patient is soiled, wash the vulva and perianal area with soap and water, rinse, and dry.	Cleansing removes large numbers of organisms that could contribute to postcatheterization infection.

(continued)

Skill Procedure 21-4. Continued

Suggested Action	Reason for Action
Don clean gloves if any bloody drainage is present.	Gloves act as a barrier against bloodborne viruses.
Wash hands.	Handwashing reduces the spread of microorganisms.
Remove the wrapper from the catheterization tray. Open and position the wrapper so it can receive soiled supplies.	Depositing used supplies helps maintain the sterility of the remaining equipment and controls the transmission of microorganisms.
Open the sterile wrap surrounding the catheterization tray as described in Chapter 16.	The sterile inner wrap protects the contents from contamination.
Don sterile gloves contained within the catheterization tray as described in Chapter 16.	Using sterile gloves maintains the sterility of the other supplies within the kit.
Remove the sterile towel from the tray and unfold it without touching any unsterile surface. Wrap the towel about both gloved hands and place it beneath the patient, as shown in Figure 21-13.	Wrapping the towel around the gloves prevents contamination while positioning the sterile towel. The towel provides a sterile area below the perineum.

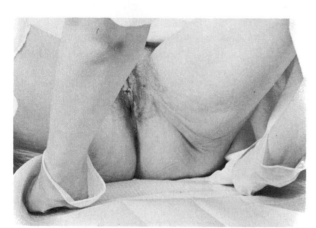

Figure 21-13 Notice how the nurse wraps the edges of a sterile towel around the gloved hands to protect them from contamination while tucking the towel under the edges of the patient's buttocks.

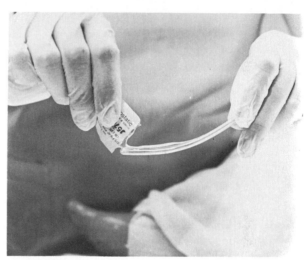

Figure 21-14 The nurse lubricates the catheter generously with prepackaged sterile lubricant found within the catheterization set.

Pour the antiseptic over the cotton balls.	All preparation of the equipment that involves two hands must be done before separating the patient's labia.
Test the balloon on the catheter by instilling the fluid from the prefilled syringe. Then aspirate the fluid back into the syringe.	Prefilling the balloon is a way of determining that the balloon is not defective before it is inserted.
Spread lubricant on the tip of the catheter for about 1½–2 in (3.5–5 cm), shown in Figure 21-14.	Lubrication eases insertion.
Place the catheterization tray between the patient's legs on top of the sterile towel.	Placing the prepared supplies near the patient helps prevent contamination.
Pick up a moistened cotton ball with the sterile forceps in the dominant hand and wipe one side of the labia majora from an anterior to a posterior direction.	The external labia is cleansed before progressing to inner areas. Wiping towards the vagina and rectum avoids introducing organisms into the urethral area. Using forceps prevents contamination of the glove on the dominant hand.

(continued)

Skill Procedure 21-4. Continued

Suggested Action	Reason for Action
Discard the soiled cotton ball within the outer wrapper of the catheterization tray. Avoid touching the sterile forceps to any nonsterile surfaces.	Discarding the soiled cotton ball confines organisms and reduces the possibility of transferring them to other equipment and supplies.
Use a separate cotton ball for the other side of the labia majora.	Using a separate cotton ball for each stroke ensures that debris will not be transferred back to the patient.
Use the thumb and fingers of the nondominant hand to separate the labia majora and the labia minora to expose the urinary meatus, shown in Figure 21-15.	The urinary meatus lies within and between the labia minora. Separation of the labia facilitates its identification.

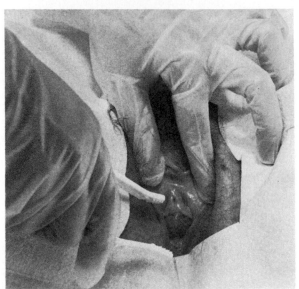

Figure 21-15 The labia minora are well spread and separated. This helps to expose the area for cleansing and for locating the urinary meatus. The nurse's forceps points to the meatus, which appears as a small dimple.

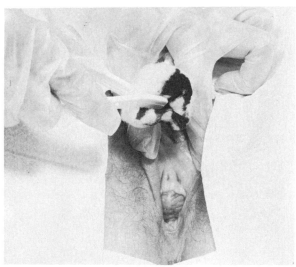

Figure 21-16 The nurse begins cleaning by starting the stroke directly above the meatus.

Consider the gloved hand that touched the patient to be contaminated.	When something sterile is touched with something nonsterile, it is contaminated. The contaminated glove cannot be used during the subsequent insertion of the catheter.
While retracting the labia with the nondominant hand, use a separate cotton ball to clean each of the labia minora as shown in Figure 21-16.	Keeping the labia separated keeps the urinary meatus from contact with skin folds that could contain organisms.
Use the final cotton ball to wipe centrally from above the urinary meatus toward the vagina as shown in Figure 21-17.	The final stroke completes the cleansing and removal of debris from around the urinary meatus.
Discard the forceps with the last cotton ball within the wrapper being used for soiled supplies.	Keeping soiled areas separate from sterile areas is one of the principles of asepsis.
With the sterile gloved hand, pick up the catheter approximately 3–4 in (7.5–10 cm) from its tip shown in Figure 21-18. Insert it into the meatus about 2–3 in (5–7.5 cm).	The female urethra is about 1½–2½ in (4–6.5 cm) in length. By advancing the catheter farther than this, the tip should be well within the bladder.

(continued)

Skill Procedure 21-4. Continued

Suggested Action	Reason for Action

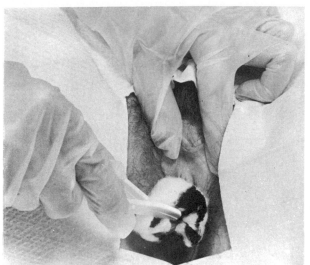

Figure 21-17 The stroke is completed in a straight line ending well beneath the meatus. One cotton ball is used for each stroke. The areas to the sides of the meatus are cleaned while keeping the labia separated.

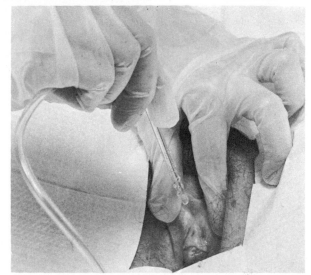

Figure 21-18 The catheter is inserted while the nurse continues to hold the labia apart.

Suggested Action	Reason for Action
Expect that urine will begin to flow when the catheter tip reaches the bladder.	If urine is in the bladder once the catheter passes the external and internal sphincters, it will drain out through the tubing.
Advance the catheter another ½–1 in (1.3–2.5 cm).	Inserting the catheter slightly farther ensures that the area of the balloon will be within the bladder rather than the urethra during inflation.
Place the outer end of the catheter within a compartment of the catheterization tray or into a sterile specimen container, shown in Figure 21-19, if it is not already connected to a drainage bag.	The bed may become wet with draining urine if the exposed end of the catheter is not in a receptacle.
Reposition the nondominant hand so as to stabilize the inserted catheter.	Once the catheter is in the bladder, retraction of the labia can be discontinued.
Use the sterile gloved hand to pick up the prefilled syringe and inflate the balloon of the catheter.	The balloon keeps the catheter retained within the bladder.
Withdraw the fluid from the balloon if the patient describes any feelings of pain or discomfort.	Incorrectly inflating the balloon while it is still in the urethra can injure the tissue.
Tug gently on the catheter after the balloon has been filled.	Applying slight tension will indicate if the catheter is well anchored in the bladder.
Connect the catheter to a urine collection bag.	Urine forms continuously and will need to be collected while it drains.
Wipe the urethra of any excess residual lubricant.	Cleaning the skin indicates a concern for the patient's comfort and dignity.
Remove gloves.	Gloves are no longer needed once the catheter has been inserted.
Follow the suggestions for anchoring the catheter and attaching the drainage bag to the bed as described later in the text.	Attaching the catheter to the skin prevents pulling on the balloon. The placement of the drainage bag should facilitate the gravity flow of urine.

(continued)

Skill Procedure 21-4. Continued

Suggested Action	Reason for Action

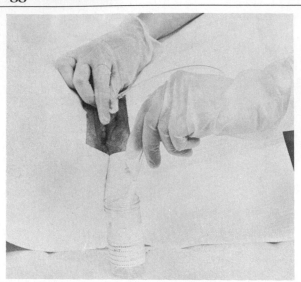

Figure 21-19 Once the urine is flowing, the nurse may allow the nondominant hand to hold the catheter securely in place while directing the urine into a sterile specimen container or the receptacle holding the catheterization equipment.

Suggested Action	Reason for Action
Remove the catheterization tray and make the patient comfortable in bed.	The nurse should restore the room to its original order.
Replace the bed to a low position.	The potential for injury is less with the bed in a low rather than high position.
Wash hands.	Handwashing should be performed after completing the care of a patient.
Record the time of the catheterization, the amount of urine removed, a description of the urine, and the patient's response to the procedure.	An accurate record is important for documenting and evaluating the patient's care.

Skill Procedure 21-5. Inserting an Indwelling Catheter in the Male Patient

Suggested Action	Reason for Action
Explain the procedure to the patient.	An explanation reduces anxiety and promotes cooperation.
Gather the following equipment: catheterization kit, cotton bath blanket, and drainage bag if it is not contained within the kit.	Organization promotes efficient time management.
Raise the bed to a high position.	Back strain and fatigue are reduced when the nurse does not bend from the waist while performing the procedure.
Pull the privacy curtains around the bed.	The patient has a right to be protected form the view of others during care.
Position the patient in a supine position.	Adequate visualization of the male urinary meatus can be obtained when the patient is flat with his legs together.

(continued)

Skill Procedure 21-5. Continued

Suggested Action	Reason for Action
Cover the patient with a bath blanket. Fold the linen to the foot of the bed.	Covering the patient shows concern for his modesty.
If the patient is soiled, wash the penis, scrotum, and perianal area with soap and water, and rinse and dry.	Cleansing removes large numbers of organisms that could contribute to postcatheterization infection.
Don clean gloves if any bloody drainage is present.	Gloves act as a barrier against bloodborne viruses.
Wash hands.	Handwashing reduces the spread of microorganisms.
Expose the genital area from beneath the bath blanket.	Exposing the patient is never done until it is necessary.
Remove the wrapper from the catheterization tray. Open and position the wrapper so it can hold soiled supplies.	Depositing used supplies helps maintain the sterility of the remaining equipment and controls the transmission of microorganisms.
Open the sterile wrap surrounding the catheterization tray as described in Chapter 16.	The sterile inner wrapper protects the contents from contamination.
Don sterile gloves contained within the catheterization tray as described in Chapter 16.	Using sterile gloves maintains the sterility of the other supplies within the kit.
Remove one sterile drape from the tray and unfold it without touching any unsterile surface. Place the towel over the thighs of the patient. Place the drape with the circular opening over the penis.	The drapes provide a sterile working area.
Pour the antiseptic over the cotton balls.	All preparation of the equipment that involves two hands must be done before touching the penis with a gloved hand.
Test the catheter balloon by instilling fluid from the prefilled syringe. Aspirate the fluid back into the syringe.	Prefilling the balloon is a way to determine that the balloon is not defective before it is inserted.
Spread lubricant over 6–7 in (15–18 cm) of the catheter.	Lubrication eases insertion. The male urethra is longer and the length of lubrication reflects this.
Place the catheter tray beside or on top of the sterile drape covering the patient's thighs.	An accessible tray prevents accidental contamination.
Lift the penis with the nondominant hand and retract the foreskin if the patient is uncircumcised.	The urinary meatus is the only opening in the penis. Retracting the foreskin helps in visualization.
Consider the gloved hand that holds the penis to be contaminated.	When something sterile touches a nonsterile area, it becomes contaminated.
Pick up a saturated cotton ball with the forceps as shown in Figure 21-20, and swab the penis in a circular manner from the meatus toward the base of the penis. Repeat using separate cotton balls.	Debris and organisms should be removed away from the direction of the meatus to decrease the potential for infection.
Deposit each used cotton ball within the plastic outer wrapper. After the final cleansing, the forceps may be discarded also.	Once cotton balls have been used for cleansing they should be contained and separated from the remaining sterile supplies.
Apply gentle traction pulling the penis straight up with the contaminated gloved hand.	Holding the penis in this manner helps to straighten the urethra.
Pick up the lubricated catheter with the sterile gloved hand and insert the catheter 6–8 in (15–20 cm) as shown in Figure 21-21.	The male urethra is longer and the catheter must be inserted farther than in a female before it reaches the bladder.
Do not force or push the catheter through the urethra. To facilitate the passage, ask the patient to breathe deeply; then rotate the catheter slightly. As an alternative, exert a bit more traction on the penis or lower the penis a bit toward the toes as shown in Figure 21-22.	Applying force can cause injury. Deep breathing and positioning techniques may help relax muscles sufficiently to facilitate catheter insertion.

(continued)

Skill Procedure 21-5. Continued

Suggested Action	Reason for Action

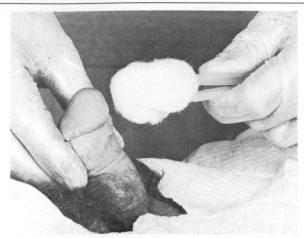

Figure 21-20 The penis is cleaned with cotton balls saturated with antiseptic, using a circular motion. The cleaning starts at the meatus.

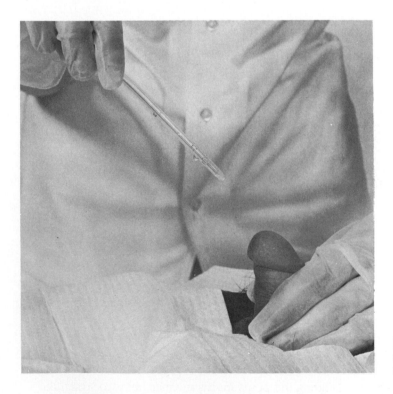

Figure 21-21 Notice that the nurse holds the penis on either side to position it straight up. With the meatus opened and well exposed, the catheter can be inserted.

Discontinue the procedure if the male has unusual discomfort or if there is continued resistance during insertion. Report the information promptly.

Expect that urine will begin to flow when the catheter tip reaches the bladder.

Continued resistance may be due to an enlarged prostate gland constricting the urethra. The bladder may need to be drained using a suprapubic catheter.

If the bladder contains urine it will drain out through the tubing once the catheter passes the external and internal sphincters.

(continued)

Skill Procedure 21-5. Continued

Suggested Action	**Reason for Action**

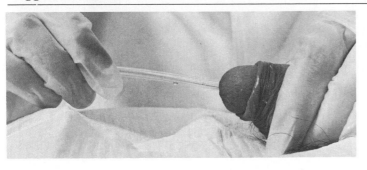

Figure 21-22 If the catheter meets mild resistance when it reaches the area of the prostate gland, lowering the penis often helps the catheter to be passed.

Suggested Action	**Reason for Action**
Advance the catheter another ½–1 in (1.3–2.5 cm).	Inserting the catheter slightly farther ensures that the balloon will be within the bladder rather than the urethra during inflation.
Place the exposed end of the catheter within a compartment of the catheterization tray or into a sterile specimen container if it is not already preconnected to a urine collection bag.	The bed may become wet with draining urine if the end of the catheter is not in a receptacle.
Reposition the nondominant hand to stabilize the catheter at the tip of the meatus.	Once the catheter is draining urine, traction on the penis can be relaxed.
Use the dominant hand to pick up the prefilled syringe and inflate the balloon.	The balloon keeps the catheter retained within the bladder.
Withdraw the fluid from the balloon if the patient describes any feelings of pain or discomfort.	Incorrectly inflating the balloon while it is still in the urethra can injure the tissue.
Tug gently on the catheter after the balloon has been filled.	Applying slight tension will indicate if the catheter is well anchored in the bladder.
Connect the catheter to a urine collection bag.	Urine forms continuously and will need to be collected while it drains.
Wipe the urethra of any excess residual lubricant.	Cleaning the skin indicates a concern for the patient's comfort and dignity.
Remove gloves.	Gloves are no longer needed once the catheter has been inserted.
Follow the suggestions for anchoring the catheter and attaching the drainage bag to the bed as described in the text.	Attaching the catheter to the skin prevents pulling on the balloon. The placement of the drainage bag should facilitate gravity flow of urine.
Remove the catheterization tray and make the patient comfortable in bed. Replace the bed to a low position.	The nurse should restore the cleanliness, safety, and comfort of the patient.
Wash hands.	Handwashing should be done after completing the care of a patient.
Record the time of the catheterization, the amount of urine removed, a description of the urine, and the patient's response to the procedure.	An accurate record is important to document and evaluate the patient's care.

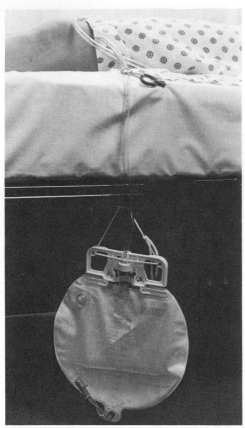

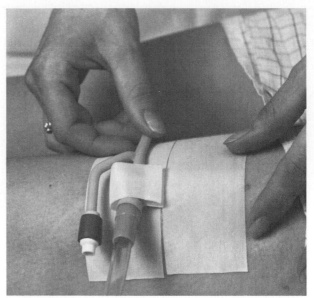

Figure 21-24 The nurse is securing an indwelling catheter on a woman's leg. The securing device is Cath-Secure, a disposable product that eliminates the use of repeated applications of adhesive. There is no chance of constriction or of contamination because the device cannot slide past the catheter lumen. A similar device for securing a catheter could be made with strips of adhesive. (Courtesy of the MC Johnson Company, Inc., Leominster, MA.)

Figure 21-23 In a closed urinary drainage system, the collection bag is attached to the bedframe below the level of the bladder. The tubing coils on the bed but hangs straight into the bag to promote gravity drainage.

on the collection bag that indicate the volume of drained urine. This helps in the routine assessment of urine. A port at the bottom of the drainage bag permits urine to be emptied without separating the connection between the catheter and the drainage tubing—hence the name closed drainage system. A *port* is an opening for instilling or removing fluid; some ports are self-sealing. To further avoid the need for separation, the drainage system may also contain a special port through which specimens may be taken or irrigations may be instilled.

To reduce the potential that the collection device will become a reservoir of pathogens, the entire drainage system is changed when the patient's catheter is changed. It may be changed more frequently, but care must be taken that the end of the catheter is not contaminated when the connection is separated.

Stabilizing the Catheter

A catheter that is not stabilized may pull on the internal sphincter, causing discomfort. Securing the catheter to the skin will prevent this from occurring.

For women the tubing should be anchored to the upper thigh, as illustrated in Figure 21-24. This prevents the

patient from lying on the tubing, yet allows freedom of movement without any pull on the catheter. For the male patient, the tubing can be secured in one of two ways. Both are illustrated in Figure 21-25. These methods of stabilizing the catheter for a male eliminate the pressure and irritation at the angle between the lower part of the penis and the scrotum.

Managing an Indwelling Catheter

Once a retention catheter has been inserted, the nurse is responsible for its daily care and maintenance. Special assessments and skills may be used to maintain its drainage and reduce the possibility of an infection. Skill Procedure 21-6 describes the actions that may be used to manage an indwelling catheter.

Irrigating an Indwelling Catheter. A catheter that drains well usually does not have to be irrigated. The usual purpose of an irrigation is to remove particles that are interfering with the drainage of urine. If the patient has a generous fluid intake (up to 2500 mL to 3000 mL daily), urine production increases and particles that may be present in urine become diluted. The catheter is irrigated naturally, avoiding any further invasive procedure.

Irrigating an indwelling catheter is sometimes necessary, however, to keep the catheter free of debris. Blood clots and mucus are especially likely to plug the catheter. A physician's order is necessary for a catheter irrigation in

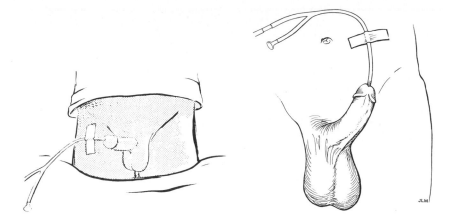

Figure 21-25 These two drawings illustrate acceptable methods for anchoring an indwelling catheter in a male patient. Both eliminate pressure and irritation at the penoscrotal angle.

most instances. There are three possible methods to irrigate a catheter. They include using an open system, using a closed system, and using a three-way catheter.

Using an Open System. If a catheter is separated from its drainage system, there is a potential for contaminating the open ends. Opening the system contributes to the incidence of bladder infections in catheterized patients. Therefore, the nurse's aseptic technique must be impeccable. Because using an open system has the greatest poten-

tial of all three for transferring organisms into the urinary tract, it is the least desirable method for irrigating a catheter. The procedure for an open system irrigation is described in Skill Procedure 21-7.

Using a Closed System. The incidence of urinary tract infections can be reduced by maintaining an intact system between the catheter and the drainage system. Catheters are now being made with a self-sealing port. The port

(Text continues on page 530)

Skill Procedure 21-6. Managing an Indwelling Catheter

Suggested Action	Reason for Action
Always perform handwashing when beginning care of a patient or after contact with heavy soiling.	Hands that contain organisms are one of the chief routes by which pathogens are spread.
Maintain a confident and reassuring attitude when caring for the patient. Handle equipment gently.	Most patients are fearful of having an indwelling catheter and may become upset if they think the nurse is unfamiliar with equipment.
Clean the perineal area, especially around the meatus, thoroughly at least two times a day and after each bowel movement.	Keeping the perineal area immaculately clean helps prevent organisms from entering the urinary system.
Use soap and water to clean the perineal area and rinse well. Many authorities recommend cleaning with an antiseptic, povidone iodine (Betadine) being a common one.	Thorough cleanliness and inhibition of bacterial growth around the meatus help prevent a urinary tract infection.
Use a separate area of the washcloth for each stroke, as described for inserting the catheter.	Cleansing from an area of less contamination to one that is greater prevents the transfer of organisms.
Avoid using powders or lotions after cleaning.	Powders and lotions are likely to trap and retain organisms.
Provide a generous fluid intake; 2500 to 3000 mL daily is an appropriate amount for most patients.	A generous fluid intake keeps urine diluted and free flowing. The prompt drainage of urine acts as a natural irrigation, preventing obstruction and infection.
Keep the tubing intact and free of kinks.	Any separation can provide an opportunity for contamination. The tubing should remain open and drain without interference.

(continued)

Skill Procedure 21-6. Continued

Suggested Action	**Reason for Action**
Encourage the patient to be up and about as ordered. The collection container may be carried as illustrated in Figure 21-26.	Encouraging ambulation helps prevent complications due to immobility and promotes feelings of independence and well-being.

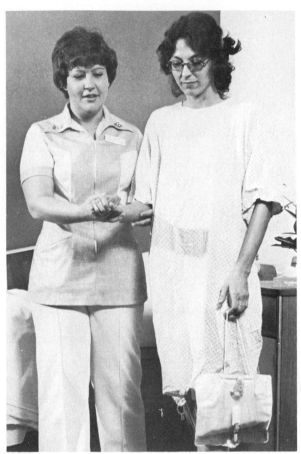

Figure 21-26 The patient is able to walk about while carrying the urine collection receptacle. Notice that the bag is held at a level lower than the bladder.

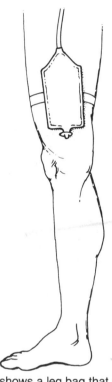

Figure 21-27 This shows a leg bag that can be worn when a patient has an indwelling catheter. It may also be used with an external catheter. This device allows an individual, male or female, to dress in usual clothing, while disguising that a catheter is draining.

Instruct the patient on the use of a drainage bag attached to the leg. This appliance is especially handy when the patient is ambulating, and it is concealed well within normal clothing. A leg bag is illustrated in Figure 21-27.	Being able to ambulate and dress normally promotes feelings of independence and self-esteem.
Note the volume and characteristics of the urine regularly and record the observations. The urine can be observed through the transparent tubing and the collecting container, as shown in Figure 21-28.	Observing urinary output and characteristics of the urine aids early detection of signs of complications. Document assessments at least every 8 hours, though observations can be made more frequently.
Empty and measure the accumulated urine as the nurse in Figure 21-29 is doing. Usually this is done every 8 hours.	Removing urine periodically without separating connections minimizes the risk of introducing pathogens into the urinary tract.

(continued)

Skill Procedure 21-6. Continued

Suggested Action	Reason for Action

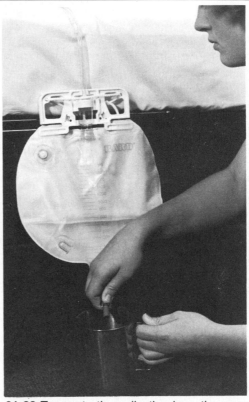

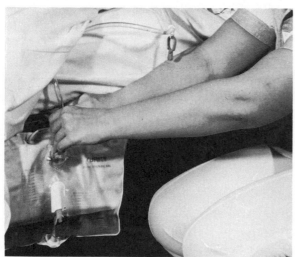

Figure 21-28 The nurse can examine the appearance of the urine through the transparent tubing and collecting bag.

Figure 21-29 To empty the collecting bag, the nurse opens the port at the bottom. This permits all the connections between the drainage device and the catheter to remain closed, yet permits the nurse to measure and dispose of accumulated urine.

Report any indications of possible problems. These may include a burning sensation and irritation at the meatus, leaking of urine around the catheter, cloudy urine, a strong odor, an elevated temperature, and chills. Also note whether the skin remains in good condition at the site where tubing is attached to it.

Reporting facilitates implementing measures that may prevent or treat early complications associated with an indwelling catheter. The nurse is held accountable for responsible care and safety of the patient.

Promote the acidity of urine. Cranberry juice and other food sources of ascorbic acid and vitamin C are usually used.

Keeping the urine acidic helps ward off bacterial growth.

Arrange for the patient to take a tub bath or shower when permitted. The catheter should be clamped temporarily if the collecting container is higher than the bladder. In a tub, the container may be hung over the side of the tub with the catheter clamped. In the shower, the collection container may be emptied and attached to the leg. Clamping is then usually unnecessary.

Using the tub or shower for personal hygiene promotes cleanliness, which, in turn, helps prevent infection. Self-care develops feelings of independence and well-being.

Teach the patient how the system works and how it is cared for.

A well-educated patient can help reduce complications by maintaining a well-functioning drainage system.

(*continued*)

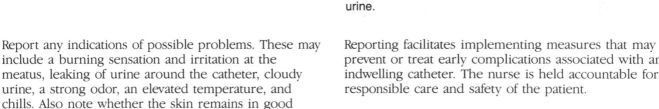

Skill Procedure 21-6. *Continued*

Suggested Action	Reason for Action
Plan on changing an indwelling catheter as necessary or as specified by agency policy. One indication that the tubing needs to be changed is that sandy particles are freed when the tubing is rolled between the thumb and fingers.	Any time an invasive procedure is performed, there is a risk of introducing pathogens. There should be an adequate reason for its change. The usual length of time between the need for catheter changes varies from 5 days to 2 weeks.
Use the following to predict the time when the next catheter change should take place. If there is crusting at the top of the catheter when it is removed, the catheter needs changing. When crusting is not present, subsequent catheters may remain in place a few days longer.	Crusting is an indication that substances in the urine are crystallizing and forming sediment. If this accumulates, it can interfere with the flow of urine. As long as no crusting is noted, it can be assumed that the catheter is functioning well and others could continue in that condition for an additional period of time.

Skill Procedure 21-7. *Irrigating an Indwelling Catheter Using an Open System*

Suggested Action	Reason for Action
Gather sterile equipment: an asepto syringe, basin, tubing protector, and gauze moistened with antiseptic. Sterile normal saline is used as an irrigating solution unless otherwise specified.	The urinary bladder is a sterile cavity. Sterile equipment and techniques must be used to prevent infection.
Clean the area where the catheter and tubing join with antiseptic, as the nurse in Figure 21-30 is doing, and disconnect the catheter and tubing.	Wiping the immediate area of the connection removes organisms from the surface.

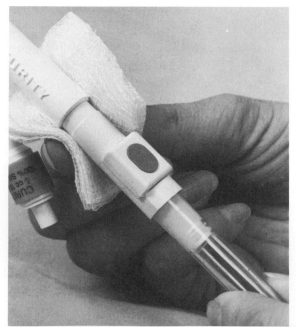

Figure 21-30 The nurse wipes the area where the catheter and the drainage tubing will be separated for irrigating purposes with sterile gauze moistened with antiseptic solution.

(continued)

Skill Procedure 21-7. Continued

Suggested Action	**Reason for Action**

Protect the separated end of the tubing with the protector, as shown in Figure 21-31. Another method would be to cover the opening with sterile gauze moistened with antiseptic. Take care to secure the gauze so it cannot accidentally slip off.

The collection system will be reconnected after irrigation. If the tip of the drainage tube has been contaminated, organisms will be introduced into the system when it is closed. The plastic guard or sterile gauze acts as a transmission barrier.

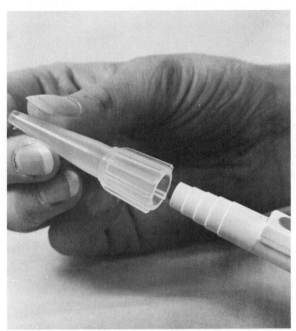

Figure 21-31 The nurse places a sterile cap on the end of the drainage tubing to protect it from contamination while irrigating the catheter. Some catheters are manufactured with a self-sealing port that provides a separate lumen through which irrigation solution may be instilled. This avoids having to open the closed system and reduces the possibility of contamination.

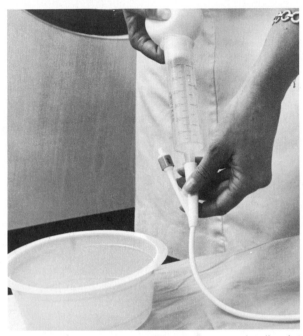

Figure 21-32 The nurse instills sterile normal saline into the catheter for irrigation. A sterile basin is ready to collect the solution, which will return by gravity once the syringe is removed.

Fill the syringe with 30 to 60 mL of solution and insert the syringe tip well into the end of the catheter.

A closely fitting connection allows fluid to move through the catheter rather than leak onto bed linen or the patient.

Gently compress the ball of the syringe to instill the irrigating solution, as shown in Figure 21-32.

The flow of fluid helps to dilute and free sediment or debris within the lumen of the catheter.

Do not apply force. Remove and replace the catheter if it cannot be irrigated.

Using a great deal of pressure may injure tissue or cause the solution to leak from the connection.

Remove the syringe when it is empty of the solution.

Suction should be avoided because the mucosa of the bladder is easily injured. Removing the syringe breaks the vacuum suction.

Allow the instilled solution to flow back by gravity into the basin. The catheter may be milked by holding and stretching sections of the catheter between the thumb and forefinger. Milk the catheter in a direction away from the bladder toward the open end of the catheter.

Milking creates slight negative pressure that facilitates the breakup of sediment that allows free drainage. Milking away from the bladder prevents debris from being forced back into the bladder.

(continued)

Skill Procedure 21-7. *Continued*

Suggested Action	Reason for Action
Connect the catheter and drainage tubing and assess for the drainage of urine into the collecting bag.	The urine should once again drain naturally by gravity.
Note the total amount of solution used for irrigating and measure the amount of solution returned in the basin.	The difference in these two amounts indicates the amount of urine that drained with the irrigating solution. In some cases there is less drainage than solution instilled. The amount that remains will eventually drain into the collection bag.
Record the fluid amounts accurately if a record is being kept. The total amount of fluid instilled is listed as intake; the solution drained is output.	When fluid balance is being assessed, both amounts must be recorded. Any amount that did not immediately drain will be calculated as output when the urine in the collecting bag is measured.
Discard the solution that has drained into the basin.	The nurse is responsible for keeping the environment clean.
Replace or protect the irrigating equipment, depending on the frequency of irrigation.	Sterile equipment that has been opened may become accidentally contaminated. Unless the nurse can be assured of its sterile condition, it should not be reused.
Record the irrigation according to agency policy.	Documentation provides a record of care and the patient's response so that evaluation can objectively take place.

avoids having to open the system for the purposes of irrigation or obtaining a sterile urine specimen. To irrigate a catheter with an access port, the nurse should:

- Perform appropriate handwashing.
- Fill a 30-mL to 50-mL syringe with irrigating solution, such as sterile normal saline.
- Attach an 18- or 19-gauge 1½-inch needle to the syringe.
- Cleanse the access port with an alcohol swab.
- Remove the cap from the needle.
- Puncture the port at approximately a 45° angle until the bevel of the needle is within the lumen of the catheter.
- Kink or clamp the drainage tubing below the access port so that the solution will move toward the tip of the catheter and not into the drainage bag.
- Gradually instill the solution.

- Remove the needle from the port when the syringe is empty.
- Release the clamped drainage tubing.
- Observe the characteristics of the fluid as it drains through the clear tubing.
- Repeat if the catheter does not appear to drain well or if a large amount of debris is present in the drainage.
- Dispose of the uncapped needle and syringe in a puncture-resistant container.
- Wash hands when completing the care.
- Record the amount of solution used for the irrigation on the fluid intake record.
- Document the procedure, the results, and the response of the patient.

Using a Three-Way Catheter. A three-way catheter shown in Figure 21-33 is another example of a closed system. The catheter gets its name from the fact that its

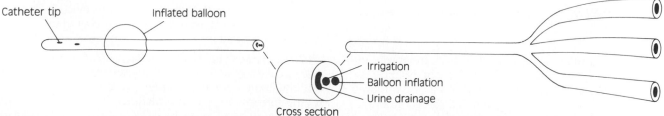

Figure 21-33 A three-way catheter is constructed so there are three distinct passages through the middle of the tubing. (Adapted from Timby BK: Clinical Nursing Procedures, p 512. Philadelphia, JB Lippincott, 1989)

external end has the two standard openings found on a Foley catheter, one for inflating the balloon and the other for drainage, plus a third opening that can be used to instill irrigating solution. Figure 21-34 shows the relationship and use of the openings on a three-way catheter.

A three-way catheter is used when the patient needs frequent intermittent or continuous bladder irrigations. A patient who has had bladder or prostate surgery is an example of a candidate for these types of irrigations. Skill Procedure 21-8 provides suggestions for providing an irrigation using a three-way catheter.

Removing an Indwelling Catheter. Catheters eventually must be removed either because their need no longer exists or because they require changing. The nurse usually removes the catheter. These techniques may be followed:

- Empty the balloon before removing the catheter. The balloon is emptied by inserting the barrel of a syringe and withdrawing the fluid that was used during balloon inflation.
- Gently pull on the catheter near the point where it exits from the meatus.
- Clean the perineum, following appropriate principles of medical asepsis.
- Inspect the catheter. Be sure it is intact. Report the situation promptly if that is not the case. Save the catheter for further inspection.
- Continue to assess the patient after an indwelling catheter is removed, focusing on the patterns of urinary elimination. The time and the amount of first voiding should be noted. Report any of the following: inability to void within 8 to 10 hours, frequency, burning, hesitation in starting the stream of urine, dribbling, cloudiness, or any other unusual color or characteristic of the urine.
- Provide a generous level of fluids similar to that when the catheter was in place.
- Record the time of catheter removal according to agency policy.

Urinary tract infections are one of the most common acquired infections. The invasive nature of a catheter is a logical explanation for this. The nurse can reduce accompanying risks by practicing principles of medical and surgical asepsis. This includes keeping the patient scrupulously clean, especially in the area of the meatus. Seeing to it that the patient has a generous fluid intake also cannot be overemphasized.

Teaching Self-Catheterization

Some patients who need frequent catheterization can learn to do so themselves. These persons usually have irreversible disease or injury conditions that interfere with bladder functioning. Intermittent catheterization has an advantage in that the catheter does not remain in place for very long at any one time. This reduces the high risk for infection.

Catheterizations that are performed in health agencies follow principles of surgical asepsis. Self-catheterization is done following principles of medical asepsis. Experience indicates that this is entirely safe.

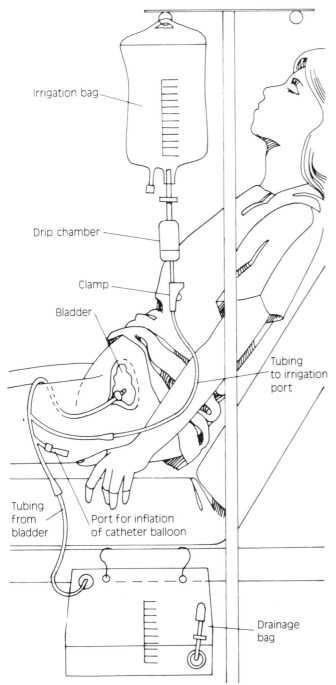

Irrigation bag

Drip chamber

Clamp

Bladder

Tubing to irrigation port

Tubing from bladder

Port for inflation of catheter balloon

Drainage bag

Figure 21-34 The irrigation solution infuses from the bag that hangs from the IV pole while fluid simultaneously drains from a port in the catheter. (Adapted from Timby BK: Clinical Nursing Procedures, p 512. Philadelphia, JB Lippincott, 1989)

Skill Procedure 21-8. Using a Three-Way Catheter for Irrigation

Suggested Action	**Reason for Action**
Explain the procedure to the patient.	An explanation reduces anxiety and promotes cooperation.
Assemble the following equipment: three-way catheter, catheterization kit, 1000- or 2000-mL bag of sterile irrigating solution, tubing for the irrigation solution, urine drainage bag if not included in the catheterization kit, and a clamp for the drainage tubing if irrigation is intermittent.	Organization promotes efficient time management.
Insert the catheter following the technique described in Skill Procedure 21-4 or 21-5.	A three-way catheter is usually inserted preoperatively or during an operative procedure. It may need to be changed postoperatively if it does not drain well.
Wash hands.	Handwashing reduces the spread of microorganisms.
Tighten the clamp on the empty tubing that will be used for delivering the irrigation solution.	Clamping the tubing prevents the solution from leaking when the tubing is inserted within the solution.
Remove the protective cap from the insertion spike on the tubing and the cover on the port of the irrigating solution without contaminating either of them.	The connecting areas are kept free of contamination to reduce the potential for infection.
Insert the spike within the solution and hang the solution from a hook or IV pole.	Hanging the solution permits the nurse to use both hands to prepare the equipment.
Squeeze the drip chamber on the solution until it is partially filled.	A partially filled drip chamber facilitates counting drops in order to regulate the rate of an instillation.
Unclamp the tubing and allow fluid to fill the empty tubing. Reclamp the tubing when all the air has been displaced.	Flushing the tubing prevents instilling air into the bladder.
Attach a piece of tape with the current date and time to the tubing.	Tubing must be replaced according to a scheduled routine established by the agency's infection control policy. Dating tubing identifies how long it has been in use.
Pull privacy curtains around the patient's bed.	The patient has a right to be protected from the observation of others.
Hang the irrigating solution from an IV pole or standard so that it is approximately 2½–3 feet above the level of the bladder.	A continuous or intermittent irrigation uses the principle of gravity.
Aseptically remove the cover on the free end of the irrigation tubing and insert it into the third port on the catheter.	All connections must be made without contaminating either opening.
Open the clamp on the irrigating tubing and regulate the rate of infusion if the irrigation will be continuous.	The physician prescribes the volume that is instilled over a period of time.
Refer to the manufacturer's instructions for the drop factor, the number of drops that equal 1 mL of solution.	The size of openings in drip chambers vary among tubing manufacturers. Therefore, the volume of a drop is not standard. Each manufacturer identifies its drop factor on the product wrapper.
For an intermittent irrigation, clamp the urinary drainage tubing below the area where it is inserted into the catheter.	Clamping allows the irrigating solution to be instilled before it is drained from the bladder.
Open the clamp on the irrigation tubing and allow the volume of solution prescribed by the physician to be instilled. Reclamp.	Intermittent irrigations are instilled in a short amount of time.

(continued)

Skill Procedure 21-8. Continued

Suggested Action	Reason for Action
Release the clamp on the drainage tubing.	The urine and irrigating solution will drain by gravity.
Record the volume of instilled solution on the fluid intake record.	The drainage bag will collect both urine and irrigation solution. The exact amount of urine is determined by subtracting the volume instilled from the total drainage.
Repeat the instillation of irrigation solution at the prescribed intervals.	Irrigation is followed by periods of drainage.
Record the procedure, characteristics of drainage, and any subjective responses of the patient.	The nurses' notations document the care and the response of the patient to his care.

The procedure for self-catheterization is essentially the same as when a nurse inserts a straight catheter. The following are some differences and points to emphasize.

- It is important to stress that thorough handwashing must be performed before self-catheterization. The catheter should be washed well in soap or detergent and water, rinsed, dried, and stored in a clean covered container. Some authorities recommend that the catheter be boiled 20 minutes between uses. Although sterile technique is not used, the importance of cleanliness and other practices of medical asepsis are important to prevent infection.
- The patient who can void should be encouraged to do so first—and then use the catheter if there is concern that the bladder has not been emptied. This may help promote at least some control over voiding. Certain patients may not be able to void, and this step can be eliminated.
- A man will find a standing or sitting position convenient for self-catheterization. A woman most often sits on a toilet seat.
- A good light is important for adequate visualization of the meatus. This is more difficult for the female than the male. While learning this procedure, women find that using a mirror helps in locating the meatus. After the technique is well learned, a mirror may no longer be necessary.
- The perineal area is cleansed well with soap and water using cotton balls. The cotton balls are not sterile and the patient does not wear sterile gloves.
- The catheter is lubricated and inserted the appropriate distance, depending on the sex of the individual.
- The patient is taught Credé's maneuver to remove as much urine from the bladder as possible before withdrawing the catheter.
- When urine flow stops, the patient pinches the catheter and gently removes it. Pinching prevents leaking of urine that may be within the catheter.
- The frequency of self-catheterization varies. At first, it may be needed every few hours. Some patients even-

tually perform self-catheterization only every 8 to 12 hours. The time interval between catheterizations depends on the amount of urinary control the patient develops.
- Patients who self-catheterize should be taught the importance of maintaining the acidity of the urine as well as taking in a generous amount of fluids.

Eliminating Urine From a Surgical Opening

At times patients require surgery to restore or maintain urinary function. The elimination of urine may be altered in some manner. Temporarily, the surgeon may insert a catheter directly through the skin into the bladder or into the kidney. The patient may eliminate urine through the catheter as well as from the urethra. The characteristics and amounts of urine are assessed separately.

Another possible alternative for urine elimination occurs when permanent reconstruction must be done. This happens most frequently when the bladder is diseased and must be removed. The surgical technique is called a urinary diversion. A *urinary diversion* is a procedure in which the ureters are surgically implanted elsewhere. They may be brought through an opening in the abdominal wall onto the skin of the abdomen. There are other surgical variations as well. An artificial opening is called a *stoma*. A urinary stoma excretes urine.

Caring for this type of patient presents many physical, emotional, psychological, social, and spiritual challenges for the nurse. A means must be provided for collecting the urine that no longer is stored and released from the bladder. It is also necessary to care for the skin around the new surgical opening; it was never designed to be in constant contact with urine. These patients are often faced with life-threatening diagnoses; they question the meaning of life and death in a highly personal way. The changes in body image can affect the patient and others with whom he shares a close relationship.

Caring for a Urinary Stoma

Though the patient with a urinary diversion is at high risk for many problems, the focus of this discussion will center on the care that is related to urine elimination. A patient with a stoma wears an appliance. An *appliance* is a plastic collecting bag. It has an opening that fits around the stoma and is attached to the skin with a special adhesive, as shown in Figure 21-35. The patient may wear a belt or use paper tape to hold the appliance in place. There can be a great deal of stress on the skin as the appliance becomes heavy with the weight of urine.

Some appliances have an opening at the bottom, to which drainage tubing can be attached. This permits drainage from the appliance during night hours. It eliminates the need for the patient to empty his collecting bag during sleeping hours.

Nursing measures for a patient with a urinary appliance include the following:

- Make sure that the opening fits the stoma. The stoma can be measured with a special tool, shown in Figure 21-36. There should be only about 1/16 to 1/8 of an inch of skin exposed around it. The less skin that is exposed, the less likely skin irritation around the stoma will be. The tissue of the stoma may be damaged if the opening is too small.
- Use a specially designed skin adhesive to attach the appliance to the skin around the stoma. A solvent is used to remove the adhesive when the appliance is changed. This reduces abrasion of the skin.
- Empty the collecting bag when it is one-third to one-half full. Urine can drain through a port provided for this purpose. This reduces stress on the skin and avoids removing the entire appliance each time urine accumulates.
- Change the appliance only when it becomes loose or uncomfortable. As long as the skin and the stoma are unaffected, and the urine is draining well, frequent changing can lead to unnecessary trauma to the skin.
- When the appliance is changed, try to do so in the morning shortly after awakening. Urinary output is normally low at this time of the day. Changing is easier

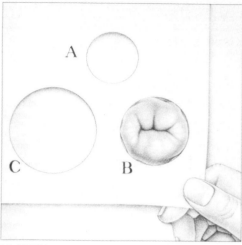

Figure 21-36 This stoma measuring card helps determine the size of the appliance that fits best. Accurate fit reduces injury to the skin and stoma, promoting extended comfort while the appliance is in place. (Courtesy of Hollister Inc, Libertyville, IL.)

when urine is not dripping in high amounts onto the skin.

- Insert a tampon a short distance into the stoma or place a folded, sterile gauze square into the stoma when changing the appliance. This absorbs urine and helps keep the area dry so the adhesive will attach well.
- Clean a reusable bag with soap or detergent and hot water. Rinse well. A half-strength solution of white vinegar or household bleach may be used for soaking the appliance in order to control odors. Commercial liquid deodorants instilled directly within the appliance are also available. Airing and exposing the appliance to sunlight may also help reduce odors.
- Keep the skin dry and clean around the stoma. Antibiotic or steroid creams may become necessary if skin irritation occurs.
- Describe specific care techniques that have been successful on the nursing care plan. This ensures continuity of care is provided by other nurses.
- Be sure the patient has a generous fluid intake, at least 2000 mL or more daily. This helps keep urine diluted and freeflowing, and it removes organisms and debris that may accumulate in the urine or around the stoma.
- Help the patient adjust his diet. For some patients, a diet with minimal amounts of certain minerals (e.g., calcium) is recommended to help prevent the formation of kidney stones. Asparagus is discouraged because it causes the urine to have a strong odor. Consuming foods high in vitamin C helps control infection because they keep the urine acidic.
- Be sure the patient understands how his urinary diversion works and what care it needs. A well-educated

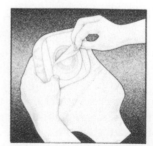

Figure 21-35 Removing the protective cover exposes an adhesive patch on an appliance. The center ring fits over the stoma. (Courtesy of Hollister Inc, Libertyville, IL.)

patient can learn to resume normal living and to care for himself safely and efficiently.

- Encourage the patient to return to his normal way of living. Clothing conceals the appliance well. Some patients benefit from visits with others who have had a similar operation.
- Consult with other health personnel who have expertise in stoma care when perplexing problems occur.

Obtaining Urine Specimens

Urine can be tested for a great many substances. The general laboratory study of urine is called a *urinalysis*. It can provide a great deal of information about the condition of the patient. The nurse may obtain and examine a sample of urine from time to time. Various techniques may be used to obtain a specimen for urinalysis. These include collecting a specimen directly from the patient as he voids it from a catheter or stoma. The skill and judgment that the nurse uses in collecting the specimen can affect the results of the analysis.

Collecting a Voided Specimen

A voided specimen is obtained by assisting a patient to a toilet or using a bedpan or urinal. The urine is voided either directly into the container or into the bedpan or urinal. Some of the urine is then poured into the specimen container. Toilet tissue should be discarded. Paper within the specimen makes urine difficult to examine. The container is properly labeled and sent to the laboratory. A note should be made if the urine contains menstrual blood. Misinterpreting that the blood is from the urinary tract can result in an inaccurate medical or nursing diagnosis.

Specimens of urine should not be allowed to stand at room temperature before they are sent to the laboratory. Bacterial growth is likely to occur as well as alter other results of the urinalysis. The usual procedure is to store a urine specimen in a refrigerator if it is not taken directly to the laboratory. Specimens that are collected from multiple voidings are either refrigerated on the nursing unit or placed in a container with a chemical preservative.

Collecting a Clean-Catch Midstream Specimen

A *clean-catch midstream specimen* is a voided specimen collected under conditions of thorough cleanliness after approximately the first 30 mL of urine have been voided. The advantage in collecting a voided specimen in this manner is that if organisms appear in the urine, they are most likely from structures such as the bladder or kidneys rather than just surface contamination. Cleansing removes organisms from the urinary meatus. Voiding moves any residual organisms present in the urethra out with the beginning stream of urine. This principle was similarly applied when a small amount of sterile solution was wasted before it was added to a sterile container, as described in Chapter 16. Catching the midstream specimen as it flows out of cleaned structures provides a more accurate analysis regarding the presence of organisms. Techniques for obtaining this type of specimen are described in Skill Procedure 21-9. Due to anatomical differences, the cleansing techniques differ somewhat, depending on whether the patient is male or female.

Collecting a 24-Hour Specimen

Some tests require that the entire volume of urine from a 24-hour period be collected. The procedure for ensuring that the test can be performed accurately is as follows:

- Instruct the patient about the importance of collecting *all* urine for a period of 24 hours.
- Have the patient void just prior to beginning the collection.
- Discard this urine because it has been formed in the urinary system before the study began.
- Add a preservative of the agency's choice to the specimen container and keep the specimen cool to decrease decomposition and odor of the urine.
- Save *all* urine for the 24-hour period; place each voided specimen into the larger container with preservative.
- Have the patient void at the exact time that the specimen collection ends. Include it with all the other collected urine. This urine completes the total produced within the urinary system during the previous 24 hours.

Obtaining a Specimen From a Catheter

A sterile specimen can be taken from a catheter at the time it is inserted. Some modifications must be made if the catheter has been in place for some time.

Obtaining a sample of urine from a drainage bag that has held accumulating urine for several hours or longer is not considered the best technique for an accurate analysis. The urine in the collecting bag is not fresh; therefore, this technique is not recommended. Separating the collecting tubing from the catheter could be done. However, a separation in a closed system increases the risk of introducing organisms. Pathogens may then travel through the tubing to the urethra and even possibly to the bladder, where an infection can occur.

The best technique for obtaining a fresh, sterile specimen from a catheter is the following:

- Clamp between the catheter and the drainage tubing, if it is not contraindicated, for approximately 15 minutes before collecting the specimen. This ensures that there will be a sufficient quantity of urine available for the specimen. A minimum of 15 mL should be collected for a urinalysis.

Skill Procedure 21-9. Collecting a Clean-Catch Midstream Specimen

Suggested action	Reason for Action
Gather equipment: cotton balls, antiseptic of the agency's choice, and a sterile specimen container. Gloves may be used if the patient cannot collect the specimen.	Following proper cleansing and collection techniques, the sample of urine is considered a sterile specimen.
Assist the patient to the bathroom or have a clean bedpan or urinal handy.	Some of the urine must be voided before it is collected.
Position the patient either on the toilet with the legs well spread or in a manner in which cleansing the urinary meatus can be performed prior to voiding.	The labia and urinary meatus of a female are best cleansed in this position. A male patient may stand or lie on his back.
Separate the labia well on a female patient, or retract the foreskin of an uncircumsized male.	Organisms are present in the tissue around the urinary meatus. By holding the tissue away from the meatus, contamination of the specimen is prevented.
Clean the area at and around the meatus in the manner described for catheterization. Use each antiseptic-saturated cotton ball once. Cleanse away from the meatus.	Precautions are used to prevent infection and to prevent organisms at and near the meatus from being washed into the specimen. This cleansing technique prevents bringing organisms to the meatus.
Have the patient void about 30 mL into the toilet, bedpan, or urinal while continuing to hold the labia apart or the foreskin in a position of retraction.	The first voided 30 mL of urine are discarded. It is expected that any organisms still located at the meatus will have been flushed away. If the labia or the foreskin fall back into place, the area at the meatus becomes contaminated.
Hold the specimen container so that the edges of the opening are not touched.	Washing is a good medical aseptic technique; however, all organisms are not removed. The specimen container should not be contaminated with these organisms.
Catch some of the urine in the container as it is being voided.	A sample of the urine released midway during voiding constitutes the specimen.
Allow the labia or the foreskin to fall back into place.	It is no longer necessary to position this tissue away from the meatus.
Instruct the patient to continue voiding into the toilet, bedpan, or urinal until the bladder is emptied.	It is unnecessary to fill the entire specimen container. Any urine remaining in the bladder after the specimen is collected can be voided and discarded.
Label the laboratory slip identifying that the urine was collected by the clean-catch midstream method and take it to the laboratory.	Urine should not be allowed to stand unrefrigerated once it has been collected.
Record on the patient's chart that the specimen was obtained and taken to the laboratory.	Written communication avoids duplication of work by documenting completed actions.

- Before the drainage system is entered, the *port*, a self-sealing access area, is cleaned thoroughly with an antimicrobial agent. This step is illustrated in Figure 21-37. Some catheters that do not contain a port must be entered through the catheter above its connection to the drainage tubing, as shown in Figure 21-38.
- A small sterile needle is inserted into the port of the catheter as shown in Figure 21-39. Urine will fill the syringe when the nurse pulls back on the plunger. The urine can be placed directly into a sterile specimen container.

Collecting a Specimen From a Stoma

If a urine specimen is needed from a patient with a stoma, two methods may be used. To obtain a fresh specimen, cleanse the area around the stoma. Hold the specimen container beneath the stoma and allow the urine to drip directly into it. Increasing the fluid intake just prior to the collection of urine is helpful when obtaining a specimen in this manner. Urine may also be collected from the appliance. Empty the urine from the appliance. Then hold the container beneath the drainage port. Since urine flows constantly from the stoma, it should not take long to collect

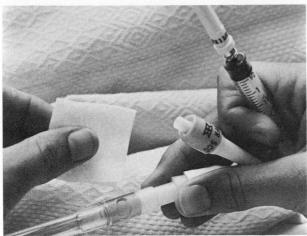

Figure 21-37 Before the closed urinary drainage system is entered to obtain a specimen, the area is thoroughly cleaned. This precaution helps decrease the chance of introducing organisms into the system.

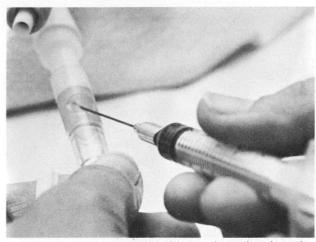

Figure 21-39 The needle is held at a slant when insertion is made through a port. A sterile 5-mL or larger syringe is used to aspirate the urine. The sample of collected urine is placed directly from the syringe into a sterile specimen container.

15 mL or more. This method avoids having to remove the appliance from the skin.

Performing Common Urine Tests

The nurse may on occasions perform certain urine tests to detect abnormal substances. This assessment is done to add to the database and provide current information about the patient's urinary function and overall state of health. These tests do not require the use of a microscope or complex methods of analysis. Performing the tests involves no additional cost to the patient. Therefore, the nurse may use independent judgment in determining when one of these tests should be performed. When they are performed on a routine basis, the order for testing is usually written by a physician.

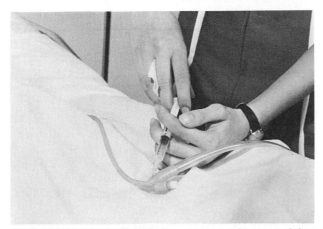

Figure 21-38 This catheter does not contain a special port through which specimens may be obtained. Instead, a small sterile needle, gauge 25, is introduced near the end of a catheter to withdraw approximately 15 mL for a urine specimen. The needle hole is so small that leakage will not occur.

The results of the test are recorded in the patient's record or on a flow sheet. They are not recorded on a laboratory form.

Testing for Sugar and Acetone

The nurse may test the patient's urine for its sugar and acetone content. If a patient is a newly diagnosed diabetic, the nurse may teach the patient urine testing before discharge. More and more diabetics, however, are learning to perform home blood testing. This method provides more accurate information about the level of glucose within the body.

To ensure accuracy for urine testing, a second voided specimen is required. A *second voided specimen* involves having the patient empty his bladder about one-half hour before the test specimen will be obtained. This provides a specimen that contains substances from the most recent kidney filtration rather than reflecting what has been excreted over the past several hours or more. The test is usually performed before meals and at bedtime when the sugar content should be at its lowest. This allows the nurse or the patient to adjust food consumption or an insulin dosage.

Several types of commercial testing kits are available. Some require using a tablet. A tablet is dropped into a sample of urine and water to test for glucose, and a drop of urine is placed onto a tablet to test for acetone. After a recommended period of time, the color changes are compared with a chart provided by the manufacturer.

Others use a strip of treated paper, as illustrated in Figure 21-40. The strip is saturated with urine. Following a specified number of seconds, its color is compared with a color chart. The particular method for testing urine depends on the agency's choice.

Strips may also be available to test urine for other sub-

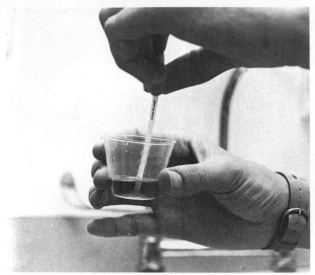
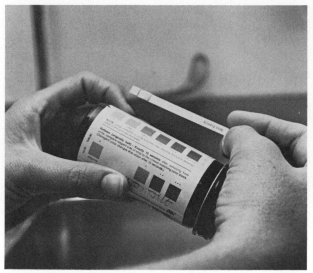

Figure 21-40 (*A*) The nurse places a specially treated strip into the urine. (*B*) After waiting the number of seconds specified by the manufacturer, the nurse compares the color of the strip with a color chart. This test measures sugar and acetone. Other strips measure other substances in urine. Be sure that the color chart and the testing materials are not outdated. Also, commercial kits vary in how they are used. Be careful not to confuse one manufacturer's materials with another's.

stances, such as albumin, blood, or bile. These tests are relatively simple and the manufacturer's instructions are easy to follow. However, accuracy is essential.

Testing for the Specific Gravity

A nurse often tests urine for its *specific gravity*. This test provides a measurement of the weight of urine as compared with the weight of water. The amount of dissolved substances in urine contributes to its higher weight. The more concentrated the urine, the higher its specific gravity will be; the more diluted, the lower its specific gravity will

be. The average normal range of specific gravity is between 1.005 and 1.025, although even wider ranges have been observed in some healthy persons.

A *urinometer* is an instrument used to measure the specific gravity of urine. Urine is placed in a cylindrical container. The calibrated urinometer, is placed in the urine. The more concentrated the urine, the higher the urinometer will rise in the urine. The reading on a urinometer should be taken at eye level, in this case at the bottom of the cup-shaped meniscus formed by the urine. This is illustrated in Figure 21-41.

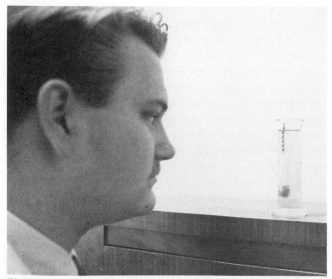

Figure 21-41 The nurse places a urinometer into a specimen of urine and reads the calibrated urinometer at eye level for an accurate determination of the urine's specific gravity.

Suggested Measures to Promote Urinary Elimination in Selected Situations

When the Patient Is an Infant or Child

Expect that characteristics of normal urine for an infant and child resemble those of an adult, except that the total amount voided in each 24-hour period is smaller. Despite the smaller amount, infants and children excrete more urine in proportion to body weight than adults. In general, the urine of infants and young children tends to be lighter in color than that of an adult.

Anticipate that voiding will occur at more frequent intervals for infants and children. A child will feel the need to urinate when about 100 to 150 mL of urine collects in the bladder. The bladder holds even less in toddlers and much less in infants.

To assess the control of urinary elimination, use the following information as a guide:

18 months old	An infant is usually aware of having a wet diaper.
2 years old	A toddler begins to cooperate with toilet training.
2½ years old	Daytime control of urinary elimination begins, although frequent accidents occur.
3 years old	Nighttime control of urinary elimination is possible for some, although accidents occur.

Expect that, despite having control at home, many children will lose this control when hospitalized. This is a reaction to the stress of being separated from a familiar environment. Regression to more infantile behavior can be considered normal unless other factors are present.

Perform a catheterization on an infant or child in a manner similar to an adult. Differences include the size of the catheter and the length it is inserted.

Obtain assistance from a parent or other staff person to immobilize the hands or body of a child who must be catheterized. The nurse will not have the ability to maintain sterile technique while trying to prevent the child from contaminating the equipment. A papoose board is often used if no other alternative is available.

Catheterization may seem similar to sexual assault to the child. It is helpful to have a parent present during the explanation and performance of this procedure.

With children who can cooperate, have them practice deep breathing exercises before catheterization. Deep breathing helps promote relaxation during the procedure.

Direct the catheter downward when catheterizing a young girl because the urethra hooks around the symphysis pubis somewhat like the letter C.

Use equipment of the agency's choice when collecting a urine specimen from an infant or young child who cannot cooperate. Most agencies have a plastic, disposable collection bag that contains an adhesive backing. It adheres to the perineal area. A diaper is placed over the collecting bag to prevent the child from dislodging it. Be sure that adhesive is applied to dry, clean skin. It has been found that for the male infant, it is easier when the penis and the scrotum are placed inside the collecting device. Some nurses use a finger cot over the penis of newborn males if a urine specimen is required.

Provide additional fluids that the child enjoys before collecting a urine specimen from children. This promotes urine production and often helps gain the child's cooperation.

When the Patient Is Pregnant or in the Early Postpartal Period

Expect that the characteristics of normal urine for a pregnant woman resemble those during nonpregnancy, except that the total amount voided in each 24-hour period increases and tends to have a lower specific gravity. Sugar in the urine during pregnancy is relatively common, but when present, the finding should be reported. Albumin in the urine is also a significant abnormal assessment to report.

Anticipate that a pregnant woman will void more frequently than usual when the enlarging uterus causes pressure on the bladder. This occurs early in pregnancy and continues until the uterus rises out of the pelvis and into the abdomen. It recurs late in pregnancy when, because of its size, the uterus again causes pressure on the bladder.

If a catheter is difficult to introduce into the bladder of a woman in labor, proceed slowly and gently and *never use force*. The difficulty is most probably due to the head of the fetus pressing on the lower bladder and urethra as the fetus descends through the birth canal.

Proceed with extreme care if a woman in the postpartum period requires catheterization. A good light is essential because the meatus may be diffi-

NURSING CARE PLAN

21-1. High Risk for Urge Incontinence

Assessment

Subjective Data

States, "I hope when this catheter comes out I don't wet myself again. I'd like to go home without wearing a leg bag or being connected to a drainage bag."

Objective Data

75-year-old woman admitted to long-term care facility for rehabilitation following repair of a fractured hip. Fracture occurred as a result of tripping on way to bathroom because of feeling an urgent need to void. Has had an indwelling catheter with continuous drainage for 4 weeks.

Diagnosis

High Risk for Urge Incontinence related to reduced bladder capacity secondary to prolonged insertion of an indwelling catheter.

Plan

Goal

The patient will be able to wait at least 3 hours between voidings without experiencing incontinence by 6/12.

Orders: 6/2

1. Before removing Foley catheter, perform bedside *cystometrogram* by instilling sterile water until the patient indicates feeling the need to void. Measure the volume instilled.
2. Remove the catheter and maintain a 3-day log of:
   - Time of each urination
   - Volume per voiding
   - Episodes of incontinence.
   - Cause of incontinence.
3. Maintain a total intake of approximately 2500 mL/day divided in the following amounts:
   - 1200 mL on day shift
   - 1200 mL on evening shift
   - 100 mL during the night.
4. When there is an urge to void, help patient to
   - Breathe deeply while waiting longer to void
   - Sing a song
   - Tell a story about her family as a distraction technique while proceeding to the toilet at a safe pace.
5. Praise every urinary elimination that occurs without incontinence. _ F. WISNIECKI, RN

Implementation (Documentation)

6/2   1000   Bedside cystometrogram performed. Felt an urge to void when 100 mL of sterile water was instilled through catheter. Reconnected to gravity drainage for 15 minutes and then catheter removed. Instructed to drink approximately one glass of fluid per hour. Explained the 3-day assessment log. Explored distraction techniques to avoid incontinence while increasing bladder capacity. _ N. ZAK, LPN

Evaluation (Documentation)

     2000   Feeling a need to void at approximately 2-hour intervals (see log for specifics). Has had two episodes of dribbling while getting onto toilet. Sings "Amazing Grace" as a distraction technique. States, "I was so hoping this wouldn't happen; I'm determined to avoid that catheter again." Praised for the two successful voidings without incontinence. Drinking fluids at scheduled intervals.

           _ S. BURKE, LPN

cult to find due to local swelling. Use care to avoid additional discomfort in the perineum.

When the Patient Is Elderly

Keep in mind that, the kidney's general level of function tends to decline with age. As a result, the system may have lost its earlier level of effectiveness in maintaining the fluid and chemical balance of the body.

Assess the urinary function of elderly patients accurately. The elderly are more prone to urinary problems due to alterations in bladder control or retention of urine. This is especially true of women who experience stress incontinence and males with an enlarged prostate gland.

Remember that urinary incontinence, a relatively common problem among the elderly, has profound psychological effects on the patient and his family. Unfortunately, in many instances, efforts to correct the situation are impossible. The best the nurse can offer in this situation is emotional support, care that minimizes dangers of complications, and physical comfort.

Expect that the incontinent elderly patient is often depressed and frustrated when there is little hope for bladder control. The shame of being unable to control urination may result in social isolation. Incontinent patients require the nurse's ingenuity in providing methods for maintaining the patient's lifestyle while disguising the loss of control.

Teaching Suggestions to Promote Urinary Elimination

Teaching opportunities are offered throughout the content of this chapter. Key points and additional information are summarized as follows:

Many people are unaware of how the urinary system operates. Sharing information with patients, especially those with alterations in urinary elimination, helps in gaining their cooperation and also helps them promote their own health and well-being.

Patients, too, should be familiar with the normal appearance of urine and with the relationship between fluid intake and urinary output. This ensures that they will recognize abnormal conditions and seek prompt health care when indicated.

Incontinent patients should be instructed that limiting fluid intake is a dangerous method to control urination. It may have an overall effect of altering the body's fluid and chemical balance, a more life-threatening condition than incontinence.

Nurses should develop detailed teaching plans for patients who will use self-catheterization, use an indwelling catheter after discharge from a health agency, or have a urinary diversion. Well-educated patients have fewer complications and enjoy physical and psychosocial well-being when they understand what has caused a problem, how it can be managed, and what self-care techniques are necessary to promote health.

Teach the family or patient to change the drainage tubing and collecting receptacle used with a catheter several times a week. The equipment can be washed thoroughly in hot, soapy water, rinsed well, and stored in a clean towel or covered container. Some prefer soaking the equipment in an antiseptic solution, but it should be rinsed well after soaking so that none of the antiseptic can reach the bladder.

Teach the patient with a stoma to be aware of weight gains or losses. This may change the size of the stoma and create an improperly fitting appliance. A decrease or increase of 5 to 10 lb may require refitting the external appliance.

Instruct the patient with a urinary diversion that sexual activity will not injure the stoma nor will pregnancy interfere with its functioning. The size of the stoma may change during pregnancy, but this may only involve a change in the size of an appliance and more frequent emptying.

Obtaining urine specimens and performing certain common tests can be carried out by most patients when they have been properly taught. Stress collecting the first voided specimen in the morning or a second voided specimen, depending on the purpose of the test. The patient may benefit from a set of written instructions for review at home.

Bibliography

Baer CL: Investigating dysuria. Nursing 19(5):108–110, 1989

Barker JC, Mitteness LS: Shedding light on nocturia. Geriatr Nurs 10(5):239–240, 1989

Brinsko V: It's in the bag. Journal of Urological Nursing 8(1):563–564, 1989

Bristoll SL, Fadden T, Fehring RJ, Rhode L, Smith PK, Wohlitz BA: The mythical danger of rapid urinary drainage. Am J Nurs 89(3):344–345, 1989

Does cranberry juice help in urinary infections? Nurses Drug Alert 12(11):87, 1988

Frank A, Murray SM: A no-guess guide for urinary color assessment. RN Magazine 51(6):46–47, 49, 51, 1988

Gurevich I: How to make every culture count. RN Magazine 51(8):49–55, 1988

Hahn K: Think twice about urinary incontinence. Nursing 18(1):65–67, 1988

Hough E: Effective management of urinary drainage systems in critical care areas. Intensive Care Nursing 5(2):82–87, 1989

Jenkins G: Clothed for continence. Geriatric Nursing Home Care 7(9):11–13, 1987

Lohr JA: The foreskin and urinary tract infections. J Pediatr 114(3):502–504, 1988

McCormick KA, Scheve AAS, Leahy E: Nursing management of urinary incontinence in geriatric inpatients. Nurs Clin North Am 23(1):231–263, 1988

Miller RH: Urinalysis: What do those numbers mean? AD Nurse 3(2):8–10, 1988

Oliver H: The treatment of choice . . . intermittent self-catheterisation. Nursing Times 84(31):70, 1988

Ouslander JG, Greengold B, Chen S: External catheter use and urinary tract infections among incontinent male nursing home patients. J Am Geriatr Soc 35(12):1063–1070, 1988

Preshlock K: Detecting the hidden UTI. RN Magazine 52(1):65–66, 68–69, 1989

Roe BH, Reid FJ, Brocklehurst JC: Comparison of four urinary drainage systems. J Adv Nurs 13(3):374–382, 1988

Sawyer DL: Potential for infection: A nursing diagnosis for the patient with an indwelling catheter. Focus on Critical Care 16(1):46–52, 1989

Sleep J, Grant A: Pelvic floor exercises in postnatal care. Midwifery 3(4):158–164, 1987

Smith DAJ: Continence restoration in the homebound patient. Nurs Clin North Am 23(1):207–218, 1988

Stark JL: A quick guide to urinary tract assessment. Nursing 18(7):57–58, 1988

Staudenmayer T: Preventing urinary tract infections. Nursing 19(4):106–107, 1989

Tunick PM: Alteration in urinary elimination. Journal of Gerontological Nursing 14(1):25–30, 46–47, 1988

22

Promoting Bowel Elimination

Chapter Outline

Behavioral Objectives
Glossary
Introduction
Reviewing Bowel Elimination
Understanding Factors Affecting Bowel Elimination
Assessing Bowel Elimination
Identifying and Relieving Common Alterations in Bowel
    Elimination
Performing Skills That Empty the Bowel
Eliminating Stool Through a Stoma
Obtaining a Stool Specimen
Suggested Measures to Promote Bowel Elimination in
    Selected Situations
Applicable Nursing Diagnoses
Teaching Suggestions to Promote Bowel Elimination
Bibliography

Skill Procedures

Promoting and Maintaining Bowel Elimination
Inserting a Rectal Tube
Inserting a Rectal Suppository
Administering a Cleansing Enema
Changing an Ostomy Appliance
Irrigating a Colostomy
Collecting a Stool Specimen

Behavioral Objectives

When the content of this chapter has been mastered, the learner will be able to:

Define terms appearing in the glossary.
List and describe the functions of the structures involved with the elimination of stool.
List at least seven factors that affect intestinal elimination.
Describe assessments that directly provide information about bowel elimination.
Discuss measures that promote and maintain bowel elimination.
Discuss five common alterations in bowel elimination; describe factors that contribute to their development and methods to help overcome them.
Describe how to remove a fecal impaction, insert a rectal suppository, and insert a rectal tube.
Demonstrate the administration of a high-volume enema and describe the differences when a hypertonic enema solution is administered.
Discuss the differences between an ileostomy and a colostomy.
Demonstrate the application of an ostomy appliance.
Identify the purpose of and describe the procedure for irrigating a colostomy.
Discuss the differences in care when a patient has a continent ostomy.
Describe the general steps for collecting a stool specimen.
List suggested measures for promoting bowel elimination in selected situations, as discussed in this chapter.
Summarize suggestions for the instruction of patients that are offered in this chapter.

Glossary

Bowel All the structures in the lower intestinal tract involved in the actual process of stool elimination.
Cathartics Drug preparations that induce emptying of the bowel. Synonym for *laxatives*.
Cleansing enema An instilled solution used to empty the lower intestine.
Colostomy An opening into the colon.
Continence The ability to control elimination.
Continent ostomy An ostomy that allows an individual to control the release of liquid stool or urine. Synonym for *Kock pouch*.
Defecation The act of eliminating stool from the bowel.
Diarrhea The passage of watery, unformed stools accompanied by abdominal cramping.
Enema The instillation of solution into the large intestine.

Enterostomal therapist A nurse who has been certified in the care of ostomates.

Excoriation A condition that occurs from chemical injury to the skin.

Flatulence An excessive amount of gas within the intestinal tract.

Flatus Expelled intestinal gas.

Gastrocolic reflex The automatic increase in peristalsis during the process of eating and drinking.

Hemorrhoids Distended veins in the rectum.

Hypertonic solution A mixture of water with a higher amount of dissolved substances than found in blood.

Ileostomy An opening into the ileum, a portion of the small intestine.

Intestinal distention A condition that results when intestinal gas accumulates and is not expelled. Synonym for *tympanites.*

Kock pouch An ostomy that allows an individual to control the release of liquid stool or urine. Synonym for *continent ostomy.*

Laxatives Drug preparations that induce emptying of the bowel. Synonym for *cathartics.*

Ostomate A person who has an ostomy.

Ostomy A surgically created opening into a body structure.

Peristalsis The rhythmic muscular contractions that move contents through the gastrointestinal tract.

Retention enema An instillation of solution that is held within the large intestine.

Suppository An oval or cone-shaped solid substance designed for easy insertion into a body cavity.

Tympanites A condition that results when intestinal gas accumulates and is not expelled. Synonym for *intestinal distention.*

Introduction

Food is digested, absorbed, and eliminated by structures in the gastrointestinal tract. Undigestible substances and some water are eliminated as stool, or feces. Just as was true of urinary elimination, the process of eliminating intestinal waste is important for life and health. Too rapid elimination may deplete the water and chemical balances of the body. Infrequent elimination may cause discomfort and abdominal distention and may lead to obstruction in bowel elimination. If uncorrected, either situation may lead to death.

The process of elimination is aided by helpful bacteria that are present in the lower intestine. These nonpathogens assist in breaking down fiber and organic material. This produces intestinal gas and contributes to the odor associated with stool. They also help in making vitamin K, necessary for blood clotting, and some B vitamins.

This chapter reviews briefly the process of intestinal elimination and discusses measures to help promote it. Nursing skills that may assist the patient with alterations in bowel elimination are also described.

Reviewing Bowel Elimination

All the structures of the gastrointestinal tract must function adequately to maintain bowel elimination. The act of elimination involves the functioning of the structures collectively referred to as the *bowel.* These structures include the large intestine, the rectum, the anal canal, and the anus.

The Large Intestine

The large intestine, also called the colon, is composed of four parts. The function of the large intestine involves the collection and excretion of intestinal wastes. However, each one of the four substructures of the colon contributes to the overall purpose.

- The ascending colon absorbs up to 800 to 1000 mL of water from intestinal wastes daily. The absorption of water accounts for the formed, semisolid nature of normal stool. When absorption does not occur properly, the stool remains soft and watery. If too much water is absorbed, the stool is dry and hard. Each area of the colon absorbs water. The water content of the stool decreases as stool moves through the bowel.
- The transverse colon transports wastes along the large intestine and continues to absorb water.
- The descending colon acts to collect forming stool.
- The sigmoid colon collects formed stool and retains it until it can be eliminated.

The Rectum, Anal Canal, and Anus

The rectum acts as a passageway for feces moving from the sigmoid colon to the anal canal. As the rectum distends with stool, pressure on nerves signals the need to have a bowel movement.

The anal canal provides a reservoir for stool prior to its elimination. It contains a ring-shaped band of muscle, called the internal sphincter. It controls filling from the intestine. The internal sphincter is not under voluntary control.

The anus is the terminal outlet of the rectum. This structure could be compared to the urinary meatus. An external sphincter is located at the anus. It can be voluntarily contracted or relaxed to control the elimination of stool from the body.

Defecation

Defecation is the act of eliminating stool from the bowel. It is facilitated by *peristalsis,* the rhythmic muscular contractions that move contents through the gastrointestinal tract. When the internal sphincter relaxes to allow stool to pass into the rectum and anal canal, the urge to have a bowel movement is recognized. The individual voluntarily relaxes the external sphincter to release stool. This process is facilitated by performing Valsalva's maneuver. This closes the glottis and increases abdominal pressure due to the contraction of pelvic and abdominal muscles.

Understanding Factors Affecting Bowel Elimination

A variety of factors influence normal intestinal elimination:

- The volume of the stool is affected by the amount of food that is consumed. A diet high in fiber and roughage produces a larger stool and promotes quicker passage through the intestinal tract. A diet low in roughage produces a smaller stool and tends to increase the time it remains within the bowel.
- The types of foods consumed also affect the characteristics of stool and associated aspects of elimination. Certain foods, such as red meat, can alter the color of stool. Some foods, such as beans, cucumbers, or cabbage, are called gas formers because they increase the volume of intestinal gas.
- Fluid intake influences elimination. A normal to above average consumption of liquids and watery foods helps keep the stool moist; a low fluid intake results in a drier stool.
- Most individuals experience an urge to defecate in association with the gastrocolic reflex. The *gastrocolic reflex* is an automatic increase in intestinal peristalsis during the process of eating and drinking. It seems to be most active when consuming the first food of the day.
- Stool is usually eliminated in a cycling pattern. The frequency of having a bowel movement varies among healthy persons. Some have one or more movements a day; others normally defecate less often. Many individuals eliminate at approximately the same time or times each day.
- Patterns of bowel elimination and the characteristics of stool are influenced by drugs and other conditions in which stool is delayed or rapidly propelled through the gastrointestinal tract.
- Defecation can be voluntarily controlled. Some delay defecation despite the urge to eliminate. This is done by contracting the external sphincter. Others force elimination despite a lack of stimulation. Either of these two responses can lead to discomfort during elimination, and can also promote the formation of hemorrhoids. *Hemorrhoids* are distended veins in the rectum. They are made worse by straining, which causes increased congestion of blood in the area.
- Nervous tension affects bowel elimination. For some, tension results in a state of increased muscle contraction. Digestion and elimination slow. For others, peristalsis becomes rapid and the individual may experience abdominal cramping and diarrhea.
- An intact spinal cord and state of alertness affect bowel elimination. Unconscious individuals or those with lower body paralysis may not be able to control or release stool voluntarily.
- Gravity, movement, and exercise facilitate muscle tone and the ease of elimination.

Assessing Bowel Elimination

The nurse generally obtains certain basic information from the patient at the time of admission. Questions about the frequency, characteristics, and consistency of the stool are asked to identify the patterns of bowel elimination that are unique to the patient. The nurse usually inquires about the date of the last bowel movement and the use of any self-administered medications or techniques for promoting bowel function.

While performing a physical assessment, the bowel sounds are auscultated. The abdomen is gently palpated, noting any tenderness or unusual enlargement. The condition of the skin around the anus may be inspected.

Noting the Characteristics of Stool

While providing care the nurse has the opportunity to assess the characteristics of the patient's stool. This adds to the initial data base of information about bowel elimination. The volume, color, odor, consistency, and shape of the stool are assessed. These characteristics are mentally compared with those of normal stool. Table 22-1 provides a description of the appearance and content of normal stool.

Tests are not routinely performed on stool. They are usually only ordered when the stool appears abnormal. A sample of any unusual stool should be saved in a covered container in case testing is necessary. There are some tests that the nurse may perform on stool, using color-coded strips similar to those described for testing urine. They are used most often to detect blood that may be hidden in the stool. The results of any laboratory tests performed on stool add to the assessment information.

Identifying and Relieving Common Alterations in Bowel Elimination

Various definitions of common problems associated with bowel elimination were provided in Chapter 18 in a discussion of the disuse syndrome of inactive patients. These terms and their definitions, though not listed again in the glossary, will be repeated to provide review and continuity within the content of this chapter.

Table 22-1. Characteristics of Normal Stool

Item	Description
Amount	The volume depends on the amount and type of food a person eats, but the average adult stool weighs 100 g to 300 g, of which about 70% is water.
Color	The stool is brown in color. It darkens with standing.
Odor	The characteristic aromatic odor of the stool varies with its *p*H, which is normally neutral or mildly alkaline. The odor is caused by bacterial action in the gastrointestinal tract.
Consistency and shape	The stool is a formed, semisolid mass, which assumes the shape of the rectum.
Components	The stool contains wastes of digestion, bile pigments and salts, intestinal secretions, leukocytes that migrate from the blood, shed epithelial cells, bacteria, inorganic material (primarily calcium and phosphates), and very small amounts of undigested material (such as seeds and fibers).

Constipation

Constipation is a condition in which the stool becomes dry and hard and requires straining in order to eliminate it. Infrequency of stool passage is a characteristic of constipation, although it is not always the main one. For example, some may be constipated yet have a daily bowel movement. Others who defecate no more than three times a week are not necessarily constipated if the stool is passed easily without discomfort. The consistency of the stool and the effort associated with bowel elimination are of more importance than the interval between defecations.

Individuals who report that they are constipated describe many symptoms that they attribute to retained stool such as headache, malaise, and anorexia. These may be coincidental or unique to some individuals. After doing an extensive study of the literature, McMillan and Williams (1989) narrowed the characteristics of constipation into a cluster of eight related signs and symptoms, listed in Table 22-2. The severity of constipation is based on the number of signs and symptoms present on the list and the intensity with which they are experienced.

Small stool volume is also associated with constipation. It is one of the characteristics on the list in Table 22-2. The bulk of the stool is related to the undigestible fiber content of the diet. Plant sources of food, especially raw fruits and vegetables, grains, and nuts, are high in fiber. The cellulose that remains as the end-product following their digestion absorbs water. This increases the quantity of stool but makes it softer and easier to pass. Burkitt (1984) compared the stools of people in North America and Europe with those in underdeveloped countries in the world. The for-

mer are known to characteristically consume low amounts of dietary fiber and likewise experience a higher incidence of constipation. In Burkitt's study there were significant differences, identified in Table 22-3, in both stool weight and transit time. Transit time is the time it takes for food to travel from the mouth to the anus.

Pseudo Constipation. Some individuals think of themselves as being constipated but do not manifest the common characteristics associated with it. They believe that bowel elimination should occur daily, even at the same approximate time. They are more likely to use various unnecessary and, in some cases, harmful self-treatments to induce a daily bowel movement. The North American Nursing Diagnosis Association has accepted the diagnostic category of Perceived Constipation, which ap-

Table 22-2 Chief Characteristics of Constipation

- Abdominal distention or bloating
- Change in amount of gas passed rectally
- Less frequent bowel movements
- Oozing liquid stool
- Rectal fullness or pressure
- Rectal pain with bowel movement
- Small volume of stool
- Unable to pass stool

From McMillan SC, Williams FA: Validity and reliability of the Constipation Assessment Scale. Cancer Nurs 12(3):183–188, 1989

Table 22-3. Comparison of Stool Weight and Transit Time

Country	Stool Weight	Transit Time
North America and Europe	80–120 g	72 hr average
Third World	300–500 g	36 hr average

From Burkitt D: Fiber as protective against gastrointestinal diseases. Am J Gastroenterol 79(4):249–252, 1984, copyright by the American College of Gastroenterology.

plies to bowel-fixated individuals who abuse laxatives or other purgatives in order to evacuate their bowel.

Chronic abuse of laxatives, enemas, or suppositories can eventually lead to actual constipation. The tone of the bowel becomes sluggish because it is repeatedly subjected to artificial stimulation.

Identifying Types and Causes of Constipation.

Once a patient's pattern of bowel elimination indicates constipation, the cause must be determined. Constipation can be best prevented and treated by understanding the circumstances that interfere with normal elimination of stool. Table 22-4 lists various types of constipation and related factors. The following also contribute to constipation:

- Certain diseases or physical conditions that cause inactivity or immobility predispose to constipation.
- An inadequate intake of food or the intake of highly processed foods with little or no fiber content lead to stools of small volume and little water content.
- A long transit time causes stool to collect and remain within the bowel. The lower bowel is able to absorb water. The stool dehydrates the longer it is retained.

Relieving Constipation. When constipation occurs, it may require the combined efforts of the physician and nurse to provide measures that restore bowel elimination. When no disease is present, the nurse can often help patients understand and use measures to overcome constipation. Normal patterns of elimination may take time to restore. Improvement has been observed among patients who make an effort to change their habits and long-held beliefs. Skill Procedure 22-1 describes common measures to help promote bowel elimination when no disease or injury process is causing it. Table 22-5 provides a recipe to help relieve constipation with food sources rather than medication.

Fecal Impaction

Fecal impaction is the retention of feces, which form a hardened mass in the rectum. The mass enlarges as more and more stool accumulates. The dry condition and increased volume make it impossible to pass normally. There is no specific length of time in which an impaction develops. Some have been known to form within 24 hours in certain individuals. The patient is likely to say he is constipated. Usually, he experiences a frequent desire to defecate but is unable to do so. Rectal pain may be present due to his unsuccessful attempts to evacuate the bowel.

A patient with a fecal impaction may expel liquid stool around the impacted mass. For the inexperienced person, it may seem as though the patient is experiencing fecal incontinence. However, this symptom in combination with a lack of normal defecation is almost a sure indication of an impaction. The nurse can easily confirm the suspicion by inserting a lubricated, gloved finger into the rectum. If the presence of hard formed stool is felt, the nurse should prepare to take measures that facilitate its removal.

Table 22-4. Types of Constipation

Type	Cause	Contributing Factors
Primary or simple constipation	Extrinsic factors	Decreased physical activity Inadequate privacy Inadequate time for defecation Inadequate dietary fiber
Secondary constipation	Pathology	Partial intestinal obstruction Hypothyroidism Spinal cord compression
Iatrogenic constipation	Consequence of other treatment	Narcotic analgesia Anticancer drug therapy, especially with Vinca alkaloids Anticonvulsants Antidepressants Tranquilizers

From Cimprich B: Symptom management: Constipation. Cancer Nurs 8(1 suppl): 39–43, 1985

Suggested Action	Reason for Action
Explore the patient's patterns of elimination to validate that the symptoms are characteristic of constipation.	Misleading literature, advertisements and long-held beliefs have caused many individuals to be bowel conscious. Some may attempt to alter bowel elimination unnecessarily.
Consume a variety of foods, but especially include fresh fruits, vegetables, and whole grains. Limit eating highly processed and refined foods.	Bulk and residue that are made up of undigestible fibers produce more feces and stimulate peristalsis.
Eat a nutritious breakfast that consists of adequate portions.	The gastrocolic reflex is more often experienced following a period of fasting.
Avoid snacking as a substitute for eating a full meal.	Snack foods are likely to lack nutrition and be low in fiber. They relieve hunger and interfere with eating patterns that promote the formation and elimination of stool.
Drink an adequate amount of fluids, preferably between 2000 and 3000 mL daily.	Dietary liquids contribute to the moisture content of stool.
Participate in some form of regular exercise.	Exercise and activity promote muscle tone and stimulate peristalsis.
A hospitalized patient should walk about the room and hallway, if possible.	The hospitalized patient who is as active as his condition permits tends to maintain normal patterns of elimination.
Respond to the urge to have a bowel movement when the stimulus is experienced.	Delaying defecation causes the absorption of more moisture from the stool. It may also cause the bowel to become insensitive to the normal urge to defecate.
Promote relaxation and privacy when there is a need to defecate.	Stress and worry, using a public toilet or one located in an unfamiliar environment, and being rushed for adequate time may disrupt normal bowel elimination.
Assume a sitting position for bowel elimination. Provide support for the feet. A short person may need a footstool. Having a patient sit on a bedpan on the edge of the bed or on a commode simulates use of the toilet. A patient who cannot be in this position will usually find it best to have the head of the bed elevated and the knees somewhat flexed.	This aids gravity and relaxation of the external sphincter so that stool can be eliminated. Contraction of muscles and the use of Valsalva's maneuver increase abdominal pressure and aid expulsion of stool.
Use laxative medications infrequently and follow labeled instructions.	Frequent use of drugs that purge the system can cause the bowel to become sluggish in responding to natural stimuli.
Select medications that promote bowel elimination appropriately. *Laxatives* are preparations that induce emptying of the bowel. Some persons use the word *cathartics* as a synonym. A drug that softens or lubricates stool may be a more desirable action.	Laxatives tend to act more harshly on the gastrointestinal system than stool softeners. Using medications without proper knowledge contributes to abuse and can increase problems associated with elimination.
Avoid using enemas or suppositories on a regular basis, and never use them when abdominal pain, nausea, or vomiting is present.	Repeated use of enemas or suppositories can have the same effect as abuse of laxatives. Their use as self-treatment for disease symptoms can cause serious complications.
Teach the patient the signs and symptoms associated with significant alterations in bowel elimination and abnormal characteristics of stool. These include change in the shape of stool, altering periods of constipation and diarrhea, and the presence of blood in the stool.	Changes in bowel elimination are significant signs of some diseases. Changes should be reported immediately so that early diagnosis and treatment can occur. The signs described are early warnings of colorectal cancer. This is one of the leading types of cancer among men and women. Assuming that these signs are due to something minor can delay the potential for cure.

Table 22-5. Recipe to Relieve Constipation

Mix the following ingredients to a pasty consistency:
    1 cup of applesauce
    1 cup of unprocessed bran
    ½ cup of 100% prune juice

Take two tablespoons at bedtime with a glass of fluid. If constipation is severe, increase to two tablespoons upon rising and at bedtime.
Refrigerate mixture in a covered container between uses.

From Behm R: A special recipe to banish constipation. Geriatr Nurs 6(4):216–217, 1985. Reprinted with permission. Copyright by the American Journal of Nursing Company.

Identifying Causes for a Fecal Impaction. Various factors predispose a person to the development of a fecal impaction.

- Constipation usually precedes an impaction. Therefore, factors that cause constipation may also cause fecal impaction.
- Conditions that cause abdominal weakness can contribute to an impaction, since the individual may lack the strength to contract his abdominal muscles in an effort to expel stool.
- Retained barium used as a contrast medium during some x-ray examinations of the gastrointestinal tract contributes to the formation of an impaction.
- Extremely fibrous foods, such as bran and fruit seeds, when consumed with an inadequate amount of fluid, have been known to cause an impaction.
- Some enteric-coated tablets have been known to cause fecal impaction. These medications are covered with a material that prevents the active ingredient from dissolving in the stomach. These drugs undergo breakdown when in the small intestine. However, some have been found to accumulate similarly to undigested substances.

Relieving a Fecal Impaction. Several measures may relieve a fecal impaction. The stool may be passed if sufficient moisture and lubrication are instilled into the rectum. An oil retention enema is often prescribed to first provide lubrication to the mass and the mucous membrane that lines the rectum. A cleansing enema may follow an oil retention enema. A discussion of enemas appears later in this chapter.

Digital removal of stool may become necessary if the administration of enemas fails to produce results. Digital removal involves inserting a gloved and well-lubricated finger into the rectum in order to break up and remove the fecal mass. This is likely to cause the patient discomfort and possible trauma to the bowel during removal. If digital removal is necessary, the following actions are suggested.

- Place the patient in a left or right Sims' position, depending on the dominant hand of the nurse. This position permits the inserted finger to follow the anatomic structure of the rectum.
- Assure the patient that the finger will be inserted gently. The anus may be very tender from the frequent attempts to evacuate the bowel unsuccessfully. If hemorrhoids are present, they may also be injured and bleed as stool in the area is manipulated.
- Place a bedpan conveniently on the bed so that pieces of removed feces can be deposited within it.
- Fold back the bed linen so that the patient is covered but there is access to the rectal area.
- Apply a clean glove for the dominant hand. The intestinal tract is not sterile so the glove is not required to be sterile.
- Lubricate the forefinger generously to reduce resistance during insertion.
- Insert the finger gently to the level of the hardened mass. The presence of the finger added to the mass usually causes discomfort for the patient.
- Slowly and carefully move the finger around and into the hardened mass to break it up. The impaction may be composed of round stonelike formations of stool that can be removed once they are broken up.
- Allow the patient intervals of rest if the impaction is large and difficult to remove. This helps avoid discomfort as well as injury to the mucous membranes.
- Make every effort to eliminate the cause and prevent the formation of another impaction.

Intestinal Distention

An excessive amount of gas within the intestinal tract is known as *flatulence.* Expelled intestinal gas is called *flatus.* When the gas is not expelled and instead accumulates, the condition is called *intestinal distention,* or *tympanites.*

Distention can be identified by inspecting and percussing a swollen abdomen. Gentle tapping with the fingers produces the drumlike sound of a tympany instrument. The abdomen can be measured for more objective assessment and evaluation. Usually the patient will describe cramping pain. If distention is sufficient to cause pressure on the diaphragm and the chest cavity, shortness of breath and dyspnea may also occur.

Identifying Causes of Intestinal Distention. The bowel normally accumulates 7 to 10 L of gas daily (Vaughn and Mencek, 1986). The largest percentage comes from swallowed air and air that is present in food. Other minor sources include gas that diffuses from the bloodstream and bacterial fermentation. All but approximately 0.5 L is absorbed through the intestinal mucosa into the bloodstream, where it is eliminated through respiration. The amount that remains within the intestine is released from the rectum usually at the time of bowel elimination.

Certain conditions predispose a person to form greater amounts of gas or interfere with its absorption. These include

- Swallowing larger than usual amounts of air while eating and drinking. Persons who are tense sometimes gulp air. Drinking through a straw contributes to air swallowing. Consumption of carbonated beverages can increase gas accumulation. Even smoking cigarettes, gum chewing, and sucking on hard candy have been implicated in swallowing air.
- Eating spicy and hot foods have been shown to shorten transit time. Therefore the opportunity for absorbing intestinal gas is reduced.
- Consuming gas-forming foods increases the volume of gas in the intestinal tract. There seems to be a wide range of reactions among individuals to foods such as onions, cucumbers, and cabbage. The human body lacks an enzyme to break down the oligosaccharide in beans to a simple sugar. Their consumption is notorious for increasing intestinal gas.
- Inactivity tends to impair the movement of gas through the intestinal tract. Activity promotes gas elimination from the rectum to the atmosphere. Lack of movement or a tight sphincter keeps gas trapped and contributes to abdominal distention and discomfort.
- Some patients experience intestinal distention after surgery in which the bowel is handled. Peristalsis slows or temporarily stops while bacteria continue to form gas. When the patient can again pass flatus, it is a positive sign that intestinal functioning is restored.
- Drugs, such as morphine, tend to decrease peristalsis and thus cause distention as well as constipation.
- The presence of a mass that obstructs the passage of stool may also interfere with the ability of the intestine to eliminate gas.

Relieving Intestinal Distention. The following are suggested nursing measures to help bring relief from intestinal distention.

- Identify the cause, when possible, and treat the condition that has contributed to the gas accumulation.
- Have the patient move about in bed and walk to help promote the movement and expulsion of the gas.
- Have the patient assume various positions to help move gas in the direction of the anus. Gas is lighter than fluids or solids, and hence will rise. Positioning the patient so that the rectum and anus are higher than the bolus of gas may help to distribute and expel the gas. These include lying prone, assuming a knee-chest position, lowering the upper body over the edge of the bed, and even a side-lying position may be effective. The nurse should use good judgment when considering positioning. The patient's comfort and safety must be primary concerns. Some consequences of these positions may be more damaging than the intestinal gas.
- Insert a rectal tube to help gas escape. The technique is described in Skill Procedure 22-2. Gas will usually follow the path of least resistance. The inserted tube provides a channel through which the gas can travel despite a contracted sphincter.
- An intestinal tube inserted through the nose may be used as a last resort. It is inserted similarly to a nasogastric tube discussed in Chapter 8. An intestinal tube is much longer in order to reach the bowel. Suction removes gas and liquid substances, thus relieving the effects of intestinal distention.

Diarrhea

Diarrhea is the passage of watery, unformed stools accompanied by abdominal cramping. Although frequent bowel movements do not necessarily mean that diarrhea is present, persons with diarrhea usually have stools frequently. This condition tends to have a sudden onset and last only a short period of time. Other associated signs and symptoms include nausea and vomiting, and the presence of blood or mucus in the stools.

Identifying Causes of Diarrhea. Various factors predispose to the development of diarrhea:

- Diarrhea may be a response on the part of the body to rid itself of some allergic substance within the intestinal tract. It may also be a natural defense for eliminating an irritating substance, such as tainted food or intestinal pathogens.
- Some individuals respond to stress with an increase in the rate of peristalsis. This shortens the time during which water can be absorbed from the stool.
- Certain dietary indiscretions cause diarrhea. Rich pastries, coffee, fruits, and alcoholic beverages may produce temporary diarrhea for some persons.
- Intentional or accidental abuse of laxatives can cause diarrhea. There seems to be an increased incidence of eating disorders, one of which involves purging the body with laxatives to compensate for eating binges.
- Intestinal diseases may be accompanied by diarrhea. Diarrhea occurs as a result of chemical and mechanical changes within the bowel. This type of diarrhea may be chronic and is less easily relieved.

Relieving the Effects of Diarrhea. The following nursing measures are recommended to help the patient who has diarrhea:

Skill Procedure 22-2. Inserting a Rectal Tube

Suggested Action	Reason for Action
Select a straight catheter according to the size of the individual. A size 22 to 32 is appropriate for an adult. A flexible hollow tube with openings along the insertion tip may also be used.	The anus is large enough to permit the insertion of a tube of this size without causing discomfort or trauma. A flexible tube prevents injury to the mucous membrane. The holes provide openings through which the gas can escape.
Close the door and pull the privacy curtains.	If the patient is tense and embarrassed, it is likely to cause discomfort while inserting a rectal tube.
Position the patient on his left side.	The position helps to facilitate the passage of the tube past the sphincters and into the rectum.
Lubricate the rectal tube generously.	Lubrication reduces friction and eases insertion.
Separate the buttocks well so that the anus is in plain view and insert the tube for about 4 to 6 inches in an adult. The tube should be inserted a shorter distance in a child.	Positioning the tube well above the sphincters stimulates peristalsis and helps prevent the tube from slipping out of place.
Tape the tube in place to the side of the buttocks or inner thigh.	This allows the patient to move and change positions without displacing the location of the tube.
Place the free end of the tube into a clean, soft towel.	The towel will absorb any stool that may also drain through the tube, yet not interfere with moving about in bed.
Leave the rectal tube in place for a period of no longer than 20 minutes.	The rectal tube can affect the ability to voluntarily control the sphincter if placement is prolonged.
Reinsert the rectal tube every 2 to 3 hours if the distention has been unrelieved or reaccumulates.	Reinserting the tube after a rest period allows gas to move in the direction of the rectum. Replacement acts to stimulate peristalsis and continues the release of gas.

- Take into consideration that diarrhea is often an embarrassing and usually painful disturbance. Listen to the patient and give him opportunities to explore possible causes.
- Reduce or remove the cause of diarrhea when possible. Explain the importance of avoiding foods and fluids that cause diarrhea.
- Temporarily limit the consumption of food. Provide clear liquids until the number of stools and the consistency improve. Follow with bananas, applesauce, and light foods. Avoid fried foods, highly seasoned foods, or foods high in roughage.
- Investigate the relationship between the side effects of medications and the occurrence of diarrhea. Consult with the physician when a prescribed drug may be a factor in diarrhea.
- Remember that a person with diarrhea often finds it extremely difficult to delay the urge to defecate. When a patient has diarrhea, the problem should be noted on the nursing care plan. The nursing orders should include instructions to watch for the patient's signal light and to answer it promptly. It may be necessary to place the bedpan within easy reach for the patient yet out of sight to prevent embarrassment.

- Use hygienic measures following each stool. Clean the patient well, and rinse and dry the area thoroughly. Use soft toilet tissues or cloths to avoid further injury to anal tissue. Apply a medicated powder or cream according to agency policy. Friction, soap residues on the skin, and watery feces irritate the skin and may lead to tissue breakdown.
- Count the number of stools that the patient excretes. Frequent diarrhea can lead to water and chemical imbalances. This can take place fairly quickly in the very young or debilitated patient.
- Consult with the physician concerning the possible use of medications to control the diarrhea or abdominal cramping.

Fecal Incontinence

Fecal incontinence is the inability to retain stool within the bowel. *Continence* is the ability to control elimination. For the most part, patients with fecal incontinence are much more devastated psychologically than those with urinary incontinence. It is difficult to disguise when stool is expelled. Incontinent patients and their families require much support and understanding.

Identifying Causes of Fecal Incontinence. Although fecal incontinence is not life threatening, identifying its cause may help resolve the condition. By obtaining a complete history from the patient about his bowel habits, possible causes for the incontinence may be determined. There are some possible factors that should be considered.

- Usually the cause of fecal incontinence is a result of disease or injury. If these are progressive or permanent types of conditions, such as damage to the spinal cord or stroke, the outlook for restoring control is doubtful.
- Determine if a fecal impaction is present. Retained stool may be the underlying problem.
- Loss of bowel control may occur for only a temporary period, for instance when associated with diarrhea. This presents less of a potential problem for eventual control.
- Some individuals may lose control of the bowel if they must wait to use a toilet.
- Taking an extremely harsh or large dosage of a laxative may result in such rapid peristalsis that loss of control is simply unavoidable.

Managing Fecal Incontinence. Nursing measures suggested for the patient with diarrhea can be used if the incontinence is due to a temporary or reversible cause. Anal control ultimately depends on proper functioning of the anal sphincter. For some patients, sphincter control can be improved. When the incontinence is likely to be a continuous problem, the following actions may be helpful:

- See to it that the patient eats regularly and has a nutritious and well-balanced diet. Eating foods that are high in bulk and fiber can help keep the stool more formed. A formed stool is more easily controlled than one that is liquid.
- Note whether there are certain times of the day when incontinence is more likely to occur, such as after breakfast or another meal. This is when the gastrocolic reflex is more likely to be activated.
- Place the patient on a bedpan shortly before a time when the individual is likely to eliminate stool. If there is no pattern, place the patient on a bedpan at frequent intervals, such as every 2 to 3 hours. Do not allow the patient to remain on the bedpan for long periods of time.
- Consult with the physician about using a suppository or an enema every 2 to 3 days. If a pattern can be established by stimulating peristalsis and emptying the lower bowel with these aids, fecal incontinence may become manageable.
- Use moisture-proof undergarments and absorbent pads as necessary to protect bed linen and clothing when incontinence is frequent. Diapering the patient should be avoided to help preserve the patient's dignity and self-esteem.

Performing Skills that Empty the Bowel

There are times when individuals may have alterations in bowel elimination, such as constipation, which must be relieved. There are also certain diagnostic examinations for which adequate inspection requires a clean bowel. The nurse may utilize various skills for removing stool from the lower bowel.

Inserting a Rectal Suppository

A *suppository* is an oval or cone-shaped solid substance designed for easy insertion into a body cavity. Examples are shown in Figure 22-1. A suppository is constructed to melt at body temperature. Because a certain amount of absorption takes place in the large intestine, some medications can be given by suppository. The most frequent reason for administering a suppository is to promote the expulsion of feces and flatus.

Suppositories have various actions. Some soften the feces; some lubricate the anal canal; some stimulate peristalsis by chemical means. Others liberate carbon dioxide, thus increasing rectal bulk to stimulate defecation. Skill Procedure 22-3 describes how to insert a rectal suppository.

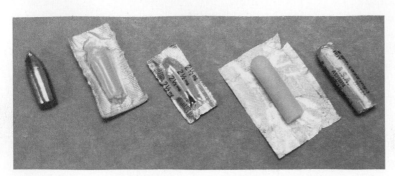

Figure 22-1 These are examples of suppositories. They are made in a variety of sizes and shapes.

Skill Procedure 22-3. Inserting a Rectal Suppository

Suggested Action	Reason for Action
Close the door and ensure privacy by pulling the curtains surrounding the bed.	Individuals are likely to be tense if concerned about unexpected interruptions.
Position the patient on his left side and drape the patient to expose only the buttocks.	Proper positioning provides an adequate view and access to the rectal area. Using the left side facilitates the use of the nurse's right hand. Reverse the position if the nurse is left-handed.
Apply a finger cot or don a clean glove on the dominant hand.	The finger cot or glove acts as a barrier from contact with stool within the rectum.
Lubricate the length of the finger and the suppository.	Lubrication reduces friction and eases insertion.
Separate the buttocks so that the anus is in plain view and have the patient take several deep breaths.	Having the patient take deep breaths helps relax the anal sphincters and makes insertion more comfortable.
Introduce the suppository beyond the internal sphincter, about the distance of the inserted finger. The suppository should be in contact with the mucous membrane and not be embedded in stool.	The suppository should be placed well into the rectum, where its effect is desired. The medication must be absorbed by melting and contact with the mucous membrane. Placement in stool slows the desired action and effect.
Instruct the patient to retain the suppository until he has an urge to defecate, usually in 15 minutes to 45 minutes.	Retaining the suppository allows time to achieve maximal results.
Allow the patient to walk about if he is ambulatory.	Walking about often helps distribute the medication and stimulate peristalsis.
Request that the patient save stool for examination.	The nurse should observe the amount and other characteristics of the stool to evaluate the effectiveness of the procedure.
Record the procedure and the results according to agency policy.	The patient's chart contains a continuous record of care and the patient's response.

Administering an Enema

An *enema* is the introduction of a solution into the large intestine. The most common type is the *cleansing enema,* which is used to empty the lower intestinal tract of feces. The most frequently used solutions are soap and water, normal saline, and highly concentrated hypertonic solutions.

Administering a Large Volume Enema. One method for cleansing the bowel involves instilling a large amount of solution. The volume of the solution distends the walls of the bowel and causes the urge to defecate. Defecation usually occurs within 5 to 15 minutes after administration. In the process of expelling the solution, any stool that is present will also be eliminated. The large volume ensures that a major area of the lower colon will be empty.

Soap and water, tap water, and normal saline are often used when administering a large volume enema. Soap solutions also act by stimulating peristalsis through chemical irritation of the mucous membranes. Too much soap or soap that is too strong can be extremely irritating. Mixing concentrated liquid soaps in prepackaged packets with 1000 mL of water provides an appropriate dilution. If the packets of soap are not available, 5 mL of mild liquid soap may be substituted.

Tap water or normal saline may be preferred for its nonirritating effect on patients with rectal diseases or for patients being prepared for rectal examinations. Tap water and normal saline appear to have about the same degree of effectiveness for cleansing the bowel. However, tap water can be absorbed through the bowel. Tap water enemas that are repeated one after the other can result in fluid imbalances.

Skill Procedure 22-4 describes the administration of a cleansing enema when a large volume of solution is used.

Instilling a Hypertonic Enema Solution. A *hypertonic solution* is a solution in which there is a higher amount of dissolved substances than that found in blood. Hypertonic solutions act on the principle of osmosis. In other words, fluid moves from an area of low concentration of substances to one in which there is a higher concentration

(Text continues on page 557)

Skill Procedure 22-4. Administering a Cleansing Enema

Suggested Action	Reason for Action
Assemble the necessary equipment. Items needed include tubing, size 26 to 32, a regulating clamp on the tubing, a container for the solution, and lubricant. Many health agencies purchase disposable enema equipment sets.	The rectum can accommodate a large tube. The container must be large enough to hold approximately 1000 mL without overflowing.
Close the clamp on the tubing between the container and the insertion tip.	If the clamp remains open, the solution will drain onto the work area.
Prepare 1000 mL of the specified solution at a temperature of 40° to 43°C (105°–110°F).	For maximal stimulation, comfort, and safety, the solution should enter the intestine at slightly higher than normal body temperature. An adult colon is estimated to hold about 750 to 1000 mL.
Plan with the patient where he will defecate. Have a bedpan, commode, or nearby bathroom ready for his use.	The patient is better able to relax and cooperate if he knows everything is ready when he feels the urge to defecate.
Position and drape the patient on his right or left side, depending on the dominant hand that will be used for instilling the enema.	The nurse should arrange the patient's position to facilitate control of the tubing and solution. Fluid will fill the colon regardless of which side the patient lies.
Drape the patient exposing the buttocks, and place a waterproof pad under him, as shown in Figure 22-2.	Providing for the patient's warmth, modesty, and possible soiling will help him relax.

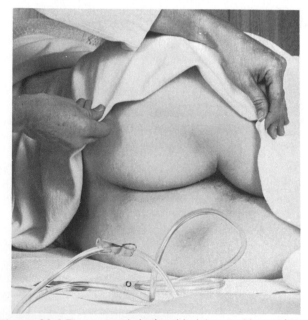

Figure 22-2 The patient is in the side-lying position and properly draped. A pad is placed under the buttocks. The solution and clamped tube are ready for insertion.

Place the container of solution so that it is between 30 and 50 cm (12–20 in) above the level of the patient's anus. The container may be hung on a standard or held in the nurse's hand at the proper height.	Gravity causes the solution to enter the intestine. The level of the container influences the rate and pressure of the instillation. The higher the container, the faster and greater the pressure will be. Elevating the container higher than this level may result in rapid distention and pressure in the intestine. This can cause too rapid expulsion of the solution, poor cleansing, and damage to the mucous membrane.

(continued)

Skill Procedure 22-4. *Continued*

Suggested Action	**Reason for Action**

Generously lubricate the end of the rectal tube for 5 to 7 cm (2–3 in), as illustrated in Figure 22-3.

Friction is reduced when the surface is lubricated, resulting in easier insertion and less likelihood of injury to mucous membrane.

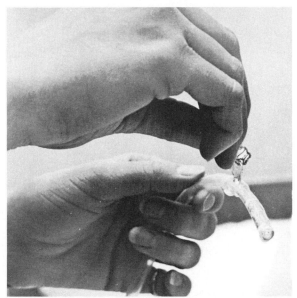

Figure 22-3 The nurse lubricates the rectal tube generously with a prepackaged lubricant of the agency's choice.

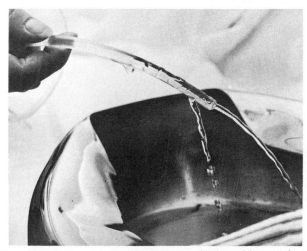

Figure 22-4 The solution is allowed to fill the tubing so that air is not introduced into the patient.

Open the clamp and fill the tubing with solution to displace the air, as the nurse in Figure 22-4 is doing.

Although allowing air to enter the intestine is not harmful, it adds to the volume within the rectum and colon. Filling the tube with solution also warms the tube.

Lift the buttock to expose the anus, as illustrated in Figure 22-5. Slowly insert the tip of the tubing 7 to 10 cm (3–4 in) with a rotating motion. Direct it at an angle pointing toward the umbilicus, as shown in Figure 22-6.

Good visualization of the anus helps prevent injury to tissues. The anal canal is approximately 2.5 to 5 cm (1–2 in) in length. The tube should be inserted past the internal sphincter. Further insertion may damage intestinal membrane. The suggested angle follows the normal anatomical contour. Slow insertion of the tube minimizes spasms of the intestinal wall and sphincters.

If the tube meets resistance while it is inserted, permit a small amount of solution to enter, withdraw the tube slightly, then continue to insert it. *Do not force entry of the tube.* Ask the patient to take several deep breaths or place warm moistened cloths over the anal area.

Resistance may be due to spasms within the intestine or failure of the internal sphincter to relax. Using these techniques may overcome the resistance. Forcing a tube may cause injury to the internal sphincter.

Release the clamp and instill the solution slowly over a period of 5 to 10 minutes.

Instilling the solution slowly helps distribute the solution to upper levels of the intestine, promoting more thorough cleansing. It avoids cramping and an urgent desire to defecate.

If the patient experiences cramping and the urge to defecate before sufficient amounts of solution have been instilled, try these techniques: instruct the patient to breathe in small, fast breaths, as if panting; slow or stop the flow of solution briefly by lowering the solution container; clamp the tubing and have the patient contract his external sphincter.

Panting helps relax muscles and promote distribution of the fluid. Reducing the volume being instilled allows time for the bowel to adjust to the distention. Tightening the external sphincter provides added control, preventing the premature expulsion of the solution.

(continued)

Skill Procedure 22-4. Continued

Suggested Action	**Reason for Action**

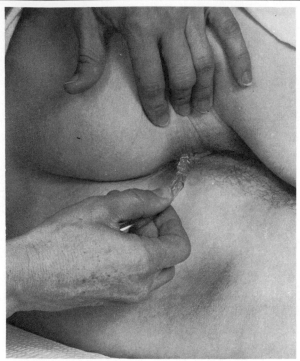

Figure 22-5 The nurse lifts the buttocks, exposes the anus, and prepares to introduce the rectal tube.

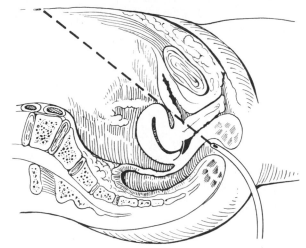

Figure 22-6 The tube is inserted so that it points toward the umbilicus and follows the normal rectal contour.

Suggested Action	**Reason for Action**
Clamp and remove the tubing after sufficient solution has been given or the patient protests that he is unable to retain more.	Clamping prevents the remaining solution from leaking onto the pad or patient.
Encourage the patient to retain the solution within the intestine for 5 to 15 minutes.	This amount of time usually allows muscular contractions to become sufficient to produce good results.
Help the patient to a sitting position on a bedpan, commode, or toilet when he experiences a strong urge to defecate.	The sitting position aids in defecation.
Prepare to siphon the enema solution if the patient cannot expel intestinal contents after an extended period of time.	The solution should be expelled and not remain within the intestine. A siphon drains a solution by gravity into a container located below the level of the solution.
To siphon, fill the enema solution container with 100 mL of warm water (105°F), fill the tube with water, clamp it, and insert it into the rectum. Allow some solution to instill and then lower the container of solution well below the level of the anus.	Lowering the container will permit fluid to drain out of the intestine and back into the container. This action is rarely necessary.
Note the amount and character of the stool and the patient's response to the enema.	If too little stool has been expelled, additional measures may be necessary to accomplish the cleansing.
Record the procedure and the results of the enema according to agency policy.	Recording provides a written means of communication among health personnel and documentation of the implemented medical and nursing orders.
Clean and dry the patient, leaving him in a position of comfort.	The patient may feel the need to rest, following what can be an exhausting experience.
Clean reusable equipment. Disposable equipment should also be cleaned; it may be given to the patient for his personal use.	Abundant bacteria in the intestine can be spread to others when equipment is not properly cared for.

tration. A hypertonic solution will draw fluid from body tissues into the bowel. This increases the fluid volume in the intestine to more than the original amount that was instilled.

Hypertonic enema solutions are available in commercially prepared, disposable containers. The total amount of solution is about 4 oz, or 120 mL. The solution also acts on the mucous membranes as a local irritant. Usually, the patient defecates after administering the enema. In many health agencies and in the home, these disposable administration sets have become the method of choice for cleansing the lower intestinal tract of feces. They are less fatiguing and distressing to patients than cleansing enemas and can be easily self-administered.

Giving a hypertonic enema solution differs from the procedure described for administering a high-volume cleansing enema in the following ways:

- The solution container comes with an attached pre-lubricated tip in the commercial sets; therefore, no additional equipment or supplies are needed.
- The entire container of solution can be warmed by placing it in another container of warm water. Some patients do not warm the container at all prior to self-administration. Since there is a low volume of solution, few experience any discomfort.
- The recommended position for the patient receiving a hypertonic enema is the knee-chest position, as shown in Figure 22-7. The position allows for good distribution of solution in the lower large intestine. However, if the patient cannot assume this position, or if the patient will be administering the enema to himself, have him lie in bed on his back or on either side.
- The prelubricated tip is inserted completely within the rectum. Disposable hypertonic enema sets are also available for children. To ensure safety, the applicator tip is shorter and there is less volume.
- Apply gentle, steady pressure on the solution container, which collapses as the solution enters the intestine. It takes about a minute or two to instill the solution and about two to eight minutes to obtain results.

Administering a Retention Enema. A *retention enema* is an instillation that is held within the large intestine. Some are retained for a period of time; others are not expelled at all. Oils, such as mineral, cottonseed, or olive oil, are usually used for retention enemas. The primary purpose of the oil retention enema is to lubricate and soften the stool so that it can be expelled more easily. Usually, 100 to 200 mL of oil are given slowly to avoid stimulating peristalsis and the desire to defecate. The effectiveness of an oil retention enema varies. Often, it becomes necessary to follow an oil enema with a cleansing enema before defecation occurs.

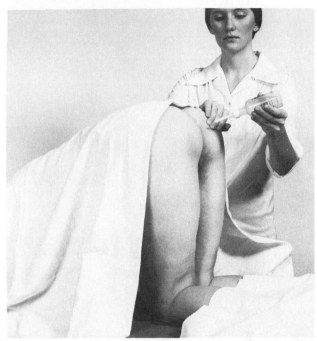

Figure 22-7 The patient is properly draped and in the knee-chest position to receive an enema using a hypertonic solution.

Giving an oil retention enema differs from administering a high-volume cleansing enema in the following respects.

- If reusable equipment is used, a size 14 to 20 rectal tube is recommended for an adult. This smaller tube helps minimize muscular contractions at the anal sphincters and thus helps a patient retain the oil. Most agencies have prepackaged oil retention enema sets that contain necessary supplies and equipment, including oil. Disposable oil retention enema sets may be similar in appearance to hypertonic enema solution sets.
- Oil is warmed only to body temperature to minimize the muscular stimulation caused by a warmer or colder solution.
- The patient is encouraged to retain the oil for at least 30 minutes before attempting to have a bowel movement. This provides time to soften and lubricate the feces.

Achieving Various Purposes With Enemas. The general purpose of an enema is to remove feces from the lower bowel. Table 22-6 lists additional types of enemas, along with their purpose and pertinent comments.

This text does not discuss each listed enema in detail because they are used very infrequently in clinical practice. Also, the nurse who is familiar with the principles and techniques for administering a cleansing enema, as described earlier in this chapter, will find that administering

Table 22-6. Special Types of Enemas

Purpose	Comments
Harris Flush To relieve distention	By holding the container of solution about 18 inches above the patient, allowing a small amount of solution (250 mL to 300 mL) to enter the intestine, and then lowering the container below the level of the patient, the intestine alternately fills and drains. It is expected that the patient will expel flatus as well as some feces, which will drain into the container when it is lowered.
Colonic Irrigation To wash out or flush the entire length of large intestine	Solution is introduced and drained from the intestine simultaneously by using two tubes. About 3000 mL to 4000 mL of solution are used.
Carminative Enema To relieve distention	An example of solution used is one of equal parts of milk and molasses.
Anthelmintic Enema To destroy intestinal parasites	Usually administered as a retention enema.
Emollient Enema To protect and soothe intestinal mucous membrane	Oils are commonly used. The enema is retained.
Nutritive Enema To supply the body with nutrients and/or fluids	Dextrose solution is commonly used. Adequate nourishment is impossible but may be used temporarily or in emergency situations. The enema is retained.

an enema for an alternative purpose may only require slight modifications in the general procedure.

Teaching the Patient to Self-Administer an Enema. The actions in Skill Procedure 22-4 can be used as a good guide to teach a patient how to administer his own enema. A common misunderstanding many people have is that the enema can be given successfully while sitting on a toilet. The enema solution cannot be distributed very well in this position unless a great amount of pressure is used to force the solution upward against gravity. The patient will usually experience a need to defecate sooner because of the pooling of solution within the rectum. Overall there will be a less than desirable cleansing effect.

Reinforce that enemas should not be taken on a routine basis. The occasional use of an enema may not be harmful. Problems arise when a patient self-administers frequent unnecessary enemas. Eventually the normal urge to defecate is absent or markedly decreased. The bowel may become completely dependent on the need for enemas to eliminate feces.

Advise patients to also refrain from automatically self-administering an enema when nausea, vomiting, or abdominal pain is present. Increasing the volume and pressure within the gastrointestinal tract may lead to severe complications of some conditions that are associated with these symptoms.

Eliminating Stool Through a Stoma

When the suffix *ostomy* is attached to a root word, it describes a surgically created opening into a body structure. The prefix that is combined with ostomy indicates the location of the artificial opening. Gastrostomy and jejunostomy were discussed in Chapter 8. A *colostomy* is an opening into the colon or large intestine. An *ileostomy* is an opening created between the ileum, which is a portion of the small intestine, and the abdominal wall. Figure 22-8 shows the locations of ostomies performed in various areas of the intestine. The word *ostomate* refers to a person on whom an ostomy has been performed. Ostomates have unique problems and needs. All members of the health-care team must participate in providing care that will meet each ostomate's optimal recovery.

Collecting Stool From an Intestinal Stoma

There are no natural sphincters in a stoma. A fairly new surgical procedure is being performed in which a type of valve is fashioned to prevent the automatic expulsion of stool or urine. This type of ostomy requires siphoning liquid at periodic intervals. However, for most ostomates, controlling the elimination of stool or urine is impossible. Most all intestinal ostomates wear an appliance to collect

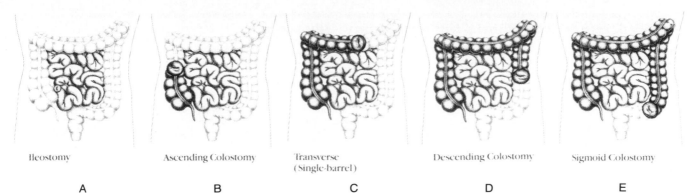

A	B	C	D	E
Ileostomy	Ascending Colostomy	Transverse (Single-barrel)	Descending Colostomy	Sigmoid Colostomy

Figure 22-8 The following anatomical drawings show the location of various ostomies. An ileostomy (*A*) produces watery or pastelike stool almost continuously. An ascending colostomy (*B*) produces watery or semisolid stool, which may be expelled frequently. A transverse colostomy (*C*) expels pastelike or semisolid stool in an unpredictable frequency. A descending colostomy (*D*) and a sigmoid colostomy (*E*) are likely to release feces that resembles normal stool. These may become regulated through colostomy irrigations. (Courtesy of Hollister Inc, Libertyville, IL.)

fecal wastes. It is fastened and worn in a manner similar to the one for a urinary diversion discussed in Chapter 21.

Stool that collects within an appliance can be emptied through an opening at the bottom without removing the appliance from the skin. Once the contents are rinsed from the appliance, it can be reclosed.

Changing an Appliance

Ostomates learn to change an appliance before being discharged from the health agency. Some appliances may require daily changing. Others may need changing every 3 to 7 days. Factors such as the location of the stoma, the consistency of the stool, and the condition of the skin affect the need for changing an appliance.

Prevention of skin breakdown is one of the biggest challenges in ostomy care. Enzymes in stool can quickly cause excoriation. *Excoriation* is the chemical injury of skin. It can be prevented by properly fitting the appliance and protecting the skin with substances that act as a barrier between the skin and fecal wastes. Barrier substances also help attach the appliance in a manner that prevents slipping. The nurse may follow the suggested actions in Skill Procedure 22-5 when changing an appliance.

Irrigating a Colostomy

The purpose of a colostomy irrigation is to remove formed stool and in some cases regulate the timing of bowel movements. It involves instilling solution through the stoma into the colon, similar to administering an enema.

This procedure is usually only necessary for individuals who have a colostomy. The stool from a colostomy can range from semisolid to the formed consistency that is passed from the rectum during normal bowel elimination. The variation depends on the anatomical location of the ostomy along the length of colon. Once an individual recovers from the operative period, stool elimination from the colostomy may be released in a cycle similar to normal bowel movements. With regulation, a patient with a sig-

moid colostomy may choose to omit wearing an appliance and may cover the stoma with only a gauze square.

An ileostomy is not irrigated, since the consistency of stool from this area of the bowel is liquid or similar to thin paste; its passage is rarely difficult. An ileostomy drains at frequent intervals and therefore regulation is not easily achieved. Some learn a degree of control, knowing that the release of stool is more apt to occur after meals.

To irrigate a colostomy, the nurse can follow the suggested actions described in Skill Procedure 22-6.

Draining a Continent Ostomy

A *continent ostomy* is a surgically created opening in which the drainage of liquid stool or urine is controlled by the patient. This technique has only recently been used for a small, selective number of patients. It was first performed on patients who required an ileostomy; it is now also being used when a urinary diversion is performed. The continent ostomy is also referred to as a *Kock pouch* after the surgeon who developed the technique. The surgeon creates a reservoir out of the ileum that collects liquid stool or urine. Just inside the stoma, a valve made of tissue retains the collection of urine or feces. The release of the liquid stool or urine takes place when the patient inserts a catheter and siphons the drainage from the internal pouch.

The advantage of this type of ostomy is that an appliance need not be worn. The disadvantage is that the patient must drain the accumulating liquid stool or urine about every 4 to 6 hours. A gravity drainage system can be used during the night.

If the patient has a continent ostomy, the following actions may be used in its care:

- Place the patient in a comfortable sitting position.
- Insert a lubricated catheter, size 22 to 28, into the stoma.
- Expect resistance after the tube has been inserted

(Text continues on page 566)

Skill Procedure 22-5. Changing an Ostomy Appliance

Suggested Action	**Reason for Action**
Prepare to change the appliance when it is one-third full or no more than one-half full.	An appliance that is allowed to become extremely full may pull away from the skin due to its weight. It will also cause obvious bulges under clothing.
Assemble the replacement appliance and any solvents, adhesives, or skin care preparations that are necessary.	There are various choices available in ostomy appliances. Each type may require different substances for removal and attachment. The skin may require special treatment from time to time, depending upon its state of impairment.
Schedule the appliance change for a time of day when there is sufficient time and the activity of the ostomy is relatively quiet. Allow a minimum of 20 minutes if there are no unusual problems.	Rushing while changing an appliance can result in poor attachment or poor placement on the skin. When there is less likelihood of stool being eliminated, the patient will feel less embarrassed and relaxed.
Remove the appliance from the skin, following the manufacturer's recommendations. Some possible methods include using a solvent, gently peeling the adhesive away from the skin in small sections, or loosening the adhesive with warm water.	Pulling adhesive from the skin can injure the tissue. Covering irritated skin with another appliance can compound the damage to the area. Taking sufficient time to do a proper job and being gentle will maintain the integrity of the skin.
Place the removed appliance into a waterproof bag.	Eventually the nurse will need to rinse the soiled appliance before disposing of it.
Wash the stoma in a circular manner with plain warm water or mild soapy water using a soft washcloth or gauze. The patient may shower or bathe without an appliance.	The area around the stoma should be cleaned of stool, skin secretions, and adhesive before a new appliance is attached. Soap may be irritating to some; rinse well if soap is used.
Explain to the patient that it is normal for the stoma to appear red. Removal of mucous and slight bleeding from the surface of the stoma is also normal. Washing should not cause pain or discomfort to the stoma. Excoriated skin may be painful during washing.	The stoma is inverted bowel that normally has a rich blood supply. Its surface is mucous membrane, which explains the presence of clear, sticky material. The bowel does not contain sensory nerves. The patient may bathe or shower without the appliance.
Inspect the condition of the skin and the stoma. Report signs of excoriation or a very dark red, blue, or swollen appearance to the stoma.	Breakdown usually occurs under the stoma where the appliance attaches to the skin. Abnormal color and size may indicate a problem with circulation of blood to the stoma.
Pat or fan the area completely dry.	Adhesive materials will not stick firmly to wet skin.
Measure and trim the opening of a disposable appliance to fit the size of the patient's stoma. Add $1/16$ to $1/8$ inch to the opening for the stoma.	Some appliance rings are custom made to fit individuals; disposable appliances must be adapted according to each patient's needs. The opening of the appliance should be just large enough to avoid pinching the stoma.
Peel the covering from the adhesive backing that will surround the stoma, as shown in Figure 22-9.	To preserve its adhesive quality, the protective cover should not be removed until ready for immediate use.
Have the patient stand or lie down in bed.	The skin should be taut when the appliance is applied. Sitting causes wrinkling of the skin.
Position the opening of the appliance over the stoma, as illustrated in Figure 22-10. Allow only a thin margin of exposed skin around the stoma.	The adhesive backing must be applied to skin, not the stoma itself. If too much skin is exposed, it may become excoriated from contact with fecal wastes.
Press the adhesive patch outward from the stoma to the skin without forming wrinkles, as shown in Figure 22-11.	Uneven application may form air pockets or wrinkles if the edges are pressed before the center areas. An appliance that is not uniformly applied may become uncomfortable or loose.

(continued)

Skill Procedure 22-5. Continued

Suggested Action	Reason for Action

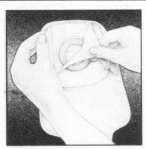

Figure 22-9 This type of appliance has a protective cover over the adhesive backing. The side strips allow the appliance to be handled while positioning the opening over the stoma. (Courtesy of Hollister Inc, Libertyville, IL.)

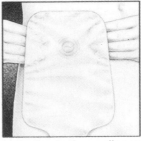

Figure 22-10 The opening in the appliance is positioned over the stoma so that only a thin margin of skin is exposed. (Courtesy of Hollister Inc, Libertyville, IL.)

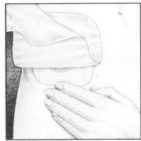

Figure 22-11 The adhesive backing is smoothed to avoid wrinkles and air pockets. The adhesive strips on the sides can be removed once the inner area is in place. (Courtesy of Hollister Inc, Libertyville, IL.)

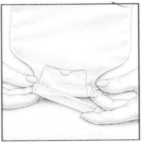

Figure 22-12 The bottom of the appliance is folded and sealed, using a clamp. This type of clamp is curved to fit flatly against the natural curve of the body so that wearing an appliance is less obvious. (Courtesy of Hollister Inc, Libertyville, IL.)

Fold and seal the bottom of the appliance with a special clamp, shown in Figure 22-12. Other types of appliances may be closed with a rubber band or other similar material.

The opening at the bottom of the appliance permits emptying without removing the appliance from the skin. Tight closure prevents leaking of the contents.

Skill Procedure 22-6. Irrigating a Colostomy

Suggested Action	Reason for Action
Obtain equipment: 500 to 1000 mL of irrigating solution, most often tap water or normal saline at 40.5°C to 43°C (105°F to 110°F); an irrigating cone or valve; tubing; lubricant; irrigating sleeve; and belt. A bedpan will be needed as a receptacle for drainage from the sleeve if the patient is confined to bed.	Organizing the equipment and having it ready helps conserve time and energy and helps make teaching effective. An irrigation is likely to use less solution than an enema. Solution may cause cramping if it is too cold. Injury to the intestinal mucosa may occur if the solution is too hot.
Fill the container with solution and expel the air from the tubing by releasing the clamp long enough to allow solution to drain through. Direct the tip into the bedpan or toilet.	Removing air from the tubing increases the potential volume of fluid that can be instilled. It prevents cramping and the discharge of gas from the stoma.
Place or hang the container of solution so that it will be approximately 12 inches above the patient's stoma.	The level of the container affects the rate and pressure during instillation of fluid.

(continued)

Skill Procedure 22-6. Continued

Suggested Action	Reason for Action
Have equipment ready for changing the appliance after the irrigating solution has been instilled and drained.	Usually the discharge of stool during the immediate postoperative period may be more liquid and unpredictable than after complete recovery. Wearing an appliance is usually necessary initially.
Place the patient in a sitting position either in bed, in a chair, or on the toilet.	This allows the patient to observe or assist with care that he will eventually be performing independently. It also promotes the drainage of the solution by gravity once it has been instilled.
Place absorbent padding on the bed or on the patient.	Irrigating solution may drip accidently. Protective covering helps avoid changing linen and clothing.
Remove the dressing or appliance. Place it within a waterproof container for wastes.	The appliance may contain residue of stool. Organisms are present in feces; the soiled equipment should be disposed of in such a way that the spread of organisms is prevented.
Secure the irrigating sleeve over the stoma and fasten it with a belt as the nurse is doing in Figure 22-13.	An irrigating sleeve is not attached with adhesive, since it is only worn for a short period of time during the irrigation.

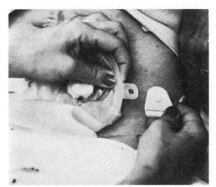

Figure 22-13 The irrigating sleeve is secured in place, using a belt that fastens around the patient's waist.

Center the opening of the sleeve, exposing the stoma as shown in Figure 22-14. The sleeve is similar to a large appliance except that there is an additional opening at the top.	The sleeve will provide a channel through which irrigating solution and stool will drain into the bedpan or toilet.
Place the lower end of the sleeve into a bedpan, commode, or toilet, as shown in Figure 22-15.	Fluid expelled during or following the irrigation will drain down the sleeve into a receptacle for wastes.
Attach a cone, if available, to the tip of the irrigation tubing. Lubricate it well.	The cone prevents injuring the bowel with the tubing. It also controls the depth of insertion, since it cannot be passed farther than the distance that matches the diameter of the stoma.
Some health agencies use other insertion devices such as tubing and a nipple valve, as shown in Figure 22-16.	The valve prevents solution from escaping from the stoma.
Gently insert the cone or tubing into the stoma at an angle that follows the natural path of the colon, as shown in Figure 22-17. The tip of the tubing should not be inserted more than 4 to 6 inches within the stoma.	Following the natural path of the colon reduces resistance during insertion and instillation of fluid.

(continued)

Skill Procedure 22-6. Continued

Suggested Action	Reason for Action

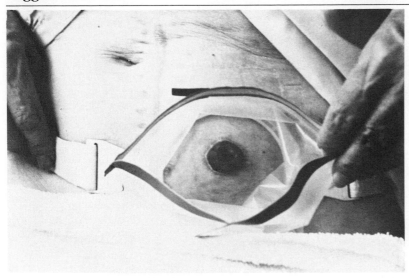

Figure 22-14 The access area of the plastic irrigating sleeve opens over the stoma.

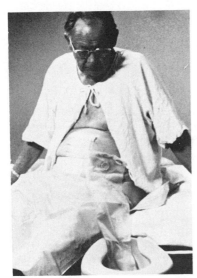

Figure 22-15 The lower end of the irrigating sleeve has been placed into a bedpan that will collect stool and irrigating solution when draining occurs.

Do not force the cone. If resistance is met, pull the cone out slightly, release a little solution, wait a minute or so, and try again. If another attempt fails, discuss the problem with a supervising nurse.

Forcing the cone may injure intestinal mucosa. Removing the cone slightly and instilling a little solution often helps overcome resistance.

Have the patient hold the cone securely, if possible, after it is in place, as shown in Figure 22-18.

Encouraging the patient to assist as much as possible helps him learn to handle the equipment and gain self-confidence in self-care.

Anticipate that not all patients will be willing to look at or assist with their care.

Patients require time to adjust to the change in body image.

(continued)

Skill Procedure 22-6. *Continued*

Suggested Action	Reason for Action

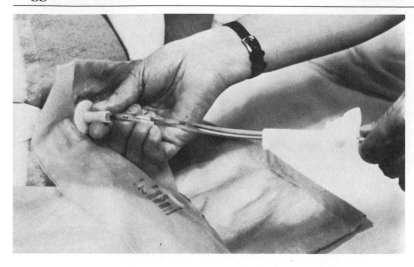

Figure 22-16 This nurse uses a calibrated tube and a valve during irrigation of a colostomy. The tube is passed through the valve for the desired length. The valve prevents the irrigation solution from leaking back onto the abdomen and side of the patient.

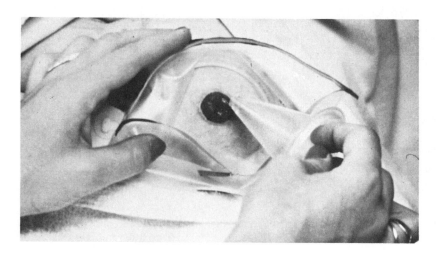

Figure 22-17 The lubricated cone is gently introduced into the stoma at an angle so that it follows the natural path of the colon.

Suggested Action	Reason for Action
Open the regulating clamp to instill the solution. Allow 5 to 10 minutes for instillation.	To aid in fluid distribution and the comfort of the patient the fluid should not be instilled too rapidly.
Clamp the tubing temporarily if the patient complains of cramping. Release the clamp and continue with the irrigation once the patient's discomfort disappears.	Stopping the instillation of fluid limits rapid bowel distention and increased peristalsis.
Discontinue the irrigation after giving the prescribed amount of solution. Pinch or clamp the tubing and remove it from the top of the irrigating sleeve.	The irrigating solution will drain from the stoma. Clamping the tubing before withdrawal prevents solution still within the tube from leaking.
Close the top of the irrigating sleeve to enclose the stoma.	The return will spill out of the sleeve opening at the top if it is not closed.
Provide the patient with reading material or supplies to perform personal hygiene while waiting for the irrigation to finish draining.	Other activities may be accomplished while the solution and stool are being expelled from the stoma.

(continued)

Skill Procedure 22-6. Continued

Suggested Action	Reason for Action

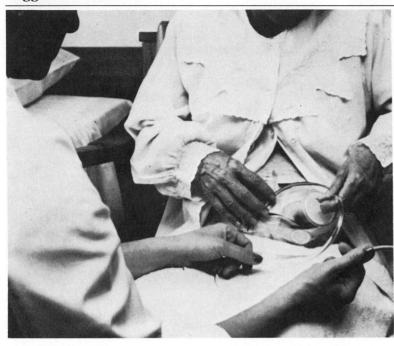

Figure 22-18 The patient holds the cone firmly as the nurse opens the flow control clamp, which allows the irrigating solution to enter the colon.

Remove the belt and sleeve when the draining has stopped. Clean the stoma with plain water or mild, soapy water. Pat the skin dry before applying an appliance, if one is needed.

Place an appliance of the patient's choice over the stoma, as shown in Figure 22-19.

By using irrigations, some ostomates can control elimination and thus avoid the need to constantly wear an appliance. Many eventually cover the stoma with only a dry dressing.

Control of elimination is not usually achieved while the patient recovers from surgery. It may occur as the patient recovers at home.

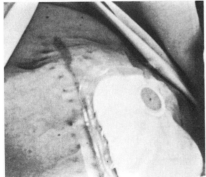

Figure 22-19 After the skin around the stoma is cleaned and dried, an appliance is placed over the stoma.

Refer the patient to an enterostomal therapist and recommend that he attend local meetings of self-help groups of ostomates.

An *enterostomal therapist* is a nurse who has been certified in the care of ostomates. Self-help groups share their knowledge and discuss common problems. They can provide support once a patient is discharged.

approximately 2 inches; this is the location of the valve that controls the retention of liquid stool or urine. Instruct the patient to take deep breaths, cough, or perform Valsalva's maneuver at this time.

- Gently advance the catheter through the valve.
- As stool or urine begins to flow through the catheter, direct it into a container or toilet that is at least 12 inches below the patient's ostomy. Expect drainage of stool to take 5 to 10 minutes; urine should drain in less time. There may be large variations in the amounts that drain in the early postoperative period. The pouch may eventually stretch to hold as much as 600 mL. The average amount that drains each time is between 200 and 250 mL.
- Remove the catheter and clean it with warm soapy water. Place it in a clean, sealable, plastic bag until its next use.
- Cover the stoma with a gauze square or a large bandage.

Plugging of the catheter may become a problem because of thick stool or mucus that blocks the drainage holes in the catheter. Suggestions for clearing the tube include the following:

- Instruct the patient to perform Valsalva's maneuver.
- Rotate the catheter tip inside the stoma.
- Milk the catheter.

If these are not successful, the catheter should be withdrawn, rinsed, and reinserted. If repeated efforts do not result in any drainage, a physician should be notified. Draining should not be delayed longer than 6 hours.

Obtaining a Stool Specimen

Information acquired from the examination of a stool specimen can add to the nurse's database assessments. They may help in making a medical or nursing diagnosis.

Stool may be analyzed to detect any number of abnor-

Skill Procedure 22-7. Collecting a Stool Specimen

Suggested Action	Reason for Action
Obtain a waxed paper container that has a cover or use the appropriate container specified by the health agency.	Stool is moist and the container should not permit saturation of fecal wastes onto the surfaces of work areas. A cover helps contain the odor and conceals the specimen.
Have the patient void into a toilet or separate receptacle before the stool specimen is collected.	Urine mixed with stool may interfere with the proper examination required for some tests.
Observe principles of medical asepsis when collecting stool.	Sterile technique is not necessary, since the stool already contains organisms. Principles of medical asepsis restrict and contain organisms, preventing their transfer to cleaner areas.
Use a clean bedpan. Avoid taking specimens from a toilet if possible.	When stool becomes mixed with water its consistency changes. Water and urine may destroy some parasites and obscure proper diagnosis.
Lift a portion of stool approximately equivalent to 1 teaspoon to 2 teaspoons, with two clean tongue depressors.	Only a small sample of stool is usually necessary for analysis. Tongue depressors provide a convenient method for removing stool from the bedpan.
Place the feces directly into the container. Discard the remaining stool.	The stool should not be allowed to remain in the bedpan where moisture may evaporate or other changes can occur.
Take care to avoid contaminating the outside of the specimen container with stool.	A clean outer surface prevents spreading organisms to individuals who handle and examine the specimen.
Wash hands thoroughly after collecting stool and handling the bedpan.	Organisms are spread easily when good handwashing is not practiced.
Label and attach the appropriate laboratory form to the specimen.	Poor identification may result in having to repeat the collection and examination.
Take the specimen directly to the laboratory. Notify the laboratory personnel as to the contents of the specimen container and the requested test.	The specimen may need to be refrigerated, kept at room temperature, or warmed until it can be examined.
Record the collection of the specimen, description of the stool, and the time it was taken to the laboratory.	Charting is a method for recording that diagnostic measures have been carried out.

Table 22-7. Special Stool Examination Techniques

Purpose of Examination	Recommended Techniques
When examining for the presence of blood	Obtain only a small amount of stool when it is being tested for blood. One common method is to use a rectal applicator or a gloved finger to swab the stool. The stool on the finger or applicator is then placed directly onto a special slide.
When examining for the presence of pinworms	Use *clear* cellophane tape. Frosted tape makes examination difficult. Place the tape directly over the anal region, remove almost immediately, and place on a slide. Be sure to collect a specimen immediately in the morning, before the patient has had a bowel movement or a bath. Pinworms tend to come to the anal canal area during the night.
When examining for the presence of parasites	See to it that the patient does not have a laxative or enema because parasites may thus be destroyed. Include some blood or mucus, when present in the stool, because parasites tend to thrive in these media.
When collecting an entire bowel movement	Rinse a bedpan and then line it with plastic material that will stick to the damp surface. Have the patient defecate, then twist and tie the plastic and place it in an appropriate container. This technique is also helpful when stools need to be weighed.
When collecting a specimen for culture purposes	Pass a sterile rectal swab beyond the internal sphincter, rotate it carefully, and place the swab in an appropriate container.
When collecting a specimen from a patient with a colostomy or ileostomy	Remove a portion of stool from the patient's collecting bag and place the stool directly into a specimen container.

mal characteristics or components. For example, feces may be examined for blood, bile, parasites, and parasite eggs. The nurse either instructs the patient in the collection of a specimen or personally obtains the specimen from a sample of the patient's stool. The technique for collecting a stool specimen depends on the purpose of the test. Skill Procedure 22-7 describes actions that pertain to any collection of stool. Table 22-7 lists particular techniques that are indicated when specific information is needed.

Suggested Measures to Promote Bowel Elimination in Selected Situations

When the Patient Is an Infant or Child

Assess the characteristics of a normal stool according to an infant's age and diet. Use Table 22-8 as a guide.

Diarrhea may rapidly become serious in infants and young children because they are especially susceptible to water and chemical imbalances.

Plan that infants and children with diarrhea are often placed in isolation to help control the spread of causative organisms. Many children with diarrhea may be placed within the same isolation room to facilitate their care. Isolation techniques are described in Chapter 17.

Compare and describe the characteristics of abnormal stool that a sick infant or child eliminates.

Be especially careful to keep infants and young children with diarrhea clean and dry because their skin is very sensitive to irritation. Change diapers as often as necessary to prevent stool from remaining in contact with the skin. Rinse soap or detergent off the skin well because remnants are irritating to the skin. Protect the skin as indicated with an ointment of the agency's choice.

Expect that rectal suppositories containing drugs are frequently prescribed for infants and children because they may have difficulty swallowing medications. Pediatric suppositories are smaller, and the dosage is reduced in comparison to adult drugs.

Use appropriately-sized equipment when giving an infant or child a cleansing enema. One guide to determine the appropriate amount of solution to use is to prepare 10 to 15 mL per kg (2.2 lb) of body weight, but no more than 300 mL. The preferred solution for a cleansing enema for a child is normal saline because it will not alter fluid distribution in the body.

Place infants and young children on a diaper or bedpan when giving a cleansing enema. Insert the tip of the tubing 2 to 4 inches only and administer the solution *slowly*.

Table 22-8. Characteristics of Infants' Stools

Ingested Substance	Appearance	Frequency
Amniotic fluid swallowed during the period before birth	Dark blackish green, sticky stool called meconium	Meconium is passed four to six times daily for 1 to 2 days after the baby is born.
Breast milk	Unformed, pastelike, bright or golden yellow	Frequency is unpredictable. Some pass stools once or twice a day and others at every feeding.
Cow's milk	Firmer consistency, yellow but not as bright as seen with breast milk	Infants fed cow's milk pass stools less often, usually one to three times a day.
Soft and solid foods	Formed, brownish color	A bowel movement once a day becomes common as the infant approaches toddler age.

Massage the abdomen gently, if this technique is not contraindicated, to help expel the enema solution.

Use child-sized disposable enema equipment. Disposable equipment for children usually contains about 70 mL (just over 2 oz) of solution. This type of cleansing enema is not ordinarily recommended for children under 2 years of age.

Use about 60 to 100 mL of oil when giving an oil retention enema to children. Place pressure on the anus or use adhesive strips to hold the buttocks together securely so that the oil will be retained.

Use child-sized equipment for infants and children who have a colostomy or ileostomy. Skin care around a stoma is especially important because of the sensitivity of a child's skin to irritation and injury.

Be especially supportive of parents whose child has a colostomy or ileostomy. Surgery of this magnitude with its continued demands for care can be very devastating to parents. It has been found that if parents accept a child's colostomy or ileostomy, so will the child.

When the Patient Is Elderly

Take into account that gastrointestinal motility, muscle tone, and digestive enzymes decrease with age. These normal aging processes tend to predispose a person to constipation.

Obtain a health history that includes a careful assessment of the elderly person's elimination patterns. When possible, practices the patient uses to promote elimination should be included in his nursing care plan, if they are safe. For example, if the patient drinks hot water or prune juice before breakfast to promote elimination, follow this routine unless it is contraindicated.

Include a dietary history when assessing the patient's elimination patterns. Many elderly persons have diets low in fiber and bulk; they tend to eat processed convenience foods. Such diets predispose the patient to constipation.

Assess intestinal elimination patterns accurately. Many elderly persons become very bowel conscious and report a problem with constipation erroneously because they lack accurate information concerning elimination.

Use a teaching program that includes bowel retraining for the elderly with constipation or incontinence. When possible, include the use of a commode, which is generally more acceptable to

Applicable Nursing Diagnoses

After assessing a patient's bowel elimination patterns, the nurse may identify these nursing diagnoses.
- Constipation
- Perceived Constipation
- Colonic Constipation
- Diarrhea
- Bowel Incontinence
- Toileting Self-Care Deficit
- Situational Low Self-Esteem

Nursing Care Plan 22-1 reflects the nursing process as it applies to a patient with Colonic Constipation. Colonic Constipation is defined as, "The state in which an individual's pattern of elimination is characterized by hard, dry stool which results from a delay in passage of food residue" (North American Nursing Diagnosis Association, 1989).

NURSING CARE PLAN

22-1. Colonic Constipation

Assessment

Subjective Data

States, "I've got a problem with constipation. I haven't had a bowel movement in 4 days even though I've felt like I need to pass stool. I sit and strain but I only pass a small amount of hard stool. I used to have a problem now and then when I was a kid; but since I'm living alone it's getting to be very frequent. Maybe its's because I don't eat regularly and when I do, it's a lot of convenience food."

Objective Data

21-year-old man recovering from a fractured ankle that occurred when he tripped on an area rug in his apartment yesterday. Plaster cast on L. leg that extends from toes to midcalf. Abdomen tympanic during percussion. Bowel sounds are hypoactive in all four quadrants.

Diagnosis

Colonic Constipation related to inadequate dietary habits.

Plan

Goal

The patient will have a bowel movement within 24 hours and list 3 ways to improve the regularity of bowel elimination by 10/25.

Orders: 10/24
1. Give oil retention enema as ordered for prn administration.
2. Give prescribed laxative at HS if no bowel movement has occurred.
3. Encourage drinking at least 8 to 10 glasses of fluid per day; avoid carbonated beverages.
4. Instruct about high fiber foods and inform that daily consumption should consist of at least 4 servings. ——————————————————— A. ZIMMERMAN, RN

Implementation (Documentation)

10/24

1300 Instructed to drink at least 5 more glasses of fluid today and 8 to 10 thereafter. Explained that soft drinks increase intestinal gas. Given paper and pencil to record his current eating pattern, food likes, and dislikes. ———— M. HASS, LPN

1330 200 mL oil retention enema administered. Instructed to remain in bed and retain solution for at least 30 minutes or longer if possible. ———— M. HASS, LPN

Evaluation (Documentation)

1400 Helped to bathroom using crutches and three-point nonweight bearing gait. Passed a moderate amount of hard stool. Blood observed on stool and toilet paper. States, "It took a lot of straining but I feel much better now." ———— M. HASS, LPN

1400 Reviewed dietary list. Noted the following: does not eat breakfast, usually eats lunch at fast-food establishment near campus, fixes frozen meals in evening, snacks on chips. ———— M. HASS, LPN

1445 Recommended eating breakfast and waiting at home a little while for urge to eliminate. Include whole grain bread/toast, cereal, fresh fruits, fruit juices, salads, and nuts or seeds as additions to diet for at least 4 servings each day. States, "I guess I could eat an apple or carrots between classes. I used to eat shredded wheat for breakfast. They sell salads where I eat lunch. I didn't realize soda pop could add to the bloating I've been feeling. Maybe I'll have to start shopping and eating a little differently from now on." ———— M. HASS, LPN

the patient than a bedpan, when helping to establish normal elimination patterns.

Advise against using routine enemas or laxatives. Fluid and chemical imbalances occur more easily in the elderly than in other adults.

Use a tightly rolled cloth, such as a towel about 4 cm (1½ in) in diameter, to help an elderly person retain a cleansing or retention enema. The roll should be placed between the buttocks with pressure on the anal area. Then, position the patient flat on his back.

Keep in mind that the skin of an elderly person is especially thin and sensitive to fecal matter. Use nursing measures to keep the patient meticulously clean and the skin well protected.

Teaching Suggestions to Promote Bowel Elimination

Key suggestions to promote intestinal elimination are included in the summary below. Information on specific conditions that affect elimination have also been added.

Problems often arise because people lack knowledge about normal bowel elimination. Sharing accurate information with patients helps promote health and well-being. Some areas include how to prevent and manage constipation, diarrhea, fecal incontinence, intestinal distention, and fecal impaction.

Although laxatives and enemas sometimes play a proper role in intestinal elimination, they are also very often abused. Teaching their proper use and the dangers of abuse is a nursing responsibility.

Individuals are often able to perform many self-care techniques when they experience alterations in bowel elimination. The nurse can use the same skill procedures described for inserting a suppository, administering an enema, ostomy care, and collection of a stool specimen when a patient needs to learn one of these skills.

The patient who has an ostomy should be told about various skin protection methods. One of the most common substances used is karaya. Vanishing cream is another inexpensive protectant. Tincture of benzoin may be sprayed or swabbed on the skin if the skin is not already irritated. It can also be used to create a tacky surface to enhance the adhesive quality of an appliance.

A plastic or paper cup placed over the stoma before spraying or swabbing the area protects the stoma and prevents fecal material from dribbling on the cleaned area.

Explain to an ostomate that odors can be controlled by keeping the appliance clean and deodorized. They may be washed between uses with soap and water and rinsed well. A white-vinegar solution, one part vinegar and three parts water, is good for removing odors. Some nurses have found that placing a deodorant tampon in the collecting bag helps absorb liquid stool and control odors. A tampon absorbs about 2 oz of fluid. Still another method found helpful to control odors is saturation of a piece of tissue with vanilla extract and placement of the tissue at the bottom of the bag. Commercial deodorants are available. Some are used in soaking solutions for the appliance; others may be placed inside while it is being worn.

Teach the ostomate the importance of a balanced and nourishing diet. Only foods that stimulate excessive peristalsis or cause gas should be avoided. Keep in mind that not all people are troubled by the same kinds of foods; some may choose to continue eating them occasionally despite the changes they cause in bowel elimination.

Instruct the ostomate patient that one way to release accumulating gas from an appliance is to prick pinholes at the upper end of the appliance. This provides a route for the escaping gas, yet prevents leakage of fecal wastes from the bottom of the appliance.

Encourage the ostomate to construct coverings for the appliance that conceal its contents if this is a concern during sexual activity. Bathing and emptying an appliance are also important before sex.

For the patient with a continent ostomy, advise that a MedicAlert ID be worn in case of a medical emergency. When a person cannot speak for himself, emergency medical personnel should be able to determine that an ostomy requires draining and continuous care.

Bibliography

Behm R: A special recipe to banish constipation. Geriatr Nurs 6(4):216–217, 1985

Burkitt D: Fiber as protective against gastrointestinal diseases. Am J Gastroenterol 79(4):249–252, 1984

Cerrato PL: Is America really constipated? RN Magazine 52(5):81–82, 84, 86, 1989

Cimprich B: Symptom management: Constipation. Cancer Nurs 8(1 suppl):39–43, 1985

Clarke B: Making sense of enemas. Nursing Times 84(30):40–41, 1988

Ellickson EB: Bowel management plan for the homebound elderly. Journal of Gerontological Nursing 14(1):16–19, 40–42, 1988

Kearns P: Exercises to ease pain after abdominal surgery. RN Magazine 49(7):45–48, 1986

Krasner D: What's wrong with this stoma? Am J Nurs 90(4):46–47, 1990

McLane AM, McShane RE: Empirical validation of defining characteristics of constipation: A study of bowel elimination practices of health adults. Classification of Nursing Diagnoses Proceedings of the Sixth Conference of the North American Nursing Diagnosis Association, 456–464, 1986

McLane AM, McShane RE: Nursing diagnosis: Colonic constipation. Classification of Nursing Diagnoses Proceedings of the Eighth Conference of the North American Nursing Diagnosis Association, 431, 1989

McLane AM, McShane RE: Nursing diagnosis: Perceived constipation. Classification of Nursing Diagnoses Proceedings of the Eighth Conference of the North American Nursing Diagnosis Association, 432, 1989

McMillan SC, Williams FA: Validity and reliability of the Constipation Assessment Scale. Cancer Nurs 12(3):183–188, 1989

McShane RE, McLane AM: Constipation: Consensual and empirical validation. Nurs Clin North Am 20(4):801–808, 1985

McShane RE, McLane AM: Constipation: Impact of etiological factors. Journal of Gerontological Nursing 14(4):31–34, 46–47, 1988

Nichols R: Simple remedies for postop gas pain. RN Magazine 49(2):42–44, 1986

Vaughn JB, Nemcek MA: Postoperative flatulence: Causes and remedies. Today's OR Nurse 8(10):19–23, 1986

Williams SG, Dipalma JA: Constipation in the long-term care facility. Gastroenterological Nursing 12(3):179–182, 1990

23

Administering Oral and Topical Medications

Chapter Outline

Behavioral Objectives
Glossary
Introduction
Receiving a Medication Order
Implementing the Medication Order
Supplying Medications
Safeguarding Medications
Calculating Dosages
Reviewing the Patient's Health History
Following Basic Guidelines for Administering
   Medications
Recording Medication Administration
Reporting Medication Errors
Administering Oral Medications
Administering Oral Medications Through a
   Nasogastric Tube
Administering Topical Medications
Overcoming Noncompliance
Suggested Measures When Administering Medications
   in Selected Situations
Applicable Nursing Diagnoses
Teaching Suggestions for the Administration of
   Medications
Bibliography

Skill Procedures

Administering Oral Medications
Administering Oral Medications Through a Nasogastric
   Tube
Applying a Transdermal Patch
Instilling Medications Into the Eye
Instilling Medications Into the Ear
Administering Nasal Medications
Administering Vaginal Medications

Behavioral Objectives

When the content of this chapter has been mastered, the learner will be able to:

Define the terms appearing in the glossary.

Identify seven components of a medication order and five types of medication orders.

Describe how medications, including narcotics, are supplied and safeguarded in health-care agencies.

Identify information about a patient that may affect medication administration.

Discuss guidelines the nurse would follow in the safe preparation and administration of medication.

List five practices that have been linked with contributing to medication errors.

Describe the recommended techniques for administering oral and topical medications.

Demonstrate the recommended procedures for administering oral medications, medications through a nasogastric tube, and topical medications.

List strategies to help overcome noncompliance in the self-administration of medication.

Describe suggested measures for administering medications to patients in selected situations, as described in this chapter.

Summarize suggestions offered in this chapter for teaching patients about medications.

Glossary

Buccal A route used for administering drugs that involves placing the medication in the mouth against the mucous membranes on the inside of the cheek.

Drug Any substance that chemically changes body function. Synonym for *medication.*

Enteric coated A covering on an oral drug that prevents it from becoming dissolved until the medication is within the small intestine.

Generic name A drug's chemical name that is not protected by a company's trademark. Synonym for *nonproprietary name.*

Individual supply A quantity of medication provided for a single patient that may last for 1 to 3 days.

Inner canthus The area of the eye near the nose.

Inunction A medication incorporated into a vehicle, such as an ointment, and rubbed into the skin.

Medication Any substance that chemically changes body function. Synonym for *drug.*

Medication administration record (MAR) A form used to schedule and document drug administration.

Medication order The directions for administering a drug. Synonym for *prescription.*

Noncompliance The failure to follow instructions.

Nonproprietary name A drug name that is usually descriptive of a drug's chemical structure and is not protected by a company's trademark. Synonym for *generic name.*

Oral medications Drugs that are swallowed or instilled through a tube leading to the stomach.

Outer canthus The area of the eye near the temple.

Prescription The directions for administering of a drug. Synonym for *medication order.*

Proprietary name The name of a drug used by the manufacturer for the product it sells. Synonym for *trade name.*

Stock supply A large quantity of a frequently prescribed drug.

Sublingual A route for administering drugs that involves placing the medication within the mouth under the tongue.

Suspension A mixture of undissolved solid particles in a liquid.

Teratogenic effects The production of abnormal structures in a developing fetus causing severe deformities.

Topical administration The application of medication to the skin or mucous membranes.

Trade name The name of a drug used by the manufacturer for the product it sells. Synonym for *proprietary name.*

Transdermal Through the skin.

Unit dose system A 24-hour supply of a medication, with each single dose labeled and packaged separately from the others.

Verbal orders Instructions given to the nurse either in a face-to-face conversation or by telephone.

Introduction

Among one of the nurse's most important responsibilities is the administration of medications. A *medication* is any substance that chemically changes body function. In this chapter, the terms *medication* and *drug* will be used synonymously.

The emphasis of this chapter is the safe preparation and administration of medications. Information concerning specific drugs is more appropriately discussed in pharmacology texts.

Receiving a Medication Order

The physician determines the patient's drug therapy. The *medication order,* or *prescription,* includes the directions for administering a drug. Clerical activities may be delegated, but the nurse is the one within a health agency who is responsible for checking, transcribing, and carrying out the medication order.

A written medication order is complete when it contains all of the following seven parts:

1. The name of the patient
2. The date and time the order is written
3. The name of the medication
4. The dosage to be administered
5. The route for administering the medication
6. The frequency of administering the medication
7. The signature of the person who has written the order

The nurse must determine that the medication order is valid by checking that all seven essential parts are included in the medication order.

Identifying the Name of the Patient. The name of the patient is ordinarily imprinted on each page of his record. His full name, including first name, middle initial, and last name, is used. If there is any chance for confusion, a second name is used instead of a middle initial. If the patient's name is not imprinted on each page of the record, the full name should be written clearly on each page. The patient's full name is also used when a nurse or other authorized person transcribes orders onto medication cards or sheets.

Noting the Date and Time of the Medication Order. The person writing the order, usually the physician, indicates the date and time it is written. This information is important and is needed when discontinuation dates and times are calculated. Dating and timing an order also help to prevent oversights and errors. The information is typically written as follows: 11/1/86 10:15 A.M.

Specifying the Name of the Medication. Each drug has both a trade, or proprietary, name and a generic, or nonproprietary, name. The *trade,* or *proprietary, name* is the name used by the manufacturer for the drug it sells. The drug's *generic,* or *nonproprietary, name* is a chemical name that is not protected by a company's trademark. For example, Demerol® is a proprietary name. It is the manufacturer's brand name for meperidine hydrochloride, the generic name.

The name of the drug must be clearly written in the medication order. Some agencies permit either name to be used, while some have a policy that only the generic name should be written when ordering a drug.

Table 23-1. Terms Used When Designating Dosage Measurements

Term	Abbreviation
Metric	
Gram	G or Gm (lower case letter may be used)
Milligram	mg
Microgram	mcg
Liter	L or l
Milliliter	ml or mL
Apothecary	
dram	ℨ
drop	gtt
grain	gr
minim	m
ounce	℥

Indicating the Dosage of the Medication. The amount of a drug represents its dosage. The dose may be written in whole numbers, decimals, fractions, or symbols. Drug measurements are indicated using terms or abbreviations in the metric or apothecary systems, which are listed in Table 23-1. For home use, dosages may be indicated by using household measurements, such as teaspoon and tablespoon, which are more easily interpreted by nonprofessionals. Table 23-2 is a list of standard weights and volumes used within each system of measurement.

Nurses may find that particular clinical agencies permit medication orders to be written only in one system of measurement, usually the metric, or both may be used. There are approximate equivalents for converting dosages ordered in one system and supplied in another. Some common equivalents are listed in Table 23-3. They are best learned and committed to memory. However, a similar table of equivalents should be available on most nursing units.

Designating the Route of Administration. The medication order designates by what manner, or route, the drug is to be administered. Table 23-4 lists and describes common routes of administration. The prescription should indicate specifically which route should be used. Some medications may be given by various routes. Meperidine hydrochloride is an example. The order should be questioned if the route is not specified.

Prescribing the Frequency of Administration. The frequency with which a medication is to be given is most commonly written in standard abbreviations, which are listed and defined in Table 23-5.

Signing the Medication Order. The laws within each state govern who may legally prescribe medications. The person authorized to write a prescription most often is the physician, but it may also be a dentist, a physician's assistant, or a nurse practitioner, depending upon the individual state's statutes. The legally authorized person's signature must appear at the end of the medication order.

Table 23-2. Weight and Volume Equivalents

Weight		Volume	
Metric System			
1 kilogram	= 1000 grams	1 liter	= 1000 milliliters, or 1000 cubic centimeters
1 gram	= 1000 milligrams		
1 milligram	= 1000 micrograms		
Apothecary System			
1 grain	= kernel of wheat	1 minim	= 1 drop
20 grains	= 1 scruple	60 minims	= 1 fluidram
3 scruples	= 1 dram	8 fluidrams	= 1 fluid ounce
8 drams	= 1 ounce	16 fluid ounces	= 1 pint
12 ounces	= 1 pound	2 pints	= 1 quart
		4 quarts	= 1 gallon
Household System			
16 ounces	= 1 pound	16 drops	= 1 teaspoon
		3 teaspoons	= 1 tablespoon
		2 tablespoons	= 1 fluid ounce
		8 fluid ounces	= 1 glassful

Table 23-3. Common Equivalents Among Systems of Measurement

Metric		Apothecary		Household
Weight				
1 kilogram			=	2.2 pounds
1 gram	=	15 grains		
60 milligrams	=	1 grain		
Volume				
4 or 5 milliliters	=	1 fluidram	=	1 teaspoon
15 milliliters	=	½ ounce	=	1 tablespoon
30 milliliters	=	1 fluid ounce	=	2 tablespoons
1000 milliliters, or 1 liter	=	32 fluid ounces	=	1 quart

Questioning a Medication Order. The nurse is expected to question any medication order that does not contain all seven parts of the order. The nurse should also clarify any aspect of the seven parts of the drug order that may seem unclear or inaccurate. For example, if the writing is not legible, if the dosage or frequency is significantly different from the usual administration, or if the appropriateness of giving a particular medication to a patient is questionable, the nurse should communicate with the person who has written the order. Medication errors are

Table 23-4. Routes for Administering Medications

Term Used to Describe Route	How Drug Is Administered
Oral Administration Given by mouth	The patient swallows the drug
Inhalation Given via the respiratory tract	The patient inhales the drug
Parenteral Given by injection	Inject the drug into:
Subcutaneous or hypodermic injection	Subcutaneous tissue
Intramuscular injection	Muscle tissue
Intracutaneous or intradermal injection	Corium (*i.e.,* upper layers of the skin)
Intravenous injection	A vein
Topical administration Given by placing on the skin or mucous membrane	
Transdermal administration	Place a unit–dose of the drug on the skin; the drug is absorbed through the skin.
Vaginal administration	Insert the drug into the vagina
Rectal administration	Insert the drug into the rectum
Sublingual administration	Place the drug under the tongue; the drug is not to be swallowed or chewed
Buccal administration	Place the drug between the cheek and gum; the drug is not to be swallowed or chewed
Inunction	Rub the drug into the skin
Instillation	Place the drug into direct contact with mucous membranes
Irrigation	Flush the mucous membranes with a drug in solution

Drugs may also be injected into the arteries, heart tissues, spinal cord, joints, and peritoneal cavity. The drugs are ordinarily administered by the physician when using these routes.

Table 23-5. Common Abbreviations Used When Prescribing Medications

Abbreviation	Meaning
a̅a̅	of each
a.c.	before meals
ad lib	freely
Aq	water
b.i.d.	twice each day
c̅	with
h	hour
h.s.	at bedtime
IM	intramuscular
IV	intravenous
OD	right eye
OS	left eye
OU	both eyes
p.c.	after meals
PO	by mouth
prn	as necessary
q3h, q4h, and so on	every three hours, every four hours, and so on
q.d.	every day
q.h.	every hour
q.i.d.	four times a day
q.o.d.	every other day
q.s.	a sufficient quantity
Rx	take
s̅	without
ss	one half
stat	at once
subq	subcutaneous
t.i.d.	three times each day
tinct	tincture

serious. A questionable medication order should *never* be implemented until after the nurse has consulted the physician or another authorized person.

Receiving Verbal Orders

Verbal orders are instructions given to the nurse either during face-to-face conversation or by telephone. These forms of communication are more likely to result in misinterpretation than those that are written. A good rule to follow is to have the order written if the doctor is present. The only exception would be during a crisis, when a delay in time or action will affect the patient's safety.

The nurse must be very careful to record the information accurately when verbal orders are received over the telephone. At the very least, the following safeguards should be used.

- Have a second nurse or staff person listen simultaneously on an extension, if possible.
- Record the message immediately on paper.
- Repeat the written information back to the physician before hanging up the phone.
- Make sure the order includes the pertinent information (drug name, dosage, route, and frequency.)
- Clarify any drug names that sound similar, such as Feldene® and Seldane®, Nicobid® and Nitro-Bid®, digitoxin and digoxin.
- Spell or repeat single numbers of dosages that could be misunderstood, such as fifteen—one, five; and fifty—five, zero.
- Remind the physician to countersign the telephone order within 24 hours or according to the agency's policy.
- Rewrite the message on the physician's order sheet. Compare the written order with the telephone message. Record the date and time. Some nurses keep their written note until the order has been countersigned.
- Indicate that the order was received by telephone. Record the name of the physician from whom it was obtained, and co-sign the order with your name and title.

Eventually telephone orders will become obsolete. With increased technology physicians will be able to transmit their orders by facsimile machines or computer modems.

Implementing the Medication Order

The nurse is held accountable for accurately interpreting the medication order so that it is implemented correctly. In order to do this, the nurse must transcribe the written order exactly as it has been originally written and schedule its administration according to the policies of the agency.

Transcribing the Medication Order

Medication orders written by the physician are copied onto the patient's medication administration record. The *medication administration record,* or *MAR,* is a form used to schedule and document drug administration. Each health-care agency adopts the format it feels will ensure the safe administration of medications. Some examples include a combination of color-coded drug cards with a medication Kardex, a hand-written list of current medications and their times for administration, or a computerized printout. To avoid medication errors, the nurse is responsible for keeping the record current. The medication administration record should be compared with the original written order to determine that they are identical.

Using a Computerized MAR. Computers are being used more and more within hospitals. They speed communication and relieve the nurse of time-consuming tasks that involve the transmission of written or phoned orders. Using a unit's terminal, the nurse can enter a new drug order into the hospital's computer. A label is immediately printed. It is attached to the current medication administration record. An example is shown in Figure 23-1. The pharmacy simultaneously receives the data. Before the drug is dispensed, the pharmacist stores the new information into the computer's memory along with all the other drugs ordered for the patient. This provides a system for double-checking and evaluating the medication order. If there are any contraindications, interactions, or omissions in the new medication request, the order will be questioned before sending the drug. If not, a day's supply of the drug is sent to the unit. The computerized MAR, shown in Figure 23-2 will continue to list and schedule the drug until it is discontinued.

Scheduling Medication Administration

When the medication order is transcribed, the nurse must schedule the administration of the drug according to the frequency with which it has been prescribed. Table 23-6 provides a list of the various types of drug orders. The type of drug order may inherently affect the scheduling and the number of times the drug may be administered.

Drugs that are ordered to be given on a routine basis may be scheduled according to a predetermined timetable set by the health agency. A drug that is ordered to be given four times a day may be scheduled in a variety of patterns. For example, it may be scheduled to be given at

8 A.M., 12 noon, 4 P.M., and 8 P.M., or
10 A.M., 2 P.M., 6 P.M. and 10 P.M., or
6 A.M., 12 noon, 6 P.M., and 12 midnight

Any of these schedules will comply with the prescribed frequency of four times a day indicated in the drug order.

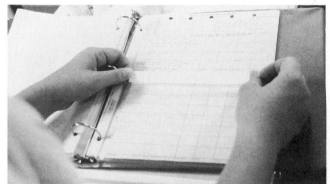

Figure 23-1 The nurse is applying a temporary drug label to the medication administration record. It identifies the medication, dosage, route, and scheduled time for administering a newly prescribed drug.

The nurse should be familiar with the policies concerning the routine times for administering medications within each agency.

Discontinuing a Medication Order

The nurse must be aware of the limitations in the length of time that a drug order is valid. The administration of some drugs must be discontinued at a specified time. Some drug orders may expire automatically according to laws and agency policies. For instance, there may be restrictions on the length of time that a narcotic, antibiotic, or anticoagulant may be administered. The date and time of the original written order will be important in determining when the drug administration must be discontinued. The date and time for the last administration of a drug should be identified on the medication record. The drug may be renewed when a new medication order is written.

It is usual to discontinue drugs the patient has been taking before surgery. After surgery, the physician writes new orders that should be followed. This practice is common also when patients are transferred to another health agency. Upon a patient's admission to a hospital, drugs that he had been taking at home are not continued unless the physician so orders. Agency policies vary about allowing the patient to keep drugs at his bedside and to take them as he would at home. The nurse must observe the policies of each particular health agency.

Supplying Medications

Medication orders are filled and the drugs are dispensed to the nursing unit by a pharmacist in the health-care facility. Drugs may be supplied to the nursing unit in several ways. An *individual supply* is a method of furnishing medications ordered for a single patient by placing enough for several days in a labeled container. The nurse then dispenses the amount needed to administer the dosage ordered. If a health agency uses the *unit dose system,* the pharmacist delivers a 24-hour supply of a patient's drugs, with each single dose labeled and packaged separately from the others. The pharmacist may also deliver a stock supply of drugs to the nursing unit. A *stock supply* is a large quantity of a frequently prescribed drug. Stock drugs may be used in emergencies when a delay in obtaining the drug may be harmful to the patient.

Safeguarding Medications

Medications can be dangerous if they are not administered in the manner in which they are prescribed. Therefore, various safeguarding mechanisms are utilized for protecting the supply from improper or illegal use.

Storing Medications

In each health agency, there is at least one area where drugs are kept in readiness for dispensing to patients. Drugs may be kept in one central area or they may be kept

MEDICATION ADMINISTRATION RECORD

SHIFT	FULL NAME/TITLE	INITIAL			
0701 - 1500	_____	____		10/02/90 00010 PHARMACY/CHART	
0701 - 1500	_____	____	TESTDP	DON'T DISC AGE: 041	
0701 - 1500	_____	____	00000000107 DEMPSEY. JAMES		
1501 - 2300	_____	____	ACCT #: 000000108 ADMIT DATE 04/21/88		
1501 - 2300	_____	____ DIAG.:	ASTHMA—EXACERBATED BY PNEUMONIA		
1501 - 2300	_____	____			
2301 - 0700	_____	____ ALL:	CODEINE	TETRACYCLINE	
2301 - 0700	_____	____			

1501 10/02/90 THRU 1500 DATE 10/03/90	1501 - 2300 0701 - 1500	2301 - 0700 1501 - 2300	0701 - 1500 2301 - 0700	COMMENTS
1 (01016) 10/01/90 1800 SOLU-CORTEF 100 MG/2ML-HYDROCORT DOSE: 100 MG. IP Q6H IP RATE = 500 MG. OVER 1 MIN. ABBOTT	1800	0000 0600	1200	
2 (03090) 09/27/90 0900 ACETAMINOPHEN EXTRA ST.CAP DOSE: 1 PO Q DAY TYLENOL			0900	
3 (04841) 10/01/90 0900 TENORMIN TAB. 50 MG. DOSE: 50 MG. PO Q DAY			0900	
4 (03096) 10/01/90 0900 LANOXIN (DIGOXIN) TAB. 0.25 MG. DOSE: 0.25 MG. PO Q DAY			0900	
5 (00543) 10/01/90 1800 BRETHINE AMP. 1 MG./ML. 1 ML. DOSE: 0.25MG SC Q6H (TERBUTALINE)	1800	0000 0600	1200	
6				
7				
8				
9				
10				
11				
12				
13				

TESTDP   DON'T DIS 00000000107 DEMPSEY. JAMES   THRU 1500 10/03/90

Figure 23-2 This computerized medication administration record is sent to the nursing unit each day. It lists all the currently prescribed medications for a patient. The nurse initials the time when a particular drug is administered and records an identifying signature at the top of the page.

Table 23-6. Types of Medication Orders

Type	Description	Example
Standing order without a termination date	A medication is given until discontinued by a physician's order. In some agencies, standing orders are automatically discontinued after a stated period of time; the order must be written again by the physician to continue the medication.	Lanoxin® 0.5 mg daily
Standing order with a termination date	A medication is given for a stated number of days or times, as ordered, and then discontinued	Diuril® 0.25 g b.i.d. × 5 days premenstrually
PRN order	A medication is given when, in the nurse's judgment, the patient needs it. The medication is discontinued in the same way as for a standing order.	Seconal® 100 mg h.s., prn
Single order	A medication is given only once, at the earliest convenience or at a specified time.	Milk of Magnesia,® 1 **3** at bedtime tonight
Stat order	A medication is given only once and immediately.	Metaraminol bitartrate (Aramine®) 4 mg IM, stat

in separate locations for more efficient administration to individual patients. For example, some hospitals have locked wall cupboards for drug storage near the entrance to each patient's room. To protect persons from drug misuse or abuse, the room, cabinet, or wall cupboard is locked, and only authorized personnel have access to the key.

Most nursing units use a portable medication cart, such as the one illustrated in Figure 23-3. It is used to store each patient's medications in a separate drawer. Each drawer is labeled with the patient's name or room number. The nurse moves the cart from room to room while dispensing medications. The cart is kept locked during periods of nonuse and whenever the nurse cannot keep it within immediate view.

Accounting for Narcotics

Narcotics are controlled substances. They must be safeguarded from possession or use by an unauthorized person. Only physicians who are currently registered with the Department of Justice, Bureau of Narcotics and Dangerous Drugs, may prescribe this category of drugs.

In health agencies, narcotics are kept in a double-locked drawer, box, or room on the nursing unit. Since narcotics are generally delivered to nursing units in stock supply, nurses are held responsible for an accurate account of their use. Federal law requires that a record be kept for each narcotic that is administered. The following information is required:

- The name of the patient who received the narcotic
- The amount of the narcotic used
- The date and hour the narcotic was given
- The name of the physician who prescribed the narcotic
- The name of the nurse who administered the narcotic.

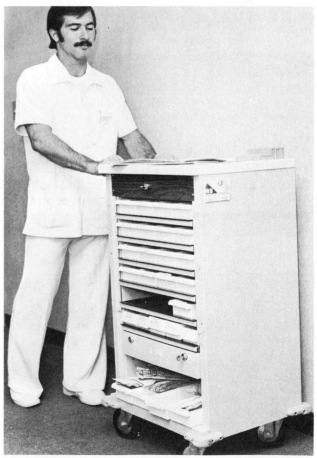

Figure 23-3 This mobile cart, along with the medication Kardex, is moved to the patient's room when medications are given. Notice that there are locked drawers on the cart. Each patient's medications are stored in a separate drawer, which is numbered according to the patient's room number. The entire cart is locked and stored in the area of the nurse's station between uses.

Any time that a full or partial dosage of a narcotic is wasted, for whatever reason, another person must witness its disposal and cosign the narcotic sheet. A narcotic may need to be discarded when it is prepared and then refused by the patient, when it is accidentally dropped, or when a patient requires a dose smaller than the amount in which the drug is supplied.

Most health agencies check narcotic supplies at the change of shifts. A nurse completing one shift checks the narcotic count with a nurse beginning the next shift. The object of the count is to verify that the number of narcotics remaining in the locked area when added to the number recorded as used equals the total amount originally supplied. Inconsistencies in the totals should be accounted for as soon as possible. An inaccurate narcotic count should be reported immediately. These special precautions are used to help control drug abuse. The nurse administering narcotics has a responsibility to see that the federal law is observed.

Calculating Dosages

It is the nurse's responsibility to administer the quantity of a drug that equals the prescribed dosage. When medications are supplied in the same dosage and system of measurement as that ordered by the physician, no calculation is required. Special formulas and mathematical computations must be used when the dosages are dissimilar.

Determining the Quantity to Administer

When dosages are supplied in a different amount but the same system and unit of measurement as that written in the medication order, the nurse must compute how much of the supplied drug to give. The following formula may be used:

$$\frac{\text{Dose Desired}}{\text{Dose on Hand}} \times \text{Quantity on Hand}$$
$$= \text{Quantity to Administer}$$

Example: 80 mg of a drug are ordered. The drug is supplied in tablets containing 40 mg per tablet. How many tablets should be administered?

Answer: $\dfrac{80 \text{ mg}}{40 \text{ mg}} \times 1 \text{ tablet} = 2 \text{ tablets}$

Note that both the supplied and ordered dosages are in the metric system of measurement. Both dosages are in milligrams, the same unit of measure. This formula can also be used to compute liquid dosages as well. It can be used to compute any problem as long as the system and the unit of measurement of the two dosages are the same.

Converting Metric Equivalents

The metric system is the most widely used for prescribing and supplying medications. At times a medication is supplied in a metric unit of measure that is different from the one prescribed. For example, the physician may prescribe 0.5 g of a drug. The drug may be supplied with a label that reads 500 mg. The nurse may follow one of the following two methods for converting one or the other of these measurements to the equivalent of the other.

1. To convert a smaller metric unit into a larger unit, move a decimal point three places to the left of the number. The resulting quantity will be smaller than the original measurement.

Example: 500 mg = ? g

Answer: 500 mg = 0.500 g or 0.5 g

2. To convert a larger metric unit into a smaller unit, move a decimal point three places to the right of the number. The resulting quantity will be larger than the original.

Example: 0.5 g = ? mg

Answer: 0.5 g = 500 mg

Once the measurements are in equivalent units of measure, the nurse will be able to determine the quantity of medication to give. In this case, the nurse has determined that the dose supplied and the dose ordered are equal. No further mathematical calculation is necessary.

Converting Between Different Systems of Measurement

When the units of measure or the systems of measurement are not the same, the nurse may be required to convert the dosages into equivalent amounts before calculating the quantity of drug to give. The equivalents in Table 23-2 and Table 23-3 may be consulted when dosages and systems differ.

Problems of this type are best computed using a ratio and proportion method. The following formula should be used:

$$\frac{\text{Known Unit of Measurement}}{\text{Known Equivalent}}$$
$$= \frac{\text{Known Unit of Measurement}}{\text{Unknown Equivalent}}$$

Example: Codeine gr ½ is ordered. It is supplied in a dosage of 60 mg per tablet. How many tablets should be administered?

Note that there are two different systems of measurement in this example. The nurse must first convert one dosage or the other to a similar system. In this case, all measurements will be converted to the metric system.

Step 1: Set up the problem by inserting the appropriate figures:

$$\frac{gr\ 1}{60\ mg} = \frac{gr\ \frac{1}{2}}{x\ mg}$$

Step 2: Cross-multiply and solve for x

$$1x = 60(\tfrac{1}{2})\ or\ 30$$
$$x = 30\ mg$$

This calculation indicates that the metric equivalent of gr ½ is 30 mg. To determine the number of 60 mg tablets to be administered, use the previous formula:

$$\frac{Dose\ Desired}{Dose\ on\ Hand} \times Quantity\ on\ Hand$$
$$= Quantity\ to\ Administer$$

Example:

$$\frac{30\ mg}{60\ mg} \times 1\ tablet = \tfrac{1}{2}\ tablet$$

Pharmacology texts can be consulted for further practice in converting dosages that are dissimilar.

Reviewing the Patient's Health History

There is certain information the nurse should know about each patient before administering any medications. This information can be reviewed in the health history obtained at the time of the patient's admission. The collected data provide a base of information related to drug therapy. The following information concerning medications should be noted.

- Nonprescription medications the patient uses, the reason, frequency, and length of time he has been using them
- Prescription medications the patient has been taking, the reason, frequency, and length of time he has been using them
- The patient's pattern for following the directions for medication use
- Any allergies the patient has to medications
- The patient's habits of daily living that may influence drug therapy, such as alcohol and caffeine consumption.

The nurse should understand the patient's diagnosis, medical plan of care, and the expected results of drug

therapy. Pharmacology texts and resources on medications provide descriptions of the medication's usual dosage range, indications for use, possible undesired effects, contraindications, symptoms of toxicity, and common routes of administration. These will be helpful when observing and evaluating the desirable and undesirable effects of the drug's action.

Following Basic Guidelines for Administering Medications

Certain guidelines apply specifically to the preparation and administration of medications. They are described later in this chapter. The following are basic actions the nurse performs when preparing and administering any medication, regardless of the route to be used.

Applying the Five Rights

For many years nurses have followed five criteria to ensure that medications are prepared and administered correctly. These criteria have been identified as the Five Rights for administering medication. They are identified in Figure 23-4. When these criteria are applied, they help to avoid potential medication errors before they happen.

Bar codes on unit doses of medication are now being used to electronically ensure that the Five Rights are being followed. Nurses use scanners, like those in department stores, while administering medications. The scanner is passed over the bar code on the drug, the patient's wristband, and the nurse's identification badge. It indicates if all the rights are correct. The nurse can then administer the medication. In addition, the scanner also electronically records the name of the nurse who administered the medication and enters the charge for the medication on the patient's account.

BE SURE YOU HAVE THE

1. **RIGHT DRUG**
2. **RIGHT DOSE**
3. **RIGHT ROUTE**
4. **RIGHT TIME**
5. **RIGHT PATIENT**

Figure 23-4 The Five Rights when giving medications.

Some nurses have added a sixth right to the list. It is the patient's right to refuse medication. The right of a rational adult patient to consent to or refuse therapy is a legal right. If the patient refuses a medication, the nurse should identify the reason for the omission of its administration in the patient's record. His refusal should also be reported to the physician or other authorized person.

Before Preparing Medications

Prior to preparing the drugs, the nurse should do the following:

- Check the patient's medication record with the original medication orders.
- Question any part of a drug order that appears inappropriate before proceeding.
- Be alert to any unusual changes, such as new additions or deletions of entries on the medication record. Errors can occur when forms are recopied or when a new medication order is transcribed.
- Question any unusual abbreviations that have been used when transcribing a medication order. Errors have occurred when the person writing the order or the one transcribing it has used unacceptable abbreviations. This practice can cause misinterpretations when administering the medication.
- Check the transcribed medication order carefully with the drug that has been supplied, as the nurse in Figure 23-5 is doing. Procedures differ. Some health agencies use a card system. Others may use a medication Kardex or a printed computerized listing.
- Organize the nursing care so that medications are given as near to the scheduled time as possible. It is common policy to give the drug no earlier or later than 30 minutes from the time specified. A medication given outside this range of time is considered a drug

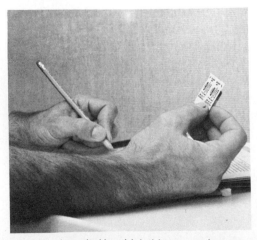

Figure 23-5 The hospital in which this nurse gives care uses a Kardex for transcribing medication orders and recording drug administration. The nurse is checking a unit dose of prepackaged medication with the patient's medication record.

error. This policy does not apply to emergency drugs. A preoperative medication should be given as closely as possible to the exact specified time because surgery is planned accordingly. This also holds true when patients are given drugs before certain diagnostic procedures.

While Preparing Medications for Administration

Safety is of the utmost importance in the preparation and administration of medications. The following guidelines are recommended when a nurse prepares medications for administration:

- Prepare medications in well-lighted conditions, and work alone without interruptions or distractions. Also, allow sufficient time so that all the drugs may be prepared without the need to leave and return to complete the task. Any circumstance that interferes with the nurse's attention and concentration can result in errors.
- Check the label of the drug container *three* times to ensure safety and accuracy:
  1. When reaching for the medication
  2. Immediately prior to pouring the medication
  3. When returning the container to its storage place.
- Do not use medications from containers with a missing or obliterated label. Guessing at the contents of a medication container is unsafe, even when one feels absolutely certain about what is inside. Return the container to the pharmacy.
- Do not return medications to a container or transfer medications from one container to another. This prevents mismatching drugs within labeled containers.
- Check expiration dates on medications, especially those that are in solution. Do not use a medication that has sediment at the bottom of the container unless the medication is to be shaken well before using. Do not use one that appears cloudy or has changed color. The potency and potential usefulness may have changed.
- Prepare medications in the order in which they will be delivered to patients. This practice helps save time when moving from patient to patient.
- Transport drugs from the area of preparation to the patient carefully and safely. Use the method of transporting provided by the agency. Identify the drugs in some manner to avoid confusing which drugs are for which patients.
- Use an individual medicine dropper for each liquid medication dispensed in this manner. Medication that remains within a dropper may contaminate other liquid medications when a dropper is reused.

While Administering Medications

Recommended guidelines when administering medications to patients include the following:

- Do not give medications that have been prepared by another person. If an error was made in preparation, the person administering the medication is responsible.
- Allow enough time to assist patients who will require help with taking medications.
- Keep all prepared medications in sight to ensure that the drugs will not be disturbed or taken by others.
- Identify the patient by checking the patient's identification bracelet, as illustrated in Figure 23-6. Also ask the patient to state his name when he is able. Be very careful when the identity of a patient is not known, when a language barrier or impediment exists, or when the patient is confused. He may respond to a name whether the name is his or not.
- Remain with the patient as he takes the medication. If there are several medications, offer each separately to the patient.
- Help the patient swallow medications without aspiration by keeping the head in a neutral or flexed position as shown in Figure 23-7.
- Do not leave medications at the bedside for the patient to take at a later time. The patient may forget to take the medication or someone else may take it.
- Omit giving a drug if the patient has symptoms suggesting an undesirable reaction to a previous administration of the drug. Report the observation immediately.
- Do not give a drug if the patient states that he is allergic to it. An allergic reaction can be serious and can even threaten the patient's life.
- Do not give a medication without further checking if the patient indicates that the drug appears different from what he has been receiving. A mistake may have been made when supplying the medication or when preparing the medication. Withholding it while checking further may avoid an error.
- Report immediately when a patient refuses a drug so that necessary adjustments in the patient's care can be made.

After Administering Medications

- Leave the patient in a comfortable position after medications have been administered.
- Check the patient in 30 minutes for desired and undesired drug effects.

Recording Medication Administration

The patient's medication record is a legal document. Medications are recorded as soon as possible after they are administered. This helps other members of the nursing and health-care team know that the patient has received the prescribed medication. The date, time, name of the drug, dosage, and route by which it was given are recorded on the medication record. The site used for an injection is recorded. The initials and signature of the nurse who administered the medication are entered in a specified area according to agency policy. Other patient information may be recorded, such as the patient's pulse rate or blood pressure, when this is indicated.

Occasionally a notation and explanation concerning drug administration should be entered on the chart. Record any medication that has been withheld and the reason for omitting the administration. An example is when drugs are withheld when a patient is fasting in preparation for a diagnostic test. Enter the administration of a drug that may be given irregularly, as needed by the patient, and explain the reason for its use.

Reporting Medication Errors

An error in medication administration occurs whenever any of the Five Rights are violated. Medications that are inadvertently omitted are also considered errors.

If a medication error occurs, the patient's condition is checked and the error is reported to the physician and the supervising nurse immediately. Health-care agencies have a special form for reporting medication errors, called an incident sheet or accident sheet. In this report, a full explanation of the situation is provided. The report serves as a method for preventing future errors by examining the practices that contributed to the error. The incident sheet

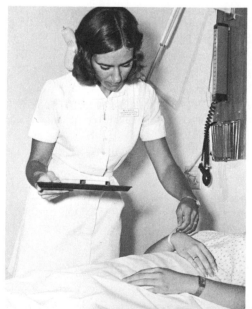

Figure 23-6 The hospital in which this photo was taken uses a card system for preparing and administering medications. The patient's name on the identification bracelet is compared with the name on the medication card, which is on the medication tray. The patient is also asked to state his name.

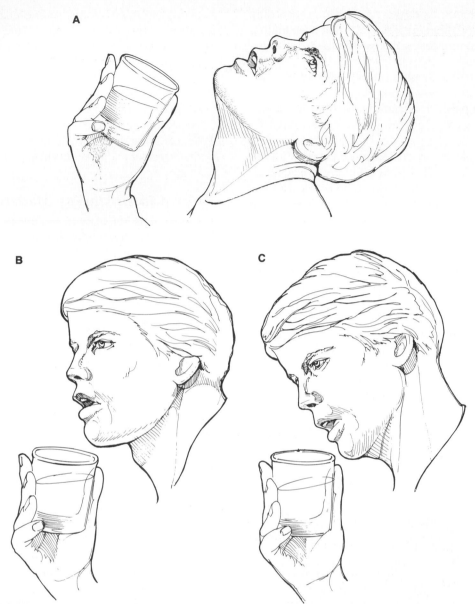

Figure 23-7 (*A*). Extending the neck interferes with swallowing oral medications. (*B*). A neutral position of the neck, or (*C*) slight flexion facilitates movement of a tablet or capsule down the esophagus. (From Lim, E: Pill-swallowing maneuver. Consultant, 27(10):55, 1987. Illustrations by Paul Singh-Roy.)

is not a part of the patient's permanent record nor should any reference be made in the chart to the fact that an incident sheet has been compiled.

Analysis of past medication errors indicates that some of the following actions are often the basis for mistakes in administering drugs:

- The nurse does not clarify an unclear medication order.
- The nurse inaccurately reads labels on medication containers.
- The nurse incorrectly calculates the quantity of the drug that is administered.

- The nurse carelessly switches medications prepared for one patient with those for another.
- The nurse does not identify patients by checking their identification and asking the patient to say his name.

Administering Oral Medications

Oral medications are those drugs administered by mouth or through a tube leading to the stomach. They are intended for absorption in the gastrointestinal tract. The oral route is the most frequently used route for medication administration. Oral medications are either solid or liquid in form.

Solid preparations of oral medications include tablets and capsules. Some tablets are scored for easy breaking if part of the tablet is needed. Certain tablets are covered with a substance that does not dissolve until the medication reaches the small intestine. These tablets are *enteric coated*. If the coating is destroyed, the medication is released in the stomach, where it is irritating to the gastric mucosa. Enteric coated tablets should never be crushed or chewed.

Liquid preparations of oral drugs include elixirs, spirits, suspensions, and syrups. The dosage of liquid medications is measured in calibrated cups. Extractors can be used to measure liquid medications, too. These devices resemble syringes and fit tightly into the neck of a bottle. The medication is withdrawn with the extractor and then the appropriate amount of the drug is placed in a cup or glass.

Skill Procedure 23-1 describes the actions that may be followed for administering medications by the oral route.

Skill Procedure 23-1. Administering Oral Medications

Suggested Action	Reason for Action
Check the medication record with the medication order.	Making sure that the information and directions are identical helps to avoid errors.
Observe medical asepsis by washing hands before preparing medications.	Handwashing removes organisms that can be transferred to patients.
Read the label of the medication container when removing the container from the shelf or drawer.	Many drugs appear similar. Reading the label verifies the contents of the container.
Check the label a second time before placing the drug into a dispensing cup.	Repetition ensures that the label has not been misread.
Pour capsules and tablets into the cap of the drug container, as illustrated in Figure 23-8. Then pour the proper amount into a medication cup.	Touching oral medications must be avoided so that organisms are not spread from the nurse's hands, which are never completely free of organisms.

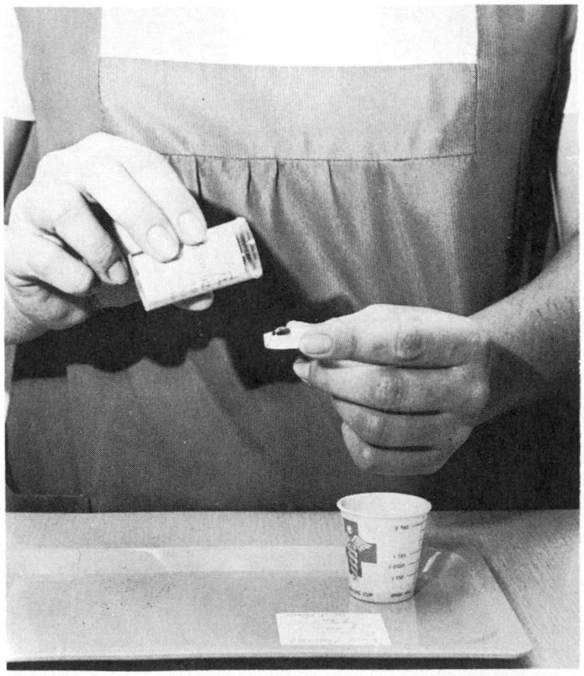

Figure 23-8 The correct number of tablets ordered for the patient is poured into the container's cap and then into the medication cup.

(*continued*)

Skill Procedure 23-1. Continued

Suggested Action	Reason for Action
Select the proper envelope of a prepackaged unit dose if this is the method of drug supply in the agency. These envelopes should be opened at the patient's bedside when the patient is given the medication.	A labeled unit dose drug is another safety check when administering medications. An unopened unit dose drug can be saved if a patient refuses the medication. This avoids wasting the drug and unnecessary expense to the patient.
Place all solid medications in the same cup with the exception of those that require special assessment of the patient prior to the administration.	Some medications should not be administered until it has been determined that the drug will not harm the patient. Separation helps to avoid administration until the assessment is made.
Read the label on the drug container a third time before returning it to its place of storage.	Attention and concentration on the label for a third time provide the opportunity for a final safety check on the contents of the container.
Place the bottle cap upside down on a working surface when preparing to pour a liquid medication.	Keeping the inner surface clean prevents contamination of the bottle cap and the contents of the container.
Use an appropriate measuring device when pouring liquids and read the amount at the bottom of the meniscus, as illustrated in Figure 23-9.	Accuracy is ensured when a calibrated cup is used and the level of the drug is observed at eye level.

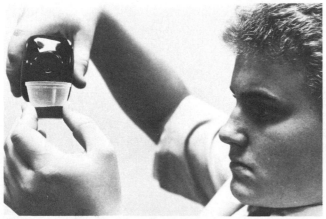

Figure 23-9 For a liquid medication, the nurse places a thumbnail at the marking on the dispensing container at the level indicated for the proper dosage. Holding the calibrated cup at eye level ensures that the amount will be read at the most accurate point of the meniscus.

Suggested Action	Reason for Action
Pour liquids from the side of a bottle opposite the label to prevent liquids from running onto the label.	A liquid that drips onto the label may lead to errors if the information becomes illegible.
Place each liquid medication in a separate container.	Mixing liquids may produce a chemical change and certainly makes the taste unpleasant.
Help the patient into a sitting position.	Swallowing is easier and safer when the patient is in a sitting position.
Identify the patient by checking the wristband and by asking the patient his name.	Using two separate methods of identification helps to ensure that the medication will be given to the patient for whom it was ordered.
Offer water before giving solid medication.	Liquids moisten the mucous membranes and help prevent oral drugs from sticking to the mouth or esophagus.

(continued)

Skill Procedure 23-1. Continued

Suggested Action	Reason for Action
Discourage liquids after the patient has swallowed cough medications.	Liquids dilute and wash cough medications from the area where they may have a local effect.
Help the patient to take the medication in amounts that he feels safe in swallowing.	A patient may prefer to swallow one medication at a time. This is probably the safest approach.
Provide the patient with a straw and encourage a generous intake of liquid, if permitted, to facilitate swallowing.	A straw may help the patient acquire a higher volume of water in the mouth without displacing the medication from its position for swallowing.
Have the patient suck on ice chips before taking a drug with an objectionable taste. Follow with warm or hot water.	Ice numbs the taste buds. Warm or hot water removes the aftertaste more quickly than does cold water.
Use other liquids or foods, such as fruit juices and applesauce, to disguise the unpleasant taste of a drug, but use them carefully.	A vehicle can lessen or overcome an unpleasant taste. However, the patient may come to dislike the vehicle due to its association with an unpleasant experience.
Offer oily medications after they have been refrigerated.	Cold oil is less aromatic and hence less objectionable than it is when administered at room temperature.
Remain with the patient until the medication is swallowed.	The nurse may need to provide assistance if the patient chokes. The nurse is responsible for documenting that the drug was taken by the patient. It is possible that a patient could discard a drug, misplace it, or accumulate many in order to harm himself.
Help the patient into a position of comfort and safety before leaving.	The position for swallowing medications need only be temporary.
Record the volume of fluid taken with the medication if the patient's intake and output are being recorded.	All liquid that is ingested or instilled is considered part of the fluid intake. Incomplete records are inadequate for accurate assessment.
Dispose or return medication administration equipment to its proper location.	Other nursing team members may need medication trays and other equipment to complete their patient care responsibilities.
Record the administration of the medication on the patient's record as soon as possible.	Records must be kept current to avoid omission or possible duplication of a medication administration.
Check the patient in 30 minutes for desired and undesired drug effects.	Pertinent assessments help to identify the patient's response to the action of a medication.

Administering Oral Medications Through a Nasogastric Tube

When a tube is used to provide nourishment, oral medications may be instilled through it. Crushed solid medications are likely to obstruct the lumen of the tube. Check with the physician and pharmacist regarding liquid forms that may be available. The pharmacist may be able to finely pulverize the solid medication and prepare a suspension. A *suspension* is a mixture of undissolved particles within a liquid. The contents must be shaken vigorously to mix the drug throughout the solution before its administration. If there is no other option than to crush solid drugs, and the feeding tube is less than a 10 French, a feeding pump should be used. Otherwise, diluting each drug to a watery consistency and rinsing the tubing before, during, and after adding medication may help to instill oral medications.

Medication should be administered separately from formula. Adding medications to tube-feeding formula is not recommended for several reasons. First, some feedings are administered slowly and continuously. An adequate dosage would not be provided with a slow infusion. Second, if the gastric residual is high, tube feedings may be postponed. Medication would not be given according to its prescribed schedule. Finally, some drugs physically interact with the formula causing problems with instillation. For instance, strongly acidic liquid medication tends to curdle the formula. Bulk-forming laxatives thicken the formula and contribute to tube obstruction.

Each medication should be instilled separately. One medication could interact with another. The nurse may see a need to withhold one particular medication once a bedside assessment takes place. If all medications are combined, the entire mixture would have to be discarded.

Enteric coated tablets or those designed for sustained release should never be crushed and administered. This interferes with their absorption and the desired therapeutic effects.

If the nasogastric tube is used for suctioning rather than nourishment, the tube must be clamped for at least one-half hour after instilling medication. If that is not done, the drugs are removed from the stomach before they can be absorbed.

To administer medications through a nasogastric tube, the suggested actions in Skill Procedure 23-2 may be followed.

Administering Topical Medications

The application of medication to the skin or mucous membranes is referred to as *topical administration*. Drugs administered topically may be placed externally or internally. Topically applied drugs may have a local or systemic effect; however, most are given in order to achieve a direct effect on the tissue to which they are applied.

Using an Inunction

A medication incorporated into a vehicle, such as oil, lotion, cream, or ointment, and rubbed into the skin is an *inunction*. This word is derived from a term that referred to the religious practice of anointing. It may be acceptable for patients to self-administer some of these medications. The nurse's role then becomes one of teaching the patient the proper technique and supervising the application. An inunction is given as follows:

- Cleanse the area of application and the hands with soap or detergent and water before applying the oil, lotion, cream, or ointment. This ensures the skin is free of debris and body oil, both of which retard absorption.
- Shake the contents of mixtures that may have become separated.
- Apply most inunctions with the fingers and hands or use a cotton ball or gauze square.
- Wear gloves if the patient has a contagious skin condition or there are breaks in the skin of fingers or hands.
- Warm the inunction if it will be applied to a sensitive area such as the face or back. This may be done by holding the container or the inunction itself in the hands or submerging a tightly closed container in warm water.
- Apply local heat to the area as ordered. This increases blood circulation, which helps absorption.

Using the Transdermal Route

The prefix trans- means across or through. The word *transdermal* means through the skin. A drug intended for application by this route enters the bloodstream after being absorbed through the skin's hair follicles and sweat glands. The most common medication administered transdermally is nitroglycerin. This drug is used primarily to control angina pectoris. Angina is chest pain caused by insufficient blood flow to the heart muscle. Scopolamine, used to relieve motion sickness, is available for transdermal application. It is generally applied in the form of a patch placed behind the ear. Estrogen, a female hormone, can be applied with a skin patch for transdermal administration. An example of a transdermal patch is shown in Figure 23-10. Skill Procedure 23-3 describes the technique to apply a transdermal patch.

Applying Nitroglycerin Ointment. Nitroglycerin is also available as an ointment. It should not be touched with the hands because it is readily absorbed through the skin. The following discussion describes directions for applying nitroglycerin ointment. Although individual manufacturers prepare the ointment slightly differently, the following can serve as general guidelines:

- Remove any previous application from the patient's skin.
- Squeeze a ribbon of ointment from the tube onto the manufacturer's application paper shown in Figure 23-11. The typical dosage is prescribed in inches or centimeters.
- Fold the paper or use an applicator to spread the measured ointment over a $2^1/_4 \times 3^1/_2$ inch (5.6 × 8.8 cm) area of the paper.
- Place the application paper containing the ointment on a clean, nonhairy surface of the skin. The upper arm, back, and chest are usual sites.
- Cover the application paper with a square of kitchen plastic wrap and secure it with tape on four sides, as shown in Figure 23-12.
- Check the patient and his vital signs approximately 30 minutes after the application to determine the response of the patient.
- Inform the physician if the patient develops a severe headache or if there is a significant lowering of the blood pressure from previous assessments.
- Rotate the sites on which the ointment is placed to prevent skin irritation.

Instilling Eye Medications

Eye medications may be applied topically either in the form of an ointment or as eyedrops. The eye is a delicate organ. It is highly susceptible to infection and injury. Direct application of a solution or ointment into the eye is not recommended because it may injure the cornea. Instead, drops and ointments are instilled into the lower conjunctival sac. Although the eye is never free of microorgan-

Skill Procedure 23-2. Administering Oral Medications Through a Nasogastric Tube

Suggested Action	Reason for Action
Compare the medication administration record (MAR) with the written order.	Rechecking the written order determines if the information was transcribed accurately.
Wash hands.	Handwashing reduces the spread of microorganisms.
Check and compare the labels on each medication at least three times with the MAR.	Reading labels ensures that the correct medication and dosage have been supplied by the pharmacy.
Prepare each drug separately.	The nurse may decide to withhold one or more medications after the bedside assessment.
Crush each solid medication and mix it with about 30 mL of warm water.	Tablets or the contents of capsules must be in a solution to move through the nasogastric tube. Warm water is more likely to help dissolve solid drugs than cold water.
Take the prepared medication, water for flushing, a clean towel, and a 30- to 50-mL syringe to the patient's bedside.	Having equipment and supplies ready saves time and energy.
Check the patient's wristband.	To avoid making a medication error, the identity of the patient receiving the drug must be verified.
Check the location of the tube following the techniques described in Chapter 8.	The nurse must verify that the end of the tube is in the stomach and not in the airway.
Help the patient into a Fowler's position. Drape the patient with a towel.	A sitting position facilitates gravity-induced movement of the medication through the tube. The towel protects the patient from becoming wet or soiled.
Instill 30 to 50 mL of water into the gastric tube.	The water clears the tube of formula that could interact with drugs. It also reduces the surface tension on the inner wall of the tube so the mixture instills easily.
Instill the medication through the tube as the water leaves the syringe. Allow the mixture to flow by gravity.	Gravity avoids the use of pressure that may cause discomfort or injure the mucosa of the stomach.
Instill 50 mL of water into the syringe before it is completely empty.	Water separates the instilled medication from the next type of drug and avoids a physical interaction within the tubing.
Instill 30 to 50 mL of water into the tubing when all the medications have been instilled.	Water flushes the medication from the tube into the stomach so that the patient receives the entire dose.
Clamp the tube while water still remains within it if the feeding is intermittent.	Maintaining fluid in the tubing prevents air from entering the stomach when subsequent fluid is instilled.
Reconnect the flushed tubing to the tube-feeding formula if nourishment is continuous.	The medication can mix with formula without problems once it is within the larger volume of the stomach.
Have the patient remain in a sitting position for about 30 minutes, or have him lie on his right side with the head of the bed slightly elevated.	These positions help the stomach to empty and prevent regurgitation and possible aspiration.
Place the patient on his left side if the medication is to remain in the stomach for a local effect.	Antacids are one type of drug that produce a desired effect when in the stomach. Lying on the left side delays movement of the stomach contents into the duodenum of the small intestine.
Record the amount of water mixed with the crushed medication and the amount used for flushing the tubing if the patient's fluid intake is being measured.	Accurate assessment depends upon accurate recording.
Record the administration of the medication as for other medications. Indicate that the drug was given through the nasogastric tube.	The record should reflect the modifications that were used while administering oral medications.

Skill Procedure 23-3. Applying a Transdermal Patch

Suggested Action	Reason for Action
Compare the MAR with the written medical order.	Rechecking the written order determines if the information was transcribed accurately.
Wash hands.	Handwashing reduces the spread of microorganisms.
Check and compare the label on the patch at least three times with the MAR.	Reading the label ensures that the correct medication and dosage have been supplied.
Check the patient's wristband.	One of the Five Rights is to administer the drug to the right patient.
Remove the patch that is currently on the skin.	The desired dosage could be exceeded if the old patch was left on the skin.
Record the date and time on the new patch.	The current date and time validate that the patch is a recent application and not one that has been unchanged.
Follow the manufacturer's suggestions for selecting an area for application.	Some patches are best applied to the arms, chest, or back. Others are recommended for behind the ear or on the abdomen below the waist.
Wash the skin with soap and water; dry well.	Adhesion is enhanced when the patch is applied to a clean, dry area of skin.
Select a nonirritated area in another location from where the previous patch was removed.	Sites should be rotated to avoid skin irritation.
Clip, but do not shave, body hair that will be covered by the patch.	Shaving creates microabrasions that could increase the rate of drug absorption. Clipping hair reduces discomfort during patch removal.
Peel the backing from the patch without touching the drug reservoir.	Contact with the hands could cause the medication to be absorbed by the nurse.
Press the adhesive side of the patch to the skin for approximately 10 seconds.	Warmth and pressure promote adhesion.
Inform the patient that bathing, swimming, and showering should not interfere with adhesion or absorption of the drug.	The outer surface of the patch is a polyester film that acts as a barrier to water. The drug flows through a membrane layer toward the skin.
Replace a loose or lost patch as soon as it is noted.	A uniform rate of absorption depends upon continuous contact between the patch and skin.
Wash hands following patient contact.	Handwashing reduces the spread of microorganisms.
Document the drug administration according to agency policy.	Most documentation systems require the nurse to initial the record to indicate the drug and the time it was given.
Record the location where the patch was applied.	Identifying the site of application helps the next nurse select an alternate location.

isms, the solutions, ointments, and equipment used to administer eye medications should be sterile. Skill Procedure 23-4 describes the technique for administering eye medications.

Instilling Ear Medications

Topical medications may be instilled into the outer, or external, ear. The outer ear is separated from the other structures of the ear by the eardrum, or tympanic membrane. Normally this barrier is intact, and clean technique is used when administering medications into the ear canal. When the eardrum has been perforated by disease, injury, or surgery, sterile technique is used since organisms have a direct passage into deeper structures. The technique for administering ear medications is described and illustrated in Skill Procedure 23-5.

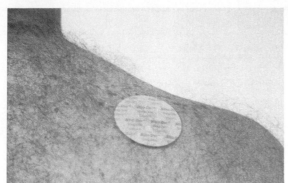

Figure 23-10 Several locations are acceptable for a transdermal patch. This one has been applied to the patient's back. The location is rotated with each application.

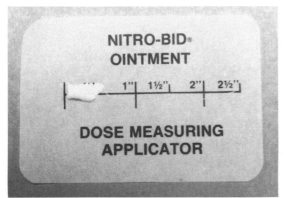

Figure 23-11 This is a nitroglycerin application paper. The words and measurements are printed backwards so they can be read correctly when applied to the patient. The dose for this patient is ½ inch.

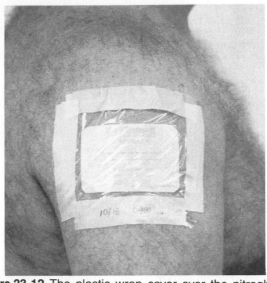

Figure 23-12 The plastic wrap cover over the nitroglycerin application paper prevents soiling clothing and promotes drug absorption.

Administering Nasal Medications

Topical medications may be dropped or sprayed within the nose. The nose is not a sterile cavity. However, because it connects with the sinuses, techniques of medical asepsis should be used. Nose drops that contain medication in normal saline solution are recommended rather than oily

---

Skill Procedure 23-4. Instilling Medications Into the Eye

Suggested Action	Reason for Action
Warm eye drops and ointments to room temperature. Roll the container between the hands for a minute or two if the medication storage area is unusually cool.	Instilling cold medication into the eye is startling and uncomfortable.
Wash hands just before administering eye medication.	Handwashing controls the spread of organisms into the patient's eye.
Position the patient supine or sitting with his head tilted back and slightly to the side into which the medication will be instilled.	Positioning in this manner allows optimal placement of the medication without excessive loss down the cheek or into the duct leading to the nose.
Clean the lids and lashes prior to instilling the medication. Use one cotton ball for each wipe.	The area around the eye should be as clean as possible to avoid introducing organisms or debris into the eye.
Move the cotton ball from the area of the eye near the nose, called the *inner canthus,* outward to the area near the temple, the *outer canthus.*	Wiping in this direction will remove secretions, residual medication from previous instillations, and organisms away from the nasal duct.
Read the label on the medication at least three times.	Ointments and containers of eyedrops look similar. The nurse must read each label carefully to avoid instilling the wrong medication.

(continued)

Skill Procedure 23-4. Continued

Suggested Action	Reason for Action
Instruct the patient to look toward the ceiling.	When the patient does not look directly at the applicator, the blink reflex is less likely to occur.
Place the thumb or two fingers of the nondominant hand below the margin of the eyelashes under the lower lid and exert pressure downward over the bony prominence of the cheek, as the nurse in Figure 23-13 is doing.	This maneuver pulls the lower lid downward and creates a pouch in the conjunctiva. This small area is a convenient pocket into which the medication may be placed.

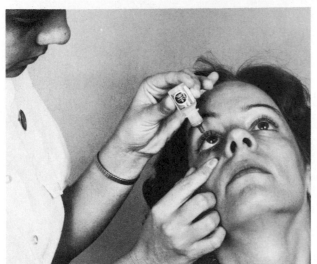

Figure 23-13 The patient tilts her head back and looks upward in preparation for receiving eyedrops. She also tilts her head slightly toward the eye receiving drops to help prevent medication from entering the duct at the inner canthus. Pressure applied downward high on the cheek exposes the lower conjunctival sac.

Suggested Action	Reason for Action
Move the medication container from below the line of vision or from the side of the eye.	Keeping the moving object out of the patient's direct vision will help to prevent him from becoming startled and moving away.
Hold the tip of the container steady above the conjunctival sac without actually touching the eye itself.	The tip of the medication container may injure the cornea or other structures if it is forced into the eye. Touching the eye contaminates the tip of the container.
Deposit the prescribed number of drops into the center of the conjunctival sac or squeeze a ribbon of ointment from the inner to the outer canthus.	Placing the drug in this manner facilitates its distribution throughout the eye when the nurse's hand is released from the patient's face.
Instruct the patient to close his eyelids gently and move the eye after the medication has been instilled.	Gently closing the eye prevents the patient from blinking eye drops out onto the cheek. Moving the eye within the orbit delivers the drug over the surface of the eye.
Apply gentle pressure over the opening to the nasolacrimal duct.	Nasal occlusion prevents systemic absorption of medication through the mucous membrane of the nose.
Provide the patient with a clean tissue to catch any medication or tears that may escape from the eye and roll down the face.	A clean tissue may be used to absorb liquids. The medication may irritate the patient's skin, and the sensation of a substance running down the cheek is unpleasant.
Instruct the patient to avoid rubbing the eyes after medication has been administered.	Pressure may cause additional irritation of the eye.

Skill Procedure 23-5. Instilling Medications Into the Ear

Suggested Action	Reason for Action
Warm the medication to room temperature.	Cold or hot medication instilled within the ear can cause discomfort, dizziness, and nausea in some patients.
Clean the outer ear with cotton balls and normal saline, if that appears necessary.	The ear canal may contain dried secretions or drainage that may interfere with the absorption of the drug.
Fill the applicator with medication.	Most ear medications are instilled using a medication dropper.
Position the patient on his side with the ear into which the instillation is to be made uppermost.	This prevents loss of any medication from the effect of gravity.
Straighten the ear canal, as illustrated in Figure 23-14. Gently pull the ear upward and backward for an adult and downward and backward for a child.	Straightening the ear canal helps the medication to reach the lowest area of the ear canal and become distributed over all the surfaces in the outer ear.

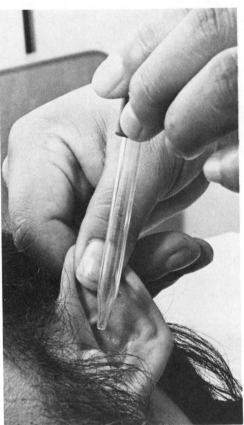

Figure 23-14 To instill eardrops in this adult patient, the nurse pulls the ear upward and backward and drops the solution along the side of the ear canal.

Hold the dropper with the tip above the ear canal.	The tip of the dropper should not touch the ear; this may cause the patient to pull away. Touching the tip to the skin contaminates the dropper.
Allow the prescribed number of drops to fall on the side of the ear canal.	When drops fall directly on the eardrum they may cause an unpleasant sensation.

(continued)

Skill Procedure 23-5. Continued

Suggested Action	Reason for Action
Encourage the patient to remain in this position for 5 minutes.	Maintaining the position allows time for medication to flow into the lowest area of the ear canal, avoiding the possibility of excessive loss from the ear.
Massage the cartilage below the opening to the ear canal.	Massage promotes the movement and distribution of the drug.
Insert cotton *loosely* within the ear canal if it is likely that the medication will drain out after the patient assumes an upright position.	The cotton wick will trap the medication within the ear canal and prevent its loss after the instillation.
Never pack cotton tightly within the ear canal.	Tightly packed cotton may interfere with drainage and could create undue pressure in the ear canal.
Wait 15 minutes between instillations if drops are to be placed in both ears.	Sufficient time must be allowed to prevent immediate loss of medication.

solutions that may be aspirated into the lungs and cause inflammation of the tissues. Skill Procedure 23-6 describes the suggested actions for instilling nasal medications.

Administering Buccal Medications

Some medications are intended to become absorbed through the blood vessels within the mouth rather than be delivered to the gastrointestinal tract. A *sublingual* administration involves placing a drug under the tongue. A *buccal* administration involves placing a drug against the mucous membranes of the cheek. These locations are shown in Figure 23-16. The patient should be instructed to allow the medication to dissolve. Eating, chewing, and smoking are contraindicated as the medication is being dissolved and absorbed.

Applying Medications to the Throat. The most frequently used method for applying topical medication to the throat is with the use of lozenges. These hard disks dissolve slowly when they are sucked, distributing the medication over the surface of the throat. Chewing or swallowing the lozenge renders it largely ineffective. The patient should not take fluids during or soon after using a lozenge. The fluids will dilute and flush the drug away and decrease its local effect.

Throat irrigants, sprays, and paints are very rarely used. The agency's procedures should be observed on those occasions when they may be ordered.

Administering Vaginal Medications

Medicated vaginal creams are ordinarily applied by using a narrow tubular applicator with an attached plunger. Suppositories that melt when exposed to body heat are also prepared for vaginal insertion. Practices of medical asepsis are used because the vagina is not sterile. The techniques in Skill Procedure 23-7 may be followed when inserting medications within the vagina.

Administering Rectal Medications

Rectal medications are used primarily for their local action. Occasionally, a medication may be given rectally for its systemic effect. Medications for rectal administration are most often in the form of a suppository, cream, or solution. The technique for inserting a rectal suppository and instilling solutions within the rectum may be reviewed in Chapter 22. Rectal creams are generally inserted using a prelubricated applicator tip attached to a tube of medication. The applicator tip is designed so that it cannot be inserted any further than safely indicated. Principles of medical asepsis should be followed when removing the applicator and storing the medication.

Overcoming Noncompliance

Noncompliance is the failure to follow instructions. One of the areas with the highest rate of noncompliance involves self-administration of medications. Despite teaching patients about self-administration of medications, studies have shown that a remarkable number of patients do not follow directions. Common reasons and suggested ways to help overcome the nonuse, misuse, and abuse of medications are described in Table 23-7. The creative nurse may find still other ways to help overcome noncompliance.

Suggested Measures When Administering Medications in Selected Situations

When the Patient Is Pregnant or Lactating

Caution pregnant women that medications should be avoided because of *teratogenic effects* on the fetus. This means that some drugs can produce abnormal structures in the developing infant causing

Skill Procedure 23-6. Administering Nasal Medications

Suggested Action	Reason for Action
Have the patient clear his nasal passages with a tissue.	Clearing nasal passages removes debris that may interfere with the instillation, distribution, or absorption of the medication.
Help the patient into a sitting position with his head tilted back if the drug is intended for the pharynx.	This position facilitates the flow of the drug downward along the nasal passages leading to the pharynx and the opening to the eustachian tube of the ear.
Have the patient lie down with his head tilted slightly backward or to the side if the drug is for the sinuses on one side of the face.	Gravity and positioning can facilitate movement of the medication toward the sinuses rather than downward toward the pharynx.
Use a rolled towel or pillow beneath the patient's neck to facilitate support and positioning.	Positioning devices help to ensure or increase hyperextension of the neck.
Remove the cover or applicator from the container of medication without touching any unclean objects in the area.	The contents of the container will become contaminated if the surfaces of the applicator or the inner cap touch areas where organisms are present.
Aim the tip of the dropper toward the upper area of the nasal passage, as shown in Figure 23-15, and squeeze the rubber cap.	The drops are more likely to flow gradually down the nasal passage than drip directly into the throat.

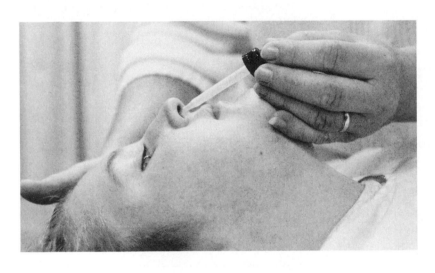

Figure 23-15 The medication in this dropper is instilled on the mucous membrane of the nasal passage where it will have a local effect. Drugs can also be absorbed systemically through the nasal mucous membranes.

Instruct the patient to breathe through his mouth as the proper number of drops are instilled.	Breathing through the nose may deliver a large amount of the medication into the respiratory passages, where it may cause coughing or aspiration into the lungs.
Help the patient to self-administer a nasal spray, if that is possible.	It is difficult to coordinate the spraying with simultaneous inhalation when two people are involved.
Place the tip of a nasal atomizer just inside the nostril.	Proper administration of the medication depends upon confining the spray within the nasal passage.
Compress the opposite nostril and instruct the patient to inhale as the container is squeezed.	Inhalation will distribute the drug within one nasal passage. No more force than that required to bring the spray into contact with the mucous membrane should be used.
Instruct the patient to remain in position for approximately 5 minutes.	Changing position may alter the movement and distribution of the medication from its intended location.

Skill Procedure 23-7. Administering Vaginal Medications

Suggested Action	Reason for Action
Ask the patient whether she needs to void prior to inserting medications within the vagina.	A full bladder may cause discomfort during insertion, or the patient may wish to get up too soon after the drug has been administered.
Provide privacy by closing the door and curtains surrounding the patient's bed.	The patient should be protected from being viewed by others during any procedure involving exposure of the genital area.
Cover the patient with a cotton bath blanket and then pull the top linen toward the bottom of the bed.	Bed linen that remains tucked around the patient interferes with inspection and access to the genital area.
Place the patient in a dorsal recumbent position with the knees flexed and slightly spread upon the bed.	This position helps when locating the vagina for proper insertion of the medication.
Remove any perineal pad that the patient may have currently in place. Use gloves or touch only the outside surface of the pad.	Patients who require vaginal medications may use a perineal pad to absorb drainage or dissolved medication. The pad should be considered contaminated with organisms.
Discard the contaminated pad into a waterproof container for disposal or pull the glove inside out over the pad and dispose of both at the same time.	Contaminated articles must be contained within a barrier that controls the spread of organisms to others.
Perform proper handwashing.	The hands should be washed after handling any soiled or contaminated articles.
Fill the applicator with cream or insert the vaginal suppository into its dispenser.	Applicators help to insert the medication deep within the vaginal canal.
Lubricate the applicator or tip of the suppository with a water-soluble lubricant.	Lubrication reduces friction as the applicator is inserted into the vagina.
Apply gloves and spread the labia in order to identify the opening to the vagina.	The opening to the vagina is best visualized when the labia are retracted.
Insert the applicator tip gently downward and backward following the contour of the vaginal wall.	The vagina is a curved cavity that may be injured unless the insertion is performed correctly.
Depress the plunger of the applicator when it has been inserted approximately 7.5 to 10 cm (3 to 4 in).	The medication is more effectively distributed and safely inserted at this distance.
Remove the applicator while keeping the plunger depressed and allow the labia to fall into place.	Preventing the parts of the applicator from moving during withdrawal prevents discomfort for the patient.
Pull the glove inside out over the applicator until it can be properly cleaned within the utility room.	The same applicator is used for repeated administrations of the medications and should be cleaned thoroughly before being stored for future use.
Apply a clean perineal pad.	A clean perineal pad absorbs vaginal drainage and prevents soiling of underclothing or bed linen.
Instruct the patient to remain lying down for at least 5 to 10 minutes, or longer if possible.	Maintaining this position allows time for the medication to become distributed at the deepest area of the vagina near the cervix.
Clean the applicator with water and soap or detergent. Dry it thoroughly, wrap, and replace it with the container of medication.	The applicator should be kept clean and ready for use at the next administration of the drug.
Perform proper handwashing before carrying out any other activities.	Handwashing is an effective technique of medical asepsis that controls the spread of organisms.

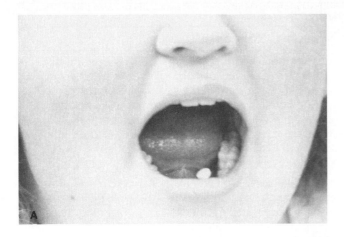

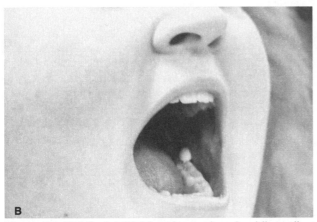

Figure 23-16 (*A*). A tablet has been placed sublingually, or under the tongue. (*B*). A tablet placed between the cheek and gum is known as buccal administration.

Applicable Nursing Diagnoses

When administering oral or topical medications, the nurse may identify these nursing diagnoses.
- Knowledge Deficit
- Impaired Swallowing
- High Risk for Aspiration
- High Risk for Injury
- High Risk for Poisoning
- Noncompliance
- Altered Health Maintenance

Nursing Care Plan 23-1 reflects the care of a patient diagnosed with Noncompliance. This diagnostic category is defined by NANDA as, "A person's informed decision not to adhere to a therapeutic recommendation" in its 1989 taxonomy.

severe deformities. The fetus is particularly susceptible to the effects of chemicals during the first 3 months of a pregnancy when the organs are developing rapidly.

Encourage a pregnant woman to discuss the effects of certain self-prescribed and prescription medications with her physician.

Explain that medications are excreted through breast milk in the lactating mother. Although many drugs appear to produce no harmful effects, certain drugs have been identified as harmful to the infant. The mother who breastfeeds an infant would be wise to discuss with the pediatrician the types of medications that may be taken safely.

When the Patient Is an Infant or Child

Be sure to check dosages carefully when administering medications to infants and children. Children respond faster and more noticeably to drugs than adults.

Use a liquid preparation of a medication when possible for a child under 5 years of age. Children have difficulty swallowing solid forms of medications.

Use a syringe without the needle or a dropper to administer liquid medications to infants and small children. Place the syringe in the side of the mouth and instill the medication in small amounts. Allow the child to swallow before administering additional medication. A dropper is illustrated in Figure 23-17.

Stimulate swallowing by gentle downward stroking motions over the larynx.

Crush or mix medications with soft foods, such as strained fruits or potatoes. Place the medication in the minimum amount of food needed.

Avoid mixing medications with formula or any essential item in the child's diet. The child may refuse foods he associates with medication.

Consider using a specially designed glass for children who fear taking a tablet or capsule. A device, illustrated in Figure 23-18, involves placing a tablet on a ledge in the glass.

When the Patient Has a Physical Handicap

Help visually impaired or blind persons organize and identify containers so that medications are taken accurately. There are pill organizers on the market with individual compartments for tablets and capsules. One is illustrated in Figure 23-19. Other techniques include identifying bottles in some way such as with rubber bands or a cotton ball taped to the bottle, using a characteristic cap, and placing each medication container in a special place and always returning it to the same place.

Table 23-7. Suggestions for Overcoming Noncompliance

Reason for Noncompliance	Ways to Help Overcome Noncompliance
Sees no value in taking medications	This attitude is most often noted among patients with chronic diseases. The following measures are suggested to help overcome it: reviewing the patient's medications and the role they play in controlling or overcoming an illness; including the patient in a plan of care in relation to taking his medications; having a written contract with the patient indicating that he will take his medications as prescribed; and seeking help from family members who can give the patient support without threats of consequences for not taking medications.
Forgets whether medications were taken	Overcoming this reason for noncompliance usually depends on developing a system of reminders with the patient. The following measures are suggested: having instructions for taking medications in writing; being sure that the patient has a clock and calendar handy for his use; keeping a diary, checklist, or record that requires the patient to make a notation each time he takes a medication rather than depending on memory; using a color-coding system as a reminder to take medications; marking medication containers with reminders, such as placing an AM on the bottom of a container and a PM on the top of it and having the patient flip the container so that the next time the medication is due is on the top; rotating places where medications are placed after taking each dose; and using an alarm, such as on a wristwatch, that is set to ring when a medication is due and reset immediately to ring when the next dose is due.
Is confused about when and how often to take medications	This common reason for noncompliance occurs especially frequently when the patient is expected to follow a complex drug program. In addition to developing a system of reminders with the patient, as described above, it is helpful to consult the patient's physician to see whether a simpler but equally effective program of drug therapy can be developed.
Feels better, no better, or worse after taking medications	The important teaching point when these causes lead to noncompliance is to be sure to explain the importance of continuing with medications for as long as prescribed, how long it may be necessary to take them before their effect is noted, and what symptoms to expect while taking medications.
Is discontented with the side effects associated with medications and the way they interfere with activities of daily living	When this cause results in noncompliance, consultation with a physician may help by finding substitute medications that produce fewer side effects or by changing a dosage, if permissible. Other suggested measures are to help the patient learn how to adjust to and cope with side effects, and be sure the patient understands the importance of drug therapy for treating his illness.
Has a variety of personal reasons, such as the cost of medications, pride, a need to be free of drug therapy, and pressure from others who use other types of medications or speak of the dangers of the prescribed medications	Helping to overcome various personal reasons for noncompliance requires individualized attention and care. Very often the nurse can seek help from others, such as from social-service personnel when the patient cannot afford prescribed medications. It is important when helping a patient to overcome personal reasons for noncompliance that the nurse give the patient ample opportunity to describe his feelings and attitudes about drug therapy and that the nurse *listen* to what the patient is saying.

Write instructions for self-administration for the hearing-impaired individual. Provide directions to a family member or friend also.

Have the patient request that the pharmacist give him a medication container cap that is not child-proof if he has difficulty removing these types of caps. This advice is not recommended if there are children in the home. In such instances, a family member must help the patient to open the container.

When the Patient Is Elderly

Take into consideration the elderly person's medical history when planning his care. Many elderly patients see several physicians who each prescribe medications. Patients may be taking nonprescrip-

NURSING CARE PLAN

23-1. Noncompliance

Assessment	***Subjective Data***
	States, "I didn't get my prescription refilled. I wasn't having any chest pain and I didn't think I needed to take my pills anymore. I figured the surgery fixed my heart."

Objective Data

63-year-old man admitted for chest pain and dyspnea. Lives with widowed sister who remains employed. Was discharged 6 weeks ago following coronary bypass surgery. Was to continue taking a beta-blocker (Tenormin® 50 mg PO daily) and a diuretic (Lasix® 20 mg PO q.o.d.) Abruptly stopped taking both medications one week ago. Pulse rate is presently 94 at rest and BP is 178/94 in R. arm while sitting.

Diagnosis

Noncompliance related to inaccurate health belief.

Plan

Goal

The patient will explain the consequences that can occur if medications are not taken by 3/7.

Orders: 3/5

1. Explain the following at separate times during the next two days:
   - The purpose for reducing myocardial oxygen consumption
   - The benefit for lowering blood pressure
   - The advantage of reducing blood volume
   - The therapeutic actions of Tenormin® and Lasix®.
2. Have patient repeat explanations and note his level of understanding; clarify any misunderstanding immediately.
3. Go over schedule of medication administration on 3/7 with patient and again with patient and his sister before discharge.
4. Advise the patient to discuss any deviations in medication schedule or dosage with his physician. —————————————————— M. MOHNEY, RN

Implementation (Documentation)

3/5

0930   Chest pain relieved by sublingual nitroglycerin administered 30 minutes earlier. Has voided 700 mL of urine in past hour following IV Lasix. Resting comfortably. Pulse = 90 bpm, BP 156/90 R. arm in semi-Fowler's position. ————
————————————————————— B. VIANNY, LPN

1000   Explained that the nitroglycerin dilates blood vessels and eases the work of the heart. Used the analogy of blowing air through a very narrow straw vs. a very wide one. Informed that one of the actions of Tenormin is to reduce blood pressure and therefore reduce the work of the heart and its need for oxygen.
————————————————————— B. VIANNY, LPN

Evaluation (Documentation)

1015   Could paraphrase explanation correctly. States, "I know people take nitroglycerin for chest pain, but I didn't know how it helped relieve it. I'd rather take a pill once a day and prevent chest pain than have to take a pill to get rid of it." ———————————————— B. VIANNY, LPN

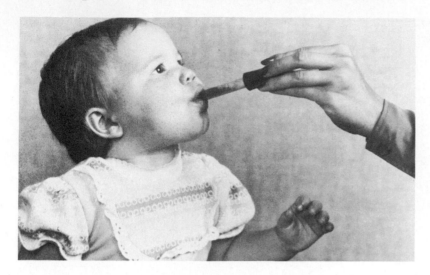

Figure 23-17 An infant receives liquid medication from a dropper that is calibrated for accurate dosage measurement. The dropper is placed beyond the sensitive taste buds on the tongue so that the child is less likely to resist taking the medication because of its taste. (Courtesy of Apex Medical Corp., Bloomington, MN.)

tion medications as well. The combination of drugs, with their potential side effects, may lead to serious complications.

Monitor the elderly person's medication carefully while taking into account the effects of aging. As a result of aging, the risk of adverse side effects and toxicity to drugs increases. Decreased gastrointestinal motility and ability to absorb drugs tend to reduce the drug action because the drugs are not being taken into the bloodstream well.

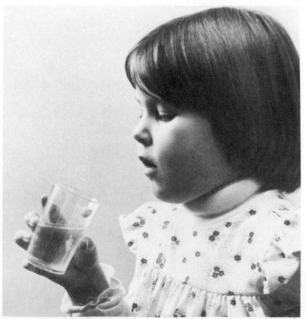

Figure 23-18 This glass has a shelf on which a tablet or capsule is placed after the glass is filled with water. Flow channels designed in the glass lift the pill, which is then carried with the water down the throat without stimulating the gag reflex. (Courtesy of Apex Medical Corp, Bloomington, MN.)

Use a pill organizer, as described earlier in this section, when the elderly patient needs help in remembering to take medications as prescribed.

Expect that a safe dosage for medications prescribed for the elderly will generally be lower than that for younger adults.

Teaching Suggestions for the Administration of Medications

Suggestions for teaching patients when giving medications have been described in this chapter. They are summarized below:

It is recommended that in addition to observing a demonstration, the patient or family member should practice in the presence of the nurse until skill for safe administration is achieved.

The patient should be taught the name of the drug, what it is for, how much to take, how long and how often he is to take the medication, what the desired and undesired effects are, and what alterations he must make in daily living, such as a dietary modification.

The nurse should teach the patient to notify his physician promptly if undesirable symptoms occur. He should also be taught not to discontinue or make any changes in his medication schedule without consulting his physician.

When a patient is to take liquid medications and the dosage is stated in teaspoons or tablespoons, he may be advised to purchase a dispenser to measure dosages accurately. The dispenser may be a special syringe, a dosing spoon like the one illustrated in Figure 23-20, or a calibrated medicine cup. It has been found that the sizes of household teaspoons and tablespoons vary considerably, with

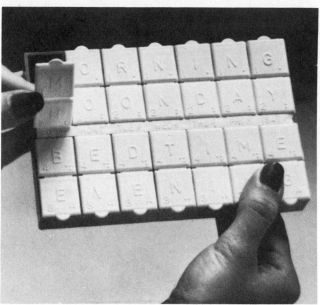

Figure 23-19 This is one type of pill organizer that many patients find helpful. The manufacturer points out that the organizer is easy to use and fill. (Courtesy of Apex Medical Corp, Bloomington, MN.)

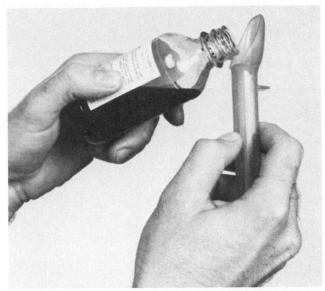

Figure 23-20 This dosing spoon has a hollow stem that is calibrated so that the prescribed amount of liquid medication can be measured accurately. When the spoon is tipped, the liquid fills the bowl of the spoon for easy administration.

the result that the patient may not take prescribed dosages accurately when using them.

It is recommended that patients taking medications over a long period of time be encouraged to carry a card or wear a bracelet that indicates special medical information. This practice helps in an emergency because health personnel are aware of what the patient is taking and can plan care accordingly. The same advice applies to individuals with allergies to medications or other substances.

Occasional treatment of minor problems with over-the-counter (OTC) drugs is a common practice. However, repetitious or long-term self-administration of OTC drugs can be dangerous. The Food and Drug Administration (FDA) attempts to protect the public by requiring truthful advertising, proper labeling, and directions for use on OTC drug packages. In an attempt to protect the individual from harm, the FDA has provided the following recommendations, which the nurse will wish to share with patients:

Tell patients:
- Don't be casual about taking drugs.
- Don't take drugs you don't need.
- Don't overbuy and keep drugs for long periods of time.
- Don't combine drugs carelessly.
- Do be cautious when using a drug for the first time.
- Do dispose of old prescription drugs and outdated OTC medications.
- Don't continue taking OTC drugs if symptoms persist.
- Don't take prescription drugs not prescribed specifically for you.
- Do read and follow directions for use.
- Do seek professional advice before combining drugs.
- Do seek professional advice when symptoms persist or return.
- Do get medical checkups regularly.

The nurse should plan to teach family members when the patient is an infant or child or when the patient is elderly and cannot assume responsibility for taking his own medications. Parents should be taught the dangers present when children are able to take medications that are not stored safely.

Problems with noncompliance often can be overcome when the patient helps prepare a plan for self-administration and when he is taught adequately about his medications and the reasons for taking them.

Bibliography

Adams C: Computer-generated medication administration records. Nursing Management 20(7):22–23, 1989

Arbeiter J: A safe way to work with the pharmacy. RN Magazine 51(10):91–92, 1988

Azzarello J: Reviewing your patient's medication regimen: A systemic approach. Home Healthcare Nurse 7(6):24–26, 1989

Carr P: The medication maze. Home Healthcare Nurse 8(1):55–56, 1990

Carr DS: New strategies for avoiding medication errors. Nursing 19(8):39–46, 1989

Cerrato PL: Drugs and food: When the dangers increase. RN Magazine. 51(11):65–67, 1988

Cobb MD: Dealing fairly with medication errors. Nursing 20(3):42–43, 1990

Cohen MR: Are errors waiting to happen? Nursing 18(9):18, 1988

Cohen MR: Better way to transcribe orders. Nursing 20(1):9, 1990

Dick L: Warning: Take only as directed. RN Magazine 52(10):83–84, 86, 88, 1989

Hahn K: About discharge medications. Nursing 18(11):89–91, 1988

Helping patients comply with drug regimens. Nurses Drug Alert 12(2):14–15, 1988

Holmes P: Modes of entry . . . new drug delivery systems. Nursing Times 84(12):34, 36, 1988

Jones IH: Code of conduct: The buck stops here . . . blindly following doctors' instructions. Nursing Times 84(17):50–52, 1988

Lim, E: Pill-swallowing maneuver. Consultant 27(10):55, 1987

McCord MA: Relating nursing diagnoses to drug therapy. Nursing 18(10):80–84, 86, 1988

McGovern K: Take the first step toward reducing medication errors. Nursing 17(12):49, 1987

McGovern K: 10 golden rules for administering drugs safely. Nursing 18(8):34–42, 1988

Murphy JI: Tube feeding problems and solutions. Advancing Clinical Care 5(2):7–11, 1990

Porterfield LM: Geriatric pharmacology. AD Nurse 3(4):12, 1988

Porterfield L: Principles of drug action. AD Nurse 3(3):11–12, 1988

Ross FM: Doctor, nurse and patient knowledge of prescribed medication in primary care. Public Health Rep 103(2):131–137, 1989

Wayland MA: Safe learning . . . helping students learn to give team medications. AD Nurse 3(3):29–30, 1988

Westfall LK: Why the elderly are so vulnerable to drug reactions. RN Magazine 50(11):39–43, 1987

Williams PJ: How do you keep medicines from clogging feeding tubes? Am J Nurs 89(2):181–182, 1989

24

Administering Parenteral Medications

Chapter Outline

Behavioral Objectives
Glossary
Introduction
Selecting Equipment for Parenteral Administration
Filling a Syringe with Medication
Reconstituting a Powdered Parenteral Medication
Mixing Two Medications in One Syringe
Cleansing the Skin at the Site of Injection
Reducing the Discomfort of an Injection
Disposing of Used Needles and Syringes
Administering an Intramuscular Injection
Administering a Subcutaneous Injection
Administering an Intradermal Injection
Administering Intravenous Medication
Suggested Measures When Administering Parenteral
    Medications in Selected Situations
Teaching Suggestions for the Administration of
    Parenteral Medications
Applicable Nursing Diagnoses
Bibliography

Skill Procedures

Locating Sites for Intramuscular Injections
Administering a Subcutaneous Injection
Using the Z-Track Technique
Administering an Intramuscular Injection
Administering an Intradermal Injection

Instilling Intravenous Medication Through a Central
    Venous Catheter
Administering Antineoplastic Drugs

Behavioral Objectives

When the content of this chapter has been mastered, the
learner will be able to:

Define the terms appearing in the glossary.
Identify parts of a syringe.
List five criteria for selecting a syringe and needle.
Identify the range of syringe and needle sizes used for
    injections by various routes.
Differentiate between an ampule and vial.
Describe or demonstrate the techniques for filling a
    syringe from an ampule, vial, or prefilled cartridge.
List the information that is generally provided on a
    medication label when a drug must be reconstituted.
Describe or demonstrate the technique for mixing med-
    ications in one syringe.
Discuss at least 10 methods for reducing the discomfort
    of an injection.
Describe how to reduce the potential for an accidental
    needle stick.
Identify five muscles commonly used for intramuscular
    injections and demonstrate how to identify their ana-
    tomical location.
Demonstrate the technique for administering intra-
    muscular, Z-track, subcutaneous, and intradermal in-
    jections.
Describe how the technique for injecting insulin and
    heparin differ from other subcutaneous injections.
List four methods of administering drugs intravenously.
Describe three types of central venous catheters.
Discuss safety techniques when working with anti-
    neoplastic drugs.
Describe modifications for giving injections to infants,
    children, or the elderly.
Discuss information that can be taught to patients who
    receive injections or administer their own parenteral
    medication.

Glossary

Ampule A glass container holding a single dose of a par-
    enteral medication.
Antineoplastic drug A medication used to treat cancer.
Bolus A single dose of medication that is administered
    intravenously in a short amount of time.
Central venous catheter Tubing that is inserted from a
    peripheral vein with the tip located in the superior vena
    cava.

603

Diluent The liquid component of a solution.

Gauge The width of a needle.

Heparin lock A device that facilitates access to the bloodstream without requiring the continuous infusion of fluids.

Insulin pen A device to administer multiple doses of insulin from a prefilled cartridge.

Intradermal injection The administration of a substance just below the epidermal layer of skin.

Intramuscular injection The administration of a medication within a muscle.

Parenteral route All methods other than oral for administering medications; the term has come to only refer to administration by injection.

Push A term used to describe the technique for administering a bolus of intravenous medication.

Reconstitution The process of adding a liquid to a powdered drug to form a solution.

Subcutaneous injection The administration of a drug between the epidermis and the muscle.

Vial A glass or plastic container of parenteral medication with a self-sealing stopper.

Wheal A raised area within the skin.

Z-track technique An injection method used to administer irritating medications into the muscle in such a way that the drug cannot leak back into subcutaneous tissue.

Introduction

The term *parenteral* refers to all routes of drug administration other than oral. It is used most commonly, however, to indicate medications that are given by injection, and is used in this manner in the text.

This chapter discusses the techniques for administering drugs within and beneath layers of skin, into muscle, and into peripheral and larger central veins. Drugs that are administered by injection must be prepared and administered following principles of surgical asepsis described in

Chapter 16. Using sterile technique minimizes the danger of injecting organisms that can lead to infection.

Selecting Equipment for Parenteral Administration

Drugs that are administered parenterally must be prepared using various types of syringes and needles. Figure 24-1 illustrates a typical example of the equipment. Note the marked areas that must be kept free of contamination.

Syringes come in various sizes and calibrations depending upon the volume and type of drug that will be administered. Figure 24-2 shows some typical syringes used to administer drugs parenterally. Syringes for medication administration generally hold amounts ranging from 1 to 5 mL. Some syringes holding the equivalent of 1 mL may be calibrated in units or in minims.

Needles are available in various lengths and gauges. The size of the needle depends upon the tissue that will be entered during the injection of the drug. Needle lengths vary from 1/2 to 2 1/2 inches. The needle *gauge* refers to the width of the needle. The common sizes of needles range from 18 through 27 gauge. The smaller the number of the gauge, the larger the lumen of the needle. An 18-gauge needle is larger than a 27-gauge needle. A needle with a large lumen is needed when the drug is thick or oily. Table 24-1 identifies common sizes of syringes and needles used for various types of injections.

The nurse must use good judgement in selecting the appropriate syringe and needle based upon several criteria that affect the administration of the medication. The following should be considered:

- The route of administration. A longer needle is required to reach deeper layers of tissue.
- The viscosity, or thickness, of the solution. Some medications are more viscous than others and require a larger lumen through which to inject the drug.
- The quantity to be administered. The larger the vol-

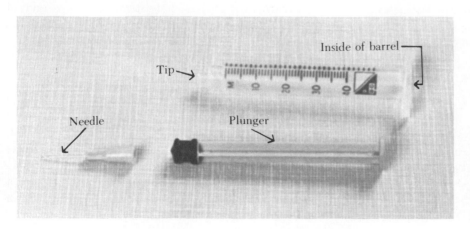

Figure 24-1 A needle and syringe have been disassembled and labeled in this illustration. The arrows indicate the areas of the equipment that must be kept free of organisms during the time of preparation and administration of parenteral drugs.

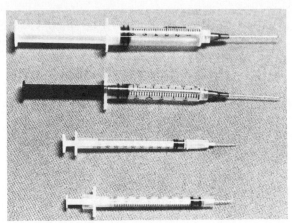

Figure 24-2 This collection of syringes shows some of the various types used for the administration of parenteral medications. Note that the syringes have the potential for holding and measuring different volumes of medication. This variety of needle lengths and gauges shows possible combinations that may be selected according to the characteristics of the medication, the size of the patient, or the site that will be used.

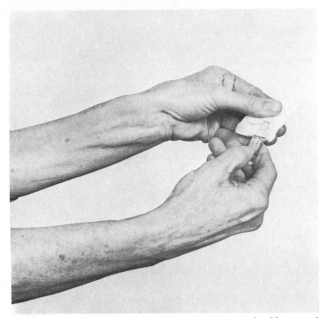

Figure 24-3 The nurse's fingers are protected with a moist pledget when the stem of the glass ampule is snapped.

ume of medication to be injected, the greater the holding capacity must be within the syringe.

- The body size of the patient. In an obese person a longer needle may be required to reach various layers of tissue than in a thin or pediatric patient.
- The type of medication. Some drugs should only be measured or administered using specific equipment. For example, insulin is most accurately prepared using a syringe calibrated in units. Drugs that are irritating to subcutaneous tissue should be administered using a long needle to ensure proper placement of the medication deep within the muscle.

Filling a Syringe With Medication

Medications for injection are usually supplied in one of three ways. They are contained in glass ampules, rubber-capped vials containing single or multiple dosages of a drug, and prefilled cartridges.

Removing Medication From an Ampule. An *ampule* is a sealed glass container that holds the usual, standard dose of a particular parenteral medication. The glass ampule must be broken in order to withdraw the drug. The ampule is opened by scoring and snapping the narrow neck of the container. To avoid a laceration or splinters of glass, the nurse should use an alcohol swab, as shown in Figure 24-3, to protect the fingers.

The ampule also is imprinted with the drug name, dosage, and volume. When a syringe is filled with a drug supplied in an ampule, the following techniques may be used.

- Assemble the needle with the syringe.
- Distribute any medication trapped in the top of the ampule into the bottom by tapping the upper area of the container.

Table 24-1. Common Sizes of Syringes and Needles

Type of Injection	Size of Syringe	Size of Needle
Subcutaneous	2, 2.5, or 3 mL calibrated in 0.1 mL	23-, 25-, or 26-gauge, 1/2- or 5/8-inch
Intramuscular	3 or 5 mL calibrated in 0.2 mL	20-, 21-, 22-, or 23-gauge, 1 1/2- or 2-inch
Intradermal	1 mL calibrated in 0.1 mL or 0.01 mL and/or in minims	25-, 26-, or 27-gauge, 1/2- to 5/8-inch
Insulin, given subcutaneously	1 mL calibrated in units	25-, 26-, or 27-gauge, 1/2- or 5/8-inch

- Score the neck of the ampule with a file.
- Protect the thumb and fingers with a gauze square or premoistened pledget.
- Snap the neck of the ampule away from the body when breaking the top free from the ampule.
- Insert the needle into the ampule, being careful not to touch the outside surface or the rim.
- Stabilize the ampule, holding it securely within the hand or inverting the ampule in the nondominant hand, as illustrated in Figure 24-4.
- Withdraw the solution into the syringe by pulling back the plunger. Keep the tip of the needle within the solution.
- Remove the syringe and tap the barrel to move any bubbles of air toward the end of the syringe.
- Expel the air bubbles and any excess medication.
- Cover the needle with its protective sheath.
- Discard the ampule and any remaining medication in a container that will not injure someone who will be disposing of nonburnable trash.
- Do not keep medications contained within an opened ampule since there is no way of ensuring the continued sterility of the drug.

Removing Medication From a Vial. A *vial* is a glass or plastic container of medication with a self-sealing rubber stopper. Medication is removed from a vial by piercing the rubber stopper with a needle following appropriate cleansing techniques.

The medication may be premixed or in powder form that will require reconstitution. The amount of drug within the vial may be enough for one dose or several doses. Any unused drug that will be administered in the future should be dated once the seal is pierced.

The following steps can be followed when removing medication from a vial:

- Remove the metal cover from the vial.
- Clean the exposed rubber cap with a swab premoistened with an antiseptic solution.
- Attach the needle to the syringe and fill the syringe with the same volume of air as the medication that will be withdrawn, as the nurse in Figure 24-5 is doing.
- Insert the needle through the rubber stopper while holding the syringe and the vial at a slightly oblique angle. Piercing the rubber stopper in this manner helps to prevent instillation of a core of rubber into the vial when the air is instilled.
- Invert the vial without touching the needle and allow the medication to enter the syringe, as illustrated in Figure 24-6.
- Remove the needle when the desired volume of medication has entered the barrel of the syringe.
- Expel any air or excess medication from the syringe, as shown in Figure 24-7.
- Cover the needle carefully with its protective sheath.

When the syringe has been filled with the correct dosage of medication, a small amount of air, approximately

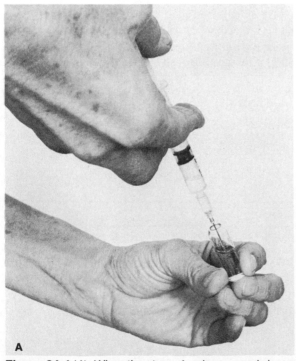
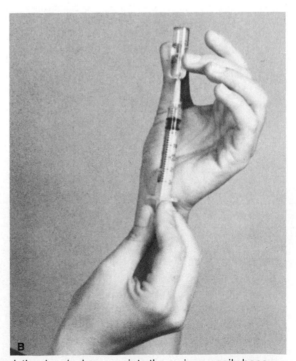

Figure 24-4 (*A*). When the stem of a glass ampule is removed, the drug is drawn up into the syringe easily because air displaces the fluid. (*B*). The ampule may be inverted when medication is withdrawn. When medication is removed in this manner, the trick is to keep the needle in the solution at all times, even as the ampule is inverted.

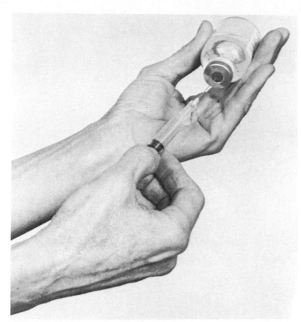

Figure 24-5 This nurse adds air to the contents of the vial, which increases pressure within the vial, making withdrawal of solution from an area under pressure easy. If air is not instilled, a partial vacuum is created in the vial as fluid is withdrawn. This makes it difficult to withdraw solution. If too much air is instilled, the pressure within the vial will propel solution into the syringe, making control and accurate filling difficult to achieve.

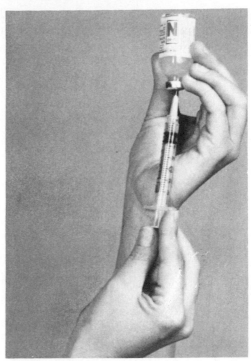

Figure 24-6 This nurse holds the inverted vial at eye level as medication is removed from the vial. Holding the vial in this manner ensures accuracy in filling the syringe with the desired volume of medication.

0.2 cc, may be pulled into the syringe. Providing an air bubble ensures that the entire dosage of medication will be administered during the time of injection. If the medication that is withdrawn can cause irritation of tissue, the needle should be removed and replaced with another sterile needle before it is inserted into the patient.

Using a Prefilled Cartridge. Some injectable medications come supplied from the pharmaceutical manufacturer in prefilled cartridges. An advantage in using a prefilled cartridge is the elimination of the time involved in transferring the drug from a medication container, such as an ampule or vial, into a syringe. A sterile needle, the size of which is appropriate for the recommended route of the drug administration, is permanently attached to the cartridge.

The name of the drug, its dosage, and volume are printed on the cartridge. The package used to store the cartridge also displays duplicate information. Both should be read and reread to make sure that the administration will provide the right drug, dosage, and route.

The nurse inserts the cartridge into a metal or plastic holder, such as the one in Figure 24-8, and screws the plunger in place. If the prescribed dosage is less than that contained in the cartridge, the unneeded portion is expelled before its administration to the patient. Some narcotics, which are controlled substances, are available in prefilled cartridges. Any narcotic that is wasted must be witnessed by another nurse. Each nurse must then cosign the narcotic record.

Most prefilled cartridges are intended for a single-unit dose of drug. Once the drug is administered, the cartridge is removed from its holder. It is discarded with the attached, uncapped needle into a puncture-resistant container.

Insulin is now available in prefilled cartridges that contain more than one dose. The prefilled cartridge is loaded into what the manufacturer calls a "pen," probably because of its similarity in appearance. An *insulin pen*, shown in Figure 24-9, is a device used to administer several doses of insulin from a single prefilled cartridge. The cartridge of insulin is replaced every seven days or sooner if the contents are used before that. The needle is removable and is changed with each use.

The insulin pen has several advantages when compared with filling a syringe from a multidose vial. First of all, diabetics often have vision problems. Many have difficulty seeing the small calibrations on an insulin syringe. The insulin pen allows the patient, a family member, or a nurse to dial a number equal to the prescribed dosage. The pen will permit only the dialed amount of drug to be injected. The potential for overdosing or underdosing is reduced. Once the pen is loaded, it can be reused for several days without having to manipulate a syringe and multidose vial each time. Only the needle has to be changed. Simplifying insulin administration may help many newly diagnosed diabetics feel more in control of the disease, and promote earlier independence and self-care.

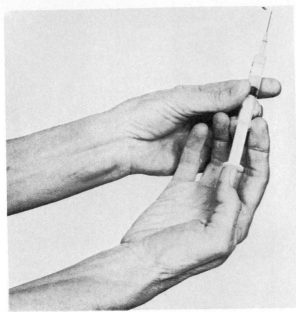

Figure 24-7 The medication has been placed within the syringe, which is held vertically—with the needle pointing upward. Air and excess medication are then removed by pressing the plunger for the necessary distance.

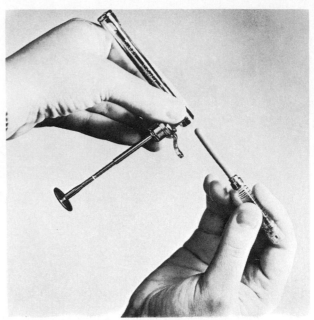

Figure 24-8 The cartridge in the nurse's right hand has been prefilled with a drug by the manufacturer. (Courtesy of Wyeth Laboratories, Philadelphia, PA.)

Reconstituting a Powdered Parenteral Medication

Some drugs intended for parenteral administration are supplied as powders. The powdered drug must be combined with a liquid or *diluent* before it can be injected. The process of adding a diluent to a powdered substance is called *reconstitution*.

The label on the drug container will provide the nurse with the following information:

- The type of diluent to add to the powder; common diluents are sterile water and sterile normal saline
- The amount of diluent to add
- The dosage of the medication per liquid volume when reconstituted
- The directions for storing the reconstituted medication.

If the reconstituted drug will be used for more than one administration of the medication, the nurse must indicate certain information on the drug label. The date, initials of the nurse who added the liquid to the powdered drug, and amount of drug per volume of solution should be indicated.

Mixing Two Medications in One Syringe

The procedure for mixing two medications in one syringe will depend on the type of containers in which the medications are supplied. The nurse must also make certain that the drugs are compatible when mixed together. It is possible for some drugs to form a solid precipitate when mixed. If this happens, the drugs must not be administered to the patient. Consulting a reference concerning drug combinations is better than having to waste expensive medication. A drug compatibility table should be available in medication preparation areas or the agency's pharmacist may be consulted.

Combining Medications From Single-Dose and Multiple-Dose Vials. The following steps may be followed when one drug is supplied in a single-dose vial and the other is contained within a multiple-dose vial:

1. Cleanse the rubber stopper on each vial with a pledget moistened with antiseptic.
2. Instill air into the single-dose vial without coating the needle with any medication.
3. Using the same syringe and needle, instill air into the multiple-dose vial.
4. Withdraw the desired volume of medication from the multiple dose vial first. This prevents mixing a second drug into the contents of a vial that may be used for subsequent administrations.
5. Reinsert the syringe and needle into the remaining vial and withdraw the appropriate volume of drug.
6. Recheck the total volume to ensure that the proper quantities have been drawn into the syringe.

Combining Drugs From Two Multiple-Dose Vials. The procedure for filling a syringe with two medications each supplied in a separate multiple-dose vial is as follows:

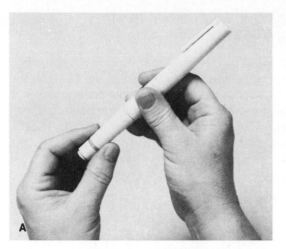

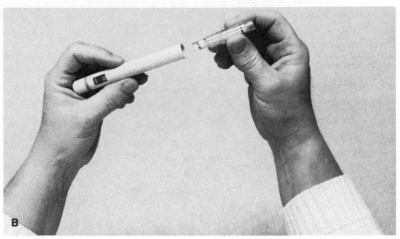

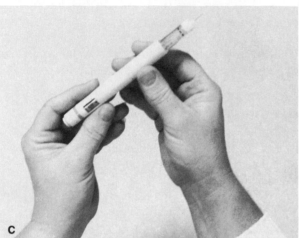

Figure 24-9 (*A*). What appears to be a fountain pen is actually a device that administers multiple doses of insulin. (*B*). The pen is loaded by inserting a prefilled cartridge of insulin. (*C*). A cap with a sterile needle is attached to the cartridge and the pen is ready to use.

1. Cleanse the rubber stopper on each vial with a pledget moistened with antiseptic.
2. Instill an amount of air comparable to the desired volume of medication into one vial without permitting the needle to come in contact with the medication.
3. Withdraw the needle and repeat the action using the second vial of medication.
4. Withdraw the desired volume of medication before removing the needle from the vial.
5. Expel all the air and any excess volume of medication so that the syringe holds the exact amount of medication needed from the first vial.
6. Change the needle and insert it into the vial containing the second medication.
7. Withdraw the desired amount from the second vial, combining both medications in the same syringe.
8. Cover the needle with a protective sheath and replace the multiple-dose vials in their storage location.

Combining Medication From an Ampule and a Vial. Combining drugs from an ampule and a vial follows the same principles and techniques as combining medications from a single-dose and multiple-dose vial. The medication in the vial is prepared and drawn into the syringe first. The medication in the ampule is drawn into the syringe after that from the vial.

Cleansing the Skin at the Site of Injection

The skin is cleansed with an antiseptic solution prior to being pierced with the needle. Using a moistened cotton ball or pledget, move in a circular pattern beginning at the point of injection outward for a distance of about 2.5 to 6 cm (1 to 2.5 inches). This technique carries debris and microorganisms away from the site of injection. Use firm pressure and friction when cleansing to help remove surface contaminants.

Reducing the Discomfort of an Injection

Following certain practices can lessen the potential for discomfort. Several techniques can greatly reduce the pain associated with an injection. The nurse may wish to utilize some of the methods included in the following list:

- Select the smallest gauge that is appropriate for the route of administration and type of medication.
- Avoid inserting a needle that is coated with irritating medication; some drugs are more prone to causing discomfort than others. The best technique is to change the needle. However, the needle can be wiped using a sterile gauze pledget. Care must be taken to avoid contaminating the needle if this method is used.
- Select a site that is presently free of irritation.
- Develop a system for rotating the injection sites when the patient is receiving frequent administration of drugs by the parenteral route.
- Numb the skin if the patient has shown an unusual sensitivity during previous insertions of a needle. Apply cold compresses or an ice cube over the area to be injected; gently tap the site of injection with the fingers several times; or spray an anesthetic, such as ethyl chloride, over the area to be injected. With the physician's approval, a small amount of local anesthetic, such as procaine hydrochloride, may be added to a medication injected intramuscularly.
- Position the patient prone with the feet pointing inward when an injection will be placed into the muscle in the buttock.
- Assist the patient to relax using deep breathing or other distraction techniques. Avoid having the patient watch the area where the needle will be placed. The mind can anticipate the entry of the needle and the imagery can intensify the discomfort.
- Insert the needle without hesitation.
- Instill the solution slowly, especially when the amount is sizable.
- Divide volumes in excess of 2.5 to 5 mL into two syringes and inject them in separate sites.
- Remove the needle rapidly to decrease the amount of medication that may spread into the surrounding tissue.
- Instill the medication by performing the Z-track or zig-zag technique discussed later in this chapter.
- Place pressure against the site of injection with a gauze pledget as the needle is withdrawn. This technique prevents pulling skin with the needle, which is an uncomfortable sensation.
- Massage the site after giving the injection unless contraindicated for the particular type of medication.

Disposing of Used Needles and Syringes

Reusable equipment is handled according to agency policy. Care must be taken to avoid needle punctures and the possible transmission of pathogens spread by blood or serum. To prevent self-injury, needles remain uncapped after their use. The entire syringe and uncapped needle are deposited in a puncture-resistant container.

Administering an Intramuscular Injection

An *intramuscular injection* is the administration of a solution containing medication into one muscle or a muscle group of the body. Since very few nerve endings are in deep muscles, irritating medications are commonly given intramuscularly. Except for medications injected directly into the bloodstream, absorption from an intramuscular injection occurs more rapidly than from other routes.

Selecting Sites for Intramuscular Injections

Various muscles may be used as sites for injection of a parenteral medication. In order to select an injection site, the nurse must know how to identify certain landmarks to avoid injuring large nerves, striking bones, or entering blood vessels. Muscles commonly used for the intramuscular administration of medications are located in the buttock, thigh, and upper arm. There are unique advantages and disadvantages associated with the muscles in each of these particular injection sites.

Using the Dorsogluteal Site. This is a common site for injecting medications into the gluteus maximus muscle in the buttock. This muscle can receive a relatively large volume of drug with minimal postinjection discomfort. If the site is not identified correctly, damage to the sciatic nerve with subsequent paralysis of the leg can result. Palpation of anatomical landmarks aids in the identification of the dorsogluteal site. This site should be avoided when the patient is under 3 years of age since the muscle is not sufficiently developed at this age.

Using the Ventrogluteal Site. The ventrogluteal site utilizes the gluteus medius and gluteus minimus muscles in the hip area. This site has several advantages over the dorsogluteal site. There are no large nerves or blood vessels in the injection area. It is generally less fatty and cleaner because fecal contamination is rare at this site. The ventrogluteal site is safe for use in children.

Using the Vastus Lateralis Muscle. This thick muscle is located in the lateral thigh. Large nerves and blood vessels are generally absent in this area. The vastus lateralis site is particularly desirable for infants and small children and other thin or debilitated individuals whose gluteal muscles are poorly developed.

Using the Rectus Femoris Muscle. This muscle is located on the anterior aspect of the thigh. The muscle is quite visible in infants and is the preferred injection site for this age group.

Using the Deltoid Muscle. The deltoid muscle is located in the lateral aspect of the upper arm. It is not often used because it is a small muscle in comparison with the others. The deltoid muscle is not capable of absorbing large amounts of solution. Damage to the radial nerve and artery is a risk when this site is used. Intramuscular injections into the deltoid muscle should be limited to 1 mL of solution. The deltoid muscle should be used only for adults. It is not sufficiently developed in infants and children to absorb medication adequately.

Skill Procedure 24-1 describes the techniques for locating and safely injecting medications intramuscularly into the various described sites.

Injecting an Intramuscular Medication

Skill Procedure 24-2 describes and illustrates how to inject medication into an intramuscular site. The suggested actions assume that the nurse observes the basic guidelines for preparing and administering medications.

Using the Z-Track Technique. The *Z-track technique,* sometimes called the *zigzag technique,* is an injection method used to administer medications that are irritating to subcutaneous tissue. However, any intramuscular injection can be given by Z-track. Patients report slightly less pain during a Z-track injection compared with the usual intramuscular injection technique. The next day reported pain is remarkably less when a Z-track injection was used.

The technique acquired its name because the tissue is manipulated somewhat like the letter "Z." Injections administered in this manner seal the medication within the muscle so that it cannot leak back through other layers of tissue following the path of the needle.

Before administering a medication using this technique, the nurse should select a needle that is long enough to reach the muscle. Depending on the patient's size and the muscle selected, the needle length may vary from 1½ inches to 2 inches or more. The original needle used to aspirate medication into the syringe must be changed. This prevents tissue contact with residue of the drug clinging to the outside of the needle.

Skill Procedure 24-3 describes and illustrates the method for administering a medication using the Z-track technique. It is assumed that the nurse observes the basic

guidelines for preparing and administering medications when following the suggested actions for using the Z-track technique.

Administering a Subcutaneous Injection

A *subcutaneous injection* involves the administration of a medication into the tissue that lies between the epidermis and the muscle. This involves a much wider area into which injected medication may be administered. The medication is absorbed fairly rapidly and begins acting within one-half hour of being administered. The equipment selected for use requires some modification from that used for intramuscular injections since the tissue is not as deep. Usually a smaller volume of medication is injected when using the subcutaneous route.

Selecting Subcutaneous Injection Sites

The sites for giving a subcutaneous injection include the upper arm, thigh, abdomen, and back. Figure 24-28 illustrates the appropriate locations of these areas.

When a patient, such as the insulin-dependent diabetic, must receive repeated subcutaneous injections, it is important to rotate the sites of injection. Rotation avoids repeated use of the same site, which can contribute to discomfort and possible tissue damage. In such cases, it is recommended that a sketch of the body be used. Each time an injection is given, the nurse indicates on the sketch exactly where the medication was injected. The sketched site is dated so that the next time an injection is given another site may be used. It is best to rotate areas of the body at the time of each injection rather than rotate among adjacent areas at the same site. The patient may also use a sketch as a record of the rotation sites he is using when self-administering the medication.

Assembling Equipment for a Subcutaneous Injection

The subcutaneous route is used to administer insulin, heparin, certain narcotics, and some immunizations. Equipment used for subcutaneous injection may depend on the type of medication that has been prescribed. Insulin is prepared in an insulin syringe that is calibrated in units. Heparin may be prepared in a tuberculin syringe or it may be supplied in a prefilled cartridge in some agencies. Most of these medication dosages are within a 1 mL volume.

A shorter needle, usually 1/2 to 5/8 inch, may be selected since the tissue into which the medication will be injected is not as deep as muscular tissue. A 25-gauge needle is most often used since the medications administered by the subcutaneous route are generally not viscous.

Skill Procedure 24-1. Locating Sites for Intramuscular Injections

Suggested Action	**Reason for Action**

The Rectus Femoris Site

Position the patient in a supine or sitting position.	The rectus femoris muscle is one of the large muscles that makes up the quadriceps group of muscles on the anterior aspect of the thigh.
Divide the thigh into thirds using the hands or subjective judgment, as shown in Figure 24-10.	The upper and lower thirds are not suitable for injecting medications.

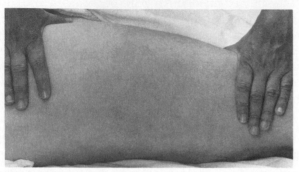

Figure 24-10 The nurse's hands can be used to divide the thigh into thirds when determining the area for injecting a drug into the rectus femoris muscle.

Inject the medication into the middle third of the thigh, as the nurse in Figure 24-11 is doing.	This site may be used as an alternative when rotating sites or when other sites show signs of irritation. It is often a convenient site for teaching patients how to self-administer injectable medication.

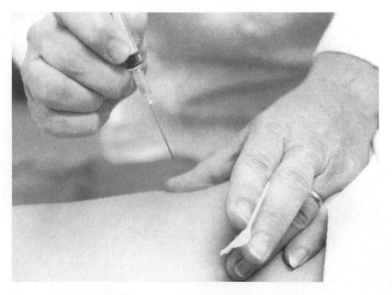

Figure 24-11 The nurse gives an intramuscular injection using the rectus femoris muscle on the front of the thigh.

The Ventrogluteal Site

Place the patient on his side with the upper knee bent and the leg placed slightly ahead of the lower leg. The patient can also be in a supine or prone position.	A side-lying position is best for exposing and palpating the anatomic landmarks prior to injecting a medication into the muscle group.
Palpate the greater trochanter at the head of the femur, the anterior superior iliac spine, and the iliac crest.	A triangular area between these structures provides the proper location for an injection.

(continued)

Skill Procedure 24-1. Continued

Suggested Action	Reason for Action

The Ventrogluteal Site

Place the palm of the hand on the greater trochanter and the index finger on the anterior superior iliac spine.

The line between these two forms one boundary of the triangle.

Move the middle finger away from the index finger as far as possible along the iliac crest, as the nurse is doing in Figure 24-12.

The line between the palm and the middle finger forms another boundary of the triangle. The iliac crest is the base of the triangle.

Inject into the center of the triangle formed by the index, middle finger, and iliac crest.

This area does not contain any major nerves or blood vessels.

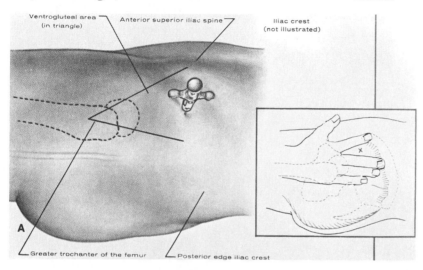

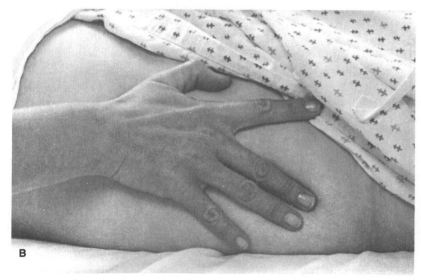

Figure 24-12 Although the side-lying position is the best to use for a ventrogluteal injection, this figure has the patient in the supine position. (*A*). The needle is in the ventrogluteal area. Notice how the nurse's palm is placed on the greater trochanter and the finger is on the anterior superior iliac spine. The middle finger is spread posteriorly as far as possible along the iliac crest. The injection is made in the middle of the triangle formed by the nurse's fingers and the iliac crest. (*B*). The ventrogluteal area is identified on a patient. (Courtesy of Wyeth Laboratories, Philadelphia, PA.)

The Dorsogluteal Site

Position the patient on his abdomen with the buttock well exposed.

The anatomy of the patient must be properly assessed in order to identify this site accurately.

Use either of the following methods to identify safe areas for injecting medication into this site:

When medication is injected into the dorsogluteal site, the sciatic nerve, trochanters of the femur, and large blood vessels must be avoided.

(continued)

Skill Procedure 24-1. Continued

Suggested Action	**Reason for Action**

The Dorsogluteal Site

• Palpate the posterior iliac spine and the greater trochanter. Draw an imaginary diagonal line between the two landmarks.

  Insert the needle superior and lateral to the midpoint of this line.

• Divide the buttock into four imaginary quadrants by drawing an imaginary vertical line through the

These methods utilize the location of anatomical landmarks to determine the safe area for injection.

Structures that may become injured can be avoided by inserting the needle into the upper outer areas of these anatomical landmarks.

The imaginary lines and various anatomical landmarks are identified in Figure 24-13.

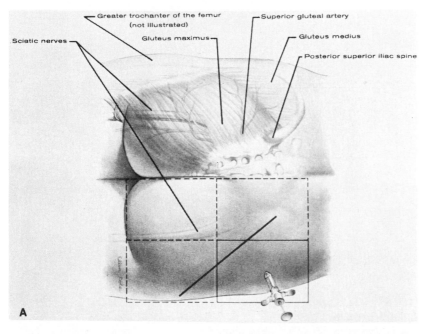

A

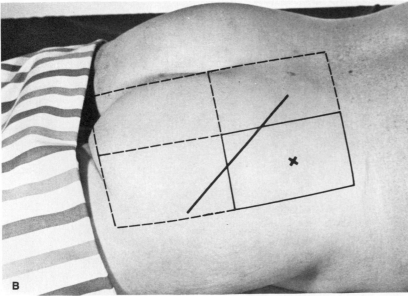

B

Figure 24-13 (*A*). The needle is in the dorsogluteal site. Notice how this site avoids entrance into any area near the sciatic nerve and the superior gluteal artery. The heavy, dark, diagonal line represents the imaginary line between the superior iliac spine and the greater trochanter. The dashed rectangular quadrants show the imaginary lines created when the buttock is divided into sectors, using the ridge of the superior iliac spine and the cleft in the buttock. The upper, outer corner of the quadrant, identified with a solid line, can be safely used for injections. (*B*). The imaginary lines indicating the dorsogluteal site are superimposed on the exposed buttock. The area identified with an X identifies the area for safe needle insertion. (Courtesy of Wyeth Laboratories, Philadelphia, PA.)

(*continued*)

Skill Procedure 24-1. *Continued*

Suggested Action	Reason for Action

The Dorsogluteal Site

bony ridge of the posterior superior iliac spine and an imaginary horizontal line from the upper cleft of the fold in the buttock.

Inject the medication in the upper outer area of the quadrant that lies superior and lateral to where the lines intersect.

The Vastus Lateralis Site

Suggested Action	Reason for Action
Have the patient lie supine or sit in a chair with the thigh well exposed.	The vastus lateralis is located on the lateral anterior aspect of the thigh.
Instruct the patient to point the toes inward.	Internally rotating the hip helps to position the leg for better exposure of the lateral aspect of the leg.
Divide the thigh into thirds to identify an imaginary rectangle.	The injection should be made into the middle rectangle of this thick muscle.

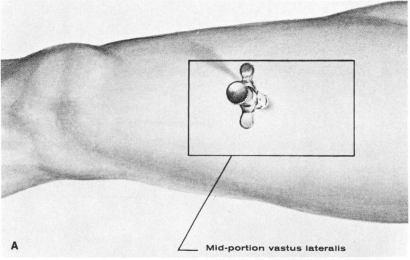

A   Mid-portion vastus lateralis

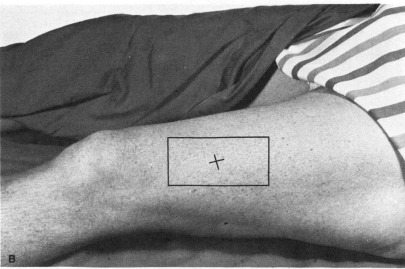

B

Figure 24-14 (*A*). The needle is in position for injecting into the center of the vastus lateralis muscle. (*B*). The same area is identified on a patient. The imaginary midrectangle can be located by positioning one hand's breadth from all four perimeters of the thigh. (Courtesy of Wyeth Laboratories, Philadelphia, PA.)

(continued)

Skill Procedure 24-1. Continued

Suggested Action	Reason for Action
The Vastus Lateralis Site	
Use the breadth of the hand as a convenient measure to divide the thigh both vertically and horizontally in the following manner:	The hand can be used to section off the perimeter of the imaginary rectangle.
• Place one hand's breadth below the greater trochanter at the top of the thigh, and a hand's breadth from the knee.	This defines the superior and inferior sides of the middle rectangle.
• Place one hand's breadth along the middle of the inner side of the thigh and one hand's breadth on the outer side of the thigh.	This defines the medial and lateral sides of the middle rectangle.
• Inject into the center of the imaginary midrectangle, as illustrated in Figure 24-14.	This area is safe for use in both adults and children.
Using the Deltoid Site	
Have the patient lie down, stand, or sit with the upper arm and shoulder well exposed.	This site is easily located in virtually all positions.
Palpate the lower edge of the acromion process and draw an imaginary horizontal line.	This forms the upper boundary of the deltoid site.
Imagine another horizontal line at the lower boundary of the axilla.	This forms the lower boundary of the deltoid site.
Inject within the center of the imaginary lines, as shown in Figure 24-15.	The deltoid muscle is much smaller than the other sites used for injections.

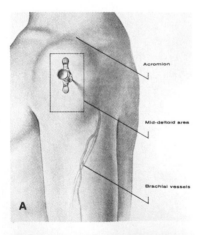

Acromion

Mid-deltoid area

Brachial vessels

A

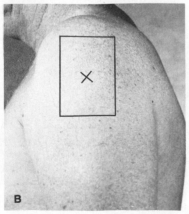

B

Figure 24-15 (*A*). The needle has been inserted in the deltoid muscle. The area for injection is bounded by the lower edge of the acromion process on the top to a point on the arm opposite the axilla on the bottom. The side boundaries are perpendicular to the lines described above about one-third and two-thirds of the way around the side of the arm, as indicated by the enclosed rectangle. (*B*). The deltoid site is identified on the arm of a patient. (Courtesy of Wyeth Laboratories, Philadelphia, PA.)

Skill Procedure 24-2. Administering an Intramuscular Injection

Suggested Action	**Reason for Action**
Evaluate the possible injection sites that may be used.	Sites that are irritated or bruised should be excluded as should any site where the anatomical landmarks cannot be easily palpated.
Select an appropriate site for the injection. The dorsogluteal site, shown in Figure 24-16, will be the example used in this procedure.	Following selective criteria in choosing a site decreases patient discomfort and possible damage to body tissues.

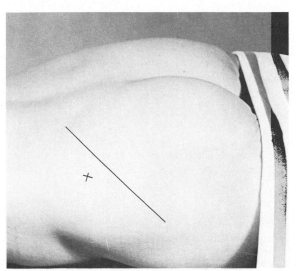

Figure 24-16 The buttock is well exposed in order to palpate and locate anatomic landmarks for determining the safe area to inject the medication. In this case, the dorsogluteal site is identified.

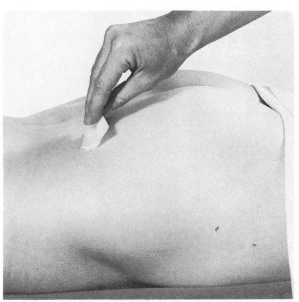

Figure 24-17 An injection site is being prepared by thorough cleansing with a swab containing an antiseptic of the agency's choice.

Using friction, cleanse the site of entry using a swab that has been premoistened with an antiseptic. Use a circular motion outward for 2.5 to 6 cm (1–2.5 in), as illustrated in Figure 24-17. Allow the skin to dry.	Cleansing the area of injection reduces the danger of forcing organisms into tissues. Introducing antiseptic into tissues with the needle causes tissue irritation. Allowing the skin to dry gives more time to inhibit the presence of organisms.
Remove the sheath protecting the needle.	Keeping the needle protected until just prior to the injection ensures its sterility.
Add a 0.2-mL bubble of air to the syringe just prior to injection.	An air bubble helps expel all the medication in the syringe and needle and reduces the possibility of pulling the drug back through the tissue as the needle is withdrawn.
Using the thumb and first two fingers, press the tissue down firmly, as illustrated in Figure 24-18.	Compression of the tissue helps to ensure that the needle will enter the muscle and not the subcutaneous layer of tissue.
Holding the syringe like a dart, insert the needle at a 90° angle quickly into the skin, as shown in Figure 24-19.	This angle facilitates needle insertion within muscle tissue. Hesitation during insertion can increase discomfort.
Continue to insert the needle firmly and steadily for almost its full length, as illustrated in Figure 24-20.	Sufficient penetration of the needle places it into the muscle.
Pull back gently on the plunger and observe the barrel of the syringe, as the nurse in Figure 24-21 is doing.	Aspiration is a method for assessing if a blood vessel has been entered.

(continued)

Skill Procedure 24-2. Continued

Suggested Action	Reason for Action

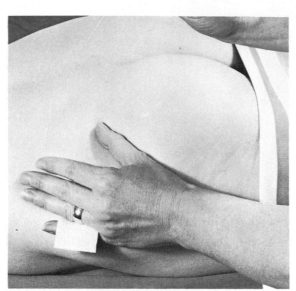

Figure 24-18 The thumb and fingers spread the skin at the injection site. The nurse is careful not to contaminate the site of entry.

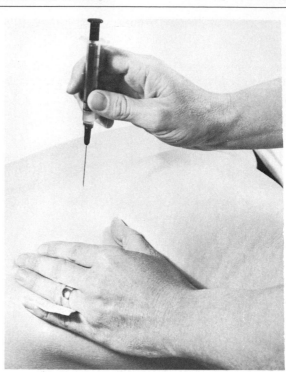

Figure 24-19 The nurse holds the syringe as a dart would be held and introduces the needle quickly.

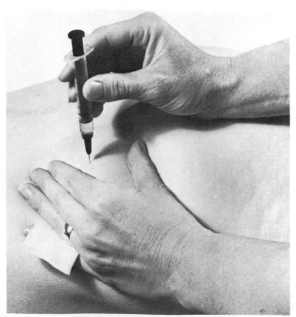

Figure 24-20 After entering the skin, the needle is introduced for almost its full length.

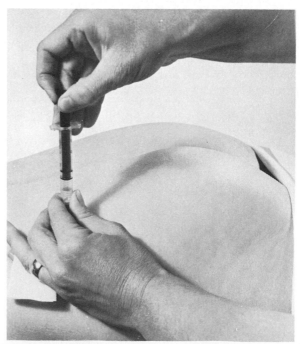

Figure 24-21 While steadying the syringe, the nurse pulls back gently on the plunger to see if blood enters the barrel of the syringe.

(continued)

Skill Procedure 24-2. Continued

Suggested Action	**Reason for Action**

Remove the syringe and needle if blood is noted, discard the medication and equipment, and prepare again.

Drugs injected intramuscularly are intended for slower absorption and may be dangerous if placed in the bloodstream, since they would be absorbed immediately.

Inject the medication slowly by pushing the plunger into the barrel, as the nurse in Figure 24-22 is demonstrating.

Slow injection allows the solution to disperse into the surrounding tissue without creating excessive pressure.

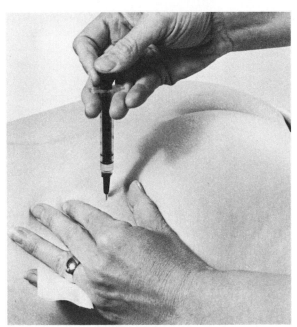

Figure 24-22 The nurse pushes the plunger its entire length. This forces the solution and the air bubble through the needle and into the muscle.

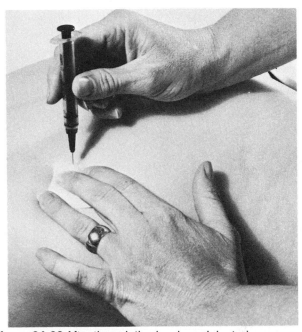

Figure 24-23 After the solution has been injected, pressure on the swab is applied against the injection site.

Withdraw the needle quickly while applying pressure against the skin surrounding the site, as shown in Figure 24-23.

Quickly withdrawing the needle while applying pressure on the injection site reduces discomfort and the risk of medication leaking into subcutaneous tissue.

Massage the injection site with the premoistened swab, as the nurse in Figure 24-24 is doing, unless this action is contraindicated.

Massaging the site helps distribute the medication and hastens absorption by increasing the blood supply to the area.

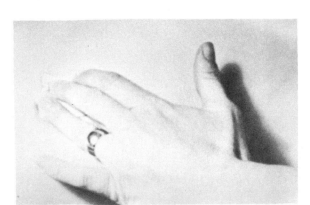

Figure 24-24 After the needle is removed, the injection site is massaged.

Skill Procedure 24-3. Using the Z-Track Technique

Suggested Action	**Reason for Action**
Replace the needle used for filling the syringe with another sterile needle that is at least 1½–2 inches long.	The needle must be free of irritating medication and long enough to be introduced deeply within the muscle.
Create an air bubble by adding 0.2 mL of air to the quantity of medication in the syringe.	The air bubble ensures that the irritating medication will be sealed into the muscle and not leak back through the path of the needle.
Select the intramuscular site where the medication will be injected. The ventrogluteal site is preferred.	A large, thick muscle should be used when irritating drugs must be injected.
Cleanse the skin over a wider area, approximately 6.5 to 8.5 cm (3–4 in).	A wider area of the skin must be manipulated, so the area that is cleansed should be of a comparable amount.
Grasp the muscle and pull it laterally about 2.5 cm (1 in), until it is taut, as the person in Figure 24-25 is doing. Continue to hold the tissue in this position.	This provides a straight path in the tissue during the time of the needle insertion, but a diagonal path when the needle is withdrawn and the tissue is released.

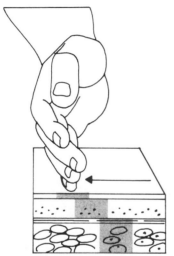

Figure 24-25 The first step in administering a Z-track injection is to pull the tissue laterally. (From Timby BK: Clinical Nursing Procedures, p 179. Philadelphia, JB Lippincott, 1989)

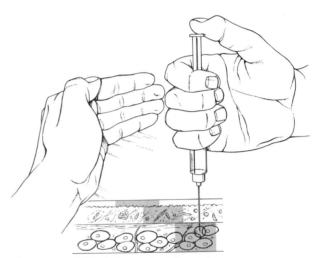

Figure 24-26 The drug is injected with one hand while the other hand stretches the tissue taut. (Adapted from Timby BK: Clinical Nursing Procedures, p 179. Philadelphia, JB Lippincott, 1989)

Insert the needle at a 90° angle using a dart-like motion.	This directs the needle tip well within the muscle.
Use the last three fingers of the hand holding the syringe to steady the barrel. Use the thumb and index finger on the same hand to aspirate.	The nondominant hand must not be released from its hold on the tissue.
Aspirate by pulling back on the plunger to identify if the tip of the needle has been placed within a blood vessel.	Medications intended for intramuscular injection should not be administered into the bloodstream.
Inject the medication with slow even pressure if no blood appears in the barrel of the syringe during aspiration, as shown in Figure 24-26.	Slow instillation allows time for the medication to become evenly distributed within the muscle.
Wait about 10 seconds with the needle still in place.	Pausing allows the medication to be distributed widely from the needle site.

(continued)

Skill Procedure 24-3. *Continued*

Suggested Action	**Reason for Action**
Withdraw the needle and immediately release the skin.	The injection track will now become a diagonal path sealing the original route of entry with layers of released tissue, shown in Figure 24-27.

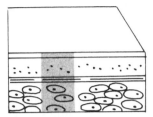

Figure 24-27 The drug is deposited within the muscle and sealed there by the diagonal recoil of the released tissue. (From Timby BK: Clinical Nursing Procedures, p 179. Philadelphia, JB Lippincott, 1989)

Apply pressure but *do not* massage the site.	Massaging the site may cause some of the trapped medication to leak from the pocket where it has been deposited and irritate surrounding tissue.

Modifying Injection Techniques

Some modifications in the injection technique are recommended when the nurse administers a subcutaneous injection. The goal is to inject into subcutaneous tissue. However, depending upon the patient's body size and layer of body fat, the angle of needle insertion or length of the needle, or both, may require some adjustments.

Authorities suggest that for a larger patient the nurse use a 90° angle for needle insertion; a 45° angle may be used when the patient is thin. Figure 24-29 illustrates needles being introduced at different angles in patients who are of different weights.

A shorter needle, for example 1/2 inch, must be inserted at a 90° angle in order to reach subcutaneous tissue in an individual of average weight. A longer needle, for example 5/8 inch, may be inserted at a 45° angle for a patient of average size.

Opinion also differs about whether the nurse should grasp the patient's tissues between the thumb and fingers or whether the skin should be stretched taut at the site of injection. The basis for the decision depends on the length of the needle and also on the body size of the patient. For a dehydrated or very thin patient and for most children and infants, grasping the tissue is preferred to stretching the skin. The nurse injecting patients in Figure 24-29 did not grasp the sites of injection. Just by changing the angle at which the needle is injected into two adult patients of different weights, one can readily reach the subcutaneous tissue with the needle.

Preparing Insulin

Insulin is a natural hormone that may not be produced by certain individuals with diabetes mellitus in sufficient amounts to meet the body's needs. Insulin must be injected since it is destroyed by digestive enzymes if given orally. It is administered using the subcutaneous route. Nurses teach newly diagnosed diabetics how to prepare insulin as well as the technique used to administer a subcutaneous injection.

Insulin is supplied in a dosage strength called a unit. The equivalent now commonly used for measuring insulin is referred to as U-100. This means that when insulin is prepared by pharmaceutical companies, the standard strength is 100 U of insulin per 1 mL. This standardization has helped to prevent dosage errors. Insulin is supplied in multiple-dose vials or prefilled cartridges.

Insulin preparations vary in onset and duration of action. The nurse must take care when reading insulin labels; many containers of insulin look similar to one another. Some preparations of insulin separate on standing and must be remixed before being drawn into a syringe.

It is common practice for one nurse to check the insulin preparation of another nurse because errors in the dosage or type of insulin can have life-threatening consequences. When teaching a patient to administer insulin, it is advantageous to also instruct a family member. Occasionally, several insulin syringes are filled at one time by a home-health nurse. The patient uses one syringe each day until the supply is replenished.

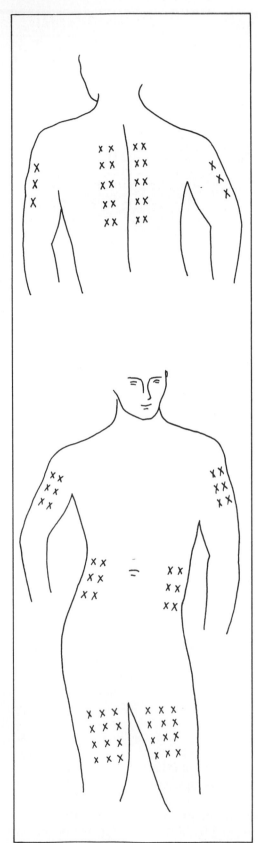

Figure 24-28 Sites on the body where subcutaneous injections can be given.

Insulins are categorized as fast, intermediate, or long acting. Intermediate and long-acting insulins are referred to as modified insulin because they contain additives that delay their absorption. Some diabetic patients use a combination of two types of insulin, each having a separate and unique time of onset and duration of action. When two types of insulin are prescribed, they are mixed in the same syringe. Combined insulins tend to bind and become equilibrated. This means that each one's unique characteristics are offset by the other. An analogy of this phenomenon would be like pouring red paint into white. In a short time neither color would be identifiable; the mixture would appear pink. If combined insulins are administered within 15 minutes of being mixed, they will still act as if they had been injected separately. Diabetics should try to duplicate the same time interval between mixing and administering their insulin each day so the pattern of glucose metabolism will not fluctuate appreciably from one day to the next.

When combining two types of insulin, the nurse can use the following sequence of actions:

1. Use an insulin syringe that is graduated in units.
2. Roll containers of insulin that have separated in solution between the palms of the hands. The container must not be shaken or the molecules of insulin protein may become damaged.
3. Cleanse the rubber stoppers on each vial with a swab premoistened with the antiseptic of the agency's choice.
4. Fill the empty syringe with the amount of air equal to the amount of medication that will be withdrawn from each vial of insulin. A portion of the total amount will be instilled into each of the containers of insulin to facilitate drug removal.
5. Inject the first portion of air into the vial of modified insulin. This is the type that has an extended time of action. Modified insulin will appear cloudy when rotated.
6. Do not permit the needle to touch the solution.
7. Inject the remainder of the air into the vial that does not contain any modifying agent; this type of insulin is referred to as Regular insulin. Regular insulin should always appear clear.
8. Fill the syringe with unmodified, or Regular, insulin with the specified number of units.
9. Request that another nurse check the type of insulin, dosage ordered, and dosage that fills the syringe before the needle is withdrawn from the vial.
10. Insert the syringe into the second vial of insulin. It is especially important that a vial of unmodified insulin not be tainted with the modified insulin. This principle is true when mixing any two drugs contained in separate multiple-dose vials.
11. Withdraw the specified number of units of modified insulin.

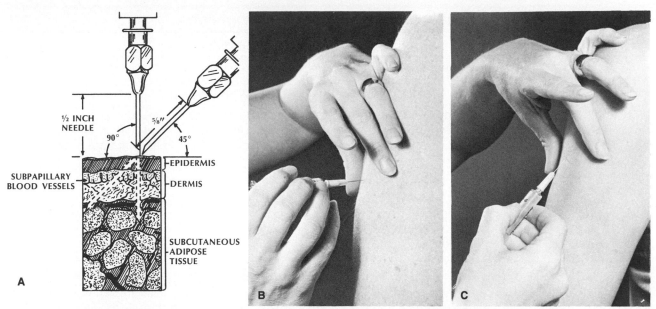

Figure 24-29 (*A*). The sketch illustrates that a ¹/₂-inch needle at a 90° angle and a ⁵/₈-inch needle at a 45° angle will be located in subcutaneous tissue. (*B*). The nurse is using a ¹/₂-inch needle. The needle is inserted at a 90° angle to inject a patient weighing 190 pounds. (*C*). It is inserted at about a 45° angle when injecting a patient weighing 120 pounds.

12. Request that the same nurse now check the second type of insulin, the dosage ordered, and the dosage within the syringe.
13. Remove the syringe from the container of insulin if the measurement is accurate, and administer the insulin.

Administering Heparin

Heparin is an anticoagulant that is frequently administered subcutaneously as well as intravenously. The unique characteristics of the drug require special techniques when using the subcutaneous route for its administration.

Heparin may be supplied in multiple-dose vials or pre-filled cartridges. The dosages are measured in tenths and hundredths of a milliliter. This is a very small volume and must be measured in a tuberculin syringe to ensure accuracy. The needle is changed following withdrawal of the drug from a multidose vial and replaced with another prior to administration.

Various techniques may be used to prevent bruising in the area of the injection. Ice may be applied to the site before administration to create vasoconstriction and reduce the possibility of bleeding at the site. The plunger is not aspirated once the needle is in place. Massaging the site is contraindicated since this can increase the tendency for local bleeding.

Injecting Medication Subcutaneously

Skill Procedure 24-4 describes how to administer a medication subcutaneously. It is assumed that the nurse observes the guidelines for preparing and administering a medication in addition to the suggested actions in the procedure.

Administering an Intradermal Injection

An *intradermal injection* involves the administration of a substance within the layers of the skin. Such an injection is placed just below the epidermis. Intradermal injections are commonly used for diagnostic purposes. Examples include tuberculin tests and allergy testing.

A common site for an intradermal injection is the inner aspect of the forearm, although other areas are also satisfactory, such as the back and upper chest. Small amounts of solution are administered, usually not more than 0.5 mL. A tuberculin syringe is used for measuring the dosage. A 25- to 27-gauge needle 1/2 inch in length is used when administering an intradermal injection.

The needle is inserted at a 10- to 15-degree angle for proper placement of medication. A small raised area, or *wheal,* such as the one shown in Figure 24-30, should appear at the injection site as the medication is instilled.

Skill Procedure 24-5 describes and illustrates how to administer an intradermal injection. It is assumed that the nurse observes the basic guidelines for preparing and administering a medication in addition to utilizing the suggested actions in the Skill Procedure.

Administering Intravenous Medication

Medications administered intravenously have an immediate effect. The intravenous route is the most dangerous route of administration. The medication is delivered directly into the bloodstream. It cannot be recalled nor can its actions be slowed. For these reasons usually only selec-

Skill Procedure 24-4. Administering a Subcutaneous Injection

Suggested Action	Reason for Action
Select an appropriate site for the injection. Refer to a site rotation guide if one is available.	The selection of a site should include consideration of how often a site has been used. Avoid using any site that appears to be bruised or swollen and tender.
Using friction, clean the skin thoroughly with a pledget moistened with an antiseptic. Allow the skin to dry.	Cleansing reduces surface contaminants. Drying prevents introducing antiseptic that may irritate the tissue. As the skin dries, the antiseptic continues to be active.
Add a bubble of air to the syringe, especially if it is critical that the entire dosage of the medication be injected.	The bubble of air ensures that all medication is released from the syringe and the needle.
Hold the skin taut over the injection site or grasp the area surrounding the injection site and hold it in a cushion manner. The choice depends on the size of the patient and the length of the needle.	Holding the tissue taut helps the nurse to be sure that the subcutaneous tissue is being entered in most well-nourished, hydrated persons. Grasping the tissue facilitates entering subcutaneous tissue when the patient is thin, dehydrated, or small.
Insert the needle to almost its full length at an angle of 45° to 90° depending on the body size and length of the needle.	Subcutaneous tissue is abundant in well-nourished persons. It is usually sparse in thin, dehydrated, or small persons.
When the needle is in place, release the grasp if the tissue has been bunched.	Injecting the solution into relaxed tissue allows the drug to enter with less discomfort.
Pull back gently on the plunger of the syringe to determine the location of the needle.	Placement is checked to assess if the needle has been inserted into a blood vessel.
Do not aspirate if heparin is being administered.	Aspiration increases the potential for causing a pocket of blood to form at the injection site. Heparin is not dangerous if absorbed into the bloodstream.
Inject the solution slowly.	Slow injection allows the solution to disperse into the surrounding tissue.
Withdraw the needle quickly while applying pressure against the injection site.	Rapid withdrawal of the needle while pressure is applied on the injection site reduces discomfort.
Massage the area where the injection was made unless contraindicated by the type of drug that has been administered.	Massaging the area of injection may help spread the medication in subcutaneous tissues and hastens absorption. Massage would be contraindicated when heparin has been injected since it will cause excessive bruising of the tissue.

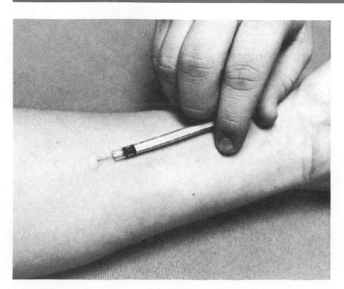

Figure 24-30 The bevel of this needle has been inserted between the layers of skin at about a 10° angle. A wheal forms as the solution is instilled. It appears to be similar in size and appearance to a mosquito bite.

Skill Procedure 24-5. Administering an Intradermal Injection

Suggested Action	Reason for Action
Select an area on the inner aspect of the forearm, about a hand's breadth above the patient's wrist.	The forearm is a convenient and easy location for introducing an agent intradermally.
Cleanse the skin with a swab moistened with an antiseptic using a circular motion outward from the site of entry.	Debris and organisms are removed from the center outward toward the periphery.
Cleanse the area with acetone if the skin is oily. Allow the area to dry.	Acetone is a defatting agent and is effective for removing oils from the skin. Allowing time for the antiseptic to dry also allows time for it to continue working.
Hold the patient's arm and stretch the skin taut with the thumb.	Taut skin provides an easier entrance into the intradermal area.
Place the syringe almost flat against the patient's skin, and insert the needle, bevel side up, at a 10° to 15° angle, as the nurse in Figure 24-31 is doing.	The intradermal area is only a short distance beneath the skin.

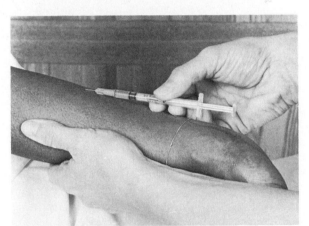

Figure 24-31 The nurse holds the needle almost parallel to the skin on the forearm when administering an intradermal injection.

Insert the needle about ⅛ inch and slowly inject the solution while watching for a small wheal to appear.	The bevel must be completely under the skin so that the solution does not leak out on the surface of the skin. If the needle is inserted too deeply, the wheal will not be seen.
Withdraw the needle quickly at the same angle at which it was inserted.	Withdrawing the needle in this manner minimizes tissue damage and discomfort for the patient.
Do not massage the area after removing the needle.	Massaging the area where an intradermal injection is given may interfere with test results.
Observe the patient's condition frequently within the first half hour after instilling an allergy test substance.	Severe allergic reactions may occur in the early period following the injection of substances to which the patient may be allergic.
Observe the area for signs of a local reaction at ordered intervals, usually in 24 hours and again in 48 hours.	The response to the injected substance must be assessed to determine future treatment. It may take 1 to 2 days for a definitive response to appear.

tively qualified nurses are permitted to administer intravenous medications. Even those who are responsible for intravenous medication administration must exercise extreme caution in preparing and instilling them.

Intravenous administration is the route chosen in an emergency when immediate action is required. However, there are many clinical situations in which drugs are administered intravenously. A number of antibiotics can be administered to a patient through the intravenous route. When access to the bloodstream already exists, the intravenous administration of medications prevents the discomfort experienced from repeated intramuscular injections. Intravenous medications can be administered continuously or intermittently.

Diluting Intravenous Medication in a Large Volume of Fluid

Medications can be added to a large volume of intravenous solution and administered slowly over a number of hours. The medication is usually added to the solution by the pharmacist. The container of solution must be labeled to show the name and dosage of the drug that has been added. Continuous infusions of intravenous medications are often regulated with an infusion pump or controller so that the prescribed amount of the medication is infused accurately.

Administering Intravenous Medications Intermittently

A medication can be administered as an intravenous bolus. A *bolus* is a single dose of medication injected directly into an intravenous line. Sometimes the term *push* is used to differentiate the technique used for rapid administration of the drug from a slower infusion. Medications may be administered intermittently through a port or chamber on an established intravenous line, through a piggy-back arrangement that is discussed in Chapter 25, or through a heparin lock.

Using an Established Intravenous Line. When medications are not added to the solution in the pharmacy, the nurse may be required to administer them while the infusion is being given. Most intravenous infusion tubing allows for a place where the drug can be added, either to a special chamber as illustrated in Figure 24-32, or at a self-sealing port in the intravenous tubing. When a drug is added to a chamber it is diluted in approximately 100 mL of the intravenous fluid. Therefore, it requires more time to infuse. When medications are instilled into a port, they may be administered all at once or slowly over a period of several minutes.

Using a Heparin Lock. Occasionally, a drug is ordered to be given intravenously at regular intervals, such

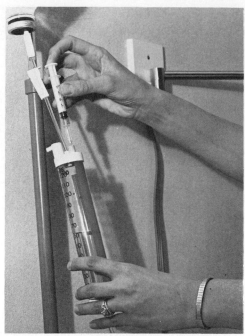

Figure 24-32 This equipment allows a drug to be injected with a needle and syringe into a chamber that is between the container of solution and the patient. The patient receives the medication more quickly than if the drug is mixed with the entire amount of solution in the bottle.

as four times a day. However, many patients do not require the additional fluid volume that would result from the continuous infusion of an intravenous solution.

Rather than having to puncture the patient repeatedly, a heparin lock is used. A *heparin lock* is a device, shown in Figure 24-33, that facilitates access to the bloodstream without requiring the continuous infusion of fluids. It is attached to a venipuncture device and contains a resealable rubber port through which heparin is instilled to keep clots from forming. Drugs are instilled through the same port at intermittent intervals. During the remaining time the port is secured to the patient's arm or hand.

When the patient has a heparin lock, the following steps may be used when instilling intermittent intravenous medications:

1. Cleanse the port using a pledget moistened with an antiseptic of the agency's choice.
2. Insert a needle and syringe containing 1 to 2 mL of sterile normal saline.
3. Aspirate the syringe to assess for the appearance of blood. A blood return indicates that the device remains located in the vein and the access line is free of any clot or occlusion.
4. Instill the sterile normal saline through the port. This will flush the venipuncture device of previously instilled heparin.

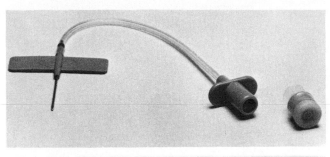

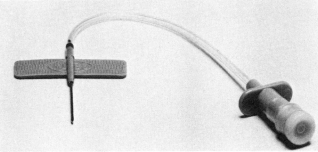

Figure 24-33 (*A*). The device in the lower right of the photo is a heparin lock. It is pictured with a winged-tip needle, or venipuncture device, also called a butterfly needle. (*B*). This photo shows the heparin lock inserted within the venipuncture device as it would appear when in use in the patient. All intravenous medications and solutions are instilled through the center of the rubber seal on the heparin lock.

5. Insert the needle that will be used to deliver the medication into the port and instill the drug over the prescribed period of time.
6. Remove the needle from the lock when the medication has been instilled.
7. Cleanse the port, insert a syringe containing 1 to 2 mL of sterile normal saline, and instill the saline solution. This will flush any remaining medication from the venipuncture device. It also prevents any drug incompatibility reactions from taking place when heparin is again instilled within the lock device.
8. Insert a syringe with 1 mL of heparin, or the amount specified by agency policy.
9. Instill the heparin solution within the lock and venipuncture device. The heparin will remain within the lumen of the needle or catheter and prevent clotting around the tip.
10. Repeat the sequence of instilling saline followed by heparin every 8 hours if medications are not instilled in the meantime.
11. Change the site of the venipuncture device and heparin lock at intervals determined by agency policy.

Some nurses use the acronym SASH to help remember the steps in giving a medication through a heparin lock. These letters represent:

S—Saline irrigation
A—Administer medication
S—Saline irrigation
H—Heparin instillation.

Using a Central Venous Catheter. Intravenous medications can be instilled into a central venous catheter as well as into a needle or short catheter in a peripheral vein. A *central venous catheter* is longer in comparison with a peripheral venous access device. The extra length is needed because it is inserted into a vein, usually the subclavian, until its distal tip is located in the vena cava.

A central catheter has several advantages over a peripheral catheter. It avoids the necessity for multiple or frequent venipunctures when drug and fluid therapy may involve an extended length of administration. Because the catheter deposits drugs into a large blood vessel with a high volume of blood, it allows irritating or highly concentrated drugs and solutions to be instilled without traumatizing the vein wall. Some have a dual use in that venous blood can be withdrawn from the catheter rather than puncturing a peripheral vein when blood tests are ordered. A central venous catheter reduces the potential for infiltration. It frees the patient's hands for movement and self-care.

Central venous catheters are made of polyvinyl chloride, polyurethane, or silicone rubber. Each substance in the list is progressively better than the former at preventing the adhesion of platelets and potential clot formation near the inserted catheter.

Central catheters may have single, double, or triple lumens, or channels. The advantage of multiple lumens is that incompatible substances or more than one solution or drug can be given simultaneously. Each infuses through a separate channel and exits the catheter at a different location. Thus, the drugs or solutions never interact with one another. When a lumen is used only intermittently, it can be capped with a heparin lock device. The unused lumen is kept patent by routine flushes with normal saline or heparinized saline.

Types of Central Venous Catheters. There are several types of central venous catheters. The type that is selected is usually determined by the anticipated duration and purpose of its use.

Short-Term Central Catheter. When a patient requires short-term therapy lasting only a few days or weeks, a polyurethane or polyvinyl chloride catheter may be inserted into a central vein. The procedure is performed in the patient's room under aseptic conditions. The skin is scrubbed, draped, and a local anesthetic is used. Placing the patient in a Trendelenburg position with a rolled towel in the middle of the back helps to fill and distend the vein so it is more easily identifiable to the physician. The physician uses a needle to pierce the skin and gain access to the vein. Once the needle is within the vein, the catheter is threaded over or through it. The catheter is advanced the appropriate length. Examples of this type of central venous catheter can be seen in Figures 8-24 and 24-34.

An air embolism must be prevented, because atmospheric air can enter the lumen of the tubing. Any air within the lumen could be pushed into the bloodstream as fluid instills. Though small bubbles of air may not be dangerous, an open line accompanied by rapid or deep ventilation potentiates the possibility of lethal consequences. Therefore, before completely withdrawing the guide needle and connecting the catheter to flushed IV tubing, the patient is instructed to exhale and hold his breath or bear down in a grunting fashion. This is repeated again any time the IV tubing or caps on the end of the catheter are changed. Clamping the catheter during these types of changes is an added safety measure to prevent an air embolism.

Once inserted, the short-term catheter is sutured to the skin. An x-ray is taken to make sure the catheter is in the desired location and has not accidentally pierced the pleura of the lung.

When the integrity of the skin is impaired, a patient is susceptible to increased risk for infection. Because a central venous catheter is not changed as frequently as a peripheral IV site, it is important to assess the area for redness, swelling, tenderness, and drainage. Transparent occlusive dressings are replacing bulky gauze dressings because they provide better observation of the site. The dressing should be dated as a reminder of when to change it.

If the catheter or any one of its ports is not needed, the lumen can be kept patent for future use. A flush solution is instilled into a capped end. It fills the lumen and prevents blood cells from collecting on the tip. The type, volume, and strength of flushing solutions varies among institutions. Follow the local policy.

Tunneled Catheters. When a central venous catheter is

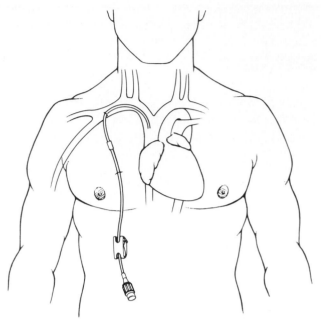

Figure 24-35 A Hickman catheter is one type of central venous catheter that is tunneled beneath the skin.

needed for longer use, risk for infection increases. Several catheters, such as the Hickman®, Broviac®, and Groshong® catheters, are inserted with a portion of the catheter tunneled from the vein through subcutaneous tissue exiting onto the skin lateral to the xiphoid process, as illustrated in Figure 24-35.

Tunneled catheters have a Dacron® cuff just above the exit site. Fibrin is deposited within the cuff. This not only helps to stabilize the catheter but acts as a barrier against organisms that may migrate from the skin to the catheter

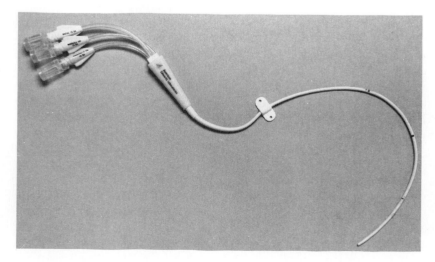

Figure 24-34 A triple-lumen central venous catheter provides three external ports to administer drugs or fluids through the internal catheter. The winged tab midway on the catheter is used to suture the catheter to the skin once it has been inserted.

track. Because of the greater complexity of insertion, tunneled catheters are inserted surgically under fluoroscopic examination. The catheter can be used immediately, but the skin will not heal completely for two to three weeks.

In addition to using the ports for administering drugs in solution, replacement fluids, and total parenteral nutrition, blood samples for laboratory tests can be drawn through the Hickman and Groshong catheters. The Broviac catheter's lumen is 1.0 mm, much smaller than either of the other two. Therefore, it should not be used to draw blood. One manufacturer has designed a fused double-lumen catheter combining the components of both the Hickman and the Broviac catheters. One port is 1.6 mm, the size of the Hickman catheter; the other is the size of the Broviac catheter. Blood can be drawn from the larger lumen rather than a peripheral site when tests are needed.

All of the tunneled catheters can be capped for intermittent use. The Hickman and Broviac catheter caps are flushed with heparinized saline. The Groshong catheter only requires flushing with sterile normal saline. This reduces the potential for altering the clotting mechanisms when the catheter is used with any frequency.

Implanted Catheter. The greatest protection against infection is provided by a central catheter that is totally implanted under the skin. This type of catheter, shown in Figure 24-36, has a self-sealing port that must be pierced with a special needle in order to instill drugs or fluids. To reduce skin discomfort, a local anesthetic is first applied topically. The port can sustain approximately 2000 punctures, making it possible for the catheter to remain in place for several years barring any complications. A dressing is applied only when the catheter is being used.

The silicone material of the catheter is associated with the lowest incidence of clot formation. It requires only monthly flushing with heparinized saline. The reduced incidence for infection, reduced thrombus formation, durability, and ease of care make this one of the best access devices for long-term drug and fluid therapy.

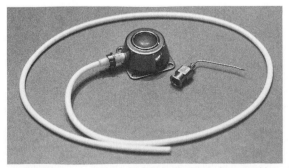

Figure 24-36 The central venous catheter is inserted into the vena cava and implanted completely beneath the skin. The needle at the right is used to pierce the skin and the soft center of the implanted port when drugs are administered.

Skill Procedure 24-6 describes how a central venous catheter is used to instill intravenous drugs.

Administering Antineoplastic Drugs. *Antineoplastic drugs* are those used to treat cancer. Nurses who care for patients with this disease in the hospital, outpatient clinics, and at home administer toxic drugs that will destroy cancerous cells so they do not continue to grow and multiply. Drug therapy, either used alone or in combination with surgery or radiation, is a valuable tool for curing cancer. Patients and nurses sometimes refer to the use of anticancer drugs as chemotherapy; some shorten the term to "chemo." Table 24-2 provides a list of several antineoplastic drugs and their classifications.

Antineoplastic drugs are toxic to both normal and abnormal cells. It has been found that these drugs can even cause adverse effects in the pharmacists who mix them and the nurses who administer them. These types of drugs can be absorbed by health-care professionals through inhalation of tiny fluid droplets of medication or dust particles on which the droplets fall. If deposited on the skin, they can be absorbed or introduced within the body on articles touched by the hands such as food, sticks of chewing gum, or cigarettes. When transferred to the caregiver, they can cause headaches, nausea, dizziness, and burning or itching of the skin. Long-term, unprotected exposure to small amounts of these drugs can lead to changes in fast-growing body cells including sperm, ova, or fetal tissue. It is important, therefore, that nurses understand safety measures for administering these drugs and how to avoid exposure and contact with hazardous material.

In most cases, drugs are reconstituted or diluted with sterile IV solutions in the pharmacy. To alert nurses who may be unfamiliar with either the generic or trade names of antineoplastic drugs, the pharmacist attaches a special label such as the one shown in Figure 24-39. The pharmacist wears protective clothing when preparing the drugs under a vertical flow containment hood or biologic safety cabinet, such as the one in Figure 24-40. Wearing a powered air purifying respirator is recommended to prevent inhalation of the drug in the absence of a safety cabinet or hood. Although gloves are worn, appropriate handwashing is always performed before and after mixing or handling these drugs. All supplies must be disposed of in leakproof, puncture-resistant receptacles. The receptacles are labeled clearly to warn others of the dangerous contents inside. Skill Procedure 24-7 provides suggested actions for the nurse who may be administering chemotherapy drugs intravenously. The nurse may instill these drugs into an existing peripheral intravenous line or through a central venous catheter. Antineoplastic drugs are administered by other routes as well. For example, some chemotherapeutic drugs are administered into the peritoneum, into the cerebrospinal fluid of the spine, into arteries, and between the pleura.

Skill Procedure 24-6. Instilling Intravenous Medication Through a Central Venous Catheter

Suggested Action	Reason for Action
Check the written medical order.	Reading the order as it was written ensures that it has been correctly transcribed on the MAR.
Read and compare the label on the drug with the MAR at least three times.	Rereading ensures that the correct drug and dosage have been supplied by the pharmacy.
Obtain the following supplies: alcohol and povidone iodine swabs, syringe with normal saline flush solution, tape, drug, filtered IV tubing, and infusion pump.	Organizing needed equipment promotes efficient time management.
Wash hands.	Handwashing reduces the transmission of microorganisms.
Prepare a 3- to 5-mL syringe with a 20-gauge, 1-inch needle with sterile normal saline.	The heparin present in the lumen must be flushed in case the drug interacts with heparin. Repeated punctures with a large or long needle can lead to leaks and the need to replace the capped end.
Insert the IV tubing within the solution containing the drug and flush the air from the tubing.	To avoid an air embolism, the air in the tubing is displaced with fluid.
Thread the flushed tubing through an infusion pump. Infusion pumps are discussed in Chapter 25.	An infusion pump provides an accurate, constant flow of fluid.
Identify the patient by reading the name on the wristband.	Checking the wristband ensures that the medication will be given to the correct patient.
Wash hands again.	Handwashing reduces the transfer of organisms to the ports of the catheter.
Have the patient turn his head away from the catheter.	Turning the head reduces the deposit of microbes that may be present in oral or respiratory areas.
Swab the port and a few inches of the catheter above the port with povidone iodine. Repeat the cleansing with an alcohol swab.	Antiseptics reduce the presence of microorganisms around the port.
If the drug solution will be instilled directly into the end of the proximal tip of the catheter, clamp the catheter.	Clamping reduces the risk of air entering the tubing and causing an air embolism.
If no clamp is available, place the patient in Trendelenburg position or have the patient exhale and hold his breath or bear down.	These alternatives raise the interthoracic pressure and reduce the potential for atmospheric air to enter the lumen of the catheter.
Insert the syringe with saline into the port shown in Figure 24-37 or catheter tip. Unclamp the tubing and instill the saline flush.	Saline displaces the heparin from the tubing and prevents any interaction between it and the drug.
Do not use force if there is any resistance. Notify the physician.	Force may rupture the catheter or dislodge a clot. Urokinase, a thrombolytic agent, may need to be instilled to restore patency.
Attach a needle to the IV tubing and insert it into the capped port if the catheter flushed easily.	A sealed port must be pierced with a needle when administering an intermittent drug solution.
If the infusion will instill through an uncapped port, clamp the catheter and attach the tubing without contaminating either ends. Unclamp the catheter.	The catheter should be clamped any time it is disconnected. Keeping the connections sterile reduces the potential for infection.
Tape the connections between the IV tubing and the catheter as the nurse is doing in Figure 24-38.	Securing the connection prevents accidental separation.
Regulate the rate of infusion according to the prescribed volume and time.	Rapid infusion can cause fluid overload or toxic drug manifestations.

(continued)

Skill Procedure 24-6. Continued

| **Suggested Action** | **Reason for Action** |

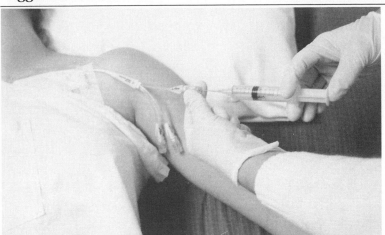

Figure 24-37 The nurse flushes the heparin from the sealed port on a triple-lumen central venous catheter.

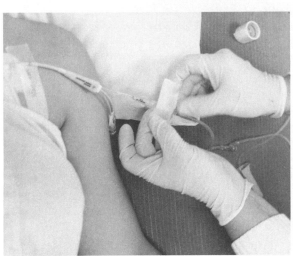

Figure 24-38 After inserting a needle, which is connected to tubing and a container of medication, the nurse tapes the needle within the port.

Suggested Action	Reason for Action
Observe the patient for any untoward effects.	A serious drug reaction is likely to occur shortly after the drug is infusing.
Wash hands.	Handwashing reduces the spread of microorganisms.
Document the administration of the drug.	Recording drug administration provides evidence that the prescribed treatment has been carried out.
When the infusion has been completed, flush the line again according to the type of central venous catheter and the agency's policy.	Flushing moves the drug within the tubing completely in the bloodstream. Catheters vary in the type and volume of solution used to maintain patency.
Discard all empty solution containers, tubing, and syringes in the appropriate waste containers.	Containment of used supplies reduces litter, the potential for accidental needle sticks, and transmission of organisms.
Record the volume of fluid that was instilled.	Parenteral as well as oral liquids are part of the patient's fluid intake.
Document the response of the patient to the infused drug solution.	The patient's record should identify his response to the prescribed treatment.

Table 24-2. Common Antineoplastic Drugs

Classification	Generic Name	Trade Name
Plant alkaloids	vincristine	Oncovin®
	vinblastine	Velban®
Antitumor	bleomycin	Blenoxane®
Antibiotics	doxorubicin	Adriamycin®
Antimetabolites	methotrexate	Mexate®
	fluorouracil	5-FU®
	6-mercaptopurine	Purinethol®
Nitrosoureas	cyclophosphamide	Cytoxan®
	streptozocin	Zanosar®
Miscellaneous	cisplatin	Platinol®
	1-asparaginase	Elspar®

Observing for Complications

The nurse should be constantly alert for signs of complications when a patient is receiving medications intravenously. Assessment of the intravenous site and complications related to the infusion of intravenous fluids is discussed in Chapter 25.

Administration of some medications into the tissues rather than the bloodstream can cause necrosis and sloughing of the tissue. Therefore, the nurse must carefully check the placement of the venipuncture device before and during medication administration.

Suggested Measures When Administering Parenteral Medications in Selected Situations

When the Patient Is an Infant or Child

Avoid the deltoid and dorsogluteal sites in infants and preschoolers because these muscles are not developed enough to absorb medications adequately.

Use a 5/8–1-inch needle in infants; in an older baby or child, a 1–1½-inch needle can be used.

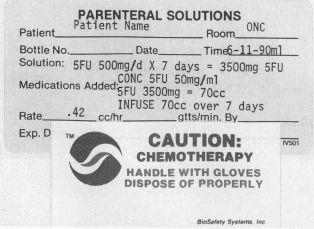

Figure 24-39 This drug label indicates that the medication is hazardous and must be handled cautiously. This particular drug is inserted within a miniature infusion pump and administered continuously over a period of a week.

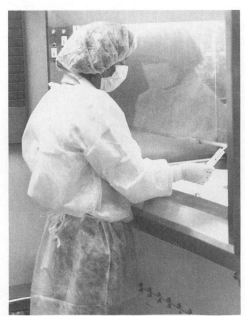

Figure 24-40 A pharmacist dons protective clothing before mixing chemotherapy drugs under a safety hood.

Skill Procedure 24-7. Administering Antineoplastic Drugs

Suggested Action	Reason for Action
Determine that the patient has been informed and given consent for the administration of chemotherapeutic drugs.	A signed consent verifies that the patient has been instructed on the risks and benefits of each drug he will receive.
Identify the patient by reading his wristband.	Proper identification prevents administering a drug to the wrong patient.
Make the patient comfortable in a reclining chair or bed.	Responding to the patient's comfort needs demonstrates care and concern.
Explain the procedure to the patient.	Cancer patients fear chemotherapy and are often very anxious and frightened.
Wash hands.	All patients, and especially cancer patients, are at risk for acquiring infections from microorganisms on the hands of caregivers.
Assess the patient thoroughly. Observe especially for signs of infection, condition of the area around the IV site, vital signs, current weight, and any effects following previous drug administration.	Cancer patients are prone to infections, damage to skin or veins from drugs, nausea and vomiting, anemia, and hair loss.
Review current, related laboratory test results such as blood cell counts, and liver and kidney function.	Drug therapy may need to be postponed if organ functions are seriously altered.
Ask the patient if he has any allergies.	Patients with a history of allergic reactions may react similarly to chemotherapy drugs.
Have emergency equipment and drugs available.	A delay in time can be life-threatening.
Administer prescribed drugs that will reduce the side effects of the drug therapy, such as something to control nausea.	It is easier to control symptoms by prevention than by medicating the patient after they occur.
Apply a scalp hypothermia cap, if ordered, 15 minutes before administering the drug, and leave it in place until one-half hour after the drug is given.	Reducing blood flow to the scalp during administration may decrease hair loss.
Read the written medical order and the drug label at least three times.	Rereading and comparing the information helps to prevent medication errors.
Calculate the dosage based on the patient's current weight and height.	Dosages are often prescribed according to weight or body surface area. Cancer patients are prone to weight loss.
Wash hands again before preparing to administer the drug.	Handwashing removes transient microbes that may have been deposited on the hands of the nurse during assessment.
Don a long-sleeved, cuffed, low-permeability gown with a closed front.	Wearing a gown prevents drug contamination on the skin or uniform.
Don one or two pairs of surgical latex, nonpowdered gloves. Cover the cuffs of the gown with the cuffs of the gloves.	Latex gloves are less permeable than polyvinyl chloride. Doubled gloves are even less permeable than a single pair. Powder from gloves could be inhaled and transfer drug residue into the nurse's lungs.
Wear a mask and goggles if there is a potential for drug splash.	A mask and goggles act as a physical barrier from contact between a splashed drug and the mucous membrane of the eyes, nose, or mouth.
Cover the work area surface with a disposable absorbent pad.	An absorbent pad will control and contain a small spill of hazardous drug.
Keep 70% alcohol and detergent available.	Alcohol inactivates the drug when poured over a small spill. After absorbing the mixture with a pad, the area of the spill is cleaned three times with detergent and finally clean water.

(continued)

Skill Procedure 24-7. Continued

Suggested Action	Reason for Action
If the medication must be withdrawn from a vial, vent the rubber stopper with a filter needle.	A vent reduces air pressure and prevents the release of droplets of the drug through the pierced stopper when the needle is withdrawn.
Express any air in the needle or syringe onto a gauze square or alcohol swab.	Releasing air bubbles into the air could result in droplet inhalation or transfer to the floor and nearby objects.
Dispose of the gauze or alcohol swab in the biohazard receptacle.	Confining hazardous wastes limits the potential for accidental exposure to others.
Check that the IV is patent and within the vein by either lowering the infusing solution or pinching the tubing and observing for a flashback of blood.	Some drugs can be toxic to the tissue if they are infused outside the vein.
Use a stopcock to instill the drug through an existing IV line.	A stopcock eliminates the need for a needle to access a port. Needles can cause an accidental puncture of the line, allowing the drug to leak from the tubing.
Attach the syringe to the stopcock and begin to instill the drug slowly.	Rapid administration may produce the onset of side effects or rupture the blood vessel into which it is being administered.
Aspirate blood frequently to verify that the drug is continuing to infuse in the vein.	Evidence of a blood return indicates that the medication is being delivered in the venous circulation.
Obtain a fluid pump or controller for a drug mixed with IV solution.	An infusion device ensures administration of a drug within the prescribed time at a precise rate.
Use tubing that contains a filter.	A filter removes contaminants and precipitants.
Make sure that Luer Lok connections, shown in Figure 24-41, have been used to join sections of IV tubing.	Luer Loks screw to lock connections in place and are less likely to pull apart and leak infusing medication.

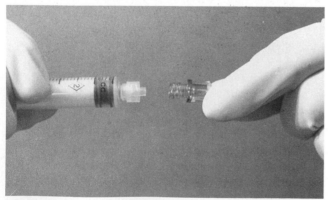

Figure 24-41 This illustrates the principle of a Luer Lock. The male and female ends are first connected. Then the outer cap is screwed over the adjacent threads. Once fastened, the connection cannot be pulled apart.

Secure the drug solution into the existing IV port.	Taping the junction of the admixture or using a Luer Lok connection helps to prevent separation of the infusing fluid and leaking of the drug.
Assess the patient to determine his response to the administration of the drug.	Drugs administered intravenously can cause rapid changes in a patient's condition.
Stop the infusion if there is any question that the drug is no longer being instilled within the vein or the patient experiences a severe reaction during its infusion.	The safety of the patient is more of a priority than continuing the drug administration.

(continued)

Skill Procedure 24-7. Continued

Suggested Action	Reason for Action
Flush the line with IV fluid between the administration of two different drugs.	Flushing prevents an interaction between two potentially incompatible drugs.
When the drug is infused, discard all disposable equipment into the biohazard container.	Preventing contact with the drug protects the safety of others.
Flush and instill heparin through any venous access device that will not be used immediately.	Flushing clears the catheter of the drug. The heparin prevents clots from forming at the tip of the catheter.
Remove gloves without touching skin or clothing. Place the gloves and removed gown in the biohazard receptacle.	Contact with skin or clothing can transfer residual drug to the nurse.
Wash hands immediately.	Gloves become more permeable the longer they are worn. Handwashing can remove any drug that penetrated the gloves.
Document pertinent assessments, the administration of the drug, and the response of the patient.	The patient's chart is a record of his care and treatment.
Wear gloves and gown and perform thorough handwashing when handling body fluids such as blood, vomitus, urine, and stool from patients who received antineoplastic drugs within the past 48 hours.	Toxic chemicals are excreted in various body fluids. Contact can transfer these chemicals to the nurse.

Use a 23- to 25-gauge needle for thin injectable drugs. A 21- or 22-gauge needle is more appropriate for thick medications like antibiotics.

Tell a child that an injection will hurt but that he can cry if he wishes. Telling a child a lie destroys confidence in the nurse.

Proceed in giving an injection without delay. Allowing a child to stall for time will not decrease his discomfort and may heighten his anxiety.

When injecting into a child's thigh, keep the knees extended because the child may flex them when the needle pierces the skin.

Ask a child to count or recite the ABCs while giving an injection. Concentrating on the task distracts the child from anticipating the pain of an injection.

Perform painful procedures such as injections in a place other than the child's room. This helps the child feel safe in his crib or bed and not associate it with being hurt.

Be sure to hug the child after an injection so the child will not assume that nurses only cause pain or that the injection was punishment for being bad.

Place a Band-Aid over the injection site and praise the child for enduring the discomfort.

Give a child an empty syringe without a needle after an injection. The child can act out his feelings with the syringe and a surrogate of himself, such as a doll or stuffed animal.

When the Patient Is Elderly

Bunch the tissue of a thin person to elevate the muscle and avoid striking bone with the needle.

Suggest that the visually impaired or blind person obtain a loading gauge to measure a dosage of an injectable medication. Diabetics often use these gauges, such as the one shown in Figure 24-42, to administer insulin.

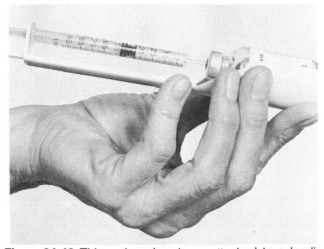

Figure 24-42 This syringe has been attached to a loading gauge. When a visually impaired person withdraws medication, the barrel on the syringe cannot be pulled back farther than the preset distance, which corresponds with the correct amount of medication. (Courtesy of George Wright Industries, Lincoln, NE.)

NURSING CARE PLAN

24-1. High Risk for Altered Protection

Assessment	**Subjective Data**
	States, "I haven't been eating much. It's difficult to swallow; as a result I'm losing weight and feeling very weak."
	Objective Data
	26-year-old man admitted with enlarged cervical and axillary lymph nodes. Medical diagnosis is Hodgkin's lymphoma. Has had a Hickman central venous catheter inserted and will begin chemotherapy. Side effect of one drug is thrombocytopenia.
Diagnosis	High Risk for Altered Protection related to debilitated state and tendency to bleed secondary to side effect of chemotherapy.
Plan	**Goal**
	Blood loss will be minimal as evidenced by normal red blood cell count and negative hemoccult tests on urine and stool throughout hospitalization.

Orders: 2/10

1. Obtain all blood samples from central line.
2. Monitor platelet count and hold chemotherapy if count is <100,000 until physician is consulted.
3. Assess skin for bruising, catheter site for bleeding, and test urine and stool for occult blood q day.
4. Avoid aspirin or products containing salicylates.
5. Use a soft bristle toothbrush or swabs for mouth care.
6. Substitute oral forms of medications rather than IM whenever possible.
7. If injections must be given, apply pressure for at least 3 minutes or longer to control bleeding. —————————————————————————— N. HURDER, RN

Implementation (Documentation)

2/10   1300   Blood for CBC and chemistry profile obtained from central venous catheter. Catheter flushed following blood draw. Results of blood tests unavailable at this time. ——————————————————————— A. VALERIONI, LPN

Evaluation (Documentation)

1330   Skin is intact except at catheter insertion site. No evidence of bleeding from site. No bruises noted on skin. Urine and stool test negative for occult blood. Has not taken any over-the-counter aspirin products in the last two weeks. Soft bristle toothbrush used for mouth care. No evidence of active bleeding from gums following mouth care. Not currently scheduled for injectable medications except those that will infuse through the central line. ————— A. VALERIONI, LPN

Teaching Suggestions for the Administration of Parental Medications

Devices such as the one in Figure 24-43 are available that help a patient learn how to self-inject medication.

Explain that when using the dorsogluteal site for an injection, discomfort can be reduced by positioning the patient on the abdomen with the feet pointing inward.

Inform patients that subcutaneous injections should be at least 1 inch apart if the same site is used more than once in the same week.

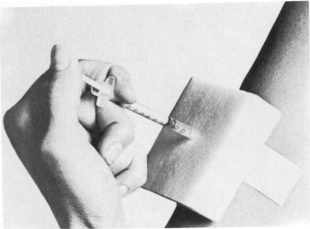

Figure 24-43 This skin and tissue simulator helps the patient who must learn self-administration of an injection. The device is made of material that resembles the "feel" of real skin and underlying tissues. (Courtesy of Meditec, Inc, Englewood, CO.)

Applicable Nursing Diagnoses

Nurses who administer parenteral medications may identify these nursing diagnoses.

- High Risk for Infection
- High Risk for Injury
- High Risk for Altered Protection
- Knowledge Deficit
- Anxiety
- Fear

Nursing Care Plan 24-1 demonstrates the nursing process as it applies to a patient with the nursing diagnosis of High Risk for Altered Protection. This category has been accepted for testing and as of 1990 does not yet appear in a published NANDA taxonomy. The current definition for this diagnosis is, "The state in which an individual experiences a decrease in the ability to guard the self from internal or external threats." This diagnosis applies to patients with immunite deficiencies, impaired healing, or altered clotting.

Inform a diabetic that storing insulin in an empty thermos protects it by providing insulation in extreme or fluctuating temperatures.

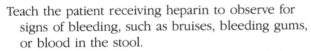

Teach the patient receiving heparin to observe for signs of bleeding, such as bruises, bleeding gums, or blood in the stool.

Recommend that diabetic patients look for solid, white particles that may adhere to their vial of insulin. This indicates a decrease in its potency. The insulin can be returned and replaced free of charge from the pharmacy where it was dispensed. Manufacturers of the insulin will reimburse the pharmacist.

Advise patients who use predrawn insulin syringes that they should be stored so the needles are upright. This prevents the suspended particles from settling at the hub and potentially obstructing the flow of insulin through the needle.

Explain to diabetics that nonrefrigerated insulin should not be used after 2 months.

If insulin is refrigerated, the diabetic should be told to wait at least 20 to 30 minutes before preparing the injection. It is less painful and becomes absorbed more quickly upon warming.

Tell a diabetic preparing for a trip to take all the syringes he will need or an additional prescription that may be required to purchase syringes in some states.

Recommend that the diabetic who is traveling by air keep his insulin with him rather than packed in a suitcase that may be lost or delayed upon arrival.

Bibliography

Barlett KA, Burgoon DJ: Venous access devices: Appropriate for home use? Home Healthcare Nurse 8(2):38–41, 1990

Bulcavage LM, Morales LS: Safety issues in the handling of chemotherapeutic agents. Emphasis Nursing 2(2):75–83, 1987

Cawley MM: Recent advances in chemotherapy: Administration and nursing implications. Nurs Clin North Am 25(2):377–392, 1990

Cohen MR: Always prepare an I.V. admixture before labeling the container. Nursing 18(3):10, 1988

DeMonaco HJ: I.V. drug delivery: New technologies for consideration. Journal of Intravenous Nursing 11(5):316–320, 1988

Garabedian–Ruffalo SM, Ruffalo RL: Compatabilities and stabilities of IV preparations. Critical Care Nurse 9(2):81–85, 1989

Hahn K: Brush up on your injection technique. Nursing 20(9):54–48, 1990

Hennesy J, O'Donnell L, Bear J: Home instructions for postchemotherapy care. Oncology Nursing Forum 15(2):201, 1988

Herget MJ, Williams AS: New aids for low-vision diabetics. Am J Nurs 89(10):1319–1322, 1989

Keen MF: Get on the right track with Z-track injections. Nursing 20(8):59, 1990

Masoorli ST, Miller KH: Putting some comfort in chemotherapy. RN Magazine 51(8):73–74, 76, 78, 1988

McConnell EA: Giving intradermal injections. Nursing 20(3):70, 1990

McGovern K: 10 golden rules for administering drugs safely. Nursing 18(8):34–42, 1988

Robertson C: The new challenges of insulin therapy. RN Magazine 52(5):34–38, 1989

Sohl L, Nze R: Working with triple lumen catheters. Nursing 18(7):50–54, 1988

Steil CF, Deakins DA: Today's insulins: What you and your patient need to know. Nursing 20(8):34–39, 1990

Testerman EJ: I.V. drug administration guidelines: A simplified format. Journal of Intravenous Nursing 11(3):188–190, 1988

Todd B: Intravenous drug hazards: Interactions, adsorption, and inadequate mixing. Geriat Nurs 9(1):20, 22, 1988

Viall CD: Your complete guide to central venous catheters. Nursing 20(2):34–41, 1990

Wachs T: Urokinase administration in pediatric patients with occluded central venous catheters. Journal of Intravenous Nursing 13(2):100–102, 1990

Walters P: Chemo: A nurse's guide to action, administration, and side effects. RN Magazine 53(2):52–60, 1990.

Wickham RS: Advances in venous access devices and nursing management strategies. Nurs Clin North Am 25(2):345–364, 1990

25

Maintaining and Restoring Fluid and Chemical Balance

Chapter Outline

Behavioral Objectives
Glossary
Introduction
Understanding Fluid Balance
Assessing Fluid Balance
Performing Physical Assessments
Common Fluid Imbalances
Correcting Fluid Imbalances
Administering Intravenous Fluids
Administering a Blood Transfusion
Understanding Electrolyte Balance
Understanding Acid–Base Balance
Suggested Measures to Promote Fluid and Chemical
    Balance in Selected Situations
Applicable Nursing Diagnoses
Teaching Suggestions to Promote Fluid and Chemical
    Balance
Bibliography

Skill Procedures

Increasing Oral Fluid Intake
Limiting Oral Fluid Intake
Starting an Intravenous Infusion
Changing Solution Containers
Changing Infusion Tubing
Adding a Piggyback Solution
Administering a Blood Transfusion

Behavioral Objectives

When the content of this chapter has been mastered, the learner will be able to:

Define terms appearing in the glossary.

List the chief functions and sources of body water and ways in which the body normally loses water.

Discuss assessment techniques for detecting fluid imbalances.

Describe how to determine fluid intake and fluid output and the usual practices involved in recording measured amounts.

Describe measures to promote fluid balance, especially ways to increase and limit oral fluid intake.

List at least six reasons for administering fluids intravenously.

Discuss five assessments that may be useful for determining a patient's response to fluid therapy.

Identify the equipment that the nurse should prepare when a patient will receive intravenous fluids.

Discuss guidelines for selecting a vein for infusing fluids.

Describe the actions involved in starting an intravenous infusion.

Calculate the infusion rates using common drop factors.

Describe the actions involved in providing the following aspects of patient care: caring for the venipuncture site, changing solution containers, changing infusion tubing, attaching a piggyback solution, and discontinuing an infusion.

Describe possible complications of intravenous infusion and the appropriate nursing response for each.

Discuss modifications in infusion equipment when administering a blood transfusion.

Describe the proper sequence of nursing actions when administering a blood transfusion.

List and describe various types of transfusion reactions; identify the nurse's actions when responding to a possible reaction.

List possible substitutes for blood and components of blood that may be infused separately.

List the primary functions of each of the following electrolytes and list several food sources that supply the body with each of them: sodium, potassium, chloride, phosphate, calcium, magnesium and bicarbonate.

List at least seven signs and symptoms that may suggest electrolyte imbalance.

Discuss measures that help prevent or correct electrolyte imbalance.

List suggested measures for promoting fluid and

chemical balance in selected situations, as described in this chapter.

Summarize suggestions for the instruction of patients offered in this chapter.

Glossary

Acid A substance containing hydrogen ions that can be liberated or released.

Acidosis A condition in which the *p*H of blood falls below 7.35.

Active transport A process requiring energy and sometimes a carrier substance to move dissolved substances through a semipermeable membrane from an area of low concentration to one that is more highly concentrated.

Air embolism A rare, but potentially deadly, complication that occurs when a large volume of air enters a vein.

Alkali A substance that can accept or bind with hydrogen ions. Synonym for *base*.

Alkalosis A condition in which the *p*H of blood measures more than 7.45.

Anion An electrolyte with a negative electrical charge.

Base A substance that can accept or bind with hydrogen ions. Synonym for *alkali*.

Blood transfusion The intravenous infusion of whole blood.

Body fluid The mixture of body water and dissolved chemicals.

Carrier substance A constituent in body fluid that helps transport a dissolved chemical compound through a semipermeable membrane.

Cation An electrolyte with a positive electrical charge.

Circulatory overload A complication caused by administering too much intravenous fluid for the patient's system to circulate and eliminate.

Colloid solution A mixture of water and molecules of suspended protein.

Crossmatching A laboratory test that determines whether blood specimens of the donor and recipient are compatible.

Crystalloid solution A mixture of water and uniformly dissolved crystals, such as salt and sugar.

Dehydration A condition that results from a low volume of body water.

Dialysis A procedure that removes water and toxic chemicals from the body when the kidneys are not functioning adequately.

Diffusion A process in which dissolved substances move passively through a semipermeable membrane from an area of higher concentration to an area of lower concentration.

Donor The person giving blood.

Drop factor The number of drops that equal one millili-

ter, determined by the manufacturer of a particular brand of IV equipment.

Edema An excess of water in the interstitial space within body tissues.

Electrolytes Chemical compounds that dissolve and separate into individual molecules, each carrying either a positive or negative electrical charge.

Extracellular fluid All body water except that contained within cells.

Fluid balance The state in which water remains in normal amounts and percentages within various locations within the body.

Fluid imbalance A condition in which the body's water is not in the proper volume or location within the body.

Fluid intake All sources of fluid consumed or instilled into the body.

Fluid output All fluid eliminated from the body, including drainage from tubes, catheters, and wounds.

Hemoconcentration A condition in which the fluid content of blood is decreased.

Hemodilution A condition in which the fluid content of blood is increased.

Hypertonic solution A mixture of water and crystals in higher concentration than found in intravascular fluid.

Hypervolemia An excess of water in the circulating blood.

Hypotonic solution A mixture of water and crystals in lower concentration than found in intravascular fluid.

Hypovolemia Below average amount of water in the circulating blood.

Infiltration The escape of an infusing solution into tissues.

Insensible water loss Water that is lost in a form that is not seen or felt.

Interstitial fluid Water surrounding the outside of cells; a subcategory of extracellular fluid.

Intracellular fluid Water located inside cells.

Intravascular fluid Water within blood known as plasma or serum; a subcategory of extracellular fluid.

Intravenous fluids Those solutions instilled within a patient's vein.

Isotonic solution A mixture of water and crystals in equal concentration to that found in intravascular fluid.

Milliequivalent The unit for measuring electrolytes. Abbreviated mEq.

Nonelectrolytes Chemical compounds that remain bound together when dissolved in a solution and cannot conduct electricity.

Osmosis The movement of water through a semipermeable membrane from an area of lower concentration of dissolved substances to higher concentration.

*p*H The hydrogen ion concentration in a fluid.

Piggyback solution A second solution joined and elevated above the primary infusion. Synonym for *secondary infusion*.

Plasma The fluid component of blood. Synonym for *serum*.

Primary infusion The first hung of two intravenous fluid containers.

Recipient The person receiving blood.

Secondary infusion A second solution joined and elevated above the primary infusion. Synonym for *piggyback solution.*

Semipermeable membrane A layer of tissue that selectively allows certain substances to move in and out.

Serum The fluid component of blood. Synonym for *plasma.*

Skin turgor The fullness of the skin in relation to underlying tissue.

Third spacing A fluid imbalance in which water becomes trapped in interstitial areas due to a loss of plasma proteins.

Typing The laboratory test that identifies the proteins on red blood cells.

Venipuncture The act of entering a vein.

Introduction

Water is one of the chief necessities of life. All the water in the body contains chemical substances. For this reason it is common to use the term *body fluid* when referring to the mixture of water and dissolved chemicals. The body normally has a remarkable ability to excrete or conserve fluid and chemicals to maintain all of the body's components in appropriate amounts. This chapter summarizes the processes involved in fluid and chemical balance, discusses common imbalances, and describes methods for restoring balance.

Understanding Fluid Balance

Fluid balance is the state in which water remains in normal amounts and percentages within various locations within the body. Healthy persons maintain fluid balance automatically. They take in a wide variety of fluids and foods in various quantities and dispose of wastes and excesses as a result of complicated chemical mechanisms. One of the most basic measures for maintaining fluid and chemical balance is consuming an adequate fluid intake and eating a nourishing diet.

Body Fluid Proportions

The human body is made up of approximately 45% to 75% water. The amount of water varies according to an individual's age, sex, and body fat composition. Table 25-1 shows a comparison of percentages based on the variables of age and sex.

Water content within the body decreases in proportion to increases in body fat. There may be wide differences in body composition among both sexes and age groups. Women tend biologically to have greater amounts of body fat. It could be said that, in general, women have less body water than men. This is reflected in the figures listed in Table 25-1.

The Main Functions of Body Water

Because the body is almost primarily a fluid structure, water plays a major role in dissolving and transporting substances. The main functions of water include:

- Transporting dissolved nutrients, oxygen, vitamins, hormones, enzymes, and blood cells within the body. These are called nonelectrolytes. They are more descriptively defined later in this chapter.
- Transporting substances called electrolytes, such as sodium, chloride, or bicarbonate. These are also discussed later in more detail. An imbalance of water often results in an imbalance of one or more electrolytes.
- Removing and transporting the wastes from metabolism, such as carbon dioxide, so that they may be eliminated from the body.
- Helping to regulate body temperature. Evaporation aids cooling; water promotes warmth by conducting heat produced by cell metabolism.
- Aiding digestion and elimination.
- Contributing the major component to the body's secretions.

From the length of this list, it is obvious that water is vital to life. Life can be sustained without food for many days;

Table 25-1. Average Water Percentages in Parts of the Body According to Age and Gender

Location of Body Water	In Infants	In Adult Males	In Adult Females	In the Elderly
In the blood (intravascular)	4%	4%	5%	5%
In tissues surrounding body cells (interstitial)	25%	11%	10%	15%
Within body cells (intracellular)	48%	45%	35%	25%
Total body water	77%	60%	50%	45%

Table 25-2. Average Adult Daily Sources of Water

Source of Water	Amount of Water (mL)
Ingested water	1200–1500
Ingested food	700–1000
Metabolic oxidation	200–400

however, an individual will die much sooner when deprived of water.

The Chief Sources of Water

The total amount of water that most adults consume is between 2000 and 3000 mL per day. A range between 1500 and 3500 mL would not be considered abnormal. Most of that amount is obtained by consuming liquid beverages and drinking water. The second largest source is from eating food, all of which contains liquid. Certain foods, such as fresh fruit, contain large quantities of water; some foods, such as cereal and dried fruits, contain little. Water is also an internal by-product from the metabolism of food. Table 25-2 lists the average amounts of water that a normal adult acquires from each of these three sources per day.

Methods of Eliminating Water

The amount of fluid that is consumed every day is similar to the amount that is eliminated. Most of the water is lost through the kidneys. Some moisture is lost in stool and in obvious perspiration from areas where the skin contains abundant sweat glands. A certain amount of water is lost in a form that cannot usually be seen or felt. This is called *insensible water loss*. It occurs from the lungs during expiration and through the skin. The amount of water loss varies among people under various circumstances. Variations include changes in environmental temperature and humidity, body temperature, and activity. A comparison of water losses under various conditions is listed in Table 25-3.

Fluid Distribution

Though body fluid is literally located throughout all the structures of the body, it is common to speak about fluid as being located in specific compartments. It should be kept in mind that these areas are not separate and distinct from one another. Water moves constantly in and about all these locations. Changes in the distribution of fluid in one area will automatically set in motion fluctuations in other areas.

Generally, body fluid is located inside and outside cells. The fluid within cells is called *intracellular fluid*. It represents the highest volume of water in the body. All the remaining fluid is called *extracellular fluid*. This category is further subdivided into *intravascular fluid*, fluid within the blood-vessel (vascular) system also known as *plasma* or *serum*, and fluid between cells, called *interstitial fluid*. Figure 25-1 illustrates the locations and percentages of fluids in the body. The proportions of fluid in each area tend to remain at a fixed amount when an individual is healthy.

When the ratio of water to dissolved substances in any body fluid location changes, water will relocate. This process restores proper proportions to maintain homeostasis. The movement and relocation of water is governed by the principle of *osmosis*. That is, water moves from an area where there is a lower concentration of dissolved substances to one where there is greater concentration. The process of osmosis is illustrated in Figure 25-2.

To redistribute itself, water moves through a *semipermeable membrane*. Cell walls and capillary walls are examples of semipermeable membranes in the body. A semipermeable membrane can be compared to openings like screened windows in a building. The windows keep birds out but let light and air in. Semipermeable membranes in the body allow substances, like water, to move in or out.

Fluid Regulation

Numerous, complex mechanisms automatically adjust the volume of fluid within the body to maintain a constant state of balance. They include the stimulation of thirst and the activation of hormones that influence kidney filtration and

Table 25-3. Average Daily Water Losses

Exit Route	Normal Loss (mL)	With Elevated Body Temperature (mL)	Following Active Exercise (mL)
Urine	1200–1700	1200	500
Feces	100–250	200	200
Perspiration	100–150	1400	5000
Insensible losses			
Skin	350–400	350	350
Lungs	350–400	250	650
Total	2100–2900	3400	6700

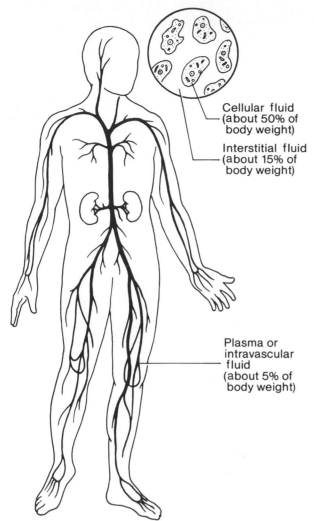

Cellular fluid
(about 50% of
body weight)

Interstitial fluid
(about 15% of
body weight)

Plasma or
intravascular
fluid
(about 5% of
body weight)

Figure 25-1 Normal distribution of fluids in the body. Amounts based on percentage of body weight.

reabsorption. A text that discusses physiology is an excellent resource for reviewing these biological functions.

However, certain circumstances can threaten the body's ability to regulate fluid amounts and distribution. When fluid losses are severely reduced or excessive, or intake is similarly affected, the body may not be able to adjust automatically to sustain the health of an individual. The nurse must be able to recognize when additional support measures may be necessary to restore fluid balance.

Assessing Fluid Balance

The nurse should become familiar with the patient's state of health, the history of his present illness, and the medical plan for therapy. Because balance is maintained when the intake of food and beverages is in proper proportion to output, anything that upsets these functions should act as a warning to the nurse. These are a few typical questions to consider:

- Has the patient's normal food and fluid intake changed? If so, for how long has it differed from usual?
- Have there been restrictions on what the patient could eat or drink?
- Has there been any unusual loss of body fluids? If so, how long has the loss been occurring?

Any situation in which the patient has lost fluids warns of imbalance. Examples include extreme perspiration, vomiting or diarrhea, wound or body drainage, and blood loss. With fever, patients lose more fluid than when their body temperature is normal, as Table 25-3 indicates. Inadequate fluid intake can result from nausea, a poorly balanced diet, an inappropriate self-restriction of fluid to control urinary

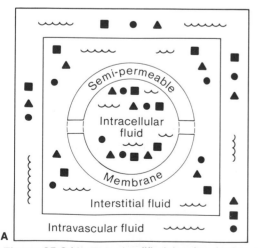

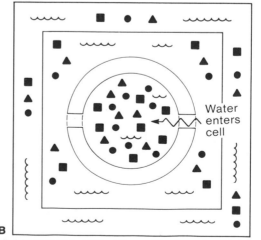

Figure 25-2 (*A*). This simplified drawing depicts a state of fluid balance in all locations of body water. Note that there is an equal ratio of dissolved substances, depicted as geometric figures, in each of the fluid areas, indicated by a wave. (*B*). When a fluid area becomes concentrated with dissolved substances, as shown within the cell of this drawing, water will move by osmosis from a less concentrated area to dilute and restore the proper proportions of water to dissolved substances. The size of the cell, in this case, will increase as more water enters through its semipermeable membrane.

incontinence, or the unavailability of food or fluids. Fluid retention is associated with kidney failure, heart failure, and some liver diseases. Imbalances also can result from the indiscriminate use of diuretic drugs, salt, and tap water enemas. In fact, it is the rare illness or indiscretion that does not threaten fluid or chemical balance.

One of the simplest methods for objectively assessing fluid balance is to compare the amount of a patient's fluid intake with fluid output. Other data that help the nurse determine the patient's fluid status will eventually be discussed.

Documenting Fluid Intake and Output

When an individual is healthy, the amount of fluid that is taken in should approximate the same amount that is lost. To determine that a balanced ratio exists, the nurse may collect data by measuring and recording various amounts of fluids.

Determining Fluid Intake.

Fluid intake is determined by measuring all sources of fluid consumed or instilled into the body. The nurse must be constantly aware of the sources of water even though they may not be in the form of food or beverages. Fluid intake includes all the liquids a patient drinks and some foods, nourishment instilled during a tube feeding or parenteral hyperalimentation, intravenous fluid administration, and irrigation solutions instilled into tubes or catheters. When there is any question about the type of fluid that should be measured, the nurse should consult with a supervising nurse or refer to agency policy.

Each agency develops a list to be used as a guide for measuring the liquids that a patient consumes from his dietary tray. An example of the amounts of liquid that common food and beverage containers hold is listed in Table 25-4. Keep in mind that these amounts may vary, depending on the sizes of containers that each agency uses. When the amount of a liquid is not known, a calibrated pitcher should be used to measure the volume. The nurse should avoid estimating an approximate amount. Too often the estimate is inaccurate.

Recording Fluid Intake.

Agency policies should be followed concerning the frequency and times of day when the amount of liquid intake is recorded. A good practice to follow is to record the amount of a patient's intake either immediately after it has been consumed or at frequent intervals during the day. Trying to recall the type and amount of fluids after several hours is likely to result in errors.

The nurse uses a form supplied by the agency for recording intake. Most hospitals have a bedside form for recording amounts throughout the day. The bedside form usually has large spaces where the time, type of fluid, and

Table 25-4. Volume Equivalents for Common Containers

Container	Volume (mL)
Teaspoon	5
Tablespoon	15
Juice glass	120
Drinking glass	240
Coffee cup	210
Milk carton	240
Water pitcher	900
Paper cup	180
Soup bowl	200
Cereal bowl	120
Ice cream cup	120
Gelatin dish	90

amount can be recorded. The agency may also require that totals from the bedside form be recorded each shift in a specific area on the patient's permanent record. At the end of each 8-hour and 24-hour period, the nurse, or someone working under the nurse's direction, totals the amount, records it, and prepares a new form for the next day. Figure 25-3 is an example of a hospital form used for a summary recording. A form used for bedside recording and other information about the oral intake of fluids can be reviewed in Chapter 8.

Determining Fluid Output.

Patients whose intake is measured and recorded ordinarily need to have fluid output measured and recorded. *Fluid output* is the sum of all the liquid eliminated from the body. Fluid output is determined by measuring urine, emesis, drainage from tubes, and the fluid drained following an irrigation. In some cases, to ensure accurate assessment of fluid loss, the nurse may be required to measure liquid stool or weigh wet linens, diapers, or dressings saturated with blood or other secretions. The weight of wet items is compared to the weight of a similar dry item. An estimate of output is based on the knowledge that one pint (475 mL) of water weighs about 1 pound (0.47 kg).

	INTAKE			OUTPUT		
	Oral.	IV	Other	Urine	NG	BM/Other
7-3						
3-11						
11-7						
TOTAL						

Figure 25-3 This hospital's form shows an example of the area where the totals from the bedside record of fluid intake and output are recorded on the patient's permanent record.

Urine is the chief source of fluid output. For accurate measurement of urine, the nurse should do the following:

- For the patient who uses the bathroom for voiding, a container, such as the one in Figure 25-4, is placed inside the toilet bowl underneath the toilet seat. The container is calibrated in milliliters to make measurement of the urine convenient.
- For the patient confined to bed, a bedpan or urinal may be used. Pour the voided urine into an appropriate measuring device provided by the agency. Place the calibrated container on a flat surface for an accurate reading.
- If the patient has a catheter, the drainage container is calibrated for easy measurement. It should be measured at least at the end of every shift. If urine output must be assessed hourly, Figure 25-5 shows a urine collection device that allows smaller volumes to be kept separate from the total amount until they have been measured.
- The contents of a leg bag can be emptied and measured using a pitcher with markings that indicate graduated amounts.
- Be sure to instruct patients who are ambulatory when their urinary output is to be measured. They will then be less likely to urinate directly into the toilet. Some patients can be taught how to measure their own urinary output. This is a good idea when the patient can be depended upon for accuracy. It helps the patient develop independence and involves him with his care.
- Teach the patient or a member of his family how to measure urinary output in home situations. Any cali-

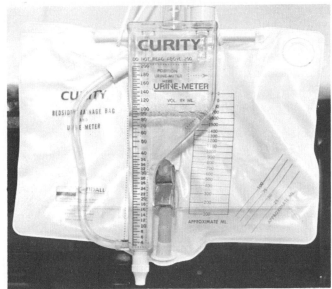

Figure 25-5 This gravity drainage container collects small amounts of urine in a separate collector. At periodic intervals, the nurse can measure and record the amount. The urine can then be added to the total being collected within the larger drainage receptacle.

brated container may be used for measuring. It is aesthetically preferable to use one that can be discarded when it is no longer necessary to measure output.

Recording Fluid Output. The nurse should follow the same practices and agency policies for recording fluid output as described for recording fluid intake. Figure 25-6 illustrates an example of one form commonly used at the

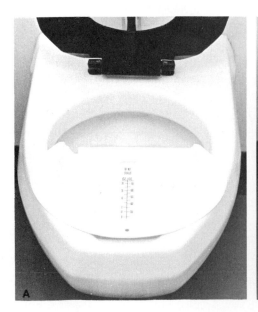

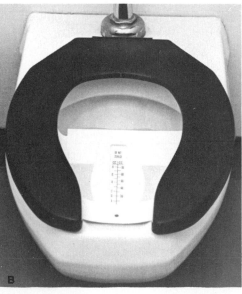

Figure 25-4 (*A*). This urine collection device, placed inside the toilet, helps maintain an accurate measurement of fluid output when the patient is able to use the toilet. (*B*). The patient can urinate into the toilet normally. The urine can remain there without the danger of accidental flushing until the amount is measured and recorded.

SHIFT	FLUID OUTPUT		OTHER	STOOLS
	URINE	EMESIS	SUCTION ☐	
7-3	175 ml 350 ml 225 ml			
8 HR.	750 ml			
3-11	250 ml 200 ml			
8 HR.	450 ml			
11-7	 200 ml			
8 HR.	200 ml			
24 HR.	1400 ml			

NAME Conrad V. Jones
ROOM 342
DATE 5-16

Figure 25-6 This is the output section of a bedside intake and output form. Note that there are three 8-hour totals as well as the 24-hour total on the form. Patients whose urinary output is measured and recorded will almost always need their fluid intake measured and recorded also. The form for recording intake is similar. It can be seen in Chapter 8.

patient's bedside for the periodic recording of measured amounts of fluid output.

Analyzing Other Measurable Data

Information taken for other purposes may help in analyzing if a patient has a fluid imbalance. The nurse may wish to evaluate the cluster of measurable data listed in Table 25-5.

Performing Physical Assessments

No single sign or symptom necessarily indicates fluid imbalance. Each deviation from normal must be analyzed for its significance and possible cause. The data in Table 25-5 lists a cluster of related data that generally accompany fluid imbalances. The following is a review of data gathered during a physical assessment of various systems of the body that may be associated with a fluid imbalance.

The Integumentary System. The nurse may observe various signs and symptoms typical of fluid imbalances when examining the skin and mucous membranes.

- The skin may appear warm, flushed, and dry when the patient is experiencing fluid deficit. It may appear cool, pale, and moist in fluid excess.
- The lips chap and a whitish coating may be present on the lips and tongue when the patient experiences a low volume of fluid. The mucous membranes may feel dry and sticky. With adequate or excess fluid, tissues will appear moist.
- The eyes appear sunken as subcutaneous tissues around them lose fluids; they may appear small with fluid excess as the surrounding tissues swell with water.
- The turgor of the skin may change with alterations in fluid volume. *Skin turgor* is the fullness of the skin in relation to the underlying tissue. With low levels of body fluid, skin can be lifted almost separately from the tissue underneath. With excessive levels of body fluid, it will be difficult to grasp the skin between the

Table 25-5. Measurable Data That May Indicate Fluid Imbalance

Type of Data	Fluid Deficit	Fluid Excess
Body weight	Recent weight loss	Recent weight gain
Blood pressure	Hypotensive	Hypertensive
Body temperature	Elevated	Normal
Pulse	Rapid, weak, thready	Full, bounding
Respirations	Rapid, shallow	Moist, labored
Specific gravity of urine	Elevated	Low
Red blood cell count	Elevated	Low
Hematocrit	Elevated	Low
Hemoglobin	Elevated	Low

forefinger and thumb. A normally hydrated person's skin should return to its original position immediately after being grasped.

- An individual with fluid excess may exhibit edema. *Edema* is an excess of fluid in the interstitial space within body tissues. It causes swelling and makes the skin appear tight. Edema is often seen around the eyes and in the parts of the body that tend to collect fluid due to gravity, such as the fingers, ankles, and feet. The patient may indicate that rings or shoes no longer fit. The impression of the weave in stockings may remain on the skin even after they have been removed for some time. The person who lies in bed may exhibit edema in the lower part of the back and buttocks. One way to assess the presence of edema is to press a finger gently into the skin. If the impression remains after pressure has been released, the condition is called pitting edema. It is illustrated in Figure 25-7.

The Gastrointestinal and Urinary Systems. These two systems are commonly affected by the patient's intake of food and fluids. Some common signs and symptoms typical of fluid imbalances include the following:

- Thirst is a common symptom when fluid intake has been low.
- The patient with a fluid deficit may expel drier stool or experience constipation. An individual with kidney failure who retains fluid, may have frequent, moist bowel movements.
- The urine is light in color and almost odorless when fluid levels are high. It is dark and has a strong odor when fluid levels are low. The nurse may wish to measure the specific gravity of urine, as discussed in Chapter 21.

The Circulatory and Respiratory Systems. These systems are also affected as a unit when the patient is experiencing fluid imbalances. This occurs because the

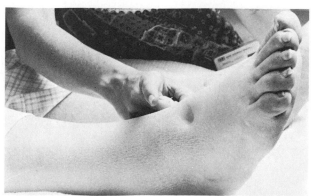

Figure 25-7 The nurse applied pressure on this patient's foot for a few seconds. The imprint in the edematous tissue demonstrates pitting edema.

heart circulates blood, which has a major fluid component, through the lungs. The following are typical of fluid imbalances:

- The lung sounds may seem wet when fluid levels are high. The patient may find it easier to breathe when sitting up rather than lying down when there is an excess of body fluid.
- The patient may experience fatigue and chest pain if the volume of blood is inadequate to supply oxygen to the heart muscle.
- The neck veins may distend from the skin when the patient is in a sitting position. This usually indicates fluid excess. When the patient has a low fluid volume, it may be difficult to distend any peripheral veins when obtaining a specimen of blood or inserting a needle for an intravenous infusion.

The Nervous System. An individual's level of consciousness often becomes affected when there are dangerous changes in the person's fluid status. The following are typical:

- Normal personality characteristics may change. The active, outgoing person may become withdrawn and quiet, or vice versa as the brain struggles to adjust to the changes in body fluid distribution.
- The person with low fluid volume is likely to seem weak, sleepy, and disoriented as the fluid imbalance worsens.
- A patient with fluid excess may appear tense and worried. Insomnia may be present.
- Eventually convulsions, coma, and death may occur with either type of fluid imbalance.

Common Fluid Imbalances

Fluid imbalance is a general term describing any of several conditions in which the body's water is not in the proper volume or location within the body. One of the locations in which fluid levels is likely to become imbalanced is the blood, or the area of intravascular fluid. When describing an imbalance in this area, certain prefixes and the suffix *emia,* referring to blood, are used in combination. When fluid is excessive in this location, the term *hypervolemia* is used to describe it. This term means that there is a high volume, or amount, of water present in the blood. *Hypovolemia* is a term that indicates a below average amount of water in blood. Other terms used to describe imbalances in the chemicals within intravascular fluid follow a similar pattern and are listed later in the chapter.

When an individual eventually experiences fluid deficits in all the areas where fluid is distributed, he is in a state of *dehydration.* The body no longer has the ability to restore fluid balance by redistributing fluid from one area to another. There simply is an insufficient supply to meet the need. An example of an individual suffering from dehydration can be seen in Figure 25–8.

Fluid imbalance can also occur when fluid becomes trapped in interstitial areas. This is called *third spacing*. It often occurs when there is a loss of proteins from the plasma of blood. This can occur suddenly when a person is burned, experiences a crushing injury, or has a severe allergic reaction. It can occur slowly with some types of kidney and liver diseases. The total volume of body fluid essentially remains the same with third spacing. However, the percentages of fluid within various compartments are changed. The percentage of water located within the interstitial space is greater than it should be, and the percentage of water in the intravascular area is lower than its normal amount. The body cannot relocate the water until the level of plasma proteins is restored to normal.

Correcting Fluid Imbalances

Certain principles help in planning actions when correcting fluid imbalances becomes a necessary part of a patient's care.

- Fluid deficits need to be corrected by replacing fluid and controlling their loss.
- Fluid excesses can be reduced by limiting fluid intake and increasing fluid loss.
- The degree and type of fluid imbalance and the body's ability to cope with them determine the type and intensity of therapy needed.

The nurse and the doctor usually work together when planning measures to correct fluid imbalances. Whenever possible, it is desirable to have the patient participate in correcting the fluid imbalance to whatever extent he can.

Several approaches are commonly used to help correct fluid imbalances. To reduce fluid deficits, oral liquid intake may be increased by providing additional servings of food and beverages during the day. Tube feedings may be used

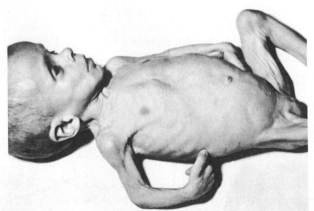

Figure 25-8 This child illustrates severe dehydration. Note the sunken eyes and poor skin turgor.

both for the benefit of fluid replacement and nourishment. Intravenous infusions are often used to increase fluid volume when there is an urgent need to do so. Infusions and transfusions are discussed later in this chapter.

To promote fluid loss, diuretic drugs may be prescribed by the physician. Some individuals with kidney failure may need temporary or permanent dialysis treatments. *Dialysis* is a procedure that removes water and toxic chemicals from the body when the kidneys are not functioning adequately.

The nurse's contribution to promoting the restoration of fluid balance includes developing and implementing a plan for increasing or limiting the intake of oral fluids.

Increasing Oral Fluid Intake

The nurse may independently order and implement measures that replace fluid loss by increasing the patient's oral fluid intake. This action has been referred to in the past as forcing fluids. Because that term conveys a negative image of the nurse-patient relationship, more nurses use the term encouraging fluids.

The specified amount the patient should take is indicated in a nursing order. An amount equal to or somewhat above the average daily requirement, for example, 3000 mL, may be an acceptable oral fluid intake goal per day. It may be helpful to specify the goal for each shift. Plan to have the patient consume more of the total amount during the day rather than during the evening and night. The techniques in Skill Procedure 25-1 may be used when increasing the daily intake of oral fluids.

Restricting Oral Fluid Intake

Though diuretic drugs may achieve dramatic results in promoting fluid loss, restricting oral fluid intake can also have a positive effect. The patient will still need to consume some liquid. Many patients can temporarily reduce their oral fluid intake to between 1000 to 1500 mL in 24 hours. In some cases, the patient's oral intake is restricted to the same volume as the urine that is excreted. Occasionally, the physician will determine the amount of fluid restriction. When the nurse must limit the intake of oral liquids, the actions in Skill Procedure 25-2 may be useful in the nursing care plan.

Administering Intravenous Fluids

Intravenous fluids are those solutions instilled within a patient's vein. They may include solutions of water and chemicals, blood, or blood products.

Policies and practices vary concerning who may administer and regulate intravenous fluids. The discussion that follows is provided to help those nurses who will be responsible for this type of clinical skill. Nevertheless, the information is recommended reading for nurses who are also assigned to care for patients receiving intravenous

Skill Procedure 25-1. Increasing Oral Fluid Intake

Suggested Action	Reason for Action
Explain the reasons for increasing consumption of oral fluids to the patient.	Obtaining and encouraging the patient's participation will ensure better achievement of the goal.
Develop a list of beverages that the patient generally enjoys drinking.	Increasing fluid intake when not feeling well is not always a pleasant or easy task.
Plan a schedule for the amount that will be consumed over a 24-hour period.	The patient should understand that the fluids can be replaced gradually.
Divide the total allotment of fluids so that the patient will drink greater amounts during the early hours of the day and less in the evening.	Larger amounts of fluid are easier to take after a night of sleep when there has been little or no fluid intake. Taking fluids in the evening tends to disturb sleep because the patient may need to void.
Set an hourly goal with the patient and provide some means of measuring the progress toward the goal. Indicate on a graph or picture when the patient moves closer to reaching the goal.	It helps to see evidence of progress toward reaching a goal. The nurse can use creativity in designing a graph or picture that illustrates the current efforts toward the goal.
Keep fluids handy at the bedside at all times and in containers the patient can handle.	Lack of accessibility can be one reason for not reaching a goal.
Offer a variety of fluids to avoid monotony and lack of interest. Change the serving glass or container frequently.	Drinking the same thing, even though it may be something the person likes, can become unpleasant after awhile.
Provide small amounts of a favorite liquid frequently. Serve the refreshment in small containers.	The patient is likely to feel defeated if the nurse brings a large volume to drink at any one time.
Serve fluids at the proper temperature.	It is unappetizing to sip drinks normally served cold when they are warm, and vice versa.
Include Jell-O, popsicles, ice cream, and sherbert as alternatives to liquid beverages.	These items are considered fluids and can be substituted for beverages consumed from a glass.
Keep an accurate record of fluid intake and output.	Records will help in evaluating the effectiveness of the plan.

fluids. All nurses may not necessarily perform venipuncture techniques, but may still be responsible for monitoring the infusion, for observing the patient, and for discontinuing the fluid therapy.

Intravenous fluid replacement is ordered by the physician. The prescribed solution is considered a medication. The specific type, volume, and rate of administration are part of the medical order. The nurse must exercise extreme caution that the correct solution is infused. This is a priority of concern since any substance that is instilled directly into the circulatory system produces a rapid effect because of its almost instant distribution throughout the body.

Purposes for Administering Intravenous Fluids

A patient may receive fluids intravenously for several reasons, including the following:

- To restore fluid balance quickly when a patient experiences a significant fluid loss

- To prevent fluid imbalance for a patient who is currently or potentially likely to experience a loss of body fluid
- To maintain fluid balance when the patient temporarily is unable to eat and drink
- To replace specific electrolytes or other chemicals such as water-soluble vitamins
- To provide some measure of nutrition
- To administer medications, such as anesthetics or antibiotics
- To establish access to the vascular system in case emergency medications may need to be administered quickly
- To replace blood cells or specific components of blood

Types of Intravenous Solutions

Intravenous fluids fall into two basic categories. They are either a crystalloid or a colloid solution. A *crystalloid solution* is a mixture of water and uniformly dissolved crystals, such as salt and sugar. A *colloid solution* is a

Skill Procedure 25-2. Limiting Oral Fluid Intake

Suggested Action	Reason for Action
Explain the purpose for restricting the intake of oral liquids.	Understanding promotes cooperation.
Indicate the total amount the patient may consume in one day, using measurements the patient will understand.	Patients are often unfamiliar with terms such as milliliters or liters. Using terms like one quart or four drinking glasses to explain the equivalent of 1000 mL may help the patient understand the extent of his limitation.
Schedule the distribution of the fluid intake throughout the 24-hour period.	It is unwise to let the patient consume the total amount early in the day and then totally restrict his intake later.
Ration the fluid so that the patient will have the opportunity to drink fluids other than at mealtimes.	Food contains liquid, and the patient's thirst may be relieved temporarily just from the water in food.
Keep fluids out of sight as much as possible.	Seeing something that is forbidden is frustrating. The patient may be tempted to drink it.
Use small containers to serve liquids.	Serving small amounts of fluid in large containers reminds him of what he cannot have.
Avoid serving foods and fluids that tend to increase thirst.	Sweet drinks and foods and dry or salty foods increase thirst.
Serve liquids at their proper temperature.	When the patient can only drink a small amount, liquids should be served so that the patient will experience the maximum pleasure with their consumption.
Offer ice chips, but calculate it as part of the total amount of fluid that the patient is allowed.	Ice appears to be greater than its actual volume. Melted ice is about one half the volume of the frozen state. It melts slowly and the patient may extend the time during which the liquid is consumed.
Use water in a plastic squeeze bottle with a spray top or an atomizer to moisten the patient's mouth.	This technique helps decrease thirst while using little fluid.
Help the patient maintain good oral hygiene.	Oral hygiene helps lubricate the lips and mucous membranes of the mouth. This relieves thirst and prevents drying and chapping of the lips.
Permit the patient to rinse his mouth with water as long as he is not tempted to swallow the water.	Keeping the mouth moist will reduced thirst.
Maintain an accurate record of the patient's fluid intake and output.	An accurate record helps in evaluating the effectiveness of the plan.
Evaluate the urinary output.	To excrete adequate amounts of toxic wastes, the patient should eliminate at least 500 mL of urine per 24 hours. Fluid restriction may need to be adjusted if the urine output is lower than this amount.

mixture of water and molecules of suspended protein. The protein does not actually dissolve. Whole blood, packed cells, plasma, and plasma proteins such as albumin are examples of colloid solutions. The substances in a colloid solution remain in the intravascular space because the protein molecules are too large to move through a semipermeable membrane.

Crystalloid solutions are further subdivided into isotonic, hypotonic, and hypertonic solutions. Each item refers to the amount of dissolved crystals present in the solution. An *isotonic solution* contains an equal amount of

dissolved crystals, as normally found in plasma. The distribution of water and chemicals will remain relatively unchanged when an isotonic solution is infused.

A *hypotonic solution* contains fewer dissolved crystals than normally found in plasma. It represents a dilute solution in comparison to the fluid within and around cells. Therefore, when infused intravenously, the water in the solution will enter through the semipermeable membrane of blood cells. The blood cells will become larger as they fill with water. This can temporarily increase blood pressure as it expands the circulating volume. Water may also pass through capillary walls and become distributed within other body cells and the interstitial spaces. This acts to equalize the ratio of water to dissolved substances throughout the body. It is, therefore, an effective mechanism for rehydrating individuals experiencing fluid deficits.

A *hypertonic solution* has a higher amount of dissolved crystals than present in plasma. It will draw water into the intravascular compartment from the more dilute areas of water within the cells and interstitial spaces. This can help to relieve edema as cells and tissues shrink and dehydrate from fluid loss. It can be expected that urine output will increase as a regulatory mechanism compensating for the added fluid volume present in the blood.

Table 25-6 provides a list of intravenous solutions that are either isotonic, hypotonic, or hypertonic. These commercially available solutions are commonly used in clinical situations in which fluid balance must be maintained or restored. The pharmaceutical companies that prepare intravenous solutions have excellent literature explaining the nature of and common indications for the solutions they prepare.

Assessing the Patient Requiring Fluid Therapy

The nurse should gather a database that can be useful for evaluating the effect and results of fluid therapy. Focus assessments should be made throughout the period of fluid replacement and continue until the patient's fluid balance is no longer an actual or potential clinical problem.

The following are observations that can help with comparative assessments:

- The patient's vital signs, including temperature, pulse, respiration, and blood pressure, should be taken prior to and at periodic intervals during fluid infusion. The variations in these physiological signs may reflect early, subtle responses of the patient to changes in fluid volume.
- The body weight should be recorded. It may be compared with the patient's admission weight or weights that have been recorded on previous days. The conditions for recording weight should be as similar as possible—same time of day, same scale, and same type of clothing.

Table 25-6. Classification of Intravenous Solutions

Solution	Components	Special Comments
Isotonic Solutions		
0.9% saline, also called normal saline	0.9 g of sodium chloride/100 mL of water	Contains amounts of sodium and chloride in physiologically equal amounts to that found in plasma
5% dextrose and water, also called D_5W	5 g of dextrose (glucose/ sugar)/100 mL of water	Isotonic when infused but the glucose is metabolized quickly, leaving a solution of dilute water
Ringer's Solution or Lactated Ringer's	Water and a mixture of sodium, chloride, calcium, potassium, bicarbonate, and in some cases, lactate	Replaces electrolytes in amounts similarly found in plasma. The lactate, when present, helps maintain acid–base balance
Hypotonic Solutions		
0.45% sodium chloride, or also called half-strength saline	0.45 g of sodium chloride/100 mL of water	A smaller ratio of sodium and chloride than found in plasma causing it to be less concentrated in comparison
5% dextrose in 0.45% saline	5 g of dextrose and 0.45 sodium chloride/100 mL of water	The sugar provides a quick source of energy, leaving a hypotonic salt solution
Hypertonic Solutions		
10% dextrose in water, also called $D_{10}W$	10 g of dextrose/100 mL of water	Twice the concentration of glucose than present in plasma
3% saline	3 g of sodium chloride/100 mL of water	The high concentration of salt in the plasma will dehydrate cells and tissue

- A record of intake and output should be collected and continued throughout the period of fluid therapy. If no prior record is available, the nurse may assess the color, odor, and specific gravity of urine.
- The nurse may selectively note physical assessments, such as the condition of skin and mucous membranes, filling of veins, and level of consciousness.
- Laboratory test results may reflect hemoconcentration or hemodilution. *Hemoconcentration* is a condition in which the fluid content of the blood is decreased; *hemodilution* is a condition in which the fluid content of the blood is increased. Cell counts and levels of serum electrolytes may appear abnormal, but this may only be a paper deficit or excess rather than an actual clinical state. In other words, when a specimen of blood is analyzed, the levels and numbers of substances within the blood sample may appear low or high in relation to the proportion of fluid that is present. Correcting the fluid imbalance often restores the reported levels of other substances found in the blood to normal ranges.

Preparing for Intravenous Fluid Replacement

Nursing units generally stock commonly used intravenous solutions and equipment within clean utility rooms or medication areas. Blood and blood products are usually stored, undergo extensive safety checks, and then are released by the laboratory or blood bank.

Preparing the solution and infusion equipment must be done while following the principles of medical and surgical asepsis. The nurse should practice good handwashing technique and be prepared to use skills that prevent the contamination of any openings or connection areas. Contamination could introduce organisms into the patient's circulatory system.

Preparing the Solution. Solutions for intravenous infusions are dispensed in bottles or in collapsible plastic bags. The variety of solutions on the market is almost without limit. Manufacturers of fluids may use different names for identical, interchangeable solutions. If a nurse has questions about the particular solution that is ordered and the name of a stocked solution, the supervising nurse, physician, or the hospital pharmacist generally is glad to interpret.

Solutions come in various volumes. They are usually in amounts of 1000, 500, 250, 100, and 50 mL. The volume that the physician orders depends on the length of time over which the fluid therapy will be required.

It is common that if a patient requires continuous intravenous therapy, an average of three 1000-mL containers of solution may be needed per day. The physician should specify the amount and sequence in which the solutions should be infused if they are different. Smaller volumes of intravenous solutions, such as 250 mL of normal saline, are used prior to and after administering blood. The amount of saline solution used may vary according to the agency's policy. Whatever the type or amount of solution, the nurse should always know which is currently being infused and which solution is to follow.

Solutions containing a medication that instills in an hour or less may be diluted in 50- or 100-mL solutions. The hospital pharmacist generally prepares the medication with the solution. Certain substances may be incompatible with various solutions. Having pharmacy personnel prepare additives decreases the likelihood of administering undesirable combinations. Any substance added to solutions should be clearly labeled on the bottle or bag. In addition, most pharmacies are equipped with a laminar airflow hood. Mixing medications and solutions under this air-filtering device reduces the danger of contamination.

Some solutions that contain medications are prepared in advance and refrigerated to slow their decomposition. If this is the case, the nurse will want to remove the solution from the refrigerator and let it warm to room temperature prior to the scheduled infusion. This can prevent the patient from feeling chilled or experiencing a change in body temperature.

Attaching Intravenous Tubing. Intravenous tubing, shown in Figure 25-9, is used to transport the fluid from the solution container to the needle or catheter within the patient's vein. Tubing comes in a variety of lengths with possibilities for additional extensions or connections. A glass container of solution requires vented tubing. Because a plastic bag collapses upon itself while the solution infuses, unvented tubing can be used.

The nurse uses a spike at the top of the tubing to pierce the container of solution, as in Figure 25-10. Just below the

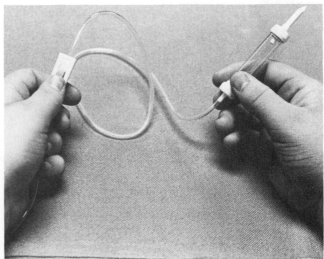

Figure 25-9 IV tubing showing spike, drip chamber, and regulator clamp.

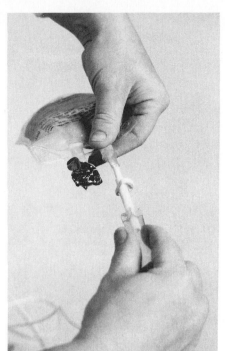

Figure 25-10 The nurse inserts the spike into the tube that extends from the bag of intravenous fluid.

spike lies the drip chamber. The drip chamber is partially filled by compressing and releasing the empty reservoir as shown in Figure 25-11. The rate of infusion can be controlled with a roller clamp that is attached to the tubing.

The nurse selects from various types of tubing when preparing to administer fluids. The type of tubing must be chosen according to the individual needs of the patient and the solution he will receive. Some types of solutions, such as blood and blood products, require unique types of tubings. Filters are sometimes incorporated within intra-

venous tubing. An IV filter tubing, shown in Figure 25-12, is used to trap undissolved particles, air bubbles, and bacteria. Agency policy indicates whether and when a filter should be used.

Using Gravity or an Infusion Device. Most intravenous solutions infuse by gravity. The bag or bottle is supported on a pole attached at the head of the hospital bed or suspended on a portable standard. Normally, the pressure in the patient's vein is higher than atmospheric pressure. Therefore, in order for the solution to infuse, it must be elevated at least 18 to 24 inches (45 to 60 cm) above the venipuncture site. The height of the solution affects the rate of flow. The higher the solution, the faster it will infuse. If the infusing fluid is lowered, the flow will become slower.

Some health agencies use an infusion pump, shown in Figure 25-13, or a volumetric controller when administering intravenous fluids. A pump uses pressure to infuse solutions. It adjusts the force needed to push fluid into the vein according to the resistance it meets. Pumps are generally more expensive to use because they require special cassettes and tubing. A volumetric controller, shown in Figure 25-14, usually uses standard IV tubing. Fluid infuses by gravity, but the controller mechanically compresses the tubing at a certain frequency to infuse the solution at a precise preset rate. Both a pump and controller sound audible and visual alarms if the infusion is not progressing at the rate intended. Interruptions in the rate of infusion can be due to an occlusion at the venipuncture site or kinked tubing. Some also indicate if air is detected within the tubing. Alarms also sound when an infusion is nearing completion. Newer controller models allow the nurse to program the rate and volume of more than one container of solution. In some cases, when one container of fluid

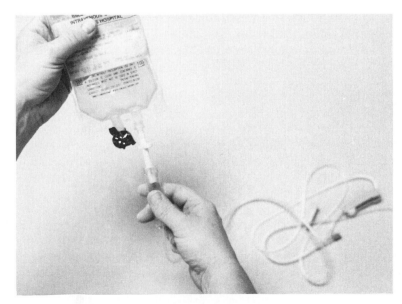

Figure 25-11 The nurse squeezes the area beneath the spike until the drip chamber is partially filled with fluid.

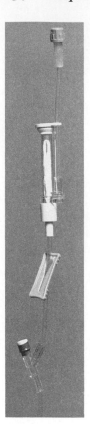

Figure 25-12 An inline filter removes air bubbles as well as undissolved drugs, bacteria, and endotoxins that are 0.22 microns or larger in size.

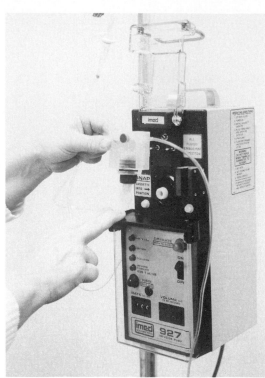

Figure 25-13 This nurse is inserting a cassette, a part of the specialized tubing needed when administering intravenous solution with an infusion pump.

finishes infusing, the controller automatically resumes the infusion of the other solution.

Selecting a Venipuncture Device. *Venipuncture* is a term that refers to the act of entering a vein. Since the circulatory system is a continuous loop, there is no means of access other than puncturing. Hollow needles are inserted through the skin and into a vein when fluids are administered intravenously.

Because venipuncture is an invasive procedure and the skin is no longer an intact barrier against pathogens, principles of asepsis are very important. Most agencies use disposable needles dispensed in sterile packages. This eliminates possible sources of contamination from reusable equipment.

When possible, the needle size should be smaller than the vein to reduce tissue damage and discomfort when it is introduced. The lower the size of gauge, the larger is the lumen of the needle. For most intravenous infusions for adults, a 20-, 21-, or 22-gauge needle is used. A size 18- or 19-gauge needle should be selected when colloid solutions are infused because a smaller needle may become plugged with the suspended proteins.

The venipuncture needle ideally should be short with a sharp bevel to pierce the skin and vein and reduce tissue damage. A bevel is the tapered tip of the needle. Figure 25-15 illustrates the bevel and lumen of a needle. Most needles used for entering a vein are 18 to 22 gauge and 1 to 1½ inches (2.5–4 cm) long. Butterfly needles, also called winged-tip or scalp vein needles, are short, thin-walled needles with plastic tabs. Many prefer to use this type of venipuncture device because of the ease of handling and stabilizing them. The needle may be found in an infusion set or preselected separately.

Plastic intravenous catheters are becoming a popular substitute for metal needles. They reduce the incidence of infiltration because the catheter is flexible rather than rigid and because the tip is blunt rather than sharp. Plastic catheters still require a metal needle for the initial venipuncture.

Two types of plastic catheters may be used. An intracath is threaded through the needle and into the vein. The needle is withdrawn from the vein and skin but remains attached to the tubing. The tip of the needle is covered so it does not puncture the tubing or the patient. An angiocath, illustrated in Figure 25-16, is a plastic catheter that surrounds the outer circumference of the needle. Once the needle pierces the vein, the catheter is threaded into the vein over the needle. The needle is then completely removed and the IV tubing is attached.

Because catheters are flexible, they are less likely to become displaced; however, they may become kinked. This type of venipuncture device may be used when:

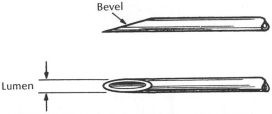

Figure 25-15 The bevel of a needle is its slanted edge, and its lumen is the space within the tubular needle shaft. The size of the lumen is indicated by the gauge size of the needle. A smaller number indicates a larger opening, whereas a larger number indicates a smaller channel.

of drug is administered intradermally, or between the layers of the skin. The technique for intradermal injections is discussed in Chapter 24. Another technique is to spray the area with ethyl chloride or inject sterile normal saline intradermally at the site of entry. The ethyl chloride cools and numbs the area, making it somewhat insensitive to pain. The saline produces sufficient pressure in the area to dull sensation, and it is less irritating to tissues than injectable anesthetics. The use of medications, excluding normal saline, should always be preceded by an inquiry about any allergies the patient may have. If the patient is sensitive to any of these substances, or ones similar to these, the medication should not be used.

Performing Venipuncture

Nurses become better skilled in performing venipunctures with continued practice and experience. Each new venipuncture provides additional challenges in site selection and insertion.

Selecting a Vein. The choice for the site of a venipuncture will vary with each patient. The following are factors that should be considered when selecting a vein:

- Superficial veins are more easily located and accessible for puncturing. Figure 25-17 identifies and shows the anatomic locations of various veins commonly used for venipuncture.
- Veins in the arm and hand are used in preference to veins in the foot or leg. This is done because circulation is often reduced in the lower extremities. It poses a potential risk of thrombus and embolus formation

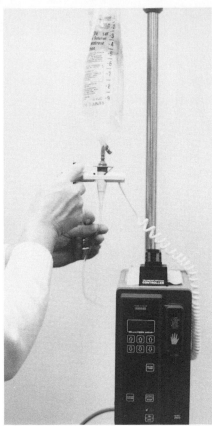

Figure 25-14 The nurse attaches a device from this volumetric infuser that monitors the drops of fluid as they fall into the drip chamber.

- An infusion is to run for an extended period of time
- The veins are unusually difficult to locate and enter
- The patient is young or active, or unable to exercise some degree of protection of the infusion site
- The solution or medication is likely to cause discomfort or damage to tissue if it does not remain within the vein.

Assembling Venipuncture Equipment. When the nurse gathers the equipment, some of which may be optional, an infusion of intravenous fluids will be started. The following items are usually necessary: gloves, a tourniquet, a pledget moistened with antiseptic to cleanse the site, a dry, sterile pledget, antiseptic ointment, a gauze square to cover the venipuncture site, and adhesive strips to secure the needle and dressing.

The nurse should use judgment and follow agency policies when collecting other equipment. For instance, an armboard may be needed to anchor the arm and hand when a patient may not be relied upon to be cautious when moving about.

Some agencies have written policies that permit the nurse to inject a small amount of local anesthetic, such as lidocaine, at the puncture site to eliminate pain. This type

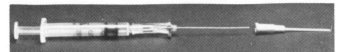

Figure 25-16 This catheter threads over the needle. After the needle and catheter have been introduced into the vein, the needle and syringe are carefully withdrawn, leaving only the catheter in place in the vein. The tubing from the intravenous solution is then connected to the catheter.

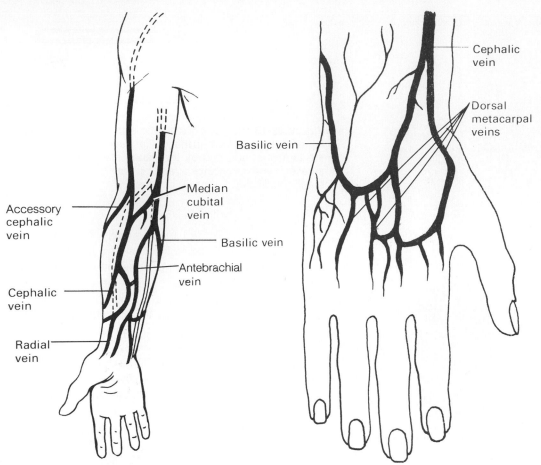

Figure 25-17 These two drawings show potentially suitable sites for introducing solutions into the veins on the forearm and on the back of the hand.

when a foreign object, such as a needle or catheter, is placed within the vein.

- Use veins in the arm or hand on the patient's non-dominant side. The patient is less likely to feel inconvenienced with restricted motion. The potential for displacing the needle or catheter will be less, since the nondominant side will be used infrequently during activities associated with daily living.
- The choices available for possible sites may be limited by the patient's condition. For example, a person with severe burns of both forearms will not have vessels available in these areas. No infusions or injections of any kind should be permitted on the same side as recent extensive breast surgery because of possible problems with circulation in the area.
- Apply a tourniquet as shown in Figure 25-18. A blood pressure cuff inflated midway between the patient's systolic and diastolic blood pressure can be substituted for a tourniquet. The blood pressure cuff is often more comfortable for the patient. It will not pinch the skin or pull hair.
- Avoid using an area of a vein that will compromise

joint movement. The antecubital veins located on the inner side of the elbow are usually very accessible and relatively easy to enter, but their use limits the patient's ability to flex his arm. This may prove to be very uncomfortable if the infusion is to take several hours' time. The metacarpal, basilic, and cephalic veins are good venipuncture sites.

- Distend and inspect the veins as the nurse in Figure 25-19 is doing. In general, when the arm is used, it is best to select a vein as low as possible on the back of the hand or on the lower forearm. The nondominant hand is the preferred first site. The forearm is used when veins on the back of the hand are unsuitable. The vein on the inner aspect of the elbow is the last to be considered but is usually quite accessible and easy to enter. Veins on the inner surface of the wrist are avoided because of the marked skin sensitivity in the area. If the vein is damaged during venipuncture or therapy, another vein higher on the arm can be used for subsequent entry. Using an area below a damaged vein would require that the fluid move through the section of injured vein. This could affect the circula-

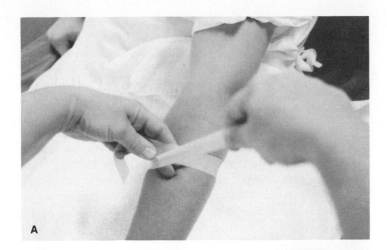

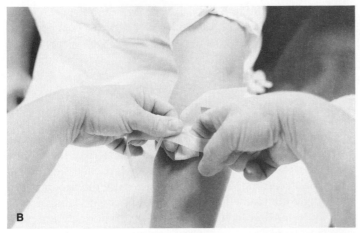

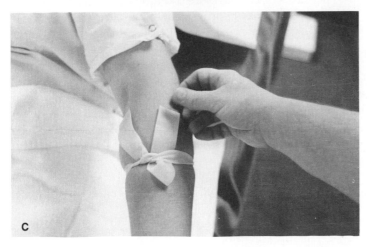

Figure 25-18 (*A*). The first step in applying a tourniquet is to pull the ends tightly in opposite directions. (*B*). One end is then tucked beneath the other. (*C*). When finished, the tourniquet remains in place. The free ends are positioned away from the area where the needle or catheter will be inserted. It is easily released by pulling up on one of the ends.

tion of the solution and reduce the body's ability to repair the tissue.

- Feel and look for an area in the vein that is fairly straight. It should approximate the length of the venipuncture device. A straight area in a vein is less likely to become accidentally perforated once the needle is inserted into it.

- Thin-walled and scarred veins should be avoided. They are difficult to enter. Scarred veins feel hard and bumpy, or cordlike, to the finger's tip. The normal vein is smooth, pliable, and resilient. Experience helps the nurse acquire skills in palpating veins to determine their general condition.

- It is recommended that a needle not be inserted into a

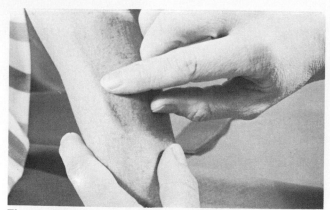

Figure 25-19 The nurse palpates veins to evaluate their use as a venipuncture site.

valve in a vein. A valve feels like a small lump. Most are found where veins branch off from each other.

- Use larger veins for infusing hypertonic solutions, those containing irritating medications, those administered rapidly, and those that are thick or sticky. Generally, the forearm veins are preferred over those on the back of hand for the types of solutions just mentioned.
- Spare sites that may be needed for subsequent infusions if the duration of fluid therapy is likely to be lengthy. Sites will need to be changed periodically. If no regard for future site selection has been made, the nurse may be forced to use sites that are less accessible, more uncomfortable, and potentially more hazardous.

Cleaning the Site. The area where the needle will be inserted is cleaned in the following manner:

- Wash the area about to be entered with soap or detergent and water if the patient's skin is soiled with drainage or body discharge.
- Use a cotton ball or gauze pledget moistened in an antiseptic for cleansing the site of entry to avoid introducing organisms into body tissue.
- Move the cotton ball or pledget in a circular motion beginning at the point of entry, and move outward in a circular motion for a distance of about 2.5 to 6 cm (1–2.5 in). This technique carries debris away from the site of injection.
- Use firm pressure when cleansing, thus creating friction. Haphazard up-and-down movements and superficial swipes with the cotton ball or pledget accomplish little.

Starting the Infusion. An intravenous infusion is most often started by a qualified nurse. If access to the vein proves unsuccessful after a limited number of attempts, the nurse may request that a physician or someone else

proficient at venipuncture, such as an anesthetist, start the infusion. Skill Procedure 25-3 describes the actions that may be followed when an infusion is begun or when the site needs to be changed during prolonged therapy.

Many health agencies have a written policy identifying the length of time that an IV may remain in its original site. A common timeframe for changing an IV site is every 48 hours. If there are complications, the site should be changed more frequently. Occasionally, there are extenuating circumstances, such as difficulty in locating additional sites because of extensive prior use, that may justify leaving an infusion longer than 48 hours at a particular site. The nurse should record the current appearance of the site and the reason for not changing it.

Calculating the Infusion Rate

It is a nurse's responsibility to calculate, regulate, and maintain the rate of flow according to the physician's order. The physician indicates the number of milliliters to be given within a period of time, such as for 1-, 8-, or 24-hour periods. The rate is then calculated by the nurse on the basis of drops of solution per minute.

There is no standard equivalent of drops per milliliter among commercially manufactured IV equipment. The size of the opening into the drip chamber of the tubing, and subsequently the size of the drop itself, varies among manufacturers. Most health agencies use the products of a single company. The nurse should become familiar with those used in each particular agency where clinical practice takes place. The more common equivalents, called the *drop factor,* are: 15 drops equal 1 mL, 20 drops equal 1 mL, and 60 drops equal 1 mL. Because blood is a colloidal solution, the drop size must be larger to permit the molecules of protein to flow through. Therefore, when blood is infused, tubing different from that used for infusing crystalloid solutions must be utilized. The drop factor when using a blood set is usually 10 drops equal 1 mL.

To determine how many milliliters of solution are to be given each hour, the nurse should use the following formula:

$$\frac{\text{Total number of mL to be given}}{\text{Total hours of infusion}} = \text{mL to be given per hour}$$

For example, a physician orders 3000 mL of solution to be infused over a 24-hour period.

$$\frac{3000 \text{ mL}}{24 \text{ hr}} = 125 \text{ mL to be infused per hour}$$

The nurse then determines the number of drops to be infused per minute. This requires using the drop factor

(Text continues on page 663)

Skill Procedure 25-3. Starting an Intravenous Infusion

Suggested Action	**Reason for Action**
Explain the purpose of the infusion and the steps that will be followed to access the vein.	The patient who understands the procedure will be better able to cooperate during and after it has been performed.
Assemble the solution and infusion equipment that will be used during the venipuncture.	This is an invasive procedure. The nurse should have all the items collected and available for use so that the procedure will not be interrupted.
If possible, have the patient on his back in bed in a low Fowler's position.	The supine position permits either arm to be used and allows for good body alignment. The low Fowler's position usually is most comfortable for the patient.
Evaluate the sites that will most likely meet the needs of the patient and circumstances of the infusion, such as the rate of flow, type of fluid, and so on.	Selection should ensure the best vein for the patient's comfort, prevention of complications, and administration of the solution.
Apply a tourniquet or sphygmomanometer by placing it 5 to 10 cm (2–4 in) above the site of entry.	Venous blood travels up the arm in the direction of the heart. In order to trap blood the tourniquet must be applied above the level of entry.
Inspect and palpate several potential venipuncture sites.	In case the initial vein is traumatized during venipuncture, the nurse should have other choices in mind.
Deflate the sphygmomanometer or loosen the tourniquet after determining the preferred site.	Prolonged interference with blood flow can cause numbness and discomfort.
Clip body hair at the site if it is excessive.	Body hair harbors organisms, and removing tape from hairy areas is uncomfortable for the patient.
Tear strips of tape for stabilizing the needle and prepare dressing material as the nurse in Figure 25-20 is doing.	Having the tape ready in suitable lengths will help prevent needle displacement.

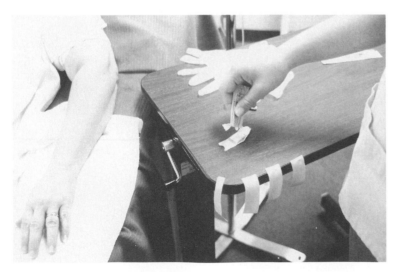

Figure 25-20 The nurse prepares all the tape and dressing supplies that will be needed before attempting to insert the needle or catheter.

Tighten the tourniquet or reinflate the sphygmomanometer when ready to proceed with the needle insertion. If a tourniquet is used, place its ends away from the site of entry.	Distention of the veins should be brief just prior to the venipuncture. The ends of the tourniquet could contaminate the area of entry if allowed to fall over the site of entry.

(continued)

Skill Procedure 25-3. Continued

Suggested Action	Reason for Action
Check for the patient's radial or brachial pulse, depending on the vein selected. If the pulse is not palpable, loosen the tourniquet.	Occluding arterial bloodflow can interfere with oxygen delivery to cells and tissues in the area.
Observe and locate the vein.	Distended veins are easier to see and enter.
Use other measures, to augment vein filling, if necessary.	These measures all use mechanisms that make the vein more elevated and distinct.

- Have the patient open and close his fist several times.
- Stroke the skin toward distal areas of the arm.
- Instruct the patient to lower his arm so it hangs momentarily.
- Apply warm compresses over the intended site of entry for 10 to 15 minutes before applying the tourniquet.
- Apply a blood pressure cuff; keep it inflated to 40 mm Hg for about 2 minutes.

Suggested Action	Reason for Action
Using friction, clean the skin *thoroughly*. Move in a circular motion at and around the site of entry with a swab moistened with an antiseptic, as illustrated in Figure 25-21.	Organisms on the skin can be introduced into the tissues or blood with the needle.

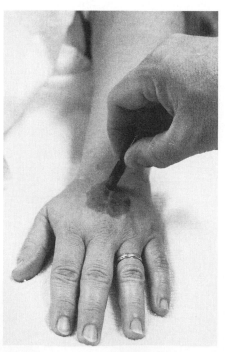

Figure 25-21 After selecting a suitable vein, the nurse cleans the prospective site of entry with a swab moistened with an antiseptic.

Suggested Action	Reason for Action
Allow the antiseptic to dry.	Injecting antiseptic irritates tissues. Drying gives the antiseptic time to reach its maximum cleansing and antimicrobial effect.

(continued)

Skill Procedure 25-3. Continued

Suggested Action	**Reason for Action**
Don clean gloves.	Gloves are a barrier against bloodborne viruses.
Use the thumb to stretch and stabilize the vein and soft tissues about 5 cm (2 in) below the intended site of entry, as illustrated in Figure 25-22.	Retraction of the vein and surrounding tissues helps straighten the vein and prevents movement of the vein as the needle is being introduced.

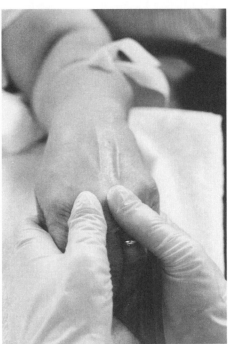

Figure 25-22 The nurse controls the position of the veins so they will not roll beneath the skin by applying slight traction with the thumb.

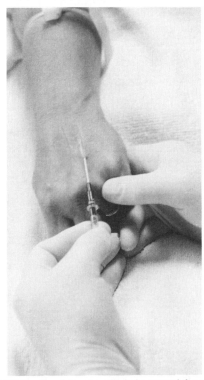

Figure 25-23 The tip of the needle is inserted through the skin and advanced. Blood appears in the needle when the vein is pierced.

Instruct the patient to take a deep breath or two while the needle is entering the skin, if no local anesthetic or other pain-relieving technique has been used.	Deep breathing helps the patient relax, which decreases his discomfort when the needle is inserted.
Enter the skin at a 45° angle while holding the needle with its bevel side up. When the needle has entered the skin, lower the angle of the needle until it is nearly parallel with the skin, at about a 10° to 15° angle.	When the bevel side is up, blood is likely to enter the needle as soon as the entry occurs, and it is less likely that the needle will be pushed completely through and out the other side of the vein.
Hold the needle bevel side down, as an alternative, when inserting a small needle into a large vein.	When the bevel side of the needle is down in a large vein, the vein is less likely to collapse on the bevel and obstruct the flow of blood through the needle.
Follow the course of the vein for a short distance to insert the length of the bevel totally within the vein, as shown in Figure 25-23.	Inserting the tip of the needle a little farther ensures placement within the inner vein wall.
Observe for a backflow of blood through the needle when the bevel is well within the vein.	The pressure of the patient's blood causes automatic backflow of blood.
Continue to palpate the vein as a guide to the angle, depth, and direction in which to thread the needle its entire length within the vein.	Having the needle placed well into the vein helps prevent dislocation of the needle. Threading helps prevent pushing the needle through the vein wall.

(continued)

Skill Procedure 25-3. Continued

Suggested Action	Reason for Action
Release the tourniquet.	The longer blood accumulates, the greater the chance of ruputuring the vein.
Apply pressure over the area of the internal tip of the venipuncture device.	This slows the backflow of blood while preparing to make the connection with the tubing.
Connect the end of the tubing to the venipuncture device, taking care to maintain sterile conditions at the connection.	A direct connection between the solution and the vein is necessary to infuse fluids.
Start the flow of solution by slowly releasing the clamp on the tubing.	The patient's blood may clot readily in the needle if the flow is not started promptly.
Remove gloves when contact with blood is no longer likely.	Tape will adhere to the gloves when proceeding to stabilize the needle and dress the site.
Place a small amount of antiseptic ointment at the entry site, if agency policy permits, as shown in Figure 25-24. Cover the area with a small, dry, sterile gauze pledget or bandage. Op-Site®, which is discussed in Chapter 20, is used to cover the point of entry in some agencies.	An antiseptic ointment and dressing placed at the needle's point of entry helps decrease the incidence of infection at the injection site.

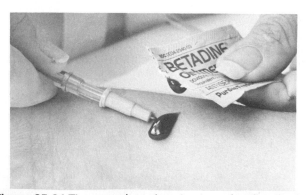

Figure 25-24 The nurse has placed a drop of antiseptic ointment at the needle's entry site.

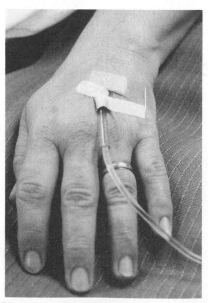

Figure 25-25 A bandaid is used as a dressing over the punctured skin. A strip of adhesive tape is placed under the needle, sticky side up, and crossed over the top of the angiocath.

Secure the needle with tape, as shown in Figure 25-25.	Securing the needle well helps prevent it from slipping out of the vein.
Incorporate a length of tubing with tape as shown in Figure 25-26. Do not encircle the arm or hand with tape.	The weight of the tubing and the movement of the patient may pull the needle out of the vein when the tubing is not well anchored. If tape encircles the hand or arm, it may cut off circulation.
Write the date, time, the gauge of the needle or catheter, and initials on the tape used for securing the needle or catheter in place.	Having information near the site of entry provides a quick reminder for when the infusion needs to be changed to another site.

(continued)

Skill Procedure 25-3. Continued

Suggested Action	**Reason for Action**

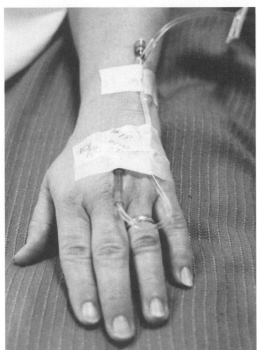

Figure 25-26 The nurse secures the tubing with more tape and records the date, time, size of the angiocath, and initials on the tape.

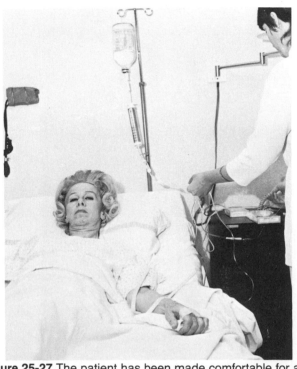

Figure 25-27 The patient has been made comfortable for an intravenous infusion. Her arm has been secured on an armboard. The nurse adjusts the flow of fluid.

Adjust the rate of flow according to the physician's order as the nurse in Figure 25-27 is doing.	The physician prescribes the rate of infusion. The nurse will need to compute the number of milliliters and drops per minute, as described elsewhere in the chapter.
Apply a tab made from tape to the tubing, indicating the nurse's initials, date, and time of initial use.	The tubing is changed at least every 48 to 72 hours. Providing identifying information helps others adhere to the policy.
Record the time, volume, solution, site, size, and type of venipuncture device in the chart.	The chart acts as a permanent record for all the care, observations, and procedures performed during the patient's stay in a health agency.

determined by the manufacturer of the IV tubing being used. The formula is as follows:

$$\frac{\text{Number of mL per hour} \times \text{drop factor}}{60 \text{ minutes}}$$
$$= \text{drops to infuse per minute}$$

For example, using the amounts in the order given in the first example in which 125 mL are to be infused every hour, assume that the intravenous equipment has a drop factor of 20 drops equal 1 mL.

$$\frac{125 \text{ mL} \times 20}{60} = 41.6 \text{ rounded to } 42 \text{ drops/minute}$$

The nurse would then count the number of drops falling into the drip chamber of the tubing per minute. By adjusting the regulator clamp, the number of drops per minute can be increased or decreased until the infusion rate matches the calculated rate.

Maintaining the Intravenous Infusion

The nurse must maintain the infusion and care for the infusion site. Some modifications may be used when providing routine care. Infusion solutions may be made portable by using a standard on wheels, shown in Figure 25-28, which promotes activity and exercise. Special gowns that snap up the entire length of the sleeve prevent dislodging the IV during the performance of personal hygiene.

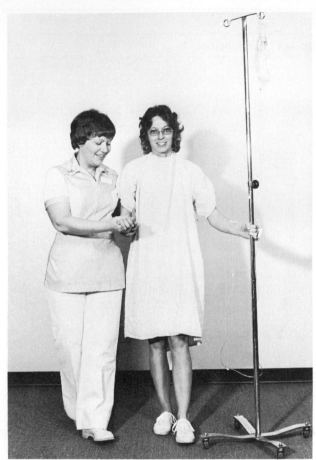

Figure 25-28 This patient is taking her first walk in her room while receiving intravenous therapy. The patient is wearing rubber-soled shoes that reduce the risk of slipping and falling.

When IV gowns are not available, the following technique may be used to change a patient gown with a closed sleeve:

- Remove the container of solution from its standard. Keep the solution above the site of the infusion or blood from the patient's vein may enter the tubing.
- Slip the sleeve over the venipuncture device, tubing, and container of solution.
- Thread the solution container and tubing from the neckline of the new gown and out the sleeve.
- Insert the patient's arm with the infusing solution through the sleeve.
- Rehang the container of solution from its standard.

Monitoring the Rate of Infusion. Maintaining the proper rate of flow is important. Too slow a flow may not meet the patient's needs for fluid. Infusing fluid too rapidly may overtax the body's ability to circulate the fluid.

The nurse should make timely observations, at least every hour, to determine that the volume of intravenous solution is infusing according to schedule. The task may be simplified by marking the container with a time strip. The

nurse should be able to tell at a glance whether the solution is being infused at the proper hourly rate. An example of a marker that can be placed on the solution container is illustrated in Figure 25-29. Some nurses mark directly on a plastic bag of solution. However, it is probably better not to use a heavy felt-tipped pen because questions have been raised about the possibility of the ink penetrating the bag and entering the solution.

The rate of flow of an intravenous infusion may be altered by several factors. These factors are listed and explained in Table 25-7

Readjusting the Rate of Flow. If an infusion is not progressing according to schedule, it may be necessary for the nurse to make adjustments in the rate. However, the volume should never be rapidly increased or decreased in a short period of time. To compensate for a deficit or

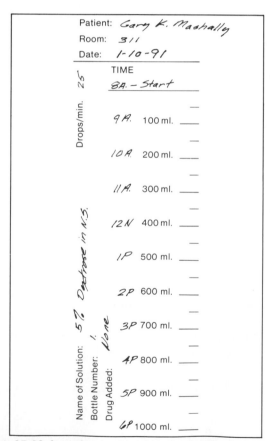

Figure 25-29 A marker is placed on the bottle of solution so that the flow rate can be easily monitored. In this example, the physician has ordered that the patient is to receive 1000 mL of solution over a 10-hour period. The agency uses equipment that has a drop factor of 15 drops equals 1 mL. The nurse adjusts the rate so that 25 drops fall per minute to infuse the solution at the rate at which it was ordered.

Table 25-7. Common Factors Affecting the Rate of Intravenous Flow

Factor	Explanation
Changing distances between the height of the container and the insertion site	Distances may change as the patient ambulates, moves to a chair, stretcher, or toilet, or alters the position of the hand in which the solution is infusing. As distances increase, the rate speeds, and as distances decrease, the rate will slow.
Occlusion of the tubing or lumen of the venipuncture device	Tubing can become compressed by the patient's weight or parts of the bed, thus slowing or stopping the rate of infusion. A blood clot, inflammation, or swelling at the tip of the needle may similarly affect the infusion rate.
Faulty regulator clamp or tampering	A faulty regulator clamp may become loose, causing an increased volume to be infused in a short time. Some patients purposely change the adjustment of the clamp, causing it to slow or infuse more rapidly.
Administration of cold fluid	Cold fluid may cause localized constriction of the blood vessels slowing the rate of infusion.
Changes in the patient's blood pressure	The fluid infuses by overcoming the venous pressure within the vessel. Changes in arterial pressure are likely to affect venous pressure, since the vascular system is a continuous loop. The rate of flow will slow or speed according to the rise and fall of blood pressure.

excess of infused volume, the rate should be adjusted over each remaining hour of administration. Even so, the increased or decreased rate should never exceed 25% of the original infusion rate. Consider the following situation.

Fluid is to infuse at a rate of 125 mL/hour or 42 drops/minute using the drop factor of 20 drops equal 1 mL. Two hours after hanging 1000 mL of fluid, the nurse notes that only 125 mL have infused instead of the scheduled 250 mL. A total of 875 mL remains in the container.

The nurse assesses the site. Pulling back on the needle a bit, rotating it, or elevating and depressing the needle, the nurse determines that the rate has slowed due to the bevel of the needle resting against the vein wall.

The nurse repositions the angle of needle placement by elevating the external hub with a small piece of gauze. The nurse must now recalculate the new rate of flow by using the following formula:

Milliliters of fluid remaining
Total hours remaining
= new volume of mL/hour

Example: $\dfrac{875 \text{ mL}}{6 \text{ hrs}}$ = 145.8 rounded to 146 mL/hour

To determine if this recalculated rate will exceed the 25% limit, the nurse would proceed to calculate as follows:

Step One: Previous volume per hour
− New volume per hour
= mL of difference

Example: 146 mL per hour (new volume)
− 125 mL per hour (previous volume)
21 mL > difference

Step Two: $\dfrac{\text{Milliliters difference}}{\text{Previous ml per hour}} \times 100$
= percentage of rate change

Example: $\dfrac{12 \text{ mL}}{125 \text{ mL}}$ = .168 × 100
= 16.8% change in infusion rate

Since this is well within the acceptable range of safety, the nurse may readjust the rate of flow using the previous formula for calculating the drops per minute in order to infuse the new volume.

Example: $\dfrac{146 \times 20}{60}$ = 48.6 rounded to 49 drops/minute (new rate)

If the difference is greater than 25%, the nurse should inform the physician of current fluid assessments such as the patient's blood pressure, pulse, respiratory rate, and current urine output. The physician may then wish to prescribe a readjustment in the volume that can be infused.

Caring for the Site. The venipuncture site is a type of open wound. It is important to inspect and dress the wound at routine intervals specified by the health agency. Some notation about its condition should appear daily in the permanent record.

A common practice is to change the dressing once in every 24-hour period. Agency policy may indicate a particular antimicrobial ointment that should be used. The principles of asepsis are no less important when changing this dressing than when changing the dressing over an incision. In fact, sterile technique is particularly important in this case, since the venipuncture site is a direct line to the bloodstream. Pathogens may be circulated easily to other parts of the body.

Changing Solution Containers. When the patient requires continuous or repeated infusions of solutions, it may become necessary to change solution containers as they become nearly empty. Also, a solution container that has been hanging up to 24 hours should be changed to

reduce the potential for growing pathogens. If a venipuncture site must be changed, it may be more convenient to change the solution container at the same time. This may not always be possible. Skill Procedure 25-4 describes the actions that should be followed when only the solution container must be changed.

Changing Infusion Tubing. Most agencies set infection-control policies that indicate the length of time that tubing may continue to be used. Tubing is usually changed at least every 48 to 72 hours. This is best done when the

Skill Procedure 25-4. Changing Solution Containers

Suggested Action	Reason for Action
Determine that the replacement solution is available about one hour before it is needed.	The replacement solution should be available before the current solution has completely infused.
Be ready to switch containers when the infusion container is empty but the drip chamber still contains fluid.	If air enters the tubing, it will have to be removed using techniques described further in this procedure.
Tighten the regulator clamp on the infusion tubing to slow the rate of infusion.	The rate should be fast enough to keep the solution infusing, but slow enough to prevent partially emptying the tubing.
Lower the empty solution container, with its tubing, from the standard. Position the container on a slant or resting on its wide base with the neck facing upward.	Keeping the opening upward will prevent any solution within the container from leaking out the punctured opening.
Pull the spike from the container, without touching the tip.	The tip will be inserted within the sterile replacement solution. Touching causes contamination.
Remove the seal from the replacement solution.	The seal protects the solution from contamination; it should not be removed until just prior to puncturing with the spike.
Immediately insert the spike into the container of the fresh solution.	Prolonged exposure of the tip to the air increases the potential for contamination with pathogens.
Hang the solution container from the infusion standard.	The height of the container should be 45–60 cm (18–24 in) above the level of the vein.
Inspect for the presence of air bubbles in the tubing and proceed to displace them from the tubing.	Air bubbles probably are not dangerous in small amounts. However, they may cause the patient to become concerned for his safety.
Displace the air bubbles by using one of the following three methods: • Move the regulator clamp below the air and tighten to stop the flow. Tap the bubbles as shown in Figure 25-30. • Milk the air in the direction of the drip chamber or the filter, or work the air upward by wrapping the tubing around a circular object as illustrated in Figure 25-31. • Another method for removing air is to insert a small-gauge needle into a rubber connection in the tubing below the air. As fluid moves the air in the direction of the needle, the bubbles will be released out the end of the needle into the atmosphere and not into the patient.	Air will rise or take the path of least resistance.

(continued)

Skill Procedure 25-4. Continued

Suggested Action	Reason for Action

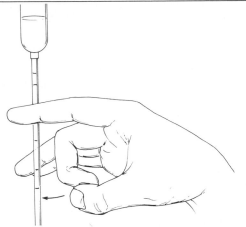

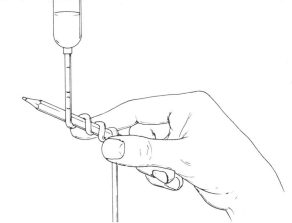

Figure 25-30 Beginning directly below the lowest level of air in the tubing, thump the tubing, proceeding upward until the air escapes from the tubing. (Adapted from Nichols AO, Day J: Pearls for Nursing Practice, p 55. Philadelphia, JB Lippincott, 1979)

Figure 25-31 Beginning below the level of air in the tubing and twisting the tubing around a pen, pencil, scissors, or other object will also displace air from the tubing. (Adapted from Nichols AO, Day J: Pearls for Nursing Practice, p 55. Philadelphia, JB Lippincott, 1979)

Loosen the regulator clamp and adjust the infusion rate to deliver the ordered volume over the prescribed amount of time.	The rate will need to be timed and readjusted once the position of the regulator clamp has been changed.
Attach a new time strip to the solution container.	A time strip aids in monitoring the progress of the infusion.
Record the volume of infused solution on the intake portion of the fluid record.	An accurate record of fluid intake and fluid output should be maintained on all patients receiving intravenous fluids.
Record the addition of new solution wherever it is designated by agency policy.	Many agencies require that a new volume of intravenous solution be recorded similarly to medications.

solution and the site are changed. However, it may be necessary to change the tubing without changing the solution container or the venipuncture device. If that is the case, the nurse may follow the actions described in Skill Procedure 25-5.

Attaching a Second Container of Solution

Occasionally, the physician will order that the infusion of a fluid be interrupted while another solution is allowed to infuse. The solution that was hung first is called the *primary infusion.* The additional container of solution is referred to as a *piggyback solution* or *secondary infusion.* It is so named because it is joined in tandem and elevated above the primary infusion, as shown in Figure 25-32. This method is often used when medication has been diluted in 50- or 100-mL volumes that infuse slowly over perhaps as much as an hour's time.

When preparing to attach a piggyback solution, the

nurse may follow the suggested actions in Skill Procedure 25-6.

Detecting Complications

Regular assessments of the site of the infusion, the equipment that is delivering the infusion, and the patient's overall responses during the fluid infusion should be made frequently. The nurse should be on the alert and be prepared to take action if any signs of complications occur when a patient is receiving intravenous fluids.

Immediately report signs and symptoms of problems with respirations, such as dyspnea, noisy breathing, and coughing. Respiratory and cardiac problems are often caused by *circulatory overload.* This is a condition that is caused by administering too much solution for the patient's system to circulate and eliminate. The flow rate should be decreased, the patient should be placed in a Fowler's position, vital signs should be

Skill Procedure 25-5. Changing Infusion Tubing

Suggested Action	Reason for Action
Obtain sterile infusion tubing like that being currently used.	The new tubing completely replaces the outdated tubing.
Tighten the regulator clamp on the replacement tubing.	The occlusion of the lumen prevents leaking.
Lower the solution container from the standard; hold it securely at an angle with the neck of the container pointing upward.	Tilting prevents solution from leaking through the already punctured seal.
Remove the outdated spike and put the fresh, sterile spike into the solution, taking care to keep the tip sterile.	All connections that will contact fluid entering the bloodstream should be kept free of contamination.
Reattach the solution container to the standard and compress the drip chamber, filling it approximately one-third full.	Squeezing and releasing the drip chamber pulls fluid from the container into the fluid reservoir.
Remove the protective cap from the end that will connect with the venipuncture device, and clear the tubing of air by loosening the regulator clamp.	Once the lumen of the tubing is no longer occluded, fluid will fill the tubing and displace the air.
Replace the protective cap and tighten the regulator clamp while preparing to disconnect the outdated tubing from the venipuncture device.	The connecting tip must remain sterile. Clamping prevents leaking of solution.
Peel back or remove the dressing if it covers the connection area between the needle or catheter and the outdated tubing.	The tubing will be changed, but the venipuncture device must remain undisturbed.
Disconnect the outdated tubing while holding the venipuncture device firmly in place. Pinch the tubing as it is removed.	Pulling may displace the venipuncture device from its position within the vein. Pinching prevents the tubing from leaking.
Remove the protective cap and attach the fresh, sterile tubing to the venipuncture device without touching the tip.	The switch in tubings must be done while maintaining sterile conditions at the tip of all connection.
Loosen the regulator clamp on the newly connected tubing.	The fluid will now continue infusing into the venipuncture device.
Time and adjust the drip rate.	The flow must be adjusted so that it continue to infuse at the prescribed rate.
Label the tubing with the current date, time, and initials.	Labeling helps determine the time for the next scheduled change.

assessed, and the physician should be notified for further orders. The complication is serious and the infusion may have to be stopped entirely.

Check for *infiltration*, which is the escape of solution into tissues. A dislodged needle or a needle that has penetrated the wall of the vein may cause fluid to pass into subcutaneous tissue. Typical signs include a slow flow rate or no flow of solution, swelling in the area of the venipuncture site, a burning sensation, local pallor of the skin, and coldness. A penlight is often helpful to detect infiltration. The light will illuminate the skin differently in the area of infiltration. Another technique is to apply a tourniquet to the arm above the venipuncture site. If infiltration is occurring, the solution will continue to flow; if the needle is in the vein, the solution will stop flowing because the tourniquet is occluding the pathway through the vein. Lowering the solution container below the infusion site is no longer a recommended technique. The needle should be removed when infiltration has occurred and a new site should be selected. The arm may be elevated. Warm compresses are placed over the area of infiltration for 20 to 30 minutes, three or four times a day, for one to two days. Notify the physician immediately if the fluid contained a drug that may cause injury to tissue. Drugs may be needed to counteract the damaging effects.

Check for phlebitis, which may occur when a solution is

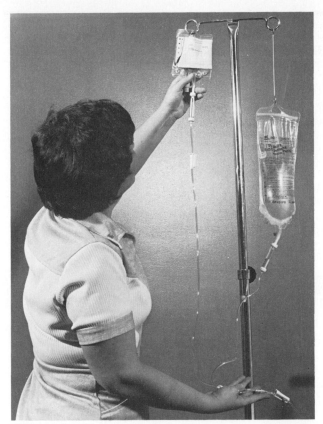

Figure 25-32 A small volume of fluid, called a piggy-back solution, is connected to the tubing on a larger volume primary infusion. Note that the small bag, which often contains a dissolved medication, is hung about 25 cm (10 in) higher on the standard than the other solution container.

particularly irritating to the vein or the venipuncture device remains in the same site for a prolonged period of time. The area will appear red, warm, swollen, and painful. The rate may slow due to localized edema. Further use of the vein should be avoided. Remove the venipuncture device. Restart the infusion in the opposite arm or hand. Apply warm compresses as described following an infiltration to promote comfort and speed the healing process. Notify the physician of the observations and actions taken.

Infection at the site may occur and could spread to other parts of the body through pathogens within the blood stream. The site may appear red and puffy. Purulent drainage may be present. The patient may have a rise in temperature and chills. Discontinue the infusion at its present site. Follow principles of asepsis when dressing the wound. Notify the physician for further orders. A culture may be necessary to identify the type of pathogens that are present. Subsequent treatment and care will depend on measures required for controlling the spread of the microorganisms.

An *air embolism* is a rare, but deadly, complication that occurs when a large volume of air enters the vein. If proper techniques are followed when tubing is attached, infusions usually do not permit lethal amounts of air to enter the patient. The minimal quantity of air that would be fatal to humans is not known, but animal experimentation indicates that it is

(Text continues on page 672)

Skill Procedure 25-6. Adding a Piggyback Solution

Suggested Action	Reason for Action
Obtain the solution and a short length of tubing designed to connect with the primary infusion.	The tubing from a piggyback solution does not need to be long, since it does not attach directly to the venipuncture device.
Remove the seal on the secondary solution container as shown in Figure 25-33 and insert the spike.	All connections are maintained in sterile condition.
Tighten the regulator clamp and gently squeeze the drip chamber.	Squeezing the drip chamber will cause fluid to enter the lower portion of the chamber.
Fill the drip chamber approximately one-third full or to the mark indicated by the manufacturer.	The drip chamber should only be partially filled so that the drops are visible as they leave the infusion container.
Remove the protective cap on the lower end of the tubing and release the regulator clamp.	As the fluid flows, air is displaced from the tubing so none will enter the patient.
Attach a short, small-gauge needle to the exposed end of the infusion tubing.	The needle will be used to pierce a port on the primary infusion tubing, completing the connection of the two.
Cleanse the port on the primary infusion tubing shown in Figure 25-34 and insert the needle as the nurse in Figure 25-35 is doing.	The port has been exposed to organisms within the environment. Cleansing removes microbes present on the surface of the port.

(continued)

Skill Procedure 25-6. Continued

Suggested Action   **Reason for Action**

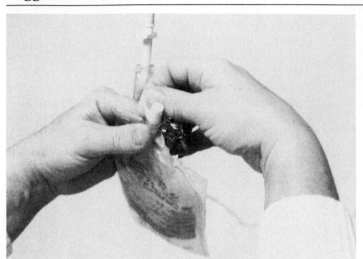

Figure 25-33 The seal is pulled from the small bag of solution.

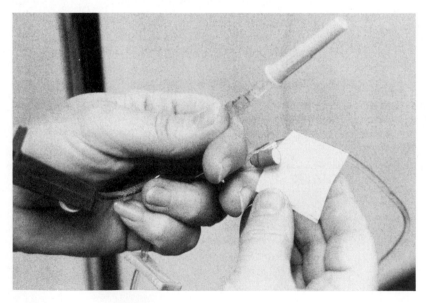

Figure 25-34 The port is cleaned by wiping it with an alcohol swab.

Hang the secondary infusion solution from the same standard as the primary set.	The solution container should be 45 to 60 cm (18–24 in) above the venipuncture site.
Lower the primary infusion approximately 25 cm (10 in) below the height of the piggyback solution, using a plastic or metal hanger.	The solution in the higher container will infuse due to greater hydrostatic pressure. When the higher container is empty, the lower container will resume infusing.
Tape the needle, shown in Figure 25-36, within the port.	Taping the needle ensures that it will not be pulled out accidentally.
Rehang the primary infusion at its original height when the piggyback solution has finished infusing and recheck the flow rate.	The infusion rate should be checked just to validate that the fluid will continue infusing at the rate at which it was ordered.

(continued)

Skill Procedure 25-6. Continued

Suggested Action	**Reason for Action**

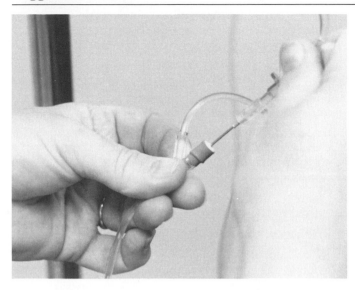

Figure 25-35 The nurse supports the port with one hand and inserts the needle through its seal.

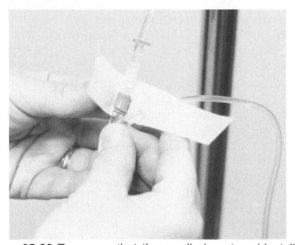

Figure 25-36 To ensure that the needle is not accidentally pulled out of the port, the nurse tapes the connection.

Allow the empty piggyback container and tubing to remain in place within the port to maintain a closed system when future intermittent infusions of the same additives will be used.	The spike should not be exposed to the environment if it will be subsequently used again.
Hang a replacement piggyback container in the following manner:	The same tubing can be used for up to 48 hours, provided it is used to deliver the exact same additives.
• Remove the spike from the empty piggyback container and insert it into the fresh solution.	
• Lower the piggyback solution below the level where it connects with the tubing from the primary solution.	Since the needle remains in the port, gravity flow from the primary infusion is used to displace the air in the secondary tubing.
• Loosen the regulator clamp on the secondary solution if it was closed.	Fluid from the primary solution will backfill the secondary tubing as long as no occlusion is present.

(continued)

Skill Procedure 25-6. Continued

Suggested Action	Reason for Action
Prepare new tubing for each different piggyback solution.	Using separate tubings will prevent possible incompatibility and precipitation from occurring.
Insert each additional needle into adjoining areas within the port.	More than one needle can be placed in the same port at one time.
Record the volume of infused solution on the bedside form for fluid intake.	Accurate records of the total volume of fluid intake and fluid output must be maintained on patients receiving intravenous solutions.
Record the administration of a piggyback solution or its intravenous medication as indicated by agency policy.	Solutions or additives are considered as medications and they may require recording in other areas within a patient's permanent record.

much larger than the quantity that could be present in the entire length of infusion tubing. The average infusion tubing holds about 5 mL of air, an amount not ordinarily considered dangerous. Patients, however, are often frightened when they see air in the tubing, and every effort should be made to keep this from happening. If a patient experienced an air embolism, the nurse would likely detect a sudden and extreme drop in blood pressure, tachycardia, cyanosis, and diminished level of consciousness. The nurse should position the patient on his left side and elevate his feet above the level of the heart. Since air rises, the air will enter the right atrium, where it will remain trapped. This position is maintained until the air can be absorbed.

Discontinuing the Infusion

When the solution has infused and no more is scheduled to follow, the nurse discontinues the infusion in the following manner:

1. Clamp the tubing and remove the tape that held the dressing and venipuncture device in place.
2. Gently press a pledget moistened with antiseptic solution over the site of entry.
3. Remove the needle or catheter by pulling it out without hesitation, following the course of the vein. If the needle or catheter is removed by twisting, raising, or lowering, it could damage the vein.
4. Apply pressure to the injection site for 30 to 45 seconds while elevating the forearm, as illustrated in Figure 25-37. This technique helps stop bleeding

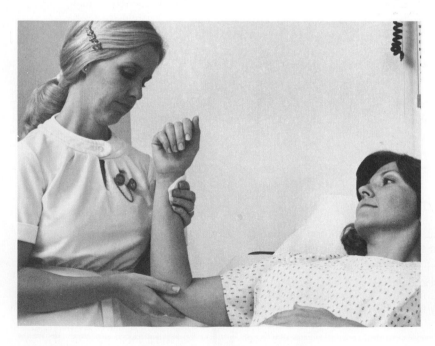

Figure 25-37 The nurse elevates the patient's forearm and places pressure at the injection site after removing the needle when discontinuing an intravenous infusion.

from the injection site. Then apply a small, dry pressure dressing.

5. Flex and extend the arm or hand several times to help the patient regain sensation and mobility in the area where the needle was located.

6. Record the amount and type of fluid infused during the current shift on the bedside fluid intake record.

7. Document and sign a notation on the patient's record concerning the time of termination, the type of fluid, and the condition of the venipuncture site.

Administering a Blood Transfusion

A *blood transfusion* is the intravenous infusion of whole blood. Most often, blood is collected from one person, called the *donor*, and given to another, called the *recipient*. Donors are screened in order to ensure that the person giving the blood is healthy and will not be endangered by the loss of a fraction of his blood volume.

Donated blood is tested for serum hepatitis and HIV antibodies to avoid the possibility of spreading these diseases from infected blood. Blood that tests positive is automatically not used. Nevertheless, the fear associated with acquiring these blood-transmitted diseases has caused many individuals in good health to have their own blood collected and stored. It is then administered at a later date if it is needed. This method has been found safe because there are no dangers of passing organisms from one person to another or receiving mismatched blood. The disadvantage is that instances are relatively rare in which it can be predicted that a person will need a blood transfusion. Blood is generally collected and stored from 21 to 35 days.

Before blood can be given to a patient, it must be determined that the blood of the donor and that of the recipient are compatible. Incompatible red blood cells can react with one another, causing clumping within the vascular system and possible death to the recipient.

Blood is categorized into four major groups—A, B, AB, and O—depending on the type of protein present on the surface of the red blood cells. In addition to the four major groups, other factors differentiate one group of blood cells from another (*e.g.*, Rh factor). The laboratory test that identifies the proteins on red blood cells is called *typing*.

The blood type of the donor and the blood type of the recipient are tested, using a test called *cross-matching*, to determine the compatibility between the two blood specimens. Though the recipient is almost always given an identical blood type during a transfusion, there may be exceptions in an emergency. Table 25-8 provides a list of blood types that are compatible.

Table 25-8. Compatible Blood Types

Recipient's Blood Type	Donated Blood Type*
A	A and O
B	B and O
AB (Universal Recipient)	AB, A, B, and O
O (Universal Donor)	O

*A recipient with Rh positive blood may receive Rh positive or Rh negative blood although it is preferred if this factor matches as well. (Rh negative means that the factor is absent from the surface of the blood cell). An Rh negative person should *never* receive Rh positive blood.

Starting a Blood Transfusion

Blood is collected and dispensed in 500-mL bottles or plastic containers. Each container is called a unit of blood. An anticalcium agent is added to the blood to prevent clotting. Blood is a colloid solution; it is not unusual for individuals to be sensitive to the various protein molecules in blood and other blood products.

Policies may vary among health agencies about the administration of a blood transfusion. In some agencies a written consent form must be signed by the patient before blood is administered. Skill Procedure 25-7 may be followed if the nurse is responsible for starting and monitoring a blood transfusion.

Infusing Blood Products

Some patients do not need all the components of whole blood. For example, one may need red blood cells but not the plasma and its contents. Packed red blood cells, which must be crossmatched, may be given. In other situations, only plasma is required. Frozen or fresh serum is particularly useful in emergencies for immediate restoration of fluid volume. Serum presents no compatibility problem, and time need not be lost typing and crossmatching blood and seeking donors. Still other patients may require only blood platelets or just albumin, a single plasma protein. These can be collected separately from whole blood and administered intravenously.

Using Blood Substitutes

Several solutions may be substituted for blood in certain situations. Plasma expanders, such as Dextran® and Hetastarch®, increase circulating volume and maintain blood pressure, but have no effect on oxygenation of cells and tissue.

Fluosol DA® and other perfluorocarbons have been tested and used on a limited basis as an artificial substitute for blood in humans. When administered to a patient, this blood substitute can carry 20 times the oxygen found in plasma; however, the patient's serum must be highly oxy-

(Text continues on page 676)

Skill Procedure 25-7. Administering a Blood Transfusion

Suggested Action	Reason for Action
Obtain a signed consent on required forms after the physician has informed the patient about the risks and benefits related to a blood transfusion.	A nurse witnesses a patient's signature but is not responsible for providing the information on which the patient must base his consent.
Obtain special blood infusion tubing with an inline filter.	The filter acts to remove clots or other large, undissolved substances before they can enter the patient's vein.
Use a needle or catheter with a large lumen, such as an 18-gauge or 19-gauge, for venipuncture.	The lumen of the venipuncture device must be large enough to permit protein molecules to pass through.
Attach the standard volume of sterile normal saline, usually 250 mL, to one extension of the blood set tubing. Tighten the clamp on the line leading for blood.	Normal saline is the only type of crystalloid solution that will not clump or cause red cells to burst. Saline is used to displace the air in the tubing, wet the filter, and begin the infusion.
Do not add medications to the saline or the blood.	Interactions can occur.
Asses the patient's vital signs, including body temperature, prior to starting the infusion.	A baseline of assessments helps to evaluate the patient's response during the infusion of blood.
Recheck the patient's armband and other identifying data again.	Doublechecking helps ensure that no errors have been made.
Select a large vein as a site for the venipuncture.	A large vein facilitates infusing a thick colloid solution in a relatively short period of time.
Use only the saline solution when beginning the infusion.	It is important to make sure that the saline is infusing well before administering the unit of blood.
Secure and stabilize the venipuncture device as the saline begins to infuse.	Although the infusion may not be lengthy, the device should be secured so it remains in the vein.
Obtain the unit of blood from the laboratory or blood bank.	Blood is kept in controlled refrigeration and released only after typing and crossmatching it with blood from the intended recipient.
Be sure to doublecheck with another person to see that all laboratory numbers on the blood identically match those of the patient. Check the labels, the blood type, and the Rh factor.	An error in compatibility can be fatal. All personnel involved in the blood transfusion must sign and cosign several forms indicating that the precautionary checks were made and that they matched.
Check to see that the blood has not passed its expiration date. Approximate shelf-life is 21 days, but 35 days is now more commonly considered the limit.	Old red blood cells tend to break down and release potassium. When this is infused, a cardiac arrhythmia or possible cardiac arrest can occur.
Plan to give the blood as soon as it is brought to the nursing unit.	Allowing blood to sit and warm may result in cell destruction or growth of pathogens.
Do not store blood in the unit's refrigerator.	The temperature of the refrigerator is not sufficiently well controlled to be safe for blood storage.
Invert the unit of blood gently several times before and during the infusion to mix the red cells evenly with the plasma. Avoid squeezing or shaking the container.	As blood sits, the plasma separates from the cells. Vigorous movement may damage the cell walls, releasing potassium.
Spike the container of blood.	Blood infuses through the remaining section of the Y-tubing.
Tighten the clamp on the tubing to the saline and release the clamp on the blood line after it has been determined that the saline is infusing well.	If blood infiltrates the tissues, it causes discoloration and irritation to tissues. If the saline is infusing well, it can be expected that the blood will also.
Inspect the commercial blood set to determine the manufacturer's drop factor.	A common drop factor for blood infusion sets is 10 drops equal 1 mL.
Regulate the infusion of blood at a slow rate of approximately 2 mL/minute.	A slow rate allows time to detect an untoward reaction before a large volume has infused.

(continued)

Skill Procedure 25-7. Continued

Suggested Action	**Reason for Action**
Increase the rate after 15 minutes to 7–9 mL/minute if the patient is not experiencing any signs of a reaction.	Incompatibility reactions, perhaps the most dangerous complication, usually occur in the first few minutes of a transfusion.
Remain with the patient from 15–30 minutes into the infusion. Make pertinent assessments of vital signs every 5–15 minutes. Observe the patient's response to the infusion.	The nurse needs to be present to detect early signs of a transfusion reaction.
Be familiar with the signs and symptoms of a reaction to the blood.	The nurse must be able to recognize the seriousness of pertinent observations.
• Hypotension, tachycardia, dyspnea, restlessness, constriction in the chest, back pain, and flushing are a few manifestations of an incompatibility reaction.	An incompatibility reaction is one of the most serious types of complications and often the earliest to appear. It is a type of allergic reaction to proteins on the red cells.
• A febrile reaction may be characterized by a sudden onset of fever with shaking chills during or following the infusion, with headache, tachycardia, and generalized muscle aches.	A febrile reaction usually is associated with an allergic reaction to foreign proteins other than the red cells in the donated blood. The reaction releases chemicals that raise body temperature.
• Fever, chills, and a drop in blood pressure may be associated with the infusion of blood contaminated with pathogens.	A septic reaction is usually associated with administering blood that has warmed either prior to its administration or has taken longer than 4 hours to infuse.
• Mild allergic reactions may be manifested by large hives, itching, and discomfort, but usually no drastic changes in vital signs.	Reactions may occur in hypersensitive persons to one or more foreign proteins within the donated blood. These reactions may be reduced by the administration of antihistamine medications.
• Moderate chilling during the reaction with little or no significant change in body temperature may just be a temporary reaction to the cold blood. However, the nurse should substantiate that conclusion with other assessments.	The blood may cause the patient to feel chilled as it enters and begins to circulate throughout the body. This is not serious as long as other signs and symptoms do not also accompany the chilling.
• Hypertension, dyspnea, moist breath sounds, distended neck veins, and a bounding pulse may indicate circulatory overload.	When a large volume of blood is administered in a short amount of time, the amount may overwhelm the cardiovascular system of some individuals.
• Tingling in the fingers, low blood pressure, cramps, and, finally, convulsions may be associated with an effect caused by the chemical added to prevent blood clotting of the stored blood.	Anticalcium agents added to prevent blood clots can lower the patient's serum calcium level. An antidote, usually calcium chloride, is given to overcome a reaction of this type.
Take the following steps if the patient has any signs or symptoms of a reaction to the blood:	
• Stop the transfusion *immediately*. Administer the normal saline solution. *Do not remove the needle from the vein.*	The blood is the usual factor in the reaction. Stopping the blood limits the escalation of the reaction. Maintaining access to the vascular system ensures that there is an open intravenous line for emergency use.
• Place the patient in a Fowler's position, unless ordered to the contrary.	A Fowler's position will help ease breathing for a dyspneic patient.
• Report all observations immediately and follow any orders the physician prescribes.	The sooner that emergency drugs and measures are provided the better the outcome will be.
• Monitor the vital signs frequently and continue to make careful observations of the patient's condition.	All collected data will aid evaluation of the patient's response throughout the reaction and its treatment.
• Send the first urine voided after a transfusion reaction to the laboratory to be examined for hematuria.	If red cells have been destroyed during an incompatibility reaction, they will appear in the urine.

(continued)

Skill Procedure 25-7. Continued

Suggested Action	Reason for Action
• Save the blood and tubing.	Most agencies require a laboratory analysis of the blood and the equipment used to administer it.
Follow an uneventful infusion of blood with an administration of a small volume of the normal saline solution.	A small volume of saline is used after the blood transfusion to flush as many blood cells as possible from the filter and tubing.
Record the volume of blood and saline that was infused on the patient's bedside fluid intake form.	A unit of blood is the equivalent of 500 mL. Any infused solution is considered fluid intake.
Record all assessments, care, and the patient's response in the permanent record.	The nurse's notations are a record of the care delivered to the patient.

genated first. It is not entirely without risk. Uses other than as a transfusion substitute have been explored. Currently there are several proposals and experimental tests being performed using Fluosol DA. Because Fluosol DA has a smaller molecular size than red blood cells, it can deliver oxygen to organs such as the brain and myocardium that are ischemic because of nearly occluded blood vessels. The same principle applies to individuals experiencing a sickle-cell crisis; the ischemic pain can be reduced or relieved by the passage of the Fluosol DA through vessels that have become obstructed by clumps of sickled red blood cells. This same chemical could improve the preservation of organs for transplantation. Another potential use is to administer Fluosol DA before cancer chemotherapy or radiation. It has been shown that hypoxic cancer cells are less affected by standard cancer treatments. By improving the oxygenation of abnormal cells, the effectiveness of the therapy could be enhanced.

Other substances are being tested to discover a safe, effective substitute for red blood cells. Hemoglobin solutions have been used successfully in animals. Attempts are being made to recycle outdated red blood cells in donated blood by sealing them within a lipid capsule. This product is referred to as microencapsulated hemoglobin. With continued research, these substances may be better for treating anemia and hypovolemia than perfluorocarbons. Finding an artificial blood substitute may eventually reduce the need to rely upon human blood donors and the risk of bloodborne viral diseases.

Understanding Electrolyte Balance

All body fluid contains chemicals called nonelectrolytes and electrolytes. *Nonelectrolytes* are chemical compounds that remain bound together when dissolved in a solution and, therefore, cannot conduct electricity. Glucose is an example of a nonelectrolyte. *Electrolytes* are chemical compounds that dissolve and separate into individual molecules, each carrying either a positive or negative electrical charge. For example, the chemical compound of salt is sodium chloride. These two molecules separate when dissolved. The sodium molecule carries a positive electrical charge while the chloride molecule carries a negative charge. In general, these separated molecules are called ions. More specifically, a *cation* is an ion with a positive electrical charge. An *anion* is an ion with a negative electrical charge.

The total cations in the body normally equal the total anions. They balance each other, as illustrated in Figure 25-38. Electrolytes are measured in *milliequivalents,* abbreviated mEq, per liter. Table 25-9 is a list of various electrolytes and the amounts that are normally found in the plasma, or serum, of blood.

Major Electrolytes and Their Chief Functions

Body fluid is figuratively an alphabet soup of electrolytes and other chemical substances. Those ions that are found in the greatest proportions in the body are called major electrolytes. There are other electrolytes, no less important, but in lesser amounts. They are called minor electrolytes. Zinc, selesium, and chromium are examples.

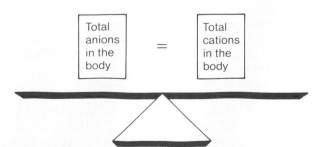

Figure 25-38 The total anions in the body are equal to the total cations in the body when they are described in milliequivalents per liter.

Table 25-9. Normal Serum Electrolyte Levels

Serum Electrolyte	Normal Level
Sodium (Na)	137–147 mEq/L
Potassium (K)	4.0–5.6 mEq/L
Chloride (Cl)	98–106 mEq/L
Phosphate (PO_4)	1.7–2.6 mEq/L
Calcium (Ca)	4.5–5.8 mEq/L
Magnesium (Mg)	1.4–2.3 mEq/L
Bicarbonate (HCO_3)	
Adult	25–29 mEq/L
Child	20–25 mEq/L

The following is a description of the major electrolytes and a brief summary of their function and food sources.

Sodium. Sodium is a cation. It is the most abundant cation in extracellular fluid. It has important functions in the body, such as helping to maintain the correct volume of body fluid, acid–base balance, and normal nervous and muscle cell activity. Sodium is found in many foods and especially in bacon, ham, processed luncheon meats, sausages, catsup, mustard, cheese and other dairy products, and table salt.

Potassium. Potassium is a cation. It is the most abundant cation in intracellular fluid. It functions in the body to help maintain proper cell activity and transmit electrical impulses, especially through the heart. Gastrointestinal secretions contain large quantities of potassium. Most fresh fruits and vegetables are rich in potassium. Especially rich food sources include bananas, peaches, figs, dates, oranges, prunes, apricots, potatoes, and tomatoes.

Chloride. Chloride is the chief extracellular anion. It is essential for the production of hydrochloric acid in gastric juices and plays a role in acid–base balance. Chloride is found in foods that are also high in sodium.

Phosphate. Phosphate is the major anion in intracellular fluid. It is important for maintaining acid–base balance, plays a role in nerve and muscle activity, and carbohydrate metabolism. It is necessary for proper cell division and for the transmission of hereditary traits. Phosphorus, from which the electrolyte phosphate derives, is found in most foods, but especially in beef, pork, and dried beans and peas.

Calcium. Calcium, the most abundant mineral in the body, forms the framework for bones and teeth. In its electrolyte form, calcium is a cation and is important for the transmission of nerve impulses, blood clotting, and muscle contraction. Calcium is found in milk, cheese, and dried beans, and, to a lesser extent, in meats and vegetables.

Magnesium. Magnesium is a cation. It is especially important for the promotion of enzyme activity. Because it is widespread and found in almost all foods, deficiencies are seldom found in persons who are eating normally.

Bicarbonate. The bicarbonate molecule is an anion that is essential for acid–base balance. Acid–base balance and its related imbalances will be discussed later in this chapter. Bicarbonate can come from food and drug sources, but it is also formed within the body.

Electrolyte Distribution

Electrolytes are distributed in different proportions in extracellular and intracellular tissue. Their proportions remain relatively constant due to the movement and relocation of various ions through the processes of diffusion and active transport. *Diffusion* is the process in which ions move from an area of greater concentration to an area of lesser concentration through a semipermeable membrane. This happens very passively with no release of energy. However, when molecules move in the opposite direction, it requires active transport. *Active transport* is a process requiring energy to move molecules through a semipermeable membrane from an area of low concentration to one that is higher. Movement of molecules may also require a carrier substance. A *carrier substance* facilitates the transfer of an electrolyte or nonelectrolyte through a semipermeable membrane. For example, insulin is the carrier substance that is needed to transfer glucose, a nonelectrolyte, through a cell's membrane.

Electrolyte Imbalances.

It is possible that an individual could suffer an excess or deficiency of any one or a combination of electrolytes. The type of electrolyte depends on the nature of the fluid loss or gain, and the individual's diet. For instance, the individual with severe diarrhea may experience a potassium deficit, since gastrointestinal secretions are high in potassium; electrolyte levels of calcium, for example, may remain normal. Table 25-10 is a list of terms used when describing specific imbalances of electrolytes.

Detecting Electrolyte Imbalances. The source of electrolytes is the food and beverages that are consumed daily. Therefore, any change in the intake of nourishment and water will probably affect the amount and balance of electrolytes. Because these electrolytes become dissolved

Table 25-10. Terms Describing Electrolyte Imbalances

Imbalance	Definition
Hypernatremia	An excess of sodium in the blood
Hyponatremia	A deficit of sodium in the blood
Hyperkalemia	An excess of potassium in the blood
Hypokalemia	A deficit of potassium in the blood
Hyperchloremia	An excess of chloride in the blood
Hypochloremia	A deficit of chloride in the blood
Hyperphosphatemia	An excess of phosphate in the blood
Hypophosphatemia	A deficit of phosphate in the blood
Hypercalcemia	An excess of calcium in the blood
Hypocalcemia	A deficit of calcium in the blood
Hypermagnesemia	An excess of magnesium in the blood
Hypomagnesemia	A deficit of magnesium in the blood

in body fluid, any condition that affects fluid loss or retention is also going to affect the balance of electrolytes. It is unlikely that a person would experience an imbalance of one kind without also experiencing an imbalance of the other.

Certain related signs and symptoms accompany abnormal levels of electrolytes. However, because each electrolyte has diverse and unique functions, it is difficult to detect an imbalance based only on physical assessment alone. The most conclusive assessment technique involves an analysis of blood in which the serum levels of electrolytes are measured.

Despite the fact that physical assessments cannot be totally relied on to detect imbalances of electrolytes, some of the following should suggest an impending electrolyte imbalance:

- Any chronic or acute loss or retention of fluid
- The recent or prolonged administration of medications, such as diuretics, that are likely to cause a change in fluid volumes or electrolyte levels
- Loss of muscle strength, twitching muscles, or leg cramps
- EKG changes, specifically changes in the normal appearance or timing of a wave and wave complexes
- Bradycardia, tachycardia, and other abnormalities of pulse rate and rhythm
- Numbness or tingling in the fingers, toes, or lips
- Confusion, disorientation, depression, seizures, or changes in levels of consciousness.

Preventing and Correcting Electrolyte Imbalances. Severe electrolyte deficits may require infusions of specific electrolytes or electrolyte solutions. Other invasive procedures, such as dialysis or the administration of certain drugs that promote electrolyte excretion, may be used when there are electrolyte excesses. Severe electrolyte imbalances can lead to death if they are not restored to balance quickly.

The following is a list of measures that may prevent or help promote normal levels of electrolytes:

- Help the patient maintain proper nutrient and fluid intake.
- Carefully assess any patient who receives medications that predispose to fluid or electrolyte imbalances.
- Provide additional dietary sources of electrolytes that are likely to be depleted. For example, the patient who routinely takes certain diuretics may be served orange juice or a banana daily to replace the potassium that may be lost in urine. A patient with diarrhea, vomiting, or excessive perspiration may benefit from drinking Gatorade, a beverage that contains a mixture of replacement electrolytes.
- Maintain accurate recordings of fluid intake and output, as well as body weight. Notify the physician early when there are significant changes in these figures.
- Communicate with laboratory personnel when the results of laboratory tests are urgently needed.
- Inform the physician when laboratory tests indicate abnormal results.
- Implement drug orders or intravenous solution administration as soon as possible when the patient is experiencing altered levels in fluid or electrolytes.

Understanding Acid–Base Balance

All body fluids are either acidic, basic, or neutral. An *acid* is defined as a substance containing hydrogen ions that can be liberated or released. An *alkali* or *base* is a substance that can accept or bind with hydrogen ions. A combination of these two tends to balance each other, resulting in a condition that is neither acidic or basic, but neutral.

The nature of the fluid can be determined by measuring its pH. The term pH is an expression of hydrogen ion concentration. The range of pH is based on a numerical scale from 1 to 14; 7 is considered neutral. A pH in the range of 1 to 7 is acid; the lowest number represents the highest acidic level. A pH above 7 up to 14 is considered basic; the highest number represents the highest basic level. The pH of pure water is 7; gastric secretions have a pH of about 1.0 to 3.0; secretions from the pancreas have a pH of about 10.

The normal pH of blood is slightly alkaline, measuring a pH in the range of 7.35 to 7.45. The pH of blood is primarily maintained by a fixed ratio between carbonic acid molecules and bicarbonate molecules. Normal acid–base balance is regulated primarily by the body's ability to retain or eliminate hydrogen ions, by carbon dioxide excretion from the lungs, and by the ability of the kidneys to excrete or reabsorb substances that influence acid–base balance.

The ratio of carbonic acid molecules and bicarbonate molecules must remain constant or the narrow range of balance will be disrupted. Death will occur rapidly when an acid–base imbalance occurs. When the levels of blood pH change, the terms acidosis and alkalosis are used to identify the altered state. *Acidosis* is the condition in which the pH of blood falls below 7.35. *Alkalosis* is the condition in which the pH of blood measures more than 7.45. Types of acidosis and alkalosis are described further in Table 25-11.

Identifying Acid–Base Imbalance

Besides various abnormal yet nonspecific signs and symptoms, an arterial blood gas analysis provides the best data for establishing that an acid–base imbalance exists. Among other data, this test measures the blood pH; the level of dissolved carbon dioxide in the blood, abbreviated PCO_2; the level of dissolved oxygen in the blood, abbreviated PO_2; and the amount of bicarbonate, abbreviated HCO_3. The normal ranges for these substances are indicated on the sample form in Figure 25-39.

Preventing and Correcting Acid–Base Imbalance

Most acid–base imbalances must be treated aggressively as soon as they are detected. Balance can be promoted by treating the metabolic or respiratory cause creating the imbalance. Some cases of acidosis may be treated by administering sodium bicarbonate intravenously. Respiratory acidosis and alkalosis can be treated by methods that restore normal respirations.

The nurse can help prevent acid–base imbalances by:

- Providing a patient with adequate fluids and nutrients
- Implementing skills that reduce the loss of fluids and electrolytes
- Ensuring adequate ventilation
- Instructing patients on the proper dosage and self-administration of medications that predispose to alterations in acids, bases, and other electrolytes.

Table 25-11. Types of Acid–Base Imbalances

Type	Description	Nursing Observation
Respiratory acidosis	Respiratory acidosis results from a respiratory phenomenon. The primary cause is a deficiency in respiratory ventilation, resulting in hypoventilation. Pneumonia, emphysema, and respiratory obstructions are common causes.	Dyspnea, hypoventilation Disorientation Drowsiness, coma Plasma pH less than 7.35
Respiratory alkalosis	Respiratory alkalosis results from increased respiratory ventilation. The primary cause is hyperventilation associated with extreme emotions, anxiety, an elevated temperature, or salicylate intoxication.	Rapid breathing Numbness and tingling of fingers, toes, and mouth Eventually convulsions Plasma pH above 7.45
Metabolic acidosis	Metabolic acidosis results from an accumulation of acid components or a decrease in alkaline components in the blood. Common causes include a decreased food intake, infections, diabetic acidosis, renal failure, and diarrhea.	Deep, rapid breathing Weakness Disorientation Coma Plasma pH less than 7.35
Metabolic alkalosis	Metabolic alkalosis results from an excess of alkaline components or a decrease in acid components in the blood. Common causes include excessive ingestion of alkalis, fluid loss from gastric suction, and therapy to increase urinary excretion.	Disorientation Muscle cramps Slow respiratory rate Stupor Plasma pH above 7.45

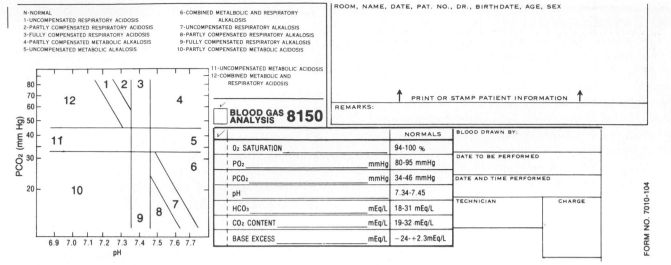

THREE RIVERS AREA HOSPITAL, 214 SPRING STREET, THREE RIVERS, MI. 49093   BLOOD GAS ANALYSIS

Figure 25-39 This hospital's laboratory form shows the normal values for substances measured during a blood gas analysis. The nomogram on the left can be used to interpret the figures. To use the nomogram, draw a line vertically from the point at the bottom of the square corresponding to the patient's measured blood *p*H. Draw a second line horizontally from the left side of the square at the point corresponding to the patient's measured PCO₂. The lines should intersect in one of the twelve sectors. The nurse can then refer to the key of numbers at the top of the form for a quick interpretation. (Courtesy of Three Rivers Area Hospital, Three Rivers, MI.)

Suggested Measures to Promote Fluid and Chemical Balance in Selected Situations

When the Patient Is an Infant or Child

Take into consideration that infants and children have a greater proportion of body water. Their mechanisms to maintain fluid balance are less well-developed than are those of adults. As a result, fluid and chemical imbalances often develop rapidly and become severe quickly. The premature infant and the newborn are especially quick to develop fluid imbalances.

Think of infants and young children as "smaller vessels with a larger spout" when compared with adults. This means that they lose water more quickly because of a comparatively large skin surface in terms of body weight than adults.

Take into consideration that normal serum electrolyte concentrations are not strikingly different among infants, children, and adults, except that bicarbonate levels are lower in the young. Children and infants tend to develop imbalances relatively quickly and easily.

Expect that signs and symptoms of fluid imbalances in general are similar in children and adults, except that behavioral changes include irritability and increased crying.

Provide children with cool drinks or popsicles on hot days when they become so involved in play that they do not take time for fluid intake.

Try to start an intravenous infusion in a treatment room rather than at a child's bedside. A child is comforted when he can think of his own room as being safe from painful procedures.

Explain the procedure for administering intravenous fluids and let the child act out the procedure on a doll. This helps decrease fear and lets the child displace and express his own feelings in a non-threatening way.

Select equipment of an appropriate size for infants

Applicable Nursing Diagnoses

Patients who have fluid, electrolyte, and acid–base imbalances are likely to have these nursing diagnoses.

- Feeding Self-Care Deficit
- Fluid Volume Deficit
- Fluid Volume Excess
- Altered Oral Mucous Membrane
- High Risk for Impaired Skin Integrity
- Knowledge Deficit
- Anxiety
- Fear

Nursing Care Plan 25-1 illustrates the nursing process as it applies to a patient with Fluid Volume Deficit. This diagnostic category is defined by the North American Nursing Diagnosis Association (1989) as, "The state in which an individual experiences vascular, cellular, or intracellular dehydration."

NURSING CARE PLAN

25-1. *Fluid Volume Deficit*

Assessment	**Subjective Data**
	States, "I've been living on the streets. I don't have a job. I haven't been able to get anything to eat in several days."
	Objective Data
	56-year-old homeless man brought to the Emergency Department after being found by police wandering and confused near Main St. Outdoor daytime temperatures have been in the 90° ranges. Height 5'10″, weight 137 lbs. States usual weight is around 160 lbs. T—100° orally, P—100 and weak, R—28. Oral mucous membranes are dry. Able to void 50 mL of dark, amber urine. BP 100/68 in R. arm while sitting up. Skin is dry and tents for >5 seconds when compressed.
Diagnosis	Fluid Volume Deficit related to inadequate oral intake and increased insensible fluid loss.
Plan	**Goal**
	The patient's oral fluid intake will be between 1500 to 3000 mL in the next 24 hours (8/15).
	Orders: 8/14
	1. Compile a list of food and fluid likes and dislikes.
	2. Provide a minimum of 100 to 200 mL/hour of preferred liquids/hour over the next 16 hours. Avoid disturbing hours of sleep.
	3. Request dietary department to send foods that are good sources of sodium, such as milk, cheese, 1 bouillon, ham, etc.
	4. Refer to Salvation Army shelter for the homeless before discharge. — R. ARMSTRONG, RN

Implementation (Documentation)		
8/14	1000	States "I like just about anything. I'm so thirsty. A big, cool glass of lemonade sounds wonderful right now." Also lists ginger ale and orange juice as favorite beverages. Dietary department notified to send sodium-rich foods for next 24 hours. Discharge planner notified for referral to Salvation Army. — L. O'CONNELL, LPN

Evaluation (Documentation)		
	1030	200 mL of orange juice provided and consumed. Weakness and tremors of the hand noted. Able to use a straw with glass. ——————— L. O'CONNELL, LPN
	1230	Ate macaroni and cheese, sausage, stewed tomatoes, and whole milk for lunch. ——————— L. O'CONNELL, LPN
	1430	Total oral fluid intake since 1000 has been 1000 mL. Urine is lighter in color. Voided a total of 600 mL since admission. Vital signs improving; see graphic sheet for specifics. Discharge planner will visit in A.M. 8/15. — L. O'CONNELL, LPN

and children when starting an intravenous infusion. Select a small needle, such as a 27-gauge or a butterfly needle. Catheters are often used because of their flexibility.

For an infant, a small armboard can be made with two tongue blades wrapped in gauze and secured with tape when a small-sized board is unavailable. Select veins for administering an intravenous infusion in the same manner as for an adult. A scalp vein is often used for an infant, although some nurses prefer peripheral veins.

Anchor a needle or catheter well for intravenous therapy. When a scalp vein is used for an infant, a protective shield can be placed over the needle.

Monitor intravenous therapy used for infants and children carefully. In terms of the flow rate and amounts of added medications and electrolytes. The margin for error is small. A controller helps considerably to maintain an appropriate flow rate and is often used for infants and children receiving intravenous therapy.

Look for reactions to solutions of intravenous medications, intravenous fluids, and blood transfusions as for an adult when caring for an infant or child. Crying and restlessness are frequently present in the child too young to describe when he feels ill.

When the Patient Is an Adolescent or Young Adult

Discourage fad or crash dieting that severely restricts the intake of food or fluids.

Explain the dangers of using starvation, self-administered laxatives, or self-induced vomiting to control weight gain.

Encourage exercise-conscious individuals to select alternative forms of active exercise when temperatures and humidity levels are extremely high.

Advise an individual who exercises during hot, humid weather to drink extra water, orange juice, or other beverages to replace fluids and electrolytes lost through perspiration.

When the Patient Is Elderly

Take into account that mechanisms of the body that maintain fluid balance become fragile with increasing age. As a result, fluid imbalances in the elderly develop relatively quickly, can become severe rapidly, and respond slowly to treatment.

Expect that the concentration of electrolytes remains essentially the same as persons grow older, except that the plasma concentration of sodium is somewhat higher in the elderly.

Explain to an elderly patient the importance of identifying all medications, both prescription and nonprescription drugs, that are taken. For example, many nonprescription drugs taken by the elderly for the relief of constipation and antacids contain magnesium. Overuse of these can lead to hypermagnesemia. Excessive self-administration of sodium bicarbonate can alter acid–base balance. Cough medicines containing ammonium chloride can affect kidney regulation of acid–base and electrolyte balance.

Expect that veins in the elderly are often hardened (sclerotic) and also fragile. Small-gauge needles, such as a 22-gauge needle, should be used for intravenous therapy and inserted, secured, and removed with care. Because the elderly person's veins are easily injured, every effort should be taken to preserve those that are available.

Inspect an IV site when leaking occurs. As individuals age, skin turgor around the venipuncture device is likely to be less than that found in younger patients.

Monitor intravenous therapy closely. The elderly are very susceptible to water and electrolyte imbalances, but measures to restore balance must be used with caution to avoid imbalances of the opposite nature.

Teaching Suggestions to Promote Fluid and Chemical Balance

Chapter 8 discussed nursing measures and described the importance of patient teaching about ways to promote proper nutrition. This chapter has explained the benefits of proper nutrition and fluid intake as they relate to fluid and chemical balance.

To the extent that a patient can understand it, information in this chapter should be shared with patients. They should know why it is so important to eat a well-balanced diet and have an adequate fluid intake. Similarly, information in this chapter will help the nurse teach patients the importance of observing special diets, or using recommended food supplements, and of increasing or limiting fluids as ordered. Patients tend to follow prescribed therapy better when they understand why their therapy is important and how it will help promote health and well-being.

Bibliography

Barry A, Miller D: Infection control in clinical nursing practice . . . intravascular (IV) tubing changes . . . site changes. Infection Control Canada 3(1):10–14, 1988

Boykoff SL, Boxwell AO, Boxwell JJ: 6 ways to clear the air from an IV line. Nursing 18(2):46–48, 1988

Burns C, Crawford M: A method for rapidly calculating intravenous drip rates. Focus on Critical Care 15(4):46–48, 1988

Chenevey B: Overview of fluids and electrolytes. Nurs Clin North Am 22(4):749–759, 1987

Francombe P: Intravenous filters and phlebitis. Nursing Times 84(26):34–35, 1988

Gasparis L, Murray EB, Ursomanno P: IV solutions: Which one's right for your patient? Nursing 19(4):62–64, 1989

Gurevich I: IV filters have proponents but avoid use if doubts exist. Hospital Infection Control 16(3):37–38, 1989

Hahn K: Monitoring a blood transfusion. Nursing 19(10):20–21, 1989

Holder C, Alexander J: A new and improved guide to IV therapy . . . protocols for intravenous therapy. Am J Nurs 90(2):43–47, 1990

In the market for an electronic infuser? Am J Nurs 88(9):1225A–1226B, 1228F, 1988

Ingbar DH: The quest for a red blood cell substitute. Respiratory Care 35(3):260–272, 1990

Innerarity SA: Electrolyte emergencies in the critically ill renal patient. Critical Care Nursing Clinics of North America 2(1):89–99, 1989

Lenox AC: IV therapy: Reducing the risk of infection. Nursing 20(3):60–61, 1990

Lichtor JL: Transfusion reactions *part 1*. Current Reviews for Nurse Anesthetists 12(3):18–24, 1989

Lichtor JL: Transfusion reactions *part 2*. Current Reviews for Nurse Anesthetists 12(4):27–32, 1989

Lorenz BL: Are you using the right IV pump? RN Magazine 53(5):31–37, 1990

Lunger DG: Potassium supplementation: How and why? Focus on Critical Care 15(5):56–60, 1988

Magdziak BJ: There's just no excuse for IV complications. RN Magazine 51(2):30–31, 1988

Matheny NM: Why worry about IV fluids? Am J Nurs 90(6):50–57, 1990

Mathewson M: Intravenous therapy. Critical Care Nurse 9(2):21–23, 26–28, 30–36, 1989

Millam DA: Managing complications of IV therapy. Nursing 18(3):34–43, 1988

Negron SB: A smart way to secure an IV. Am J Nurs 89(5):687, 1989

Poyss AS: Assessment and nursing diagnosis in fluid and electrolyte disorders. Nurs Clin North Am 22(4):773–783, 1987

Rithalia SVS: Never mind the volume, what about the flow rate? Intensive Care Nursing 4(3):128, 1988

Ryan KA: Standardized care plans for IV therapy. Journal of Intravenous Nursing 12(2):94–98, 1989

Sabo CE, Michael SR: Managing DKA and preventing a recurrence. Nursing 19(2):50–56, 1989

Sherman JE, Sherman RH: IV therapy that clicks. Nursing 19(5):50–51, 1989

Sommers M: Rapid fluid resuscitation: How to correct dangerous deficits. Nursing 20(1):52–60, 1989

Sumner J: Preserving IV power if fluids are restricted. RN Magazine 51(8):26–28, 1988

Spotlight on acid–base balance. Nursing 20(3):32 HH, 32 JJ, 1990

Sprauve D: Fluids, electrolytes, and acid–base balance. Nursing 20(3):103, 105–107, 1990

Stromberg C, Wahlgren J: Saving money with effective in-line filters. Intensive Care Nursing 5(3):109–113, 1989

The well-dressed peripheral IV site. Emergency Medicine 20(7):63, 67, 1988

Thurkauf GE: Understanding the beliefs of Jehovah's Witnesses. Focus on Critical Care 16(3):199–204, 1989

Tietjen SD: Starting an infant's IV. Am J Nurs 90(5):44–47, 1990

Wandel JC: The use of postural vital signs in the assessment of fluid volume status. J Prof Nurs 6(1):46–54, 1990

26

Caring for the Mechanically Immobilized Patient

Chapter Outline

Behavioral Objectives
Glossary
Introduction
General Purposes for Mechanical Immobilization
Using Splints
Using Supportive Devices
Caring for the Patient Who Has a Cast
Caring for the Patient in Traction
Using a Continuous Passive Motion Machine
Suggested Measures Related to Mechanical
    Immobilization in Selected Situations
Applicable Nursing Diagnoses
Teaching Suggestions Related to Mechanical
    Immobilization
Bibliography

Skill Procedures

Providing Basic Cast Care
Petaling a Cast Edge
Caring for the Patient in Traction
Using a Continuous Passive Motion (CPM) Machine

Behavioral Objectives

When the content of this chapter has been mastered, the
learner will be able to:

Define the terms appearing in the glossary.
List at least five general purposes for mechanical immo-
    bilization devices.
Identify four types of splints and indicate the reason for
    their use.
Describe the technique for applying a splint in an emer-
    gency and measures that should be included with its
    use.
Demonstrate the application of a triangular sling.
Identify three types of casts and the body areas they
    generally enclose.
List advantages and disadvantages of two types of mate-
    rials used for constructing a cast.
Describe the nurse's responsibilities when assisting
    with the application of a cast.
Discuss methods for supporting and ensuring thorough
    drying of a wet plaster cast.
Describe the initial assessments that should be made
    after a cast has been applied.
Discuss the immediate and continuing care of a patient
    with a cast.
Identify measures that may be used to keep a cast clean,
    repair cast edges, and maintain cast structure when a
    window has been cut.
Discuss two methods for removing a cast.
Describe potential changes in a body part that may be
    expected when a cast is removed and methods for
    assisting the patient to adjust to those changes.
Describe observations that the nurse may use to deter-
    mine that traction is being properly maintained.
Describe the care that should be provided for a patient
    in traction.
Discuss the uses and advantages of a continuous passive
    motion machine.
List suggested measures that apply to the care of patients
    requiring mechanical immobilization, as described
    in this chapter.
Summarize suggestions for patient teaching offered in
    this chapter.

Glossary

Bivalved cast A cast that has been cut into two separate
pieces.
Body cast A rigid mold that encircles the trunk of the
body.
Brace A device that supports weakened body structures
during weight bearing.
Cast A solid mold of a body part.
Closed reduction Realignment of broken bone ends with-
out making a surgical incision.
CPM machine An electrical device that exercises joints.
Cravat binder A piece of cloth folded into a strip of a
desired width to support a joint.

Cylinder cast A rigid mold that encircles an arm or leg.

Fracture A break in the continuity of a bone.

Hip spica cast A rigid mold that encircles one or both legs and the lower trunk.

Immobilizer A cloth or foam splint used to limit movement and pain in an injured body part.

Inflatable splint An immobilizing device that produces its effect by surrounding an injured body part with air. Synonym for *pneumatic splint.*

Manual traction Pulling on a part of the body using an individual's hands and muscular strength.

Mechanical immobilization Restricted movement as a result of the application of a splint, cast, or traction.

Molded splint A plastic immobilizing device that is bent to fit the contour of a body part.

Open reduction Realignment of broken bone ends through an incision.

Pneumatic splint An immobilizing device that produces its effect by surrounding an injured body part with air. Synonym for *inflatable splint.*

Petals Strips of adhesive tape used to repair rough or crumbling edges of a cast.

Reduction Repositioning of a broken bone into its proper alignment.

Skeletal traction Pulling effect applied directly to the skeletal system by attaching wires, pins, or tongs into or through the bone.

Skin traction Pulling effect applied indirectly to the skeletal system by attaching equipment and weight to the skin.

Sling A muslin binder that elevates and supports an injured area.

Splint A device that immobilizes and protects an injured part of the body.

Stockinet Stretchy fabric that is knitted in a tube.

Traction Equipment attached to the bed and patient to produce pull and counterpull on a particular part of the body.

Traction splint Metal immobilizing device that also applies a pulling effect on an injured body part.

Window A square piece removed from a cast.

Introduction

Some patients are inactive and physically immobile due to an overall debilitating condition. The patient who is mechanically immobilized is in a somewhat different situation. *Mechanical immobilization* is the restriction of movement as a result of the application of a splint, cast, or traction. Any apparatus of this type temporarily confines or limits otherwise active individuals.

These forms of treatment cover, attach to, and confine areas of the body for varying periods of time. For these reasons, they require specialized skills to accomplish their intended purpose yet avoid injury to body structures during their use. This chapter will describe the techniques for caring for individuals who require mechanical immobilization.

General Purposes for Mechanical Immobilization

Most individuals for whom mechanical immobilization is used have sustained trauma to the musculoskeletal system. These injuries are painful and do not heal as rapidly as those of the skin or soft tissue. They require a period of inactivity during the time that new cells are restoring the integrity of the damaged structures.

Splints, casts, traction, and similar devices in this category may be applied to accomplish any one or a combination of the following:

- Relieve pain and muscle spasm
- Support and align damaged tissues
- Reposition injured and healing musculoskeletal structures
- Maintain functional positions until healing is complete
- Allow activity while restricting movement of an injured area
- Prevent further structural damage and deformity.

Using Splints

Splints are devices that immobilize and protect an injured part of the body. They come in a variety of designs depending upon the need for their use.

Ambulances stock *inflatable splints,* also called *pneumatic splints,* which become rigid when filled with air. The injured body part is inserted into the deflated splint. The splint molds to fit the injured part and prevents movement when inflated. These splints also control bleeding and swelling by virtue of the pressure they exert. Emergency vehicles also carry traction splints made of metal. They are not as easily applied as an inflatable splint. They require special instruction prior to their use to avoid injuring structures even further. A *traction splint* is applied in such a way as to immobilize and pull on muscles that are in a state of contraction. Both pneumatic and traction splints are intended for very brief periods of use immediately after an injury occurs, until some other form of treatment can be provided.

Cloth and foam splints, called *immobilizers,* are used frequently to limit motion in the area of a painful but healing injury, such as in the neck and knee. This type can be removed for brief periods allowing for dressing and hygiene needs. Velcro or buckle closures permit them to be adjusted to fit a body part of almost any shape and size.

Molded splints are made from plastic, like the one

shown in Figure 26-1. They are used by patients with chronic injuries or diseases when prolonged support and inactivity are necessary to prevent further damage and pain. They maintain the body part in a functional position to prevent contractures and muscle atrophy during the period of disuse.

Applying an Emergency Splint

Whether one is using a manufactured splint or an improvised splint made from common articles in an emergency, several important techniques should be followed:

Avoid changing the position of an injured part of the body even if it appears grossly deformed. Moving damaged structures can increase the severity of the injury.

Leave a high-top shoe or a ski boot in place if an injured ankle is suspected. The footwear can act as a splint to limit movement of the ankle and reduce pain and swelling.

Select a splint or substituted splint material that will not permit movement of the body part once it is applied. Examples that may be adapted for use include flat boards of lumber, tree limbs, broom handles, rolled layers of newspaper, rolled blankets, or pillows.

Apply the splinting device so that it spans the injured area from the joint above the injury to beyond the joint below the injury. For instance, if the lower leg has been injured, the splint should be long enough to restrict movement of the knee and ankle.

Inflate a pneumatic splint to the point that it can be indented only 1.3 cm (1/2 in) with the fingertips. Avoid inflation longer than 30 to 45 minutes, or circulation in the area may be affected.

Use an uninjured area of the body adjacent to the injured part if no other sturdy material is available. For example, an injured arm can be immobilized to the chest; one finger can be secured to the one beside it.

Cover any open wounds with clean material to absorb blood and prevent the entrance of dirt and additional pathogens.

Apply soft material over any area of the body that may be subject to pressure or rubbing by areas on an inflexible splint.

Use tape or wide strips of fabric in several areas to confine the injured part to the splint so it cannot be moved. Narrow cord can create a tourniquet effect, especially if it encircles swelling tissue.

Assess the color and temperature of fingers or toes to evaluate if blood flow is adequate. Loosen the attached device if the digits appear pale, blue, or cold.

Elevate the entire length of the immobilized part, if that is possible, so that the lowest point is higher than the heart. Elevation will reduce the rate of swelling.

Provide for the individual's warmth and safety and seek assistance in transporting the injured person to a health agency.

Using Supportive Devices

While injured body structures are healing, supportive devices are used, thus enabling an individual to move about with less pain and without the need for a more confining device.

Braces

Braces are designed to support weakened structures during weight bearing. For this reason they are made of sturdy materials, such as metal and leather. When custom made for the leg, they are incorporated into a shoe. Some back braces are cloth with metal staves, or strips, that are sewn within the fabric of the brace. The nurse must take care that a back brace is not applied upside down. Any improperly applied or ill-fitting brace can cause discomfort, deformity, and pressure sores.

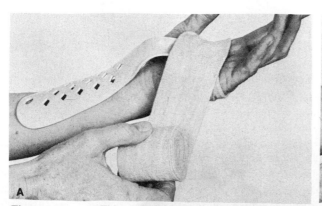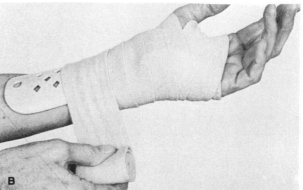

Figure 26-1 (*A*). This patient is securing a molded plastic splint that spans the hand, wrist, and forearm. Notice that the Ace bandage anchors the splint with a circular turn in the palm of the hand. (*B*). The patient proceeds to unroll the bandage up the forearm.

Slings

Slings are muslin binders that elevate and support an injured area. They are frequently used to position an arm across the chest, but they may also be used to suspend a leg when a patient is confined to bed.

Commercial arm slings are available, but they are more costly than triangular pieces of muslin cloth. Slings come in various sizes. A common size for an adult triangular sling is made by cutting a 1 meter (36 to 40 inch) square in half diagonally.

A triangular sling used to support the arm is applied as follows.

1. Place the open triangle on the patient's chest with the base of the triangle along the length of the patient's chest on the unaffected side, as shown in Figure 26-2.
2. Place the upper end of the base of the triangle around the back of the neck on the unaffected side.
3. Place the apex or point of the triangle under the affected arm.
4. Place the lower end of the base of the triangle across the affected arm.
5. Tie the two ends of the base of the triangle in a knot at the side of the neck, as illustrated in Figure 26-3. A knot should not be tied over the cervical spine in back of the neck because it may create pressure on the bony prominences and cause discomfort to the spine.
6. Be sure the hand is higher than the elbow in the sling to prevent swelling in the hand.
7. Fold and secure the material at the elbow on the affected side neatly. A pin may be used behind the sling so that it is out of sight, to secure the material.

A triangular sling is a versatile item. It may be converted

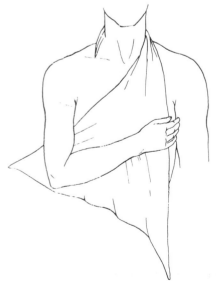

Figure 26-2 The points of a triangular piece of fabric are positioned in these locations prior to fashioning a sling.

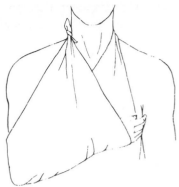

Figure 26-3 When a sling has been properly applied and fastened, the knot is at the side of the neck, the hand is elevated higher than the elbow, and all the loose ends have been secured.

into a cravat binder, shown in Figure 26-4, and used in several different ways. A *cravat binder* is a piece of cloth folded into a strip of a desired width. It may be used as a temporary measure to support a joint, as a tourniquet to control severe bleeding, or as a binder around the head.

Casts

A *cast* is a solid mold of a body part. It is used to immobilize an injured structure that has been placed in correct anatomical position. Casts are used chiefly when an individual has sustained a *fracture,* which is a break in the continuity of a bone. The broken ends of the bone are repositioned when the doctor performs a procedure called a *reduction.* A *closed reduction* means the bone is realigned without making a surgical incision. During an *open reduction,* an incision is made and the bone ends are repositioned under the doctor's direct view. In addition to the use of a cast, sometimes repositioned bone is held in place internally with the use of metal devices, such as nails, wires, screws, pins, or rods.

Types of Casts. There are basically three types of casts. They are classified according to their shape and the area in which they are applied. They are categorized into cylinder casts, body casts, and hip spica casts. The materials and principles involved in cast applications permit many variations in the three general types.

A *cylinder cast* is a rigid mold that encircles an arm or leg, leaving the toes or fingers exposed. It can be applied to enclose varying lengths of an extremity, such as a short leg cast or a long leg cast. However, following the initial reduction, the cast will extend to include joint areas above and below the broken bone. This prevents movement of the repositioned bone ends so that healing will take place with the bone in correct alignment. As healing progresses, the cast may be trimmed or shortened.

A *body cast* is simply a larger form of a cylinder cast. Instead of encircling an extremity, a body cast encircles

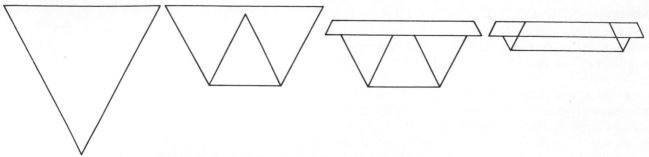

Figure 26-4 Left to right, a cravat is being made from a triangular binder or sling.

the trunk of the body. It generally extends from the nipple line on the chest to the hips. For some individuals with spinal problems, the body cast may extend from the occiput and chin areas to the hips with modifications made for exposing the arms. This type of cast may be cut in two and worn like a clam shell. This design permits one half of the cast to be removed while the patient is lying either prone or supine so that bathing and skin care can be provided.

A *hip spica* is a type of cast that encircles one or both legs and the lower trunk. It is usually used when a fracture has occurred in the femur close to the hip joint. A hip spica may be strengthened by attaching a bar spanning a cast area on one leg to a cast area on the other leg. This type of cast is trimmed in the anal and genital areas to provide room for the elimination of urine and stool. However, the patient is unable to sit during elimination. The nurse must protect the cast from soiling using plastic wrap and provide a fracture bedpan. A hip spica cast is very heavy, hot, and frustrating because it limits movement and changing positions.

Cast Construction. At one time casts were made only from plaster of paris, which was embedded in gauze strips and rolls and hardened as it dried. There have always been disadvantages in using this material. Though plaster casts are inexpensive and become rigid eventually, they are heavy, dry slowly, and soften if they become wet.

Technological advancements have now created alternative substances that are being used as cast materials. Casts are being made of fiberglass and also polyurethane. They are marketed under a variety of names. The chemical substances in these cast materials are incorporated within widely woven rolls that become more porous than plaster, letting air in and moisture out.

These newer cast materials tend to be strong, are lighter in weight, dry within 5 to 15 minutes, and will not soften when wet. Some have mistakenly interpreted this to mean that they could swim and shower with a synthetic cast. Unfortunately, the cast will not decompose but the person's skin underneath may, because the moisture does not evaporate easily. Each of these two materials used in cast construction are more expensive than plaster. For some, the advantages of their use may outweigh the added cost.

Applying a Cast. The nurse prepares the patient and assists the doctor when a cast is applied. The patient should be informed by the doctor that a cast is necessary. If a choice of cast materials is possible, the doctor may permit the patient to select the type that will be used.

Preparing the Skin. Since the skin will be covered for weeks or months, it is important that the skin is clean and protected. The nurse may prepare the skin in the following way:

- Remove clothing that will interfere with the cast application.
- Provide the patient with prescribed pain medication if he is experiencing discomfort.
- Wash the area thoroughly with warm water and soap or detergent. Some agencies use special antimicrobial cleansers to reduce the number of surface organisms.
- Wait to cleanse the area if the patient is uncomfortable and will be eventually anesthetized.
- Note any cuts or abrasions that may become infected once the cast is applied. Under the cast it will be warm, dark, and moist—a perfect environment for pathogen growth.
- Cover the skin with *stockinet,* stretchy fabric that comes knitted in a tube. The purpose of the stockinet is somewhat analogous to wearing stockings inside shoes. It protects the skin and absorbs moisture. Cut the stockinet much longer than the intended length of the cast. It will eventually be folded back making a smooth, cushioned edge at each end of the cast.
- Smooth any wrinkles in the stockinet and make sure it is not too tight.
- Cut thick pieces of felt for placement over and around bony prominences, such as the ankle, knee, elbow, and wrist.
- Wrap the entire area with cotton padding.
- Explain that as a plaster cast is applied, the sensation of heat will be felt. Steam or heat waves may even be seen rising from the surface of the wet cast.

Assisting with Application of the Cast. The nurse should have the following items ready for the doctor: strips and rolls of cast material, a source of water for wetting the cast material, gloves if the doctor prefers, and knife or scissors. The doctor may wish to help himself to the cast materials, wetting them as needed while the nurse maintains the body part in position. At other times special tables with supports and slings may be used to maintain the patient's position. This frees the nurse to anticipate and provide the doctor with wetted cast materials. Synthetic cast materials dry so quickly that once the cast application begins everyone must work quickly and in a coordinated manner.

The nurse must take care when disposing of the water used to wet the plaster rolls and strips. Since the plaster in the water can ruin plumbing pipes, the water should be emptied in a sink that contains a special trap.

Handling and Drying a Wet Cast.

Casts made of the newer synthetic materials dry quickly. Drying of fiberglass casts may be facilitated with the use of a special ultraviolet lamp. These casts become rigid so quickly that the patient may bear weight within 15 to 30 minutes after application.

On the other hand, plaster casts may remain wet for 24 hours to 48 hours depending upon the level of humidity in the air. During this period the cast is vulnerable to becoming misshaped. At worst this could change the alignment of the repositioned bone. At the least, indentations can eventually rub internally and form pressure areas on the skin underneath.

Any wet plaster cast should be supported on pillows so that it is cushioned rather than pressed against a firm surface. The nurse should only use the palms of the hands to move and reposition the cast while it is wet. This technique can be seen in Figure 26-5.

Ordinarily, the air circulation in the room is adequate for drying the layers of plaster. A fan may hasten drying. To facilitate air drying, the cast should not be covered with bed linen or clothing. The patient's position should be changed every few hours to dry all the surfaces and depths of the cast. Plastic liners on pillows protect the pillow from becoming moist and musty, but may interfere with evaporation of water from the cast.

Using heat to dry the cast is not generally advisable. However, if a form of heat is applied, such as with a light within a cradle, it should not be covered nor used for an extended period of time. These precautions should be followed so that the patient will not become burned. Often attempts to use heat to dry the cast result in drying the surface but not the inner areas. This can lead to cracking of the plaster material.

Assessing the Patient Who Has A Cast.

Because most casts are applied after an injury and surgical procedure, the nurse may expect that the area will swell and bleed. These are the two immediate problems about which the nurse must be concerned. Swelling is especially serious since the cast is rigid and will not expand as the area within the cast becomes larger. The cast can have a tourniquet effect. If tissue becomes damaged due to a lack of adequate blood supply, amputation may be necessary. Nerves may also be damaged by a constricting cast. However, neurologic signs are not likely immediately after the cast has been applied. Neurologic assessment is discussed later in Skill Procedure 26-1.

Assessment is somewhat difficult because the nurse will be unable to see directly beneath the cast. However, certain physical assessment techniques may be used to detect early complications in the area where the cast has been applied.

Evaluating Swelling and Circulation.

One assessment technique for determining the extent and effects of swelling and circulation involves performing the blanching test, as the nurse in Figure 26-6 is doing. Swelling affects blood flow. The nurse compares the appearance of and sensation in the fingernails or toes to determine if

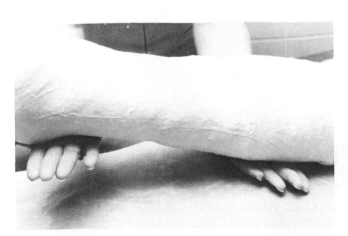

Figure 26-5 A damp cast should be handled with the palms of the hand to help prevent dents and flat spots.

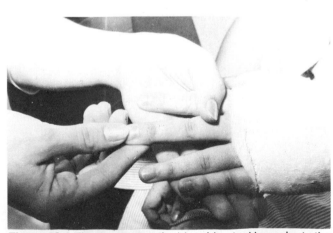

Figure 26-6 The nurse uses the blanching test to evaluate the adequacy of blood flow. The nail is compressed and the rate of color return is noted. The nail in an uncasted area is also assessed and the two are compared. (From Farrell J: Illustrated Guide to Orthopedic Nursing, 3rd ed, p 61. Philadelphia, JB Lippincott, 1986)

circulation is impaired. A radial or pedal pulse may or may not be palpated depending upon the length of the cast. In most cases, the area in which these arteries are located will be covered by the cast. All assessments are compared with duplicate assessments on the same area on the opposite side of the body, if that is possible. If that cannot be done, the nurse must mentally compare the assessment data with similar assessments performed on other individuals who have had casts. This assessment is performed at least every hour, or more frequently, for the first 24 hours after the cast application and then every 4 hours for another 2 to 3 days. After that, assessments should be made at least once on each shift throughout the patient's stay in the health agency. Performing this technique is discussed further in Skill Procedure 26-1.

Detecting and Evaluating Bleeding. Since cast materials are constructed of porous gauze rolls, strips, or tape, it is logical that the cast will absorb blood and other drainage. The volume and the rate of the drainage may be evaluated by inspecting all surfaces of the cast. It is more likely that bleeding will be evident in the area of a surgical incision. However, blood may drain toward the lower surfaces of a cast under the influence of gravity.

The nurse should inspect all surfaces of the cast. Venous and capillary bleeding is characterized by a reddish brown appearance. When blood is observed on the cast, the nurse should circle the drainage on the cast. The circled margin is dated, the time indicated, and the initials of the nurse should appear on the cast. A description of the assessed size of the drainage area should also be noted in the patient's record with related data, such as the patient's blood pressure, pulse rate, and level of consciousness. These data add to the basis for evaluating the significance of the blood loss.

At 1- to 3-hour intervals, the nurse should inspect the previously circled margin and draw another line if the bleeding has extended beyond the previous line. A comment should follow in the nurse's notes as to whether the bleeding line remains the same or has changed.

The nurse should never hesitate to notify a physician if swelling or bleeding continues to increase. In fact, the nurse would be held accountable and more than likely negligent if these observations went unreported and the patient experienced complications. A cast may need to be cut or removed if the patient's safety or life is endangered.

Caring for the Patient Who Has a Cast

Special skills must be used when the patient has a cast. Skill Procedure 26-1 describes nursing measures that may be used during the time that a cast is applied.

Maintaining a Cast

A cast must continue to remain intact and rigid during the full time it is applied. Plaster casts are more likely to weaken, crack, and crumble. At times the only alternative will be to add more strips or rolls of plaster or change the cast completely. The nurse can use various techniques that will maintain the cast or repair it temporarily.

Keeping a Cast Clean. Most casts are either white or semiclear in appearance. Many people, especially children and adolescents, use the cast medium to display signatures, graffiti, and drawings.

With wear, casts are bound to appear soiled. Those who are concerned about the appearance of a soiled cast may be helped by using various measures. Wetting the plaster can weaken the cast. However, the cast can be cleaned with a damp cloth and a little cleanser. It can be whitened with shoe polish used sparingly. An oversized knee sock, leg warmer, or narrow tube knit fabric can be used to cover a cast and add to its appearance.

Repairing Cast Edges. Cast edges may become sharp and cause skin abrasions or pressure sores. If a cast edge begins to crumble, it can irritate the skin within the cast. This may tempt the patient to insert objects for scratching. The nurse can repair cast edges by applying petals made from tape. The steps for petaling a cast can be found in Skill Procedure 26-2.

Replacing a Cast Window. Sometimes it may become necessary to cut a square piece, called a *window,* out of a cast. A window facilitates inspection of an area without removing the entire cast. An example of a window is shown in Figure 26-11. A window may also permit various treatments, such as application of medication or a dressing, to be performed.

Once a window has been cut, the piece of plaster should not be thrown away. It should be replaced in its original site and secured with tape or a length of roller bandage. If the windowed area remains open, the tissue inside has a tendency to bulge through the window. This may lead to uneven pressure on the skin, possible skin breakdown, or pressure on nerves.

Removing a Cast

A cast may need to be removed or split as an emergency measure if swelling becomes severe. The cast may also be removed when it will be replaced by another or when sufficient healing has occurred.

The physician usually uses an electric cast cutter to separate and remove the cast. In an emergency, the nurse could wet the cast and cut through the softened areas with sturdy scissors. In some agencies, there may be a written

Skill Procedure 26-1. Providing Basic Cast Care

Suggested Action	**Reason for Action**
Remove residue of plaster from the skin with a wet wash cloth.	When plaster is used, it is likely that it may drip and stick to various areas of the skin. It is especially annoying to a patient when it remains between toes, where it often cannot be reached.
Elevate the extremity in a cast, as one authority states, "the higher the better." Each distal joint should be higher than the preceding one. Pillows with a waterproof covering or a sling, like the one illustrated in Figure 26-7, may be used to help elevate a cast.	Elevating an area in a cast helps promote venous circulation and prevent problems of tissue edema and pressure caused by swelling under the cast.

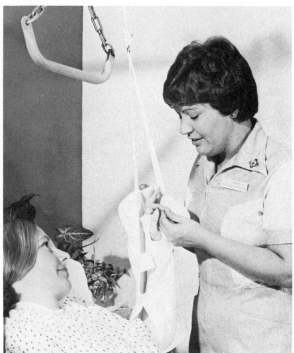

Figure 26-7 Slings may be used to suspend and elevate extremities that have been placed in a cast. The arm is well elevated at a comfortable height and allows the patient some degree of movement in bed.

Place ice bags next to a wet cast, especially over the area of an incision, to help control swelling and bleeding.	Cold causes vasoconstriction, which reduces the loss of fluid from within capillaries into the tissue spaces.
Expose the cast directly to the air.	A cast produces heat as it dries. If the cast is covered, moisture accumulates and evaporation is delayed.
Do not allow anything to rest on a wet cast and do not allow a wet cast to be placed on a flat, hard surface. Pillows are used under a cast, allowing it to dry on a soft surface. Bed linens should not be allowed to rest on the cast. A wet cast should be handled with the palms of the hands, not the fingers.	A wet cast dents and flattens easily. This is likely to cause pressure on tissues under the cast in dented and flattened areas. Handling a wet cast with the fingers causes dents in the cast.

(continued)

Skill Procedure 26-1. Continued

Suggested Action	**Reason for Action**
Support bed linens over a cradle or high footboard if the patient with a leg cast feels chilled. Linens can also be supported on straps extended from opposite sides of the bed between side rails.	Linens may become moist when they are in contact with a wet cast. As long as linens do not interfere with air circulation around the cast, the nurse may cover the patient.
Change the patient's position every 1 to 2 hours.	Repositioning helps to expose all the surfaces to air in order to dry the cast evenly and completely.
Use heat to facilitate drying a plaster cast only in rare circumstances. *Do not overdo.* Cradles with lights should not be covered with linens in this situation.	The heat may dry the surface but not the interior, leading to cracking. The skin under the cast may burn if too much heat is used. Covering a cradle over a wet cast may not allow moisture to evaporate easily.
Watch for signs and symptoms of excess pressure on tissues under the cast.	A cast is a hard, rigid object that can interfere with blood flow, nerve function, and skin integrity.
The following assessment techniques should be used frequently:	Frequent assessments help in identifying problems before they escalate.
1. Use inspection and palpation to test for swelling, paleness, cyanosis, and coolness, of the skin.	These signs and symptoms are typical of poor circulation. It could be due to a cast that is too tight if the opposite area of the body does not appear similar.
2. Pinch the nailbeds and then release the pressure to test for the return of blood flow into the nail. Perform the same assessment on the opposite hand or foot.	The color in the nailbeds should go from white to pink immediately when circulation is good. The color change in patients with dark skin is less pronounced but observable.
3. Take pulse rates near casted areas to the extent the cast permits.	If no pulse can be felt, the cast may be interfering with arterial flow, which must bring oxygen to cells and tissue.
4. Ask the patient if there is sensation in the fingers or the toes. Ask the patient to describe any unusual feelings, such as numbness or tingling. Touch the exposed skin areas with objects of varying temperatures and textures if the patient describes unusual changes. This helps validate the ability of the patient to identify and discriminate sensations.	Pressure on nerves, cells deprived of oxygen, or tissue spaces filled with fluid may dull or alter the sensations a patient feels.
5. Ask the patient to move his fingers and toes to test for movement. It is insufficient to check only a few fingers or toes or for him just to be able to wiggle them. The nurse in Figure 26-8 is assessing the patient's ability to move all the fingers on the arm that has been placed in a cast.	Normally, all toes and fingers should move with ease. The patient should be able to flex and extend the fingers or toes. If not all move or the movements are not normal, there could be pressure on one or more nerves that could result in permanent deformity.
Watch for spots on the cast due to bleeding. Venous blood normally is dark red, then turns brown, and stops within a relatively short time.	Some bleeding can be expected after an open reduction. The nurse uses assessment to determine if the patient is losing arterial blood or if the blood loss is excessive.
Draw a ring around an area of drainage on the cast and add the date, time, and initials.	Encircling a stain on a cast with a line makes it simple to compare findings when drainage continues.
Feel for hot spots over the surface of the cast.	When inflammation is present from phlebitis or a pressure sore, the cast generally feels warmer in the affected area than other parts of the cast.
Inspect for drainage, other than blood, due to an infection or necrotic tissue from an advanced pressure sore. Sniff the cast edge if an odor is not obvious. If an infection or sloughing tissue is present, the drainage is more likely to be brownish in color and will have a foul odor.	An infection can lead to serious weakening or delayed healing if it extends to the depth of the bone. A pressure sore may extend more widely and deeply if the cast remains in place. The earlier these signs are detected and treated, the better the outcome will be.

(continued)

Skill Procedure 26-1. Continued

Suggested Action   **Reason for Action**

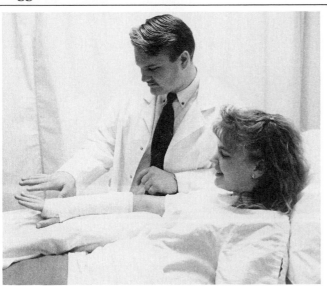

Figure 26-8 The patient is asked to demonstrate motion in all fingers and to extend them.

Perform and document all these assessments regularly. A patient with a new cast should be assessed at least every hour for 24 hours and then every 4 hours for another 2 or 3 days. After that, the cast should be checked several times a day. Less frequent checking of a cast may be safe in *some* situations. Report *promptly* when abnormal signs and symptoms are noted.

Nurses are legally responsible for monitoring the condition of a patient in a cast. The consequences of delaying or not reporting significant assessments are too serious to allow one to take that responsibility lightly.

Change a casted patient's position frequently. Even patients with small casts tend to move little and must be encouraged to move about as much as permitted.

Encouraging mobility helps to prevent the many problems that are associated with the disuse syndrome, as described in Chapter 18.

Turn a patient to his unaffected side when moving him. Support a dry cast under joint areas.

Handling a cast under a joint gives good support and helps to prevent cracking the cast if it is wet or weak.

Use range-of-motion exercises for unaffected joints, and use a trapeze on the bed when possible to promote activity. Isometric exercises may be used for strengthening muscle groups under a cast.

Exercising not only promotes well-being but is also important to keep muscles in shape for eventual ambulation or activities of daily living.

Elevate the head of the bed on blocks when a patient is in a body cast. Provide prism glasses to help him read.

Elevation helps breathing, facilitates digestion and elimination, and helps him to be stimulated by activity in the environment. Prism glasses permit a patient to read while lying flat.

Inspect the edges of the cast for rough areas or chipping plaster.

Rough areas can cause skin abrasion or breakdown. Crumbs of plaster can fall into a cast and cause discomfort and itching.

Apply petals of tape to rough and crumbling cast edges in the manner described in Skill Procedure 26-2.

Petals are trimmed strips of tape inserted over the edges of a cast to smooth and repair cast edges temporarily to protect the integrity of the skin.

Rub skin areas near the edge of the cast with alcohol. Apply lotion sparingly to exposed areas if the skin appears dry. Caution the patient not to insert objects, such as straws, eating utensils, bobby pins, combs, toothbrushes, and coat hangers when the skin itches.

Alcohol helps to keep the skin clean and in good condition. Lotion tends to build up and become sticky. Objects inserted under a cast may fall inside or cause an alteration in the integrity of the skin.

(continued)

Skill Procedure 26-1. Continued

Suggested Action	Reason for Action
Remove crumbs and debris within the cast with a vacuum cleaner hose, hair dryer hose on a cool setting, or with a bulb syringe.	Air may be used to blow particles out or move them so that the patient does not experience as much discomfort or itching. Air will not damage the skin.
Protect the cast from becoming wet when tending to hygiene needs such as bathing or elimination. Use plastic wrap in the perineal area.	When a plaster cast absorbs moisture, the cast becomes soft. Plastic and plastic wrap are barriers to water and other forms of liquid, such as urine.
Provide general nursing care that is conducive to well-being, such as providing stimuli, movement, personal hygiene, nourishing diet with abundant sources of calcium for healing, sufficient fluids, comfort, and adequate rest and sleep.	Keeping the body in good physical condition promotes healing and helps to reduce the potential for complications.

Skill Procedure 26-2. Petaling a Cast Edge

Suggested Action	Reason for Action
Trim any frayed areas from the edge of the cast.	Loose and hanging pieces will not feel comfortable even if covered by petals of tape.
Stretch the stockinet from under the cast so that it extends higher above the cast edge.	The stockinet should not be allowed to slip beneath or become wrinkled inside the cast.
Fold the stretched stockinet over the trimmed cast edge and secure it in place temporarily with a strip of tape.	The stockinet may slip back within the cast if it is not secured in place.
Cut several strips of 1- or 2-inch-wide adhesive tape.	Adhesive tape is structurally tougher and more durable than other types of tape.
Trim the end of the strips to form curves or points, as shown in Figure 26-9. Some nurses prefer to trim both ends of the tape.	The trimmed end(s) will fit the contour of a circle more easily without wrinkling than a flat edge on the tape. It is more important that the inner side of the tape does not wrinkle than the part that will extend over the outside of the cast.

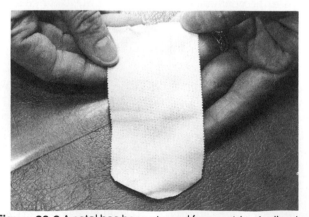

Figure 26-9 A petal has been shaped from a strip of adhesive.

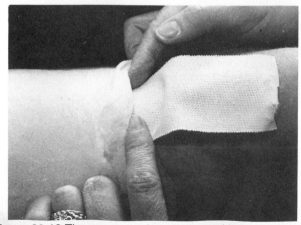

Figure 26-10 The rounded edge of the petal is placed under the cast's edge. The opposite end is brought up over the edge of the cast.

Slip half of the trimmed end of the tape on the inside of the cast with the sticky side facing the stockinet as the nurse is doing in Figure 26-10.	The side that contains the adhesive must be applied to the cast and not the skin.

(continued)

Skill Procedure 26-2. Continued

Suggested Action	Reason for Action
Press the tape to make contact with the inner side of the cast. Take care that it remains smooth.	If the tape does not remain flat, it can cause irritation, discomfort, and even contribute to forming a pressure sore.
Hold the inserted end in place while bringing the opposite end over the edge of the cast. Press it into place.	Secured tape will be less likely to come loose.
Repeat using as many strips as necessary next to one another to cover the entire cast edge or just the rough and crumbling areas.	This technique acquired its name because, when finished, the tips of the tape resemble the petals of a flower extending from its center.

policy approving the use of a cast cutter by a qualified nurse.

A cast cutter is a noisy instrument that can be frightening to a patient. There is a natural expectation that an instrument sharp enough to cut a cast would be sharp enough to lacerate several layers of skin and tissue. However, when used properly, an electric cast cutter should leave the skin intact.

When the cast is removed, the cutter is moved along medial and lateral sides of the cast in order to bivalve it. A *bivalved cast* is one that has been split in two. After one-half of the plaster shell has been removed, the stockinet and whatever padding was used prior to the cast application can be cut away with scissors.

Care Following Cast Removal

The patient should be prepared for the expected change in the appearance of the body part that has been enclosed as well as the potential decrease in functional use. Many assume that the body part will look the same and be capable of its previous motion and strength. That, however, is rarely the case.

The muscle will usually have become smaller and

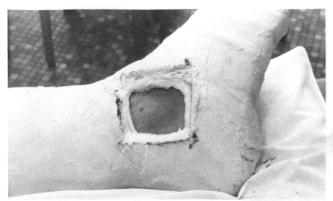

Figure 26-11 A square window has been cut from a cast to assess the skin underneath. (From Farrell J: Illustrated Guide to Orthopedic Nursing, 3rd ed, p 62. Philadelphia, JB Lippincott, 1986)

weaker with the period of disuse. The skin will be pale and waxy looking. It may contain scales or patches of dead skin. The joints may be limited in their range of motion.

The skin may be washed as usual with soapy warm water but the semiattached areas of loose skin should not be forcibly removed. Lotion applied to the skin may add moisture and prevent rough edges from catching on clothing.

The area may swell once the support of the cast has been removed. Therefore, the patient may need to elevate a leg periodically or continue to wear a sling while upright. Crutches, a cane, or a brace may be needed until muscle strength and joint movement return with gradual progressive exercise or physical therapy.

Caring for the Patient in Traction

Traction is the application of equipment to the body to provide pull and counterpull on a particular part of the skeletal system. The pull is achieved by using weights in the form of sandbags or metal disks; the counterpull is almost always produced exclusively by the patient's own body weight.

Traction is usually applied and used while a patient is confined in bed. Occasionally it may be possible to apply traction within the construction of a cast. This is the exception rather than the rule. Traction is generally applied by using slings, ropes, pulleys, and weights. The nurse must be aware of the various types of traction, the principles for maintaining their effect, and measures that will ensure that the patient receives proper nursing care.

Types of Traction

The three general types of traction are manual traction, skin traction, and skeletal traction.

Manual traction is the pull on a body part using an individual's hands and muscular strength. This type of traction is most often used during the reduction of a fracture. It may also be used when replacing a dislocated bone end into its original position within a joint.

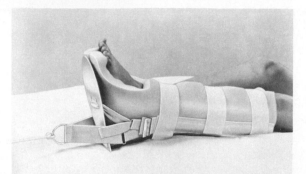

Figure 26-12 Buck's traction can be applied to one or both legs. The nurse must especially assess mobility and sensation of the involved leg and toes, since the function of the peroneal nerve may be affected by the compression of traction equipment. (Courtesy of Patient Care Systems, Division of Zimmer, Charlotte, NC.)

Skin traction is a pull applied indirectly to the skeletal system by attaching equipment and weight to the skin. There are various names for commonly applied forms of skin traction. Figure 26-12 shows a leg in Buck's traction. A child who does not weigh very much could not provide much counterpull with this type of skin traction. To compensate for that factor, an infant or young child may be placed in Bryant's traction, shown in Figure 26-13, to take advantage of the additional influence of gravity. Figure 26-14 shows another type of skin traction. It is applied to the skin at the chin and back of the neck but its effect is intended for the musculoskeletal structures around the cervical vertebrae.

Skeletal traction is a pull applied directly to the skeletal system by attaching wires, pins, or tongs into or through the bone. Figure 26-15 shows tongs inserted into burr

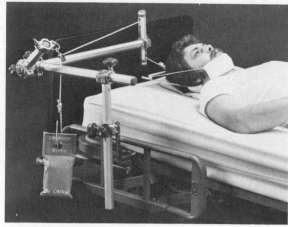

Figure 26-14 A cervical halter, a type of skin traction, is being used on this patient. Any use of a pillow or elevation of the top end of the bed frame must be specified by the physician in a written medical order. (Courtesy of Patient Care Systems, Division of Zimmer, Charlotte, NC.)

holes within superficial layers of the cranium. They are not deep enough to enter the area of the meninges beneath the cranium. Figure 26-16 is an example of skeletal traction in which a wire has been inserted through a bone in the lower leg. The numbers of ropes, pulleys, and weights may appear frightening to the patient, his family, and even the nurse. However, most of this equipment, with the exception of what is attached to the bone, is being used to suspend the leg and balance the pull when the patient moves horizontally or vertically in bed.

A traction cart, similar to a dressing cart, is usually available on nursing units. It contains the various equipment that would be needed when assisting with the application of traction.

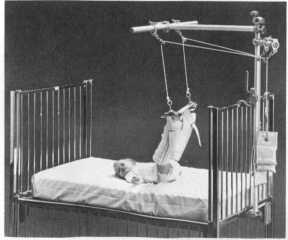

Figure 26-13 Bryant's traction is used in children who are 1 to 3 years old or who weigh less than 18 kg (40 lb). It must always be applied to both legs, even if pathology only exists in one. (Courtesy of Patient Care Systems, Division of Zimmer, Charlotte, NC.)

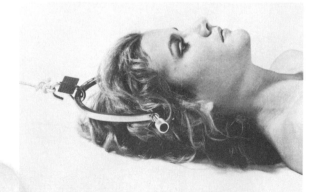

Figure 26-15 These tongs are located within burr holes in the cranium. If they should become displaced, the nurse should apply manual traction to the head and neck to prevent motion until assistance arrives and a replacement can be made. (Courtesy of Patient Care Systems, Division of Zimmer, Charlotte, NC.)

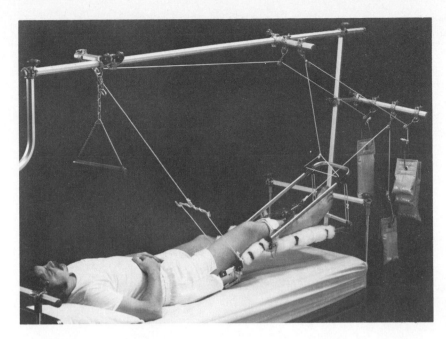

Figure 26-16 Skeletal traction is applied through a bone. A wire has been inserted through this patient's proximal tibia. The insertion site serves as a potential port of entry for pathogens (Courtesy of Patient Care Systems, Division of Zimmer, Charlotte, NC.)

Maintaining Traction

The nurse must make various focus assessments to determine that the pull and counterpull are being maintained. The nurse should:

- Evaluate if the directions of the pull and the counterpull are in opposite but straight lines.
- Check that the patient or other objects are not interfering with the ratio of pull to counterpull. This may occur if the patient rests his weight against the lower area of the bed frame. Bed linen or blankets may also get caught in the traction line and interfere with the ratio of pull to counterpull.

- Examine all the ropes to determine that they move freely through the pulleys.
- Inspect the weights to determine that they are the amount ordered by the physician and that they hang free from the floor.

The patient in traction is relatively immobile because he is confined to bed. The nurse must provide care while maintaining the mechanical equipment. Various observations and actions must be carried out to ensure that complications do not occur. Skill Procedure 26-3 may be used as a general guide for the care of patients in traction.

Skill Procedure 26-3. Caring for the Patient in Traction

Suggested Action	Reason for Action
Inspect the mechanical equipment used to apply traction.	All the equipment should be in good repair and applied securely to the bed and the patient.
Provide a trapeze if the type of traction allows the patient to raise his body weight.	A trapeze may facilitate exercise, self-care and nursing care.
Position or reposition the patient so that his body is in the center of the bed and the body part in traction is in the same line of pull.	The body must be maintained in good alignment and provide adequate counterpull in relation to the pull of the traction.
Avoid tucking top sheets, blankets, or bedspreads beneath the mattress.	Coverings can interfere with the pull produced by the traction equipment.
Instruct the patient and assigned nursing personnel as to the length of time the patient must be attached to the traction equipment.	Traction is almost always meant to be applied continuously. Exceptions may be made when a patient in skin traction receives physical therapy.

(continued)

Skill Procedure 26-3. Continued

Suggested Action	**Reason for Action**
Identify the positions the patient may assume.	Most patients must lie flat and cannot even roll to either side without changing the direction of pull.
Wash the posterior areas of the body and rub bony prominences by depressing the mattress enough to insert a hand.	The patient should not turn to the side. Some types of traction may permit the patient to raise himself off the bed by using a trapeze.
Make the bed by removing bottom sheets from the head to the foot of the bed. Remake the bed by applying the linens in the reverse direction.	The technique for making an occupied bed must be modified since the traction patient cannot roll from side to side.
Use some type of pressure-relieving device on the bed, such as one of the examples discussed in Chapter 20.	Being restricted to a supine position creates the potential for pressure sores over the scapulae and coccyx.
Apply elbow and heel protectors, if necessary.	Friction and shearing forces may be reduced, thereby decreasing the potential for skin breakdown.
Omit using a pillow if the patient is in neck or head traction, unless specifically ordered by the physician.	Elevating the head may alter the line of pull.
Use a fracture bedpan for bowel elimination if elevating the hips alters the line of pull.	A fracture bedpan can be inserted without appreciably raising the patient's hips off the bed.
Encourage active range-of-motion and isometric and isotonic exercise as much as possible.	Body areas that are unrestricted by traction should be kept flexible and in good tone. Isometric exercise may be performed on the areas where motion is restricted.
Encourage frequent dorsiflexion of any unrestricted lower extremities.	It may be impossible to provide a footboard because it may interfere with the ratio of pull to counterpull.
Inspect the skin where pins, wires, or tongs have been inserted. Look for redness, tenderness, swelling, and drainage.	Piercing the skin alters the skin's barrier to organisms. Pathogens may begin colonizing open skin areas and can then extend into the bone.
Cleanse the skin areas around the insertion points of skeletal traction using soap or an antimicrobial solution.	Cleansing removes the numbers of organisms present around an open area. Antimicrobial agents interfere with pathogen growth.
Apply and change dressings around skeletal traction insertion sites.	Dressings may be used to cover open areas and maintain antimicrobial agents next to the skin.
Cover any sharp points on traction equipment, such as the ends of pins, wires, or tongs, with pieces of cork, eraser, or folded gauze squares.	Sharp points may scratch or puncture caregivers, or tear clothing and linen.
Assess the color, temperature, and mobility of all areas where traction is applied.	If applied improperly, traction may interfere with the function of nerves and circulation of blood.
Insert padding material inside slings if they become wrinkled.	A wrinkled sling may occlude blood flow through an area or lead to skin breakdown. Padding helps to cushion and distribute the pressure.
Record the frequency of bowel movements and request an order for a stool softener or other measure to assist with bowel elimination when necessary.	Immobility and embarrassment about using a bedpan can easily lead to constipation.
Move the patient, bed and all, out into the hall or lounge area. Rearrange the position of the bed within the room.	Monotony and confinement can lead to depression due to social isolation.
Allow the patient to schedule his own activities and decorate the room with assorted items. Be flexible in enforcing rules regarding visitors.	When a patient feels some control over his life and lifestyle, depression may not be quite so severe.

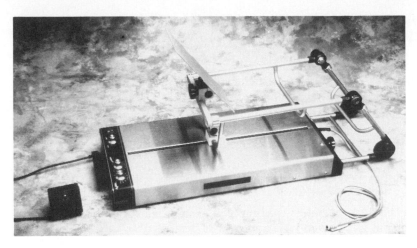

Figure 26-17 The CPM machine slides a preset distance forward and backward within the middle track. The movement causes flexion and extension of the joint. (Stryker Model 326-1 Leg Exerciser, Courtesy of Stryker Instruments, Kalamazoo, MI.)

Using a Continuous Passive Motion Machine

Many individuals whose mobility and comfort have been compromised by arthritis undergo artificial joint replacement surgery. Postoperative exercise is essential to restore function. However, pain often interferes with active exercise among even the most cooperative patients. As a result of discomfort, many resist achieving the degree of motion, frequency, or duration of prescribed exercise. Now, however, postoperative recovery and rehabilitation are being improved with the use of a continuous passive motion (CPM) machine shown in Figure 26-17.

A *CPM machine* is an electrical device that passively exercises the joint. The machine can be used almost immediately after surgery. It can be adjusted to repeatedly move the joint a preset number of degrees of flexion and back to extension again. Machines can produce anywhere from 0° to 110° of motion 2 to 10 times per minute. Initially, the machine settings are regulated at very low speeds and degrees of movement. It is common to begin with 5° or 10° of flexion cycling 2 times per minute. The adjustments are progressively increased each subsequent day as the patient's tolerance builds. Skill procedure 26-4 describes how to use a CPM machine.

Several advantages have been identified with the use of a CPM machine. Besides restoring and increasing range of motion, the movement prevents pooling of venous blood. Reducing stasis of blood decreases the risk of forming blood clots. Wound healing is accelerated by facilitating the circulation of synovial fluid about the joint. Using the machine tends to speed the time when active exercise and weight bearing can begin.

The CPM machine is also being used in burn rehabilitation. Burn patients generally have normal joint structure and function. However, they frequently develop loss of joint flexibility and movement, when scar tissue causes skin contraction and muscle shortening. Exercise limits these undesirable consequences of the healing process. Like orthopedic patients, the burn patient's active exercise is often not sufficient or frequent enough to provide optimal results. The CPM machine can supplement or substitute for active exercise.

Suggested Measures Related to Mechanical Immobilization in Selected Situations

When the Patient Is an Infant or Child

Carefully assess an infant or small child who has just had a plaster cast applied. The heat produced by a drying cast can alter a small individual's body temperature in a short amount of time.

When the cast extends to the perineal area, protect it well with plastic material to help keep the cast clean, dry, and free of odors when the child cannot control elimination.

Help children adjust to wearing a cast by making it attractive. Most children enjoy drawing or coloring pictures on the cast. A foot cast may be colored to look like a sneaker, and so on.

Check a child in traction frequently. His smaller body weight and increased activity level may lead to improper positioning.

Provide and change mobiles or other visual stimuli frequently to reduce sensory deprivation.

Help parents to select safe toys that will stimulate and hold a child's attention. Pull-string toys that randomly reproduce sounds or words are examples that may be useful.

Take special precautions when helping an immobilized child to eat. A supine position can interfere with swallowing and digestion. Aspiration of food is also a potential risk.

Skill Procedure 26-4. Using a Continuous Passive Motion (CPM) Machine

Suggested Action	Reason for Action
Explain the purpose, application, and use of the CPM machine to the patient.	Keeping a patient informed reduces anxiety and promotes cooperation.
Develop a schedule with the patient to use the machine for at least six periods per day.	Exercise should alternate with periods of rest and the performance of other daily activities such as hygiene, elimination, active exercise, and progressive ambulation.
Assess the patient's need for analgesic medication before using the CPM machine.	Pain is easier to control before it intensifies with exercise.
Instruct the patient on techniques for muscle relaxation and pain control such as deep breathing, listening to audiotapes, watching television, or applying an ice bag.	The effect of medication can be augmented or substituted with nonpharmacologic techniques. Narcotic analgesics depress respirations and increase the risk of pulmonary complications.
Secure a length of sheepskin or soft flannel cloth onto the horizontal bars of the CPM machine to form a sling.	The sling elevates and supports the leg while using the machine.
Assess for the presence and quality of peripheral pulses, capillary refill, edema, temperature, sensation, and mobility of the toes in the affected extremity.	The nurse is accountable for assessing the cardiovascular and neurologic condition of the operative extremity. Abnormalities should be reported before using the CPM machine.
Compare neurovascular assessments with those in the unaffected extremity.	Similar findings may indicate deficits that existed before the operative procedure.
Empty any wound drainage container. Change or reinforce the dressing.	Motion tends to increase drainage from the wound, especially in the early postoperative period.
Position the patient flat or slightly elevate the head of the bed.	The patient may tolerate the exercise longer if in a comfortable position.
Place the CPM machine on the bed and position the patient's foot so it rests against the support plate.	The foot should be supported in a neutral position avoiding plantar flexion.
Check that the knee joint corresponds to the hinge at the top of the frame. Figure 26-18 illustrates correct positioning.	The machine must be adjusted to bend and straighten the leg at the knee joint.

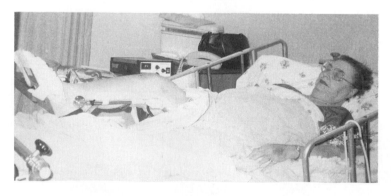

Figure 26-18 A patient who has had a total knee replacement uses a CPM machine. The monitor displays the degree of flexion produced by the machine.

Use Velcro or canvas straps to secure the leg within the fabric cradle of the machine.	Straps ensure that the leg will not roll from or drop out of the machine causing pain or trauma.
Adjust the machine to begin exercising the joint at a low degree of motion and cycles per minute.	Low settings are used initially each time the machine is used to minimize discomfort and gradually increase the patient's tolerance for movement.

(continued)

Skill Procedure 26-4. Continued

Suggested Action	Reason for Action
Turn on the machine and observe the patient's response to the passive movement.	Exercise may need to be postponed temporarily if analgesia has not taken effect yet.
Readjust the alignment of the leg or position of the machine for optimal comfort.	Minor repositioning may enhance the patient's comfort and tolerance of the exercise.
Gradually increase the degree of motion and cycles per minute until reaching the prescribed amount.	Beginning each use of the machine at the lowest settings allows time to adapt before reaching the current day's goal.
Remind the patient to take deep breaths every hour.	Secretions tend to pool with infrequent changes of position. Atelectasis occurs because of hypoventilation.
At the end of a period of exercise, turn the machine off with the leg in an extended position.	It is easier to support and remove the leg while it is in an extended position.
Release the straps from around the leg. Support the joints beneath the knee and ankle and lift the leg from the cradle.	Joint support reduces pain during movement.
Remove the machine from the bed. Encourage the patient to perform isometric and active exercises.	Active exercises are more easily performed once the joint has been limbered through passive exercise.
Record the length of time the patient used the CPM machine and the maximum degree of flexion and cycles per minute.	Appropriate documentation aids in evaluating the progress of the patient.

Caution children who begin progressive ambulation once a cast or traction is removed to do so slowly. Falling can lead to reinjury.

When the Patient Is Elderly

Selectively group patients of similar ages. Long-term confinement can be emotionally distressing when there are extremes in interests or lifestyles among those who must share a room.

Implement preventive measures to maintain skin integrity early during the period of mechanical immobilization. Skin breakdown is more easily prevented than treated.

Encourage an elderly person to perform as many of the activities of daily living as possible. Aging individuals are especially depressed by continuing losses of independence.

Provide a variety of methods for orienting patients, such as large numbered calendars and clocks. When one day is so similar to the next, a patient may become temporarily disoriented to the date and time.

Maintain arm strength by encouraging various upper extremity exercises. The elderly may become extremely weak with prolonged immobilization, which may slow eventual ambulation efforts.

Anticipate that an elderly person may require home care, delivered meals, or extended care in a nursing home or adult foster care home. Begin discussing referrals early if the family cannot provide the care following discharge.

Applicable Nursing Diagnoses

Nurses who care for mechanically immobilized patients commonly identify these nursing diagnoses.
* Altered Tissue Perfusion
* High Risk for Injury
* High Risk for Disuse Syndrome
* High Risk for Impaired Skin Integrity
* Impaired Physical Mobility
* Activity Intolerance
* Bathing/Hygiene Self-Care Deficit
* Pain

Nursing Care Plan 26-1 has been developed to illustrate the nursing process applied to a patient with Impaired Physical Mobility. NANDA (1989) defines this diagnostic category as, "A state in which the individual experiences a limitation of ability for independent physical movement."

NURSING CARE PLAN

26-1. Impaired Physical Mobility

Assessment	**Subjective Data**
	States, "I wish I could just get up and move around. My hip hurts and I feel so scared about walking."
	Objective Data
	70-year-old man admitted for a L. total hip replacement done on 2/7. Must maintain limited flexion of operative hip and continuous abduction of operative leg. Scheduled for physical therapy instruction on performing a three-point partial weight-bearing gait 2/10.
Diagnosis	Impaired Physical Mobility related to restricted positioning, limited weight bearing, pain, and fear.
Plan	**Goal**
	The patient will ambulate 6 feet with the assistance of a walker by 2/10.

Orders: 2/9

1. Instruct and supervise dorsiflexion, plantar flexion, and quad-setting exercises of both legs q 1 hour while awake.
2. Maintain abduction wedge between legs to keep knees apart at all times while in bed.
3. Keep bed flat or with slight elevation (30°–45°) of head.
4. Encourage use of PCA pump at frequent intervals to control pain.
5. Transfer from bed to standing position at the bedside following these directions:
   a. Slide affected L. leg to edge of bed; remove abduction wedge.
   b. Have patient use trapeze or elbows and hands to slide buttocks and legs perpendicular to bed. Remind to avoid leaning forward and praise efforts at moving.
   c. Lower unaffected R. foot to floor and help with lowering affected L. foot keeping knees apart.
   d. Apply safety belt around waist.
   e. Brace feet and pull forward on belt.
   f. Stand at bedside putting only partial weight on L. leg.
   g. Reverse actions for returning to bed. ———————————— D. FENTON, RN

Implementation (Documentation)

2/9

	0730	Positioned from back to R. side with abduction wedge between legs. F. CLINTON, LPN
	0930	Positioned on back with head of bed raised 45° for breakfast. Active isotonic and isometric exercises done. Assisted with bathing legs and back. Having sharp, throbbing pain in L. hip. Encouraged to use PCA pump. Pain reduced following administration of morphine by PCA pump. ———————— F. CLINTON, LPN
	1000	Assisted to transfer out of bed and stand at bedside following procedure outlined in written plan of care. ———————————— F. CLINTON, LPN

Evaluation (Documentation)

	1030	Follows directions well when transferring from bed. Needs frequent reminding to lean backward. Alternated full weight bearing on R. leg with partial weight bearing on L. States, "That was easier than I imagined." Assisted back to bed keeping knees apart and hips slightly flexed. Abduction splint reapplied. ————————————————————————————— F. CLINTON, LPN

Teaching Suggestions Related to Mechanical Immobilization

All patients should understand the purposes of the treatment and the methods for maintaining the equipment. Many teaching suggestions have already been described throughout this text. When the patient will be leaving the health agency and providing self-care, the importance of comprehensive teaching becomes a priority for preventing complications.

Identify foods that are a source of complete protein. Indicate the type and amounts of foods that will supply at least three servings from the milk group each day, and foods that are sources of vitamin D. Bone healing requires additional nutrients and calcium, and the body requires vitamin D to use calcium.

Discourage patients from snacking frequently on high-calorie foods. It is easy to add additional weight while physical activity is restricted. Weight gain can cause a body cast to become tight. Added weight may increase the stress on weak joints, muscles, or healing bones once mobility is resumed.

Patients who are discharged wearing a cast need written and oral instructions about how to keep the cast clean and dry. They should be taught very carefully about symptoms they can expect to experience and which ones should be reported *promptly* if they occur. Patients sent home with wet casts are especially in need of instructions about how to detect evidence of excessive pressure from casts and how to care for their casts.

Teach the patient to avoid getting his cast wet. Good protection from rain and from water may be obtained by placing waterproof material around the cast. A hair dryer on a warm setting works well when a small part of the cast accidentally becomes wet.

Provide phone numbers of the nursing unit, emergency room, or doctor's office for the patient or family members. Explain that they should call promptly if any untoward signs or symptoms appear.

Bibliography

Birdsall C: How do you use the continuous passive motion device? Am J Nurs 86(6):657–658, 1986

Ceccio CM, Horsosz JE: Teaching the elderly amputee to meet the world. RN Magazine 51(9):70–72, 74, 76–77, 1988

Ceccio CM: Rx: Home care. Keeping pin sites problem-free. RN Magazine 51(2):70, 1988

Continuous passive motion, an innovative concept enhancing the healing process of bone fractures. Canadian Operating Room Nursing Journal 7(6):14–15, 1989

Feller NG, Stroup K, Christian L: Helping staff nurses become mini-specialists . . . cast care. Am J Nurs 89(7):991–992, 1989

Frary TN: Tips on cast application. Journal of the American Academy of Physician Assistants 2(1):64–66, 1989

Hansell MJ: Fractures and the healing process. Orthopedic Nursing 7(1):43–50, 1988

Jones IH: Making sense of traction. Nursing Times 86(23):39–41, 1990

Jones–Walton P: Effects of pin care on pin reactions in adults with extremity fracture treated with skeletal traction and external fixation. Orthopedic Nursing 7(4):29–33, 1988

Keenan K: Clinical validation of the etiologies and defining characteristics of the nursing diagnosis impaired mobility. 8th Conference Classification of Nursing Diagnosis Proceedings ():291–295, 1989

Krug BM: The hip: Nursing fracture patients to full recovery. RN Magazine 52(4):56–61, 1989

Lessons from a patient . . . the immobile patient. AD Nurse 2(6):11–13, 1988

McGough CE: Introduction to CPM . . . continuous passive motion. J Burn Care Rehabil 9(5):494–495, 1988

Milde FK: Impaired physical mobility. Journal of Gerontological Nursing 14(3):20–24, 38–40, 1988

Morris L, Kraft S, Tessem S, Reinisch S: Nursing the patient in traction. RN Magazine 51(1):26–31, 1988

Morris L, Kraft S, Tessem S, Reinisch S: Special care for skeletal traction. RN Magazine 51(2):24–29, 1988

Olson B, Ustanko L: Self-care needs of patients in the halo brace. Orthopedic Nursing 9(1):27–33, 52, 1990

Peters VJ, Fox JM: Knee surgery clears a hurdle. RN Magazine 51(7):20–25, 1988

Redheffer G: Treating wounds on the scene *part 1*. Nursing 19(7):51–57, 1989

Redheffer G: Treating wounds on the scene *part 2*. Nursing 19(8):47–51, 1989

Redheffer GM, Bailey M: Assessing and splinting fractures. Nursing 19(6):51–59, 1989

Rubin M: The physiology of bed rest. Am J Nurs 88(1):50–55, 57–58, 1988

Sica S, Davis D, Grechis K: Immobility syndrome: Use it or lose it: AD Nurse 2(6):6–10, 1987

Sumchai AP, Sternbach GL, Laufer M: Cervical spine traction and immobilization. Topics in Emergency Medicine 10(1):9–22, 1988

Total knee replacement. Orthopedic Nursing 6(6):57–59, 1987

27

Promoting Cardiopulmonary Functioning

Chapter Outline

Behavioral Objectives
Glossary
Introduction
Clearing the Airway
Suctioning the Airway
Relieving Airway Obstruction
Caring for the Patient With an Artificial Airway
Restoring Cardiopulmonary Function
Suggested Measures to Promote Cardiopulmonary
  Function in Selected Situations
Applicable Nursing Diagnoses
Teaching Suggestions to Promote Cardiopulmonary
  Function
Bibliography

Skill Procedures

Promoting Postural Drainage
Suctioning the Upper Airway
Dislodging an Object from the Airway
Suctioning Secretions from a Tracheostomy
Providing Tracheostomy Care
Administering Oxygen
Maintaining Water-Seal Drainage
Performing Cardiopulmonary Resuscitation

Behavioral Objectives

When the content of this chapter has been mastered, the learner will be able to:

Define the terms appearing in the glossary.

Describe at least two methods for thinning respiratory secretions.

Discuss methods of providing added moisture to air.

Explain the advantages and disadvantages of using warmed and cooled humidity.

Explain how postural drainage, percussion, and vibration are used and how they are carried out.

Identify the indications for suctioning the airway and describe the actions that should be followed.

Describe how to collect a sputum specimen.

List the signs of sudden airway obstruction and describe recommended techniques for dislodging an object from the airway.

Discuss various methods for maintaining an open airway. Describe the insertion and care of devices used within the mouth and nose.

Describe how to remove secretions from a tracheostomy and care for the inner cannula.

Identify two methods for administering an inhaled drug.

List basic information the nurse should know prior to administering oxygen.

Describe how oxygen equipment is assembled and prepared.

Discuss the care that should be provided when oxygen is administered by nasal cannula, nasal catheter, mask, tent, or into a tracheostomy.

Identify the purpose of using water-seal drainage and describe the care that is required to maintain its effectiveness.

Explain how to administer cardiopulmonary resuscitation to adults, indicate when it is and is not used, and describe how and when to use a self-inflating bag and mask.

List suggested measures for promoting cardiopulmonary functioning in selected situations, as described in this chapter.

Summarize suggestions for patient teaching offered in this chapter.

Glossary

Aerosolization The process of suspending droplets of water in a gas.

Airway The passages through which air from the atmosphere moves to and from the lungs.

Atomization The process of producing rather large droplets of water.

Cardiopulmonary Pertaining to the circulatory and respiratory systems.

Cardiopulmonary resuscitation A combination of techniques to open and maintain a good airway and provide artificial ventilation and circulation. Abbreviated CPR.

Cracking A technique that briefly releases oxygen within a tank to clear the outlet of dust and other debris.

Crepitus A crackling sound heard coming from within tissue.

External cardiac compression The rhythmic administration of pressure on the chest wall as a substitute for normal heart contractions.

Heimlich maneuver The technique for administering abdominal or chest thrusts to clear an object from the airway.

Hemothorax A condition in which blood fills the pleural space.

Humidification Adding moisture to the air.

Hypoxemia A condition in which there is a less than adequate level of oxygen in the blood.

Hypoxia A deficiency of oxygen in inspired air. It also describes a condition in which the tissues and cells are experiencing an inadequate supply of oxygen.

Intermittent positive-pressure breathing A mechanical means for administering gases or drugs above atmospheric pressure. Abbreviated IPPB.

Nebulization The process of transforming a liquid into a mist or fog of fine droplets.

Percussion A technique for loosening respiratory secretions by striking the chest with rhythmic gentle blows using a cupped hand.

Pneumothorax A condition in which atmospheric air enters the pleural space.

Postural drainage A technique for removing secretions from air passageways by placing the patient in various positions that utilize gravity.

Rescue breathing Artificial ventilation of the lungs using the rescuer's breath.

Suctioning A procedure in which a catheter is used to clear the airway of secretions.

Tracheostomy An artificial opening into the trachea.

Transtracheal method Administration of oxygen through a tiny catheter inserted directly into the trachea.

Vibration A technique for loosening respiratory secretions using firm, strong, circular hand movements to produce wavelike tremors.

Introduction

The word *cardiopulmonary* refers to the circulatory and the respiratory systems. The act of respiration involves the exchange of gases: oxygen from inhaled air and carbon dioxide from cellular waste are exchanged. These two substances, along with other nutrients and wastes, are transported by the circulatory system. Cell life cannot exist without the coordinated functioning of the cardiopulmonary system.

This chapter describes various skills for promoting and assisting cardiopulmonary functioning. It includes emergency measures to use when these systems become impaired and, in some cases, fail.

Most measures described in this chapter will require a physician's order. Recording is done according to agency policy and should include the patient's reaction to whatever type of intervention is used.

Clearing the Airway

The *airway* includes the passages through which the air from the atmosphere moves to and from the lungs. Any situation that narrows the passageways can interfere with optimal ventilation and the transportation of oxygen to the blood and cells of the body.

The nurse can utilize various skills to keep the airway clear. Methods to encourage coughing and deep breathing as techniques for promoting ventilation were discussed in Chapter 19. These measures should be reviewed since they are basic to maintaining cardiopulmonary functioning.

Liquefying Secretions

The respiratory tract is lined with mucous membrane. This tissue keeps the passageways moist and sticky so that nongaseous particles are trapped before falling into delicate smaller structures within the lungs. Dry air or a reduced volume of body water can alter the moist condition within air passages. The mucous membrane can become dehydrated, causing mucus to become thicker than usual. Trapped particles will then tend to remain within the lungs because the mucus is too thick to be raised. The airway will not be easily cleared. This can lead to narrowing of the passageways and a decreased volume of exchanged gases.

To avoid this, the nurse should keep the patient well hydrated. This may be done by encouraging an adequate fluid intake. This will balance the body's needs with its supply. Mucus produced when the body is well hydrated ordinarily should be thin enough to be removed by clearing the throat or coughing.

Providing Humidification

Measures are available for providing *humidification,* that is, adding moisture to the air that the patient breathes. *Atomization* refers to the production of rather large droplets. *Nebulization* is the production of a mist or fog. Suspending the droplets in a gas is called *aerosolization.* These processes have the effect of delivering and distributing moisture directly within the respiratory tract rather than indirectly through the processes of body fluid distribution.

Machines that add moisture to air increase humidity to the air within the room. They can be connected to hoods or tents, which deliver the moisture in the immediate area of the patient's nasal passages. They may also be connected directly to tubes within the airway.

Warmed Air Inhalation. Steam vaporizers are now virtually obsolete. These provide humidification by transforming water from a liquid state to a gas by boiling. Machines of this type always pose the potential for accidental scalding and tend to elevate body temperature or interfere with its regulation.

However, the therapeutic effect of warmed, moist air is still desirable. Warm, moist air soothes inflamed and irritated mucous membranes and loosens respiratory secretions. The inhaled air, carrying minute droplets of water, brings moist heat to the respiratory tract. This produces the same results as when moist heat is applied locally to other parts of the body.

Health agencies now use various humidification techniques in which beads of moisture are produced without excessive heat being used to produce steam. Those that warm as well as moisten the air may be selectively controlled within a preset temperature range. Usually a setting close to body temperature is used. These machines now contain automatic regulators that turn the heating element on and off according to the desired levels. Alarms sound if overheating occurs. These humidifiers are far superior to the types that boiled water continuously.

Cool Mist Inhalation. For those who may not benefit from the warming of inhaled air, a mist humidifier may be prescribed. It aerates the water, making fine droplets of moisture that the patient breathes along with the air in the atmosphere. Humidification is always necessary when the patient is receiving oxygen since increased percentages of oxygen dry the mucous membranes.

Humidification of this type is not warmed; in fact, it may be cooled with ice to an approximate temperature of 21°C or 70°F. The patient may become chilled and wet. The patient should be protected from drafts and from chilliness with appropriate coverings. Absorbent fabrics such as cotton bath blankets and towels may be used to collect condensation accumulating around the patient. Clothing and bed linen should be changed as it becomes necessary. The nurse should check the fluid and ice levels on each shift and refill as indicated.

Administering Postural Drainage

Postural drainage is a technique for clearing secretions from air passageways by placing the patient in various positions. Gravity is used to help promote drainage. It is often recommended for the patient with considerable heavy respiratory secretions who finds it difficult to raise the material by coughing only. Skill Procedure 27-1 describes the actions that may be used when the patient requires postural drainage.

Using Percussion and Vibration

Many patients, especially those with chronic pulmonary diseases, have difficulty raising mucus from the respiratory tract even with postural drainage. To enhance postural drainage, or if postural drainage does not seem effective, percussion and vibration may be ordered. *Percussion* is the technique of striking with rhythmic gentle blows using a cupped hand. *Vibration* is the technique of using firm, strong, circular movements with open hands to produce wavelike tremors. Both of these actions are intended to cause thick secretions to break loose from within the airway.

When percussion and vibration are performed, the patient is placed in various positions, such as the sides, back, and abdomen, so that all areas over both lungs can be percussed and vibrated. Percussion and vibration are continued for about 15 minutes if the patient tolerates the therapy well. Figure 27-2 illustrates how to percuss and vibrate the chest wall.

With the break up of mucus, the patient can more easily raise and expectorate it. Other procedures may be performed in conjunction with percussion and vibration to clear the airway effectively. Areas over the spine, liver, kidneys, abdomen, breasts, clavicle, and sternum should not be percussed or vibrated because of the danger of injuring tissues.

Suctioning the Airway

Sometimes coughing may be inadequate or the patient too weak to expectorate or swallow raised mucus. *Suctioning* is a procedure in which a catheter is used to remove secretions from the airway. The nurse may use suctioning to remove secretions from the upper airway in the area of the oropharynx and nasopharynx or deeper within the trachea and bronchi. Suctioning the lower airway through a tracheostomy will be discussed later in this chapter.

Assembling Suction Equipment

The source of suction may be a wall unit or a separate portable machine. Usually a pressure of 100 to 140 mm Hg using a wall unit or a low setting, usually 10 to 15 mm Hg, using a portable suction machine is sufficient enough to remove secretions from an adult without damaging the tissue severely.

A suction catheter is made of flexible plastic or rubber. Catheters are available in a variety of sizes. The size selected should allow for the passage of air around the outside of the catheter. An adult is likely to require a size 14 to 18 French while catheters in smaller sizes, indicated

Skill Procedure 27-1. Promoting Postural Drainage

Suggested Action	**Reason for Action**
Plan to use postural drainage before meals and before bedtime. Postural drainage is usually ordered two or four times each day.	Some positions for postural drainage are uncomfortable and may produce nausea and vomiting when therapy is carried out soon after eating.
Administer prescribed medications that act to dilate respiratory passages before starting therapy.	Medications that dilate the respiratory passageways promote a larger area for more effective drainage.
Be familiar with the positions that the patient can and cannot safely assume.	Patients with certain illnesses (*e.g.,* some heart diseases) may not be able to assume certain positions with safety.
Have paper tissues and a waterproof container for raised secretions available for the patient.	The patient can be expected to cough and raise wet secretions cleared from the airway during and after postural drainage.
Know what areas of the lungs are to be drained and position the patient accordingly. Place the patient with the affected area uppermost. Various positions are illustrated in Figure 27-1.	Secretions move in the respiratory tract by gravity. Placing the patient so that secretions can drain from the lower areas of the lungs to larger upper air passages promotes more efficient removal.

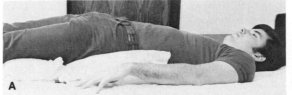
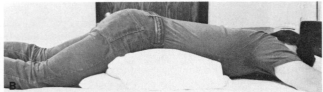

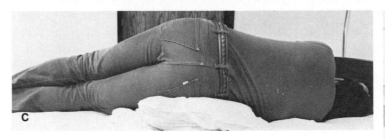

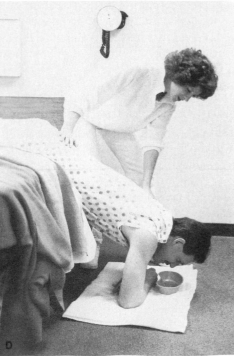

Figure 27-1 (*A*). The lower front portions of both lungs can be drained by elevating the hips while the patient is on his back. (*B*). The lower portions of both lungs can be drained by elevating the hips while the patient is on his abdomen. (*C*). The lateral portions of the lungs can be drained by elevating the hips while the patient is on his right, and then his left, side. (*D*). This position allows for good drainage from the trachea. A Fowler's position will help drain the upper anterior portion of the upper lobes. Having the patient lean over the bed helps drain the posterior portions of the upper lobes.

Allow the patient to remain in one position for 15 to 30 minutes, or for as long as 45 minutes if the patient can tolerate it and the desired effect is being achieved.	It takes time for thick secretions to drain from the respiratory tract.

(*continued*)

Skill Procedure 27-1. *Continued*

Suggested Action	Reason for Action
Assess the patient frequently for fatigue, faintness, a rapid pulse rate, dyspnea, and chest pain.	These signs are associated with untoward effects of postural drainage.
Stop the therapy and report any unusual effects associated with the procedure.	The nurse is responsible for the safety of the patient.
Continue to observe the patient and collect data.	The nurse should continue adding assessments to determine if the problems are related to the procedure or some other cause.
Encourage the patient who is not experiencing any undesirable effects to cough and expectorate as the procedure progresses.	Coughing helps to raise secretions that drain and accumulate in upper respiratory passages.
Describe the volume and characteristics of the secretions raised as well as the patient's overall response to the procedure.	The effectiveness of the measure may be evaluated on the basis of the nurse's recorded description in the patient's permanent record.
Dispose of moist tissues and raised secretions.	Retained secretions often contain pathogens. Proper disposal controls the spread of organisms to others.
Provide equipment for oral hygiene.	Oral hygiene may need to be provided more frequently for the patient who raises and expectorates respiratory secretions.

by lower numbers, should be used for children. Suction catheters have a series of holes located along the sides of the insertion tip. This design allows the removal of larger amounts of secretions during a short amount of time. A vent or Y-connector at the upper end of the catheter permits creation of a vacuum once the catheter is in its proper location. The secretions are pulled into the catheter and tubing and deposited within a receptacle attached to the suction unit.

Assessing the Need for Suctioning

Suctioning should never be performed routinely. This procedure can cause injury to respiratory passageways, remove oxygen as well as secretions, cause bradycardia and hypotension, and often causes the patient to feel apprehensive and frightened. Some criteria that indicate a need for suctioning include ineffective coughing and expectoration; dyspnea; cyanosis of the skin, lips, and nailbeds; moist breath sounds heard on auscultation with a stethoscope; rattling sounds heard without a stethoscope; vibrations felt over areas where secretions are moved about during respiration; and tachycardia. The nurse should note these focus assessments before, during, and after the suctioning procedure. Repeated suctioning should be avoided and frequent suctioning should always be performed after providing the patient with periodic rest and oxygenation.

Performing Nasopharyngeal or Oropharyngeal Suctioning

The nurse may choose to suction the upper airway either through the nose or mouth or both. However, separate catheters should be used for each.

Agencies differ as to the recommendation for medical or surgical asepsis when performing oropharyngeal and nasopharyngeal suctioning. One rationale is that if the tip of the catheter will not be passed further than the pharynx, a place where organisms are ordinarily found in larger numbers, the procedure may follow principles of medical asepsis or clean technique. Others feel that any patient who requires suctioning already is susceptible to infection. Therefore, it is better to be overly cautious when it comes to his protection. The nurse should follow the policies developed by the health agency.

Clean gloves may be worn as a transmission barrier to protect the nurse from pathogens present in the patient's secretions. If sterile gloves are used, they protect both the nurse and the patient from contact with pathogens. A basin of normal saline should be available for rinsing the lumen of the catheter. If the agency procedure specifies that sterile technique be used, the solution and the basin should be sterile. The catheter may be dipped into the saline solution or coated with water-soluble lubricant prior to insertion within the nose; it need not be lubricated, other than with saline, prior to insertion within the mouth.

Skill Procedure 27-2 describes the actions involved in using suctioning for clearing the upper airway of secretions.

Collecting a Sputum Specimen

A patient who accumulates copious amounts of secretions within the respiratory tract, called sputum, will more than likely need to have it analyzed by the laboratory of the health agency. The nurse is responsible for collecting the specimen. It is not uncommon for the physician to request

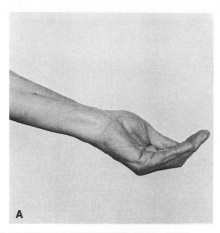

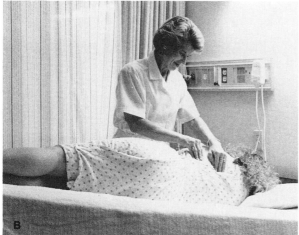

Figure 27-2 (*A*). When performing percussion, the hand is cupped as if to carry water. (*B*). The cupped hand is struck rhythmically over areas of the chest and back. The sound is similar to galloping horses.

that three different specimens be obtained to ensure adequate test results.

A specimen is best obtained early in the morning because a higher volume of secretions is likely to have accumulated throughout the night. Another time that may provide a better opportunity for collecting specimens would be following respiratory therapy treatments, postural drainage, and percussion and vibration.

The patient should be instructed that the specimen consist of material coughed up from the respiratory tract and not saliva that is present in the mouth. Special mucus traps are available for use with suction catheters if a specimen must be obtained using the suction catheter.

The following steps are used to collect a sputum specimen:

1. Encourage the patient to have a generous fluid intake and have him breathe humidified air when possible. These measures help to prevent the sputum from becoming sticky and difficult to raise.
2. Use a large-mouthed sterile container that has a secure cover and have the patient expectorate directly into it.

3. Avoid contaminating the inside of the container by exposing it to air unnecessarily or touching it.
4. Avoid collecting a specimen after the patient eats. Food particles in the specimen make examination difficult.
5. Assess the volume and other characteristics of the sputum that will be sent to the laboratory. Some sputum specimen containers are calibrated, making measurement easy. Another technique is to fill an identical container with water to the level of the sputum expectorated and then measure the amount of water.
6. Handle sputum specimens carefully and observe aseptic techniques to avoid spreading organisms to the hands, linens, and personal care items. Sputum should be considered highly contaminated.
7. Provide the patient with the opportunity for mouth care following the raising of sputum.
8. For best results, label and send the sputum specimen to the laboratory within an hour of collecting it.

Relieving Airway Obstruction

The airway may be occluded suddenly by an aspirated object or food. Cardiopulmonary function may also become compromised if the tongue or swelling closes off the passageway for air through the trachea and bronchi. Various measures may be used to promote air exchange.

Assisting the Individual With a Blocked Airway

Certain measures are helpful in an emergency to assist a victim who is choking on a foreign object. In adults, the foreign object is most often a piece of food. In children, in addition to food, the object may be a large piece of gum, buttons, marbles, deflated balloons, or removable parts from toys.

Signs of Sudden Airway Obstruction. The nurse should be able to differentiate distress due to an airway obstruction from a heart attack. The symptoms are somewhat similar. If the symptoms occur at the time of eating, aspiration of food into the airway is a real possibility. The following signs are typical when a victim is choking on a foreign object:

- Grasping for the throat with the hands, as illustrated in Figure 27-5. This is the universal sign of choking.
- Spontaneous efforts to cough and breathe.
- Producing a high-pitched sound while inhaling indicates that air passageways are almost totally blocked.
- Turning pale and then blue.
- Being unable to speak, breath, or cough indicates a total block.
- Collapsing and becoming unconscious. The victim
(Text continues on page 713)

Skill Procedure 27-2. Suctioning the Upper Airway

Suggested Action	Reason for Action
Assess the patient to determine the need for suctioning.	Suctioning should be done only when secretions are accumulating and the patient is not able to clear his own air passages.
Explain the purpose and plan for suctioning to the patient.	The patient who understands the measures that will be provided can tolerate and cooperate with the procedure.
Gather the equipment that will be needed for suctioning, such as catheter, extension tubing, suction unit, basin of normal saline, gloves, and lubricant.	The patient who cannot breathe well may be extremely anxious. Disorganization may tend to heighten the patient's anxiety.
Attach the suction machine to the wall outlet or power source. Set the pressure gauge, as the nurse in Figure 27-3 is doing, according to the age and size of the patient.	A wall unit may be regulated at 100 to 140 mm Hg for an adult or a low setting, approximately 10 to 15 mm Hg, using a portable machine. Follow agency recommendations when a written policy specifies pressure ranges for upper airway suctioning.

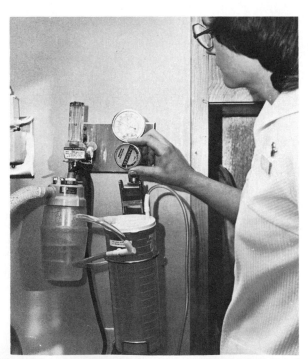

Figure 27-3 The nurse begins the suctioning procedure by turning on the suction machine and checking to see that it is working properly.

Provide privacy by closing the room door and pulling the cubicle curtains surrounding the bed.	The patient should be protected from the view of others when any procedure is carried out.
Protect the front of the patient's bed clothes and pillow with clean towels.	Towels are easily removed and laundered.
Place the patient in a semi-Fowler's position.	A semi-Fowler's position aids breathing and passage of the catheter.
Inspect the condition of the nares if the catheter will be inserted through the nose.	The catheter is more easily passed through a nostril that is not narrowed or partially obstructed as a result of a deviated nasal septum.

(continued)

Skill Procedure 27-2. Continued

Suggested Action	**Reason for Action**
Preoxygenate the patient with 100% oxygen for 1 to 2 minutes.	This provides a potential extra reserve of oxygen within the blood to compensate for the volume of oxygen that will be removed during suctioning.
Open the package containing the catheter without touching the tip to any unsterile equipment or articles. Attach the catheter to the tubing that extends from the suction unit.	The suction tip should be kept sterile prior to placing it within the patient.
Check to see that there is suction by placing a thumb over the vent, as the nurse in Figure 27-4 is doing.	When the vent is closed, the pressure gauge should register at the level previously set.

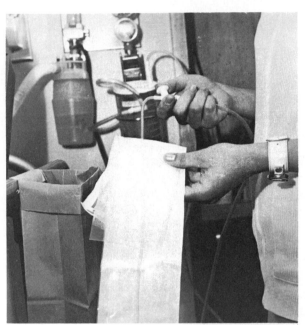

Figure 27-4 The suction catheter is sterile when dispensed in its plastic bag. The top is turned down sufficiently enough to connect the catheter with the suction machine. The nurse checks to see that there is suction by placing a thumb over the vent, as shown. When the thumb is off the valve, there will be no suction through the catheter.

Don a sterile or clean glove on the dominant hand.	The hand that will hold the catheter should be covered with a glove that acts as a transmission barrier.
Measure the distance from the tip of the nose to the tip of the patient's earlobe without actually touching the catheter to the patient's face.	The length between these two structures is approximately the distance to the pharynx.
Turn on the suction machine with the nondominant hand.	The hand that will be used during direct contact with the patient should not touch the pressure gauge, which is neither clean nor sterile.
Test the suction by pulling normal saline through the suction catheter.	It is better to identify mechanical problems before the suction catheter is inserted.
Lubricate the suction tip by coating it with water soluble lubricant or wetting it with the rinsing solution.	Lubrication reduces friction and facilitates the ease of insertion. To avoid injury, the catheter should never be forced through a body structure.

(continued)

Skill Procedure 27-2. Continued

Suggested Action	Reason for Action
Follow the floor of the nose or the side of the mouth during insertion.	These techniques help to reduce the potential for sneezing or gagging during insertion.
Expect that the patient may cough. Encourage the patient to cough if this does not occur as a reflex action.	Coughing helps to break up and raise thick secretions to a level where they may be reached by the suction catheter.
Turn the patient's head to the side and stop the catheter insertion if it appears that vomiting may occur.	There is a danger of aspiration if the patient should vomit. Interrupting the insertion may allow time for the feeling to pass.
Occlude the vent or exposed tip of the Y-connector once the end of the catheter is in the desired location.	Suction should never be applied during insertion of the catheter, only during its removal.
Rotate or twist the catheter as it is being removed.	This helps to remove secretions from all the surface areas of the airway.
Release the finger from the vent if the catheter seems to resist removal. This is more likely to occur when suctioning structures deeper than the pharynx.	Spasms may occur. The patient should still be able to breathe when the suction is not being applied. Relaxation will eventually counteract the spasm and the catheter will be released.
Observe the patient's response during suctioning. An assistant may be desired especially to assess the pulse of a patient who is elderly or has a history of heart disease. Watch the heart rate and rhythm on a cardiac monitor, if that is in use.	Temporary reduction of oxygen levels within the blood as well as stimulation of the vagus nerve during the insertion of the catheter can cause bradycardia or other dangerous arrhythmias.
Complete the process in no more than 15 seconds from the time of the insertion of the catheter to its removal.	Suctioning that extends beyond this period of time may remove significant amounts of oxygen needed by the cells and tissues of the body.
Rinse the secretions from the tubing by inserting the catheter in the basin of normal saline and applying suction.	The protein in mucus may dry and obstruct the tubing.
Repeat suctioning if assessments indicate that secretions are still present, but allow a 2- to 3-minute rest period and reoxygenation in between.	Repeated attempts at suctioning fatigue the patient and can lower the amount of oxygen in the blood to dangerous levels.
Pull the glove on the dominant hand inside out over the catheter and dispose of both when suctioning is completed.	Enclosing the contaminated catheter within the soiled side of the glove helps to control the spread of microorganisms.
Turn off the suction machine.	The suction machine need only be operational during the time of the procedure.
Reassess the patient.	The nurse should collect data similar to that gathered before suctioning to evaluate the response of the patient to the procedure.
Provide mouth care.	Oral hygiene measures will remove unpleasant tastes and mouth odors related to the cleared respiratory secretions.
Record pertinent assessments and a description of the suctioning procedure in the chart.	The permanent record should reflect the quality and standards of care provided for the patient as well as his unique responses.
Empty the container that holds the suctioned secretions.	The container holding suctioned secretions supports the growth of pathogens and is aesthetically unpleasant to observe.

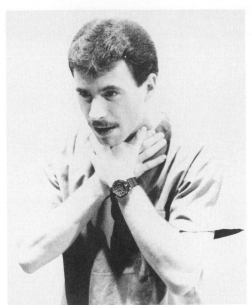

Figure 27-5 The victim who has aspirated an object into the airway and experiences airway obstruction should grasp the throat, signaling the universal sign for choking.

will die unless the foreign body is removed to allow for air exchange in the lungs.

Dislodging an Object From the Airway. If it is determined that the victim is indeed choking and there is poor or absent air exchange, action should be taken immediately to dislodge the foreign object. A series of manual thrusts is recommended to remove a foreign object on which a victim is choking. For infants younger than 1 year of age, a combination of back blows and chest thrusts is advised. The sequence of recommended actions for an adult is described and illustrated in Skill Procedure 27-3.

Caring for the Patient With an Artificial Airway

Various tubes and hollow devices may be inserted into the nose or mouth of an unconscious or critically ill patient to maintain an open airway. Simpler types, such as the oral airway shown in Figure 27-9, hold the tongue forward so that it cannot obstruct the air passages. An oral airway or nasopharyngeal airway, placed in upper airway structures, may be inserted by a qualified nurse. An endotracheal tube, inserted into the trachea using a laryngoscope as a guide, is generally the responsibility of a physician, nurse anesthetist, or certified critical care personnel. The physician usually inserts a tracheostomy tube, which is introduced through an incision in the lower neck.

Inserting and Maintaining an Artificial Upper Airway

An artificial airway is placed within the patient's nose or mouth to maintain an open upper airway. The nurse may use the following description as a guide for inserting and providing care for the patient with an oral airway device. Modifications that apply to a nasopharyngeal airway are found at the end of the discussion.

1. Position the patient on his back with his neck hyperextended, if this is not contraindicated.
2. Perform good handwashing technique.
3. Insert the thumb and index finger into the patient's mouth to separate the teeth and spread the jaw.
4. Use a tongue blade as an additional measure, if needed, to open the mouth and depress the tongue.
5. Hold the airway so that the curved tip points upward toward the roof of the mouth.
6. Guide the airway to the back of the mouth while

Skill Procedure 27-3. Dislodging an Object From the Airway

Suggested Action	Reason for Action
Ask if the patient can speak.	Speech is only possible when air moves from the lower areas of the lungs through the vocal cords. If the victim can speak, either the airway is only partially occluded or something else is causing the symptoms.
Encourage forceful coughing.	Coughing increases intrathoracic pressure and can sometimes force a foreign object into a larger air passage so that breathing can resume.
Avoid attempts to assist the victim as long as there is adequate air exchange.	Attempts to assist may lead to unnecessary injury to the victim.
Call for emergency assistance if the victim continues to be unsuccessful in his efforts to relieve a partial obstruction.	The assistance of emergency personnel may become necessary if the situation becomes prolonged or progresses to a complete obstruction.

(continued)

Skill Procedure 27-3. *Continued*

Suggested Action	Reason for Action
Review the "Suggested Measures to Promote Cardiopulmonary Functioning in Selected Situations" at the end of this chapter if the victim is an infant under the age of 1.	Altering the position of infants and administering back blows are additional techniques used to dislodge an object from the airway of victims under the age of 1.
Prepare to perform the *Heimlich maneuver,* also called abdominal thrusts, if the victim has an ineffective cough, increased respiratory difficulty, or cannot exchange any air.	The Heimlich maneuver must be performed when the victim's own efforts to relieve the obstruction are unsuccessful.
Stand behind the victim and allow him to lean over with his head lower than his chest, as illustrated in Figure 27-6.	This positioning increases intrathoracic pressure and allows gravity to help in the removal of an aspirated object.

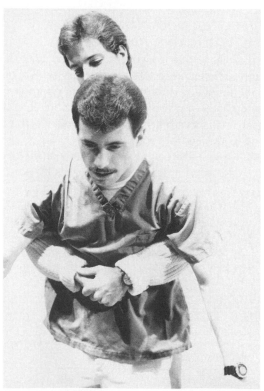

Figure 27-6 The rescuer positions himself behind the victim.

Alternatively, get behind the victim who is sitting in a chair.	This alternative position may be used when the weight of a victim cannot be supported by the rescuer.
Bring the arms around the victim's abdomen.	The hands must be below the lungs in order to elevate the diaphragm.
Make a fist, the thumb tucked inside, with one hand and grab the fisted hand with the other.	Using a fist and the combined effort of the strong muscles of the arms helps to provide enough pressure to force out air trapped below the object.
Place the flat side of the clasped fist against the victim's abdomen between the lower end of the sternum and above the navel, not on the lower sternum or the rib cage.	Proper hand placement is necessary to prevent injury to abdominal and thoracic organs.

(continued)

Skill Procedure 27-3. Continued

Suggested Action	**Reason for Action**
Press the clasped fist into the victim's abdomen with a forceful thrust. Do not squeeze, but rather carry out the maneuver in an upward direction.	With sufficient force, the trapped air may cause enough pressure to dislodge the object from the airway.
Repeat this action 6 to 10 times until there is restoration of breathing or the victim becomes unconscious.	Efforts should be continued even if they are not successful the first time.
Follow by sweeping the throat or administering rescue breaths or cardiopulmonary resuscitation as described in the following section and in more detail in Skill Procedure 27-8 when a victim cannot breathe and the heart has stopped beating.	When the conscious victim becomes unconscious, further actions are necessary to help restore breathing and circulation.

When the Victim is Unconscious

Place the victim in a supine position.	A supine position is the preferred position for an unconscious victim in order to place the hands properly and administer abdominal thrusts.
Kneel over the victim placing one leg on each side of the victim's hips facing toward the head.	Working directly over the victim provides the best use of the rescuer's body mechanics and strength.
Place the hands on top of each other in the midline between the victim's rib cage and navel and administer a forceful upward thrust with the heel of the bottom hand.	Positioning the hands in this manner facilitates applying force to the center of the abdomen without encircling the victim's abdomen.
Perform six to ten repeated abdominal thrusts if the object does not become dislodged.	Continuing efforts must be made to restore breathing despite initial unsuccessful attempts.
Open the unconscious victim's mouth and sweep the throat is illustrated in Figure 27-7. Take care to avoid driving the object deeper within the airway.	If the object is not too low in the respiratory tract, a sweeping action with a finger will sometimes help to bring it to the mouth for removal.

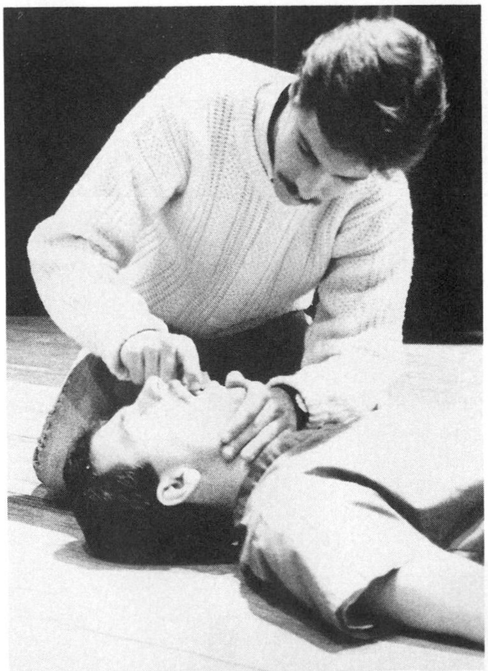

Figure 27-7 A hooked index finger can be used to remove a foreign object lodged in the mouth or throat.

(continued)

Skill Procedure 27-3. *Continued*

Suggested Action	Reason for Action

When the Victim is Unconscious

Tilt the head upward and lift the chin to open the airway.	Adjusting the position of the head will move the tongue from the airway and may permit partial air exchange.
Administer two rescue breaths into the victim's mouth and observe if the chest rises during the ventilation attempts.	Seeing the chest rise provides evidence that air is passing through the airway and filling the lungs.
Continue with rescue breathing, administering one breath every 5 seconds on anyone over 8 years of age. Faster rates, listed in Table 27-3, must be administered to infants and children.	Efforts must continue to revive the patient when no spontaneous breathing is occurring.
Begin cardiac compressions at a rate of 80 to 100 per minutes with two breaths administered between every 15 compressions on victims who are 8 years old or older when a pulse cannot be felt.	When there is no pulse, the rescuer must include cardiac compressions to provide resuscitation.
Continue with resuscitation efforts until the victim responds or the rescuer becomes exhausted.	Resuscitation efforts should be continued while waiting for assistance.

When the Victim Is Obese or Pregnant

Stand behind the victim with arms under the victim's axillae. Place the clasped fist on the middle of the victim's sternum, not at the lower end of the sternum or at the edge of the rib cage, as illustrated in Figure 27-8.	This position helps prevent injury to the sternum, ribs, and organs located within the thoracic cavity.

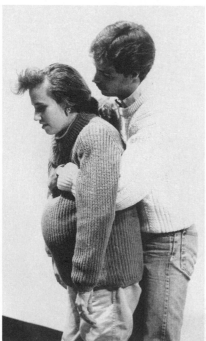

Figure 27-8 These two people demonstrate how the hands are positioned higher when the victim is pregnant or obese.

(continued)

Skill Procedure 27-3. Continued

Suggested Action	Reason for Action
When the Victim is Obese or Pregnant	
Administer six to ten chest thrusts rather than abdominal thrusts.	Chest thrusts provide an alternative method for relieving an obstruction from a victim with an enlarged abdomen without injuring a fetus or enlarged abdominal organs.
Continue with resuscitation efforts, as described earlier and in Skill Procedure 27-8, if the victim fails to breathe spontaneously and has no pulse.	Additional measures must be performed when attempts to free an object from the airway prove unsuccessful.

keeping the tongue forward and below the oral airway.

7. Turn the airway within the mouth until it is positioned over the top of the tongue following its natural contour.
8. Secure the flange of the exposed end of the airway to the skin in the area of the lips using tape.
9. Perform oropharyngeal or nasopharyngeal suctioning as necessary to clear secretions from the natural and artificial airway.
10. Remove the oral airway briefly every 4 hours.
11. Assess the condition of the mouth and tongue.
12. Provide mouth care and skin care to the taped area and lips.
13. Rinse and clean the oral airway.
14. Reinsert the oral airway if the patient remains unconscious.

A nasopharyngeal airway may be used rather than an oral airway. It is inserted similarly to a nasopharyngeal catheter; however, the airway is secured in place rather than removed. The alternate nostril should be used when a nasopharyngeal airway is removed, cleaned, and reinserted every 8 hours.

Caring for the Patient With a Tracheostomy

A *tracheostomy* is an artificial opening into the trachea. A hollow device is inserted into the opening and the patient breathes through it. The tube has an inner and an outer cannula or, more simply, a tube within a tube. The outer cannula rests in the patient's trachea and the inner cannula fits into the outer cannula to form one opening, through which the patient breathes.

Some tracheostomy tubes have an inflatable cuff. One is illustrated in Figure 27-10. The cuff is filled with air so that secretions from the upper air passages cannot pass around the cannula and be aspirated. The cuff also helps hold the cannula in place. It prevents oxygen that the patient may be receiving from leaking out rather than being delivered to the lungs. Unless the cuff is of a type that is very pliable and soft, it should be deflated at regular intervals. If this is not done, the cuff may cut off the blood supply to the area and cause injury to tissue. An experienced nurse is ordinarily responsible for inflating and deflating a tracheostomy cuff.

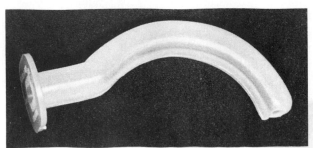

Figure 27-9 A plastic disposable airway may be inserted through the mouth, following the contour of the mouth and upper respiratory tract. When in place, the oral airway holds the tongue so that it cannot drop back into the throat. It can be suctioned easily if secretions accumulate.

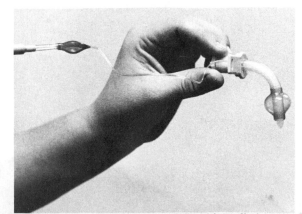

Figure 27-10 This nurse holds an inflatable cuffed tracheostomy tube in the direction in which it would be located in the patient.

Removing Secretions From a Tracheostomy. Secretions may accumulate within the lower respiratory air passages. To remove these secretions, suctioning may be performed by inserting a suction catheter through the tracheostomy tube. This procedure *must* be performed following the principles of sterile technique. Many factors affect the potential for infection in a patient with a tracheostomy, such as the extended presence of an artificial object in the trachea, altered skin integrity due to the incision and opening for the tracheostomy tube, and the limited ability of the patient to remove the build up of secretions naturally.

The procedure for removing secretions from a tracheostomy is somewhat similar to the skills involved in suctioning the upper airway. Skill Procedure 27-4 de-

scribes and illustrates the special adaptations that may be performed when suctioning a tracheostomy.

Providing Tracheostomy Care

The inner cannula should be cleaned regularly to help prevent infection. Most agencies specify that cleansing should be performed at least once every 8 hours. The inner cannula must be removed in order to clean it. Cleansing should be performed in a short amount of time since secretions may accumulate and dry on the surface of the outer cannula, which remains in place. This can interfere with the ability to reinsert the inner cannula. It may ultimately require replacement of the entire equipment within the surgical opening or risk endangering the patient's life. A duplicate set of sterile equipment should be

---

Skill Procedure 27-4. Suctioning Secretions From a Tracheostomy

Suggested Action	Reason for Action
Assess for evidence of mucus accumulating in the patient's respiratory tract, such as noisy, moist, and labored respirations, and increased pulse and respiratory rates.	Noisy, moist, and labored respirations indicate that mucus is accumulating in the respiratory tract, putting extra stress on the cardiopulmonary system.
Help the patient into a Fowler's position, if permitted.	The patient can ventilate more fully in this position.
Encourage and help the patient to cough up respiratory secretions, to see whether this will clear the respiratory tract.	Suctioning, which is irritating to mucous membranes, should be avoided when the patient can successfully cough up secretions.
Wipe away secretions coughed out through the tracheostomy tube.	The secretions below the tracheostomy tube will not be expectorated from the mouth.
Use wipes that are free of lint around the tracheostomy opening.	Inhaled lint irritates the respiratory passages and may cause undue coughing.
Give the patient 100% oxygen for 1 to 2 minutes before suctioning.	Giving oxygen before suctioning prevents depletion of the supply to the cells. Suctioning removes oxygen, as well as debris, from the respiratory tract.
Attach a sterile catheter to the tubing leading from the suction source. The catheter should be about half the diameter of the tracheostomy tube.	If the catheter is too small, suctioning will be ineffective. If the catheter is too large, it may injure tissue and totally obstruct the airway.
Don a sterile glove on the dominant hand. Touch the catheter only with a sterile, gloved hand.	Sterile technique is used to help prevent introducing organisms into the patient's respiratory tract.
Lubricate the catheter with fresh, sterile, normal saline for each pass of the catheter. Bacteriostatic water is usually not recommended.	Lubricating the catheter decreases irritation to mucous membranes. The preservative used in bacteriostatic water is irritating to mucous membranes.
Test the catheter with the saline to be sure it is patent and working properly.	Potential mechanical difficulties should be identified before inserting the suction catheter.
Instill 4 to 5 mL of fresh, sterile normal saline into the tracheostomy tube if mucus is sticky and crusty material is present.	The normal saline helps liquefy sticky mucus and thus makes it easier to remove it with the suction catheter.
Insert the catheter carefully and slowly about 15 to 25 cm (6–10 in) into the inner cannula and into the respiratory passage without covering the vent on the tubing.	Respiratory membranes can be easily injured when a catheter is inserted carelessly. Having suction on while inserting the catheter removes valuable amounts of oxygen unnecessarily.

(continued)

Skill Procedure 27-4. *Continued*

Suggested Action	**Reason for Action**
Have the patient turn his head to the side opposite where the catheter is to be located. To suction the left bronchus, instruct the patient to turn his head to the right, and vice versa.	Turning the head will provide easier access for placement of the catheter within one or the other bronchi.
Occlude the vent and gently twist and rotate the catheter, as the nurse is doing in Figure 27-11, while removing it slowly from the respiratory tract.	Twisting the catheter improves the removal of the secretions from the circular surfaces of the air passages.

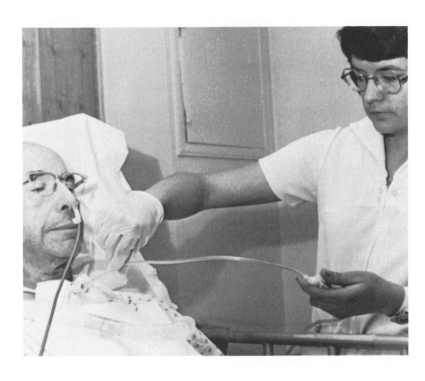

Figure 27-11 After donning a sterile glove, the suctions the patient.

Apply suction for only 10 seconds and never more than 15 seconds at one time. Then allow a rest period of 2 to 3 minutes between suctions, and preoxygenate the patient again.	Suctioning removes oxygen as well as secretions from the respiratory tract. The patient suffers an insufficient supply of oxygen when suctioning is prolonged.
Flush the catheter with sterile normal saline between passes with the catheter.	Rinsing the catheter prevents inefficient application of suction from partially obstructed tubing.
Suction the inner cannula as often as necessary to keep it open and free of mucus. This may be as often as every 5 to 10 minutes when the tracheostomy has been first performed. It *may* be as infrequent as three or four times every 24 hours.	Suctioning must be performed as often as necessary to keep the respiratory tract clear and open. Excessive suctioning irritates mucous membranes.
Oxygenate the patient after suctioning has been completed.	Giving the patient oxygen after suctioning restores the depleted supply within the blood.
Dispose of the glove and the catheter after suctioning.	To maintain sterile technique, this equipment must not be reused.
Restock additional sterile gloves and suction catheters as the supply is used.	A tracheostomy may require frequent and, in some cases, immediate suctioning to maintain adequate ventilation.

kept at the patient's bedside so that everything is ready if the tracheostomy tube must be replaced.

When the inner cannula is cleaned, the stoma is also cared for, the dressing around the stoma is changed, and the ties securing the tracheostomy tube are changed as well. Dressings and tapes are a source of infection when they are not properly cared for and should be changed when they become soiled or damp. Skill Procedure 27-5 provides a description of the actions for providing tracheostomy care.

Restoring Cardiopulmonary Function

Heart diseases and pulmonary diseases are two of the leading causes of disability and death in the United States. Measures must often be implemented that either temporarily or permanently help to restore the functions of the cardiopulmonary system when it becomes impaired or ceases to operate. This may be done by administering prescribed inhaled medications, providing oxygen, main-

Skill Procedure 27-5. Providing Tracheostomy Care

Suggested Action	Reason for Action
Assemble equipment, which generally comes already prepared, with various items that will be needed.	Disorganization will interfere with completing tracheostomy care within a minimal safe period of time.
Obtain a waterproof receptacle for holding contaminated and soiled items.	Care must be taken to keep items containing organisms separate from clean and sterile areas within the work space.
Open the tracheostomy care set following the principles of surgical asepsis described in Chapter 16.	Contamination of the contents of the set could lead to the spread of organisms within the patient's respiratory tract.
Add sterile hydrogen peroxide to one basin and sterile normal saline or sterile water to a second basin within the set.	These solutions must be added before sterile gloves are donned to avoid contaminating the hands.
Remove the dressing from around the stoma and place it within the container for soiled items.	A soiled dressing contains pathogens and should be suitably contained to control the spread of organisms.
Wash hands thoroughly and don sterile gloves.	Even though the hands were washed prior to opening the equipment set, they must be rewashed after handling the soiled dressing.
Clean around the stoma with a sterile swab moistened with sterile hydrogen peroxide. Follow with a second swab moistened in the saline.	Cleaning the stoma removes secretions and organisms that could cause an infection.
Discard both swabs with the soiled dressing following their use.	Each swab should be used only once to avoid reintroducing organisms into a cleaned area.
Remove the inner cannula by unlocking it from its position within the outer cannula, as the nurse in Figure 27-12 is doing.	Most twist free for removal; however, individual manufacturers vary in the methods used for securing the two tubes.
Deposit the inner cannula in the basin of hydrogen peroxide.	Hydrogen peroxide is an antimicrobial agent and also loosens protein substances. It is an ideal solution for removing secretions from the surfaces of the cannula.
While holding the cannula, insert a brush or sterile pipe cleaner through the center of the cannula. Scrub the outer surfaces also.	The bristles help to mechanically remove debris that the peroxide is unable to loosen chemically.
Rinse the cannula in the basin of sterile normal saline or sterile water.	Rinsing removes remnants of undiluted hydrogen peroxide that may irritate the tissue within the respiratory tract.
Drain or dry the cannula using a gauze square and reinsert it within the outer cannula.	The inner cannula should be replaced within 5 minutes of being removed.
Secure the inner cannula in place.	If the cannula is not secured, it could be expelled if and when the patient coughs.

(continued)

Skill Procedure 27-5. Continued

Suggested Action	Reason for Action

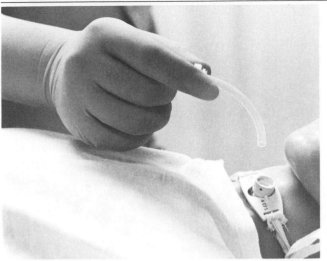

Figure 27-12 The nurse removes the inner cannula only for regular cleaning. The outer cannula remains in place within the tracheostomy. Note that the tracheostomy ties have been secured at the side of the neck, where the knot or bow is less likely to cause pressure.

Suggested Action	Reason for Action
Place a sterile dressing over the stoma incision and under the exposed areas of the tracheostomy tube.	Special dressings that resemble miniature pants protect the incision from organisms and absorb secretions.
Fold a gauze square to fit over the stoma incision using material that does not fray, if special tracheostomy dressings are not available.	Fiber particles that may fall into the respiratory tract can irritate the tissue.
Remove the gloves and deposit them in the container holding the soiled dressing and swabs.	The contaminated gloves and other soiled articles may be discarded for eventual burning to destroy any pathogens that may be present.
Thread clean tracheostomy ties through the slits on each side of the outer cannula before removing the soiled ties.	The tracheostomy tube is only held in place by the ties. Removing one set before the other is secure creates a potential for displacement.
OR	
Seek the assistance of another person who will stabilize the tracheostomy tube while one set of ties is removed and replaced with another.	With the help of another person, the tube can be held in place when the ties are removed. This provides more room for threading the clean ties.
Secure the ties in place at the side of the neck.	A knot in the back of the head may cause pressure and irritation.
Check to see that the ties allow adequate blood flow.	The ties should not be so tight that they impair the circulation of blood.
Remove all soiled equipment from the room to designated areas in a utility room.	A new sterile equipment tray should be obtained each time tracheostomy care is provided.

taining water-seal drainage, and administering cardiopulmonary resuscitation.

Administering Inhaled Medications

Drugs that help to restore cardiopulmonary functions can be given by any route. However, some that are particularly useful to the pulmonary system, and indirectly to the heart, are administered by inhalation. Much of the absorption occurs on the surfaces of lung tissue. Because of the large surface area in the lungs, absorption after inhalation generally is rapid. Drugs commonly used are antibiotics, expectorants, and those that help to dilate the bronchioles and bronchi.

Before drugs can be inhaled, they must be vaporized to

permit entry into the body with each inspiration. Drugs intended for administration by inhalation are added to a vehicle such as water. The mixture is then processed into droplets. The finer the particles, the farther they will travel into the respiratory tract.

Using a Hand-Held Inhaler. A spray may be produced in several ways. When a hand-held inhaler is compressed, air is forced through the container holding the drug in solution. The increased pressure in the unit then forces solution into a narrow channel. The force breaks the larger droplets of fluid into a fine mist. The mist is inhaled through the mouth. If the inhalation is intended to produce effects in the nasal passage as well as in the remainder of the respiratory tract, the patient closes his mouth while he breathes and inhales the substance through his nose. Commercially prepared nebulizers with medications are available. This type is being used by the patient in Figure 27-13.

Providing Aerosol Treatments. Drugs can be inhaled using a machine that mixes oxygen or compressed air with a drug. A device of this kind is shown in Figure 27-14. This method of administration is valuable for patients who may be required to inhale a drug several times a day.

A common means to administer oxygenated air and a

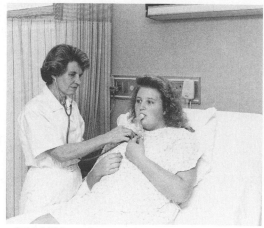

Figure 27-14 This patient receives an aerosol treatment. The nurse assesses the patient's lung sounds.

nebulized drug using a machine is by *intermittent positive-pressure breathing,* usually abbreviated IPPB. Using this method, a machine provides a specific amount of air and medication under increased pressure. IPPB forces deeper inspiration by positive pressure inhalation and permits the patient to exhale normally. The amount of pressure varies according to the patient's tolerance and needs. Usually, IPPB therapy is ordered to be used two to four times daily for 15 to 20 minutes each time.

There are many models of IPPB machines on the market. The one illustrated in Figure 27-15 is portable and especially useful for home use. In many health agencies, respiratory technicians are responsible for administering IPPB therapy. The nurse will wish to become familiar with the machine used in each agency of clinical practice so as to understand the exact nature of the therapy the patient receives.

Providing Oxygen Therapy

Oxygen is essential for life. When the body is deprived of adequate amounts of oxygen, hypoxia and hypoxemia can occur within a relatively short time. *Hypoxia* is defined as a deficiency in the amount of oxygen in inspired air; it has also come to mean a condition in which cells and tissues are experiencing an inadequate supply of oxygen. *Hypoxemia* is a condition in which there is a less than adequate level of oxygen in the blood.

Oxygen therapy is provided when the cardiopulmonary system is functioning poorly either because ventilation is inadequate or the circulatory system is impaired, or both. For example, when the lungs are diseased, oxygen is added to inhaled air so that the blood receives sufficient oxygen. Certain heart conditions impair the ability to circulate blood through the lungs. Oxygen therapy is then used to ensure that the tissues will be adequately supplied. The higher concentration of oxygen compensates for the limited transfer of oxygen to the blood.

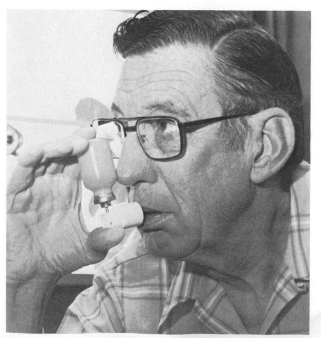

Figure 27-13 The patient uses a nebulizer, which can be purchased in most drugstores with a physician's prescription. He is about to place the mouthpiece into his mouth. Then, by pressing his fingers and thumb together on the nebulizer, the drug will be nebulized and inhaled into his respiratory passage.

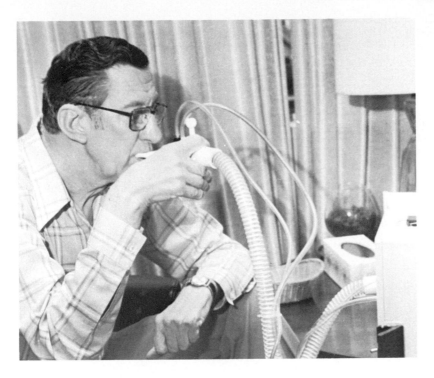

Figure 27-15 The patient holds the mouthpiece securely between his lips as he gives himself intermittent positive-pressure breathing therapy. The pressure forces deep inspirations but allows the patient to exhale normally.

Basic Guidelines for Administering Oxygen.
Certain basic guidelines should be observed when administering oxygen therapy:

Oxygen therapy is prescribed by the physician, except in certain emergency situations when experienced nurses are permitted to use independent judgment. The physician's order will specify the method of administration and the amount of oxygen to be given. Prior to 1983, physicians ordered the amount of oxygen in liters per minute, such as "3 L/min." Since that time, the Joint Commission of the Accreditation of Healthcare Organizations (JCAHO) has required that the amount of oxygen be prescribed on a percentage basis rather than as liters per minute. Table 27-1 may be used to convert the liter flow rate to its equivalent percentage using various delivery methods. The nurse administers oxygen just as cautiously as administering a medication, observing the same precautions and attention to accuracy as when giving a drug.

Patients suffering from insufficient oxygen often feel as though they are suffocating and are unable to breathe. They are usually restless, worried, and frightened. Respirations are characteristically achieved with great effort. It is a terrifying experience to be unable to breathe adequately. The patient needs support and the comfort of feeling that everything possible is being done.

Oxygen therapy must sometimes be instituted with such speed that there is little time for explaining procedures to the patient. However, some concurrent instruction is generally possible. After the patient is out of immediate danger, he should be told about the equipment and measures being used in his care.

The patient's responses to oxygen therapy are most accurately determined by laboratory examinations of the patient's arterial blood. Observations of the patient are also important for judging responses prior to and concurrent with oxygen therapy. These observations should include changes in the coloring of the patient's skin and nailbeds, changes in the vital signs and the nature of respirations, and level of consciousness.

Oxygen becomes progressively toxic at high concentrations. Signs of oxygen toxicity include a dry cough that may eventually become moist as lung damage occurs, chest pain felt beneath the sternum, nasal stuffiness, nausea and vomiting, and restlessness. The lungs and brain may become damaged, but unfortunately signs of injury to these structures may not be identified as early as other signs.

Oxygen supports combustion and, hence, must be used with great care. The following recommendations are offered to help avoid fires:

- "NO SMOKING" signs should be placed in prominent places and the patient and his visitors should be taught the importance of this regulation.

- Electrical devices, such as razors, radios, and television sets, should be removed or checked *carefully*

Table 27-1. Conversion Equivalents for Oxygen Therapy

Delivery Method	L/min	Equivalent Percentage
Nasal Cannula	2	28
	4	36
	6	44
Simple Mask	5	40
	6–7	50
	7–8	60
Partial Rebreather Mask	6	35
	8	45–50
	10	60
Non-rebreather Mask	6	55–60
	8	60–8
	10	80–90
Venturi Mask		
Color code: Blue	4	24
Color code: Yellow	4	28
Color code: White	6	31
Color code: Green	8	40

to be certain they are not sources of any sparks. All electrical equipment used with the patient's care, such as suctioning equipment, should be in good working order and properly grounded.

- Electrical signal devices should be checked for safety or removed from the room. A simple hand bell may be used instead.

- Oil and alcohol for backrubs are generally not used because of the fire danger they present. Lotions are used instead. No petroleum products should be used for lubricating the lips.

- Oil and grease should not be used near oxygen gauges and outlets because of the danger of their igniting spontaneously.

- There should be no open flames in the presence of oxygen. For example, candles may not be used during religious ceremonies for the sick when oxygen is in use.

- Fire extinguishers should be readily available wherever oxygen is being used and personnel should be familiar with their use.

- If oxygen is delivered from a tank, the tank should be secured properly to its stand to prevent accidents.

- Precautions should be used concerning static electricity. Fabrics that generate static electricity should not be used in the presence of oxygen. Some agencies require nurses working around oxygen to wear cotton uniforms and undergarments to help avoid static electricity.

Oxygen is delivered to the respiratory tract artificially under pressure. Therefore, excessive drying of mucous membranes lining the respiratory tract occurs unless the oxygen is humidified. Because oxygen is only slightly soluble in water, it can be passed through solutions with little loss. Tap or distilled water is generally used for this purpose. Some authorities recommend that the solution be warmed to between 52 and 54 °C (125 to 130 °F) to improve the humidification of the oxygen. The exact method of moisturizing oxygen depends on the agency's equipment. One type appears in Figure 27-16. The humidifying solution is attached below the flow meter. It may need to be refilled from time to time.

In many health agencies, oxygen is piped into each patient unit and is immediately available from an outlet in the wall. The oxygen is supplied from a central source through a pipeline, usually at 50 to 60 lbs/square inch of pressure. A specially designed flowmeter is attached to the wall outlet. The flowmeter opens the outlet and a valve makes regulation of the oxygen flow possible. Oxygen is compressed and dispensed from a steel tank when oxygen is not piped into the room.

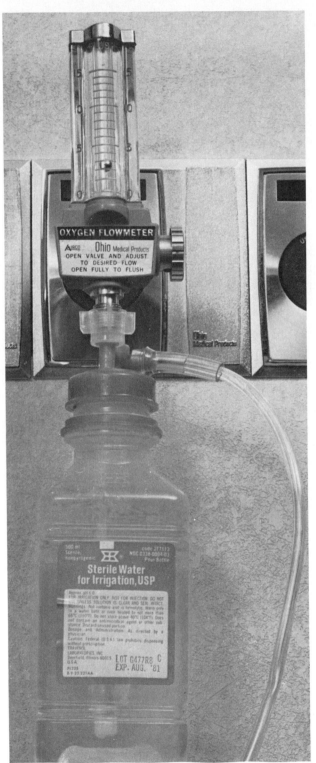

Figure 27-16 This is an oxygen flowmeter. A valve controls the amount of oxygen in liters per minute that the patient will receive. The oxygen bubbles through the humidifier bottle before being delivered to the patient.

Handling an Oxygen Tank. A few health agencies, such as nursing homes, may provide oxygen by tank rather than by piped-in wall units. Many are utilizing small individual tanks of oxygen for those patients who require it. However, when a large tank is the only source of supply, the nurse must be aware of its potential hazards when handling the equipment.

Tanks of oxygen are delivered with a protective cap to prevent accidental force against the tank outlet. When a standard, large tank is full, its contents are under more than 2000 lb of pressure per square inch. Force accidentally applied to a partially opened outlet could cause the tank to take off like a rocket, with disastrous results. The tank should be transported carefully while strapped onto a wheeled carrier.

When oxygen is dispensed from a tank, the tank should be handled as follows.

- Check to see that the tank contains oxygen. Gases other than oxygen are used in many health agencies. Administering the wrong gas is a serious error!
- "Crack" the tank. *Cracking* is a term that refers to releasing oxygen briefly in order to clear the outlet of dust and other debris before the regulator is applied. Use two hands to "crack" a tank so that opening it can be well controlled. Turn the wheel of the tank valve slightly so that a small amount of oxygen may be released. The force with which the oxygen is released from the opening causes a loud hissing sound, which may be frightening. It is recommended that oxygen tanks be "cracked" away from the patient's bedside unless he has been prepared for the noise with a proper explanation.
- Attach a humidifier to the tank and fill it with water according to the manufacturer's directions.
- Check to see that the tank is stabilized at the patient's bedside in a properly fitting stand so that there is no danger of the tank's tipping and possibly causing injury. The equipment is now ready to deliver oxygen to the patient.

Methods for Delivering Oxygen. Oxygen can be delivered to a patient in several ways. The oxygen may be administered with a nasal cannula, nasal catheter, mask, tent, and even into a tracheostomy. The doctor indicates the method for delivering the oxygen in the medical order. Basically all facilitate providing the oxygen directly to structures involved in breathing. Some methods of delivering oxygen are more efficient in providing higher concentrations of oxygen to the patient than others. This may become a critical criterion for selecting a particular delivery method when the patient is severely hypoxemic.

Using a Nasal Cannula. The simplest way to administer oxygen is through a cannula. A cannula is a hollow tube. A nasal cannula is a disposable plastic flexible tube with protruding prongs. The prongs are inserted into the patient's nostrils. The tube is then positioned over the ears and under the chin. The cannula can be self-adjusted to fit the patient comfortably without occluding the supply of oxygen. The patient in Figure 27-17 receives oxygen by nasal cannula. A cannula's advantage is that it does not interfere with eating, drinking, or talking.

It is generally recommended that no more than about 7 L of oxygen be delivered per minute through a cannula. Amounts higher than 7 L are too drying to mucous membranes. In most instances, 2 to 4 L/minute is a common prescription.

The nasal cannula is frequently the method used to administer oxygen to patients with chronic lung diseases. The respiratory center in the brain is generally stimulated by rising levels of carbon dioxide. However, the respiratory center of patients with chronic pulmonary diseases adapts to elevated levels of carbon dioxide in the blood. The stimulus to breathe then comes from sensing a low level of oxygen. If high percentages of oxygen are administered to chronic lung disease patients, respirations slow and the patient may even stop breathing. Because a cannula can deliver supplemental oxygen at low percentages, it is often the preferred method of administration.

Many home-care patients who require oxygen therapy also use a nasal cannula for its administration. The oxygen is supplied through the cannula from an oxygen tank. Smaller, more portable cannisters can be filled from the larger tank reservoir. The smaller containers of oxygen can be held in the hand, strapped to the back, or fastened to a wheelcart that can be pulled or easily pushed about.

The Nasal Catheter. A nasal catheter is a very efficient means of administering oxygen. It, too, allows a patient to eat and talk normally. It is generally somewhat less comfortable than a nasal cannula since it is inserted through a nostril into the nasopharynx and secured to the nose with tape. It is not intended to be removed for extended periods during the day. As is true of oxygen given through a cannula, oxygen has a very drying effect on mucous membranes when it is administered through a catheter at more than 7 L/minute.

Using an Oxygen Mask. Various types of masks for administering oxygen are available. One type is a simple, plastic, disposable one. It allows some room air to enter the mask. The air mixes with the oxygen so that dangerously high levels of oxygen are not inhaled by the patient.

Another type is the Venturi mask, shown in Figure 27-18. It allows air to enter the mask and exhaled carbon dioxide to leave the mask at special ports. It can supply up to 40% oxygen; the level of oxygen in the atmosphere is nearly 20%.

Two types of masks have a reservoir bag. The patient breathes oxygen from the bag through the mask. One is the partial rebreathing mask, which provides a moderately high concentration of oxygen. It allows some room air to enter the device but eliminates carbon dioxide so that the patient does not rebreathe his own exhaled car-

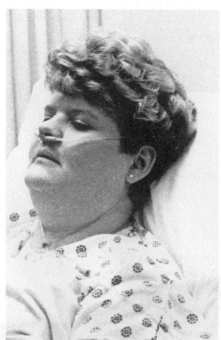

Figure 27-17 This shows how a nasal cannula is secured so that the prongs remain in the nostrils.

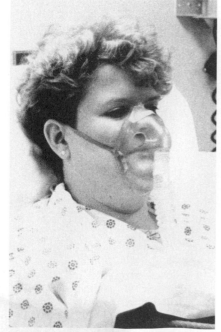

Figure 27-18 This photo shows a patient with a disposable oxygen mask in place. Most patients find the elastic strap to be most comfortable when placed just above the ears and around the back of the head.

bon dioxide. The partial rebreathing mask is most often used for patients who are seriously ill and in need of fairly high concentrations of oxygen. An example is a patient acutely ill with pneumonia.

The second type of mask with a reservoir bag is a nonrebreathing mask, which provides the patient with the highest concentration of oxygen. It allows little or no air to enter the reservoir bag and exhaled air to leave the mask. A nonrebreathing mask is most often used for patients with smoke inhalation or carbon monoxide poisoning who require very high concentrations of oxygen.

A disadvantage of all oxygen masks is that they interfere with eating and talking. If a patient is taking nourishment by mouth, the mask needs to be removed and a cannula or catheter used while the patient eats.

In general, masks are uncomfortable for most patients. They tend to irritate the skin where they rest on the face. Another disadvantage is that they often aggrevate feelings of claustrophobia (fear of enclosed areas).

Using an Oxygen Tent.

An oxygen tent is a light, portable structure made of clear plastic and attached to a motor-driven unit. The motor circulates air in the tent. A thermostat in the unit keeps the tent at a comfortable temperature for the patient. The tent fits over the top part of the bed so that the patient's head and chest fit inside of it. Oxygen is supplied to the tent through a special opening.

The tent is seldom used now for adults because other methods for delivering oxygen have been found to be more efficient, very handy, and less cumbersome. However, the nurse may still find tents being used with children, who are less likely to keep a cannula, catheter, or mask in place. Tents may also facilitate the combination of oxygen and humidification therapy for children with croup, bronchitis, and other respiratory conditions. The tent permits unrestrained movement and is less likely to cause excessive dryness of mucous membranes. A face tent or face hood may be placed over the head of small infants and children who are not likely to move about in bed.

Using Transtracheal Oxygen.

Some patients continue to need oxygen even after being discharged from a hospital or nursing home. Most wear a nasal cannula that is connected to a portable reservoir of oxygen. Many patients feel self-conscious using oxygen in public; others are bothered by skin and mucosal irritation from the cannula.

Transtracheal delivery of oxygen is now being used with selected patients in lieu of receiving oxygen by nasal cannula. The *transtracheal method* involves administering oxygen through a tiny catheter inserted directly into the trachea. The catheter is about the diameter of a 16-gauge angiocath but longer.

The tracheal opening is not used immediately for oxygen administration. The incision must mature for approximately a week. A stent, a temporary tube similar in size to the eventual transtracheal catheter, is placed within the incision. Its only function is to keep the incision from closing while the wound edges heal. Once healing begins, a guide wire is inserted through the stent and the stent is removed. The catheter is then threaded over the guide wire. The catheter is held within the trachea by a necklace-type chain that encircles the neck. The small device is not very noticeable and can even be covered by a collar or other accessories such as a scarf or tie. Patients are able to speak and consume food and fluids as usual.

Because the oxygen is being delivered constantly to the lower airway, patients can usually achieve the same level of oxygenation with half the liter flow required with a cannula. Depending on the volume and consistency of mucus production, catheters may need to be cleaned and replaced several times a day or as little as once a week.

Using a Tracheostomy Collar or T-Piece.

Several devices, such as the T-piece shown in Figure 27-19 permit oxygen and humidification to be delivered directly to a tracheostomy. It is common for the water used for humidification to condense within the tubing. Therefore, these devices need to be removed, drained, and replaced frequently.

Skill Procedure 27-6 provides a summary of the care that should be provided when the patient receives oxygen therapy by various common methods of delivery. Whenever implementing the actions that are described, it is assumed that the nurse will have provided an explanation (Text continues on page 732)

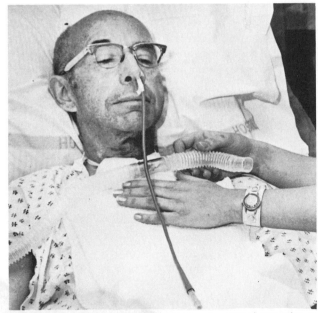

Figure 27-19 The large plastic tubing fastened over the tracheostomy is called a T-piece. It supplies moisturized air or oxygen to the patient. The tube in the patient's nostril is a gastric gavage tube, used to give this patient nourishment and oral medications.

Skill Procedure 27-6. Administering Oxygen

Suggested Action	Reason for Action
Observe practices of medical asepsis.	The upper respiratory passages are not considered sterile.
Assist the patient into a position of comfort, usually a variation of a Fowler's position.	Fowler's position reduces the effort of breathing by promoting more area for lung expansion.
Check the flow meter and level of fluid for humidification frequently during the course of time that the patient receives oxygen therapy.	The nurse must administer the prescribed amount of oxygen while ensuring its proper humidification. Administering too little or too much oxygen may endanger the patient's life.
Provide special hygiene measures for the nose and mouth that keep the tissues moist, lubricated, fresh, and clean during the course of therapy.	Oxygen is drying to mucous membranes. The patient may mouth breathe and be too fatigued to take adequate fluids or initiate hygiene measures independently.

Care When Using a Nasal Cannula

Attach the nasal cannula to the humidified oxygen source. Start the oxygen at the rate that will deliver the prescribed percentage of oxygen, usually 2 to 4 L/min.	Starting oxygen and making certain that the apparatus is functioning properly are less frightening, safer, and more comfortable for the patient than starting oxygen after the cannula is in place.
Determine that the oxygen is flowing by placing the prongs of the cannula in a glass of water.	The oxygen should form bubbles when the prongs are submerged in water.
Dry the cannula well before applying it to the nose.	Large droplets of inhaled moisture may cause choking. A wet cannula next to the skin is likely to feel uncomfortable.
Place the prongs of the cannula in the nostrils. Secure the cannula in place.	Oxygen is delivered from the tips of the prongs into the nose efficiently when the cannula is in a good position on the patient.
Instruct the patient to breathe through his nose.	Oxygen may be lost and never reach the lungs in sufficient therapeutic amounts when the patient mouth breathes.
Move the cannula slightly from time to time. Use small gauze squares to pad areas where the cannula tends to create pressure and irritate the skin.	While still having the cannula in place, changing the position and cushioning helps relieve pressure and aid absorption of moisture from next to the skin.
Remove and clean the nasal prongs on the cannula every 8 hours or more often if indicated.	Soiled prongs are uncomfortable and unpleasant for the patient.
Cleanse the nostrils around the cannula as necessary.	Accumulated secretions at the nostrils are uncomfortable for the patient and will irritate the skin and mucous membrane.

Care When Using a Nasal Catheter

Attach the catheter to the humidified oxygen source and start the oxygen at the prescribed rate. Usually 5 to 7 L/minute are used.	Starting oxygen and seeing to it that the apparatus is functioning properly are less frightening, safer, and more comfortable for the patient than starting oxygen after the catheter is in place.
Test that oxygen is moving through the catheter by placing the catheter tip in water.	When oxygen flows through the catheter, bubbles form in the water.
Drain the catheter well and then lubricate the tip with a water-soluble lubricant. A size 10 or 12 catheter about 40 cm (16 in) long is usually used for adults.	Lubricants reduce friction and thus minimize irritation to nasal membranes. Oily substances, if aspirated into the lungs, can be harmful. Petroleum-based products pose a potential fire hazard.

(continued)

Skill Procedure 27-6. Continued

Suggested Action	**Reason for Action**

Care When Using a Nasal Catheter

Measure the distance from the tip of the nose to the tip of the ear lobe.

This distance is the length at which the tip will be located in the upper pharynx when properly inserted.

Inspect the nares and insert the catheter through the side that is straighter.

Insertion of a tube is more easily performed in a nasal passage that is open and straight.

Assess the position of the catheter by depressing the tongue with a tongue blade and adjust the position as necessary. The placement of the catheter is illustrated in Figure 27-20.

A catheter inserted too far may cause the patient to gag or result in delivering oxygen to the gastrointestinal tract. Oxygen escapes when the catheter is not inserted far enough.

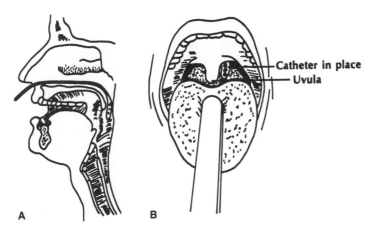

Catheter in place
Uvula

A   B

Figure 27-20 (*A*). This side view shows the correct location of a nasal catheter in the nose and the pharynx. (*B*). To make sure the catheter is placed properly, it is necessary to ask the patient to open his mouth. The tip of the catheter should be located just below the uvula.

Secure the nasal catheter to the nose in the same manner that a nasogastric tube is secured. The technique for taping can be reviewed in Chapter 8.

The nasal catheter should be secured so that it cannot become displaced. Positioning the catheter so that it extends in a straight line from the nose prevents pressure sores from forming at the nostril.

Attach the lower length of tubing to the patient's gown while providing sufficient slack to accommodate moving.

The attachment of a device in the nose should not interfere with movement or changing head positions.

Check the flow of oxygen regularly and maintain it at the prescribed rate.

Too little or too much oxygen is equally undesirable.

Remove and clean the catheter at least every 8 hours, or more often if indicated.

A soiled catheter is uncomfortable and unpleasant.

Clean the nostrils and alternate the nostril used when replacing the nasal catheter.

Oxygen can dry the mucous membranes and their protective secretions. Replacing the catheter within the same nostril can cause ulcerations within the mucous membrane.

Check regularly to see that the catheter is not kinked or otherwise obstructed by the patient or hospital equipment, such as parts of the bed.

A blocked catheter will decrease or halt the flow of oxygen.

(continued)

Skill Procedure 27-6. *Continued*

Suggested Action	Reason for Action
Care Using a Face Mask	
Attach the tubing from the face mask to the source of oxygen.	Oxygen must be humidified; moisture may be present from the patient's exhalations, but humidity is also usually added.
Flood the mask with oxygen at a rate of 8 to 15 L initially.	When the mask is placed over the patient's face, the patient can feel fearful of suffocating unless sufficient levels of oxygen are immediately available.
Adjust the mask in place to cover the nose and mouth. Fill open spaces between the skin and the mask with gauze.	More accurate concentrations of oxygen can be delivered when a mask conforms to the face and potential sites for leakage are sealed.
Regulate the flow of oxygen at the prescribed rate once the mask has been in place for several minutes.	The administration of oxygen must continue at the prescribed rate once a sufficient level has been achieved.
Use a mask with a reservoir bag to deliver oxygen ordered above 60% concentration.	It is difficult to achieve an oxygen concentration above 60% without using a reservoir bag.
Encourage the patient to breathe normally and help him to relax if he seems to struggle while receiving oxygen.	Support and instructions from the nurse may relieve anxiety and restore a more normal pattern to breathing.
Assess that the reservoir bag used for delivering oxygen does not collapse more than halfway during inspiration.	Oxygen flows directly into the bag and sufficient amounts may be available at the time of each breath.
Remove and clean the mask at least every 8 hours, or more often as indicated.	Moisture may accumulate within the mask, making it uncomfortable and unpleasant to the patient.
Wash the face and dry it well each time the mask is removed.	Evaporation is reduced in the area where the mask is applied. Skin care is essential to remove accumulated secretions and maintain cleanliness.
Care When Using an Oxygen Tent	
Inspect the tent for tears, nonfunctioning zippers, or ports in need of repair.	Oxygen will escape from the tent through any opening.
Place the tent over the upper portion of the bed.	Only the nose and mouth must be exposed to the oxygen. Covering the upper body provides room for movement and lessens feelings of claustrophobia.
Flood the tent with oxygen to achieve the desired level prescribed.	Each time the tent is opened, it will take an increased volume of oxygen to restore the concentration to its prescribed amount.
Tuck all the edges of the tent securely beneath the mattress. Use a bath blanket to enfold the edge of the tent that covers the upper body of the patient.	Oxygen can leak out through open spaces.
Check the level of oxygen in the tent using an oxygen analyzer. Fill and maintain the liquid used for humidification. Regulate the temperature setting that will be maintained within the tent.	Enclosing an individual can be hazardous if the amount of oxygen, the humidity, and environmental temperature within the tent are not adequate for safety.
Supply the patient with a device for summoning the nurse.	The patient may feel anxious within the tent and must know that it is possible to call someone to come to his assistance.
Care Using Transtracheal Oxygen	
Assess the skin around the catheter daily.	Redness, swelling, or purulent drainage suggests the presence of an infection.

(continued)

Skill Procedure 27-6. *Continued*

Suggested Action	Reason for Action

Care Using Transtracheal Oxygen

Suggested Action	Reason for Action
Clean the edges of the tracheal opening with hydrogen peroxide on cotton-tipped applicators until the incision is healed completely.	Hydrogen peroxide mechanically removes debris, such as dried serum, from wounds.
While bathing, use a mild soap such as Ivory to wash the skin where the catheter is inserted once healing is complete.	Mild soap is nonirritating but removes body oil, dirt, and transient organisms.
Apply a nasal cannula before beginning catheter cleaning. Connect the oxygen tubing from the transtracheal catheter to the cannula.	The cannula provides an alternate method of delivering oxygen while the catheter is removed.
Instill 1.5 mL of sterile normal saline directly into the opening of the catheter.	The saline liquefies mucus that collects within or near the tip of the catheter.
Encourage the patient to forcefully cough after taking several deep breaths.	Coughing can loosen mucus that coats the outer surface of the catheter that lies within the trachea.
Insert a cleaning wire within the catheter and withdraw it; repeat two more times.	The cleaning wire loosens secretions that adhere to the inner surface of the catheter.
Clean the removed wire brush with soap and water. Store it in a clean towel or container.	Cleaning follows principles of medical asepsis.
To replace a catheter, apply water-soluble lubricant to a new or clean catheter. Unfasten the current catheter from the chain necklace.	The lubricant reduces friction during insertion. Retained water-soluble lubricant will not cause lipid pneumonia.
Remove the current catheter and replace it with the new or clean one. Reattach the chain necklace to the catheter. Connect the oxygen tubing to the transtracheal catheter.	If replacement is delayed more than 30 minutes, the opening may seal.
Clean the removed catheter with soap and tepid water. Dry the catheter and store in a clean place for future use.	Hot water is damaging to the plastic component of the transtracheal catheter.
Avoid reusing cleaned transtracheal catheters after three months.	Catheters tend to become brittle with extended use.

Using a Tracheostomy Collar or T-Piece

Suggested Action	Reason for Action
Attach the device to the neck so that it covers the tracheostomy opening.	An individual with a tracheostomy does not breathe through his nose or mouth, but through the stoma.
Regulate the flow rate of oxygen.	The flow rate must be set at the amount necessary to deliver the percentage of oxygen prescribed by the physician.
Regulate the temperature of the humidified gas.	Warming the nebulized fluid increases the amount of moisture present in the oxygen.
Use large tubing from the oxygen source to the patient.	Condensation occurs less rapidly when the diameter of the tubing is increased.
Assess frequently for the accumulation of condensation within the tracheostomy collar or T-piece.	The fine mist droplets in the nebulized fluid tend to become larger as condensation occurs.
Remove the collar or T-piece frequently to drain the tubing.	Moisture can be aspirated. The wet condition within the tubing can support the growth of pathogens.
Suction the tracheostomy and provide tracheostomy care as frequently as necessary when moisture accumulates.	The moisture increases the potential for such complications as aspiration, skin breakdown, and infection.

of its use and implemented safety precautions related to the environment and the source of the oxygen supply.

Maintaining Water-Seal Drainage

There may be times when a lung partially or completely collapses. When this happens, the pleural space fills with air, called a *pneumothorax,* or it fills with blood, called a *hemothorax.* It is possible that both may be present at the same time.

The lung collapses due to the loss of negative pressure within the pleural space. The atmospheric air, which is higher in pressure, moves into and remains within the pleural space. The lung is no longer able to expand completely during each inhalation. Gas exchange is severely impaired.

Water-seal drainage may be instituted to remove the accumulated air or blood and gradually re-expand the collapsed lung. When water-seal drainage is used, the nurse must understand the equipment and the measures necessary for maintaining its care.

Many types of commercially manufactured systems, such as the one in Figure 27-21, are being used now for water-seal drainage and have replaced the use of glass bottles. Regardless of what type is used, the nurse can expect that one or two large catheters will extend from the upper or lower chest of the patient. The catheter(s) will drain into a collection chamber. The system is designed to prevent atmospheric air from re-entering the pleural space by partially filling one of the chambers in the drainage device with water; hence, the term

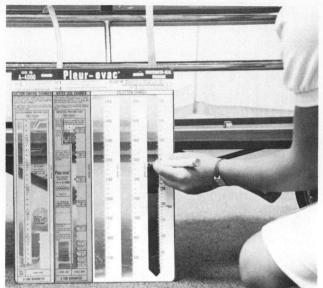

Figure 27-21 This is a commercial water-seal drainage system. This model contains chambers for drainage, water-seal, and suction, if that is prescribed.

water-seal drainage. A vent will be located in the system to permit air from within the pleural space to escape. As the air and blood drain from the pleural space, the lung will gradually re-expand. Suction may or may not be applied. When suction is used, it can speed the evacuation of fluid or air.

Skill Procedure 27-7 provides suggested actions for maintaining water-seal drainage.

Skill Procedure 27-7. Maintaining Water-Seal Drainage

Suggested Action	Reason for Action
Place the patient in Fowler's position or turned somewhat toward the side on which the chest tube has been inserted.	Gravity will help to move secretions in the direction of the drainage tube.
Assess the patient's lung sounds, vital signs, color, and effort of breathing.	A baseline of assessments can be used to mark the progress of the patient's response to treatment.
Expect that no lung sounds will be heard over the areas in which the lung is deflated.	Air will only be moving in the functioning areas of the lung.
Inspect all connections to determine that they are secure and airtight. Tighten or tape connections, as the agency policy indicates.	Air must be prevented from entering the system or the lung will continue to remain collapsed. Connections may be taped to ensure that they will not separate.
Inspect the fluid level in the water-seal chamber and keep it filled to the 2 cm level.	Water must be present to prevent atmospheric air from entering the drainage system. It may slowly evaporate.
Pinch off the tubing leading to the suction control chamber, if it is being used, to inspect the level of water. Keep the water level at 20 cm.	When suction is operating there may be so much bubbling that it may be difficult to assess the water level.
Adjust the amount of suction.	Suction should be adjusted to produce constant gentle bubbles in the fluid in the suction control chamber.
Observe the nature and amount of drainage in the collection chamber.	The characteristics of the drainage indicate the volume and type of drainage being removed from the pleural space.

(continued)

Skill Procedure 27-7. *Continued*

Suggested Action	Reason for Action
Report bright red bleeding or a volume that exceeds 100 mL/hour.	Bleeding is expected immediately following insertion, but it should be dark red and the volume should gradually decrease.
Mark the levels of drainage on the collection chamber. Initial, date, and mark the time of the levels.	Marking and timing the drainage level aids objective assessment and promotes accurate recording and calculation of fluid output.
Do not empty the collection container routinely.	Emptying the collection chamber increases the risk that air will enter the pleural space when the equipment is disconnected.
Observe that the level of water in the water-seal chamber rises and falls in synchrony with the patient's respirations.	As the pressures within the thorax change with breathing, the level of the water will coincide with those changes.
Become concerned if the fluid fails to rise and fall within the water-seal chamber during ventilation.	Failure of the water to fluctuate can be a welcome sign that the lung is expanded. Or, it may mean that the tubing is occluded.
Report constant bubbling in the water-seal chamber.	Constant bubbling may mean that an air leak is present. Periodic bubbling may occur as a result of the suction pulling air through the water-seal fluid.
Clamp the tubing for an instant using a hemostat close to the chest insertion site if constant bubbling is observed in the water-seal chamber.	If bubbling continues, the air leak exists below the level of the clamp.
Release and reclamp the hemostat at increasing increments down the length of the tube until the bubbling stops.	When the bubbling stops, it can be assumed that the air leak is between the clamp and the last location that was assessed.
Tape the tubing in the area of the air leak.	The tape will seal the air leak and re-establish the full function of the water-seal drainage system.
Keep the drainage device level below the area of the chest. Chest tubes may be curled on the bed but should hang straight into the collection chamber.	Straight gravity drainage helps maintain continuous movement of fluid into the collection chamber.
Avoid kinks in the drainage tube(s) or obstruction from the body weight of the patient.	If the tubing is occluded, drainage will not occur and pressure will build within the pleural space.
Encourage coughing and deep breathing at least every 2 hours.	Coughing and deep breathing aid in removing secretions from the upper airway and help force more air and drainage out from between the pleural space.
Encourage the patient to move about in bed, ambulate if allowed, and exercise the shoulder on the side of the drainage tube(s).	Inactivity should be avoided. Patients have a tendency to hold their shoulder rigid on the side of the chest tube(s). Exercise maintains the joint's range of motion.
Assess the skin area around the insertion site. Feel and listen for air crackling in the tissues.	Air may escape into the tissue around the insertion site rather than through the tubing. The crackling sound is called *crepitus*.
Milk the tubing only if absolutely necessary to remove secretions that interrupt drainage.	Stripping the tubing creates a dramatic increase in negative pressure that may injure pleural membranes. This action should never be performed routinely.
Do not clamp the tubing for an extended period of time. Temporary clamping may be indicated when the entire drainage device will be changed, but this should be accomplished within 2 minutes.	When air in the pleural space has no route for escape, it can compress the re-expanding lung causing increased tension within the pleural space.
Insert an accidentally disconnected chest tube into a container of water rather than clamping the tubing.	A partial pneumothorax is better than a tension pneumothorax.

(continued)

Skill Procedure 27-7. Continued

Suggested Action	Reason for Action
Disconnect the tube leading to the suction source to transport a patient. Keep the drainage collector below the level of the patient.	Drainage will be temporarily removed by gravity only.
Continue to assess lung sounds, vital signs, and the effort of breathing throughout the time that water-seal drainage is used.	Periodic documentation should record the progress of the patient and the effectiveness of the treatment.

Administering Cardiopulmonary Resuscitation

Cardiopulmonary resuscitation, commonly abbreviated CPR, consists of techniques to open and maintain a good airway and provide for artificial ventilation of the lungs and circulation of the blood. It is performed on a person who has suffered sudden and unexpected failure of the cardiopulmonary system. The term *rescue breathing* is sometimes used for artificial ventilation. It means using the rescuer's breath to revive someone who is unable to breathe for himself. *External cardiac compression* is the rhythmic administration of pressure on the chest wall as a substitute for normal heart contractions.

The ABCs of Basic Life Support.
The procedure of cardiopulmonary resuscitation is often described as the ABCs of basic life support.

- A is for Airway
- B is for Breathing
- C is for Circulation

The letter A means that the respiratory tract must be opened so that air can enter and leave the victim's lungs. The letter B means that if the victim does not start to breathe spontaneously after the airway is opened, artificial ventilation must be started. The letter C means that if the victim is pulseless, artificial circulation must be started along with rescue breathing.

The carotid artery is recommended for checking the pulse of an adult. It is an easily accessible artery when clothing about the neck is removed. Arteries in the extremities may be pulseless, but a pulse may still be felt at the large carotid artery, even when the heartbeat is of poor quality. A femoral artery is satisfactory but is ordinarily not as accessible as the carotid.

Indications for Cardiopulmonary Resuscitation.
When no breathing or pulse can be felt and signs of death are not pronounced, resuscitation efforts are made. However, it is not generally administered when prolonged cardiac arrest is suspected, such as when the person has been found dead, and signs indicate that he has been dead for some time.

Dilemmas occur when it is established that a person is terminally ill. If the person is a patient in a health agency, it is more than likely that there will be technology and personnel available at the time of death to revive the patient successfully. The choice as to whether cardiopulmonary resuscitation will be performed, in this situation, is usually discussed with the patient and the family. The wishes of the individuals involved are recorded on the patient's permanent record and on the nursing Kardex so that all personnel are aware of the directives concerning resuscitation.

Performing Cardiopulmonary Resuscitation.
Skill Procedure 27-8 describes and illustrates CPR for adults using either one or two rescuers. Administering CPR can be tiring and, when possible, it is better to have two rescuers who can switch responsibilities from time to time.

Before starting cardiac compressions, it is particularly important to be sure the victim is pulseless. If a pulse is present and compressions are given, the victim may develop a potentially fatal cardiac arrhythmia. Table 27-2 lists common errors when giving CPR and the effects of these mistakes on the victim. Various modifications in CPR techniques should be made depending upon the age of the victim. The differences are listed in Table 27-3.

Using a Self-Inflating Breathing Bag and Mask.
Several self-inflating breathing bags and masks are on the market. A popular example is the Ambu bag, shown in Figure 27-27. It is used in emergency situations for artificial ventilation and, in such instances, replaces giving mouth-to-mouth ventilation. The bag is compressed by the rescuer to force air into the lungs. It self-inflates during the time the rescuer releases pressure, allowing exhalation to occur. Oxygen need not be used but, in many situations, it is added to enrich the air.

The recommended procedure for using a self-inflating breathing bag and mask is as follows:

- Stand at the head of the patient if he is on a bed, or kneel at his head if he is on the floor. This positioning facilitates handling the bag and mask.

(Text continues on page 739)

Skill Procedure 27-8. Performing Cardiopulmonary Resuscitation

Suggested Action	Reason for Action
Two Rescuers	
Place the victim on a flat, firm surface, such as the floor, ground, or a board. The legs may be slightly elevated.	During cardiac compression, the firm surface on which the victim lies prevents dissipation of pressure on the sternum. Lying flat with the legs slightly elevated promotes blood flow to the brain.
Place one rescuer on one side of the victim's head; this rescuer will provide artificial ventilation. Place the second rescuer on the victim's opposite side near his chest; this rescuer will provide artificial circulation, if needed.	Having the rescuers positioned as described allows for maximum efficiency when assessing the victim and administering artificial ventilation and circulation.
First Rescuer	
Attempt to arouse the victim by shaking and shouting.	Stimulating the patient may restore consciousness.
Send someone to notify emergency personnel if the victim does not respond.	Advanced life support techniques may be needed if basic efforts to restore breathing and circulation are ineffective.
Tilt the head back by lifting the chin and pushing down on the forehead. This is illustrated in Figure 27-22.	Tilting the victim's head backward opens the airway by extending the neck and lifting the tongue from the throat.

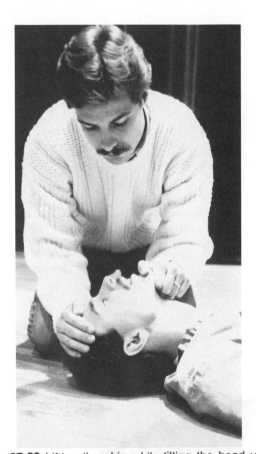

Figure 27-22 Lifting the chin while tilting the head usually facilitates breathing by opening the airway.

(continued)

Skill Procedure 27-8. Continued

Suggested Action	**Reason for Action**

First Rescuer

If the airway does not open with the above maneuver, the jaw thrust method should be used. Move to the top of the victim's head and place the fingers behind the victim's jaws. Push the jaw forward. This may be followed by slightly tilting the head backward; use the thumbs to retract the lower lip. This is illustrated in Figure 27-23.

This technique may be attempted secondarily when tilting the head and lifting the chin does not open the airway; it should be the method of choice when the victim has a possible neck injury.

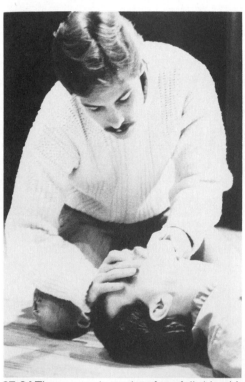

Figure 27-24 The rescuer is ready to forcefully blow his breath into the victim's mouth. Notice that the rescuer has pinched the nose shut so that air does not escape.

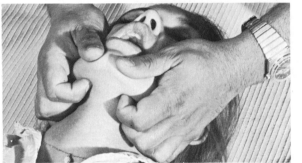

Figure 27-23 In this case, the rescuer opens the victim's airway by pushing the jaw forward while tilting the head back.

Remove any objects or vomited substances within the mouth.

Loose objects or liquid substances can be forced further within the airway as resuscitation efforts continue.

After the airway is open and cleared, listen for breathing and watch to see whether the chest or abdomen is rising and falling.

If the patient is breathing, there is no need to administer artificial ventilation.

While keeping the head tilted backward pinch the victim's nose shut with a finger and thumb from the hand that is on the victim's forehead, as illustrated in Figure 27-24.

Keeping the head tilted backward helps maintain an open airway. Pinching the nose shut allows maximum ventilation with no loss of air through the nostrils.

Prepare to administer two rescue breaths into the mouth of the victim.

Air delivered from the rescuer to the victim has an adequate amount of oxygen to sustain life.

(continued)

Skill Procedure 27-8. *Continued*

Suggested Action	Reason for Action

Second Rescuer

Take a deep breath, seal your lips around the victim's widely open mouth, and blow a forceful breath lasting 1 to 1½ seconds. Lift your face away from the victim and allow him to exhale passively. The chest should visibly rise and then fall. A pocket mask, shown in Figure 27-25, can be substituted for direct mouth-to-mouth breathing.

The force of rescue breathing needs to be sufficient so that the chest visibly rises when air is forced into the victim's mouth and then visibly falls with the victim's passive exhalation. The rescuer will note resistance in his own airway and can hear and feel air leave the victim when rescue breathing is given properly.

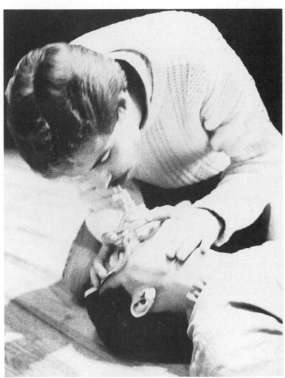

Figure 27-25 Ventilations can be effectively administered by mouth to mask. When properly positioned over the mouth and nose, an airtight seal is formed. A strap can be used to hold the mask in place if there is no other rescuer available to perform compressions.

Repeat this procedure once more.

Giving breaths that last 1 to 1½ seconds after taking the time for a full breath will prevent distention of the stomach with air, which could lead to vomiting and aspiration of vomitus.

OR

Cover the victim's nose with your mouth and administer the ventilations, if it is impossible to develop a good seal around the victim's mouth. Open the victim's lips between rescue breaths to allow the escape of air.

This technique may be used on an adult when the rescuer cannot develop or maintain an airtight passage into the respiratory tract.

Feel for a carotid pulse by lightly pressing two fingers into the groove between the trachea and the muscles at the sides of the neck.

The carotid artery is a large vessel and is likely to produce more obvious pulsations than could be felt at other peripheral sites on an adult.

(continued)

Skill Procedure 27-8. Continued

Suggested Action	Reason for Action
First Rescuer	

Suggested Action	Reason for Action
Continue with one rescue breath every 5 seconds, each lasting 1 to 1½ seconds, as long as the adult victim shows respiratory inadequacy.	A minimum of 12 regularly spaced rescue breaths per minute has been found to supply any victim over the age of 8 with sufficient oxygen to maintain cell integrity.
Continue to tilt the victim's head backward during all artificial ventilation.	Keeping the head tilted throughout artificial ventilation helps maintain an open airway.
Check for the presence of a pulse every few minutes. If the victim is pulseless, prepare to coordinate administering ventilations with cardiac compressions.	Resuscitation must provide ventilation and circulation when the victim's own cardiopulmonary system no longer functions.

Suggested Action	Reason for Action
Second Rescuer	

Suggested Action	Reason for Action
Place the width of the heel (the part near the wrist) of one hand over the long axis of the lower half of the sternum, but about 3.75 cm (1½ inches) from the xiphoid process.	Keeping off the xiphoid process at the tip of the sternum prevents possible liver injury and internal hemorrhaging.
Place the second hand over the first hand; the fingers should interlock. Bring the shoulders directly over the hands and keep the elbows and arms straight. This is illustrated in Figure 27-26.	Interlocking the fingers helps keep them off the victim's ribs, where pressure may cause fractures. This position, with the elbows and arms straight, allows for best exertion of pressure on the sternum over the heart.

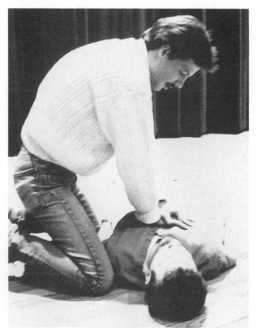

Figure 27-26 The rescuer compresses the victim's chest, forcing blood from the heart into the vascular system. Note that the rescuer's fingers are interlocked, his elbows are straight, and his shoulders are positioned over the victim's chest for most effective compression.

(*continued*)

Skill Procedure 27-8. *Continued*

Suggested Action	**Reason for Action**

Second Rescuer

Exert pressure on the sternum by rocking forward slightly so that pressure is applied almost vertically downward. Depress the sternum a minimum of 4 to 5 cm (1½–2 in) on anyone over the age of 8 and then relax pressure immediately, but without using a bouncing movement.	Depressing the sternum causes the heart to be compressed and forces blood into the aorta and pulmonary arteries. Relaxation of pressure allows the heart to expand and refill.
Keep the hands in proper position and on the victim's chest wall between compressions so that the heart can fill with blood.	Keeping the hands in place over the sternum helps to administer regular and even compressions.
Allow a pause after each five compressions to permit the administration of a rescue breath that lasts 1–1½ seconds.	A brief pause during ventilation further prevents the possibility of inducing vomiting or aspiration.
Continue with compressions and relaxations at a rate of 80 to 100 per minute as long as the victim's heart does not beat spontaneously.	A compression rate of 80 to 100 per minute will maintain adequate blood pressure and flow to maintain cell integrity for all victims except infants up to 1 year of age. A faster rate, identified in Table 27-3, is necessary for infants.
Check the effectiveness of CPR after the first minute and then regularly every few minutes by noting whether the pupils respond to light, pulsation is at the carotid artery, and the victim shows improvement in skin color.	When pupils constrict in the presence of light, adequate blood flow with oxygenated blood is reaching the brain. The carotid artery is large, centrally located, and ordinarily readily accessible. Color and pulsation will return spontaneously when the victim's heart begins to beat on its own.
Enlist assessment assistance from the rescuer providing ventilations or a third person so that CPR is never interrupted longer than 7 seconds.	CPR should be performed without interruptions in order to facilitate the maximum oxygenation and circulation for the victim.

One Rescuer

The procedure of CPR is as described previously when there is only one rescuer to perform artificial ventilation and circulation, *except:*

- When no one is available to assist, the rescuer should begin resuscitation efforts for a full minute and call for emergency assistance. If circumstances are such that this is impossible, resuscitation should be uninterrupted.
- Administer two rescue breaths after each 15 cardiac compressions. Repeat this pattern for a total of four cycles per minute. The same rates of compression apply whether CPR is performed by one or two rescuers.

- Place the mask firmly over the patient's nose and mouth with the rescuer's thumb placed near the patient's nose and the index finger near the patient's chin. The other fingers should be used to hold the patient's chin up and back to keep an open airway. Otherwise, place the victim's head over a rolled towel to hyperextend the neck. Proper patient positioning, hand placement, and application of equipment are illustrated in Figure 27-28.
- Spread the edges of the mask laterally if there is difficulty in getting the bag to fit tightly. When the mask returns to its normal shape, the victim's tissues will be gathered into the mask on his face and the seal will usually be tighter.
- Do not use straps to keep the mask in place. They get in the way if the victim vomits or needs to be suctioned.
- Squeeze the bag to force inhalation and quickly release pressure on the bag to allow for exhalation.
- Compress the bag at the average normal respiratory rate unless the victim's condition indicates otherwise.

Discontinuing Cardiopulmonary Resuscitation. CPR is discontinued when a person begins breathing

Table 27-2. Common Errors During Cardiopulmonary Resuscitation

Error	Effect
The airway is not patent.	Air cannot enter the lungs in sufficient quantity to sustain life when the airway is not open.
The head is tilted back too far and with too much force when a cervical injury is present.	The head tilt may cause damage to the victim's spinal cord in the area of the injury. A modified jaw thrust is recommended, in which the head is maintained in a neutral position rather than tilted backward.
The seal made by the rescuer's mouth over the victim's mouth or nose is broken.	Sufficient air will not enter the victim's lungs when the seal formed by the rescuer's mouth is not maintained.
The rescue breaths are of insufficient force to cause the victim's chest to rise with each one.	When the victim's chest does not visibly rise and fall with each complete rescue breath, sufficient air for adequate ventilation is not entering the lungs.
Artificial ventilation is too forceful or it is administered when there is an airway obstruction.	There will be distention of the stomach if artificial ventilation is too forceful. This occurs more commonly in children than in adults. The danger is that distention tends to cause vomiting and predisposes the victim to aspiration. It also causes the diaphragm to rise and interfere with proper artificial ventilation and circulation.
The fingers of the rescuer rest on the ribs of the victim during compression.	Pressure on the rib cage may result in fractures of the ribs.
The xiphoid process is depressed during cardiac compression.	Depression of the xiphoid process may lacerate the liver and cause internal hemorrhaging.
Some pressure is maintained between cardiac compressions on the victim's chest wall.	When there is not complete relaxation after each cardiac compression, the heart cannot adequately fill with blood.
The sternum is depressed less than the recommended distance.	Blood flow and pressure will be insufficient to maintain cell integrity.
The rescuer administering cardiac compression is not properly positioned directly over the victim and/or has his elbows bent.	The thrust of compression will be ineffective when the rescuer is improperly positioned. Also, the rescuer will tire more quickly.
Sudden, irregular, or jerking movements are made during cardiac compressions.	Sudden, irregular, and jerking movements tend to cause injuries and are ineffectual for maintaining good blood flow and pressure.
CPR is interrupted for more than 7 seconds. If a victim *must* be intubated or moved, the interruption should not exceed 30 seconds.	Ventilation and circulation quickly become inadequate, and cell integrity suffers, when CPR is interrupted.

and his heart starts beating. If the victim does not respond to resuscitation, remains unconscious, and has pupils that are dilated even in the presence of light for as long as 30 minutes, further resuscitation efforts will probably be to no avail. However, the final decision about further resuscitation efforts is left up to the physician or the leader of the resuscitation team. In the meantime, the victim is given resuscitation until the rescuer is exhausted and cannot continue. Some persons have been reported to have survived without permanent brain damage even after signs of death were present for as long as an hour or two. This has been found to be the case especially with children involved in cold water drownings and others suffering from hypothermia.

Suggested Measures to Promote Cardiopulmonary Function in Selected Situations

When the Patient Is an Infant or Child

Assess infants and small children carefully because they cannot communicate in the same manner as an adult. Flaring of the nostrils, a grunt on exhalation, restlessness, and poor skin color are typical signs of a need for oxygen in youngsters.

Be prepared to use an isolette or oxygen hood when an infant needs oxygen therapy. An isolette fits over the crib. It is transparent, permitting the

Table 27-3. Differences in CPR Among Infants, Children, and Adults

Technique	Infant (≤1 year of age)	Child (1–8 years of age)	Adult (≥8 years of age)
Rescue breaths			
Initial	2 breaths	2 breaths	2 breaths
Subsequent breaths	1 every 3 seconds	1 every 4 seconds	1 every 5 seconds
Rate	20/minute	15/minute	12/minute
With chest compressions: One Rescuer	1 breath/5 compressions	1 breath/5 compressions	1 breath/5 compressions
Two Rescuers			2 breaths/15 compressions
Duration	1–1½ seconds	1–1½ seconds	1–1½ seconds
Compressions			
Location	In the midline, one finger's width below the nipples	Two finger widths above the tip of the sternum	Two finger widths above the tip of the sternum
Hand use	Two fingers (or, in neonates, encircle the infant's chest with both hands and compress the sternum using both thumbs)	Heel of one hand	Two hands
Rate	At least 100/minute	80–100/min	80–100/min
Depth	½–1 in	1–1½ in	1½–2 in

(With permission of the American Heart Association: Standards and guidelines for cardiopulmonary resuscitation and emergency cardiac care. JAMA 255:2841–3034, 1986.)

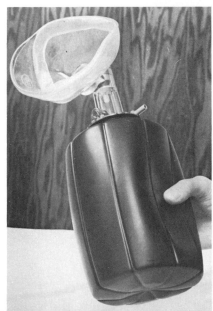

Figure 27-27 This is a self-inflating breathing bag and mask. The mask is made of transparent plastic so that the rescuer can better observe the victim.

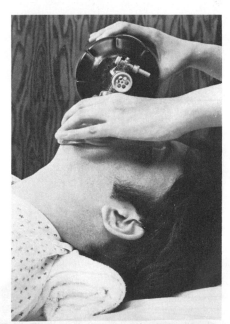

Figure 27-28 The mask is properly applied over the victim's nose and mouth, and the rescuer is ready to use the right hand to compress the bag. Note that the victim's head is placed over a rolled towel to help keep his airway open.

Applicable Nursing Diagnoses

Patients with cardiopulmonary problems may develop these nursing diagnoses.
- Ineffective Breathing Patterns
- Ineffective Airway Clearance
- Impaired Gas Exchange
- Decreased Cardiac Output
- Altered Tissue Perfusion
- High Risk for Suffocation
- Activity Intolerance

Nursing Care Plan 27-1 has been developed to illustrate how the nursing process applies to a patient with Ineffective Airway Clearance. This diagnostic category is defined in the NANDA taxonomy (1989) as, "A state in which an individual is unable to clear secretions or obstructions from the respiratory tract to maintain airway patency."

infant to be seen. Portholes are provided through which care and therapy are given. Warmed oxygen and humidity can be easily supplied to an isolette. An oxygen hood provides similar therapy but only covers the infant's head.

Be prepared to use a croupette for youngsters requiring humidified air for inhalation. A croupette has a metal frame, over which a tent is constructed with plastic sheets and linen and into which humidified air is supplied. In some instances, oxygen may also be added to the humidified air in a croupette.

Place infants and young children in the various positions for postural drainage while holding them on the lap over the thighs when they cannot maintain proper positioning in bed.

When percussing the chest wall of an infant, consider using a nursing nipple instead of a cupped hand. The rim of the nipple is petaled with adhesive tape in the same manner as a cast is petaled, as described in Chapter 26. The petaling provides sturdiness to the rim. Some nurses have found that a tennis ball cut in half is effective for percussing the chest wall of a young child.

When vibrating the chest wall of an infant or young child, consider using the handle of an oscillating electric toothbrush rather than the hands.

Take sufficient time to explain about a tracheostomy that is to be performed on an infant or child. Having a tracheostomy can be an extremely frightening experience for parents as well as for children.

Plan to have someone in attendance with infants and children who have a tracheostomy because they cannot signal for help and may try to remove the cannula. Restraining the elbows may be necessary

in some situations but restraining does not replace the need to stay with young patients at all times.

When the victim is an infant or child, use emergency measures to relieve choking as described earlier in this chapter, with the following important differences:

- For evidence of choking, note whether a child too young to speak can cry. If the airway is open, the child will be able to cry; if the airway is obstructed by a foreign object, the child will not be able to cry.

- Place an infant on his abdomen while he is resting on the rescuer's forearm. Position the head of the victim lower than the rest of the body to administer four back blows with the heel of the hand between the shoulder blades when the victim is under 1 year of age, as illustrated in Figure 27-29. Otherwise, a young child can be placed crosswise over the rescuer's thighs with the head lower than the rest of the body. Having the head lower than the rest of the body permits gravity to assist in removing a foreign object from the respiratory tract.

When an infant is on his back or on the rescuer's thighs with the head lower than the rest of his body, administer chest thrusts to the middle of the sternum at about the level of the nipples, well away from the lower end of the sternum. The thrusts are administered with two fingers, as illustrated in Figure 27-30.

Avoid using abdominal thrusts in infants and children because of the danger of injuring internal organs. Use chest thrusts instead.

Give CPR to infants and children in the same manner as for adults, applying the modifications listed in Table 27-3 and the following suggestions:

- Use a brachial artery to check for the pulse on an infant, as illustrated in Figure 27-31. This site is

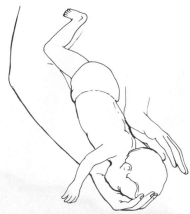

Figure 27-29 When administering a back blow, the infant rests on the forearm of the rescuer while his head is supported in the rescuer's hand.

NURSING CARE PLAN

27-1. *Ineffective Airway Clearance*

Assessment	***Subjective Data***
	States, "I've had such a hard time breathing this past week. I stayed home from work. Most of the time I slept in my recliner chair. I couldn't even eat or drink much."

Objective Data

48-year-old man with a history of smoking 2 packs of cigarettes per day admitted with possible bacterial pneumonia. T—101° (oral) P—100. Breathing is rapid (30/min) and shallow. Uses accessory muscles and demonstrates nasal flaring. Bronchial breath sounds and inspiratory gurgles heard in distal R. upper lobe both anteriorly and posteriorly; all other areas of lungs sound clear. Has a persistent cough but does not raise sputum. Skin is hot and dry. Urine is a dark concentrated amber color.

Diagnosis

Ineffective airway clearance related to weak cough and retained secretions.

Plan

Goal

The patient's lungs will sound clear throughout by 12/4.

Orders: 12/1

1. Auscultate lungs $\bar{q}$ shift, and before and after coughing or other respiratory therapy.
2. Elevate head of bed at all times.
3. Maintain 2000–3000 mL fluid intake of patient's choice (avoid milk) for 24 hours.
4. Instruct to take 3 deep breaths in through nose and out mouth, lean forward, and cough forcefully. Repeat $\bar{q}$ 1–2 hr while awake.
5. Perform oral/pharyngeal suctioning if secretions are loosened but not expectorated. ——————————————————— L. HOWARD, RN

Implementation (Documentation)

12/1   0730   Continues to demonstrate effort at breathing. Sitting upright, nostrils flare, and physical activity is limited. Lungs clear except for inspiratory gurgles in RUL. Receiving 36% O_2 per nasal cannula at 4 L/min. IV of 1000 mL of 5% D/W $\bar{c}$ 800 mg of aminophyllin infusing at 30 mL per hour through infusion pump. Respiratory department contacted concerning new order for aerosol therapy. Instructed on deep breathing and coughing technique. ——————— A. SANTINI, LPN

Evaluation (Documentation)

0800   Breathing and coughing performed 3 times with no change in lung assessments. Able to drink a pot (240 mL) of hot tea with sugar and lemon. ———————————————————————————————— A. SANTINI, LPN

1000   Able to raise a small amount of tenacious, purulent sputum following breathing and coughing. Specimen sent to laboratory for culture and sensitivity. Lung sounds remain unchanged. ——————————— A. SANTINI, LPN

recommended by the American Heart Association. The apical pulse, which can be heard with a stethoscope or felt with a fingertip at a point under the nipple line and just to the left of the sternum, is recommended by some authorities. It is suggested that agency policy be observed if there is a question about where to obtain a pulse rate on an infant.

• Tilt the head of an infant or young child backward to open the airway very gently and without exaggeration. The neck is pliable and can be injured with relative ease.

• If the child is small, the rescuer should cover both the mouth and nose with his mouth when adminis-

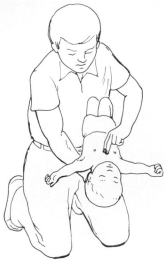

Figure 27-30 How to administer a chest thrust to an infant.

tering artificial ventilation. Some authorities recommend covering the mouth of the rescuer with a hankerchief while administering rescue breathing.

- Use rescue breaths smaller than those for an adult but deep enough to make the chest wall rise.

Teaching Suggestions to Promote Cardiopulmonary Function

Teaching suggestions for helping patients promote cardiopulmonary functioning are summarized below.

Patients using oxygen at home should be taught to use safety precautions, as described in this chapter, to prevent accidents with fire. Oxygen is safe to use when its characteristic of supporting combustion is respected at all times.

Patients using oxygen at home should have careful instructions about safe amounts to use. Many persons are likely to think that if a small amount is helpful, larger amounts may be even more helpful. The dangers of using other than prescribed amounts should be carefully explained.

Steam vaporizers may still be used in some homes.

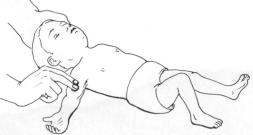

Figure 27-31 How to obtain a pulse rate at the brachial artery on an infant.

Patients and parents of children should be taught about the dangers of burns because steam humidifiers become very hot.

Some patients are discharged with a tracheostomy in place. The home care of a tracheostomy is similar to care given in a health agency. If a reusable inner cannula is used, the patient should be instructed to have several on hand so that, while cleaning one, another one is in place.

A patient with a tracheostomy who uses a reusable cannula should be taught how to clean it and maintain his care as follows:

- Use a small brush or pipe cleaner while scrubbing the cannula with soap or detergent and water.

- Rinse the cannula well after scrubbing it and boil it for 8 to 10 minutes, or place it in 70% alcohol for disinfection for 20 minutes or longer. Be sure to rinse the cannula well with sterile water because alcohol is irritating to mucous membranes.

- Clean cannulas are best stored in a sterile, covered jar.

- The patient with a tracheostomy should be instructed about reporting symptoms that indicate an infection. He should also be taught the urgency of obtaining immediate medical attention if the outer cannula becomes obstructed or is dislodged.

Many lives are saved when persons at the scene of an emergency are familiar with how to administer CPR and how to relieve choking on a foreign object. Nurses are looked to as examples and sources for information. They should teach people the importance of enrolling in classes, now offered by a variety of community organizations, to learn proper techniques.

It is better to prevent choking than to have to handle an emergency when it occurs. In addition to helping people learn how to remove a foreign object from respiratory passages, the following measures should be taught concerning how best to prevent choking and how to signal for help when choking:

Do not talk or laugh with food in the mouth.

Cut food into small pieces and chew it well.

Make sure dentures fit well to prevent choking.

Do not drink alcoholic beverages in excess. Choking is more common when the alcohol blood level is excessive.

When choking, grasp the throat with both hands to signal for help.

Take special precautions with infants and children to prevent choking. Keep small objects, such as small toys or parts of them, coins, safety pins, nuts or popcorn, away from infants and small children. Their natural curiosity often leads to emergency situations because they tend to place objects in the mouth without realizing the dangers of choking.

Bibliography

Bolgiano CS, Bunting K, Shoenberger MM: Administering oxygen therapy: What you need to know. Nursing 20(6):47–51, 1990

Britt J: What to do when your patient codes. Nursing 20(1):42–43, 1990

Carroll P: Safe suctioning. Nursing 19(9):48–51, 1989

Carroll PF: Good nursing gets COPD patients out of hospitals. RN Magazine 52(7):24–28, 1989

Carroll PF, Maher VF: Quick review of a code's legal aspects. Nursing 20(5):38–39, 44, 1990

Centala M, Paige J, Wros PW: One way to avoid resuscitation roulette. Am J Nurs 90(6):29–30, 1990

Ellstrom K, Bella LD: Understanding your role during a code. Nursing 20(5):36–44, 1990

Erickson RS: Mastering the ins and outs of chest drainage *part 1.* Nursing 19(5):36–44, 1989

Grandstrom D, Wierzbicki LA: A better way to deliver long-term oxygen therapy. RN Magazine 52(9):58–62, 65, 67, 1989

Hahn K: Tips for giving oxygen therapy. Nursing 20(2):70, 1990

Heimlich HJ, Patrick EA: The Heimlich maneuver: Best technique for saving any choking victim's life. Postgrad Med 87(8):38–48, 53, 241–244, 1990

Jones S, Clark V: Dos and Don'ts of a code: Dealing with cardiac arrest. AD Nurse 4(2):10–16, 1989

Juip M, Harned JC: Giving mouth-to-mouth ventilations. Nursing 18(12):48–49, 1988

Konz CM: Action STAT! Emergency intubation. Nursing 20(2):33, 1990

Makrevis CS: Be prepared: Call mock codes. RN Magazine 53(1):19–20, 22, 1990

Miracle VA, Allnutt DR: How to perform basic airway management *part 1.* Nursing 20(4):55–60, 1990

Miracle VA, Allnutt DR: Using a manual resuscitator correctly *part 2.* Nursing 20(5):49–51, 1990

Sheard T: Going face to face with fear . . . giving mouth-to-mouth resuscitation . . . fears about AIDS. Nursing 20(4):43, 1990

Wesmiller SW, Hoffman LA: Interpreting your patient's oxygenation status. Orthopedic Nursing 8(6):56–60, 1989

Wesmiller SW, Hoffman LA, Wiseman M: Understanding transtracheal oxygen delivery. Nursing 19(12):43–47, 1989

Willens JS, Copel LC: Performing CPR on adults. Nursing 19(1):34–43, 1989

Willens JS, Copel LC: Performing CPR on children. Nursing 19(2):57–64, 1989

Willens JS, Copel LC: Performing CPR on infants. Nursing 19(3):47–53, 1989

Unit V

Nursing Skills
Used During a
Dying Experience

28

Caring for Terminally Ill and Grieving Individuals

Chapter Outline

Behavioral Objectives
Glossary
Introduction
Examining Attitudes and Responses to Dying
Preparing to Provide Terminal Care
Informing the Dying Patient
Identifying Patterns of Emotional Reactions
Supporting Options for Care
Responding to Emotional Needs
Meeting Spiritual Needs
Attending to Physical Needs
Recognizing the Signs of Approaching Death
Summoning the Family
Helping Arriving Relatives
Confirming Death
Nursing Responsibilities After the Patient's Death
Understanding the Grieving Process
Suggested Measures for Terminally Ill or Grieving
  Patients in Selected Situations
Applicable Nursing Diagnoses
Teaching Suggestions Involving Terminally Ill and
  Grieving Individuals
Bibliography

Skill Procedures

Performing Postmortem Care
Facilitating the Process of Grieving

Behavioral Objectives

When the content of this chapter has been mastered, the learner will be able to:

Identify and describe the stages of dying, as described by Dr. Elisabeth Kübler-Ross.

Describe the options for care that are generally available to patients with a terminal illness.

Describe nursing measures that may be useful when meeting the emotional needs of dying patients.

List common fears shared by many dying individuals.

Discuss approaches for meeting the dying patient's spiritual needs.

Identify unique physical problems of dying patients and nursing interventions that may be useful.

List various signs associated with approaching death.

Describe approaches for informing and supporting a family member when death is near.

Describe the nursing responsibilities associated with care of the body and patient's belongings.

Discuss typical grief reactions and methods that help others to resolve the loss of a loved one.

Describe the nursing measures that may facilitate grieving a perinatal death.

List suggested measures for the care of the terminally ill patient in selected situations as described in this chapter.

Summarize suggestions for patient and family teaching as offered in this chapter.

Glossary

Active euthanasia The deliberate ending of the life of an individual who is suffering from an incurable condition.

Anticipatory grief The grief that begins when learning that a death will occur.

Autopsy An examination of the organs and tissues of a human body following death.

Avoidance A technique used to separate oneself from situations that are threatening or unpleasant.

Brain death A term meaning that there is no evidence of brain functioning in an individual who is being kept alive with life support machines.

Denial A psychological technique in which an individual does not believe certain information to be true.

Euthanasia A term meaning an easy death.

Grief The physical and emotional feelings related to separation and loss.

Grief work Activities that lead to resolving a loss. Synonym for *mourning*.

Hope The ability to cling to the possibility of a positive outcome in spite of overwhelming odds.

Hospice An organization dedicated to providing care and services exclusively to dying patients and their families.

Living will A written statement describing the wishes of the writer concerning his medical care when his death becomes inevitable.

Mourning Activities that lead to resolving a loss. Synonym for *grief work.*

Paranormal experience One that is not considered humanly possible and resembles something supernatural.

Passive euthanasia Using techniques that relieve pain but that do not delay natural death from occurring.

Pathological grief Actions that indicate an individual is not accepting the reality of a death.

Perinatal death The death of an infant that occurs prior to, during, or shortly after birth.

Postmortem care Care of the body after death.

Shroud A garment for enclosing a dead body.

Symbolic language Communication that involves terms or statements that carry a double meaning.

Terminal illness One from which recovery is beyond reasonable expectation.

Thanatologist One who studies death and dying.

Tolerance A condition in which a person requires more of a drug to achieve a similar effect once obtained with a lower dosage.

Introduction

Scientific technology, improved nutrition, and advancements in health care have all added increased years to life expectancy. Figure 28-1 shows the gradual increases added to human life over the past 40 years. Life expectancy continues to lengthen year by year. Yet death is a certainty. The only unknowns are when, where, and how death will occur. Nurses and other health personnel are probably involved more than any other group with individuals who experience impending death.

Death may be sudden and unexpected for some; but it may be somewhat predictable for individuals with a termi-

nal illness. A *terminal illness* is one from which recovery is beyond reasonable expectation. The condition that contributes to death may be a disease or it may be the result of injury. Information compiled in Table 28-1 shows the current leading causes of death in the United States.

When a patient is dying, the nurse is faced with dual responsibilities. The dying patient requires holistic care in perhaps the fullest meaning of the term. At the same time, those individuals who have developed a significant relationship with the dying patient, which may include family, friends, and even health-care staff, will need support. All will be dealing with grief. *Grief* encompasses the physical and emotional feelings related to separation and loss.

This chapter will deal with many aspects of the dying and grieving experience. The unique emotional, spiritual, and physical problems of the terminally ill will be discussed. Approaches that are helpful in dealing with anticipatory grief will also be described. *Anticipatory grief* is the grief that begins when learning that a death will occur.

Examining Attitudes and Responses to Dying

It is difficult to deal with any problem that does not seem to be a reality. Death seems to be one of those unrealistic events. It is not unreasonable to understand the futility that individuals feel when dealing with the certainty of approaching death.

People are not usually prepared for death. Most individuals have been sheltered from death by institutions that provide care for the terminally ill or that relieve the family's involvement by arranging the funeral.

Table 28-1. Leading Causes of Death in the United States*

1	Heart diseases
2	Cancer
3	Cerebrovascular diseases
4	Accidents
5	Chronic lung diseases
6	Pneumonia and influenza
7	Diabetes mellitus
8	Suicide
9	Chronic liver diseases and cirrhosis
10	Atherosclerosis
11	Kidney diseases
12	Homicide
13	Perinatal conditions
14	Septicemia
15	Congenital defects

* Ranking based upon information compiled for the year 1984 by The National Center for Health Statistics, U.S. Department of Health and Human Services, Hyattsville, MD.

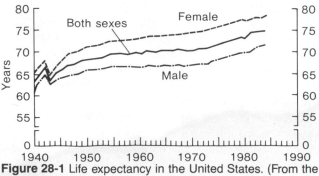

Figure 28-1 Life expectancy in the United States. (From the National Center for Health Statistics, U.S. Department of Health and Human Services, Hyattsville, MD)

Life-sustaining advancements occur now with such frequency as to make death seem as though it could be postponed almost indefinitely. Transplant procedures provide dying individuals with not only a new healthy organ but also a second chance at life. Critical care techniques literally snatch many a person from almost guaranteed death. The examples go on and on.

As a result of the lack of experience with death, most individuals react somewhat instinctively when personally involved with impending death. Some common reactions of patients, family members, and health-care professionals are recognized:

Denial: denial is a psychological technique in which an individual does not believe certain information to be true. This approach is difficult to sustain as accumulating evidence tests its logic.

Avoidance: avoidance is a technique used to separate oneself from situations that are threatening or unpleasant. Health-care personnel are more often inclined to use this approach since the dying person represents a personal defeat.

Hope: hope is the ability to cling to the possibility of a positive outcome against overwhelming odds. This human quality helps individuals to endure a hardship while believing that it will ultimately be resolved.

Most individuals prefer to put thoughts of death "in the closet." They prefer to think and deal with death only when it becomes absolutely necessary to do so. However, this approach does not always provide the best resources for dealing with death and dying. More and more individuals, called *thanatologists,* are studying death and dying and encouraging others to do so.

Preparing to Provide Terminal Care

Each nurse will more than likely become involved with the care of a terminally ill patient. Personal values and attitudes are closely associated with the quality of care that a nurse provides. Since the subject of death is not one that most nurses have thought about, it is best to take the opportunity to explore various aspects of death and dying before being faced with the actual experience. This intellectual approach may help to resolve future conflicts before becoming emotionally involved.

Exploring Feelings About Death

Since nurses are a product of their culture, it is not difficult to understand that they would share similar values. In our culture, youth, health, and productivity are valued in contrast to aging, illness, or retirement. Most individuals are strongly dedicated toward life and the future. We live in a death-denying society. For these reasons, nurses may ex-

perience difficulty when caring for individuals who are chronically ill, elderly, or approaching death.

One's personal feelings about death and dying are particularly important to understand before providing terminal care. The nurse who neglects to do so is in a questionable position to be able to meet the needs of terminally ill patients and their families. The easy way is to avoid involvement and remain detached. Sadly enough, the dying person and the family are often emotionally abandoned. They are left to face a very frightening situation alone while the nurse performs care like an unfeeling robot.

Discussing ideas with others is one of the most effective ways of developing insight about death and dying. This can be done in a formal conference with other health or nursing personnel; it can be done informally through discussions with friends, family, counselor, or clergyman. Some even propose that it is beneficial to write one's own hypothetical obituary as a method for provoking thought and discussion.

The answers to the following questions often help a nurse to clarify personal feelings about death and dying:

- What is my concept of death?
- Who or what has contributed to my feelings about death?
- What kinds of goals or experiences are especially important to me before I die?
- Would I want to know that my condition is terminal?
- If I could control the events that lead to my death, what would I want them to be?
- Whom would I want to have present during my terminal illness?
- Where would I prefer to die?
- What fears do I have about death?

Developing a Support System

The nurse is often looked to as the source of strength during a period of crisis. However, there may be times when the nurse may feel the need to ventilate frustration and receive support rather than always give it. Most nurses find their coworkers extremely empathetic and comforting. The nurse must never feel that the burden of care depends on only one person. Other health-team members include the physician, pharmacist, psychologist, social worker, dietitian, clergyman, and others. All are allies who may provide help that complements and supplements the nursing care of the terminally ill patient and his family. When nurses feel a sense of support, they are better able, in turn, to support others.

A support system begins by developing an environment in which nurses know they can turn to each other. It includes being able to share daily work problems, sadness, and humor—and, possibly most of all, being able to share themselves and their personal feelings. Nonverbal communication techniques such as touch in the form of a pat on the back or a hug are often helpful. Weeping, laughing, and also being silent together can be comforting and supportive. Peer support works best when nurses not only reach out for support they need but also readily say, "How can I help you?"

Examining Euthanasia

When caring for a terminally ill patient, a nurse must often deal with ethical and legal issues about ending life or prolonging it by artificial means. *Euthanasia* literally means an easy death. The term has also come to mean mercy killing. The use of euthanasia is generally considered when death is inevitable and life-saving measures are of questionable benefit. *Passive euthanasia* refers to using techniques that relieve pain but that do not delay natural death from occurring. *Active euthanasia* is the deliberate ending of the life of an individual who is suffering from an incurable condition; this form of euthanasia is illegal.

Despite a hopeless situation, the patient and the family remain the focus of attention. They are the ones who should control decisions affecting medical care. They often need time to work through their feelings. At one time the medical emphasis was on extending the quantity of life no matter what the cost. Today, there is a greater concern about providing quality and dignity to the dying patient's life. Each set of circumstances is unique. What may be reasonable or ordinary care for one individual may be unreasonable or extraordinary to another. The important factor is that communication occurs.

Decisions are often made about whether to implement resuscitative procedures for a terminally ill patient. The nurse should make sure that the following protocols have been followed when a "Do not resuscitate," or DNR, order has been given.

- The patient and his family must understand the terminal nature of the condition.
- The patient and his family should receive explanations of the possible alternatives for treatment and the options that are available.
- Some notation about the discussion with the patient or the family should be documented in the progress notes.
- The patient makes the decision, if he is rational and capable of doing so; or,
- The family members all decide after substituting their judgment for what they believe would be the wishes of the patient.
- The order must be written on the patient's permanent record. A verbal order or a telephone order is not sufficient.
- The order should be reviewed periodically and changed at any time the patient or the family decides otherwise.

Following a Living Will

A *living will* is a written statement describing the wishes of a person concerning his medical care when his death is near. The person who signs a living will contemplates his own philosophy of living and dying while still enjoying health. The written document helps guide the family and health workers to understand and implement an individual's wishes if he is unable to participate in the decision-making process.

A living will may specify the desire for life-sustaining measures or opposition to these. Generally a living will describes a desire to avoid being kept alive by artificial means or use of heroic measures when there is no reasonable expectation of recovery. An organization called Concern for Dying has prepared a living will form and offers it to anyone upon request. It is illustrated in Figure 28-2.

A nurse may sometimes disagree personally with the wishes identified by another individual who writes a living will. However, the right of a competent, rational, adult to make certain decisions about his own eventual terminal care is increasingly accepted. Though not all states consider a living will legally binding, many court decisions have upheld medical care that has followed the use of a living will. The nurse is advised to follow the physician's orders and local laws when using life-prolonging measures for a terminally ill person.

Requesting Organ Donations

Body organs, such as the kidneys and heart, and tissues, such as skin and bone, may be needed for transplants. Organs cannot legally be bought or sold. Donations remain the one and only method by which organs are available for transplants. They must be voluntarily given. Before death, patients may grant this permission. However, in many states, after the patient's death the next of kin still must sign a permit and have it properly witnessed before tissue or organs may be removed from the body. Figure 28-3 is an example of an organ donation form. Hospitals may develop their own form using a similar format.

Nurses may find that they are involved in asking patients or their families about the eventual donation of organs. Those who are involved in requesting organ donations must be sensitive, compassionate, and articulate. Care must be taken that no one feels that another patient is being treated preferentially at the expense of the donor. It is not uncommon for those approached as potential donors to feel victimized and extremely distraught. No one should feel coerced into agreeing to organ donations or made to feel guilty for refusing.

There is not an adequate supply of organs in comparison to their need. To compensate for this, legislation concerning organ procurement has been enacted. Federal law now requires that hospital personnel actively seek out and request organs for transplantation. Table 28-2 provides age

To My Family, My Physician, My Lawyer and All Others Whom It May Concern

Death is as much a reality as birth, growth, maturity and old age—it is the one certainty of life. If the time comes when I can no longer take part in decisions for my own future, let this statement stand as an expression of my wishes and directions, while I am still of sound mind.

If at such a time the situation should arise in which there is no reasonable expectation of my recovery from extreme physical or mental disability, I direct that I be allowed to die and not be kept alive by medications, artificial means or "heroic measures". I do, however, ask that medication be mercifully administered to me to alleviate suffering even though this may shorten my remaining life.

This statement is made after careful consideration and is in accordance with my strong convictions and beliefs. I want the wishes and directions here expressed carried out to the extent permitted by law. Insofar as they are not legally enforceable, I hope that those to whom this Will is addressed will regard themselves as morally bound by these provisions.

Signed_____

Date _____

Witness_____

Witness_____

Copies of this request have been given to _____

_____

_____

_____

IMPORTANT

Declarants may wish to add specific statements to the Living Will to be inserted in the space provided for that purpose above the signature. Possible additional provisions are suggested below:

1. a) I appoint _____
   to make binding decisions concerning my medical treatment.
   OR
   b) I have discussed my views as to life sustaining measures with the following who understand my wishes

   _____,
   _____,
   _____.

2. Measures of artificial life support in the face of impending death that are especially abhorrent to me are:
   a) Electrical or mechanical resuscitation of my heart when it has stopped beating.
   b) Nasogastric tube feedings when I am paralyzed and no longer able to swallow.
   c) Mechanical respiration by machine when my brain can no longer sustain my own breathing.
   d) _____

3. If it does not jeopardize the chance of my recovery to a meaningful and sentient life or impose an undue burden on my family, I would like to live out my last days at home rather than in a hospital.

4. If any of my tissues are sound and would be of value as transplants to help other people, I freely give my permission for such donation.

CONCERN FOR DYING
250 West 57th Street, New York, N.Y. 10019

Figure 28-2 This living will has been prepared and is distributed by an organization called Concern for Dying.

criteria when considering the use of various organs. Once removed, organs must be transplanted within a certain time to ensure their function. There is more latitude with donated tissue. Most can be removed up to 24 hours, some even 36 hours, after circulation has ceased. Table 28-3 provides recommended timelines for use of donated body parts.

Lobbyists are encouraging legislation that would allow automatic removal of organs without requiring any permission from the patient or his family. So far this has been passed in a few states, but it has been generally limited to the removal of corneas. The nurse will want to prepare for this aspect of care of the terminally ill by becoming acquainted with local laws and agency policies concerning organ donation.

Informing the Dying Patient

Arguments can be made for both concealing and revealing the truth about a terminal condition. However, there is growing evidence that most individuals wish to be informed when their condition is terminal. One poll showed that up to 90% of adults surveyed said they would want to know when their illness is probably terminal. In general, health practitioners support the position that patients should be told. This is usually the responsibility of the attending physician. When patients are informed, it is also important that they understand that no one is giving up on the treatment of the condition nor the quality of care they will receive.

Many have observed that most patients realize even

Organ Procurement Agency of Michigan

𝒪𝓡𝓜

Subsidiary Of
TRANSPLANTATION SOCIETY OF MICHIGAN
2203 Platt Road, Ann Arbor, Michigan 48104

1-800-482-4881   (313) 973-1577   Detroit—464-7988

ANATOMICAL GIFT DONATION STATEMENT

I understand that in the present state of medical practice, several organs and tissues are being removed from persons who have died unexpectedly, and are being used for transplantation to living persons or for medical or scientific research. I understand that organs are removed after my relative has died, and before the organs suffer any damage, (usually within eight [8] hours) and that this gift authorizes all examinations of the body which are necessary to assure the medical acceptability of the gift.

I appreciate the benefits that come from organ donation and also understand the criteria used in determining death in the case of decedent. I am the surviving:

(1) _____ Spouse
(2) _____ Adult son or daughter
(3) _____ Mother or Father
(4) _____ Adult brother or sister
(5) _____ Guardian of the patient at the time of death
(6) _____ Other person authorized or obligated to
             dispose of the body

_____
          Relationship

Relatives or persons in a class before my class are not available to sign this form (or have already signed such a form). I have no knowledge that during his or her lifetime the decedent, _____, was opposed to or said things against making an anatomical gift or organ donation such as the one described below. I do not know of any relative or person in a class before mine who is opposed to this gift, nor do I know of any person in the same class as myself who is opposed to this gift.

I hereby make the following anatomical gift from the body of _____:

( ) Any needed organs or parts, or
( ) Only the following organs or parts:

_____
(Please specify the organ(s) or part(s))

The specified organ(s) and/or part(s) may be used for any of the purposes allowed by law, i.e. transplantation, therapy, medical research and education.

WITNESSES:

_____

_____
          Name

_____

_____
          Relation

_____
          Date

Figure 28-3 This is a sample of the type of form that is used when seeking permission for organ donation.

without being told that they are suffering from an incurable illness. The nonverbal communication of the patient's family and the health personnel speak louder than words. Patients often feel even more isolated, lonely, and rejected when the truth is withheld, especially when they are told falsehoods.

In some situations, the decision is made to withhold information from the patient. At times, this is valid. Some people indicate that they simply do not want to know. When this is the case, the person's wishes should be respected. When the patient's mental condition is such that he cannot comprehend, trying to help him understand may serve no good purpose.

Informed patients usually react negatively to the news at first. Despite this, studies have shown that there are several advantages when the truth is revealed. These include:

- Maintaining all relationships with the patient on the basis of honesty rather than sustaining the false pretense that recovery will occur.
- Providing the patient with the opportunity to complete unfinished business. That is, to put his legal and personal affairs in order and accomplish any remaining tasks or goals.
- Facilitating the use of still unidentifiable inner resources that have been demonstrated to prolong life. This has often been called the "will to live."
- Promoting more meaningful communication between the patient, family, and health care personnel.
- Resolving grief earlier and more effectively. Grief is resolved better when individuals feel free to say and do things with the dying patient that they would later regret not having done.

Identifying Patterns of Emotional Reactions

Although every person provided with the knowledge of impending death responds in his own distinctive way, studies have shown that there is a common pattern. Dr. Elisabeth Kübler-Ross, a recognized authority on the subject, has described stages that a dying person experiences. These stages are listed and described in Table 28-4.

Not all persons go through the stages in the same order. Also, a person may skip one stage or fall back a stage. Stages may overlap. The length of any stage may range from a few hours to months. Nevertheless, knowing about these stages is valuable when trying to understand and help patients and their families cope with dying.

Kübler-Ross and others have offered suggestions on how to help patients through stages of dying, as follows:

- Accept any manner in which the patient responds.
- Provide a nonjudgmental atmosphere in which the patient can express his feelings freely.
- Be ready to *listen,* especially at night when patients tend to awaken and want to talk.
- Work to understand the patient's feelings. His feelings, not the nurse's, should take precedence.
- Provide the patient with a broad opening for communication, such as, "Do you want to talk about it?" By not defining "it," the nurse allows the patient to choose the topic that he wishes to discuss.

Supporting Options for Care

Any competent adult has the right to request aggressive treatment or refuse therapy and all variations in between. The patient may select continuous hospitalization, extended care in another health agency, home, or hospice care.

Coordinating Home Care

In most early cases, the terminally ill patient remains at home and the family assumes responsibility for his care.

Table 28-2. Criteria for Acceptable Organ Donation According to Age of the Donor*

Organ	Age Range
Kidney	6 months–55 years
Liver	< 50 years
Heart	< 40 years
Pancreas	2–50 years
Corneas	Acceptable at any age
Skin	15–74 years

*Guidelines established by the Organ Procurement Agency of Michigan, Ann Arbor, MI

Table 28-3. Organ Removal and Use Timelines

Organs	Removal to Transplant Time
Heart and lung	Within 2 hours
Heart	Within 3–4 hours
Liver	Within 8–12 hours
Pancreas	Within 24 hours
Kidneys	Within 72 hours
Tissues	
Bones, dura mater, arteries, veins, heart valves, cartilage, ligaments, skin, and corneas	Within 6–36 hours after circulation has ceased; If freeze dried or fresh frozen, can be transplanted up to 5 years after removal.

From Howard S: How do I ask? Requesting tissue and organ donations from bereaved families. Nurs 89 19(1):70–73, 1989

Table 28-4. Stages of Dying According to Kübler-Ross

Stage	Typical Emotional Response	Typical Comment
First stage	Denial	"No, not me." The patient may think there has been a mistake.
Second stage	Anger	"Why me?" The patient's hostility may be directed toward family members, friends, or health workers.
Third stage	Bargaining	"Yes, me, but . . . " The bargain may be a promise to God, if the patient is a religious person, in exchange for more time; or a person may say he will do anything in exchange for such experiences as seeing a child graduate from school or enjoying his next birthday.
Fourth stage	Depression	"Yes, me." The patient feels sadness and often cries, as though he is mourning his own death.
Fifth stage	Acceptance	"I am ready." The comment is characterized by a positive feeling and a readiness for death. This stage is usually peaceful and tranquil.

The patient may travel to and from the health agency for periodic outpatient treatment and evaluation.

Some health agencies offer services and equipment for home care. The nurse in the hospital can often anticipate special services needed by the family and assist in obtaining them. Occasionally, a hospital provides nursing staff members or community health nurses who make visits to the home to provide support and continuity of care.

In order to be successful, several conditions should preferably exist when the terminally ill person is cared for at home:

- The family and the patient should prefer home care to other options.
- The family and the patient should be aware of the patient's diagnosis and prognosis.
- There should be support systems available, such as professional personnel to call for consultation and to help with care as necessary.
- Special equipment needed for the patient should be available.
- One person should be ready and able to assume primary responsibility for the patient's care.

It has been shown that, in general, terminally ill patients cared for at home, compared with patients receiving care in a health agency, enjoy greater emotional comfort and dignity. Their families adjust better to their dying and death. When the terminally ill patient is surrounded by his family members and is in a familiar environment, he usually feels more secure. He can enjoy following his own routines, have food that he likes, and can continue to function to some degree in his family role. Family members have more opportunity to communicate and demonstrate their love and affection without feeling intimidated by the presence of strangers. Guilt feelings may be lessened by having family members care for the person. Children can participate more extensively in the last days and can be helped to understand death with less fear. Because the process of dying generally is a gradual one, family members can have the opportunity to work through some of the beginning phases of grieving that are often more difficult when the patient is in a health agency.

Facilitating Extended Care

The nurse realizes that in some instances the care needed by dying patients is too complex or demanding for family members. Families may have neither the physical nor the emotional strength to deal with the terminally ill person in the home. Care must be taken that the family is not made to feel guilty about not having the ill person at home.

When a family's situation does not permit home care, using an extended-care facility may be justified. The family should be encouraged to drop by various facilities and inspect the physical environment and evaluate the quality of care. If the agency seems pleasant, they should ask about its licensure, the services provided, and the costs involved. A social worker may be helpful in explaining how insurance and Social Security benefits may be applied to the costs of care.

Encouraging Hospice Care

Dr. Cicely Saunders of England is given credit for developing special-care facilities for the terminally ill called a *hospice*. She defined a hospice as a way station where terminally ill persons can live out their final days with dignity and meaningfulness in a caring environment. The concept is based on the shelter provided for weary travelers going from one destination to another. On a more allegorical level, the dying are on a journey to another destination as well.

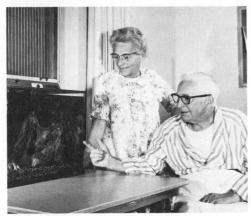

Figure 28-4 These patients visit an aquarium in the lounge of a hospice unit within a hospital. The homelike atmosphere provides an opportunity for pleasant diversion and social interaction.

Hospice care emphasizes helping the patient *live* until he dies, with his family with him, and helping the family return to normal living after the patient's death. Hospice personnel consider their patient to be the terminally ill person and his family. The care they offer emphasizes preserving a bond between the patient and his family and helping them to be prepared so that death can more readily be accepted as a normal part of life.

In the United States a hospice may be a separate facility; it may be a special unit in a hospital, as shown in Figure 28-4, or it may be services provided in the home. Hospice care workers are volunteers with various backgrounds and skills. They are specially prepared and committed to assist dying individuals and their families. They focus all their attention entirely on the needs of terminally ill patients. Every effort is made by hospice personnel to carry out any of the patient's last wishes. Figure 28-5 is an example of the flexibility and individuality given the care of hospice patients compared with traditional patient care.

Most hospices offer regularly scheduled visits, day or night care provided irregularly when called for, or optional 24-hour care if and when it is needed. Families are encouraged to care for the dying person as much as possible in order to keep the family unit intact.

The hospice movement has spread in the United States. Programs are being developed in many parts of the country. There is reason to believe that the movement will continue to grow.

Many hospice organizations provide programs for family members. Individual counseling programs are sometimes offered to family members before and after the death of a loved one as well as group meetings in which families help each other. Family members who have been in these programs have generally reported appreciating the opportunity to participate, and have found the programs to be valuable in the grieving process.

Protecting the Patient From Fraudulent Treatment

One of the dangers upon learning that a condition is terminal is that patients become desperate to prolong their life. They may reject current, acceptable methods of treatment and seek quasi-scientific or unproven approaches for treatment. The patient should be cautioned to

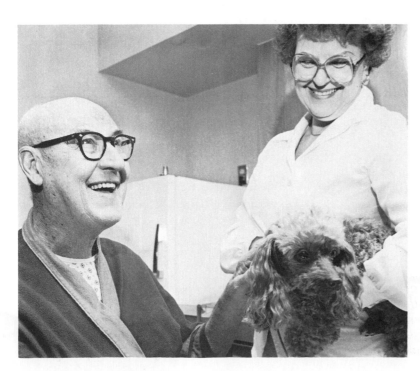

Figure 28-5 This hospice patient appears to enjoy the company of his dog. Policies in hospices are much less restrictive than in most other health agencies.

be suspicious of the following characteristics of individuals or centers that claim to cure a terminal illness:

- Those who provide the treatment are not usually medical doctors.
- The explanation for the treatment's effect is usually based upon some proposed theory rather than upon a proven principle.
- The method of treatment and the research behind its development have not been published in scientific journals to be evaluated by other professionals in the field.
- The treatment location is usually outside of the United States.
- The providers of the treatment may claim to be discriminated against by various regulatory agencies within the United States.
- Long-term studies and statistics concerning the past use of the treatment may be vague, incomplete, or nonexistent.
- The administrators of the treatment may refuse to share information or allow on-site inspection by other accepted authorities on the disease.
- The costs for the treatment are generally high and they are not usually covered by insurance or other medical assistance plans.

Participating in Experiments

There are various institutions in the United States where research on certain diseases is being conducted. Some terminally ill patients may be referred to these places.

The projects undergoing research have been scrutinized by scientific agencies before they are approved and funded. When the experiments have been proposed for humans, the research has generally already progressed through several phases of animal experimentation with somewhat predictable success.

There is a distinction between participating in fraudulent methods of treatment and taking part in a scientific experiment. Some of the characteristics of scientific research include:

- There are no guarantees or claims that the experimental methods will cure the illness.
- Usually the participant is not charged for the treatment. In fact, the participant may be paid for his participation throughout some studies.
- The research is conducted by a team of medical doctors and other highly qualified scientists.
- Statistics are extensive, well documented, and open for inspection at any time.
- The treatment center is usually associated with a prestigious university, teaching hospital, or research institution.
- The patient is provided with detailed information on which to base his decision to participate.

- A consent form, such as the one in Figure 28-6, is provided to identify the rights and duties of the researcher and the participant.

Responding to Emotional Needs

The patient who is dying requires emotional support perhaps more than at any other time during his life. It is also a time when others find support most difficult to give. The patient's helpless feelings cause him naturally to depend upon others to provide him with a sense of being safe, secure, loved, and worthwhile. The nurse can help the patient and his family by sustaining realistic hope, understanding common fears, facilitating communication, and helping the family accept reality.

Sustaining Realistic Hope

Hope may fluctuate with circumstances surrounding the illness. Yet hope always involves a positive rather than negative outlook. Realistic hope involves a wish for something that is more than likely possible.

The patient, the family, and health-care personnel will all manifest some degree of hope. However, the hope expressed by these various people may not be altogether realistic nor in agreement with one another. For example, as the patient begins to face impending death, he may hope for a quick end to his suffering. The family may still be hoping for a miraculous cure. Realistic hope should be supported. A comment such as, "we will continue to do everything we can and we hope you are right about your expectations," may help in situations when the nurse recognizes unrealistic hope. This comment neither shatters hope nor supports its unrealistic aspects.

Errors in judgment about recovery sometimes are made. Some may recall from personal experiences or publicized reports about people whose illnesses were considered terminal but who survived and lived for many years. Also, during the course of an illness medical progress may bring forth a means of saving a life. Many diabetics, for example, faced certain premature death until insulin was discovered. Hence, there is good reason to remain hopeful while caring for terminally ill patients.

Understanding Common Fears

Fears are as varied as attitudes toward death. Both may change from time to time as a terminal illness progresses. Most fear death because it represents a force over which there is no control. However, it is understandable that many choose to fight it. Some look forward to death as a relief from earthly suffering and sorrow. Still others feel so depressed and desperate that they have suicidal tendencies. Generally, by relieving an individual's fears concerning death, the nurse can facilitate moving to the stage of acceptance in which the patient can die in peace and dignity.

RESPONSIBLE INVESTIGATOR:

TITLE OF PROTOCOL:

TITLE OF CONSENT FORM (*if different from protocol*):

I have been asked to participate in a research study that is investigating (*describe purpose of study*). In participating in this study I agree to (*describe briefly and in lay terms procedures to which subject is consenting*).

I understand that

a) The possible risks of this procedure include (*list known risks or side effects; if none, so state*). Alternative treatments include (*list alternative treatments and briefly describe advantages and disadvantages of each; if none, so state*).

b) The possible benefits of this study to me are (*enumerate; if none, so state*).

c) Any questions I have concerning my participation in this study will be answered by (*list names and degrees of people who will be available to answer questions*).

d) I may withdraw from the study at any time without prejudice.

e) The results of this study may be published, but my name or identify will not be revealed and my records will remain confidential unless disclosure of my identity is required by law.

f) My consent is given voluntarily without being coerced or forced.

g) In the event of physical injury resulting from the study, medical care and treatment will be available at this institution.

For eligible veterans, compensation (damages) may be payable under 38USC 351 or, in some circumstances, under the Federal Tort claims Act.

For non-eligible veterans and non-veterans, compensation would be limited to situations where negligence occurred and would be controlled by the provisions of the Federal Tort Claims Act.

For clarification of these laws, contact the District Counsel (213) 824-7379.

_____

DATE

_____
PATIENT OR RESPONSIBLE PARTY

_____
PATIENT'S SOCIAL SECURITY NUMBER

_____
AUDITOR/WITNESS

_____
INVESTIGATOR/PHYSICIAN REPRESENTATIVE

Figure 28-6 This is an example of a form containing the specific areas of information discussed when obtaining an individual's consent for participation in human research. (From Purtillo RB, Cassel CK; Ethical Dimensions in the Health Professions, p 60. Philadelphia, WB Saunders, 1981)

These are common fears associated with the process of dying.

Abandonment. Any threatening and unknown experience produces fear. It can be reduced when it is shared with another. Many dying patients feel isolated and alone. Encouraging the family to be present and involved relieves the feeling of separation from others. The nurse in Figure 28-7 uses touch to communicate closeness to a patient.

Extreme Pain. Discomfort that cannot be relieved is both physically and emotionally exhausting. Measures for controlling pain are discussed later in this chapter.

Loss of Control. This fear may be related to the inability to control bodily functions, such as fecal or urinary elimination, diminished intellectual capacity, or the inability to maintain a previously held role within the family unit.

Dependence. Most adults resent having to depend on others for measures that once were performed independently.

Body Alterations. Some terminal illnesses must be treated by the surgical removal of body structures. Drug therapy too may cause hair loss or other changes in the patient's overall appearance. The patient may feel that he will repulse others.

Loss of Dignity. The use of highly technical equipment sometimes is associated more with the care of machines than with the patient. Dying patients fear being treated as an object rather than as a person.

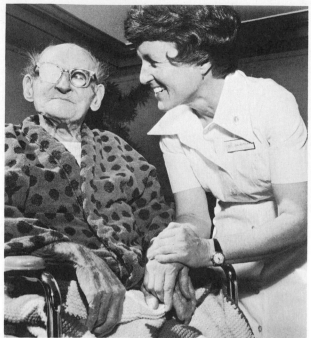

Figure 28-7 Touch is an important method of communicating. Notice that the nurse holds the man's hand in hers as she enjoys a pleasant moment with this terminally ill patient.

Financial Ruin. Medical expenses are bound to accumulate during a lengthy or catastrophic illness. The potential for leaving one's family penniless is a common fear.

Facilitating Communication

Sometimes a patient verbalizes statements that mask his true feelings. Or, he may talk in symbolic language. *Symbolic language* is a means of communication using terms or statements that carry a double meaning. The comments may be made to determine if others can tolerate talking about a certain subject. They may also be used as a substitute for thoughts that are too frightening to discuss. Children may draw symbolic pictures that convey a message since their ability to verbalize is not as finely developed.

Open communication between the nurse, the patient, and the family can help individuals to cope and deal with the reality of the issues concerning death. The nurse may need to interpret what a patient may be trying to say abstractly. Nonverbal communication often conveys messages more clearly than verbal communication. Methods for promoting effective communication and providing emotional support can be reviewed in the Skill Procedures found in Chapter 2. In summary, the nurse may wish to:

- Listen to what is being said. It is possible that the patient is sending a mixed message. There may be important clues about feelings or ideas that he is too frightened to express openly.
- Paraphrase, or restate, what may be the message.

- Provide time for the patient to perceive, confirm, or deny the interpretations.
- Pace, but do not press the patient to communicate. Too slow a response may be equated with disinterest. Firing questions may be associated with insensitivity.
- Be honest rather than clinical in communicating with a patient. When a relationship is based on trust, shortcomings are easily tolerated.

Accepting Reality

Eventually it becomes apparent that death will not be delayed much longer. The patient and family often find comfort in knowing that the patient's wishes have been followed, that the dying patient's discomfort is eased, and that there has been an opportunity to express how meaningful and appreciated the dying person has been.

Sometimes it must be explained to the family that patients may prolong dying while awaiting a sign that others are prepared to accept the loss. This has been described as "waiting for permission" to die. Death often occurs peacefully and shortly after a significant family member indicates that it is okay to "let go." Letting go can be a devastating experience. Many are afraid that it will be interpreted as giving up or demonstrating that they no longer care. By having this phenomenon, which has been identified in various studies on the dying experience, explained to them family members may feel less guilty.

Meeting Spiritual Needs

Attitudes toward death are influenced by various cultural factors, religion being one of them. Some patients, especially those with strong religious beliefs, may be ready to enter another life to which they look forward with joy. They believe that their death will be followed by great reward and peace for having lived a good and faithful life. Others may believe that death may involve some form of punishment; and perhaps others may believe that when life ends so does all form of existence.

Many terminally ill patients find great comfort in the support they receive from their religious faiths. It is important to help in obtaining the services of a clergyman as each situation indicates. However, it must be remembered that a religious faith is not an insurance policy guaranteeing security from the sorrow, fear, and loneliness of dying. The clergyman's visit does not replace the kind words and the gentle touch of the nurse. Rather, the minister, rabbi, or priest should be considered as one of the team assisting the patient to face terminal illness.

Nondenominational chapels are available in some health agencies. They may be used by the patient, when he is able, or by his family members. Figure 28-8 illustrates a chapel, which a patient's husband and a nurse are using for a private discussion and contemplation.

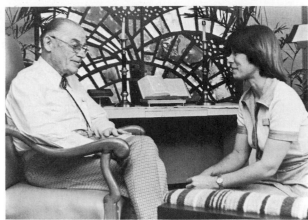

Figure 28-8 A chapel is open and available in some health agencies. Here, a family member talks with a nurse about his terminally ill wife.

Attending to Physical Needs

Unless death occurs suddenly, the nurse has an important responsibility in helping to meet the patient's physical needs at the same time as other needs are being met. The physical care generally includes actions that prevent debilitation and provide comfort.

Providing Nourishment

The patient who is terminally ill usually has little interest in nourishment. The physical effort of eating or drinking may simply be too great for him. Or, nausea and vomiting may interfere with adequate food consumption. Poor nutrition leads to exhaustion, infection, and other complications such as the development of pressure sores. When the patient is unable to take fluids and food by mouth, intravenous therapy, hyperalimentation, or tube feedings may be used to maintain nutrition and fluid intake.

When death is pending, normal activities of the gastrointestinal tract decrease. Offering the patient large quantities of food may only predispose him to distention and added discomfort.

If the swallowing reflex is present, offering sips of water at frequent intervals is helpful. As swallowing becomes difficult, aspiration may occur when fluids are given. The patient may suck on gauze soaked in water or on ice chips wrapped in gauze without difficulty because sucking is one of the last reflexes to disappear as death approaches.

Withholding food and fluids is now being considered when there is a request to withdraw life support systems from hopelessly ill or irreversibly comatose patients. This action would be considered a form of passive euthanasia.

Maintaining Elimination

Some patients may be incontinent of urine and feces. Others may need to be observed for retention of urine and for constipation, all of which are uncomfortable. Cleansing enemas may be ordered. It should be remembered that, if the patient is taking little nourishment, there may be only small amounts of fecal material in the intestine.

Catheterization at regular intervals, or an indwelling catheter, may be necessary for some patients. If the patient is incontinent of urine and feces, care of the skin becomes particularly important to prevent odors and decubitus ulcers. Waterproof bedpads are easier to change than all of the bed linens.

Administering Hygiene

The dignity of a patient is largely influenced by the image that he feels he projects to others. It is especially important to keep the dying patient clean, well groomed, and free of unpleasant odors.

If the patient is taking food and fluids without difficulty, oral hygiene is similar to that offered other patients. As death approaches, the mouth usually needs additional care. Mucus that cannot be swallowed or expectorated may need to be removed. The mouth can be wiped out with gauze, or suctioning may be necessary. Positioning the patient on his side helps in keeping the mouth and the throat free of accumulated mucus.

The mucous membranes should be kept free of dried secretions. Lubricating the mouth is helpful as well as comfortable for the patient.

Sometimes, secretions from the eyes accumulate. The eyes may be wiped clean with tissues or cotton balls moistened in normal saline. If the eyes are dry, it is usually because they tend to stay open. A lubricant in the conjunctival sac may be indicated to prevent friction and discomfort.

As death approaches, the patient's temperature usually is elevated, but as his circulatory system fails, the skin usually feels cold to the touch and the patient often perspires profusely. Sponging him and keeping him dry often promote relaxation and quiet sleep as well as cleanliness. A complete bath may be tiring and cause extreme discomfort.

Open lesions may be a source of offensive odors as dead tissue and bacterial growth accumulate within the wound. Little information is available in the literature about controlling wound odors. Some success has been achieved when yogurt or buttermilk is applied to the wound after cleansing. The wound is then irrigated to remove the dairy product used. Another possible solution involves using enzymatic ointments that debride the wound. Masking the odor with room deodorizers is not usually an adequate solution.

It is important to keep the bed linens and bed clothing dry by bathing the patient and changing linens as necessary. Using light bed clothing and supporting it so that it does not rest on the patient's body usually give additional comfort. The patient often is restless and may be observed to pick at his bed linen. This may be because he feels too warm.

The dying patient's hair should be kept clean and groomed. Dry shampoos may be used. A male patient who has preferred to be clean shaven should have that practice continued throughout his remaining life.

Positioning the Patient

Good nursing care provides for proper positioning of the patient and includes frequent changes in position although the patient may appear to be unconscious. Poor positioning without adequate support is fatiguing as well as uncomfortable.

When dyspnea is present, the patient will be more comfortable when supported in the semi-sitting position. Noisy breathing frequently is relieved when the patient is placed on his side. This position helps to keep the tongue from obstructing the respiratory passageway.

Controlling the Patient's Pain

The goal is to keep a patient free from pain yet not dull his consciousness or ability to communicate. When a terminally ill patient is discharged for home care, his medication is often changed from a parenteral route of administration to an oral route. It is important that the dosage prescribed for the oral route be comparable to the injected dosage in order to control pain at a similar level. Table 28-5 provides a list of equivalents that should be matched when the routes of administration of the same drug are changed.

It is expected that the dosage will need to be increased as the pain becomes more severe and tolerance develops. *Tolerance* is a condition in which the body requires more of a drug to achieve an effect once obtained with a lower dosage.

When pain is intense, relief is more difficult to obtain with irregular administration of drugs. Therefore, it is better to try to control pain when it is minimal rather than wait until it is excruciating. Peaks and valleys of pain can be reduced by administering pain-relieving drugs on a routine schedule throughout the 24-hour period rather than just when it becomes absolutely necessary to do so.

Some individuals are now being provided with patient-controlled analgesia, or PCA, pumps. These allow a patient to self-administer a preset volume of pain-relieving medication. Controls prevent overdosing. Once a patient administers a dose, he cannot do so again for a certain period of time. The dosage and the time can be varied. A pump allows administration of small doses as frequently as every 5 minutes. Self-administration promotes a balance of drug administration according to the patient's level of discomfort. The patient feels a sense of control.

Some nurses are concerned that the patient will become addicted to the pain medication, which is generally a narcotic, such as morphine. This development is expected. Since death is near, the possibility of addiction should not stand in the way of pain control.

Unfortunately, though tolerance develops to the pain-relieving quality of the drug, tolerance to other drug actions do not appear as quickly. Therefore, respirations may become slower and constipation is more likely with regular use of these drugs.

Sometimes pain is intensified by fear and anxiety. Other medications may be given for very anxious or depressed patients. Supplemental techniques such as imagery, biofeedback, and relaxation may be useful in potentiating the effect of the drug. Persons working with the terminally ill have noted that patients experiencing a warm supportive relationship require less pain-relieving drug therapy.

Protecting the Patient From Harm

The terminally ill patient may be very restless at times. The use of siderails on the bed is indicated. Restraining the patient is undesirable but may be necessary in some instances. The patient's relatives may offer to remain with him so that he does not injure himself. However, family members should not be left with the complete burden of the patient's safety. The patient should be checked frequently because his welfare is still the nurse's responsibility. Well-meaning but unprepared, fatigued, and

Table 28-5. Dosage Equivalents for Equianalgesia*

Drug	Dosage by Intramuscular Route (mg)	Dosage by Oral Route (mg)
Morphine sulfate	10	60
Dilaudid (hydromorphone)	1.5	7.5
Demerol (meperidine hydrochloride)	75	300
Codeine sulfate	130	200
Talwin (pentazocine)	60	180
Darvon (propoxyphene hydrochloride)	240	500

*Prepared August 1986, by Margo McCaffrey, RN, MS, FAAN, based primarily on information distributed by Analgesic Study Section, Sloan Kettering Institute for Cancer Research, New York, NY.

stressed family members sometimes misjudge the patient's need for safety precautions. The guilt, if some unexpected occurrence results in injury, is an unfair price for family members to pay.

Modifying the Environment

Nursing time is economized if the hospitalized terminally ill patient is in a room close to the nursing station. This arrangement is convenient for giving nursing care and for observing him at frequent intervals.

Having familiar objects in view can help to make the patient feel more comfortable and secure. The family may be encouraged to make his room meaningful to him. Pictures, books, and other significant objects can be very important. Whether the patient is at home or in a health agency, it is desirable to have the environment reflect his preferences. Once the environment is pleasing to the patient, it can remain thus unless he chooses to make alterations. In this way, the patient is being given some degree of control over his environment when he has lost control of most other aspects of daily living. The home environment is generally not difficult to maintain according to the patient's wishes.

It is not necessary that the patient remain in his room at all times. If his condition permits, trips outside are a pleasant change, as Figure 28-9 illustrates.

Normal lighting should be used in the patient's room. Terminally ill patients often complain of loneliness and various fears precipitated by poor vision, all of which are exaggerated by darkening the room. The room should be well ventilated and the patient protected from drafts.

When conversing at the patient's bedside, it is preferable to speak in a normal tone of voice. Whispering may be annoying to the patient and may make him feel that secrets are being kept from him. It generally is believed that the sense of hearing is the last sense to leave the body. Many patients retain this sense almost to the moment of death. Therefore, care should be exercised concerning topics of conversation. Even when the patient appears to be unconscious, he may hear what is being said in his presence. It generally is comforting to the patient for others to say things that he may like to hear. Even when he cannot respond, it is kind and thoughtful to speak to him. It also remains important for the nurse to explain to the patient what care will be given so that the patient does not misunderstand the actions or become fearful.

Involving Family Members in the Patient's Care

It is helpful to remember that family members are in the process of having to make tremendous adjustments during the patient's terminal illness. There are instances when the nurse must focus more on the needs of the relatives than the patient.

Family members often appreciate helping with the patient's care. They feel helpless and welcome the opportunity to assist. Their cooperation helps to maintain a family bond, as Figure 28-10 illustrates. Allowing relatives to help with the patient's care serves other purposes. Family members often find that helping with care improves their ability to cope with the situation. It also helps to begin and promote the grieving process, which is discussed later in this chapter.

However, the nurse needs to check on the patient frequently to determine his condition as well as the relatives' ability to cope with the situation. The nurse should explain that the family can call for nursing assistance at any time. Family members also need to know that when members leave or are too tired to give care a nurse will intervene. The nurse should be sensitive to the amount of care and involvement the family can assume. Expecting relatives to accept undue responsibility for the patient's care is unkind.

Recognizing the Signs of Approaching Death

Most persons die gradually over a period of hours or days. Human cells cease to live when there is a lack of sufficient oxygen. The capacity of tissues varies as to the length of time they can live with insufficient oxygen. During the process of dying, there are signs that usually indicate clearly that death is imminent.

Paranormal Experiences May Be Described. A *paranormal experience* resembles something supernatural. Patients may relate visions of having seen, talked with, or been in the presence of family members or friends that have died. Or, they may describe having been visited

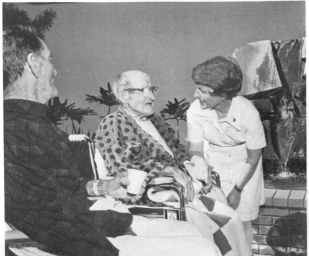

Figure 28-9 The terminally ill patient need not be confined to bed and a room. These patients are enjoying being outdoors on a patio.

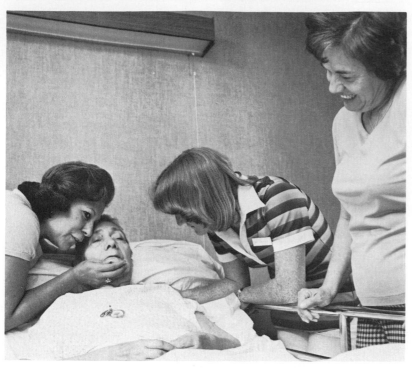

Figure 28-10 This dying patient is being visited by her daughters. They also help with her care as they continue to preserve the family unit during a terminal illness.

by a religious figure, such as an angel. Some speculate that these are guides who go with the spirit on its transference to another dimension.

Motion and Sensation Are Gradually Lost. This usually begins in the extremities, particularly the feet and legs. The normal activities of the gastrointestinal tract begin to decrease, and reflexes gradually disappear. The jaw and facial muscles relax and the patient's expression, which may have appeared anxious, becomes peaceful. The eyes may remain partly open.

Although the Patient's Temperature Usually Is Elevated, He Feels Cold and Clammy. This begins with his extremities and the tip of the nose. It reflects the beginning of circulatory collapse.

Respirations May Be Noisy and the "Death Rattle" May Be Heard. These occurrences are due to an accumulation of mucus in the respiratory tract when the patient is no longer able to raise and expectorate sputum. Cheyne-Stokes respirations occur commonly.

Circulation Fails and the Blood Pressure Falls. The patient's skin becomes cyanotic, gray, or pale. The pulse becomes irregular, weak, and rapid.

Pain, if Present, Subsides. As the patient's level of consciousness changes, the brain may no longer perceive pain.

The Patient's Mental Condition Usually Deteriorates. Such terms as being mentally "fuzzy" or "clouded," confused, and disoriented are often used to describe mental deterioration. Eventually, complete unconsciousness and coma ordinarily occur, but some patients may remain conscious until death. The amount of mental alertness varies among patients, which is important to remember when giving care.

Summoning the Family

Although signs of approaching death are appearing, the nurse should realize that no one can predict the amount of time before death actually occurs. However, it is important to make the family aware that the end is near. The nurse may wish to use some of the following suggestions to communicate this information to the family:

- Give your name, title, and indicate from where the call is being made.
- Determine the identity of the person who has answered the phone.
- Explain that you are calling because the patient's condition has worsened.
- Speak in a calm and controlled voice. The next of kin should feel that health personnel are in command of the serious nature of the patient's condition.
- Use short sentences to provide small bits of information. It is difficult to follow lengthy or technical explanations with any kind of understanding when under stress.

- Pause to allow the receiver of the call time to comprehend.
- Inform the family member of the care that is being provided at the moment. It should not appear as if the patient or his care is being abandoned.
- Urge the individual to come at once to the health agency.
- Document the time and the individual to whom the information was communicated.

The physician should be responsible for informing a patient's nearest relative if a death has occurred. This information is usually delayed until after the family member arrives in order to avoid precipitating any desperate acts, such as suicide, or contributing to a traffic accident.

Helping Arriving Relatives

Relatives of the dying patient should be met by the nurse who informed them by telephone. When everyone has the benefit of continuity in the communication, there is less confusion. If it is not possible for the nurse to meet with the family, some other designated support person should be available. The family should not be left alone; however, they may appreciate being shown to a room or area that provides privacy.

There may be a variety of emotional reactions expressed at this time. It is important that the individuals not feel inhibited because they are in the presence of strangers. It is not unusual for family members to weep and sob uncontrollably. However, the genuineness of their grief should not be misinterpreted if there is not a great display of emotions. In this culture, men are encouraged to control their feelings. If the family has had a period of time to anticipate the patient's death, much of the emotion may already be spent.

Expect a rather severe emotional reaction if the dying person has been a victim of a sudden and unexpected accident. These family members have not had the opportunity to prepare for the loss. They are especially in need of emotional support that includes allowing them to express their grief and listening to them as they vent their feelings.

Confirming Death

The patient must be pronounced dead by a physician. Generally the nurse can determine that a patient is dead when there is no evidence of pulse, respirations, or blood pressure. The pupils will become dilated and fail to respond to light. These were at one time the traditional signs of death.

In the case of extensive use of artificial means for maintaining life support, other criteria have been adopted in order to redefine death. New assessments are now used to declare individuals "brain dead." *Brain dead* means that

despite the fact that the heart is beating and ventilation is occurring mechanically, the brain is no longer functioning. Brain wave activity is determined by electroencephalography. Recordings are taken over a period of 24 hours to validate the conclusion before any life-support measures are discontinued.

Obtaining Permission for an Autopsy

An *autopsy* is an examination of the organs and tissues of a human body following death. A coroner has the right to order that an autopsy be performed if the death involved a crime, was of a suspicious nature, or occurred without any medical consultation prior to the death. Otherwise, an autopsy cannot be performed without the written consent of the next of kin.

It is generally the physician's responsibility to obtain permission for an autopsy. It involves the same delicate communication as when requesting organs for transplant. When permission is being sought, the nurse often can assist by helping to explain the reasons for an autopsy. This requires tact and compassion. Many relatives will find comfort when they are told that an autopsy may help to further the development of medical science as well as to establish proof of the exact cause of death.

Issuing a Death Certificate

The laws of this country require that a death certificate be issued for each person who has died. The laws specify the information that is needed. Death certificates are sent to local health departments, which use the information to compile statistics that make up the information in Figure 28-1 and Table 28-1. These statistics become important in identifying trends, needs, and problems in the fields of health and medicine.

The mortician assumes responsibility for handling the death certificate and filing it with the proper authorities. The physician's signature is required on the certificate, as are those of the pathologist, the coroner, and others in special cases. The death certificate also carries the mortician's signature and, in some states, his license number.

Nursing Responsibilities After the Patient's Death

The nurse is still involved with both the patient and the family even after death occurs. Sometimes, relatives are not present at the bedside at the time of death. It is customary for the relatives to view the body when they arrive. It is kind to ask relatives if they wish to be alone during viewing. Often they do, but the nurse should accompany them if that is their wish. Other special approaches will be discussed later concerning the death of an infant.

Nurses are often confused about the effect that showing their own emotions will have on the family. The current feeling is that it is only human for nurses to become involved and attached to patients and their families. Many families are touched that the nurse has also shared their loss. Therefore, nurses should not fight to control expressing how they feel. Words of comfort are hard to come by. Speaking sincerely is always a good guide. Many times, just listening and allowing persons the time to reminisce or express their emotions is the best course of action.

The survivors of a sudden death should especially be encouraged to view the body. Seeing and touching the body confirms the reality of death. The nurse can clean and cover mutilated areas; however, most families tend to ignore the evidence of trauma and relate to the dead individual as if the injuries were not there. Sedating survivors is not recommended because it delays the normal grieving process.

Accounting for Valuables

Each agency has policies about the care of valuables when patients are admitted to the institution. Those valuables that the patient has chosen to keep with him—for example, a ring, a wristwatch, or money—require careful handling after death. Occasionally, the patient's family may take the valuables home when death becomes imminent. This should be noted on the form that the agency specifies. If valuables are still with the patient at the time of death, they should be identified, accounted for, and sent to the appropriate department for safekeeping until the family claims them. If it is impossible to remove jewelry, such as a wedding ring, the fact that it remains on the body should be noted. As a further safeguard, the article should be secured with adhesive so that it cannot slip off and be lost. Loss of valuables is serious and may result in a lawsuit. The nurse owes it to the patient's family as well as to the agency to use every precaution to prevent loss and misplacement of valuables.

Performing Postmortem Care

After the physician has pronounced the patient dead, the nurse is responsible for postmortem care. *Postmortem care* literally means caring for the body after death. The body is cleaned, identified, and prepared in a manner that will enhance its appearance at the time of visiting at the funeral home. The nurse will be guided by local procedure. Although these procedures vary among agencies and morticians, the actions in Skill Procedure 28-1 may be used as a common guide.

Understanding the Grieving Process

Grieving is a painful yet normal experience that facilitates the resolution of a death. Some compare this to emotional healing. The activities that lead to resolving the loss are called *grief work* or *mourning.*

Each culture has its rituals associated with death, burial, and mourning. These traditions help to facilitate grieving. They provide a means for attending to those who have been touched by death and who deserve special compassion and understanding. Unfortunately, many cultural traditions have been abbreviated or abandoned in recent years. This has led to ineffective grieving and, for some, a pathological state. It is important for nurses to understand the physical and emotional effects of grieving that are experienced by surviving individuals. Further, nurses should share with others the methods that will facilitate the grief process.

Identifying Common Grief Reactions

The normal grieving process may extend on the average from 6 months to 2 years. When anticipatory grieving has occurred, the mourning period may be shorter. Regardless of its length, all individuals tend to experience similar reactions. These grief reactions have been studied by noted authorities, such as Eric Lindemann, George L. Engel, and others. In separate studies most have found that grieving involves both physical and emotional reactions. These results support the concept that the mind and the body are truly interrelated.

Common Physical Reactions. Grieving individuals may experience various physical symptoms, such as anorexia, tightness in the chest and throat, difficulty breathing, lack of strength, and sleep pattern disturbances. Some claim to see, hear, or feel the continued presence of the deceased. It is not understood yet if these should be considered paranormal experiences or if they are simply the result of wishful thinking.

Despite an inability to connect these physical manifestations to any identifiable pathology, studies have shown that the incidence of death is higher among individuals who have lost a spouse in the previous 6 months to a year. It may really be possible to die of a "broken heart."

Common Emotional Reactions. There are several emotional phases through which grieving individuals pass. They have been identified by various individual researchers. The list in Table 28-6 shows those described by Engel.

Comforting Grieving Individuals

Each individual grieves differently depending upon the significance of the dead person, the amount of anticipatory grieving, the mode of death, and their own network of support. The nurse can perform some of the techniques in Skill Procedure 28-2 when facilitating the grief process. The suggested actions may also be useful to others who may be influential in helping grieving individuals to resolve their loss.

Skill Procedure 28-1. Performing Postmortem Care

Suggested Action	Reason for Action
Transfer any patient who shared a room with the deceased temporarily to another location.	The patient may be upset by witnessing the activities surrounding the death. The family will appreciate privacy with the body.
Notify the nursing administration office and the health agency switchboard.	Calls concerning the dead patient's condition should be screened. Supervisors may adjust staffing patterns when the nurse is involved with postmortem duties.
Contact any individuals involved in organ procurement.	Organs must be removed and preserved prior to embalming. The usefulness of some organs is related to the speed with which they are removed from the body.
Inform the designated mortician that the patient has died.	The mortician may indicate that the body will be removed from the nursing unit or from the morgue.
Assemble equipment for cleaning, wrapping, and identifying the body.	The body is prepared in a clean condition before it is transferred to the mortuary.
Determine that the family and clergyman have spent all the time they want with the body.	Many individuals request that certain religious services be performed before the body is removed from the room.
Place the body supine with the arms extended at the side or folded over the abdomen.	A normal anatomic position prevents discoloration of the skin from pooling blood in the areas visible in the casket.
Remove hairpins or clips.	Hard objects about the face can scratch the tissue and detract from its appearance when the body is viewed at the funeral home.
Close the eyelids by applying gentle pressure in the lowered position.	The eyes may not be easily closed if the time between death and preparation of the body is prolonged.
Replace or retain dentures within the mouth. If the dentures are not in the patient's mouth, label and send them with the body.	Dentures maintain the natural contour of the face. They may be difficult to insert several hours after the body has been transferred.
Use a small towel under the chin to close an open mouth.	If the mouth is allowed to remain open, it may be difficult to close later.
Apply gloves and remove soiled dressings or other infected sources of pathogens.	Live pathogens may continue to be present in drainage from areas of the body even though the patient is dead.
Leave all equipment in place and attached if a coroner suspects that the patient is a victim of a crime.	The equipment may become part of the evidence that establishes that a crime was committed.
If a patient died of natural causes, remove venipuncture devices, indwelling catheters, and monitor leads.	Only the body should be delivered to the mortician for burial care.
Dispose of all contaminated and soiled articles in appropriate containers.	A container acts as a transmission barrier to control the spread of organisms.
Remove gloves and discard them with contaminated articles.	The gloves are considered a source of pathogens if they have handled heavily soiled or contaminated drainage.
Wash the hands thoroughly.	Although gloves were worn, the hands should be washed in order to ensure cleanliness.
Cleanse any obviously soiled areas of the body, such as feces that may have been expelled.	The body is completely washed by the mortician and so a complete bath is not required before transferring the body.
Apply disposable pads in the perineal area.	Stool or urine may be released after death has occurred, when the sphincter muscles relax.

(continued)

Skill Procedure 28-1. Continued

Suggested Action	Reason for Action
Attach an identification tag either to the ankle or the wrist. If the wrist is used, pad the area first. Leave the agency identification bracelet intact.	The importance of proper and complete identification of the body cannot be overstressed. Mistakes cause embarrassment and additional sorrow. Padding avoids damaging visible tissue if the identification is applied too tightly. The hospital bracelet ensures proper identification if the tag is lost.
Remove or make an inventory of the valuables still attached to the body.	All personal valuables must be accounted for.
Wrap the body with a *shroud,* a garment for enclosing a dead body.	The shroud covers the patient and preserves the dignity and respect due the body from any unauthorized onlookers.
Attach an identification tag to the shroud.	This prevents having to unwrap the body in order to make proper identification.
Transport the body to the morgue as shown in Figure 28-11 or await the arrival of the mortician's assistants.	The body may be held temporarily in the morgue or transferred directly from the unit.

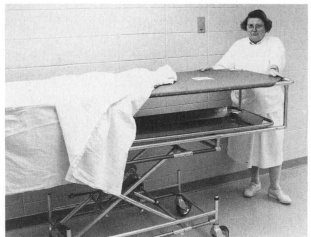

Figure 28-11 The patient's body is transported to the morgue on a special cart. Once the cart is covered by the drape, visitors and other patients are unaware that a body lies underneath.

Lock removed articles in a safe and note their placement on the permanent record.	Valuable belongings of the patient must be safeguarded for proper return to the family.
Complete the patient's permanent record indicating in what manner the body was removed.	The permanent record should reflect where and to whom the body was transferred.
Notify housekeeping to prepare the patient unit for terminal disinfection.	The unit must be cleaned and restored to readiness for subsequent patient use.

Identifying Pathological Grief

Pathological grief involves actions that indicate an individual is not accepting a death. These activities tend to be categorized as bizarre or morbid behavior. Examples include retaining all of the deceased's possessions as if in readiness for use, refusing to leave the house to attend the funeral or any other activity, attempting to make contact with the deceased through various forms of spiritualism, and, in rare instances, keeping a dead body within a residence for an extended period after death.

Table 28-6. Stages of Grief According to Engel

Stage	Description
Shock and Disbelief	Shock and disbelief are characterized by a refusal or inability to accept the fact that a loved one is about to die or has died. They are a form of denial.
Developing Awareness	This stage is characterized by physical and emotional responses. The grieving person may feel sick or experience pain; he may feel emptiness or show anger and cry.
Restitution	The stage of restitution is characterized as a period during which the loss is recognized. It is time in which one accepts the reality of the death.
Idealization	During the idealization stage, the grieving individual often exaggerates the good qualities of the person. Eventually the deceased is viewed in a more realistic perspective.

Grieving in Special Circumstances

Grief is a process that is generally experienced somewhat commonly among all individuals. However, when the loss involves a suicide or the death of a child, there are unique problems for the survivors.

Grieving a Suicide. Survivors of a suicide are not only saddened by the loss but they suffer extreme guilt for not anticipating the despair felt by the dead individual. The guilt may be further reinforced if a vindictive note was left.

Many may also be angry at being publicly embarrassed, yet feel uneasy about expressing it. Instead of using communication with support persons to resolve the death, the survivor may avoid any discussion of the death with others. It has also been found that many fear that they may also end their own life some time in the future. A professional grief counselor may be extremely helpful when individuals are tormented by these feelings.

Grieving a Perinatal Death. A *perinatal death* is the death of an infant that occurs prior to, during, or shortly after birth. This type of death requires special techniques that facilitate grief since the parents literally have no past memories to share about the child. The nurse and those associated with the grieving couple must guard against giving the impression that the baby and his unique identity never existed.

Researchers have found that ignoring the death is extremely traumatic although it is done in the spirit of attempting to shelter and protect the parents. Some suggestions that nurses can use when there is a perinatal death include the following.*

Remove any trappings that may interfere with expressing sincere feelings about the baby's death. For example, wearing a lab coat or stethoscope or sitting behind a desk create distance and physical barriers that are nonverbally inconsistent with expressing empathy.

Speak aloud the most important words. Say "death," "dead," "baby," "your son," or "your daughter." Avoiding the use of certain words may communicate to the bereaved person that you are uncomfortable.

Listen. The parents need to talk about their loss and express a variety of intense feelings. Be willing to allow them to do so without judgment and without trying to minimize their loss.

Refer to the baby by its name or the pronoun referring to its gender. This reinforces that the baby was a unique individual.

Offer the parents the opportunity to see and hold the infant. Many parents are unaware that this is even possible. They tend to fantasize, often unrealistically, for the rest of their lives about how the baby looked.

Prepare the couple who wish to see the baby for its appearance. They may expect to see something quite different. Explaining that the baby may be discolored, stiff, macerated, or that there are certain defects helps to lessen any shock that would otherwise ultimately occur.

*Portions adapted from Grief notes© 1986 with permission of Steven and Naomi Shelton, East Lansing, MI.

Skill Procedure 28-2. Facilitating the Process of Grieving

Suggested Action	Reason for Action
Express words that convey sympathy with an individual's loss. Speak from the heart.	Communication, even if it is not the most articulate, is better than ignoring an individual who is experiencing pain.
Demonstrate feelings and emotions. Do not hold back tears and sadness if they are sincerely felt.	Showing emotional involvement indicates to the family that the deceased person was meaningful and adds dignity to the memory of the deceased.
Use spontaneous touching such as a handshake, a hand on the arm, or embrace as a comforting gesture.	Grieving individuals miss being touched. Touching may be done in ways that are not sexually suggestive.
Answer any questions the individuals may have had about the treatment and the response of the patient.	Family and friends are often troubled by the fantasy that an individual was in extreme pain or had an awareness of dying.
Expect that the same questions may be asked several times by grieving family and friends.	It is difficult to comprehend information when in a distraught frame of mind. Many facts or the sequence of events may seem distorted and in need of clarification.
Mention names of nurses and doctors that were with the patient at the time of death.	Families need assurance that their loved one was not alone at the time of death. Later the family may want to talk personally with those who were present.
Encourage the family members to view, touch, and talk to the dead body.	Seeing and touching the dead individual makes the death real.
Discourage the self-administered use of alcohol or drugs.	Abused substances can suppress grief and contribute an unreal quality to the circumstances surrounding the death and memorial service.
Listen as the grieving individual discusses the death and the significance of the loss.	Repetition helps to reinforce the order of events and personal meaning of the loss.
Encourage individuals to talk about the deceased even though grieving individuals may cry.	Suppressing talk of the deceased implies that the event never occurred or that the death is easily forgotten.
Tolerate expressions of anger and guilt.	Normal grieving involves verbalizing helpless feelings and regrets concerning the deceased.
Help the mourner to list areas where assistance is needed, such as in making funeral arrangements or calling friends.	Listing specifics helps others to understand where their efforts are most appropriately needed.
Caution the survivor to make life changes slowly, such as taking an expensive trip or moving in with another relative.	Some may act impulsively and eventually regret making various financial or social decisions.
Suggest that others invite the survivor out for social activities both in mixed or solitary company.	The survivor should be made to feel valued as an individual and not be ignored because he is no longer coupled in a former relationship.
Caution a survivor from seeking a substitute for the deceased individual too quickly.	New relationships are important but none can ever be duplicated. Alienation or divorce can compound the loss felt through death.
Send cards, make phone calls, or spend time with the survivor on significant anniversary dates and holidays.	The grieving individual is likely to feel more depressed on the date of a wedding anniversary or birthday.

Wrap the baby in a warm blanket, not a towel or pathology drape. The message that is conveyed is that this infant was a person and is therefore deserving of being treated with dignity and respect.

Carry the body of the baby as if it was alive. The nurse sets an example that the baby is lovable and can be touched and held as closely as any other infant.

Offer to unwrap the infant or encourage the parents to hold the baby and do so. This relieves any future doubts about the severity of any disfigurement. Most parents somehow ignore defects, if there are any, and find comfort in discussing the baby's resemblance to other live children or relatives.

Point out the aspects of the baby that are normal. This helps the parents to keep the presence of any defects in perspective.

Allow the family time to be alone with the infant if they feel they do not require the nurse's presence. Parents may feel inhibited from communicating or examining the baby thoroughly when in the presence of the nurse.

Encourage young siblings to describe or draw a picture of the dead brother or sister. This provides the child with information to work on later. It also helps others know what impressions seem important to them.

Avoid bombarding the bereaved parents into making decisions. People who are in shock have great difficulty making decisions. They tend to be overly passive and may later deeply regret a decision they felt pressured into. Allow them ample time for consideration. It is seldom absolutely necessary to hurry the family. Many decisions and procedures can wait.

Encourage delaying any memorial service until the mother can be discharged to participate. Funerals and memorials facilitate grieving.

Help the family to seek the help of a supportive person who can make telephone calls for the family. "Telling the story" again and again can be very draining.

Discourage disposing of all the furniture, layette, and gifts at home before the mother's discharge from the hospital. This may be done to shield the mother from going home to a houseful of sad reminders. However, emptying the house tends to communicate a message that it is better to act as if the baby was never expected.

Avoid sex-role stereotyping. You may find that you are inviting the father to be strong, and denying the impact of his loss, while you are more understanding of the mother's expressions of her feelings.

Expect that family members will find different ways of experiencing and expressing their grief. People grieve at varying paces, too. It is not unusual for bereaved parents to be affected for years following the loss. One parent may feel things very intensely, while the other may "shut down" for a time. These roles may switch occasionally.

Encourage communication about the death between father and mother even though it causes painful feelings to surface. Silence about such an emotional incident is often misinterpreted as lack of concern or value for the lost child.

Avoid suggesting that the death of a child is a predictor of future emotional problems or divorce. If after becoming familiar with the aspects of normal grief there is concern that the family needs outside help, suggest that option and offer to help them find the appropriate resource.

Share the intense feelings that you are experiencing personally as a result of assisting the grieving family. Helpers need to have their own sources of support.

If the family prefers not to see the body of the dead infant, other alternatives for realizing the loss may be made available. These help to provide the parents with some tangible token that represents the existence of the infant. Some examples include taking photographs, providing a lock of hair, and supplying footprints and handprints of the infant. These could also be given to parents who view the baby. If the photographs are refused, they may be kept with the permanent record. The parents should be informed that they may have them at any time in the future. Some hints regarding photography include the following:

- The pictures should be similar to other infant photographs; they should not appear to document pathology.
- Drape a blanket to cover any pathology of the head that may be distressing to the parents.
- Place a nurse's hand within the photograph if the infant weighs under 2000 g or 5 lbs. This provides some perspective on the child's size.
- Position a hand or hands of the infant outside the blanket. Validating that an infant has the appropriate number of fingers reinforces the normal aspects of the dead infant.

Recognizing Signs of Grief Resolution

Mourning is not finished immediately after a funeral. It may take longer for some than for others. However, one sign that grief is becoming resolved is when an individual is able to talk about the dead person without becoming emotionally overwhelmed. Another sign is that the grieving individual describes the good and bad qualities of the deceased. It is common in the early stages of grief to idealize a dead individual to a point near perfection. A more realistic concept of a person's memory indicates that there has been some progress toward adjustment.

Suggested Measures for Terminally Ill or Grieving Patients in Selected Situations

When the Patient Is an Infant or Child

Be familiar with how children understand death. The following guidelines are offered.

Infants and Toddlers. Infants and toddlers generally have not enough life experience to have formulated a concept of death.

Three- to Five-Year-Old Children. Children between these ages usually consider death similarly to the loss of an object. They may be curious about death but often view it as reversible. Fear is usually associated with separation from parents rather than fear of death.

School-Age Children. School-age children generally see death as a permanent situation.

Ten- to Twelve-Year-Old Children and Adolescents. Children in this age range view death very much as adults do. Teenagers in particular often consider death an injustice because they yearn to continue with life and are saddened about leaving loved ones.

Be prepared to observe that most children become aware of the fact that they are terminally ill. Therefore, in general, authorities recommend that children be told about their prognosis in language they can understand. Just as with adults, being told the truth appears to help prevent feelings of fear, of being deserted and alone, and of suffering guilt when they believe that death is a punishment.

Expect that when the primary caretaker, usually the mother, has trouble accepting the reality of her child's impending death, the child may turn to a mother substitute, generally the nurse, for help and the emotional support he needs.

Understand that the death of a child represents an event that is out of sequence with the normal pattern of life and will therefore be more difficult to accept.

Expect that parents often suffer serious guilt feelings when a child dies. They almost always believe they neglected to do something. They may become hostile toward health personnel as their psychological pain reaches high levels. These feelings may be part of anticipatory grief and they eventually change, especially when psychological support is present. Allowing parents to participate in the care of a terminally ill child to the extent that they wish has been found to be helpful in promoting the resolution of grief.

When the Patient Is Elderly

Do not expect that an elderly patient will have a peaceful and accepting attitude toward death. Just as no two lives are the same, death also is an individualized experience.

Include the elderly person in as many aspects of his care as possible so that he has a feeling of dignity and of having at least some control over his destiny.

Applicable Nursing Diagnoses

Nurses who care for dying patients, their family, and friends frequently identify these nursing diagnoses.

- Social Isolation
- Altered Role Performance
- Altered Family Processes
- Spiritual Distress
- Ineffective Individual Coping
- Ineffective Family Coping: Disabling (or Compromised)
- Decisional Conflict
- Hopelessness
- Powerlessness
- Fear
- Dysfunctional Grieving
- Anticipatory Grieving

Nursing Care Plan 28-1 applies the components of the nursing process to a patient who is diagnosed with Hopelessness. The North American Nursing Diagnosis Association in its 1989 taxonomy defines this diagnostic category as, "A subjective state in which an individual sees limited or no alternatives or personal choices available and is unable to mobilize energy on (his) own behalf." Lynda Carpenito (1989) further explains that, "Hopelessness differs from powerlessness in that a hopeless person sees no solution to his problem and/or way to achieve what is desired, even if he has control of his life. A powerless person may see an alternative or answer to the problem, yet be unable to do anything about it because of lack of control and resources."

Recognize that the elderly may not always consider nursing measures as helpful, especially if they wish to die. More so than with younger adults, their dignity is often destroyed when they feel that technology and machines are taking over the ownership of their body.

Teaching Suggestions Involving Terminally Ill and Grieving Individuals

Unusual equipment or drugs may be used in the treatment of some illnesses. The patient and the family need to have frequent explanations for whatever is done and why. This demonstrates respect for the patient and the family. It helps to relieve fears and feelings of guilt that are common during the time a loved one is dying.

Demonstrate measures that the family members are capable of carrying out for the dying patient. Most

NURSING CARE PLAN

28-1. Hopelessness

Assessment

Subjective Data

States, "It doesn't matter what's done or not done anymore. One of these days you won't be able to stop the infections."

Objective Data

26-year-old man about to be discharged from acute care hospital after successful treatment of pneumocystis pneumonia secondary to HIV infection. During interview patient made little eye contact; stared out window. Will be followed up with home health care. Significant other expressed, "I'm afraid he'll just stop eating and taking his medications."

Diagnosis

Hopelessness related to eventual terminal outcome of illness.

Plan

Goal

The patient will identify one future related goal and participate in one goal-directed activity by time of discharge.

Orders: 1/14

1. Reinforce at appropriate times that although his illness is terminal his current health status is stable.
2. After periodic physical examinations, verbalize normal as well as abnormal findings.
3. Present reality, during interactions, that each day provides an opportunity that can be used or ignored.
4. Explore with patient the goals he hoped to accomplish before his illness.
5. Ask patient to identify those goals that he could achieve in the next year.
6. Encourage patient to develop a daily schedule and set aside time for working toward at least one goal. —————————————————————————— E. HILLYARD, RN

Implementation (Documentation)

1/15

0800   Head-to-toe assessment performed. Stated that lungs sound clear and heart rate is normal at 78 beats/min. Skin is intact. Discussed that there has been a ½ lb. weight loss since yesterday. Indicated that date of discharge remains unchanged. Offered one can of Ensure as dietary supplement. Encouraged to perform oral hygiene and use mycostatin mouthwash to prevent yeast infection. _ T. ROMIG, LPN

Evaluation (Documentation)

0830   Stated, "I think mouthcare and anything else is futile. What a time for me to get sick. I'm a writer . . . or should I say, I was a writer. A publisher was interested in an idea I had; but it's past the deadline I was given." Encouraged to contact the publisher by phone before being discharged tomorrow. ———— T. ROMIG, LPN

relatives may fear they may harm the patient although they wish to help. Careful explanations are important so that family members understand how to carry out safe and considerate care. Teaching also includes keeping the family informed about the patient's condition.

Explain that it is healthy to talk with children and other family members about death and personal wishes for terminal care. Open communication prepares individuals to deal with death as a realistic part of life.

Inform patients of organizations that may provide as-

sistance with organ or body donation and forms
for living wills.

Encourage individuals to use all of life's opportunities to say and do meaningful things with one
another so that there are few regrets or guilt
when death is imminent.

Refer individuals to support groups within the community or to printed resources, such as the selective listings in the bibliography, that may help
them to understand and deal with their own personal grief.

Bibliography

Allen A: A bright side of death . . . organ procurement. Journal of Post Anesthesia Nurses 5(1):56–59, 1990

Beaton JI, Degner LF: Life & death decisions: The impact on nurses. Canadian Nurse 86(3):18–19, 21–22, 1990

Blunt KL: Starting a loss and grief group *part 1*. Journal of Urological Nursing 9(1):829–831, 1990

Carpenito LJ: Nursing Diagnosis: Application to Clinical Practice, 3rd ed. Philadelphia, JB Lippincott, 1989

Cecchini JAL: Reach out and touch . . . dealing with dying patients and their families. Imprint 27(1):73, 1990

Collins S: Sudden death counseling protocol. Dimensions in Critical Care Nursing 8(6):375–382, 1989

Corcoran DK: Helping patients who have had near-death experiences. Nursing 18(11):34–39, 1988

Darden J: Dying at home. AD Nurse 3(1):21–22, 1988

Dugan DO: Symbolic expressions of dying patients: Communications, not hallucinations. Nurs Forum 24(2):18–27, 1989

Giordano MS: What required–request law means to you. Am J Nurs 89(10):1296–1297, 1989

Howard S: How do I ask? Requesting tissue or organ donations from bereaved families. Nursing 19(1):70–73, 1989

Koch P: Diary of a hospice nurse. NursingLife 7(6):40–50, 1987

McConnell EA: Do you really know what's troubling your patient? Nursing 20(2):43, 1990

Norris MKG: Myths and facts . . . about organ and tissue transplants. Nursing 19(7):30, 1989

Leslie HW, Battenfield S: Donation, banking, and transplantation of allograft tissues. Nurs Clin North Am 24(4):891–905, 1989

Odam RJ: The process of dying *part 2*. Geriatric Nursing Home Care 8(1):11, 1988

Pohlman KJ: Pain control: Euthanasia or criminal act? Focus on Critical Care 17(3):260–261, 1990

Saufl N, Garmon J: Organ donations—facts and fallacies. Journal of Practical Nursing 39(4):17–21, 1989

Schwartz EA: Your Jewish patient is dying. AD Nurse 4(1):12–17, 1989

Snyder LA, Peter NK: How to manage organ donation. Am J Nurs 89(10):1294–1299, 1989

Snyder R, Westerfield J: Should nurses pronounce death? Nursing 20(6):41, 1990

Stephany T: Supplies for home care of the terminally ill. Home Healthcare Nurse 8(1):53–54, 1990

Stockdale L, Hutzenbiler T: How you can comfort a grieving family. NursingLife 6(3):23–26, 1986

Ufema J: Insights on death & dying. Nursing 18(10):97–98, 1988

Appendix. North American Nursing Diagnosis Association (NANDA) List of Accepted Nursing Diagnoses

Activity Intolerance
*Activity Intolerance, High Risk for
Adjustment, Impaired
Airway Clearance, Ineffective
Anxiety
*Aspiration, High Risk for
Body Image Disturbance
*Body Temperature, High Risk for Altered
Breastfeeding, Effective
Breastfeeding, Ineffective
Breathing Pattern, Ineffective
Communication, Impaired Verbal
Constipation
Constipation, Colonic
Constipation, Perceived
Decisional Conflict (Specify)
Decreased Cardiac Output
Defensive Coping
Denial, Ineffective
Diarrhea
*Disuse Syndrome, High Risk for
Diversional Activity Deficit
Dysreflexia
Family Coping: Compromised, Ineffective
Family Coping: Disabling, Ineffective
Family Coping: Potential for Growth
Family Processes, Altered
Fatigue
Fear
Fluid Volume Deficit
*Fluid Volume Deficit, High Risk for
Fluid Volume Excess
Gas Exchange, Impaired
Grieving, Anticipatory
Grieving, Dysfunctional
Growth and Development, Altered
Health Maintenance, Altered
Health Seeking Behaviors (Specify)
Home Maintenance Management, Impaired
Hopelessness
Hyperthermia
Hypothermia
Incontinence, Bowel
Incontinence, Functional
Incontinence, Reflex
Incontinence, Stress
Incontinence, Total
Incontinence, Urge
Individual Coping, Ineffective
*Infection, High Risk for
*Injury, High Risk for

Knowledge Deficit (Specify)
Noncompliance (Specify)
Nutrition: Less than Body Requirements, Altered
Nutrition: More Than Body Requirements, Altered
Nutrition: Potential for More Than Body Requirements, Altered
Oral Mucous Membrane, Altered
Pain
Pain, Chronic
Parental Role Conflict
Parenting, Altered
*Parenting, High Risk for Altered
Personal Identity Disturbance
Physical Mobility, Impaired
*Poisoning, High Risk for
Post-Trauma Response
Powerlessness
Protection, Altered
Rape–Trauma Syndrome
Rape–Trauma Syndrome: Compound Reaction
Rape–Trauma Syndrome: Silent Reaction
Role Performance, Altered
Self-Care Deficit, Bathing/Hygiene
Self-Care Deficit, Feeding
Self-Care Deficit, Dressing/Grooming
Self-Care Deficit, Toileting
Self-Esteem, Chronic Low
Self-Esteem, Situational Low
Self-Esteem Disturbance
Sensory/Perceptual Alterations (Specify)
   (visual, auditory, kinesthetic, gustatory, tactile, olfactory)
Sexual Dysfunction
Sexuality Patterns, Altered
Skin Integrity, Impaired
*Skin Integrity, High Risk for Impaired
Sleep Pattern Disturbance
Social Interaction, Impaired
Social Isolation
Spiritual Distress (Distress of the Human Spirit)
*Suffocation, High Risk for
Swallowing, Impaired
Thermoregulation, Ineffective
Thought Processes, Altered
Tissue Integrity, Impaired
Tissue Perfusion, Altered (Specify)
   (renal, cerebral, cardiopulmonary, gastrointestinal, peripheral)
*Trauma, High Risk for
Unilateral Neglect
Urinary Elimination, Altered
Urinary Retention
*Violence, High Risk for: Self-Directed or Directed at Others

* These diagnoses have changed terminology from "Potential for" to "High Risk for."
   From the North American Nursing Diagnosis Association. Classification of Nursing Diagnoses, Proceedings of the Ninth Conference. Philadelphia, JB Lippincott, 1990.

Index

Page numbers followed by *d* indicate displays; page numbers followed by *f* indicate figures; page numbers followed by *t* indicate tables; nursing diagnoses are capitalized.

Abandonment, fear of, dying and, 759, 760f
Abbreviations, 63t
  for dosage measurements, 574t
  in patient records, 62–63
  used in prescribing medications, 576t
Abdomen, quadrants of, 293, 293f
Abdominal cavity, paracentesis and, 317, 318f
Abdominal distention, 293
  postoperative, 449t
Abdominal plain film (kidneys, ureters, and bladder x-ray; KUB), 311
Abdominal thrusts (Heimlich maneuver), 714f, 714–715
Abduction, 167t, 410–412f
Abrasion, 458t
Abscess, 460
Acceptance, dying and, 756t, 760
Accidents
  incident sheet and, 81, 81f
  steps to follow after, 233–235, 236f
Accountability, demonstrated by nursing practice, 11, 14
Accreditation, patient records and, 55
Accuracy, assessment and, 41
Acetic acid, wound care and, 474t
Acetone, testing urine for, 537–538, 538f
Acid, 678. *See also* Acid-base balance; Acid-base imbalances
Acid-base balance, 678–679, 679t

disorders of. *See* Acid-base imbalances
  patient teaching to promote, 682
Acid-base imbalances, 679
  identifying, 679, 680f
  nursing diagnoses for, 680
  preventing and correcting, 679
  types of, 679, 679t
Acid-fast bacillus (AFB) isolation, 357, 359–360t
Acidosis, 679
  metabolic, 679t
  respiratory, 679t
Acne, 118
Active euthanasia, 752
Active exercise, 168t, 170, 377
Active listening, 9
Active transport, 677
Activities of daily living, 9
Activity, 158. *See also* Exercise(s)
  blood pressure and, 260
  body temperature and, 244
  leisure-time, 170, 172
  promoting, before surgery, 432
  pulse rate and, 253–254
Activity–exercise pattern, 42t
Activity Intolerance, nursing care plan for, 173
Actual health problem, 46
Acupressure, 180
Acupuncture, 180

Acute illness, 36
Adduction, 167t, 410–412f
Admission(s), 205–209
  admitting department and, 206, 206f
  helping patient undress and, 207
  information gathering and, 207–208
  nursing diagnoses and, 215
  patient orientation and, 206–207
  patient teaching and, 215
  preparing patient's room for, 206
  procedures for
    elderly patients and, 214–215
    infant or child and, 212–214
  psychiatric, types of, 205t
  skill procedure for, 209
  valuables and clothing and, 207, 208f
Admitting department, 206, 206f
Adolescent
  physical assessment of, 298
  promoting fluid and chemical balance in, 682
  promoting personal hygiene in, 118–119
  terminal illness in, 772
Adult protective services, 203t
Adventitious lung sounds, 287, 289–290
Advocacy, 19
Aerobic exercise, 170
Aerobic microorganisms, 329
Aerosolization, 705
Aerosol treatments, 722, 722f, 723f

AFB (acid-fast bacillus) isolation, 357, 359–360t
Affective domain, 27, 27t
Against medical advice (AMA), 210–211
Age. *See also* Adolescent; Child; Elderly patient; Infant; Young adult
  blood pressure and, 260
  body temperature and, 243–244
  care provided throughout life cycle and, 19, 19f
  external cardiac compression and, differences in, 741t
  life expectancy and, 34
  natural body defenses and, 330
  pulse rate and, 253
  as risk factor
    for exercise, 166
    surgical, 429t
  sleep needs and, 190t, 191
Agency accreditation, patient records and, 55
Air, microorganisms and, 329
Airborne transmission, of pathogens, 355t, 357
Air embolism, intravenous fluid administration and, 669, 672
Air-fluidized bed, 382t, 382–383, 383f
Airway, 705–720
  artificial, 713–720, 717f
    inserting and maintaining, 713, 717
    tracheostomy and. *See* Tracheostomy
  clearing, 705–706
    humidification and, 705–706
    liquefying secretions and, 705
    percussion and vibration and, 706, 709f
    postural drainage and, 706, 707f, 707–708
  obstruction of. *See* Airway obstruction
  suctioning, 706, 708–709
    assembling equipment for, 706, 708
    assessing need for, 708
    collecting sputum specimens and, 708–709
    nasopharyngeal, 708
    oropharyngeal, 708
    skill procedure for performing, 710f, 710–712, 711f
Airway obstruction, 709–713
  dislodging objects and, 713
    skill procedure for, 713–717, 714–716f
  postoperative, 448–449t
  signs of, 709, 713, 713f
Albuminuria, 503
Alcohol, disinfection/sterilization with, 341
Alcohol abuse, as surgical risk factor, 429t

Alcohol bath, 492, 494
Alignment, 161t, 376
Alkali (base), 678. *See also* Acid-base balance; Acid-base imbalances
Alkalosis, 679
  metabolic, 679t
  respiratory, 679t
Allergy, to contrast media, 311
Alpha-tocopherol (vitamin E), 128t
Altered Comfort: Pain, nursing care plan for, 196
Altered Oral Mucous Membrane, nursing care plan for, 51
Alternating air mattress, 381, 382t
AMA (against medical advice), 210–211
Ambulatory (outpatient) surgery, 428
American Association of Critical-Care Nurses, 13
American College of Nursing Practice, 14
American Nurses Association (ANA), 5, 7, 13
Amniocentesis, 317–318
Ampule
  combining medication from ampule and vial and, 609
  removing medication from, 605f, 605–606, 606f
ANA (American Nurses Association), 5, 7, 13
Anaerobic microorganisms, 329
Anal canal, 544
Analgesia, patient-controlled (PCA), 180, 182f, 762
  skill procedure for, 183–186
Analysis, 44
Anecdotal note, 80
Anesthesia, 428
  types of, 428
Anger, dying and, 756t
Angiography, 312–313
Anion, 676
Anorexia, 130
  overcoming, 131
Antibiotics, 332
Anticipatory grief, 750
Anticoagulants, 447t, 624
Antiembolism stockings, 434, 436
  skill procedure for using, 438, 438f
Antihelminthic enema, 558t
Antimicrobial (anti-infective) agents, 331–332
Antineoplastic drugs, intravenous administration of, 629, 632f, 632t
  skill procedure for, 633–635, 634f
Antiperspirants, 87
Antiseptics (bacteriostatic agents), 332
Anuria, 502
Anus, 544

Anxiety. *See also* Fear(s); Stress
  exercise and, 162, 166
  nursing care plan for, 216
  pain and, 177
  separation, hospitalization and, 204, 205f
Apical pulse rate, 256, 258f
Apical-radial pulse rate, 257, 258f
Apnea, 195, 259
Apothecary system, 574t, 575t
Appetite
  anorexia and, 130
    overcoming, 131
  cachexia and, 129
Appliance
  intestinal stoma and, 559
    skill procedure for changing, 560–561, 561f
  for oral irrigation, 99
  urinary stoma and, 534
Arrhythmia, 255
  sinus, 255
Art, 4
Arteries, organ donation and, 755t
Arteriosclerosis, 260
Artificial airway, 713–720, 717f
  inserting and maintaining, 713, 717
  tracheostomy and. *See* Tracheostomy
Artificial eye, care of, 107, 113f
Ascending colon, 544
Ascorbic acid (vitamin C), 128t
Asepsis
  medical (clean technique), 330–340, 331d
    antimicrobial agents and, 331–332
    cleaning supplies and equipment and, 338–339
    description of, 330–331
    disinfection or sterilization and, 339–341, 340t
    disposing of needles and sharp objects and, 336, 338, 339f
    gloves and, 336
    hair and shoe covers and, 336
    handwashing and, 332, 332d, 333f, 333–334, 334f
    masks and, 336, 337f, 337–338, 338f
    patient teaching for, 351
    protective eyewear and, 336, 339f
    surgical scrub and, skill procedure for, 335f, 335–336
    terminal disinfection and, 339
    uniform and hospital garments and, 332, 334
  surgical (surgical technique), 331, 341–349
    adding sterile items to sterile field and, 343–344
    creating sterile field and, 342–343, 343f

donning and removing sterile gloves and, 345, 347–349
donning sterile gown and, 344–347
patient teaching for, 351
principles of, 341–342, 342t
Asphyxiation, preventing, 232, 235t
Aspiration, tube feedings and, 150t
Assault, 75–76
Assessment, 41–44, 276–298. *See also* Examination(s); Special procedures; Tests
accuracy and, 41
of blood pressure. *See* Blood pressure, measuring
of body composition, 166, 169f
of body temperature. *See* Body temperature
of bowel elimination, 545
of cardiovascular system, 290–291, 291f, 294t
casts and, 689
database and, 41, 42t, 43f
data collection and, 41
of fitness, 166, 169
of fluid balance. *See* Fluid balance, assessing
focus, 41
of gastrointestinal system, 293, 293f, 294t
of hearing, 284–285, 286t, 294t
information gathering and, 277–278
intravenous fluid administration and, 651–652
of learner, 26–27
of learning needs, 26
of lung sounds. *See* Lung sounds, assessing
of mental status, 280–281, 294t
of motivation to learn, 27
of musculoskeletal system, 294, 294t
need and problem recognition and, 41, 44
of need for suctioning, 708
nutritional, 126, 128–129
organizing data and, 41
of pain, 178t, 178–180, 179f
of patient requiring fluid therapy, 651–652
of patient with cast, 689
physical. *See* Physical assessment
of respiratory system. *See* Respiratory system, assessing
of skin and related structures, 87, 286, 287t, 294t
of sleep, 193
of touch, 285–286
of urinary elimination, 502–503
of vision, 282, 284, 285f, 294t
of vital signs. *See* Vital signs
Assessment skills, 8–9

Assignment sheets, 68–69, 70f
Assistance, signaling for, 227
Association of Operating Room Nurses, 13
Atelectasis, 377
postoperative, 447t
Atherosclerosis, 260
Atomization, 705
Atony, 376
Atrophy, 376
Attention span, short, patient services for patient with, 30
Audiologist, 285
Auditors, 55
Auscultation, 280, 282f
Autologous donation, 430, 430t
Autonomy, 14
Autopsy, 765
obtaining permission for, 765
Avoidance, dying and, 751
Avulsion, 458t
Awareness, developing, death and, 769t
Axilla, 242
Axillary crutches, 419
measuring patient for, 420
Axillary temperature, 242, 246
measuring with glass thermometer, skill procedure for, 250–251, 251f
normal, 244

Bacillus(i)
acid-fast, isolation and, 357, 359–360t
Döderlein, 476
Backrub, 90
skill procedure for giving, 98f, 98–99, 99f
Bacteriocide (disinfectant; germicide), 332
Bacteriostatic agents (antiseptics), 332
Balance, 161t
Bandages, 484–489. *See also* Dressings
applying, 484
skill procedure for, 489
bandaging techniques and, 484–485, 486–488t
fabrics for, 484, 485f, 485t
purposes of, 484
roller, 484–485
removing, 485
wrapping techniques for, 486–488, 486–488f
Bargaining, dying and, 756t
Barium enema (lower gastrointestinal x-ray), 312
Basal metabolic rate (BMR), 244
Base (alkali), 678. *See also* Acid-base balance; Acid-base imbalances
Base of support, 161t, 162f

Basic care, 203
Basic Four, 126, 129f
Basic life support, ABCs of, 734. *See also* Cardiopulmonary resuscitation
Bath/bathing, 88–89. *See also* Tepid sponging
alcohol bath, for reducing elevated temperature, 492, 494
bed bath
assisting with, skill procedure for, 90
complete, procedure for giving, 91–94, 92f, 93f
cool water bath, for reducing elevated temperature, 492, 494
modifications of bath procedure and, 95t
sitz bath, 495–496
skill procedure for, 88–89
Bathing/Hygiene Self-Care Deficit, nursing care plan for, 118
Battery, 75–76
Bed, 219. *See also* Mattress
adjustable, 378
air-fluidized, 382t, 382–383, 383f
circular, 382t, 384, 384f
low air-loss, 382, 382t, 383f
making
occupied bed and, skill procedure for, 224f, 224–225
unoccupied bed and, skill procedure for, 220–223, 221–223f
mattress overlays and, 380–382
moving patient up in, skill procedure for, 392–394, 392–394f
oscillating support, 382t, 383f, 383–384
overbed table and, 223, 225f
pillows and, 219, 221, 221f, 223, 378
siderails and, 380
transferring patient to chair from. *See* Transferring, from bed to chair and back to bed
turning patient in, skill procedure for, 385–391, 385–391f
Bed board, 378
Bed linen, contaminated, caring for, 364, 366, 367f
Bedpan, 505
placing and removing, skill procedure for, 507f, 507–509, 508f
Bedside stand, 223, 225
Belching, 130
Betadine (povidone-iodine), wound care and, 474t
Bias, 55
Bicarbonate, function of, 677
Bichloride of mercury, disinfection/ sterilization with, 341

Binders, 484
  application of, 485, 488
    four-tailed binder and, 488, 488f
    Scultetus binder and, 488, 490f
    skill procedure for, 489
    straight binder and, 488
    T-binder and, 485, 488, 488f
  cravat, 688f, 687
  fabrics for, 484, 485f, 485t
  purposes of, 484
Biofeedback, 180
Biopsy, 315
Biorhythms, 186, 189
Biotin (vitamin H), 128t
Birth. *See* Childbirth
Bivalved cast, 695
Bladder, urinary, 502
  bladder retraining and, 506, 509
  catheterization of. *See* Urethral
      catheterization
  cystoscopy and, 315–316
Bladder retraining, 506, 509
Bleeding
  casts and, detecting and evaluation,
      693
  postoperative, 447t
Blind patient. *See* Visually impaired
      patient
Blood. *See also* Bleeding
  body water in, 641t, 642, 642t, 652
  contamination of, pathogen transmis-
      sion by, 355t
  cross-matching, 673
  fluid imbalances and, 646t
  hemoglobin and
    fluid imbalances and, 646t
    microencapsulated, 676
  infection control and, 367, 369f
  pH of, 679. *See also* Acid-base bal-
      ance; Acid-base imbalances
  predonating, 429–430, 430t
  red blood cell count and, fluid imbal-
      ances and, 646t
  typing, 673, 673t
  volume of, pulse rate and, 254
Blood/body fluid precautions, 357,
      360–361t
Blood components, pulse rate and, 254
Blood glucose
  capillary, 318
    glucometer and, skill procedure for
        using, 318–321, 319–321f
  elevated, tube feedings and, 150t
Blood plasma (intravascular fluid; se-
      rum), 286, 641t, 642, 643t
Blood pressure, 259–270
  in adults, 261t
  in children, 261t
  death and, 764
  diastolic, 259

equipment used to obtain, 262–265,
      263f, 264f, 264t
  factors influencing, 260
  fluid imbalances and, 646t
  high, 260–261
    follow-up for first occasion of, 262t
    as risk factor for exercise, 166
  Korotkoff's sounds and, 265, 266f,
      266t
  low, 261–262
  measuring, 265–270
    in infants, 269–270, 270f
    palpation for, 266, 269
    skill procedure for, 267–269, 268f
    at thigh, 266
  normal, 260, 261t
  pulse pressure and, 262
  systolic, 259
Blood products, infusing, 673
Blood substitutes, infusing, 673, 676
Blood sugar. *See* Blood glucose
Blood supply, healing and, 459
Blood transfusions, 673, 673t, 676
  administering, skill procedure for,
      674–676
  blood products and, 673
  blood substitutes and, 673, 676
BMR (basal metabolic rate), 244
Body alterations, fear of, dying and, 759
Body build, pulse rate and, 253
Body cast, 687–688
Body composition, 162
  measuring, 166, 169f
Body fluid(s), 641. *See also* Electrolyte
      balance; Electrolyte imbal-
      ances; Fluid balance; Fluid
      imbalances
  blood/body fluid precautions and,
      357, 360–361t
  examinations of, 316–321
  extracellular, 642, 643f
  interstitial, 641t, 642, 643f
  intracellular, 641t, 642, 643f
  intravascular (plasma; serum), 641t,
      642, 643f
Body Image Disturbance, nursing care
      plan for, 453
Body mechanics, 160–162, 162f
  proper body mechanics and, skill
      procedure for using, 163–165f,
      163–166
  terminology of, 161t
Body position. *See* Position(s);
      Positioning
Body temperature, 242f, 242–253
  axillary, 242, 246
    measuring with glass thermometer,
        skill procedure for, 250–251,
        251f
    normal, 244

death and, 764
  elevated. *See* Fever
  factors influencing, 243–244
  fluid imbalances and, 646t
  low, 246, 494
    postoperative, 450t
  measuring with electronic thermome-
      ter, skill procedure for, 252f,
      252–253
  measuring with glass thermometer,
      skill procedure for, 248f, 248–
      251, 249f, 251f
  normal, 244
  oral, 242, 246
    measuring with glass thermometer,
        skill procedure for, 248f, 248–
        249, 249f
    normal, 244
  pulse rate and, 254
  raising, hyperthermia pads for, 495,
      495f
  rectal, 242, 246
    measuring with glass thermometer,
        skill procedure for, 249–250
    normal, 244
  reducing
    cool water or alcohol bath for, 492,
        494
    hypothermic blanket for, 494
  selecting site for obtaining, 246
  subnormal, 246
  thermometer and. *See* Thermometer
Body water. *See* Fluid balance, body
      water and
Body weight. *See* Obesity; Weight
Boiling water, disinfection/sterilization
      with, 340t, 341
Bolus, intravenous medications and, 626
Bolus feeding, 141
  administering, skill procedure for,
      145f, 145–146
Bone(s). *See also* Musculoskeletal
      system
  density of, exercise and, 162, 169f
  fractures of, 687
    open and closed reduction of, 687
  inactivity and, 376, 376f
  organ donation and, 755t
Bowel, 544
Bowel elimination, 543–570
  assessing, 545
  constipation and. *See* Constipation
  defecation and, 544–545
  diarrhea and. *See* Diarrhea
  enemas and. *See* Enema
  exercise and, 162
  factors affecting, 545
  fecal impaction and, 547, 549
  fecal incontinence and, 377, 551–552
  intestinal distention and, 549–550

large intestine and, 544

maintaining, skill procedure for, 548

nursing diagnoses for, 568

obtaining stool specimen and, 566–570, 567t

  skill procedure for, 566

promoting

  in elderly patient, 568, 570

  in infant or child, 567–568, 568t

  patient teaching for, 558, 570

  skill procedure for, 548

  in terminally ill patient, 761

rectal suppositories and, 552, 552f

  inserting, skill procedure for, 553

rectum, anal canal, and anus and, 544

self-administration of enema and, patient teaching for, 558

through stoma. *See* Stoma, intestinal

Braces, 686

Bradycardia, 254–255

Bradypnea, 259

Breast self-examination, 281f

Breathing. *See also* Respiration(s); Respiratory rate

characteristics of, 259

deep-breathing exercises and, 432

  skill-procedure for performing, 432–433, 433f

intermittent positive-pressure breathing (IPPB), 722, 723f

rescue, 734. *See also* Cardiopulmonary resuscitation

  age differences in, 741t

stertorous, 259

Breathing bag and mask, self-inflating, 734, 739, 741f

Bridges (dental), care of, 99, 101, 106f

Bronchial lung sounds, 287, 290f

Bronchoscopy, 315

Bronchovesicular lung sounds, 287, 290f

Bronchus(i), bronchoscopy and, 315

Brushing, of teeth, 96

  skill procedure for, 102, 102f, 103f

B scan (obstetric sonogram), 315

Buccal medication administration, 575t, 594, 597f

Burn(s), preventing, 232, 235t

Burning, on urination, 503

Cachexia, 129

Calciferol (vitamin D), 128t

Calcium

  dietary, 125t

  function of, 677

Callus, 115

Calories, 124

Canadian (Lofstrand) crutches, 419, 420f

Canes, 419

Cannula, 317

  nasal, oxygen therapy using, 725–726, 726f

   conversion equivalents for, 724t

   skill procedure for administering, 728

Carbohydrates, 124

Cardiac compression, external, 734. *See also* Cardiopulmonary resuscitation

  age differences in, 741t

Cardinal signs. *See* Body temperature; Pulse; Pulse rate; Respiration(s); Respiratory rate; Vital signs

Cardiopulmonary, definition of, 705

Cardiopulmonary functioning, 704–745. *See also* Cardiovascular functioning; Circulatory system; Lungs; Lung sounds; Respiration(s); Respiratory system; *headings beginning with term* Heart

administering inhaled medications and, 721–722

  aerosol treatments and, 722, 722f, 723f

  hand-held inhaler and, 722, 722f

airway and. *See* Airway; Airway obstruction

cardiopulmonary resuscitation and. *See* Cardiopulmonary resuscitation

exercise and, 162

maintaining water-seal drainage and, 732, 732f

  skill procedure for, 732–734

nursing diagnoses for patients with problems in, 742

oxygen therapy and. *See* Oxygen therapy

patient teaching to promote, 744–745

promoting, in infant or child, 740, 742f, 742–744, 744f

Cardiopulmonary resuscitation (CPR), 734–740

ABCs of basic life support and, 734

age differences in, 741t

discontinuing, 739–740

  errors in, 740t

indications for, 734

performing, 734

  skill procedure for, 735–738f, 735–739

self-inflating breathing bag and mask and, 734, 739, 741f

Cardiovascular functioning

assessing, 290–291, 291f, 294t

  heart sounds and, 290–291, 291f

inactivity and, 376

postoperative problems and, 447–448t

Caries, 94

Caring, 9

Caring skills, 9

Carminative enema, 558t

Carrier substance, 677

Cartilage, organ donation and, 755t

Case management (nurse-managed care), 38

Case method, 37

Cast(s), 687–695

applying, 688–689

  assisting with, 688–689

  skin preparation for, 688

bivalved, 695

bleeding and, detecting and evaluating, 690

body, 687–688

cast care and, skill procedure for providing, 691f, 691–694, 693f

construction of, 688

cylinder, 687

hip spica, 688

maintaining, 690

  edge repair and, 690

  keeping cast clean and, 690

  window replacement and, 690, 695f

patient assessment and, 689

petaling edges of, 692

  skill procedure for, 694f, 694–695

removing, 690–695

  care following, 695

swelling and circulation and, evaluating, 689, 689f, 690

wet, handling and drying, 689, 689f

Cast cutter, 695

CAT (computerized axial tomography; CT), 313, 313f

Category isolation. *See* Infection control, category isolation and

Cathartics (laxatives), 548

Catheter. *See also* Central venous catheter; Urethral catheterization; Urinary catheters

Catheter/catheterization, 514

Catheterization. *See also* Central venous catheter; Urethral catheterization; Urinary catheters

Cation, 676

CDC (Centers for Disease Control), 355, 356, 364

Celsius (centigrade) thermometer, 242–243, 243t

Center of gravity, 161t, 162f

Centers for Disease Control (CDC), 355, 356, 364

-centesis, meaning of, 311

Centigrade (Celsius) thermometer, 242–243, 243t

Central venous catheter, 627–629
  implanted, 629, 629f
  instilling intravenous medication
        through, skill procedure for,
        630–631, 631f
  short-term, 627–628, 628f
  tunneled, 628–629, 628f
Cerebrospinal fluid, lumbar puncture
        and, 316–317, 317f
Cerumen, 86
Ceruminous glands, 86
Chair(s)
  in patient's room, 225
  transferring patient from bed to. *See*
        Transferring, from bed to
        chair and back to bed
Change of shift reports, 68, 69f
Chart. *See* Patient records
Charting, 48–49, 54. *See also* Patient
        records; Recording
  computerized, 60–61, 61f, 62f
    protecting patient records and, 61
  by exception, 60
  focus, 59
  narrative, 59
  PIE, 59–60, 60f
  SOAP, 58, 59
  SOAPIE, 58, 59
  SOAPIER, 58, 59, 59t
Checklists, 67
  for perative routine, 441, 444f
Chemical(s), disinfection/sterilization
        with, 340t, 341
Chemical balance. *See* Acid-base bal-
        ance; Acid-base imbalances;
        Electrolyte balance; Electrolyte
        imbalances
Chemical environment, microorganisms
        and, 329
Chemotherapy, antineoplastic drugs
        and, intravenous administra-
        tion of, 630, 633, 633f, 633t
  skill procedure for, 634–635, 636f
Chest x-rays, 311
Cheyne-Stokes respirations, 259, 764
Child. *See also* Adolescent; Infant
  admitting and discharging, 212–214
  bowel elimination in, promoting,
        567–568
  cardiopulmonary functioning in, pro-
        moting, 740, 742f, 742–744,
        744f
  comfortable and safe environment
        for, promoting, 235–238, 237f
  examination of, assisting with,
        318–322
  exercise in, promoting, 172
  fluid and chemical balance in,
        promoting, 680–682
  healing in, promoting, 497

inactivity in, preventing, 423–424
infection control and, 372
mechanical immobilization of, 699,
        701
medication administration and, 597,
        600f
  parenteral medications and, 632,
        635
nutrition in, promoting, 154, 156
patient services for, 28–29
personal hygiene in, promoting, 117
physical assessment of, 296
preoperative and postoperative care
        in, 452
sleep in, promoting, 195–197
terminal illness in, 772
urinary elimination in, promoting,
        538–539
vital signs in, obtaining, 271–272
Childbirth
  death of infant at, grieving, 769–771
  family birthing units and, 202
  urinary elmination following, promot-
        ing, 539, 541
Chloride
  dietary, 125t
  function of, 677
Choice, patient's right to, 17
Cholecystography, 310, 312
Chronic illness, 36
Cigarette smoking, as risk factor
  for exercise, 166
  surgical, 429t
Circadian rhythm, 186
Circular bed, 382t, 384, 384f
Circular turn, roller bandages and, 486,
        486f
Circulatory overload, intravenous fluid
        administration and, 667–668
Circulatory system. *See also* Cardio-
        pulmonary functioning; Car-
        diovascular functioning
  casts and, evaluating, 689, 689f, 693
  death and, 764
  fluid imbalances and, 647
Circumduction, 409, 409f, 413f
Clean-catch midstream urine specimen,
        535
  collecting, skill procedure for, 536
Cleaning. *See also* Cleansing; Disinfec-
        tion; Sterilization
  of equipment, 211, 338–339
    thermometers and, 246, 247, 247f
  of patient room, 211
  of supplies, 338–339
Cleansing
  of eyes, 101
    skill procedure for, 106
  of hands. *See* Handwashing
  of skin

at injection site, 609
prior to surgery, 436
at venipuncture site, 658
Cleansing enema, 553
  administering, skill procedure for,
        554–556, 554–556f
Clean technique. *See* Asepsis, medical
Clear liquid diet, 133t
Client, 16. *See also* Patient(s)
Closed reduction, 687
Closed wound, 457, 458t
Clothing. *See also* Gloves; Gown;
        Uniform
  asepsis and, 332, 334
  handling, 207, 208f
  isolation, 363–364, 364f
  removing
    helping patient with, 207
    skill procedure for, 365f, 365–366,
        366f
Codeine sulfate, dosage for equi-
        analgesia, 762t
Codes of ethics, 13, 78, 78d
Cognitive domain, 27, 27t
Cognitive–perceptual pattern, 42t
Cold applications, 490–494
  cold compresses and, 491
    applying, skill procedure for,
        493–494
  cool water or alcohol bath and, 492,
        494
  ensuring safe temperatures for, 491,
        491t
  hypothermic blanket and, 494
  ice bag, 491, 492f
Cold compresses, 491
  applying, skill procedure for,
        493–494
Collaborative problem, 46
Colloid solutions, 649–650
Colon (large intestine), 544
  sigmoidoscopy and, 315
Colonic Constipation, nursing care plan
        for, 569
Colonic irrigation, 558t
Colostomy, 559. *See also* Stoma,
        intestinal
Coma. *See* Unconscious patient
Comfort, promoting
  elderly patient and, 239
  helpless patient and, 239
  infant or child and, 235–238, 237f
  patient teaching for, 197, 239
Comforting skills, 9
Commission on aging, 203t
Commode, 505
Communicable diseases, 354
  preventing spread of. *See* Infection
        control
Communication, 21–23

barriers to therapeutic relationship and, 22
listening in, 22–23
nonverbal, 21–22
of nursing care plan, 48
promoting, 23
skill procedure for, 23–24
silence in, 22
techniques for, 21t
with terminally ill patient, 760
touch in, 22, 22f
verbal, 21, 21t
written forms of, 66–67
Competency, 77
Complications
of intravenous fluid administration, 667–669, 672
of intravenous medication administration, 633
postoperative, 444
cardiovascular, 447t
gastrointestinal, 448–449t
mucous membranes and, 450t
musculoskeletal, 450t
nutritional, 450t
respiratory. *See* Respiratory system, postoperative complications and
skin and, 450t
urinary tract and, 449t
of tube feedings, 141, 144, 150–151t, 152
Compresses, cold, 491
applying, skill procedure for, 493–494
Computerized axial tomography (CAT; CT), 313, 313f
Computerized charting, 60–61, 61f, 62f
protecting patient records and, 61
Concurrent disinfection, 339
Condom, applying, 296f, 297
Condom catheter
applying, skill procedure for, 512–514, 513f
constructing, 512
Conferences, 69
Confidentiality, 79
Consent
informed, 76–77
for surgery, obtaining, 436, 439f
Constipation, 377, 546–547
causes of, 547
characteristics of, 546, 546t
postoperative, 449t
pseudo, 546–547
relieving, 547, 549t
promoting and maintaining bowel elimination and, skill procedure for, 548
tube feedings and, 150t

Constitutional signs/symptoms, 278
Consultation, with patient and team members, 49
Contact isolation, 356, 359t
Contact lenses, 107, 107f
caring for, 107
skill procedure for, 109–112f, 109–113
types of, 108t
Contact route, of pathogen transmission, 355t
Contagious diseases, 354
preventing. *See* Infection control
Contamination, 330
of food, water, drugs, or blood, pathogen transmission by, 355t
linen, equipment, and supplies and, 364, 366, 367f
Continence, 551
Continence techniques, 509, 510t
Continent ostomy (Kock pouch), draining, 559, 566
Continuing education, 13, 13f
Continuity of care, 38, 209
patient record and, 54–55
Continuous-monitoring devices, for body temperature, 251
Continuous passive motion (CPM) machine, 699, 699f
skill procedure for using, 700f, 700–701
Continuous tube feeding, 141
administering, skill procedure for, 147–149, 148f, 149f
Continuum, 35
Contract, 20
Contractures, 376
postoperative, 450t
Contrast medium, 311
allergy to, 311
Control, loss of, dying and, 759
Contusion, 458t
Convalescent diet, 133t
Cool mist inhalation, 706
Cool water bath, 492, 494
Coping mechanisms, 25, 25t
Coping strategies, 25
Coping–stress-tolerance pattern, 42t
Corneas, organ donation and, 755t
Costs. *See also* Financial issues
health promotion and, 35
Coughing, to raise secretions, 434
teaching, skill procedure for, 435f, 435–436
Counseling skills, 9
CPM (continuous passive motion machine), 699, 699f
skill procedure for using, 700f, 700–701
CPR. *See* Cardiopulmonary resuscitation

Cracking, of oxygen tank, 725
Crackles (rales), 289
Cradle, 382
Cravat binder, 687, 688f
Credé's maneuver, 510, 510f
Cross-matching, 673
Crutches, 419–421
axillary, 419
measuring patient for, 420
crutch walking and, preparing for, 420–421
crutch-walking gaits and, 421–423t, 422f, 423f
Lofstrand (Canadian), 419, 420f
platform, 419, 420f
types of, 419, 420f
Crystalloid solutions, 649, 650–651, 651t
hypertonic, 651, 651t
hypotonic, 650–651, 651t
isotonic, 650, 651t
CT (CAT; computerized axial tomography), 313, 313f
Culture, 23
eating habits and, 123
illness and, 23–24
pain and, 177
patient services and, 31
Curative nursing care, 7
Cutaneous triggering, urinary incontinence and, 509–510
Cyanocobalamin (vitamin B_{12}), 127t
Cylinder cast, 687
Cystoscope, 312
Cystoscopy, 315–316

Dakin's solution (sodium hypochlorite), wound care and, 474t
Dangling, 417–418, 418f
Darkness, microorganisms and, 329
Darvon (propoxyphene hydrochloride), dosage for equianalgesia, 762t
Data, 41
analyzing, 44
collection of, 41
for research, patient records and, 55
objective and subjective, 41
Database
adding to, 41
gathering, 41
for problem-oriented record, 56–57
Database assessment, 41
dB (decibels), 108
Deaf patient
medication administration and, 598
patient services for, 30
Death and dying
attitudes and responses to, 750–751
autopsy and, 765

Death and dying (*continued*)
  confirming death and, 765
  death certificate and, 765
  emotional needs and
    acceptance of reality and, 760
    facilitating communication and, 760
    fears and, 758–760
    responding to, 758–760
    sustaining realistic hope and, 758
  emotional reactions to, 755, 756t
  extended care and, 756
  family and
    involving in patient care, 763, 764f
    summoning, 764–765
    supporting, 765
  grieving and. *See* Grieving
  home care and, 755–756
  hospice care and, 203t, 756–757,
    757f
  informing patient and, 753–755
  nursing diagnoses for, 772
  nursing responsibilities after death
    and, 765–766
  organ donations and, requesting,
    752–753, 754f, 755t
  patient teaching for, 772–774
  physical needs and, 761–763
    elimination and, maintaining, 761
    environmental modification and,
      763, 763f
    hygiene and, 761–762
    involving family members in pa-
      tient care and, 763, 764f
    nourishment and, providing, 761
    pain control and, 762, 762t
    patient positioning and, 762
    protecting patient from harm and,
      762–763
  postmortem care and, 766
    skill procedure for performing,
      767–768, 768f
  preparing to provide terminal care
    and
    euthanasia and, 752
    feelings about death and, 751
    living wills and, 752, 753f
    support system and, 751–752
  protecting patient from fraudulent
    treatment and, 757–758
  research and, participation in, 758,
    759f
  right to die and, 79
  signs of, 763–764
  spiritual needs and, 760, 761f
Death certificate, 765
Debridement, 460
Debris, healing and, 460
Decibels (dB), 108
Decisional Conflict, nursing care plan
    for, 323

Decubitus ulcers (pressure sores), 377,
    460–463
  causes of, 460, 461f
  classification of, 462–463f, 462–463t
  patients at risk for, 461, 464t
  postoperative, 450t
  preventing, 461
    skill procedure for, 465–467, 466f
  signs of, 460–461, 462–463t
  treating, 461
Deep-breathing exercises, 432
  skill procedure for performing,
    432–433, 433f
Defecation, 544–545. *See also* Bowel
    elimination; Constipation;
    Diarrhea
Defendant, 74
Defenses, natural, against microorga-
    nisms, 329t, 329–330
Dehiscence, postoperative, 450t
Dehydration, 647–648, 648f. *See also*
    Fluid imbalances
  as surgical risk factor, 429t
Deltoid muscle, for injections, 611
  locating, skill procedure for, 616,
    616f
Demerol (meperidine hydrochloride),
    dosage for equianalgesia, 762t
Denial, dying and, 751, 756t
Dental caries, 94
Dental plaque, 94
Dentures, care of, 99, 101, 106f
Deodorants, 87
Dependence, fear of, dying and, 759
Depilatory, 440
Depression, dying and, 756t
Descending colon, 544
Dextrose and water solution, intra-
    venous, 651t
Dextrose in saline solution, intravenous,
    651t
DHealing, bandages and binders and.
    See Bandages; Binders
Diabetes mellitus
  personal hygiene in patient with,
    119
  preoperative and postoperative care
    in patient with, 452
Dialysis, 648
Diaphragmatic respiration, 257
Diarrhea, 550–551
  causes of, 550
  relieving, 550–551
  tube feedings and, 150t
Diastole, 259
Diastolic pressure, 259
Diathermy, 497
Diets. *See also* Nutrition
  prescribed, 132, 133t
Diffusion, of electrolytes, 677

Dignity
  loss of, dying and, 759
  preservation of, 19
Dilaudid (hydromorphone), dosage for
    equianalgesia, 762t
Diluent, 608
Dilution, of medications
  diluent and, 608
  in large volume of fluid, for intra-
    venous administration, 626
Direct contact, pathogen transmission
    by, 355t, 356
Directed donation, 430, 430t
Disbelief, death and, 769t
Discharge, 209–215, 213f
  leaving against medical advice and,
    210–211
  nursing diagnoses and, 215
  patient teaching and, 215
  procedures for
    elderly patients and, 214–215
    infant or child and, 212–214
  skill procedure for, 214
Disease. *See* Illness
Disease-specific isolation, 356
Disinfectant (bacteriocide; germicide),
    332
Disinfection, 339–341
  concurrent, 339
  disinfectants and, 332
  methods of, 340t, 340–341
  preparing for, 339–340
  terminal, 339
Disorientation, postoperative, 451t
Disposal
  of contaminated trash, burnable, 364
  of feces, infection control and, 367
  of needles, syringes, and sharp ob-
    jects, 336, 338, 339f, 610
  of urine, infection control and, 367
Distal, definition of, 168t
Distention
  abdominal, 293
    postoperative, 449t
  intestinal. *See* Intestinal distention
Disuse syndrome, 375
  preventing, 377–378
Diuresis (polyuria), 503
Diversional items, in hospital, 225
Document(s)
  legal, patient records as, 55
  signing, infection control and, 370,
    370f
Documenting. *See* Charting; Patient
    records; Recording
Döoderlein bacilli, 476
Donor. *See also* Organ donation
  blood transfusions and, 673
    predonation and, 429–430, 430t
Dorsal recumbent position, 306, 306f

Dorsiflexion, 376
Dorsogluteal site, for injections, 610
    locating, skill procedure for, 612–613, 614f
Dosage. *See also* Medication(s), dosage of
    megadoses of vitamins and, 126
Double-bagging technique, 364
Douche (vaginal irrigation), 476, 478, 480
    administering, skill procedure for, 480–481
Drain(s), 480–482, 481f, 482f
Drainage. *See also* Secretions
    from lesions, terms describing appearance of, 286
    postural, 706
        skill procedure for promoting, 707f, 707–708
Drainage/secretion precautions, 357, 360t
Draping, of patient, 305
Dressings, 463, 467–470. *See also* Bandages
    changing
        organizing equipment and supplies for, 470
        preparing patient for, 468, 470
        skill procedure for, 468–470, 469f, 471–474, 471–474f
    gauze, 463, 467
        changing, skill procedure for, 471–474, 471–474f
    hydrocolloid (occlusive), 467–468, 468f
        changing, skill procedure for, 468–470, 469f
    purpose of, 463
    securing, 482–483, 483f
    transparent, 467, 467f
    wet to dry, applying, 482
Droplet spread, pathogen transmission by, 355t, 357
Drowning, preventing, 232, 235t
Drug(s)
    abuse of, as surgical risk factor, 429t
    prescribed. *See* Medication(s); Medication administration; Medication order
Dry heat, disinfection/sterilization with, 340t, 341
Dura mater, organ donation and, 755t
Dying. *See* Death and dying
Dyspnea, 259
Dysrhythmia, 255
Dysuria, 503

Ear(s), 107–108, 113, 113t, 114f. *See also* Hearing; Hearing impaired patient

    assessing, 284–285, 286f, 294t
    hearing aid insertion and, skill procedure for, 114
    irrigation of, 476
        skill procedure for, 478–479, 479f
Ear medications, 590
    instilling, skill procedure for, 593f, 593–594
Eating habits, culture and, 123
ECG (EKG; electrocardiography), 311, 313, 314f
    stress, 169, 169f
Echography (ultrasonography), 315
    obstetric, 315
Edema, 286
    fluid excess and, 647
Education, for nursing, 11–13, 12t
Eductation. *See also* Patient teaching
EEG (electroencephalography), 313–314
Efflurage, 98f
Egg-crate foam mattress, 381
EKG (ECG; electrocardiography), 311, 313, 314f
    stress, 169, 169f
Elderly patient
    admitting and discharging, 214–215
    bowel elimination in, promoting, 568, 570
    comfortable and safe environment for, promoting, 239
    examination of, assisting with, 322
    exercise in, promoting, 173–174
    fluid and chemical balance in, promoting, 682
    healing in, promoting, 497–499
    inactivity in, preventing, 424–425
    mechanical immobilization of, 701
    medication administration and, 598, 600
        parenteral medications and, 635, 635f
    obtaining vital signs in, 274
    patient services for, 29
    personal hygiene in, promoting, 119–120
    physical assessment of, 298
    preoperative and postoperative care in, 454
    promoting nutrition in, 156
    sleep in, promoting, 197
    terminal illness in, 772
    urinary elimination in, promoting, 541
Electrical impulses, examinations of, 313–314
Electrical injuries, preventing, 230, 234t
Electrocardiography (ECG; EKG), 311, 313, 314f
    stress, 169, 169f

Electrodes, 313
Electroencephalography (EEG), 313–314
Electrolyte(s), 676
    distribution of, 677
    functions of, 676–677
Electrolyte balance, 676f, 676–678, 677t
    bicarbonate and, 677
    calcium and, 677
    chloride and, 677
    disorders of. *See* Electrolyte imbalances
    electrolyte distribution and, 677
    magnesium and, 677
    phosphate and, 677
    potassium and, 677
    promoting
        in adolescent or young adult, 682
        in elderly patient, 682
        in infant or child, 680–682
        patient teaching for, 682
    sodium and, 677
Electrolyte imbalances, 677–678, 678t
    detecting, 677–678
    nursing diagnoses for, 680
    preventing and correcting, 678
    tube feedings and, 150t
Electromyography (EMG), 314
Electronic blood pressure meters, 264–265
Electronic thermometer, 243, 244f
    assessing body temperature using, skill procedure for, 252f, 252–253
Elimination. *See also* Bowel elimination; Urinary elimination
    pattern of, 42t
Emboli/embolism, 376
    air, intravenous fluid administration and, 669, 672
    avoiding, 434, 436
        antiembolism stockings and, 434, 436, 438, 438f
        leg exercises for, 434, 436–437, 437f
    pulmonary, postoperative, 448t
Emesis (vomitus), 130
EMG (electromyography), 314
-emia, meaning of, 647
Emollient, 119
Emollient enema, 558t
Emotion(s), 17. *See also* Anxiety; Emotional responses; Fear(s); Stress
    blood pressure and, 260
    body temperature and, 244
    isolation and, 370
    pulse rate and, 254
    sleep and, 191–192

Emotional responses. *See also* Anxiety; Emotion(s); Fear(s); Stress
  to death and dying, 750–751
  grieving and, 766, 769t
  to illness, 24t, 24–25, 25f, 25t
  postoperative, 451t
  to terminal illness, 755, 756t
    responding to emotional needs and, 758–760
Emotional services, 17–18
Emotional support
  for family of dying patient, 765
  for nurse providing terminal care, 751–752
  providing, skill procedure for, 26
  surgery and, 430–431
Emotional well-being, 33
Empathy, 9
Endorphins, 180, 181
Endoscopy, 315–316
  percutaneous endoscopic gastrostomy and, 144
Enema, 553, 557
  antihelminthic, 558t
  barium, 312
  carminative, 558t
  cleansing, 553
    administering, skill procedure for, 554–556, 554–556f
  colonic irrigation, 558t
  emollient, 558t
  Harris flush, 558t
  hypertonic solution and, 553, 557, 557f
  large volume, 553
  nutritive, 558t
  purposes of, 557–558, 558t
  retention, administering, 557
  teaching patient to self-administer, 558
Energy, 161t
Enteric precautions, 357, 358–359t
Enterostomal therapist, 565
Enuresis, 197
Environment, 218
  microorganisms and, 329
  modifying, terminally ill patients and, 763, 763f
  nursing diagnoses for patients at risk from hazards in, 237
  sleep and, 191
Environmental psychologist, 218
Equipment
  cleaning, 211, 338–339
  contaminated, caring for, 364, 366, 367f
  for dressing change, 470
  for examination
    caring for, 310
    preparing, 303t, 303–304, 304f

  for isolation room, 362–363, 363f
  for parenteral medication administration, 604f, 604–605, 605f, 605t
  for subcutaneous injections, 622
  for suctioning, 706, 708
  for venipuncture, 654–655
    assembling, 655
    selecting, 654–655, 655f
Erect position, 305
Errors, medication, reporting, 583–584
Eructation, 130
Escherichia coli, 328
Ethics, 78–80
  allocation of scarce resources and, 79
  codes of, 13, 78, 78d
  confidentiality and, 79
  dilemmas and, 78
  right to die and, 79
  truth-telling and, 79
  whistle-blowing and, 79
Ethics committees, 79–80
Ethyl alcohol, disinfection/sterilization with, 341
Ethylene oxide gas, disinfection/sterilization with, 340t, 341
Etiology, 44
Euthanasia, 752
  active and passive, 752
Evaluation, 49–51
  consulting with patient and team members and, 49
  revising plans and, 49–51
Evisceration, postoperative, 450t
Exacerbation, 36
Examination(s). *See also* Assessment; Physical assessment; Special procedures; Tests
  advancements in, 310
  assisting with, 301–324
    in elderly patient, 322
    in infant or child, 318–322
  of body fluids, 316–321
  breast self-examination and, 281f
  to detect radiation, 314–315
  documenting, 308, 310
  of electrical impulses, 313–314
  endoscopic, 315
    percutaneous endoscopic gastrostomy and, 144
  equipment for
    caring for, 310
    preparing, 303t, 303–304, 304f
  of feces, 567t
  fluoroscopic, 311
  nursing diagnoses for patients undergoing, 322
  patient positioning for, 305–307t
  patient teaching for, 322–324
  preparing patient for, 304
  reporting and, 308, 310

  sonographic, 315
  supplies for
    caring for, 310
    preparing, 303t, 303–304
  of urine, 503, 506t
  x-ray. *See* X-ray examinations
Examination gloves. *See* Gloves
Excoriation, 559
Exercise(s), 158
  active, 168t, 170, 377
  aerobic, 170
  assessing fitness and, 166, 169
  benefits of, 162, 166
  blood pressure and, 260
  body temperature and, 244
  deep-breathing, 432
    skill procedure for performing, 432–433, 433f
  isometric, 170, 416–417
  isotonic, 170
  Kegel, 509, 511
  lack of, nursing diagnoses for, 172
  leisure-time activities and, 170, 172
  passive, 168t, 170, 377
  promoting
    in elderly patient, 173–174
    in infant or child, 172
    in pregnant patient, 172–173
    before surgery, 432
  pulse rate and, 253–254
  range-of-motion (ROM)
    basic guidelines for using, 403, 405, 406
    performing, skill procedure for, 407–416, 407–416f
  regular, 170, 170d, 171f
    program for, 171–172
  risk factors for, 166
Exhalation, 256
Expectoration, 297
Expiration, 256
Extended-care facilities, 202–203, 204f
  guidelines for selecting, 204d
  for terminally ill patients, 756
Extension, 167t, 408, 408f, 410f, 414f
External cardiac compression, 734
  age differences in, 741t
External hemorrhoids, 293
External respiration, 256
External rotation, 167t, 409, 409f, 413f
Eye(s), 101, 106–107. *See also* Vision; Visually impaired patient
  artificial, 107, 113f
  assessing, 282, 284, 285f, 294t
  cleansing, 101
    skill procedure for, 106
  eyeglass care and, 101, 106–107, 109–113
  irrigation of, 475–476
    skill procedure for, 477f, 477–478

Eye fatigue, 101
Eye medications, 588, 590
 instilling, skill procedure for, 591–592, 592f
Eye patches, promoting nutrition and, 156
Eyewear
 care of, 101, 106–107
  skill procedure for, 109–112f, 109–113
 contact lenses
  skill procedure for caring for, 109–112f, 109–113
  types of, 108t
 protective, asepsis and, 336, 339f

Face mask. *See* Oxygen mask
 oxygen therapy using, 726f, 726–727
  administering, skill procedure for, 720
  conversion equivalents for, 724t
Fahrenheit thermometer, 243, 243t
Falls
 preventing, 229–230, 233f, 234t
 risk factors for, 232d
False imprisonment, 77, 211
Family
 of dying patient
  involving in care, 763, 764f
  summoning, 764–765
  supporting, 765
 of surgical patient, assisting, 444, 446
Family birthing units, 202
Fats, dietary, 124–125
Fear(s). *See also* Anxiety; Stress
 dying and, 758–760
 pain and, 177
 as surgical risk factor, 429t
Febrile. *See also* Fever
 definition of, 244
Fecal impaction, 377, 547, 549
 causes of, 549
 relieving, 549
Fecal incontinence, 377, 551–552
 causes of, 552
 managing, 552
Feces (stool), 377. *See also* Bowel elimination; Constipation; Diarrhea; Fecal impaction; Stool specimens
 characteristics of, 545, 546t
 collecting, from intestinal stoma, 559
 disposal of, infection control and, 367
 examination of, 567t
 of infant, characteristics of, 568t
 water loss in, 642, 642t
Feedings. *See* Nutrition
Feelings. *See* Emotion(s); Emotional responses

Feet, care of, 114–115, 115f
Female, adult, physical assessment of, 298
Fever (pyrexia), 244, 245t. *See also* Hyperthermia
 constant, 245t
 cool water or alcohol bath for reducing, 492, 494
 crisis and, 245t
 intermittent, 245t
 invasion (onset) of, 244
 lysis and, 245t
 remittent, 245t
Field of vision, 87
Figure-of-eight turn, roller bandages and, 487, 487f
Financial issues
 fear of financial ruin, dying and, 760
 health promotion and, 35
 reimbursement and, 55, 203
Fingernails
 care of, 113–114
 healthy, characteristics of, 87
Fires, preventing, 230–232, 232f, 233t, 234t
First intention healing, 458–459
Fissure, 286
Fitness, 159
 assessment of, 166, 169
 fitness tests and, 169, 169f, 170t
Five Rights of medication administration, 581f, 581–582
Flatulence, 549
Flatus, 130–131, 549
Flexibility, exercise and, 162
Flexion, 167t, 407–411f, 414f, 415f
Floor, of patient's room, 218
Flossing, of teeth, 96, 99
 skill procedure for, 102–103, 103f
Flow sheets, 67–68
Fluid(s)
 body. *See* Body fluid(s); Electrolyte balance; Electrolyte imbalances; Fluid balance; Fluid imbalances
 intravenous. *See* Intravenous fluid administration
 sleep and, 192
Fluid balance, 639–676
 assessing, 643–647
  circulatory system and, 647
  determining fluid intake and, 644, 644t
  determining fluid output and, 644–645, 645f
  gastrointestinal system and, 647
  integumentary system and, 646–647, 647f
  measurable data and, 646, 646t
  nervous system and, 647

 recording fluid intake and, 644, 644f
  recording fluid output and, 645–646, 646f
  respiratory system and, 647
  urinary system and, 647
 body fluid and, 641
  distribution of, 642, 643f
  regulation and, 642–643
 body water and, 641
  elimination of, 642, 642t
  functions of, 641–642
  proportions of, 641, 641t
  sources of, 642, 642t
 disorders of. *See* Fluid imbalances
 promoting
  in adolescent or young adult, 682
  in elderly patient, 682
  in infant or child, 680–682
  patient teaching and, 682
Fluid imbalances, 647–676, 648f
 blood transfusions and. *See* Blood transfusions
 increasing oral fluid intake and, 648
  skill procedure for, 649
 intravenous fluid administration and. *See* Intravenous fluid administration
 nursing diagnoses for, 680
 postoperative, 450t
 restricting oral fluid intake and, 648
  skill procedure for, 650
Fluid intake
 determining, 644, 644t
 increasing, 648
  skill procedure for, 649
 measuring, 132, 132f
 recording, 132, 132f, 644, 644f
 restricting, 648
  skill procedure for, 650
Fluid output
 determining, 644–645, 645f
 recording, 645–646, 646f
Fluid Volume Deficit, nursing care plan for, 681
Fluoroscopy, 311
Fluosol DA, 673, 676
Foam mattress, 380–381, 382t
Focus assessment, 41
Focus charting, 59
Folic acid (vitamin B$_9$), 127t
Follow-up
 for first occasion of high blood pressure, 262t
 for problem-oriented record, 58–59, 59t
Foods. *See also* Nutrition
 basic food groups and, 126, 129f
 contamination of, pathogen transmission by, 355t

Foods (*continued*)
  junk, 126
  providing, 132–133
    helping patient to eat and, skill procedure for, 135
    serving and removing trays and, skill procedure for, 134
  sleep and, 192
Foot, care of, 114–115, 115f
Footboard, 379
Foot drop, 376
Foot splints, 379, 380, 381f
Forceps, transfer, 343–344, 345f
Foreign objects, in airway, dislodging, 713
  skill procedure for, 713–717, 714–716f
Formal teaching, 27
Four-point gait, 421t, 422f
Four-tailed binder, applying, 488, 488f
Fowler's position, 384, 395
  skill procedure for positioning patient and, 398–399, 399f
Fracture, 687. *See also* Cast(s); Splints
  open and closed reduction of, 687
Fraudulent treatment, protecting patient from, 757–758
Full liquid diet, 133t
Functional incontinence, 504t
  nursing approaches for, 510t
Functional method, 37
Furnishings, in patient's room, 219–225

Gaits, crutch-walking, 421–423t, 422f, 423f
Gallbladder, cholecystography and, 312
Gas
  intestinal, 130–131, 549
  in stomach, relieving, 131
Gastric analysis, 316
Gastric gavage, 136–141. *See also* Nutrition, tube feedings and
Gastric residual, 145
Gastrocolic reflex, 545
Gastrointestinal system. *See also* Bowel; Bowel elimination; Stomach
  assessing, 293, 293f, 294t
  fluid imbalances and, 647
  inactivity and, 377
  lower gastrointestinal x-ray and, 312
  postoperative problems and, 449t
  upper gastrointestinal x-ray and, 311–312
Gastrostomy, 144, 152, 153f
  percutaneous endoscopic, 144
Gate-control theory of pain, 181
Gauze dressings, 463, 467

changing, skill procedure for, 471–474, 471–474f
Gender
  blood pressure and, 260
  body temperature and, 244
  pulse rate and, 253
General anesthesia, 428
Generalist, 87
  physical assessment by, 282t
Generic (nonproprietary) drug names, 573
Genitourinary system. *See also* Urinary tract
  assessing, 293, 294t
Genupectoral (knee-chest) position, 307, 307f
Germicide (bacteriocide; disinfectant), 332
Germ theory, 34–35
Gingivitis, 94
Glands
  ceruminous, 86
  sebaceous, 86
  thyroid, scan of, 314–315
Glasgow Coma Scale, 292
Gloves
  asepsis and, 336
  for isolation, 364, 364f
  sterile, donning and removing, 345
    skill procedure for, 347–349, 348f, 349f
Glucometer, skill procedure for using, 319–321, 319–321f
Gluteal setting, 416–417
Glycosuria, 503
Goal (objective), 47
  establishing, 47
Good Samaritan laws, 74
Gown
  for isolation, 363
  sterile, donning, 344–345
    skill procedure for, 346f, 346–347
Granulation tissue, 458
Gravity, 161t
  intravenous infusions and, 653
  specific, 538
    testing urine for, 538, 538f
Grief, 750. *See also* Grieving
  anticipatory, 750
  pathological, 769
  resolution of, 771
Grief work, 766
Grieving, 766, 769–771. *See also* Grief
  comforting and, 766, 770
  facilitating, skill procedure for, 770
  grief resolution and, 771
  patient teaching for, 772–774
  patterns of, 766, 769t
    emotional reactions and, 766, 769t

physical reactions and, 766
  perinatal deaths and, 769–771
  suicide and, 769–771
  terminally ill patient and
    elderly, 772
    infant or child, 772
Gurgles (rhonchi), 289

Hair. *See also* Integumentary system
  care of, 115–117
    grooming and, 115, 117
    shampooing and, 116, 116f, 117
  healthy, characteristics of, 87
  removing prior to surgery, 436, 439–440, 440f
Hair covers, asepsis and, 336
Hammock effect, 381
Handicapped patient, administering medications to, 597–598, 601f
Hand rolls, 379, 379f
Handwashing, 332
  guidelines for, 332d
  isolation and, 363
  skill procedure for, 333f, 333–334, 334f
Harris flush, 558t
Healing, 456–499
  cold applications and. *See* Cold applications
  of decubitus ulcers (pressure sores). *See* Decubitus ulcers
  factors affecting, 459–460
  heat applications and. *See* Heat applications
  inflammatory response and, 457–458
  irrigation and. *See* Irrigation
  mechanisms of, 458–459, 459f
    first intention healing and, 458–459
    second intention healing and, 459
    third intention healing and, 459
  nursing diagnoses for patients with problems related to, 497
  promoting
    in elderly patient, 497, 499
    in infant or child, 497
    patient teaching and, 499
    in unconscious patient, 497
  sutures and staple removal and, 483–484, 484f
  types of wounds and, 457, 458t
  wound care and. *See also* Bandages; Binders; Dressings; Wound care
Health, 32–38. *See also* Illness; Wellness
  continuity of care and, 38
  emotional, 33
  healing and, 460
  as personal responsibility, 34

physical, 33
  as resource, 34
  restoration of, as nursing skill
      objective, 7
  as right, 34
  social, 33–34
  spiritual, 34
  wellness and, 35–36
Health care, 4
  continuum of, 38
  at home, 202
  patient record as permanent account
      of, 54
  for terminally ill patient, 755–756
  for terminally ill patients, 755–756
  trends in delivery of, 202–204
Health-care record. *See* Patient records
Health-care system, 37
Health-care team, 37, 37f
  consulting with, 49
Health history, 277
  reviewing, medication administration
      and, 581
Health-illness continuum, 35f, 35–36
Health patterns, functional, 42t
Health-perception/health-management
      pattern, 42t
Health practitioners, 4. *See also*
      Nurse(s)
  patient record and, 54
Health problems. *See* Problem(s)
Health promotion, 7
  as nursing skill objective, 7
  trends in, 34–35
Health-Seeking Behaviors, nursing care
      plan for, 297
Hearing
  assessing, 284–285, 286f, 294t
  normal, characteristics of, 87
Hearing aid, skill procedure for inser-
      tion of, 114
Hearing impaired patient
  medication administration and, 598
  patient services for, 30
Heart. *See also* Cardiopulmonary func-
      tioning; Cardiopulmonary re-
      suscitation; Cardiovascular
      functioning
  organ donation and, 755t
Heart murmurs, 291
Heart sounds, 290–291, 291f
  normal and abnormal, 291
Heart valves
  heart sounds and, 290, 291f
  organ donation and, 755t
Heat, disinfection/sterilization with, 340t,
      341
Heat applications, 490, 491, 494–497
  electrical heating pads and, 494–495

heat lamps and, 497
  hot water bottles and, 495
  hyperthermia pad and, 495, 495f
  light bulbs and, 497
  moist packs and, 496–497, 496f
  safe temperature for, 491, 491t
  sitz baths and, 495–496
  soaks and, 496
  uses of, 491
Heating pads, 494–495
Heat lamps, 497
Height, assessing, 278, 278f
Heimlich maneuver (abdominal
      thrusts), 714f, 714–715
Help, signaling for, 227
Helpless patient, promoting comfortable
      and safe environment for, 239
Hem-, meaning of, 316
Hematocrit, fluid imbalances and, 646t
Hematuria, 503
Hemoccult test, 316
Hemoconcentration, 652
Hemodilution, 652
Hemoglobin
  fluid imbalances and, 646t
  microencapsulated, 676
Hemorrhage, postoperative, 447t
Hemorrhoids, 545
  external, 293
Hemothorax, 732
Henderson, Virginia, 4–5, 5t, 6t
Heparin, subcutaneous injection of, 623
Heparin lock, intravenous medication
      administration and, 626, 627,
      627f
Hepatitis B, infection control and, 367
Heredity, as risk factor for exercise, 166
Hiccups (singultus), postoperative, 448t
Hierarchy, 36
  of needs, 36, 36f
High-level wellness, 36
High Risk For Altered Protection, nurs-
      ing care plan for, 636
High Risk For Infection, nursing care
      plan for, 371
High Risk For Trauma, nursing care
      plan for, 238
High Risk For Urinary Incontinence,
      nursing care plan for, 540
High-risk nursing diagnosis, 46d
Hip spica, 688
History, 277
  reviewing, medication administration
      and, 581
Holism, 17, 17f
Holistic nursing, 17
Home-health aid, 203t
Home health care, 202
  for terminally ill patients, 755–756

Homemaker services, 203t
Hope, dying and, 751
  sustaining realistic hope and, 758
Hopelessness, nursing care plan for, 773
Horizontal recumbent position, 306
Hospice, 203t, 756–757, 757f
Hospital
  admission to. *See* Admission(s)
  discharge from. *See* Discharge
  leaving against medical advice,
      210–211
    reactions to hospitalization and,
      204–205
  room in. *See* Patient room
  stress-producing events in, 189t
Hospital garments, asepsis and, 332, 334
Host, 328
  susceptible, 329–330
Hot moist packs, 496–497, 496f
Hot water bottle, 495
Household measurement system, 574t,
      575t
Human response patterns, 44t
Humidification, 705–706
  cool mist inhalation and, 706
  warmed air inhalation and, 706
Humidity
  of patient's room, 219
  relative, 219
Hydrocolloid (occlusive) dressings,
      467–468, 468f
  changing, skill procedure for,
      468–470, 469f
Hydromorphone (Dilaudid), dosage for
      equianalgesia, 762t
Hygiene, 86. *See also* Oral hygiene;
      Personal Hygiene
Hyperalimentation, parenteral, 153, 153f
Hypercalcemia, 678t
Hyperchloremia, 678t
Hyperextension, 167t, 407, 407f, 410f,
      413f, 415f, 416f
Hyperkalemia, 678t
Hypermagnesemia, 678t
Hypernatremia, 678t
Hyperphosphatemia, 678t
Hypertension, 260–261
  follow-up for first occasion of, 262t
  as risk factor for exercise, 166
Hyperthermia, 244. *See also* Fever
  nursing care plan for, 273
Hyperthermia pad, 495, 495f
Hypertonic solutions, 553
  for enema, 553, 557, 557f
  intravenous, 651, 651t
Hyperventilation, 259
Hypervolemia, 647. *See also* Fluid
      imbalances
Hypnosis, 180

Hypocalcemia, 678t
Hypochloremia, 678t
Hypokalemia, 678t
Hypomagnesemia, 678t
Hyponatremia, 678t
Hypophosphatemia, 678t
Hypostatic pneumonia, 376
Hypotension, 261–262
   postural (orthostatic), 261
     checking for, 262
Hypothermia, 246, 494
   postoperative, 451t
Hypothermic blanket, 494
Hypotonic solutions, 650–651, 651t
Hypoventilation, 259
Hypovolemia, 647. *See also* Fluid
     imbalances
Hypovolemic shock, postoperative, 447t
Hypoxemia, 722
Hypoxia, 722

Ice bag, 491, 492f
ICN (International Council of Nurses),
     78
Idealization, death and, 769t
Identity, loss of, hospitalization and, 205
Ileostomy, 559. *See also* Stoma,
     intestinal
Illiterate patient, patient services for, 30
Illness, 36. *See also* Health; *specific*
     disorders
   acute, 36
   body temperature and, 244
   causes (etiology) of, 44
   chronic, 36
   exacerbation of, 36
   germ theory of, 34–35
   health-illness continuum and, 35f,
     35–36
   infectious. *See* Infection(s); Infection
     control
   lifestyle and, 34–35
   natural body defenses and, 330
   pathophysiology of, 46
   patient's response to, 23–25
   prevention of, as nursing skill
     objective, 7
   remission of, 36
   sleep and, 192
   terminal. *See* Death and dying;
     Terminal illness
Immediate care centers, 202
Immobilization, mechanical. *See*
     Mechanical immobilization
Immobilizers, 685
Impaired Physical Mobility, nursing care
     plan for, 702
Impaired Swallowing, nursing care plan
     for, 155

Impaired Tissue Integrity, nursing care
     plan for, 498
Implementation, 48–49
   charting care and, 48–49
   observations and, 48
Imprisonment, false, 77, 211
Inactivity, 374–425. *See also* Mechanical
     immobilization
   bed and
     protective bed devices and,
       380–382
     specialty, 382t, 382–384
   dangers of, 375–377
     to cardiovascular system, 376
     to gastrointestinal system, 377
     to integumentary system, 377
     metabolic, 377
     to muscular system, 375–376
     psychosocial, 377
     to respiratory system, 376–377
     to skeletal system, 376, 376f
     sleep pattern and, 377
     to urinary system, 377
   disuse syndrome and, preventing,
     377–378
   maintaining joint mobility and, 403,
     405–406
     range-of-motion exercises and, skill
       procedure for performing,
       407–416, 407–416f
   nursing diagnoses for, 425
   positioning devices and, 378–380
   positioning of patient confined to bed
     and, 384, 395
     skill procedure for, 396–399,
       396–399f
   preparing patient for walking and,
     416–421
   preventing
     in elderly patient, 424–425
     in infant or child, 423–424
     patient teaching for, 425
   as risk factor for exercise, 166
   transferring patients and, 395, 399,
     402
     to and from chair, skill procedure
       for, 404–405, 404–406f
     to and from stretcher, skill pro-
       cedure for, 400f, 400–401, 401f
   turning and moving patient and, 384
     moving patient up in bed and, skill
       procedure for, 392–394, 392–
       394f
     turning patient and, skill procedure
       for, 385–391, 385–391f
Incentive spirometry, 434, 434f
Incident sheet, 80, 81f
Incision, 458t
Incontinence. *See* Fecal incontinence;
     Urinary incontinence

Independence, promotion of, 19, 20f
Indirect contact, pathogen transmission
     by, 355t, 356
Individual supply, of medications, 577
Ineffective Airway Clearance, nursing
     care plan for, 743
Infant
   admitting and discharging, 212–214
   blood pressure in, assessing, 269–
     270, 270f
   bowel elimination in, promoting,
     567–568, 568t
   cardiopulmonary functioning in, pro-
     moting, 740, 742f, 742–744,
     744f
   comfortable and safe environment
     for, promoting, 235–238, 237f
   death of, grieving, 769–771
   examination of, assisting with,
     318–322
   exercise in, promoting, 172
   fluid and chemical balance in,
     promoting, 680–682
   healing in, promoting, 497
   inactivity in, preventing, 423–424
   infection control and, 372
   mechanical immobilization of, 699,
     701
   medication administration and, 597,
     600f
     parenteral medications and, 632,
       635
   nutrition of, promoting, 154, 156
   patient services for, 28–29
   personal hygiene and, promoting, 117
   physical assessment of, 296
   preoperative and postoperative care
     in, 452
   sleep in, promoting, 195–197
   terminal illness in, 772
   urinary elimination in, promoting,
     538–539
   vital signs in, obtaining, 271–272,
     272f
Infection(s)
   healing and, 460
   infectious period and, 354
   infectious process cycle and, 330,
     330f
   intravenous fluid administration and,
     669
   patients at risk for, nursing diagnoses
     for, 351
   preventing spread of, 232
   respiratory, postoperative, 448t
   of urinary tract, postoperative, 449t
Infection control, 353–372, 357f
   category isolation and, 356–357
     AFB (acid-fast bacillus), 357,
       359–360t

blood/body fluid precautions and, 357, 360–361t
contact, 356, 359t
drainage/secretion precautions and, 357, 360t
enteric precautions and, 357, 358–359t
respiratory, 357, 358t
strict, 356, 358t
contaminated linen, equipment, and supplies and, 364, 366, 367f
disease-specific isolation and, 356
excretions and secretions and, handling of, 367
human contacts and, providing, 370
with infant or child, 372
in intensive care unit, 372
isolation garments and, 363–364, 364f
removing, skill procedure for, 365f, 365–366, 366f
isolation room and
equipment for, 362–363, 363f
preparation of, 362
pathogen transmission and, limiting, 355, 355t, 356f
patient's feelings about, 370
patient teaching for, 372
patient transport and, 369, 369f
progress toward, 354–355
protective (reverse) isolation and, 357, 361, 362t
reading materials and, 369–370
sensory stimulation and, providing, 370
signing documents and, 370, 370f
transmission barriers and, 361
universal precautions and, 357, 361d
vaccines and, 354
wristwatches and, 367, 369
Infectious period, 354
Infectious process cycle, 330, 330f
Infiltration, intravenous fluid administration and, 668
Inflammatory response, 457–458
Inflatable (pneumatic) splints, 685
Informal teaching, 27
Information
informing patient about surgery and, 428–429
informing patient about terminal illness and, 753–755
patient's right to, 16
truthfulness and, 79, 753–755
Information gathering, 277–278
admission and, 207–208
skill procedure for, 209
health history and, 277
height and weight and, 278, 278f
patient examination and. *See* Physical assessment

signs and symptoms and, 278
vital signs and, 277–278
Informed consent, 76–77
Infradian rhythm, 186
Infrared lamps, 497
Infusion. *See* Blood transfusions; Intravenous fluid administration; Intravenous medication administration
Infusion devices, 653–654, 654f, 655f
Infusion rate
calculating, 658, 663
monitoring, 664, 664f, 665t
readjusting, 664–665
Inhalation, 256
cool mist and, 706
medication administration by, 575t
aerosol treatments and, 722, 722f, 723f
hand-held inhaler and, 722, 722f
measurement systems and, 574, 574t, 575t
warmed air and, 706
Inhaler, hand-held, 722, 722f
Injection(s). *See also* Syringe
discomfort of, reducing, 610
intradermal, 623, 624f
administering, skill procedure for, 625, 625f
intramuscular, 610–611
administering, skill procedure for, 617–619, 617–619f
deltoid muscle for, 611, 616, 616f
dorsogluteal site for, 610, 613–615, 614f
locating sites for, skill procedure for, 612–616, 612–616f
rectus femoris muscle for, 611, 612, 612f
vastus lateralis muscle as site for, 610–611, 615–616, 615f
ventrogluteal site for, 610, 612–613, 613f
Z-track (zigzag) technique for, 611, 620f, 620–621, 621f
subcutaneous, 611–623
administering, skill procedure for, 624
equipment for, 611
heparin administration by, 623
insulin preparation and, 621–623
modifying injection techniques for, 621, 623f
selecting site for, 611
Injury. *See also* Trauma; Wound
extent of, healing and, 459
healing and. *See* Healing; Wound care
inflammatory response to, 457–458
Insecurity, hospitalization and, 204
Insensible water loss, 642, 642t

Insomnia, 193–195
postoperative, 449t
Inspection, 279, 279f
Inspiration, 256
Instillation, drug administration by, 575t
Insulator, 490
Insulin, preparing for subcutaneous injection, 621–623
Insulin pen, 607, 609f
Insurance
liability, 80
Medicare, 203
Integument, 86
Integumentary system, 86. *See also* Hair; Mucous membranes; Nails; Skin
fluid imbalances and, 646–647, 647f
inactivity and, 377
Intellectual ability, assessing, 294t
Intensive care unit, infection control in, 372
Intermediate care, 203
Intermittent positive-pressure breathing (IPPB), 722, 723f
Intermittent pulse, 255
Intermittent tube feeding, 141
administering, skill procedure for, 146–147, 147f
Internal respiration, 257
Internal rotation, 167t, 409, 409f
International Council of Nurses (ICN), 78
Interstitial fluid, 641t, 642, 643f
Intestinal distention (tympanites), 549–550
causes of, 549–550
relieving, 550
rectal tube and, skill procedure for inserting, 551
Intestine, large, 544
Intracellular fluid, 641t, 642, 643f
Intradermal injections, 623, 624f
skill procedure for administering, 625, 625f
Intramuscular injections. *See* Injection(s), intramuscular
Intravascular fluid (plasma; serum), 641t, 642, 643f
Intravenous fluid administration, 648–673
attaching second container of solution and, 667, 669f
skill procedure for, 669–672, 670f, 671f
attaching tubing for, 652–653, 652–654f
changing solution containers and, 666
skill procedure for, 666–667, 667f
changing tubing and, 666–667
skill procedure for, 668

Intravenous fluid administration
(*continued*)
complications of, 667–669, 672
discontinuing, 672f, 672–673
gravity and infusion devices for,
653–654, 654f, 655f
infusion rate and
calculating, 658, 663
monitoring, 664, 664f, 665t
readjusting rate of flow and, 664–
665
maintaining infusion and, 663–667,
664f
patient assessment and, 651–652
purposes of, 649
solutions for. *See* Solution(s),
intravenous
starting infusion and, skill procedure
for, 659–553f, 659–663
venipuncture and, 654–658
caring for site of, 665–666
cleaning site for, 658
device for, selecting, 654–655, 655f
equipment for, 655
vein for, selecting, 655–658,
656–658f
Intravenous medication administration,
623–637
antineoplastic drugs and, 629, 632f,
632t, 633–635, 634f
administering, skill procedure for,
633–635, 634f
central venous catheter and, 627–629,
628f, 629f, 630–631, 631f
instilling medication through, skill
procedure for, 630–631, 631f
complications of, 632
diluting medication in large volume
of fluid and, 626
established intravenous line and, 626,
626f
heparin lock and, 626, 627, 627f
intermittent, 626–629
Intravenous pyelography (IVP), 312
Intravenous tubing
attaching, 652–653, 652–654f
changing, 666–667
skill procedure for, 668
Introductory phase, of nurse-patient
relationship, 20, 20f
Inunction, 575t, 588
Invasion
of fever, 244
of privacy, 77
Invasive procedures, 302
Involuntary psychiatric admission, 205t
Iodine
dietary, 125t
radioactive, 314

IPPB (intermittent positive-pressure
breathing), 722, 723f
Iron, dietary, 125t
Irrigation, 470, 475–480
colonic, 558t
of colostomy, 559
skill procedure for, 561–565,
563–565f
drug administration by, 575t
of ear, 476
skill procedure for, 478–479, 479f
of eye, 475–476
skill procedure for, 477f, 477–478
of indwelling catheter. *See* Urethral
catheterization, catheter irrigation and
of nasogastric tube, skill procedure
for, 151f, 151–152, 152f
oral, appliances for, 99
solutions used for, 470, 474t
vaginal (douche), 476, 478, 480
skill procedure for, 480–481
of wound, skill procedure for,
475–476
Isolation. *See also* Infection control
nursing diagnoses for, 370
Isolation garments, 363–364, 364f
removing, 364
skill procedure for, 365f, 365–366,
366f
Isolation room
equipment for, 362–363, 363f
preparing, 362
Isolation techniques, 354
Isometric exercises, 170, 416–417
Isotonic exercises, 170
Isotonic solutions, 650, 651t
IVP (intravenous pyelography), 312

Jejunostomy, 152–153, 153f
Joint mobility, maintaining, 403,
405–406
exercise and, 162, 407–416, 407–416f
Junk food, 126

Kardex, 66–67, 68f
Kegel exercises, 509, 511
Kidneys, 501
organ donation and, 755t
Kidneys, ureters, and bladder x-ray (ab-
dominal plain film; KUB), 311
Knee-chest (genupectoral) position, 307,
307f
Knowledge Deficit, nursing care plan
for, 350
Kock pouch (continent ostomy), drain-
ing, 559, 566
Korotkoff's sounds, 265, 266f, 266t

KUB (abdominal plain film; kidneys,
ureters, and bladder x-ray),
311

Laceration, 458t
Lactated Ringer's solution, 651t
Lactating patient
administering medications to, 594–
597
nutrition in, promoting, 156
Lacto-ovovegetarians, 126
Lactovegetarians, 126
Language, symbolic, 760
Large intestine (colon), 544
sigmoidoscopy and, 315
Laser, 446
Laser surgery, 446, 451–452
benefits of, 446, 451
safety and, 451–452
Lateral position, 384
skill procedure for positioning patient and, 396–397, 397f
Laws, 74–77
assault and battery and, 75–76
false imprisonment and, 77
Good Samaritan, 74, 75t
health-related, 10–11
informed consent and, 76–77
invasion of privacy and, 77
nurse practice acts, 10–11, 74
nurses' employment and, 74, 75t
patients' rights and, 75, 76d
protecting nurses, 74
slander and libel and, 77
wills and, 77
Lawsuits, 74–75
causes of, 75d
defense techniques and, 80, 81f, 82d
preventing, 80
Laxatives (cathartics), 548
Learning capacity, assessment of, 27
Legal documents, patient records as, 55
Leg exercises, to prevent blood clots,
434
teaching, skill procedure for, 436–
437, 437f
Legislation. *See* Laws
Lesion, 286. *See also* Wound; Wound
care
drainage from, terms describing
appearance of, 286
healing of. *See* Healing; Wound care
Liability, 74
Liability insurance, 80
Libel, 77
Licensing, 12, 13–14
Life cycle, care provided throughout,
19, 19f

Life expectancy, health promotion and, 34

Lifestyle, illness and, 34–35

Life support, basic, ABCs of, 734. *See also* cardiopulmonary resuscitation

Ligaments, organ donation and, 755t

Light diet, 133t

Lighting, of patient's room, 218–219

Linen, contaminated, caring for, 364, 366, 367f

Line of gravity, 161t, 162f

Lipping, 343, 345f

Liquid diet
   clear, 133t
   full, 133t

Listening, 22–23
   active, 9

Lithotomy position, 306, 307f

Liver, organ donation and, 755t

Living will, 77, 752, 753f

Local anesthesia, 428

Local signs/symptoms, 278

Lofstrand (Canadian) crutches, 419, 420f

Loneliness
   hospitalization and, 204
   isolation and, 370

Loss of control, fear of, dying and, 759

Loss of dignity, fear of, dying and, 759

Low air-loss bed, 382, 382t, 383f

Lower gastrointestinal x-ray (barium enema), 312

Lumbar puncture (spinal tap), 316–317, 317f

Lumen, 515

Lungs. *See also* Cardiopulmonary functioning
   insensible water loss through, 642, 642t
   organ donation and, 755t

Lung sounds
   abnormal (adventitious), 287, 289–290
   assessing, 287
      abnormal sounds and, 287, 289–290
      normal sounds and, 287, 290f
      skill procedure for, 288–289
   bronchial, 287, 290f
   bronchovesicular, 287, 290f
   tracheal, 287, 290f
   vesicular, 287, 290f

Lying down posture, 159, 161f

Magnesium
   dietary, 125t
   function of, 677

Mainframe computer, 60

Malaise, 458

Malnutrition, 124
   postoperative, 450t

Malpractice, 75

Mandatory nurse practice act, 74

Mantra, 190

Manual traction, 695

MAR (medication administration record), 576–577
   computerized, 577, 577f, 578f

Mask. *See also* Oxygen mask
   asepsis and, 336
   for isolation, 363
   self-inflating breathing bag and mask and, 734, 739, 741f
   skill procedure for using, 337f, 337–338, 338f

Maslow, Abraham, 6t, 36

Masses, abnormal, characteristics of, 294t

Mattress, 219, 378
   air
      alternating, 381, 382t
      static, 381, 382t
   foam, 380–381, 382t
   water, 381–382, 382t

Mattress overlays, 380–382

Meals on Wheels, 203t

Measurement systems, 574t, 575t
   converting between, 580
   metric equivalents and, 580
   thermometers and
      centigrade (Celsius), 242–243, 243t
      Fahrenheit, 243, 243t

Meatus, urinary, 502

Mechanical immobilization, 684–703
   braces and, 686
   casts and. *See* Cast(s)
   continuous passive motion machine and, 699, 699f
      skill procedure for using, 700f, 700–701
   of elderly patient, 701
   of infant or child, 699, 701
   nursing diagnoses for, 701
   patient teaching for, 703
   purposes of, 685
   slings and, 687, 687f, 688f
   splints and, 685–686, 686f
      emergency, applying, 686
   traction and. *See* Traction

Mechanical soft diet, 133t

Mediation(s), noncompliance and, 597
   nursing care plan for, 599
   overcoming, 598t

Medical asepsis. *See* Asepsis, medical

Medical care, 4

Medical treatments, natural body defenses and, 330

Medicare, 203

Medication(s), 573. *See also* Medication administration
   antibiotic, 332
   anticoagulant, 447t, 624
   antimicrobial (anti-infective), 331–332
   antineoplastic, intravenous administration of, 630, 633, 633f, 633t
      skill procedure for, 634–635, 636f
   contamination of, pathogen transmission by, 355t
   diluting in large volume of fluid, for intravenous administration, 626
   dosage of, 574
      amount to administer and, determining, 580
      calculating, 580–581
      measurement systems and, 574, 574t, 575t
         converting between, 580
         metric equivalents and, 580
      for pain control, 762, 762t
      terms used to designate, 574t
   names of
      generic (nonproprietary), 573
      trade (proprietary), 573
   narcotic, accounting for, 579–580
   over-the-counter, 601
   for pain control. *See also* Patient-controlled analgesia
      in terminally ill patients, 762, 762t
   pulse rate and, 254
   radiopharmaceutical, 314
   sleep and, 192
   storing, 577, 579, 579f
   supplies of, 577
   as surgical risk factor, 429t
   syringes and. *See* Syringe

Medication administration, 572–601
   buccal, 575t, 594, 597f
   to elderly patient, 598, 600
   Five Rights for, 581f, 581–582
   frequency of, 574, 576t
   health history and, reviewing, 581
   to infant or child, 597, 600f
   by inhalation, 575t, 721–722
      aerosol treatments and, 722, 722f, 723f
      hand-held inhaler and, 722, 722f
   intravenous. *See* Intravenous medication administration
   measurement systems and, 574, 574t, 575t
   medication errors and, reporting, 583–584
   medication order (prescription) and. *See* Medication order

Medication administration (*continued*)
noncompliance and, 594
overcoming, 598t
nursing diagnoses for, 597
oral. *See* Oral medication administration
parenteral. *See* Injection(s); Intravenous medication administration; Parenteral medication administration; Syringe
patient teaching for, 600–601, 601f
to physically handicapped patient, 597–598, 601f
to pregnant or lactating patient, 594–597
preparing medications and
procedures before, 582, 582f
procedures during, 582
procedures during, 582–583, 583f, 584f
procedures following, 583
recording, 583
rectal, 594
route and, 574, 575t. *See also specific routes*
sublingual, 575t, 594
to throat, 594
through nasogastric tube, skill procedure for administering, 589
topical. *See* Topical medication administration
transdermal, 575t, 588, 591f
skill procedure for applying patch and, 590
vaginal, 575t, 594
skill procedure for, 596
Medication administration record (MAR), 576–577
computerized, 577, 577f, 578f
Medication errors, reporting, 583–584
Medication order (prescription), 573–577
abbreviations used in, 574t, 576t
administration route and, 574, 575t
date and time of, 573
discontinuing, 577
dosage and, 574, 574t, 575t
drug name and, 573
frequency of administration and, 574, 576t
patient's name and, 573
PRN, 579t
questioning, 575–576
scheduling medication administration and, 577, 579t
signing, 574
single, 579t
standing, with and without termination date, 579t
stat, 579t

transcribing, medication administration record and, 576–577
computerized, 577, 577f, 578f
verbal, 576
Meditation, 186
Membranes
mucous. *See* Mucous membranes
semipermeable, 642
Menadione (vitamin K), 128t
Mental status
assessing, 280–281, 294t
death and, 764
postoperative disorientation and, 451t
Meperidine hydrochloride (Demerol), dosage for equianalgesia, 762t
Metabolic acidosis, 679t
Metabolic alkalosis, 679t
Metabolism, inactivity and, 377
METHOD acronym, discharge and, 210
Metric system, 574t, 575t
converting metric equivalents and, 580
Microabrasion, 439
Microencapsulated hemoglobin, 676
Microorganisms, 327–351. *See also* Bacillus(i)
aerobic, 329
anaerobic, 329
asepsis and. *See* Asepsis
characteristics of, 328–329
infectious process cycle and, 330, 330f
natural body defenses against, 329t, 329–330
factors weakening, 329–330
Micturition. *See* Urinary elimination; Urination
Middle ear inflammation, tube feedings and, 150t
Military time, 63, 66, 66f, 66t
Minerals, dietary, 125, 125t
Mobility. *See* Inactivity; Mechanical immobilization
Molded splints, 685–686, 686f
Monitoring
of body temperature, continuous-monitoring devices and, 251
of infusion rate, 664, 664f, 665t
Mood. *See also* Emotion(s)
assessing, 294t
Morphine sulfate, dosage for equianalgesia, 762t
Motivation
to learn, assessment of, 27
sleep and, 191
Mourning, 766. *See also* Grief; Grieving
Mouth
care of. *See* Oral hygiene
mucous membranes of, tube feedings and, 150t

Movement(s). *See also* Inactivity; Mechanical immobilization
terms used to describe, 167–168t
Mucoid, definition of, 286
Mucopurulent, definition of, 286
Mucous membranes. *See also* Integumentary system
healthy, characteristics of, 87
natural body defenses and, 330
oral and nasal, tube feedings and, 150t
postoperative complications and, 450t
structure and functions of, 86
Mucus, 86, 286
Murmurs, 291
Muscle(s). *See also* Musculoskeletal system
inactivity and, 375–376
intramuscular injections and. *See* Injection(s), intramuscular
of pelvic floor, strengthening, 509, 511
strength of
exercise and, 162, 509, 511. *See also* Exercise(s)
postoperative muscle weakness and, 450t
Musculoskeletal system, 159. *See also* Bone(s); Muscle(s)
assessing, 294, 294t
postoperative problems and, 450t
Myelography, 313

Nails. *See also* Integumentary system
care of, 113–115, 115f
healthy, characteristics of, 87
NANDA (North American Nursing Diagnosis Association), 44
NAPNES (National Association for Practical Nurse Education and Services), 78
Narcolepsy, 195
Narcotics, accounting for, 579–580
Narrative charting, 59
Nasal cannula, oxygen therapy using, 725–726, 726f
administering, skill procedure for, 728
conversion equivalents for, 724t
Nasal catheter, oxygen therapy using, 726
administering, skill procedure for, 728–729, 729f
Nasal medications, 591, 594
administering, skill procedure for, 595, 595f
Nasogastric tube, 133–134. *See also* Nutrition, tube feedings and

administering oral medications through, 587–588
skill procedure for, 589
National Association for Practical Nurse Education and Services (NAPNES), 78
National Federation for Licensed Practical Nurses (NFLPN), 78
National Federation of Licensed Practical Nurses, 13
National League for Nursing, 13
Nausea, 130
overcoming, 131
postoperative, 448t
tube feedings and, 150t
Nebulization, 705
Nebulizer, 434
Need(s), 7d, 36, 41, 44
of dying patient
emotional, 758–760
physical. *See* Death and dying, physical needs and
spiritual, 760, 761f
hierarchy of, 36, 36f
recognizing, 41, 44
Needles, disposing of, 336, 338, 339f, 610
Negligence, 75
Nervous system
assessing, 292f, 292–293, 294t
fluid imbalances and, 647
Neutral position, 406
NFLPN (National Federation for Licensed Practical Nurses), 78
Niacin (vitamin B₃), 127t
Nightingale, Florence, 4, 5t, 6t, 11
Nitroglycerin ointment, applying, 588, 591f
Nocturia, 503
Noise, controlling, 226, 226t
Noncompliance, 594
nursing care plan for, 599
overcoming, 598t
Nonelectrolytes, 676
Nonpathogens, 328
Nonproprietary (generic) drug names, 573
Nonrapid eye movement (NREM) sleep, 191, 191f, 192t
Nonverbal communication, 21–22
North American Nursing Diagnosis Association (NANDA), 44
Nose. *See also headings beginning with term* Nasal
care of, 113
mucous membranes of, tube feedings and, 150t
Notes
anecdotal, 80
nursing, 56, 58f

progress
of physician, 56, 57f
for problem-oriented record, 58–59, 59t
Nourishment. *See* Nutrition
NREM (nonrapid eye movement sleep), 191, 191f, 192t
Nurse(s). *See also* Nursing; *headings beginning with term* Nursing
laws affecting. *See* Laws
licensing of, 12, 13–14
patients' expectations of, 17
preparing to provide terminal care. *See* Death and dying, preparing to provide terminal care and
signaling, 227
Nurse-managed care (case management), 38
Nurse-patient (therapeutic) relationship, 19–21
communication barriers to, 22
phases of, 20–21
Nurse practice acts, 10–11, 74
mandatory, 74
permissive, 74
Nursing
definition of, 4–5, 7, 7d
holistic, 17
practical, 11
responsibilities of, 12t
primary, 37–38
professional, responsibilities of, 12t
registered, 11
responsibilities of, 12t
team, 37
technical, responsibilities of, 12t
Nursing care
curative, 7
preventive, 7
rehabilitative, 7
supportive, 9, 10f
Nursing care plan, 47–48, 66, 67d, 67f
for Activity Intolerance, 173
for Altered Comfort: Pain, 196
for Altered Oral Mucous Membrane, 51
for Anxiety, 216
for Bathing/Hygiene Self-Care Deficit, 118
for Body Image Disturbance, 453
for Colonic Constipation, 569
communicating, 48
for Decisional Conflict, 323
for Fluid Volume Deficit, 681
goal establishment and, 47
for Health-Seeking Behaviors, 297
for High Risk For Altered Protection, 636
for High Risk For Infection, 371

for High Risk For Trauma, 238
for High Risk For Urinary Incontinence, 540
for Hopelessness, 773
for Hyperthermia, 273
for Impaired Physical Mobility, 702
for Impaired Swallowing, 155
for Impaired Tissue Integrity, 498
for Ineffective Airway Clearance, 743
for Knowledge Deficit, 350
for Noncompliance, 599
priority setting and, 47, 48t
for problem-oriented record, 57
revising, 49–51
for Unilateral Neglect, 424
writing nursing orders and, 47–48
Nursing diagnosis(es), 44t, 44–47, 45f, 46d
actual, potential, and possible health problems and, 46
admission, transfer, referral, and discharge and, 215
bowel elimination and, 568
collaborative problems and, 46–47, 47f
data analysis and, 44
for death and dying, 772
determining patient problems and, 44
for fluid, electrolyte, and acid-base imbalances, 680
for inactive patients, 425
lack of exercise and, 172
making, 44, 46d
for mechanically immobilized patients, 701
for medication administration, 597
for parenteral medication administration, 637
for patient, with cardiopulmonary problems, 742
for patient at risk for infection, 351
for patient in isolation, 370
for patient requiring frequent assessment of vital signs, 272
for patient requiring help with personal hygiene, 117
for patients who feels unrested or is at risk from environmental hazards, 237
for patient undergoing surgery, 452
for patient undergoing tests and examinations, 322
for patient with healing problems, 497
for patient with urinary elimination problems, 539
during physical assessment, 296
sleep and relaxation problems and, 195
writing, 44, 46, 46f

Nursing implementation, 48–49
  charting care and, 48–49
  observations and, 48
Nursing Kardex, 66–67, 68f
Nursing notes, 56, 58f
Nursing orders
  for hygienic care, 88
  writing, 47–48
Nursing practice, 3–14
  accountability in, 11, 14
  autonomy of, 14
  commitment to career and, 13
  continuous learning and, 13, 13f
  definable role of, 10–11
  educational preparation for, 11–13,
    12t
  ethical codes and, 13
  excellence in, recognition of, 14
  organizations dedicated to, 13
  responsibility in, 11
  self-regulation of, 13–14
  theories and, 4, 5t, 6t
  unique competencies of, 11
  unselfish service and, 11
  value to society, 11
Nursing process, 11, 39–51, 40f
  assessment in, 41–44
  characteristics of, 40–41
  diagnosis in, 44t, 44–47, 45f
  evaluation in, 49–51
  implementation in, 48–49
  levels of responsibilities for, 12t
  planning in, 47–48
  skill procedure for using, 50
Nursing Research, 10
Nursing skills
  basic, 8–9
  basis for, 9–10
  objectives of, 7–8
  patient services and, 21–25
Nursing team, 37
Nursing theories, evolution of, 4, 5t, 6t
Nutrition, 122–157
  basic food groups and, 126, 129f
  culture and eating habits and, 123
  diets and, prescribed, 132, 133t
  fluids and. *See* Fluid intake
  food and, 132–133
  gastric gavage and, 136–141
    skill procedure for, 136–144
  gastrostomy and, 144, 152, 153f
  hyperalimentation and, parenteral,
    153, 153f
  inadequate, as surgical risk factor,
    429t
  jejunostomy and, 152–153, 153f
  Meals on Wheels and, 203t
  microorganisms and, 329
  natural body defenses and, 330
  nutritional needs and, 123–126

patient teaching to promote, 157
postoperative problems and, 450t
problems influencing eating and,
    120–132
promoting
  in blind patient, 156
  in elderly patient, 156
  in infant or child, 154, 156
  in patient with eye patches, 156
  in pregnant or lactating patient, 156
  teaching suggestions for, 157
for terminally ill patient, 761
total parenteral (TPN), 153, 153f
tube feedings and
  administering, skill procedure for,
    145f, 145–149, 147–149f
  bolus, 141
  continuous, 141
  inserting, maintaining, and remov-
    ing nasogastric tube and, skill
    procedure for, 136–141, 136–
    141f
  intermittent, 141
  irrigating nasogastric tubes and,
    skill procedure for, 151f, 151–
    152, 152f
  nasogastric tubes and, 133–134
  problems with, 141, 144, 150–151t,
    152
  small diameter tube and, skill pro-
    cedure for inserting, 142–144,
    143f
  tube patency and, 144, 151t
vegetarianism and, 126, 130t
weight gain or loss and, promoting,
    129–130
Nutritional assessment, 126, 128–129
Nutritional–metabolic pattern, 42t
Nutritive enema, 558t

Obesity, 129
  dislodging object from airway and,
    skill procedure for, 716f, 716–
    717
  preoperative and postoperative care
    and, 452, 454
  as risk factor
    for exercise, 166
    surgical, 429t
Objective (goal), 47
  establishing, 47
Objective data, 41
Observations, nursing implementation
    and, 48
Obstetric sonogram (B scan), 315
Occlusive (hydrodolloid) dressings,
    467–468, 468f
  changing, skill procedure for, 468–
    470, 469f

-occult, meaning of, 316
Occupational Safety and Health Admin-
    istration, 367
Odors
  controlling, 226, 226t
  from wound, 761
-ogram, meaning of, 310–311
-ography, meaning of, 310
Older Americans' ombudsman, 203t
Oliguria, 503
Open reduction, 687
Open wound, 457, 458t
Operating room, 427
Oral hygiene, 94, 96, 99, 101
  benefits of, 94, 96, 101f
  denture and bridge care and, 99, 101,
    106f
  flossing and, 96, 99
    skill procedure for, 102–103, 103f
  oral irrigating appliances and, 99
  skill procedure for giving, 104f, 104–
    105, 105f
  tooth brushing and, 96
    skill procedure for, 102, 102f, 103f
Oral medication administration, 575t,
    584–585
  skill procedure for administering,
    585f, 585–587, 586f
  swallowing of medications and, 584f
  through nasogastric tube, 587–588,
    589
Oral temperature, 242, 246
  measuring with glass thermometer,
    skill procedure for, 248f, 248–
    249, 249f
  normal, 244
Orders
  nursing
    for hygienic care, 88
    writing, 47–48
  of physician, 55–56, 56f
Orem, Dorothea, 5t, 6t
Organ donations
  criteria for, 755t
  organ removal and use timelines and,
    755t
  requesting, 752–753, 754f
Organization (process), 41
Organizations, committed to nursing
    practice, 5, 7, 13, 14, 44, 78
Orientation
  neurological assessment and, 292
  of patient, hospitalization and, 206–
    207
Orthopnea, 259
Orthostatic (postural) hypotension, 261
  checking for, 262
Oscillating support bed, 383f, 383–384
-oscopy, meaning of, 311
Osmosis, 642, 643f

Osteoporosis, 162, 169f
Ostomate, 559
Ostomy, continent (Kock pouch), draining, 559, 566
-ostomy, meaning of, 559
OTC (over-the-counter) drugs, 601
Otolaryngologist, 285
Outpatient, 202
Outpatient (ambulatory) services, 202
Outpatient (ambulatory) surgery, 428
Overbed table, 223, 225f
Overflow incontinence, 504t
  nursing approaches for, 5010t
Over-the-counter (OTC) drugs, 601
Oxygen mask, oxygen therapy using, 726f, 726–727
  administering, skill procedure for, 730
  conversion equivalents for, 724t
Oxygen tank, 725
  cracking, 725
Oxygen tent, oxygen therapy using, 727
  administering, skill procedure for, 730
Oxygen therapy, 722–732
  administering, skill procedure for, 728–731, 729f
  basic guidelines for administering, 723–724, 724t, 725f
  conversion equivalents for, 724t
  face mask and, 726f, 726–727
    administering oxygen with, skill procedure for, 730
    conversion equivalents for, 724t
  nasal cannula and, 725–726, 726f
    administering oxygen with, skill procedure for, 728
    conversion equivalents for, 724t
  nasal catheter and, 726
    administering oxygen with, skill procedure for, 728–729, 729f
  oxygen tanks and, handling, 725
  oxygen tent and, 727
    administering oxygen with, skill procedure for, 730
  T-piece and, skill procedure for administering oxygen with, 731
  tracheostomy collar and, skill procedure for administering oxygen with, 731
  transtracheal oxygen and, 727
    administering, skill procedure for, 731

Pack(s), hot, 496–497, 497f
Packing, of wounds, 482
Pain, 176–186
  acute, 177
    patient-controlled analgesia and, 180, 182f, 183–186
    relieving, skill procedures for, 181–186
  assessment of, 178t, 178–180, 179f
  blood pressure and, 260
  characteristics of, 176–177, 177f
  chronic, 177
    acupuncture and acupressure and, 180
    biofeedback and, 180
    hypnosis and, 180
    placebos and, 180, 182
    transcutaneous electrical nerve stimulation and, 182, 186, 187–188
  death and, 764
  definition of, 176
  fear of, dying and, 759
  gate-control theory of, 181
  intermittent, 177
  intractable, 177
  nursing care plan for, 196
  phantom limb, 176
  postoperative, 450t
  psychogenic, 177
  referred, 177
  relieving
    guidelines for, 179–180
    patient-controlled analgesia and, 180, 182f, 183–186
    skill procedures for, 181–186
    in terminally ill patients, 762, 762t
  threshold for, 176
  tolerance of, 176
Palpation, 279–280, 280f, 281f
  measuring blood pressure by, 266, 269
Palpitation, 254
Pancreas, organ donation and, 755t
Pantothenic acid, 128t
Paracentesis, 317, 318f
Parallel bars, 418, 418f
Paranormal experiences, death and, 763–764
Parenteral hyperalimentation, 153, 153f
Parenteral medication administration, 575t, 603–638
  disposing of used needles and syringes and, 610
  in elderly patient, 635, 635f
  equipment for, 604f, 604–605, 605f, 605t
  filling syringes and, 605–607, 605–608f
  in infant or child, 632, 635
  injections and. *See* Injection(s); Syringe
  intradermal injections and, 623, 624f
    skill procedure for administering, 625, 625f
  intravenous. *See* Intravenous medication administration
  mixing two medications in one syringe and, 608–609
  nursing diagnoses for, 637
  patient teaching for, 636–637, 637f
  prefilled cartridges and, 607, 608f, 609f
  reconstituting powdered medications and, 608
  reducing discomfort of injections and, 610
  skin cleansing for, 609
Parotitis, postoperative, 449t
Passive euthanasia, 752
Passive exercise, 168t, 170, 377
Patency, of nasogastric tube, 144, 161t
Pathogens, 328. *See also* Microorganisms
  transmission of
    barriers and, 361
    limiting, 355, 355t, 356f
    routes for, 355t
Pathological grief, 769
Pathophysiology, 46
Patient
  activity or emotional status likely to influence vital signs and, 274
  admitting. *See* Admission(s)
  dignity of
    loss of, dying and, 759
    preservation of, 19
  discharging. *See* Discharge
  draping, 305
  identification of, 227
    medication administration and, 573
  orienting, hospitalization and, 206–207
  preparing for examination, 304
  psychological implications of isolation and, 370
  referring, 209, 212f
  safety of. *See* Safety
  transferring between units or agencies, 208–209, 210f
    skill procedure for, 211
  unable to cooperate, obtaining vital signs in, 272, 274
Patient(s), 16
  access to records, 61
  adolescent. *See* Adolescent
  consulting with, 49
  dignity of, preservation of, 19
  dying. *See* Death and dying
  elderly. *See* Elderly patient
  expectations of, 16–17
  female, physical assessment of, 298
  informing
    about surgery, 428–429
    of terminal illness, 753–755

Patient(s) (*continued*)
  noncompliance of, 597
    nursing care plan for, 599
    overcoming, 598t
  outpatient (ambulatory), 202, 428
  pediatric. *See* Adolescent; Child;
      Infant
  positioning. *See* Positioning
  pregnant. *See* Pregnant patient
  receiving following surgery, 443
    skill procedure for, 445–446
  referring, 46
  response to illness, 23–25
  rights of. *See* Patient rights
  transport of, infection control and,
      369, 369f
  truth-telling and, 79
    about terminal illness, 753–755
  uniqueness of, 19
Patient advocate, 19
Patient care. *See also* Patient services
  continuity of, 209
  patterns for administering, 37–38
    case method and, 37
    functional nursing and, 37
    nurse-managed care and, 38
    primary nursing and, 37–38
    team nursing and, 37
Patient-controlled analgesia (PCA), 180,
    182f, 762
  skill procedure for, 183–186
Patient education. *See* Patient teaching
Patient records, 53–71. *See also* Chart-
    ing; Recording
  abbreviations in, 62–63, 63t
  charting methods and, 59–61
  checklists and flow sheets and, 67–68
  computerized, protecting, 61
  making entries on, 63
    skill procedure for, 64–65
  military time in, 63, 66, 66f, 66t
  patient access to, 61
  problem-oriented, 56–59
  traditional, 55–56
  uses for, 54–55
Patient rights, 16–17, 33, 75, 76d
  to be heard, 17
  to be informed, 16–17
  to choose, 17
  to die, 79
  health as, 34
  Patient's Bill of Rights and, 61, 76d
  to safety, 17
Patient room, 217–226
  cleaning, 211
  furnishings in, 219–225
  humidity, temperature, and ventila-
      tion of, 219
  isolation
    equipment for, 362–363, 363f

  preparing, 362
  lighting and, 218–219
  noise in, controlling, 226, 226t
  odors in, controlling, 226, 226t
  preparing, 206
    following surgery, 441
  privacy in, 226, 226t
  walls and floors of, 218
Patient's Bill of Rights, 61, 76d
Patient services, 15–31. *See also* Patient
    care
  for blind or visually impaired patient,
      29–30
  characteristics of, 19, 19f, 20f
  components of, 17f, 17–19
  for deaf or hearing impaired patient,
      30
  for elderly patient, 20
  health promotion and, 35
  for illiterate patient, 30
  for infant or child, 28–29
  nurse-patient relationship and, 19–21
  nursing skills related to, 21–25
  for patient from different culture, 31
  patients' expectations of, 16–17
  patient teaching as, 25–28
  for patient who cannot speak, 30–31
  for patient with short attention span,
      30
  recipients of, 16
  for unconscious patient, 31
Patient teaching, 25–28
  admission and, 215
  assessing learning needs and, 26
  for comfort, relaxation, and sleep,
      197
  discharge and, 215
  formal and informal, 27
  for infection control, 372
  learner assessment and, 26–27
  learning principles and, 27, 29d
  for mechanical immobilization, 703
  medical and surgical asepsis and, 351
  for medication administration, 600–
      601, 601f
  obtaining vital signs and, 274–275
  for parenteral medication administra-
      tion, 636–637, 637f
  personal hygiene and, 120
  physical assessment and, 298
  to prevent inactivity, 425
  to promote bowel elimination, 570
    self-administration of enema and,
        558
  to promote cardiopulmonary func-
      tion, 744–745
  to promote comfortable and safe
      environment, 239
  to promote fluid and chemical
      balance, 682

  to promote fluid and electrolyte
      balance, 682
  to promote healing, 499
  to promote nutrition, 157
  to promote urinary elimination, 541
  self-catheterization and, 531, 533
  skill procedure for, 28
  special procedures and, 302–303
  surgery and, 454
  teaching methods and, 27
  for terminally ill or grieving individ-
      uals, 772–774
  tests and examinations and, 322–324
  types of learning and, 27, 27t
PCA (patient-controlled analgesia), 180,
    182f, 762
  skill procedure for, 183–186
PDT (photodynamic therapy), 451
PEG (percutaneous endoscopic gastros-
    tomy), 144
Pelvic floor muscles, strengthening, 509,
    511
Pen, insulin, 607, 609f
Pentazocine (Talwin), dosage for equi-
    analgesia, 762t
Percussion, 279, 280f
  to loosen secretions, 706, 709f
Percutaneous endoscopic gastrostomy
    (PEG), 144
Perinatal death, grieving, 769–771
Perineal care, 90
  administering, skill procedure for, 97
Periodontitis, 94, 96
Peripheral pulses, 256, 256f
Peristalsis, 544
Permissive nurse practice act, 74
PERRLA, 284
Personal-care supplies, 225
Personal hygiene, 85–120
  assessment of skin and related struc-
      tures and, 87
  backrub and, 90
    skill procedure for giving, 98f,
        98–99, 99f
  bathing and. *See* Bath/bathing
  ear and hearing aid care and, 107–
      108, 113, 113t, 114f
  eye and visual aid care and. *See*
      Eye(s); Eyewear
  fingernail care and, 113–114
  foot and toenail care and, 114–115,
      115f
  hair care and, 115–117
    grooming and, 115, 117
    shampooing, 116, 116f, 117
  mucous membranes and, structures
      and functions of, 86–87
  natural body defenses and, 330
  nose care and, 113
  ordering and recording care and, 88

patient requiring help with, nursing diagnoses for, 117
patient teaching for, 120
perineal care and, 90
  skill procedure for, 97
postoperative, 450t
promoting
  in adolescent, 118–119
  in elderly patient, 119–120
  in infant or child, 117
  in patient with diabetes mellitus, 119
  teaching suggestions for, 120
shaving and, 90, 94
  skill procedure for, 100f, 100–101
skin and
  healthy, 87
  structures and functions of, 86–87
teeth and mouth and. *See* Oral hygiene
tepid sponging and, 89–90
  skill procedure for, 95–96
for terminally ill patient, 761–762
Personal space, hospitalization and, 205
Perspiration, water loss in, 642, 642t
Petaling, casts and, 692
  skill procedure for, 694f, 694–695
Petrissage, 99f
pH, 679. *See also* Acid-base balance; Acid-base imbalances
Phantom limb pain, 176
Phenol, disinfection/sterilization with, 341
Phlebitis, 376
  intravenous fluid administration and, 668–669
Phosphate, function of, 677
Phosphorus, dietary, 125t
Photodynamic therapy (PDT), 451
Physical assessment, 278–298, 282t
  of adolescent, 298
  of adult female, 298
  auscultation in, 280, 282f
  of cardiovascular system, 290–291, 291f, 295t
  of elderly patient, 298
  of genitourinary system, 293, 294t, 295t
  of infant or child, 296
  inspection in, 279, 279f
  methods of, 279–280
  of musculoskeletal system, 294, 295t
  of neurologic system, 292f, 292–293, 295t
  by nurse generalist, 282t
  nursing diagnoses during, 296
  ofgastrointestinal system, 293, 293f, 295t
  palpation in, 279–280, 280f, 281f

percussion in, 279, 280f
performing, skill procedure for, 283–284
purposes of, 278–279
of respiratory system, 286–290, 287f, 295t
of sensory-perceptual status, 280–282, 284–286, 294–295t
of skin, 286, 287t, 295t
Physically handicapped patient, administering medications to, 597–598, 601f
Physical services, 17
Physical well-being, 33
Physician's orders, 55–56, 56f
Physician's progress notes, 56, 57f
PIE charting, 59–60, 60f
Piggyback (secondary) infusion, 667, 669f
  adding, skill procedure for, 669–672, 670f, 671f
Pillows, 219, 221, 221f, 223, 378
Placebos, 180, 182
Plaintiff, 75
Plantarflexion, 376, 376f
Plaque, dental, 94
Plasma (intravascular fluid; serum), 286, 641t, 642, 643f
Platform crutches, 419, 420f
Pleural cavity, thoracentesis and, 317, 317f
Pleural rub, 290
Plume, lasers and, 451
Pneumatic (inflatable) splints, 685
Pneumonia, hypostatic, 376
Pneumonitis, postoperative, 447t
Pneumothorax, 732
Podiatrist, 114
Poisoning, preventing, 232, 235t
Polyuria (diuresis), 503
POR. *See* Problem-oriented record
Port, 524
Position(s), 305
  erect, 305t
  knee-chest (genupectoral), 307, 307f
  lithotomy, 306, 307f
  prone, 384
    skill procedure for positioning patient and, 397–398, 398f
  recumbent
    dorsal, 306, 306f
    horizontal, 306
  Sims', 307, 307f
  sitting, 305, 305f
  supine, 384
    skill procedure for positioning patient and, 396, 396f
  terms used to describe, 167–168t
  Trendelenburg, postoperative shock and, 447t, 457f

Positioning
  for examination, 305–307t
  of patient confined to bed, 384, 395
    skill procedure for, 396–399, 396–399f
  terminally ill patients and, 762
Positioning devices, 378–380
Postmortem care, 766
  skill procedure for performing, 767–768, 768f
Postoperative care. *See* Surgery, postoperative care and
Postpartal period, promoting urinary elimination in, 539, 541
Postural drainage, 706
  skill procedure for promoting, 707f, 707–708
Postural (orthostatic) hypotension, 261
  checking for, 262
Posture, 159–160
  blood pressure and, 260
  lying down, 159, 161f
  sitting, 159, 160f
  standing, 159, 160f
Potassium
  dietary, 125t
  function of, 677
Povidone-iodine (Betadine), wound care and, 474t
Practical nursing, 11
  responsibilities of, 12t
Prefilled cartridges, 607, 608f, 609f
Pregnancy. *See also* Childbirth
Pregnant patient
  administering medications to, 594–597
  amniocentesis and, 317–318
  dislodging object from airway in, skill procedure for, 716f, 716–717
  exercise in, promoting, 172–173
  nutrition in, promoting, 156
  urinary elimination in, promoting, 539, 541
Premature contraction, 255
Preoperative care. *See* Surgery, preoperative care and
Prescription. *See* Medication order
Pressure sores. *See* Decubitus ulcers
Preventive nursing care, 7
Primary infusion, 667, 669f
Primary nursing, 37–38
Principles, as basis for nursing skills, 10
Priorities, setting, nursing care plans and, 47, 48t
Privacy
  confidentiality and, 79
  in hospital
    decreased, 204–205
    providing, 226, 226t
  invasion of, 77
PRN medication order, 579t

Problem(s), 44
  actual, potential, and possible, 46
  collaborative, 46
  determining, 44
  recognizing, 41, 44
Problem list, for problem-oriented
    record, 57
Problem-oriented record (POR), 56–57
  database for, 56–57
  initial plan and, 57
  problem list for, 57
  progress notes and follow-up and,
    58–59, 59t
Proctoscopy, 315
Prodromal signs/symptoms, 278
Product, 16
Professional nursing, responsibilities of,
    12t
Progress notes
  physician's, 56, 57f
  for problem-oriented record, 58–59,
    59t
Projectile vomiting, 130
Pronation, 168t
Prone position, 384
  skill procedure for positioning pa-
    tient and, 397–398, 398f
Propoxyphene hydrochloride (Darvon),
    dosage for equianalgesia, 762t
Proprietary (trade) drug names, 573
Prosthesis, 107
  eye, care of, 107, 113f
Protective eyewear, asepsis and, 336,
    339f
Protective (reverse) isolation, 357, 361,
    362t
Protective restraints, 77, 227–229, 229f,
    230f
  for infant or child, 237, 237f
  skill procedure for applying, 231
Protein(s), 124
Protein complementation, 124, 130t
Proteinuria, 503
Proximal, definition of, 168t
Psychogenic pain, 177
Psychological status. *See also* Emo-
    tion(s); Emotional responses;
    Mental status; Mood
  postoperative, 451t
Psychological support. *See* Emotional
    support
Psychologist, environmental, 218
Psychology, 17–18
Psychomotor domain, 27, 27t
Psychosocial changes, inactivity and, 377
Public health codes, 10–11, 74
  mandatory nurse practice acts and, 74
  permissive nurse practice acts and, 74
Pulmonary embolism, postoperative,
    448t

Pulse, 253–256
  bounding or full, 255
  feeble, weak, or thready, 255
  fluid imbalances and, 646t
  intermittent, 255
  peripheral, 256, 256f
  rhythm of, 255
  selecting site for measurement of,
    255–256, 256f
  volume of, 255, 255t
Pulse deficit, 256
Pulse pressure, 262
Pulse rate, 253
  abnormally rapid, 254
  abnormally slow, 254–255
  apical, 256, 258f
  apical-radial, 256, 258f
  normal, 253–254, 254t
  radial, 256
    assessing, skill procedure for, 257,
    258f
Pulse rhythm, 255
Pulse volume, 255, 255t
Puncture (tap), 311
  lumbar, 316–317, 317f
Puncture wound, 458t
Purulent, definition of, 286
Push, intravenous medication adminis-
    tration and, 626
Push-ups, 417, 417f
Pyelography
  intravenous (IVP), 312
  retrograde, 312
Pyorrhea, 94, 96
Pyrexia. *See* Fever; Hyperthermia
Pyridoxine (vitamin B₆), 127t
Pyuria, 503

Quadrants, of abdomen, 293, 293f
Quadriceps setting, 416
Queckenstedt's test, 316

Radial pulse rate, 256
  assessing, skill procedure for, 257, 256f
Radiation, 314
  examinations detecting, 314–315
Radionuclide (radioisotope), 314
Radionuclide scan, of thyroid, 314–315
Radiopharmaceuticals, 314
Rales (crackles), 289
Range of motion (ROM), 162
Range-of-motion (ROM) exercises
  basic guidelines for using, 403, 405,
    406
  skill procedure for performing, 407–
    416, 407–416f
Rapid eye movement (REM) sleep, 191,
    191f, 192t

RDAs (Recommended Dietary Al-
    lowances), 126
Reacting (recovery) room, 428
Readiness, for learning, assessment of,
    27
Reading material, 225
  infection control and, 369–370
Receiving room, 427
Recipient, blood transfusions and, 673
Recommended Dietary Allowances
    (RDAs), 126
Reconstitution, of powdered parenteral
    medications, 608
Record(s). *See* Patient records
Recording (documenting), 54. *See also*
    Charting; Patient records
  examinations and, 308, 310
  of fluid intake, 644, 644f
  of fluid output, 645–646, 646f
  of hygienic care, 88
  of medication administration, 576–
    577, 583
    medication administration record
    and, 576–577, 577f, 578f
Recovery (reacting) room, 428
Rectal medication administration, 575t
Rectal suppositories, 552, 552f
  inserting, skill procedure for, 553
Rectal temperature, 242, 246
  measuring with glass thermometer,
    skill procedure for, 249–250
  normal, 244
Rectal tube, skill procedure for insert-
    ing, 551
Rectum, 544
  proctoscopy and, 315
Rectus femoris muscle, for injections,
    611
  locating, skill procedure for, 611,
    611f, 612f
Recumbent position
  dorsal, 306, 306f
  horizontal, 306
Recurrent turn, roller bandages and,
    487, 488f
Red blood cell count, fluid imbalances
    and, 646t
Reduction
  of fractures, open and closed, 687
  or fractures, 687
Referral, 209, 212f
  nursing diagnoses and, 46
Referred pain, 177
Reflexes
  death and, 764
  gastrocolic, 545
Reflex incontinence, 504t
  nursing approaches for, 510t
Regeneration, 458
Regional anesthesia, 428

Registered nursing, 11
Regulation, of nursing practice, 13–14
Regurgitation, 130
Rehabilitation, 7
Rehabilitative nursing care, 7
Reimbursement
    Medicare and, 203
    patient records and, 55
Relationship, 16, 19
    nurse-patient (therapeutic), 19–21
        communication barriers to, 22
        phases of, 20–21
Relative humidity, 219
Relaxation, 186. *See also* Rest; Sleep
    nursing diagnoses for patients with
            problems related to, 195
    patient teaching for, 197
    promoting, 186
        skill procedure for, 190
REM (rapid eye movement sleep), 191,
        191f, 192t
Remission, 36
Reporting
    change of shift reports and, 68, 69f
    examinations and, 308, 310
    medication errors and, 583–584
Rescue breathing, 734. *See also* Cardio-
        pulmonary resuscitation
    age differences in, 741t
Research
    as basis for nursing skills, 10
    data collection for, patient records
            and, 55
    participation in, by terminally ill
            patients, 758, 759f
Reservoir, infectious process and, 330
Residential care, 203
Resolution, 458
    of grief, 771
Resource(s), 34
    health as, 34
    scarce, allocation of, 79
Respiration(s), 257–259
    assessing, 259
        skill procedure for, 260
    characteristics of, 259
    Cheyne-Stokes, 259, 764
    death and, 764
    diaphragmatic, 258
    external, 257
    fluid imbalances and, 646t
    internal (tissue), 258
    thoracic, 258
Respiratory acidosis, 679t
Respiratory alkalosis, 679t
Respiratory isolation, 357, 358t
Respiratory rate
    abnormally rapid, 258–259
    abnormally slow, 259
    assessment of, skill procedure for, 260

normal, 258, 258t
Respiratory system. *See also* Airway;
        Airway obstruction; Cardio-
        pulmonary functioning; Lungs;
        Respiration(s); Respiratory rate
    assessing, 286–290, 287f, 294t
        abnormal lung sounds and, 287,
            289–290
        auscultation and, 287–289
        normal lung sounds and, 287, 290f
        respiratory rate and, 258t, 258–259,
            260
    fluid imbalances and, 647
    inactivity and, 376–377
    postoperative complications and,
            432–434, 448–449t
        deep-breathing exercises and,
            432–433
        incentive spirometry and, 434, 434f
        raising secretions and, 434–436
Respite care, 203t
Responsibility
    demonstrated by nursing practice, 11
    health as, 34
    for nursing process, levels of, 12t
Rest, 218. *See also* Relaxation; Sleep
    nursing diagnoses for patients feeling
            unrested and, 237
Restitution, death and, 769t
Restraints, protective, 77, 227–229, 229f,
        230f
    for infant or child, 237, 237f
    skill procedure for applying, 231
Retching, 130
Retention enema, 557
Retinol (vitamin A), 127t
Retrograde pyelography, 312
Reverse (protective) isolation, 357, 361,
        362t
Rhonchi (gurgles), 289
Riboflavin (vitamin B$_2$), 127t
Rights
    of medication administration, 581f,
        581–582
    of patients. *See* Patient rights
Ringer's solution, 651t
    lactated, 651t
    wound care and, 474t
Risk
    for altered protection, nursing care
            plan for, 637
    for developing decubitus ulcers
            (pressure sores), 461, 464t
    from environmental hazards, nursing
            diagnoses for, 237
    high-risk nursing diagnosis and, 46d
    for infection
        nursing care plan for, 371
        nursing diagnoses for, 351
    for trauma, nursing care plan for, 238

for urinary incontinence, nursing
        care plan for, 540
Risk factors
    for exercise, 166
    for falls, 232d
    surgical, 428, 429t
Roentgenogram, 311. *See also* X-ray ex-
        aminations
Roentgenography. *See* X-ray examina-
        tions
Roentgen rays, 311
Role–relationship pattern, 42t
Roller bandages, 484–485
    removing, 485
    wrapping techniques for, 486–488,
        486–488f
ROM (range of motion), 162
ROM (range-of-motion) exercises
    basic guidelines for using, 403, 405,
        406
    skill procedure for performing, 407–
        416, 407–416f
Room. *See also* Isolation room; Patient
        room
    operating, 427
    receiving, 427
    recovery (reacting), 428
Rooming in, 213
Rotation, 167t, 407, 407f, 411f, 412f,
        415f
    external, 167t, 409, 409f, 413f
    internal, 167t, 409, 409f
Rounds, 69, 71
Roy, Sister Callista, 5t, 6t
Rub (lung sound), 290

Safety, 218, 227–233
    drowning and asphyxiation and,
            preventing, 232, 235t
    electrical injuries and, preventing,
            230, 234t
    falls and
        preventing, 229–230, 233f, 234t
        risk factors for, 232d
    fires and, preventing, 230–232, 232f,
            233t, 234t
    infections and, preventing spread of,
            232
    lasers and, 451–452
    patient identification and, 227
        medication administration and, 573
    patient record and, 54–55
    patient's right to, 17
    poisoning and, preventing, 232, 235t
    promoting
        elderly patient and, 239
        helpless patient and, 239
        infant or child and, 235–238, 237f
        patient teaching and, 239

Safety (*continued*)
  protecting terminally ill patients from
      harm and, 762–763
  restraints and, 227–229, 229f, 230f
    applying, skill procedure for, 231
  scalds and burns and, preventing,
      232, 235t
  signaling for assistance and, 227
  steps to follow when accidents occur,
      233–235, 236f
Saline solution
  intravenous, 651t
    half-strength, 651t
  wound care and, 474t
Sandbags, 378–379
Sanguineous, definition of, 286
Scalds, preventing, 232, 235t
Scars, 286, 458
Science, 4
Scientific knowledge
  as basis for nursing skills, 9–10
  health promotion and, 35
-scope, meaning of, 311
Scultetus binder, applying, 488, 490f
Sebaceous glands, 86
Sebum, 86
Secondary (piggyback) infusion, 667,
      669f
  adding, skill procedure for, 669–672,
      670f, 671f
Second intention healing, 459
Secretions. *See also* Drainage
  infection control and, 367
  liquefying, 705
  raising, 434
    skill procedure for, 435f, 435–436
  removing from tracheostomy, 718
    skill procedure for, 718–719, 719f
Self-catheterization, patient teaching for,
      531, 533
Self-examination, of breast, 281f
Self-image, 9
Self-inflating breathing bag and mask,
      734, 739, 741f
Self-perception/self-concept pattern, 42t
Self-regulation, of nursing practice,
      13–14
Selye, Hans, 6t
Semipermeable membrane, 642
Sensory alteration, 227
  death and, 764
  sensory stimulation and, skill pro-
      cedure for promoting, 228
Sensory deprivation, 227
Sensory overload, 227
Sensory-perceptual status, assessing,
      280–282, 284–286, 294–295t
  hearing and ears and, 284–285, 286f,
      294t
  mental status and, 280–281, 294t

smell and, 286, 295t
taste and, 286, 295t
touch and, 285–286, 295t
vision and eyes and, 282, 284, 285f,
    294t
Sensory stimulation, isolation and, 370
Separation anxiety, hospitalization and,
    204, 205f
Sepsis, 330
Serosanguineous, definition of, 286
Serous, definition of, 286
Serum (intravascular fluid; plasma),
    286, 641t, 642, 643f
Services, 16. *See also* Patient care;
    Patient services
Sex. *See* Gender
  blood pressure and, 260
  body temperature and, 244
  pulse rate and, 253
Sexuality–reproductive pattern, 42t
Shampooing, 117
  skill procedure for, 116, 116f
Sharp objects, disposing of, 336, 338,
    339f, 610
Shaving, 90, 94
  skill procedure for, 100f, 100–101
Shearing force, decubitus ulcers and,
    460
Shock
  emotional, death and, 769t
  hypovolemic, postoperative, 447t
Shoe covers, asepsis and, 336
Sickness. *See* Illness
Siderails, 380
Sigma Theta Tau, 14
Sigmoid colon, 544
Sigmoidoscopy, 311, 315
Signs, 278
  constitutional, 278
  of decubitus ulcers, 460–461,
      462–463t
  of impending death, 763–764
  local, 278
  prodromal, 278
  systemic, 278
  vital. *See* Body temperature; Pulse;
      Pulse rate; Respiration(s); Res-
      piratory rate; Vital signs
Silence, in communication, 22
Sims' position, 307, 307f
Single medication order, 579t
Singultus (hiccups), postoperative,
    448t
Sinus arrhythmia, 255
Sitting down posture, 159, 160f
Sitting position, 305, 305f
Sitz baths, 495–496
Skeletal system. *See* Bone(s)
Skeletal traction, 696, 696f
Skilled nursing care, 203

Skin. *See also* Integumentary system
  assessing, 87, 286, 287t, 294t
  broken, natural body defenses and,
      330
  cleansing
    at injection site, 609
    prior to surgery, 436
    for venipuncture, 658
  decubitus ulcers (pressure sores)
      and. *See* Decubitus ulcers
  healthy
    caring for, 87
    characteristics of, 87
  insensible water loss through, 642,
      642t
  organ donation and, 755t
  postoperative complications and, 450t
  preparing for cast, 688
  structure and functions of, 86
  turgor of, fluid imbalances and,
      646–647
Skin traction, 696, 696f
Slander, 77
Sleep, 186
  age variations in need for, 191
  assessment of, 193
  biologic cycles and, 186, 189
  disorders of, 193–195
  exercise and, 162
  factors influencing, 191–192
  inactivity and, 377
  loss of, effects of, 192–193
  need for, age variations in, 190t
  nonrapid eye movement (NREM),
      191, 191f, 192t
  normal, 189–191, 190t
  nursing diagnoses for patients with
      problems related to, 195
  postoperative sleeplessness and,
      449t
  promoting, 193
    in elderly patient, 197
    in infant or child, 195–197
    patient teaching and, 197
    skill procedure for, 194
    teaching suggestions for, 197
  rapid eye movement (REM), 191,
      191f, 192t
  stages of, 191, 191f, 192t
Sleep apnea, 195
Sleeplessness, 193–195
  postoperative, 450t
Sleep pattern disturbance, inactivity
    and, 377
Sleep–rest pattern, 42t
Sleep talking, 195
Sleepwalking, 195
Slings, 687, 687f, 688f
Smell. *See also* Odors
  assessing sense of, 286

Smoking, as risk factor
  for exercise, 166
  surgical, 429t
Snoring, 195
Soaks, 496
SOAP charting, 58, 59
SOAPIE charting, 58, 59
SOAPIER charting, 58, 59, 59t
Social services, 18
Social stigma, 34
Social well-being, 33–34
Society, value of nursing practice to, 11
Sociology, 18
Sodium
  dietary, 125t
  function of, 677
Sodium chloride solution. *See* Saline
    solution
Sodium hypochlorite (Dakin's solution),
    wound care and, 474t
Soft diet, 133t
  mechanical, 133t
Solution(s)
  Dakin's (sodium hypochlorite),
      wound care and, 474t
  dextrose and water, intravenous, 651t
  dextrose in saline, intravenous, 651t
  intravenous, 649–651, 651t
    colloid, 649–650
    crystalloid, 649, 650–651, 651t
    hypertonic, 651, 651t
    hypotonic, 650–651, 651t
    isotonic, 650, 651t
    preparing, 652
  Ringer's, 651t
    lactated, 651t
    wound care and, 474t
  saline. *See* Saline solution
  sterile, pouring, 343, 345f
Somnambulism, 195
Sore throat, tube feedings and, 150t
Sound waves, examinations using, 315
Space, personal, hospitalization and, 205
Spasticity, 406
Specialists, 87
Special procedures
  assisting with, 302–310, 308f
    caring for equipment and supplies
        and, 310
    equipment and supply preparation
        and, 303t, 303–304, 304f
    patient instruction and, 302–303
    patient positioning and draping
        and, 305–307t
    patient preparation and, 304
    recording and reporting data and,
        308, 310
    skill procedure for, 309–310
    test requirements and, carrying
        out, 303

understanding patient, illness, and
    plan of care and, 302
  understanding procedure and, 302
  work area preparation and, 304
  invasive, 302
  patient teaching for, 302–303
Special therapeutic diet, 133t
Specific gravity, 538
  testing urine for, 538, 538f
Specimens, 308. *See also* Stool speci-
    mens; Urine specimens
  infection control and, 367
    collecting and transporting, skill
        procedure for, 368
  sputum, collecting, 708–709
Speech, patient services for patient who
    cannot speak and, 30–31
Sphygmomanometer, 262–264, 263f,
    264f, 264t
  coin-operated, 265
Spica, hip, 688
Spica turn, roller bandages and, 487,
    487f
Spinal tap (lumbar puncture), 316–317,
    317f
Spiral-reverse turn, roller bandages and,
    486, 486f
Spiral turn, roller bandages and, 486,
    486f
Spiritual needs
  spiritual services and, 18f, 18–19
  of terminally ill patients, 760, 761f
Spiritual well-being, 34
Spirometry, incentive, 434, 434f
Splints, 685–686, 686f
  emergency, applying, 686
  immobilizers, 685
  inflatable (pneumatic), 685
  molded, 685–686, 686f
  traction, 685
Sponging, 89–90
  tepid, skill procedure for, 95–96
Spore, 329
Sputum, 297
Sputum specimen, collecting, 708–709
Stamina, exercise and, 162
Standing medication order, with and
        without termination date, 579t
Standing posture, 159, 160f
Staples, 484
  removing, 483–484, 484f
Static air mattress, 381, 382t
Stat medication order, 579t
Steam, disinfection/sterilization with,
    340t, 341
Step-down unit, 208
Sterile field, 342–344
  adding sterile items to, 343–344,
      344f, 345f
  creating, 342–343, 343f

Sterile gloves, donning and removing,
    345
  skill procedure for, 347–349, 348f,
      349f
Sterile gown, donning, 344–345
  skill procedure for, 346f, 346–347
Sterile technique. *See* Asepsis, surgical
Sterilization, 339–341
  by agency, 343, 344f
  commercial, 343, 344f
  methods of, 340t, 340–341
  pouring sterile solutions and, 343,
      345f
  preparing for, 339–340
  transfer forceps and, 343–344, 345f
Stertorous breathing, 259
Stethoscope, 264, 265f
Stimulation, sensory, isolation and, 370
Stimulus(i), 227
Stirrups, 306
Stockinet, casting and, 688
Stockings, antiembolism, 434, 436
  skill procedure for using, 438, 438f
Stock supply, of medications, 577
Stoma, 533
  intestinal, 558–566, 559f
    changing appliance and, 559, 560–
        561, 561f
    collecting stool from, 558–559
    colostomy irrigation and, 559, 561–
        565, 563–565f
    draining continent ostomy and,
        559, 566
    enterostomal therapist and, 565
  urinary, 533, 534f, 534–535
    collecting urine specimens from,
        536–537
Stomach
  gastric analysis and, 316
  gastric gavage and, 136–141. *See also*
      Nutrition, tube feedings and
  gastric residual and, 145
Stool. *See* Feces
Stool specimens, 566–567
  collecting, skill procedure for, 566
  examination techniques for, 567t
Storage, of medications, 577, 579, 579f
Straight binder, applying, 488
Stress. *See also* Anxiety; Fear(s)
  events in hospital producing, 189t
  exercise and, 162, 166
  pulse rate and, 254
Stress electrocardiogram, 169, 169f
Stress incontinence, 502, 504t
  nursing approaches for, 510t
Strict isolation, 356, 358t
Stridor, 259
Subcutaneous injections. *See* Injec-
    tion(s), subcutaneous
Subjective data, 41

Sublingual medication administration, 575t, 594

Substance abuse, as surgical risk factor, 429t

Suctioning
of airway. *See* Airway, suctioning
of secretions from tracheostomy, 718
skill procedure for, 718–719, 719f

Suffering, relief of, as nursing skill objective, 7–8, 8f

Sugar
blood, 318
elevated, tube feedings and, 150t
glucometer and, skill procedure for using, 318–321, 319–321f
urine, testing for, 537–538, 538f

Suicide, grieving and, 769

Supination, 168t

Supine position, 384
skill procedure for positioning patient and, 396, 396f

Supplies
cleaning, 338–339
contaminated, caring for, 364, 366, 367f
for dressing change, 470
for examination
caring for, 310
preparing, 303t, 303–304
of medications, 577
personal-care, 225
sterilized
by agency, 343, 344f
commercially, 343, 344f

Support, emotional
for nurse providing terminal care, 751–752
providing, skill procedure for, 26
surgery and, 430–431

Support, base of, 161t, 162f

Supportive nursing care, 9, 10f

Suppositories, rectal, 552, 552f
inserting, skill procedure for, 553

Surgery, 426–454
ambulatory (outpatient), 428
anesthesia and, 428
asepsis and. *See* Asepsis, surgical
blood for, predonating, 429–430, 430t
complications of, 444, 447–451t
respiratory, preventing, 432–436, 433f, 434f
consent for, 436, 439f
elective, 427t
emergency, 427t
fracture reduction and, 687
informing patient about, 428–429
laser, 446, 451–452
benefits of, 446, 451
safety and, 451–452
locations for, 427–428, 428t

nursing diagnoses for patients undergoing, 452
optional, 427t
patient teaching for, 454
postoperative care and, 441, 443–446
complications and, 444, 447–451t
diabetes mellitus and, 452
elderly patient and, 454
family assistance and, 444, 446
infant or child and, 452
obese patient and, 452, 454
patient's room and, preparing, 441
planning, 443–444
receiving patient and, 443, 445–446
skill procedure for, 445–446
postoperative pain and, 449t
preoperative care and, 431–441
activity and exercise and, promoting, 432
avoiding thrombi and emboli and, 434, 436–438, 437–439f
consent and, obtaining, 436, 439f
diabetes mellitus and, 452
elderly patient and, 454
infant or child and, 452
obese patient and, 454
preoperative routine and, 440–441, 442f, 442–443
preparing patient and, skill procedure for, 442f, 442–443
respiratory complications and, preventing, 432–436, 433f, 434f
surgical site and, preparing, 436, 439, 440f
preoperative routine for, 440–441
checklist for, 441, 444f
skill procedure for, 442f, 442–443
psychological support and, 430–431
required, 427t
risk factors for, 428, 429t
surgical site and, preparing, 436, 439, 440
covering prepared area and, 440, 441f
hair removal and, 436, 439–440, 440f
skin cleansing and, 436
thrombi and emboli and, avoiding, 434, 436
antiembolism stockings and, 434, 436, 438, 438f
leg exercises and, 434, 436–437, 437f
urgent, 427t

Surgical asepsis. *See* Asepsis, surgical

Susceptible host, 329–330

Suspension, 587

Sutures, 484
removing, 483–484, 484f

Sweating, water loss and, 642, 642t

Swelling, casts and, evaluating, 689, 693

Swing-through gait, 423f, 423t

Swing-to gait, 423t

Symbolic language, 760

Sympathy, 9

Symptoms, 278
constitutional, 278
of impending death, 763–764
local, 278
prodromal, 278
systemic, 278

Syndrome, 375

Syringe. *See also* Injection(s)
disposing of, 610
filling, 605–607
removing medication from ampule and, 605f, 605–606, 606f
removing medication from vial and, 606–607, 607f, 608f
mixing two medications in, 608–609
from ampule and vial, 608–609
from single-dose and multiple-dose vials, 608
from two multiple-dose vials, 608–609
prefilled cartridges and, 607, 608f, 609f

Systemic signs/symptoms, 278

Systole, 259

Systolic pressure, 259

Table, over bed, 223, 225f

Tachycardia, 254

Tachypnea, 258–259

Talwin (pentazocine), dosage for equianalgesia, 762t

Tap (puncture), spinal, 311, 316–317, 317f

Tapotement, 99f

Taste, assessing, 286

T-binder, applying, 485, 488, 488f

Teaching. *See* Patient teaching

Team
consulting with, 49
health-care, 37, 37f

Team nursing, 37

Technical nursing, responsibilities of, 12t

Technology, health promotion and, 35

Teeth
care of. *See* Oral hygiene
healthy, characteristics of, 87

Telephone, exchanging information by, 71, 71f

Temperature. *See also* Cold applications; Heat; Heat applications
body. *See* Body temperature
of patient's room, 219

TENS (transcutaneous electrical nerve stimulation), 182, 186

skill procedure for operating unit and, 187–188
Tension reduction, exercise and, 162, 166
Tepid sponging, 89–90
  skill procedure for, 95–96
Teratogenic effects, 597
Terminal (computer), 60
Terminal disinfection, 339
Terminal illness, 750. *See also* Death and dying
  in adolescent, 772
  in child, 772
    school-age, 772
      ten- to twelve year old, 772
      three- to five-year old, 772
  in elderly patient, 772
  in infant, 772
  patient teaching for, 772–774
  in toddler, 772
Terminating phase, of nurse-patient relationship, 20–21
Terminology
  for appearance of drainage from lesions, 286
  of body mechanics, 161t
  for body positions, 167–168t
  describing tests, 310–311
  for dosage measurements, 574t
  for movements, 167–168t
Tests. *See also* Special procedures
  advancements in, 310
  carrying out requirements of, 303
  nursing diagnoses for patients undergoing, 322
  patient teaching for, 322–324
  terms describing, interpreting, 310–311
Thanatologists, 751
Theory, 4, 5t, 6t
  gate-control, of pain, 181
  germ, 34–35
Therapeutic diet, 133t
Therapeutic (nurse-patient) relationship, 19–21
  communication barriers to, 22
  phases of, 20–21
Thermometer, 242–243, 243t
  centigrade (Celsius), 242–243, 243t
  continuous-monitoring devices and, 251
  disposable, single-use, 247
  electronic, 243, 244f
    assessing body temperature using, skill procedure for, 252f, 252–253
  Fahrenheit, 243, 243t
  glass, 243, 243f
    measuring body temperature using, skill procedure for, 248f, 248–251, 249f, 251f

heat-sensitive patch or tape as, 247, 251, 254f
  keeping clean, 246, 247f
    skill procedure for, 247
  tympanic, 251, 253, 254f
Thiamine (vitamin B₁), 127t
Thigh, obtaining blood pressure at, 266
Third intention healing, 459
Third spacing, 648. *See also* Fluid imbalances
Thirst, postoperative, 449t
Thoracentesis, 311, 317, 317f
Thoracic respiration, 257
Three-Minute Step Test, 169, 170t
Three-point gait, 421t, 422f
Threshold, for pain, 176
Throat
  applying medications to, 594
  sore, tube feedings and, 150t
Thrombophlebitis, 376
  postoperative, 447–448t
Thrombus(i), 376
  avoiding, 434, 436
    leg exercises for, 434, 436–437, 437f
Thyroid scan, 314–315
Tilt-table, 313, 417
Time of day
  blood pressure and, 260
  body temperature and, 244
  military time and, 63, 66, 66f, 66t
  pulse rate and, 253
Tissue
  granulation, 458
  type of, healing and, 459–460
Tissue respiration, 257
Tobacco use, as risk factor
  for exercise, 166
  surgical, 429t
Toenails
  care of, 114–115, 115f
  healthy, characteristics of, 87
Toileting, 503–506
  assisting patient to bathroom and, 504–505
  bedpan and, 505
    placing and removing, skill procedure for, 507f, 507–509, 508f
  commode and, 505
  promoting urinary elimination and, 504
  urinal and, 505–506
Tolerance
  of pain, 176
  pain medications and, 762
Tone, exercise and, 162
Tonus, 376
Topical anesthesia, 428
Topical medication administration, 575t, 588–594

buccal, 575t
  ear medications and, 591, 593f, 593–594
  eye medications and, 588, 590, 592f
  instillation and, 575t
  inunctions and, 575t, 588
  irrigation and, 575t
  nasal, 591, 594, 595, 595f
  rectal, 575t
  sublingual, 575t
  transdermal, 575t, 588f, 588–590, 591f
  vaginal, 575t
Tort, 75
Total incontinence, 504t
  nursing approaches for, 510t
Total parenteral nutrition (TPN), 153, 153f
Touch
  assessing, 285–286
  in communication, 22, 22f
T-piece, oxygen therapy using, 727, 727f, 732
  administering, skill procedure for, 731
TPN (total parenteral nutrition), 153, 153f
Trachea, bronchoscopy and, 315
Tracheal lung sounds, 287, 290f
Tracheostomy, 717f, 717–721
  removing secretions from, 718
    skill procedure for, 718–719, 719f
  tracheostomy care and, skill procedure for providing, 720–721, 721f
  tracheostomy collar and, oxygen therapy using, 727, 732
    administering, skill procedure for, 731
Traction, 695–697
  maintaining, 697
  manual, 695
  patient care and, skill procedure for, 697–698
  skeletal, 696, 696f, 697f
  skin, 696, 696f
Traction cart, 696
Traction splint, 685
Trade (proprietary) drug names, 573
Training effect, pulse rate and, 253–254
Transcutaneous electrical nerve stimulation (TENS), 182, 186
  skill procedure for operating unit and, 187–188
Transdermal medication administration, 575t, 588, 591f
  transdermal patch and, skill procedure for applying, 590
Transducer, 315
Transfer (between units or agencies), 208–209, 210f

Transfer (*continued*)
  nursing diagnoses and, 215
  skill procedure for, 211
Transfer forceps, 343–344, 345f
Transferring, 395, 399, 402
  basic guidelines for, 395
  from bed to chair and back to bed,
      395, 399, 402, 402f
    skill procedure for, 404–405,
        404–406f
    when patient can assist, 395, 399,
        402, 402f, 403f
    when patient cannot assist, 402–
        403
  to and from stretcher, 395
    skill procedure for, 400f, 400–401,
        401f
Transmission barriers, 361
Transparent dressings, 467, 467f
Transport, active, 677
Transtracheal oxygen, 727
  skill procedure for administering,
      730–731
Transverse colon, 544
Trapeze, 380, 381f
Trash, burnable, contaminated, dispos-
      ing of, 364
Trauma, 457. *See also* Injury; Wound
Trendelenburg position, postoperative
      shock and, 447t, 447f
Triggering, cutaneous, urinary inconti-
      nence and, 509–510
Trocar, 317
Trochanter rolls, 379, 379f
Truth-telling, 79
  about terminal illness, 753–755
Tubing, intravenous
  attaching, 652–653, 652–654f
  changing, 666–667, 668
Tunneled central venous catheter,
      628–629, 628f
Turgor, 286
Turning, 384
  skill procedure for, 385–391,
      385–391f
Two-point gait, 421t
Tympanic thermometer, 251, 253, 254f
Tympanites. *See* Intestinal distention

Ulcer(s)
  decubitus (pressure sore). *See*
      Decubitus ulcers
  of skin, 286
Ulceration wound, 458t
Ultradian rhythm, 186
Ultrasonography (echography), 315
  obstetric, 315
Ultraviolet lamps, 497

Unconscious patient
  dislodging object from airway in, skill
      procedure for, 715f, 715–716
  Glasgow Coma Scale and, 292
  healing in, promoting, 497
  patient services for, 31
Uniform, asepsis and, 332, 334
Unit dose system, 577
Universal Neglect, nursing care plan for,
      424
Universal precautions, 357, 361d
Upper gastrointestinal x-ray, 311–312
Ureters, 501–502
  cystoscopy and, 315–316
Urethra, 502. *See also* Urethral catheter-
      ization
  cystoscopy and, 315–316
Urethral catheterization, 514–533
  catheter insertion and, 515
    in female patient, skill procedure
        for, 516–520, 516–520f
    in male patient, skill procedure for,
        520–523, 522f, 523f
  catheter irrigation and, 524–525,
      530–531
    skill procedure for, 528f, 528–530,
        529f, 532–633
    three-way catheter and, 530f, 530–
        533, 531f
    using closed system, 525, 528f,
        528–530, 529f
    using open system, 525, 528f, 528–
        530, 529f
  catheter management and, 524–525
    skill procedure for, 525–528, 526f,
        527f
  catheter removal and, 531
  catheter stabilization and, 524, 524f,
      525f
  closed drainage system and, 515, 524
  indications for, 514
  preparing for, 515
  self-catheterization and, 531–533
  types of catheters and, 514–515, 515f
  urine specimens and, obtaining, 535–
      536, 537f
Urge incontinence, 504t
  nursing approaches for, 510t
Urinal, 505–506
Urinalysis, 535. *See also* Urine testing
Urinary bladder. *See* Bladder, urinary;
      Urethral catheterization
Urinary catheters. *See also* Urethral
      catheterization
  external, 511–512, 512f
    applying, 511–514, 513f
    condom catheters, 512
  indwelling, 515, 515f
  intermittent straight catheterization
      and, 512

  obtaining urine specimens from,
      535–536, 537f
  retention, 515
  straight, 515
Urinary diversion, 533
Urinary elimination, 500–541. *See also*
      Urinary incontinence; Urine
  catheterization and. *See* Urethral cath-
      eterization; Urinary catheters
  factors influencing, 502
  nursing diagnoses for patients with
      problems related to, 539
  promoting, 504
    in elderly patient, 541
    in infant or child, 538–539
    patient teaching and, 541
    in pregnancy or early postpartal
        period, 539, 541
    in terminally ill patient, 761
  from surgical opening, 533–535
    stoma care and, 534f, 534–535
  toileting and. *See* Toileting
Urinary frequency, 503
Urinary incontinence, 377, 503,
      506–511
  bladder retraining and, 506, 509
  continence techniques and, 509, 510t
  Credé's maneuver and, 510, 510f
  cutaneous triggering mechanisms
      and, 509–510
  functional, 504t
    nursing approaches for, 510t
  keeping patient dry and, 511
  managing, skill procedure for, 511
  overflow, 504t
    nursing approaches for, 510t
  reflex, 504t
    nursing approaches for, 510t
  strengthening pelvic floor muscles
      and, 509, 511
  stress, 502, 504t
    nursing approaches for, 510t
  total, 504t
    nursing approaches for, 510t
  urge, 504t
    nursing approaches for, 510t
Urinary meatus, 502
Urinary retention, 503
  postoperative, 449t
Urinary suppression, 502
Urinary tract, 501–502. *See also* Blad-
      der, urinary; Genitourinary
      system; Urethra
  assessing function of, 502–503
  fluid imbalances and, 647
  inactivity and, 377
  postoperative problems and, 449t
  pyelography and
    intravenous, 312
    retrograde, 312

Urinary tract infections, postoperative, 449t
Urinary urgency, 503
Urination (micturition; voiding), 502.
    See also Urinary elimination;
    Urinary incontinence; Urine
Urine, 501. *See also* Urine specimens
  characteristics of
    abnormal, 503
    normal, 506t
  disposal of, infection control and, 367
  examining, 503, 506t
  residual, 503
  specific gravity of, fluid imbalances
    and, 646t
  water loss in, 642, 642t
Urine specimens, 535–537
  collecting
    from catheter, 535–536, 537f
    clean-catch midstream specimens
      and, 535, 536
    skill procedure for, 368, 536
    from stoma, 536–537
    voided specimens and, 535
  second voided specimen, 537
  transporting, skill procedure for, 368
  24-hour, 535
Urine testing, 535, 537–541
  for specific gravity, 538, 539f
  for sugar and acetone, 537–538, 538f
Urinometer, 538, 538f
Uterus
  pregnant, amniocentesis and,
    317–318
  sonography and, 315

Vaccines, 354
Vaginal irrigation (douche), 476, 478, 480
  skill procedure for, 480–481
Vaginal medications, 575t, 594
  administering, skill procedure for, 596
Validation, 41
Valsalva's maneuver, 416, 545
Valuables
  accounting for, following death, 766
  handling, 207, 208f
Value–belief pattern, 42t
Values, 34
Value system, 34
Vastus lateralis muscle, for injections, 610–611
  locating, skill procedure for, 613–615, 615f
Vectorborne transmission, of pathogens, 355t
  disposing of burnable trash and, 364

Vegetarianism, 126, 130t
Vehicle of transmission, 330
Vehicle route, of pathogen transmission, 355t
Vein(s)
  organ donation and, 755t
  for venipuncture, selecting, 655–658, 656–658f
Venipuncture. *See* Intravenous fluid administration, venipuncture and
Ventilation, of patient's room, 219
Ventrogluteal site, for injections, 610
  locating, skill procedure for, 611–612, 613f
Verbal communication, 21
Verbal orders, 576
Vesicular lung sounds, 287, 290f
Vial(s)
  combining medication from ampule
    and vial and, 609
  multiple-dose
    combining medications from sin-
      gle-dose vial with, 608
    combining medications from two
      multiple-dose vials and, 608–
      609
  removing medication from, 606–607, 607f, 608f
Vibration, to loosen secretions, 706
Vision. *See also* Visually impaired
    patient
  assessing, 282, 284, 285f, 294t
  field of, 87
  normal, characteristics of, 87
Visiting Nurses' Association, 203t
Visual acuity, 87
Visually impaired patient
  medication administration and, 597, 601f
  patient services for, 29–30
  promoting nutrition in, 156
Vital signs, 240–275, 277–278. *See also*
    Body temperature; Pulse; Pulse
    rate; Respiration(s); Respira-
    tory rate
  frequency of obtaining, 270
  measuring
    in elderly patient, 274
    in infant or child, 271–272, 272f
    nursing diagnoses for, 272
    patient teaching for, 274–275
    in patient who cannot cooperate, 272, 274
    in special situations, 274
    when patient's activity or emotional
      status is likely to affect vital
      signs, 274
  recording, 166, 169, 270–271, 271f
Vitamins, 126, 127–128t
  megadoses of, 126

Voiding. *See* Urinary elimination;
    Urination
Volumetric controller, 654, 655f
Voluntary psychiatric admission, 205t
Vomiting, 130
  controlling, 131
  postoperative, 448t
  projectile, 130
  tube feedings and, 150t
Vomitus (emesis), 130
von Bertalanffly, Ludwig, 6t

Waffle-shaped foam mattress, 381
Walkers, 419, 420f
Walking
  canes and, 419
  crutches and. *See* Crutches
  with nurse, 418–419, 419f
  in one's sleep, 195
  parallel bars and, 418, 418f
  preparing inactive patient for, 416–418
  walkers and, 419, 420f
  walking belts and, 418, 418f
Walking belts, 418, 418f
Walls, of patient's room, 218
Warmed air inhalation, 706
Warmth. *See also* Heat; Heat
    applications
  microorganisms and, 329
Water
  body. *See* Fluid balance, body water
    and
  boiling, disinfection/sterilization with, 340t, 341
  contamination of, pathogen transmis-
    sion by, 355t
  microorganisms and, 329
  need for, 124
Water mattress, 381–382, 382t
Water-seal drainage, 732, 732f
  skill procedure for, maintaining, 732–734
Weight. *See also* Obesity
  assessing, 278, 278f
  fluid imbalances and, 646t
  gain in, promoting, 129–130
  loss of
    promoting, 130
    tube feedings and, 150t
Well-being, 33
  emotional, 33
  physical, 33
  social, 33–34
  spiritual, 34
Wellness, 35–36. *See also* Health
  health-illness continuum and, 35f, 35–36
  hierarchy of needs and, 36, 36f
  high-level, 36

dex

ursing diagnosis, 46d
, 625, 626f
neeze, 289–290
Whistle-blowing, 79
Will, 77
  living, 77
Window, in cast, 690, 695f
Working phase, of nurse-patient
    relationship, 20
Wound, 286, 457. *See also* Healing;
    Injury; Wound care
  closed, 457, 458t
  debridement of, 460
  dehiscence of, postoperative, 450t
  evisceration of, postoperative, 450t
  infection of, postoperative, 450t
  odor from, 761
  open, 457, 458t
Wound care, 463–470. *See also* Healing
  drains and, 480–482, 481f, 482f

dressed wound and, 463
dressings and. *See* Bandages;
    Dressings
packing and, 482
for terminally ill patient, 761
undressed wound and, 463
Wristwatches, infection control and, 367,
    369

X-ray(s), 311
X-ray examinations, 311–313
  angiographic, 312–313
  of chest, 311
  cholecystography, 312
  computerized axial tomographic, 313,
      313f
  contrast medium and, 311
  gastrointestinal
    lower (barium enema), 312

upper, 311–312
of kidney, ureters, and bladder (ab-
    dominal plain film; KUB), 311
myelography, 313
pyelography
  intravenous, 312
  retrograde, 312

Yoga, 186
Young adult, promoting fluid and chem-
    ical balance in, 682

Zinc, dietary, 125t
Z-track (zigzag) technique, for intra-
    muscular injections, 617
  skill procedure for using, 621f, 621–
      622, 622f